3932   374/14.   ED 30

4

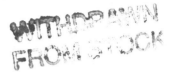

THE FABER
MEDICAL DICTIONARY

The Editor

★

SIR CECIL WAKELEY, Bt.

K.B.E., C.B., LL.D., M.Ch., D.Sc., F.R.S.E., F.R.A.C.S., F.A.C.S., F.R.S.A., F.Z.S.

Fellow of King's College, London

President of the Royal College of Surgeons of England. Senior Surgeon and Director of Surgical Studies, King's College Hospital. Surgeon to the Royal Masonic Hospital and Belgrave Hospital for Children. Consulting Surgeon to the West End Hospital for Nervous Diseases and to the Royal Navy. Examiner in Surgery to the University of Cambridge. Formerly Examiner in Surgery to the Universities of London, Glasgow, Sheffield, Durham, Bristol, Wales and the National University of Ireland. Vice President of the Imperial Cancer Research Fund and the British Empire Cancer Campaign

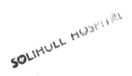

THE FABER
MEDICAL DICTIONARY

Edited by

SIR CECIL WAKELEY, Bt.

FABER AND FABER LIMITED
24 Russell Square
London

First published in 1953
by Faber and Faber Limited
24 Russell Square London W.C.1
Printed in Great Britain by
Purnell and Sons Limited
Paulton (Somerset) and London

FOREWORD

THERE is in my opinion need for a concise and comprehensive medical dictionary, and when I was asked some years ago if I would edit such a work I gladly consented. It has, however, proved to be a difficult task, which would have been impossible had it not been for all the kind help which I have received from numerous friends.

It was hoped to publish this dictionary just after the Health Service came into being, because it was felt that medical men and women and nurses in the service required an up-to-date and reliable medical dictionary. This was not to be, however, because of the meticulous care that has been taken over the proofs and the constant addition of new material, especially with regard to new pharmaceutical preparations.

I have to thank the Staff of the School of Pharmacy, University of London, for help and suggestions regarding entries on Chemistry and Pharmaceutical Chemistry. Mr. James Cleugh, M.A., St. Andrews, has supervised and corrected all the Greek and Latin derivations. Professor Wood Jones and Miss Jessie Dobson have helped me with the anatomical nomenclature and eponyms. Surgical registrars at King's College Hospital have given me constructive and stimulating criticisms and also helped in the proof reading. Miss Katharine Watson, of the staff of Messrs Faber and Faber, has proved a tower of strength throughout the whole period during which the book has been compiled. She assembled the initial material and tirelessly typed and retyped every card on which each entry in this dictionary has been made. A card index system proved invaluable in the composition of the work, for it made revision and the addition of new names easier. During all the months of hard work, including the reading of highly complicated proofs, I have never known Miss Watson's good-humoured patience to falter and I can never thank her enough for her valuable help.

In order to make doubly sure that the entries were as correct as they could be made, the proofs were re-checked by an entirely fresh team of helpers, Dr. E. A. Gates, O.B.E., M.D., Dr. J. G. Bate, M.B., Ch.B. and Miss Jean Cunningham, B.A., S.R.N., S.C.M., to whom I should also like to express my sincere thanks.

It is hoped that this medical dictionary will prove to be of real value, not only to the medical, dental and nursing professions, as a whole, but also to thousands of the laity who are working in the Health Service and require a dictionary to explain briefly the many and varied medical and surgical terms.

CECIL WAKELEY

Royal College of Surgeons of England
Lincoln's Inn Fields
London W.C.2
July 1953.

A NOTE ON
PRONUNCIATION AND DERIVATION

PRONUNCIATION

THE great majority of medical terms are of Latin or Greek origin. It cannot be laid down that there is an absolutely correct way of pronouncing them. A full phonetic guide to pronunciation is, therefore, not employed in this dictionary.

Pronunciation of consonants presents no difficulties. English and American readers should sound these as they would if the word were of English origin. For example in ABDUCENT the c is to be sounded exactly as in RECENT; though in Latin it would be correct to sound it like K.

The only guidance needed by the reader is (a) on the syllable or syllables stressed in ordinary usage, (b) whether the vowels are to be pronounced "short" or "long".

Syllables to be stressed are indicated, where necessary, by a dot at the end of the syllable. Thus ABDU·CENT.

Where there can be any doubt of the natural pronunciation of a vowel, the sign ˘ is used to indicate a short vowel, and the sign ¯ to indicate a long one. Thus ABDŪ·CENT.

Short	Ă	as	in	BAD
Long	Ā	as	in	BAKE
Short	Ĕ	as	in	BED
Long	Ē	as	in	BEET
Short	Ĭ	as	in	BID
Long	Ī	as	in	BILE
Short	Ŏ	as	in	BOG
Long	Ō	as	in	BOTH
Short	Ŭ	as	in	BUT
Long	Ū	as	in	BOOT or (with a preceding y sound)

as in BEAUTY, according to the reader's natural choice.

When two adjacent vowels form a diphthong and are pronounced as one, the sign ⁔ is placed over them. Thus ANAE·MIA.

If these simple rules are followed, the reader will be conforming to the customary pronunciation. Care has been taken not to pepper the dictionary with unnecessary signs.

DERIVATION

The source from which a word derives is given between brackets, following the word itself. The language of the source is shown as follows: G. for Greek; L. for Latin; L.L. for late Latin; Fr. for French; Ger. for German; It. for Italian; Sp. for Spanish. The source-word is printed in *italic*, and its English equivalent in ordinary type. When the main word in black type is itself a foreign word, it is not printed again between the brackets.

C.W.

A

α. First letter of the Greek alphabet. See alpha.

A. Symbol for argon.

A°. Abbreviation for Angström unit.

A². Abbreviation for aortic second sound.

AA, aa (G. *ana.*). 'Of each' in the writing of prescriptions.

Aaron's sign (Aaron, C.D., U.S. physician, born 1866). Pain in epigastric or praecordial region felt on pressure over McBurney's point, in appendicitis.

ääs·mus (G. *aasmos*, breathing out). Asthma.

A.B.A. Syn. for Injectio benzocainae. (Benzocaine 3, benzylalcohol 5, ether 10, in sterile olive oil *q.s.* to 100.)

abactē·rial (G. *a*, neg.; *bakterion*, small rod). Free from bacteria.

abac·tio (L.L.). Induced abortion.

Abadie's sign[1] (Abadie, C.A., French ophthalmologist, 1842–1932). Spasm of levator palpebrae superioris muscle; seen in primary toxic goitre.

Abadie's sign[2] (Abadie, J., French neurologist, born 1873). Insensitivity to pressure of Achilles tendon; found in tabes dorsalis.

abaissement (Fr.). Lowering, especially depression of a cataract below the line of vision in the operation of couching.

ăbālienā·tion (L. *abalienatio*, a legal transfer of property). Mental derangement.

abaptis·ton (G. *abaptistos*, not to be plunged). A trephine designed so that it cannot enter the brain.

abaragnō·sis (G. *a*, neg.; *baros*, weight; *gnosis*, knowledge). Loss of power to recognize weight.

abartic·ular (L. *ab*, from; *articulus*, joint). Distant from a joint.

abarticulā·tion (L. *ab*, from; *articulatio*, jointing, from *artus*, joint). Dislocatio f a joint.

abǎ·sia (G. *a*, neg; *bǎsis*, step). Unsteadiness of gait or inability to walk because of defective co-ordination.

ăbătardissement (Fr.). Degeneration of a breed.

abate. To curtail or lessen.

abate·ment. The lessening of a pain or reduction of a symptom.

abattoir (Fr.). A public slaughter-house for cattle.

abax·ial (L. *ab*, away from; *axis*, axis). Situated apart from the axis of any section or organ of the body.

Abbé condenser (Abbé, E. K., German physicist, 1840–1905). Mirror and a number of achromatic lenses placed beneath the microscope stage so as to give powerful illumination.

Abbe's operation (Abbe, R., U.S. surgeon, 1851–1928). 1. Lateral anastomosis of the intestine with catgut rings. 2. Cutting through a stricture of the oesophagus by means of the sawing action of a string, one end of which passes through the mouth and the other through an opening in the stomach. **A.'s catgut rings:** heavy catgut rings used to support ends of intestine being stitched together.

Abbot's paste (Abbot, W., English physician, 1831–1900). A paste containing arsenic acid, morphine and creosote.

Abbott's method[1] (Abbott, A.C., U.S. bacteriologist, 1860–1935). A method of staining the bodies of bacteria red and spores blue.

Abbott's method[2] (Abbott, E. G., U.S. surgeon, 1870–1938). A way of treating scoliosis by means of overcorrection of deformity by pulling on the spine with bandages and then applying pressure by means of a plaster jacket to fix spinal column in correct position.

abbrē·viate (L. *brevis*, short). To make short.

A.B.C. liniment. Syn. for linimentum aconiti oleosum. Liniment of aconite, liniment of belladonna and liniment of chloroform in equal parts.

A.B.C. powder. Boric acid, bismuth subnitrate and calomel in equal parts. Dusting powder.

A.B.D. capsules. Capsules containing vitamins A, B_1, B_2 and D.

Abderhalden's reaction (Abderhalden, E., Swiss physiologist, 1877–1950). A serum reaction resting upon the hypothesis that the blood reacts to a foreign protein entering the bloodstream by a protective ferment which disintegrates the protein.

abdō·men (L.). The belly; the cavity between the diaphragm and the pelvis.

abdō·minal. Pertaining to or connected with the abdomen. **Abdominal regions** are three upper in the epigastric zone, the left and right hypochondriac and epigastric; three middle in the mesogastric zone, the left and right lumbar and umbilical; three lower in the hypogastric zone, left and right inguinal and hypogastric. **Abdominal reflex:** reflex in which stroking of the skin of the abdominal wall leads to contraction of the underlying muscles.

abdō·mino·antē·rior (L. *abdomen*; *anterior*, foremost, from *ante*). With the abdomen forwards; describes position of foetus *in utero*.

abdō·minocentē·sis (L. *abdomen*; G. *kentēsis*, puncture). Surgical puncture through the abdominal wall.

abdō·minocys·tic (L. *abdomen*; G. *kustis*, bladder). Pertaining to the abdomen and the gallbladder.

abdō·minogen·ital (L. *abdomen*; *genitalis*, generative). Pertaining to the abdomen and genitalia.

abdō·minopostē·rior (L. *abdomen*; *posterior*, hindmost, from *post*). With the abdomen turned backwards; describes position of foetus *in utero*.

abdō·minō·scopy (L. *abdomen*; G. *skopein*, to inspect). Examination of the abdomen; inspection of abdominal organs with the endoscope.

abdō·minoscrō·tal. Pertaining to abdomen and scrotum.

abdō·minothorǎ·cic (L. *abdomen*; G. *thōrax*, chest). Relating to both abdomen and thorax.

abdō·minovagī·nal (L. *abdomen*; *vagina*, sheath). Relating to both abdomen and vagina.

abdō·minovesi·cal (L. *abdomen*; *vesica*, bladder). Relating to abdomen and bladder.

abduce (L. *ab*, from; *ducere*, to lead). To draw away.

abdū·cens (L. *abducere*, to draw off). Term applied to muscles and nerves drawing a part away from the median line of the body. **A. muscle:** external rectus muscle of the eye. **A. nerve:** sixth cranial nerve. **A. oris:** the caninus muscle.

abdū·cent (L. *abducere*, to draw off). Drawing away, or drawing out.

abduct (L. *abducere*, to draw off). To draw away from the median line.

abduc·tion (L. *abducere*, to draw off). 1. Drawing a part away from the axis of the body. 2. Separation of the parts of a fractured bone from each other.

Abée's support (Abée, E., German physician, 1843–1913). An appliance fixed over the breast to calm an over-active heart.

Abegg's rule (Abegg, R., Danish chemist, 1869–1910). All atoms have the same number of valences.

Abel's bacillus (Abel, R., German bacteriologist, 1868–1942). The *Klebsiella ozaenae*.

Abelin's reaction (Abelin, I., Swiss physiologist, born 1883). A test for the presence of arsphenamine in the urine.

abentĕ·ric (L. *ab*, from; G. *enteron*, intestine). Situated in a region other than the intestine.

abepithy·mia (L. *ab*, off; G. *epithumia*, desire). Paralysis of the solar plexus.

Abercrombie's degeneration (Abercrombie, J., Scottish physician, 1780–1844). Amyloid degeneration.

Abernethy's fascia (Abernethy, J., British surgeon, 1764–1831). A layer of areolar tissue covering the external iliac artery. **A.'s operation:** Ligation of the external iliac artery, with a curving incision from a point one inch within and above the anterior superior spine to a point one and a half inches above and outside the centre of the inguinal ligament. **A.'s sarcoma:** A fatty tumour generally situated on the trunk of the body.

aber·rans. Vas aberrans, *q.v.*

aber·rant (L. *ab*, from; *errare*, to wander). Atypical; departing from the usual course.

aberrā·tion (L. *abberatio*, a diversion). 1. Variation from the normal. More specifically: 2. Foetal deformity. 3. Any defect in focus or refraction of a lens. 4. Mental disorder of an unspecified kind.

aberrŏ·meter (L. *ab*, from; *errare*, to wander; G. *metron*, measure). An instrument used to measure errors in experiments.

abevacuā·tion (L. *ab*, from; *evacuatio*, an emptying). Excessive or deficient evacuation.

abey·ance. Suspended activity.

abĭă·trophy (G. *a*, neg.; *bios*, life; *atrophia*, pining). Premature loss of vitality.

ă·bient (L. *abire*, to go away). Evading the source of stimulation.

Abies (L., fir). A genus of coniferous trees, including the *A. canadensis*, which yields oil of hemlock.

ă·bietic acid. A stable acid resin $C_{19}H_{29}COOH$, related to phenanthrene. It is the principal constituent of colophony resin.

ăbīochem·istry (G. *a*, neg.; *bios*, life; Arab, *kimia*). Inorganic chemistry.

ăbīogen·esis (G. *a*, neg.; *bios*, life; *genesis*, generation). Spontaneous generation of living from non-living matter.

ăbiolŏ·gical (G. *a*, neg.; *bios*, life; *logos*, treatise). Pertaining to the study of inanimate things.

ăbiŏ·logy. The study of inanimate things.

ăbionar·ce (G. *a*, neg.; *bios*, life, *narkē*, stupor). Inaction due to physical weakness.

ăbiophysiŏ·logy (G. *a*, neg.; *bios*, life; *phusiologia*, natural philosophy). The study of inorganic processes in animate matter.

ăbi·osis (G. *a*, neg; *bios*, life). Absence of life. (Hence **abiotic.)**

ăbiŏ·trophic. Pertaining to abiotrophy.

ăbiŏ·trophy (G. *a*, neg.; *bios*, life; *trophē*, nutrition). Premature senescence or death of cells and tissues due to some unknown, intrinsic cause.

ăbir·ritant (L. *ab*, from; *irritare*, to stimulate). A drug used for the relief of irritation. (Hence **abirritation**, lowered response to stimulation; **abirritative**, soothing.)

ăbī·uret (G. *a*, neg.; biuret). Non-response to the biuret test, *q.v.*

ablactā·tion (L. *ab*, from; *lactare*, to give milk). Weaning.

ablastē·mic (G. *a*, neg.; *blastēma*, an offshoot). Nongerminal.

ablă·stin. An antibody developed in rats with *Trypanosoma Lewisi.*

ablate (L. *ab*, from; *latus*, carried). To take away or cut off.

ablā·tio, ablātion. Detachment; removal of a part; e.g. **a. retinae:** detachment of the retina.

a·blephă·ria (G. *a*, neg.; *blepharon*, eyelid). Congenital absence of the eyelids or of the palpebral fissure. (Hence **ablĕpharous**, having no eyelids.)

ablep·sia (G. *a*, neg.; *blepsis*, sight). Blindness. (Also called **ablepsy.)**

ab·luent (L. *ab*, from; *luens*, washing). A detergent agent for cleansing.

ablū·tion. 1. The act of washing or cleansing the body. 2. Detachment of chemical impurities by washing.

abmor·tal (L. *ab*, from; *mortalis*, dying). Situated apart from an injured area.

abner·val. Passing through muscle from a nerve, e.g., an electric current.

abneu·ral (L. *ab*, from; G. *neuron*, nerve). Away from the neural axis.

abnor·mal (L. *ab*, from; *norma*, rule). Not normal; departure from the usual condition.

abnormă·lity. Property of being abnormal.

abocclū·sion (L. *ab*, from; *occludere*, to shut together). Dentition in which teeth in lower and upper jaws do not meet.

aboiement (Fr.). Making barking sounds.

abolumă·nia (G. *a*, neg.; *boule*, will; *mania*, madness). Mental disturbance characterized by indecision and weakness of will.

abo·masum (L. *ab*, from; *omasum*, paunch). Fourth and actually digestive stomach of a ruminant. (Hence **abomasitis**, inflammation of the abomasum.)

abor·al (L. *ab*, from; *os*, mouth). Pertaining to regions away from the mouth.

abori·ginal (L. *ab*, from; *orīgo*, beginning). Indigenous to an inhabited place.

abort (L. *aboriri*). 1. To miscarry. 2. To check or prevent the full development of, e.g., a disease.

abor·ticide (L. *abortus*, abortion; *caedere*, to kill). Agent which produces abortion by killing the foetus.

abortifă·cient (L. *abortio*, abortion; *facere*, to make). 1. Producing abortion. 2. An agent, e.g. drug, producing abortion.

abor·tin. A glycerine extract of the *Brucella abortus*, formerly used in the diagnosis of contagious abortion in cattle.

abortion (L. *abortio*). Expulsion of a not yet viable foetus, i.e. in the human species before the end of the seventh month of pregnancy. Syn. miscarriage. **A., accidental:** a. caused by an accident. **A., artificial:** deliberately induced a. **A., contagious:** a disease of cattle due to the *Brucella abortus*. **A., criminal:** illegally produced a. **A., incomplete:** an a. in which the placenta is retained. **A., missed:** retention of a dead foetus. **A., therapeutic:** a. deliberately produced in order to save the mother's life.

abor·tionist. One who unlawfully induces abortion.

abor·tive. 1. Preventing development of a disease. 2. Abortifacient.

abor·tus fever. Undulant fever, *q.v.*

abrā·chia (G. *a*, neg.; *brakhiōn*, arm). Congenital absence of both arms.

abrā·chiocephā·lia (G. *a*, neg.; *brakhiōn*, arm; *kephalē*, head). Congenital absence of arms and head.

abrā·chioce·phalus (G. *a*, neg.; *brakhiōn*, arm; *kephalē*, head). An armless and headless monster.

abrā·chius (G.). A foetus born with no arms.

abrade (L. *abradere*, to rub off). To remove or roughen by friction.

Abrami's disease. Widal-Abrami's disease, *q.v.*

Abrams' reflex (Abrams, A., U.S. physician, 1864–1924). Contraction of the lung following upon stimulation of the chest wall. **A.'s heart reflex:** contraction of the myocardium occurring when the skin of the praecordial region is irritated. **A.'s treatment:** the percussing of the seventh cervical spine in the treatment of thoracic and abdominal aneurysm.

abrā·sio cor·nĕae (L.). The rubbing away of the superficial layers of the cornea.

abrā·sio den·tium (L.). The wearing away of teeth.

abrā·sion (L. *abradere*, to rub off). A wearing away or excoriation of skin or mucous membrane by means of a physical agent.

abrā·sive. Causing abrasion.

abrā·sor. An instrument used in abrading.

abrĕăc·tion (L. *ab*, away; *re*, again; *agere*, to act). Elimination of an emotional repression by re-living in imagination the experience which originally gave rise to it.

Abrikossoff's tumour (Abrikossoff, A. J., Russian pathologist, born 1875). A tumour made up of cell groups having the appearance of primitive myoblasts. It is also called myoblastoma.

abrō·sia. Fasting.

abruptio placentae (L.). Premature separation of the placenta.

A·brus (G. *habros*, delicate). Syn. jequirity, bumble beads, prayer beads. The seeds of *Abrus precatorius* contain abrin, a mixture of two poisonous proteins. Formerly used in dilute form for trachoma.

abscess (L. *abscessus*, a departure). The sequence of local changes which follows the introduction of some infective agent into the tissues. Commonly applied to a collection of pus forming in a tissue space as a result of such infection. Alveolar a.: collection of pus at the alveolar margin resulting from infection of the tissues surrounding a dental root. Amoebic a.: abscess, usually in the liver, caused by entamoeba histolytica, *q.v.* Anorectal a.: abscess in the connective tissue surrounding the anal canal. Apical a.: abscess at the apex of the root of a tooth. Appendicular a.: collection of pus originating in an infection of the vermiform appendix. Bartholinian a.: abscess arising in a Bartholin's gland. Blind a.: abscess which resolves without discharging its contents. Brodie's a.: chronic abscess, usually in the marrow cavity of a bone. Cerebral a.: abscess in the substance of the brain. Cholangitic a.: abscess in a biliary passage. Cold a.: abscess which shows few signs of inflammation, usually applied to a tuberculous abscess. Collar-stud a.: small superficial abscess communicating by a sinus with a larger, more deeply seated one. Dental a.: abscess connected with a tooth. Embolic a.: abscess caused by an infected embolus. Encysted a.: abscess in which the contents are walled off by a condensation of surrounding connective tissue. Epidural, extradural a.: abscess lying between the dura mater and a cranial bone. Fixation a.: abscess produced artificially, usually by injection of a chemical irritant, in order to localise a diffuse infection. Intradural a.: abscess between the dura mater and the brain. Ischiorectal a.: abscess in the ischio-rectal fossa. Lacrimal a.: abscess in or surrounding the lacrimal sac. Lumbar a.: see psoas abscess. Lung a.: see pulmonary abscess. Mammary a.: an abscess in breast tissue. Mastoid a.: abscess in the air cells of the temporal bone. Mediastinal a.: suppuration in the connective tissue of the mediastinum. Metastatic a.: secondary abscess, usually resulting from embolic dissemination of the contents of a primary abscess. Miliary a.: abscess of minute size. Palmar a.: abscess in the connective tissue of the palm of the hand. Parametric a.: abscess in the broad ligament of the uterus. Pelvic a.: suppuration in the pelvic peritoneum. Perinephric a.: abscess in the tissue surrounding the kidney. Peritonsillar a.: abscess surrounding the tonsil, syn. quinsy. Periurethral a.: abscess surrounding the urethra. Pott's a.: tuberculous abscess of bone. Psoas a.: abscess, usually tuberculous, arising in lumbar vertebrae and tracking down the sheaths of the psoas major muscle. Pulmonary a.: abscess in the lung. Pulp a.: abscess, 1. of dental pulp; 2. of pulp of a finger. Pyaemic a.: abscess resulting from circulation of septic material in the bloodstream. Retrocaecal a.: abscess behind the caecum. Retromammary a.: abscess between the breast and the chest wall. Retropharyngeal a.: suppuration in connective tissue surrounding the pharynx. Root a.: abscess surrounding the root of a tooth. Spinal a.: abscess due to bony necrosis of a spinal vertebra. Sterile a.: abscess in which no micro-organisms can be demonstrated. Stitch a.: abscess at the site of a suture. Subdiaphragmatic a.: see subphrenic abscess. Subdural a.: abscess beneath the dura mater. Subperiosteal a.: abscess between periosteum and bone. Subphrenic a.: abscess situated immediately below the diaphragm. Tropical a.: usually applied to a liver abscess due to entamoeba histolytica.

abscïs·sa (L. *ab*, from; *scindere*, to cut). The horizontal co-ordinate in diagrams.

abscï·ssion (L. *abscissio*). Removal of a part by cutting away.

abscon·sio (L. *abscondere*, to hide). Bone cavity receiving the head of another bone.

absence (L. *absentia*). Loss, or partial loss, of consciousness for a short period.

Absidia corymbifera. A pathogenic fungus, capable of causing mycosis in man.

absinth(e) (Fr.). 1. The plant *Absinthium*, or wormwood. 2. Essence of wormwood. 3. A liqueur distilled from wine and wormwood.

absinthin. A poisonous principle, $C_{20}H_{28}O_4$, obtained from wormwood.

absinthism. Addiction to absinthe.

absinthium (G. *apsinthion*, wormwood). An infusion from the leaves and tops of *Artemisia absinthium*, used as a gastric tonic, heart stimulant and anthelmintic.

absolute (L. *absolvere*, to free). Unlimited. Perfect. A. alcohol: alcohol containing less than 1 per cent (by weight) of water. A. temperature: fundamental temperature scale. A. values: actual numbers, opposed to percentages, as of cell types in a blood count.

absorb (L. *absorbere*, to suck up). 1. To suck up or draw in gases, liquids, heat or light. 2. To remove agglutinins from a serum.

absorbefā·cient (L. *absorbere*, to suck up; *facere*, to make). Causing absorption.

absor·bent (L. *ab*, from; *sorbere*, to suck). 1. Taking up, imbibing. 2. Any agent which does this.

absorptiŏ·meter (L. *absorbere*, to suck up; G. *metron*, a measure). 1. An instrument for determining the solubility of a gas in a liquid. 2. An instrument for comparing the optical densities of two or more liquids.

absorp·tion (L. *absorptio*). 1. The taking up of one substance into another. 2. The process by which water, salts and the food elements formed during digestion pass from the gastro-intestinal tract through the mucosa cells into the lymph- or blood-stream. 3. The taking up of waste products from the tissues. 4. A process in immunology whereby agglutinins may be removed from a serum. A. band, or a. line: a dark band or line in the spectrum due to absorption of light rays (wave-lengths) on their passage through a solid, liquid, or gas.

absorp·tive. Capable of absorbing.

abster·gent (L. *abstergere*, to wipe). 1. Detergent. 2. A cleansing agent.

ab·stinence (L. *abstinere*, to refrain). The action or practice of refraining from the use of food, liquor or sexual intercourse.

ab·stract (L. *abstrahere*, to draw off). 1. In pharmacology, a preparation made by mixing a powdered extract of a vegetable substance with lactose in such proportion that one part of the final product represents two parts of the drug from which the abstract was made. 2. Summary or précis.

abstrac·tion. 1. Distillation. 2. Absent-mindedness. 3. The process of forming an abstract idea.

abū·lia (G. *a*, neg.; *boulē*, will.) Loss or defect of will-power.

abuse (L. *abusus*). Misuse; over-use.

abut·ment. A support to sustain lateral stress.

A.C. Abbreviation for alternating current.

a.c. Abbreviation of 1. *ante cibum* (L.), before food; 2. air conduction (of sound).

a.-c. interval. The small interval between the auricular and carotid waves, seen in the tracing of the jugular pulse.

Acā·cia¹. Genus of mimosa type trees, some of which yield gum arabic and others catechu.

acā·cia² (Syn. *Acaciae gummi*). A dried exudate from stem and branches of *A. senegal* and other species, almost completely soluble in water. Used for intravenous injection to raise blood pressure after loss of blood. It serves as an emulsifying agent.

acalcerō·sis (G. *a*, neg.; *khalix*, pebble). Lack of calcium in the body.

acalcū·lia (G. *a*, neg.; L. *calculare*, to calculate). Lack of power to work out even simple arithmetical calculations.

Acă·lypha (Syn. Indian Acalypha; Mukta-Jhuri). A gastro-intestinal irritant can be made from the fresh or dried entire plant. It has been employed as a substitute for ipecacuanha.

acamp·sia (G. *a*, neg.; *kamptein*, to bend). Rigidity of a joint or other part.

acanthaesthē·sia (G. *akantha*, thorn; *aisthēsis*, feeling). Sensation as of a pricking with needles; usually a perverted sensibility.

Acanthia lectularia. The common bed-bug. Syn. Cimex lectularius.

Acanthocĕ·phala (G. *akantha*, thorn; *kephalē*, head). An order of nemathelminthes, comprising various species parasitic in the intestines of fish, birds and other vertebrates, characterized by a more or less spindle-shaped form, absence of an alimentary canal and the presence of a proboscis.

acan·thoid. Spinous.

acan·thokeratoder·mia (G. *akantha*, thorn; *keras*, horn; *derma*, skin). Hyperkeratosis of hands and feet.

acanthō·ma (G. *akantha*, thorn). Squamous-celled carcinoma of the skin. **A. adenoides cystica**: see epithelioma, adenoid cystic. **A. verrucosa seborrhoeica**: senile warts.

acanthō·sis (G. *akantha*, thorn). Any skin disease characterized by hypertrophy of the prickle-cell layer, with or without hyperkeratosis of the epidermis. **A. nigricans**: a skin disease characterized by hypertrophy of the prickle-cell layer, melanin deposition in the cells of the basal layer and hyperkeratosis, leading to pigmented warty elevations occurring especially at the axillae, breasts and umbilicus, about the genitalia, the angle of the mouth and round the anus. When the disease develops after the fortieth year it is commonly associated with carcinoma of the intestinal tract; when it occurs in earlier life it is sometimes associated with obesity, diabetes, or some other endocrine disturbance.

acap·nia (G. *a*, neg.; *kapnos*, smoke). A condition of diminished carbon dioxide in the blood.

Acarapis woodi. A honey-bee mite, the cause of Isle of Wight disease.

acap·sular (G. *a*, neg.; L. *capsula*, a small box). Without a capsule.

acar·dia (G. *a*, neg.; *kardia*, heart). Congenital absence of the heart. (Hence **acardiac**, having no heart.)

acardi·acus. A monster foetus with no heart, and often attached to another foetus.

acardiohāe·mia (G. *a*, neg.; *kardia*, heart; *haima*, blood). Lacking blood in the heart.

acardiotrō·phia (G. *a*, neg.; *kardia*, heart, *trophē*, nutrition). Atrophy of the heart.

acari·asis (G. *akari*, mite). Infestation with mites, or a disease caused by mites or ticks.

acă·ricide (G. *akari*, mite; L. *caedere*, to kill). A mite-destroying agent.

Acari·na (G. *akari*, mite). An order of arachnida comprising ticks and mites.

acarophō·bia (G. *akari*, mite; *phobos*, fear). Crazy fear of the itch; sometimes imaginary affection of itch.

Acarus (G. *akari*, mite). Mite or tick; a parasite of man and animals. Causing scabies, *q.v.*

acarotox·ic (G. *akari*, mite; *toxikon*, poison). Destructive to mites and ticks.

acă·ryote (G. *a*, neg.; *karuon*, nut.). Non-nucleated.

acatalep·sia (G. *a*, neg.; *katalēpsis*, comprehension). Lack of understanding. (Hence, **acataleptic**, mentally deficient, uncertain.)

acatamathe·sia (G. *a*, neg.; *katamathesia*, understanding). Inability to comprehend a situation, sounds or objects.

acataphā·sia (G. *a*, neg.; *kataphāsis*, affirmation). Inability to connect words in complete sentences.

acatapŏ·sis (G. *a*, neg.; *kata*, down; *pŏsis*, a drinking). Difficulty in swallowing.

acatastă·sia (G. *a*, neg.; *katastăsis*, stability). Deviation from the normal.

acathar·sia (G. *a*, neg.; *katharsis*, evacuation). Failure to achieve purgation.

acathex·ia (G. *a*, neg.; *kathĕxis*, retention). Lack of power to retain normally the body's secretions. (Hence **acathectic**.)

acau·dal, acau·date (G. *a*, neg.; L. *cauda*, tail). Tail-less.

acau·line (G. *a*, neg.; L. *caulis*, stem). Without a stem.

acaulinō·sis. A fungus disease, characterized by a discharging eruption, with crusts.

A.C.C. Abbreviation for anodal closing contraction.

accelerans (L. *accelerare*, to hasten). Quickening. **A. nerve**: the cardiac sympathetic nerve which quickens the heart-beat.

accelerā·tion. 1. Rate of change of velocity. 2. Quickening, as of the pulse rate.

accĕ·lerator. Term applied to certain nerves and muscles which speed up functions.

accen·tuation (L. *accentus*, accent). Increased distinctness, or intensity of sound; intensification.

accen·tuator. Any substance which intensifies the action of a tissue stain.

acceptor (L. *accipere*, to take). A substance which unites with oxygen or hydrogen in an oxidation-reduction mechanism.

access (L. *accessus*). Attack of a disease.

acces·siflexor. Term applied to accessory flexor muscles.

accession. Beginning, as of a disease.

accessory. Term applied to organs which are supplementary in function to the principal. **A. nerve**: the eleventh cranial nerve. **A. food factors**: older term for vitamins.

accident (L. *accidere*, happen). An unforeseen event, especially one causing an injury.

acciden·tal. 1. Due to an accident. 2. Having no essential connection with other conditions and/or symptoms. **A. haemorrhage**: bleeding from the placental site before the birth of the child when the placenta is in the upper uterine segment, the result of disease (toxaemia of pregnancy, etc.) rather than of accident. **A. images:** after-images. **A. murmur:** a heart murmur not due to an organic lesion of the heart.

acciden·talism. A theory of medicine which treats disease as an accidental modification of health, attending only to the symptoms of the patient and ignoring aetiology and pathology.

acci·piter (L., hawk). A bandage for the face, with tails resembling the claws of a hawk.

acclīmatizā·tion (L. *ad*, to; G. *klima*, region). Process of becoming accustomed to environmental factors, such as the climate of a country to which an individual or plant has been moved.

accommodā·tion (L. *accommodare*, to fit). The mechanism of contraction of the ciliary muscle, resulting in an increase of thickness and decrease of equatorial diameter of the lens, by which the converging power of the eye is increased so that a distinct image is still retained. **A. spasm:** spasm of the ciliary muscle.

accŏm·modative. Pertaining to accommodation.

accommodŏ·meter. Apparatus for determining the accommodative power of the eye.

accouchée (Fr.). A woman delivered of a child.

accouchement. Childbirth. **A. forcé:** rapid and forcible delivery of the child.

accoucheur (Fr.). Obstetrician.

accoucheuse (Fr.). Midwife.

accrē·tion (L. *ad*, to; *crescere*, to grow). 1. Abnormal adherence, e.g., of the two layers of the pericardium. 2. The accumulation of foreign matter in a space. 3. The mode by which crystalline substances increase in bulk.

accū·mulator. Apparatus for storing electricity.

A.C.D. Abbreviation for absolute cardiac dullness.

acē·dia (G. *a*, neg.; *kēdos*, care). Mental disorder characterized by melancholy.

A.C.E. mixture. A chloroform mixture consisting of dehydrated alcohol 1, chloroform 2, and ether 3 parts.

acen·tric (G. *akentros*, not central). Of the periphery.

acephā·lia, acephaly (G. *a*, neg.; *kephalē*, head). Congenital absence of the head.

acephalobrā·chia (G. *a*, neg.; *kephalē*, head; *brakhiōn*, arm). Congenital absence of head and arms.

acephalobrā·chius. A monster foetus without head and arms.

acephalocar·dia (G. *a*, neg.; *kephalē*, head; *kardia*, heart). Absence of head and heart.

acephalocar·dius. A monster with neither head nor heart.

acephalochei·ria (G. *a*, neg.; *kephalē*, head; *kheir*, hand). Absence of head and hands.

acephalochei·rus. A monster foetus with neither head nor hands.

acē·phalocyst (G. *a*, neg.; *kephalē*, head; *kustis*, bladder). A hydatid cyst having no daughter cysts and not producing scolices or heads.

acephalogas·ter (G. *a*, neg.; *kephalē*, head; *gastēr*, belly). Monster characterized by absence of head and belly.

acephalopŏ·dia (G. *a*, neg.; *kephalē*, head; *pous*, foot). Absence of head and feet.

acephalopŏ·dius. A monster foetus with no head and no feet.

acephalorrhă·chia (G. *a*, neg.; *kephalē*, head; *rhakhis*, spine). Absence of head and spine.

acephalostō·mia (G. *a*, neg.; *kephalē*, head; *stoma*, mouth). Absence of head, with mouth-like opening on the superior aspect.

acephalothorā·cia (G. *a*, neg.; *kephalē*, head; *thōrax*, chest). Absence of head and chest.

acephalothor·us. A monster foetus with neither head nor thorax.

acē·phalous (G. *a*, neg.; *kephalē*, head). Headless.

acephalus (Pl. acephali). A monster characterized by complete absence of the head and usually of the upper extremities as well.

aceratō·sis (G. *a*, neg.; *keras*, horn). Deficiency of horny tissues.

acer·vulus (L. *acervus*, a heap). The gritty matter lying within or near the pineal body.

acē·scence (L. *acescere*, to turn sour). 1. Sourness. 2. Turning sour.

acestō·ma (G. *akestos*, curable). An accumulation of granulations.

acetabulec·tomy (L. *ăcētābŭlum*, socket of hip-bone [literally vinegar cup]; G. *ektomē*, excision). Excision of the acetabulum with the rest of the hip joint.

aceta (L. *acetum*, vinegar). Solutions of medical substances in dilute acetic acid.

acetă·bulum (L.). A cup-shaped depression on the external surface of the innominate bone. **A. humeri:** the glenoid cavity.

acetă·ldehydase. An enzyme oxidizing acetic aldehyde to acetic acid.

acetal·dehyde. An oxidation product of ethyl alcohol, CH_3CHO.

acetă·mide. CH_3CONH_2. Deliquescent crystals made by the interaction of ammonia and acetyl chloride.

acetă·nilide. $C_6H_5NCOCH_3$. An antipyretic prepared by acetylation of aniline.

acetarsol. $CH_3CONHC_6H_3(ON)AsO(OH)_2$ 3-acetyl-amino-4-hydroxyphenyl arsonic acid. Contains 27% As. and is used in the treatment of amoebiasis, yaws, lambliasis and early syphilis.

acetar·sone. Acetarsol, *q.v.*

acetate (L. *acetum*, vinegar). Salt of acetic acid.

acē·tic. Pertaining to vinegar. **A. acid:** a colourless crystalline acid, CH_3COOH.

acē·tify. To turn into vinegar.

aceti·meter. A device for ascertaining the amount of acetic acid in a fluid.

aceto-acetic acid. $CH_3CO.CH_2.COOH$. An intermediary product of fatty acid oxidation. See also ketonuria.

Acetobac·ter (L. *acetum*, vinegar; G. *baktron*, a stick). Generic term for bacilli producing acetic fermentation of sugars.

acē·tomorphine. Heroin.

acetonā·sthma (L. *acetum*, vinegar; G. *asthma*). Asthmatic attack due to acidosis.

ă·cetone. Dimethyl ketone $CH_3.CO.CH_3$. Colourless volatile solvent. Hence, **acetonaemia:** a morbid state characterized by the presence of acetone in the blood.

acetonū·merator (L. *acetum*, vinegar; *numerus*, number). An apparatus for estimating the amount of acetone in the urine.

acetonū·ria. Excess of acetone in the urine. See also ketonuria.

ă·cetophene·tidin. An acetyl compound of phenetidin, $CH_3CONH.C_6H_4.OC_2H_5$. White tasteless crystals. Used in temperature reduction and to soothe pain. The safest of antipyretics, rarely producing rash or cyanosis. Syn. phenacetin.

aceto-soluble. Soluble in acetic acid.

ă·cetous. Resembling or relating to vinegar.

ă·cetum (L.). Vinegar; an impure, dilute acetic acid yielded by acetous fermentation of wine or other fruit juices. In pharmacology, a solution of the active principles of certain drugs in dilute acetic acid. **A. cantharidini:** Cantharidin 1 in an acetic acid solution q.s. to 2,000. **A. digitalis:** Digitalis leaves 1, dilute acetic acid (6 per cent) 9, alcohol (90 per cent) 1. Macerate 5 days. **A. ipecacuanhae:** Contains 5 per cent w/v of liquid extract of ipecacuanha in alcohol, water and acetic acid. Alkaloid content, 0.1 per cent.

A. odoratum (Syn. toilet vinegar): Acetic acid 1 in 8 with odorants. **A. officinale**: Vinegar of white wine, with about 6 per cent of acetic acid. **A. scillae**: Squill 10 per cent w/v macerated in dilute acetic acid.

acetyl. Monovalent radical of acetic acid, CH_3CO.

acetyl-β-methylchŏ·line. $(CH_3)_3NCH_2CH(CH_3)$- $OCOCH_3(CH_3)_3OH$. Cardiac depressant and vasodilator effective by oral administration.

Acetylarsan. A proprietary preparation used for the treatment of syphilis.

acetylā·tion. The process of introducing an acetyl radical into an organic molecule.

acetylchŏ·line (L. *acetum*, vinegar; G. *kholē*, bile). An active ester of choline; $CH_3.CO.CH_2CH_2N(CH_3)_3$ OH, a substance produced by mediating impulses at the myoneural junction from parasympathetic postganglionic fibres; also produced by stimulation of sympathetic preganglionic fibres.

acĕ·tylene. A colourless explosive gas, C_2H_2, formed by the action of water on calcium carbide. Possesses anaesthetic properties.

acetylsalicȳ·lic acid. An acetyl compound of salicylic acid, $CH_3.CO_2.C_6H_4.COOH$. A widely used antipyretic and analgesic substance of special value in treatment of acute rheumatism.

ACH index. An index used in estimating bodily nutrition, based on measurements of chest depth, width of hip, and girth of arm.

achalā·sia (G. *a*, neg.; *khalan*, to relax). Failure of the mechanism producing relaxation of a sphincter (especially cardiac or anal sphincter), leading to dilatation and muscular hypertrophy of the part immediately above the sphincter (oesophagus, rectum).

Achalme's bacillus (Achalme, P., French physician, born 1866). The *Clostridium perfringens*.

Achard-Castaigne method (Achard, E. C., French physician, 1860–1941; Castaigne, J., French physician, born 1871). The methylene blue test for renal permeability.

Achard-Thiers syndrome (Achard, E. C., French physician, 1860–1941. Thiers, J., French physician). See Cushing's basophilism syndrome.

ache. Continuous pain.

achei·lia (G. *a*, neg.; *kheilos*, lip). Congenital absence of one or both lips. (Hence, **acheilous**, having no lips).

achei·ria (G. *a*, neg.; *kheir*, hand). Congenital absence of one or both hands. (Thus, **acheirus**, a foetus born without hands.)

Achilles tendon. The tendon of the gastrocnemius and soleus muscles. **A. t. reflex**: see under ankle jerk.

achil·lobursi·tis. Inflammation of a bursa at the Achilles tendon.

achillodȳ·nia. Pain located in the Achilles tendon, caused usually by achillobursitis.

achillŏ·tomy. Subcutaneous division of the Achilles tendon.

achlorhȳ·dria (G. *a*, neg.; *khlōros*, green, *hudōr*, water). Absence of hydrochloric acid in the gastric secretion.

achlorŏp·sia (G. *a*, neg.; *khloros*, green; *opsis*, vision). Inability to perceive the colour green.

achŏ·lia (G. *a*, neg.; *kholē*, bile). Absence of biliary secretion. (Hence **acholic**, free from bile.)

acholū·ria (G. *a*, neg.; *kholē*, bile; *ouron*, urine). Absence of bile pigment in the urine. For **acholuric jaundice**, see under jaundice.

achondroplā·sia (G. *a*, neg.; *khondros*, cartilage; *plassein*, to form). A congenital condition characterized by disordered endochondral bone formation, resulting in stunted growth of long bones and of the cranial base. Syn. See also trident hand.

achondroplă·stic. Pertaining to achondroplasia.

ā·chor (G. *akhōr*, dandruff). 1. An acuminate pustule. 2. Crusta lactea, *q.v.*

Achorion (G. *akhōr*, dandruff). A genus of trichophyton fungi. **A. Schönleinii**: the fungus causing favus in man.

achrĕ·stic (G. *a*, neg.; *khrēstos*, useful). Unable to use the body's anti-anaemic principle. See anaemia.

achrŏ·acyte. A lymphocyte. **Achroacytŏ·sis**: excessive development of the body's lymph cells.

achroi·ocythē·mia. Lack of haemoglobin in erythrocytes.

achrŏ·ma, achrŏ·mia (G. *a*, neg.; *khrōma*, colour). Lack of colour, albinism.

achromā·sia (G. *a*, neg.; *khrōma*, colour). 1. Lack of pigment in the body. 2. Absence of staining reaction in a cell.

achrŏ·mate. A colour blind person.

achromat·ic (G. *a*, neg.; *khrōma*, colour). 1. Colourless. 2. Not staining readily. 3. Not breaking up light into coloured rays. **A. lens**: a combination of lenses of varying refraction, in which chromatic aberration is corrected by bringing two spectral colour rays to a common focus.

achrŏ·matin. The non-staining parts of the cell nucleus.

achrŏ·matism. 1. Absence of chromatic aberration. 2. Absence of colour.

achromatŏ·lysis (G. *a*, neg.; *khrōma*, colour; *lusis*, a loosing). See under plasmolysis.

achromā·tophil (G. *a*, neg.; *khrōma*, colour; *philein*, to love). Not being readily stained.

achromatophi·lia. Resistance to staining.

achromatop·sia (G. *a*, neg.; *khrōma*, colour; *opsis*, sight). Total colour blindness.

achromatŏ·sis, achrŏ·mia. Any condition characterized by absence or deficiency of natural pigment. **Achromatous**: colourless. **Achromatū·ria**: colourless urine.

achrŏ·mic. Without colour.

achrŏ·mobacter. Member of the family achromobacteriaciae, saprophytic micro-organisms usually found in water, soil and milk and characterised by an inability to produce pigment.

achromoder·mia (G. *a*, neg.; *khrōma*, colour; *derma*, skin). Absence of cutaneous pigment.

achromotrī·chia (-k-) (G. *a*, neg.; *khrōma*, colour; *thrix*, hair). Absence of pigment in the hair.

Achucárro's method (Achucárro, N., Spanish histologist, 1851–1918). A silver-tannin method of impregnating connective tissue in histology.

achy·lia (G. *a*, neg.; *khulos*, juice). Deficiency or absence of pepsin and hydrochloric acid from the gastric juice.

achylia gastrica (G. *a*, neg.; *khulos*, juice; *gastēr*, belly). Disorder of gastric secretory function, characterized by total absence of free hydrochloric acid, pepsin and other enzymes in the gastric juice. **A. gastrica haemorrhagica**: the disease accompanied by occult blood in the stomach.

aci·cular (L. *acus*, needle). Needle-shaped.

acid, acidum (L. *acidus*). 1. Any substance which yields hydrogen ions when dissolved in water. Substances in which hydrogen can be replaced by a metal or basic radical. 2. Substance having a sour taste.

acid, normal. See under normal acid.

acid-albumin. A protein which is soluble in acid and gives acid reactions.

acidaminū·ria. Presence of excessive amounts of amino acids in the urine.

acidāe·mia (L. *acidus*, acid; G. *haima*, blood). Uncompensated acidosis.

acid-fast. Applied to micro-organisms which are not easily decolorized by mineral acids when stained, e.g. the tubercle bacillus.

acid-forming. Applied to foods having a considerable acid residue.

acidification (L. *acidus*, acid; *facere*, to make). The act of making acid.

aci·dify. To render acid.

acidi·meter (L. *acidus*, acid; G. *metron*, measure). An instrument for determining the amount of free acid in a solution.

acidi·metry. Determination of the amount of free acid in a solution.

aci·dity (L. *acidus*, acid). 1. Sourness. 2. Excess of hydrogen ions in aqueous solution. **A., actual:** a. with reference to the amount of ionized hydrogen (dissociated acid) present. **A., total:** a. with reference to both dissociated and undissociated acid present.

acidocytō·sis. Presence in the blood of an excessive proportion of eosinophile leucocytes.

acidology (G. *akis*, bandage; *logos*, treatise). Science of surgical appliances.

aci·dophile. Being readily stained by acid dyes. See also eosinophile.

acido-resistant. Capable of resistance to decolorization by acids.

acidō·sis. Disturbance of the acid-base equilibrium, characterized by presence of abnormal amounts of ketone bodies, *q.v.*, or other acids in the body, due either to accumulation of these acids or to loss of alkali.

aci·dulate. To render acid.

ā·cies (L.). Border or margin.

acini·tis. Inflammation of the acini of a gland.

acino-tubular (L. *acinus*, berry or grape; *tubulus*, dim. of *tubus*, tube). Characterized by having tubular acini.

ă·cinous. Like a grape.

ă·cinus (L. grape; pl. *acini*). 1. A round or oval structure with a narrow lumen lined with granular cells. 2. One of the minute berry-like beginnings of the excretory ducts of a racemose gland. Syn. alveolus. 3. A lobule of the liver.

ackee poisoning. Poisoning with ackee, the fruit of *Blighia sapida*; characterized by acute abdominal pain and vomiting, followed after a short time by convulsions and coma. Syn. vomiting sickness of Jamaica.

aclă·stic (G. *a*, neg.; *klaein*, to break). Not refracting.

acleistocar·dia (G. *a*, neg.; *kleiein*, to close; *kardia*, heart). Imperfect closure of the foramen ovale.

acme (G. *akmē*, point). Crisis, or the critical stage of a disease.

acne (G. *akmē*, point). Inflammatory disease of the sebaceous glands. **A. agminata:** see acnitis. **A. atrophica:** a form of a. necrotica. **A. indurata:** a form of a. vulgaris, characterized by the formation of hard red or purple nodules around the sebaceous glands, which remain for a long period as indurated swellings. **A. necrotica:** a form of a. vulgaris, characterized by indolent papules and pustules which leave on healing a small depressed permanent scar. **A. rosacea:** see under rosacea. **A. scrofulosorum:** a papulo-necrotic tuberculide, *q.v.*, of the skin, characterized by deep-seated acne-like eruptions, mostly on the extensor surfaces of the limbs. **A. vulgaris:** an inflammatory disease of the sebaceous glands, characterized by comedo formation and acuminate papulo-pustules, usually affecting individuals in the post-pubertal period.

acneform, acnē·iform. Resembling acne.

acnē·mia (G. *a*, neg.; *knēmē*, leg). 1. Atrophy of the calves of the legs. 2. Congenital absence of the legs.

acni·tis (G. *akme*, point). A papulo-necrotic tuberculide, *q.v.*, of the skin, characterized by acne-like papules on the face, which tend to become pustulous and to develop into small ulcers. Syn. miliary disseminated lupoid of the face; acne agminata.

acoe·lomate. Not having a coelom.

acŏ·logy (G. *akos*, cure; *logos*, treatise). The science of therapeutics.

ă·colous (G. *a*, neg.; *kōlon*, limb). Without limbs.

acŏ·mia (G. *a*. neg.; *komē*, hair). Baldness.

ă·conite (L. *aconitum*). The poisonous dried root of the *Aconitum napellus*, used as an anodyne, diaphoretic and diuretic.

aconitina. Syn. acetylbenzoylaconine. $C_{34}H_{45}O_{11}N$, used externally in neuralgia, avoiding mucous membranes and raw skin. Very small doses may be given internally as a depressant, calmative and diaphoretic. Rarely used because of powerful cardiac action.

Aconitum. A genus of poisonous ranunculaceous herbs.

aconurē·sis (G. *acōn*, unwilling; *ourēsis*, urination). Involuntary passing of urine.

acoprō·sis (G. *a*, neg.; *kopros*, excrement). Absence of faeces from the intestinal tract.

ă·cor. Acidity or bitterness.

acorē·a (G. *a*, neg.; *korē*, pupil). Absence of the pupil of the eye.

acoria. See under akoria.

acor·mus (G. *a*, neg.; *kormos*, trunk). A monster foetus without a trunk.

acos·mia (G. *a*, neg.; *kosmos*, order). Irregularity in the course of a disease or syndrome.

Acosta's disease. Hypobaropathy, *q.v.*, first described by a Jesuit priest named d'Acosta, who wrote of it in the sixteenth century, after he had visited Peru.

acouaesthē·sia (G. *akouein*, to hear; *aisthesis*, sensation). Acoustic perceptiveness.

acou·meter (G. *akouein*, to hear; *metron*, measure). An instrument for measuring the power of hearing.

acous·ma (G. *akousma*, a thing heard). An auditory hallucination.

acousmatagnō·sis (G. *akousma*, a thing heard; *a*, neg.; *gnosis*, knowledge.) Inability to recognize sounds, owing to mental disorder.

acous·tic (G. *akoustikos*, of or for the sense of hearing). Relating to the ear or to acoustics.

acou·stics. The science of sound.

acquired (L. *acquirere*, to obtain). Applied to diseases, habits, etc., not congenital, but obtained after birth.

ă·cral (G. *akros*, extreme). Relating to the extremities.

acrā·nia (G. *a*, neg.; *kranion*, skull). Congenital partial or complete absence of the skull. Hence **acrānial**, having no skull; **acrā·nius**, a monster foetus with no skull or an incomplete one.

acrā·sia (G. *a*, neg.; *krasis*, combination). Intemperance or lack of self-control.

acrā·tia (G. *a*, neg.; *kratos*, power). Loss of strength; weakness.

acraturē·sis (G. *akratēs*, uncontrolled; *ourēsis*, urination). Difficult urination owing to bladder weakness.

Acrel's ganglion (Acrel, O., Swedish surgeon, 1717–1807). A ganglion situated on the extensor tendons of the wrist.

Acremonium. A genus of fungi, which causes **acremoni·osis** in man. The infection is characterized by fever and swellings.

acribō·meter (G. *akrībes*, exact; *metron*, measure). An instrument for measuring minute objects.

acrid (L. *acer*, sharp). Pungent.

ă·cridine. $CH:(C_6H_4)_2:N$; parent substance of a class of dyes and chemotherapeutic drugs.

acriflā·vine. An orange-red or red crystalline odourless powder consisting of a mixture of the hydrochloride of 2:8-diamino-10-methylacridinium chloride and diaminoacridine dihydrochloride, the latter being present to the extent of about one-third. It is used for the prevention of wound sepsis for it is markedly antiseptic and is non-irritant.

ă·crimony (L. *acrimonia*, sharpness). An acrid property.

acri·tical (G. *a*, neg.; *krisis*, crisis). Without a crisis.

acritochrō·macy (G. *a*, neg.; *krites*, a judge; *khroma*, colour). Colour blindness.

acro-aesthē·sia (G. *akros*, extreme; *aisthesis*, sensation). Increased sensitivity especially to pain in the distal parts of the limbs.

acro-anaesthē·sia (G. *akros*, extreme; *anaisthesia*, anaesthesia). Anaesthesia in the distal parts of the limbs.

acro-arthrī·tis (G. *akros*, extreme; *arthron*, joint). Arthritis of the distal parts of the limbs.

acro-asphyx·ia (G. *akros*, extreme; *a*, neg.; *sphuxis*, throbbing). Asphyxia of the distal parts of the limbs, e.g. 'dead' fingers and toes.

acro-atax·ia (G. *akros*, extreme; *a*, neg.; *taxis*, arrangement). Ataxia of the extremities.

ă·croblast (G. *akros*, extreme; *blastos*, germ). A body or group of bodies in the spermatid from which arises the acrosome. Syn. archoplasm.

acrobў·stiolith (G. *akrobustia*, prepuce; *lithos*, stone). A calculus of the prepuce.

acrobysti·tis. Inflammation of the prepuce.

acrocephā·lia, acroce·phaly (G. *akros*, extreme; *kephalē*, head). Congenital malformation of the head, the upper part being cone-shaped. Hence **acrocephă·lic**, being affected with acrocephalia.

acroce·phalosyndactў·lia, acroce·phalosyndactyly (G. *akros*, extreme; *kephalē*, head; *sun*, with; *daktulos*, finger). Congenital malformation characterized by acrocephalia and syndactylism of hands and/or feet. Syn. Apert's syndrome.

acrochor·don (G. *akros*, extreme; *khordē*, string). Pendulous growth on eyelids or neck.

acrocinē·sis (G. *akros*, extreme; *kinēsis*, movement). Excessive freedom of movement.

acrocontrăc·ture (G. *akros*, extreme; L. *contrahere*, to contract). Contracture of the foot or hand.

acrocyanō·sis (G. *akros*, extreme; *kuanos*, blue). Cyanosis of the distal parts of the limbs and of other peripheral parts of the body, such as nose and ears.

acrodermati·tis (G. *akros*, extreme; *derma*, skin). Dermatitis of the extremities. **A., chronic atrophic:** (Herxheimer) a chronic disease of the skin, affecting especially the upper limbs, characterized by erythematous patches or nodular infiltration, followed by general atrophy of the skin. **A. perstans:** a chronic disease of the skin affecting especially the thenar and hypothenar eminences of the hands and feet, characterized by the development of numerous pustules in a dermatitic area.

ă·crodont (G. *akros*, extreme; *odous*, tooth). Having the teeth firmly soldered to the jawbones instead of inserted into the alveoli. This condition is found in lizards.

acrodў·nia (G. *akros*, extreme; *odunē*, pain). See pink disease.

acrŏ·genous (G. *akros*, extreme; *gennan*, to produce). Apical increase of growth.

acrogē·ria (G. *akros*, extreme; *gĕron*, old man). Premature ageing of the skin of the extremities.

acrohyperhydrō·sis (G. *akros*, extreme; *hyper*, over; *hudor*, water). Excessive perspiration of the extremities.

acrohypother·mia (G. *akros*, extreme; *hypo*, under; *thermē*, heat). Excessive coldness of the extremities.

acrohў·sterosalpingec·tomy (G. *akros*, extreme; *hystera*, uterus; *salpiggion*, tube; *ektomē*, excision). Removal of both Fallopian tubes and fundus of uterus.

acromā·nia (G. *akros*, extreme; *mania*, madness). Madness characterized by great motor activity.

acromasti·tis (G. *akros*, extreme; *mastos*, breast). Inflammation of the nipple.

acromĕ·galy, acromegā·lia (G. *akros*, extreme; *megas*, great). Morbid condition due to an adenoma of the eosinophilic cells of the anterior part of the pituitary gland in adult life, causing overproduction of the growth hormone; characterized by over-growth of the distal parts of the limbs, of chin, ears and usually of the heart, sometimes leading to bitemporal hemianopia or optic atrophy, owing to pressure of the enlarged gland on the optic chiasm, and sometimes also to diabetes mellitus. Hence **acromegăl·ic**, pertaining to acromegaly.

acromegalo-gigant·ism. Gigantism caused by affection with acromegaly during the period of life between puberty and maturity.

acromĕ·galoidism. A condition like acromegaly, but not caused by imbalance of the pituitary gland.

acromĕ·lic (G. *akros*, extreme; *melos*, limb). Relating to the distal part of a limb.

acrometagĕ·nesis (G.). Over-growth of the hands and/or feet.

acrō·mial (G. *akros*, extreme; *ōmos*, shoulder). Relating to the acromion.

acromī·cria (G. *akros*, extreme; *mikros*, small). 1. Abnormal smallness of the extremities. 2. Sometimes used as a synonym for pituitary dwarfism.

acrō·mioclavi·cular (G. *akros*, extremity; *ōmos*, shoulder; L. *clavicula*, dim. of *clavus*, key). Relating to both the acromion and the clavicle.

acrō·miocor·acoid (G. *akros*, extremity; *ōmos*, shoulder; *korax*, raven; *eidos*, form). Relating to both the acromion and the coracoid process.

acrō·miohū·meral (G. *akros*, extreme; *ōmos*, shoulder; L. *humerus*, upper arm bone). Relating to both the acromion and the humerus.

acrō·mion (G. *akros*, extreme; *ōmos*, shoulder). The triangular process at the summit of the scapula.

acrō·mioscă·pular. Relating to both the acromion and the scapula.

acrŏm·phalus (G. *akros*, extremity; *omphalos*, navel). 1. The centre of the umbilicus, to which the cord is attached. 2. Abnormal projection of the umbilicus. 3. The remnant of the umbilical cord attached to the child.

acromycō·sis (G. *akros*, extremity; *mukēs*, fungus). Mycosis of the limbs.

acroneurō·sis (G. *akros*, extreme; *neuron*, nerve). Neurosis of the limbs.

ă·cronyx (G. *akros*, extreme; *onux*, finger-nail). Ingrowing of a nail. Syn. onyx incarnatus.

acro-oedē·ma (G. *akros*, extreme; *oidēma*, swelling). Chronic swelling of an extremity, often due to an injury.

ă·cropachy (-k-) (G. *akros*, extreme; *pakhus*, thick). Clubbed finger.

ă·croparaesthē·sia (G. *akros*, extreme; *para*, amiss; *aisthēsis*, feeling). Paraesthesia of the distal parts, e.g. the fingers, sometimes with angiospasm leading to gangrene.

acroparā·lysis (G. *akros*, extreme; *paralusis*, paralysis). Paralysis of the distal parts of the limbs.

acrŏ·petal (G. *akros*, extremity; L. *petere*, to seek). Rising towards the peak.

acrophō·bia (G. *akros*, summit; *phobos*, fear). Neurotic fear of being at a great height.

acroposthi·tis (G. *akroposthia*, prepuce). Inflammation of the prepuce.

ă·croscleroder·ma (G. *akros*, extreme; *sklēros*, hard; *derma*, skin). See under sclerodactylia.

acrosclerō·sis (G. *akros*, extremity; *sklēros*, hard). Hardening of the extremities.

ă·crose. $CHOH.(CHOH)_3CHO.CH_2OH$. An aldohexose formed by the action of sodium hydroxide solution on formaldehyde.

ăcrosome (G. *akros*, extreme; *sōma*, body). 1. The apical body situated at the anterior end of the spermatozoon. 2. Formerly, the granule within the acroblast from which the acrosome arises.

acrotĕ·ric. Relating to the outside.

ăcrotism (G. *a*, neg.; *krotein*, to beat). Pulselessness.

ăcro·trophoneurō·sis (G. *akros*, extreme; *trophē*, nourishment; *neuron*, tendon). Trophic disturbance of the distal parts.

A.C.S. Abbreviation for anodal closing sound.

A.C.T.H. Adrenocorticotrophic hormone. Hormone of the anterior lobe of the pituitary body which controls the function of the adrenal cortex.

actin (G. *aktis*, a ray). A protein concerned in muscular contraction.

acti·nic (G. *aktis*, ray). Producing chemical change by action of light. A. rays: any rays producing actinism.

acti·niform. Like a ray.

ac·tinism (G. *aktis*, a ray). The property of radiant energy which produces chemical changes.

acti·nium. A radio-active element. Symbol Ac.

Ac·tinobaci·llus. A genus of the family Bacteriaceae. A. lignieresi: causes actinobacillosis in domestic animals, and occasionally in man.

ăc·tinochĕ·mistry. Chemistry dealing with the action of light rays.

ăc·tinodermati·tis (G. *aktis*, ray; *derma*, skin). Dermatitis due to ultra-violet or other rays.

actinō·meter (G. *aktis*, ray; *metron*, measure). An instrument for measuring the strength of actinic rays.

Actinomy̅·cēs (G. *aktis*, ray; *mukēs*, mushroom). A genus of higher bacteria forming a septate branched mycelium (syn. ray-fungus) reproducing by spores and producing radiating forms in the living body. Also classified as a genus of hyphal fungi. Responsible for the formation of numerous antibiotic substances.

Ac·tinomycetā·ceae. A systematic family of the Actinomycetales.

Ac·tinomycetā·lēs. An order of organisms in the Schizomycetes class.

actinomycō·sis (G. *aktis*, ray; *mukēs*, mushroom). A chronic disease due to infection with one of the Actinomyces fungi, characterized by chronic suppuration, formation of granulation tissue and frequently of sinuses affecting especially the jaw, neck, intestines and lungs.

ăc·tinoneuri·tis (G. *aktis*, ray; *neuritis*). Neuritis caused by radio-active rays.

ăct·inothĕ·rapy (G. *aktis*, ray; *therapeia*, treatment). Treatment with ultra-violet rays.

ăc·tinotoxae̅·mia (G. *aktis*, ray; *toxaemia*). Toxaemia resulting from tissue destruction through radio-active rays.

action (L. *actio*, from *agere*, to do). Performance of a function. A. current: the electrical current associated with neural, muscular, glandular or other tissue activity. A. potential: the electrical changes in living tissue which can be recorded by a galvanometer.

action-tremor. Rhythmical tremors of the limbs, or incoordination of movement caused by disturbance of the function of the cerebellum. Seen in ataxia.

activate. To render active.

active (L. *activus*, from *agere* to do). 1. Characterized by action; not passive. 2. Energetic, e.g. active treatment.

actor. Any substance capable of partaking of both primary and secondary chemical reactions.

actual (L. *actus*, from *agere*). Real.

actuā·tion (L. *actus*, from *agere*, to do). Bringing into action; impulsion.

ăcuclosure (L. *acus*, needle; *claudere*, to shut). The stopping of haemorrhage by the use of a needle.

acū·ity (L. *acus*, needle). Acuteness; clearness. A. meter, an instrument, of great range and sensitivity, for determining the precise degree of deafness.

acū·minate (L. *acuminare*, to sharpen). Tapering to a sharp point.

acupre·ssion, acupre·ssure (L. *acus*, needle; *pressura*, pressure). Compression of a bleeding vessel by means of needles inserted on either side.

acupunc·ture (L. *acus*, needle; *pungere*, to pierce). Puncture of the skin or tissue by one or more needles, practised for the relief of pain (counter-irritation), for the withdrawal of tissue fluid, or to effect coagulation of blood in an aneurysm.

ăcusection. Cutting with an electrosurgical needle.

acu·sticus (G. *akoustikos*, of the sense of hearing). The auditory or eighth cranial nerve.

acute (L. *acutus*, sharp, from *acuere*). 1. Sharp; severe. 2. Said of an illness characterized by rapid onset, short course and pronounced symptoms.

acutor·sion (L. *acus*, needle; *torsio*, a wringing). Twisting an artery with a needle in order to control haemorrhage.

acyanŏp·sia (G. *a*, neg.; *kuanos*, blue; *opsis*, vision). Inability to perceive blue colours.

acyē·sis (G. *a*, neg.; *kuēsis*, conception). 1. Female sterility. 2. Absence of pregnancy.

acys·tic (G. *a*, neg.; *kustis*, bladder). Absence of the bladder.

acystiner·via (G. *a*, neg.; *kustis*, bladder; L. *nervus*, nerve.) Absence of nerve stimulus in the bladder.

Acys·tospori·dia. An order of animal parasites.

A.D. Abbreviation for anodal duration.

ad. Latin preposition meaning 'to'.

ad-. Prefix signifying toward, nearness, intensification.

·ad. Suffix expressing direction toward, e.g., caudad, towards the tail.

adactў·lia (G. *a*, neg.; *daktulos*, finger). Congenital absence of fingers or toes. Hence adăc·tylous, lacking fingers or toes.

Adair-Dighton syndrome (Dighton, C. A. Adair, contemporary British physician). A hereditary syndrome characterized by blue sclerotics, fragilitas ossium and deafness.

Adalin. A proprietary preparation of carbromal.

adaman·tine (G. *adamantinos*, hard as steel). Relating to the enamel of the teeth.

adaman·tinocarcinō·ma (G. *adamas*, a hard substance; *karkinos*, a sore). An adamantinoma which has become malignant.

adamantinō·ma (G. *adamas*, a hard substance). A neoplasm derived from the enamel organ of a developing tooth.

adaman·toblast (G. *adamas*, a hard substance; *blastos*, germ). An epithelial cell from which the enamel of the teeth is developed. Syn. ameloblast.

adamas dentis (G. *adamas*, a hard substance; L. *dens*, tooth). The enamel of the teeth.

Adami's theory (Adami, J. G., Canadian pathologist, 1861-1926). A hypothesis for the explanation of heredity. It resembles Ehrlich's theory of immunity.

Adamkiewicz's demilune cells (Adamkiewicz, A., Austrian pathologist, 1850-1921). Peculiar crescent-shaped nerve corpuscles lying beneath the neurilemma of medullated nerve fibres. They stain yellow by safranin. A.'s test: a sulphuric acid and glacial acetic acid test to detect the presence of proteins.

Adam's apple. The prominentia laryngea.

Adam's operation (Adams, W., English surgeon, 1820-1900). 1. Osteotomy of the neck of the femur by means of a saw in cases of ankylosis of the hip joint. 2. Multiple subcutaneous divisions of the palmar fascia for Dupuytren's contraction. 3. Excision of a triangular wedge of the lower lid for ectropion.

B

4. Correction of the nasal septum by means of flat, parallel-bladed forceps in cases of deflection of the septum. 5. Shortening of the round ligaments in cases of prolapsus uteri. A.'s saw: a small, straight saw for the performance of osteotomy.

Adams-Stokes disease (Adams, R., Irish physician, 1791–1875; Stokes, W., Irish physician, 1804–78). Syncope with or without convulsions and associated with bradycardia and heart block.

adaptā·tion (L. *adaptare*, to fit). 1. Structural or functional change in an organ, whereby it becomes better suited to its environment. 2. The process by which visual perception becomes possible after sudden change from light to dark, or dark to light, surroundings.

adapter. 1. A connecting part. 2. Tubing for connecting chemical appliances, or a device to join parts of surgical instruments to each other.

adaptō·meter (L. *adaptare*, to fit; G. *metron*, measure). An instrument for estimating the time of retinal adaptation to darkness.

adax·ial (L. *ad*, to; *axis*). Directed towards the axis.

adde. Latin for add.

ad. def. an. Abbreviation for L. *ad defectionem animi*, a Ciceronian phrase meaning (without *ad*) 'want of courage', but used in medical terminology to mean 'to the point of fainting'.

ad. deliq. Abbreviation for L. *ad deliquium*, meaning 'to fainting'.

ad. grat. acid. Abbreviation for L. *ad gratam aciditatem*, to a pleasing acidity.

ă·ddict (L. *addicere*, to abandon). A person who habitually takes drugs, especially narcotic drugs, or alcohol.

addic·tion. Neurotic habitual indulgence in some bad habit, or habitual use of some drug or of alcohol.

addictō·logy. The science of treating persons addicted to drugs or alcohol.

addisin. A substance present in the normal gastric juice of man. Extract of this substance from the gastric juice of the hog has been successfully used in the treatment of pernicious anaemia.

Addison's disease (Addison, T., English physician, 1793–1860). A disease, usually having a fatal termination, characterized by severe anaemia, digestive disturbances and a peculiar bronze coloration of the skin. The cause is hypofunction of the suprarenal glands, due to tuberculous infiltration.

Addison's planes (Addison, C., English anatomist, 1869–1951). Planes used in the topography of the thorax and abdomen.

additive (L. *addere*). Being added.

addū·cens (L. *adducere*, to lead to). A muscle drawing part towards the median line. A. oculi: the internal rectus muscle of the eye.

adduct. To draw towards a part or towards the median line of a body.

adduc·tion. Any movement by which a part is drawn towards another, or towards the median line of the body.

adduc·tor. Term applied to any muscle (e.g. a. hallucis) effecting adduction.

adelomor·phous (G. *adēlos*, not evident; *morphē*, form). Not having a clearly defined form; applied to the central or chief glands of the gastric mucosa.

adĕl·phia (G. *adelphos*, brother). A double monster characterized by union of the upper parts of the two organisms.

aden (G. *adēn*, gland). 1. A gland. 2. A bubo.

Aden fever. See dengue.

adenăl·gia (G. *adēn*, gland; *algos*, pain). Glandular pain.

ă·denase. An enzyme of the spleen, pancreas and liver, which hydrolyzes adenine to hypoxanthine.

adendrī·tic (G. *a*, neg.; *dendron*, tree). A nerve cell lacking in dendrons.

adenĕc·tomy (G. *adēn*, gland; *ektomē*, excision). Excision of a gland.

adenemphrax·is (G. *adēn*, gland; *emphraxis*, stoppage). Obstruction of a gland.

adē·nia (G. *adēn*, gland). Hyperplasia of the tissues of the lymphatic glands.

adĕ·niform (G. *adēn*, gland; L. *forma*, shape). Shaped like a gland.

adenine. A purine base, 6-aminopurine, derived from nucleic acids.

adeni·tis. Inflammation of a lymph node.

adeno-acanthō·ma. Carcinoma of the endometrium containing squamous epithelium.

adeno-an·giosarcō·ma. An angiosarcoma in which glands have become affected.

adĕ·noblast (G. *adēn*, gland; *blastos*, germ). 1. A cell possessing glandular functions. 2. An embryonic cell from which gland tissue is derived.

adenocarcinō·ma (G. *adēn*, gland; *karkinos*, a sore or ulcer). A carcinoma derived from glandular epithelial cells, usually of columnar type, the glandlike arrangement of which reproduces to some extent that of the organ from which the tumour arises.

ă·denocele (G. *adēn*, gland; *kēlē*, tumour). Cystic tumour containing adenomatous elements.

adenocellulī·tis (G. *adēn*, gland; L. *cellula*, dim. of *cella*, cell). Inflammation of a lymph node involving surrounding cellular tissue.

ă·denochondrō·ma (G. *adēn*, gland; *khondros*, cartilage). Tumour composed of glandular and cartilaginous tissue.

ă·denochon·drosarcō·ma (G. *adēn*, gland; *khondros*, cartilage; *sarx*, flesh). Tumour composed of adenomatous and sarcomatous tissue.

ă·denochrome (G.). The colouring matter of the suprarenal glands.

adenocyst (G. *adēn*, gland; *kustis*, bladder). Cystic lymphatic gland; glandular cyst.

ă·denocystō·ma (G. *adēn*, gland; *kustis*, bladder). A cystic adenoma.

ă·denocyte (G. *adēn*, gland; *kutos*, a container). The mature secretory cell of a gland.

ă·deno-epithelliō·ma. A tumour made up of glandular and epithelial tissue.

ă·denofibrō·ma (G. *adēn*, gland; *fibra*, fibre). Benign neoplasm composed of adenomatous and fibrous tissue.

ă·denofibrō·sis. Fibroid change in a gland.

ă·denohypersthē·nia (G. *adēn*, gland; *huper*, over; *sthenos*, strength). Excessive activity of a gland.

ă·denohypŏ·physis. The glandular, anterior part of the hypophysis.

adenoid (G. *adēn*, gland; *eidos*, form). Glandlike.

adenoid vegetations, ă·denoids. Hypertrophy of the lymphatic tissue in the nasopharynx. Hence **adenoidism**, the presence of adenoids; and **adenoiditis**, inflammation of an adenoid.

adenoidec·tomy (G. *adēn*, gland; *eidos*, form; *ektomē*, excision). The surgical removal of adenoids.

ă·denolipō·ma (G. *adēn*, gland; *lipos*, lard). Neoplasm composed of adenomatous and lipomatous tissue.

ă·denŏ·lipomatō·sis (G. *adēn*, gland; *lipos*, lard; *omos*, shoulder). Condition characterized by presence of multiple lipomata in the region of the neck, axillae and groins.

ă·denŏ·logy (G. *adēn*, gland; *logos*, discourse). Knowledge of the glands.

ă·denolymph·ocele (G. *adēn*, gland; *lymphocele*). Cyst of a lymph node.

adenō·ma (G. *adēn*, gland). A benign epithelial tumour of glandular structure closely resembling that of the gland from which it arises. **A., basophile:** see Cushing's syndrome. **A. sebaceum:** a chronic disease of the skin, characterized by firm reddish nodules due to overgrowth of sebaceous gland and sometimes also of fibrous and/or vascular tissue; occurring mainly on the face in a symmetrical pattern. Syn. Pringle's naevus. See also epiloia, tuberous sclerosis. **A., toxic:** see goitre, secondary toxic.

ăˈdenomalăˈcia (G. *adēn*, gland; *malakia*, softness). Softening of a gland.

ăˈdenomatōˈsis (G. *adēn*, gland). Any condition characterized by generalized hyperplasia of lymph nodes.

adenomyōˈma (G. *aden*, gland; *mus*, muscle). Growth of endometrial tissue within the myometrium; usually a simple hyperplasia but may become malignant.

ăˈdenomȳˈosarcōˈma (G. *adēn*, gland; *mus*, muscle, *sarx*, flesh). Adenosarcoma in which there is striated muscle.

ăˈdenomyosīˈtis. Inflammatory hypertrophy of the uterus.

ăˈdenomyxōˈma (G. *adēn*, gland; *muxa*, mucus). A tumour composed of adenomatous and myxomatous tissue.

ăˈdenomy̆xˈosarcōˈma (G. *adēn*, gland; *muxa*, mucus; *sarx*, flesh). A tumour composed of adenomatous, sarcomatous and myxomatous tissue.

adenonˈcus (G. *adēn*, gland; *ongkos*, bulk). Enlargement of a gland.

adenonēūˈral. Relating to a gland and a nerve.

adenŏˈpathy (G. *adēn*, gland; *pathos*, disease). Any disease of a gland or a lymph node.

adenopharyngīˈtis (G. *adēn*, gland; *pharugx*, pharynx). Inflammation of the tonsils and pharynx.

adenosarcōˈma (G. *adēn*, gland; *sarx*, flesh). Sarcoma developing in the fibrous stroma of a gland.

ăˈdenosarˈcorhabˈdomȳōˈma (G. *adēn*, gland; *sarx*, flesh; *rhabdos*, rod; *mus*, muscle). A tumour composed of adenomatous, sarcomatous and rhabdomyomatous tissue.

adenosclerōˈsis (G. *adēn*, gland; *sklērosis*, hardening). Hardening of a gland.

adenŏˈsinase. An adenosine-splitting enzyme.

aděˈnosine diphosˈphate and a. triphosˈphate. Mononucleotides, an important source of energy for the contraction of muscles.

adenŏˈsis. Any disease of a gland.

ăˈdenosīˈtis. Inflammation of glandular tissue.

aděˈnotome (G. *adēn*, gland; *tomē*, a cutting). An instrument for removing adenoids.

adenylˈic acid. A mononucleotide formed from adenosine diphosphate by elimination of phosphoric acid as a result of muscle contraction.

adephăˈgia (G. *adēn*, enough; *phagein*, to eat). Voracious appetite.

ăˈdeps (L. *adeps*). 1. Lard. 2. Animal fat. 3. Fat. **A. lanae:** wool fat. **A. lanae hydrosus:** lanoline.

aderˈmia (G. *a*, neg.; *derma*, skin). Absence of the skin.

aderˈmin. A pyridine derivative that is a dietary essential. Pyridoxin; Vitamin B₆; 2-methyl-3-hydroxy 4:5-(hydroxy-methyl)-pyridine. Prevents nutritional deficiencies in which muscular weakness and rigidity are prominent.

adermogěˈnesis (G. *a*, neg.; *derma*, skin; *genesis*, origin). Deficient development of the skin.

adermotrŏˈphia (G. *a*, neg.; *derma*, skin; *trophē*, nourishment). Atrophy of the skin.

Adexolin. A proprietary preparation of vitamins A and D.

adhere (L. *adhaerere*). To hold together.

adhēˈsion (L. *adhaerere*). 1. The attractive force between two different bodies that are in contact. 2. The union of two surfaces or parts. 3. Abnormal fibrous union of two surfaces as a result of inflammation.

adhesiŏˈtomy. The surgical removal of adhesions.

adhēˈsive (L. *adhaerere*). Sticky; adherent. **A. pericarditis:** see pericarditis, adhesive.

adhib. Abbreviation for L. *adhibendus*, to be used.

adiabăˈtic (G. *a*, neg.; *dia*, through, *bainein*, to go). In physics, a term applied to phenomena which are not accompanied by the production or loss of heat.

adiactïˈnic (G. *a*, neg.; *dia*, through; *aktis*, a ray). Not permeable by actinic rays.

adiadochokinēˈsis (G. *a*, neg.; *diadochos*, succeeding; *kinēsis*, movement). Inability to perform quickly alternating movements of hands, fingers or toes; usually a sign of cerebellar disorder.

adiaemorˈrhysis (G. *a*, neg.; *dia*, through; *haima*, blood; *rhusis*, flow.) A stoppage of blood circulation.

Adiănˈtum (G. *a*, neg.; *diantos*, capable of being wetted). A genus of ferns, of which the true Maidenhair is rarely found in the British Isles.

adiaphorēˈsis (G. *a*, neg.; *diaphorein*, to sweat out). Deficiency of perspiration. Hence **adiaphoretic**, to diminish perspiration.

adiăˈstolē (G.). Absence of the cardiac diastole.

adiatherˈmic (G. *a*, neg.; *dia*, through; *thermē*, heat). Impervious to heat.

Adie's syndrome (Adie, W. J., British neurologist, 1886–1935). A pathological reaction in which the pupil on the side affected contracts and dilates more slowly than the other.

adipecˈtomy. The surgical excision of fat masses.

ăˈdipocele (L. *adeps*, fat; G. *kēlē*, hernia). A true hernia with hernia sac, containing only fatty tissue.

ăˈdipocere (L. *adeps*, fat; *cera*, wax). The wax-like substance formed from fatty tissue after death. It is especially noticeable in human bodies buried in moist places.

adipŏˈgenous (L. *adeps*, fat; G. *gennan*, to produce). Producing fatty tissue.

adipohepăˈtic (L. *adeps*, fat, G. *hepar*, liver). Characterized by fatty degeneration of the liver.

adipŏˈmeter (L. *adeps*, fat; G. *metron*, measure). An instrument for measuring the thickness of the skin and subcutaneous fat.

ăˈdiponecrōˈsis (L. *adeps*, fat; G. *nekros*, corpse). Necrosis of the fatty tissues.

ăˈdipose (L. *adeps*, fat). Fat.

adipōˈsis (L. *adeps*, fat). Obesity. **A. dolorosa:** a condition characterized by the presence of painful or tender lipomata, usually affecting females. Syn. Dercum's disease. **A. tuberosa simplex:** See Anders's disease.

adipŏˈsitas, adipŏˈsity (L.). Obesity, fatness.

adiposīˈtis. Inflammation of adipose tissue.

adiposūˈria (L. *adeps*, fat; G. *ouron*, urine). Lipuria, *q.v.*

adipˈsia (G. *a*, neg.; *dipsa*, thirst). Absence of thirst.

ăˈditus (L. *aditus*, from *adire*). An entrance.

adjuncˈtion. The joining of two or more medicines in the treatment of a disease.

adjustˈment. The changes undergone by an organism in adapting itself to changing conditions.

adˈjuvant (L. *adjuvare*, to aid). A medicament added to a prescription to assist the action of another drug.

Adler's test (Adler, O., German physician, born 1879). A benzidine test for the presence of blood.

Adler's theory (Adler, A., Austrian psychiatrist, 1870–1937). The theory that people develop neuroses in order to compensate for some form of inferiority.

ad lib. (L. *ad libitum*). At pleasure.

admov. Abbreviation for L. *admove*, *admoveatur*, let there be added.

admēˈdial. Located in the neighbourhood of the median plane.

adˈnate (L. *ad*, towards; *natus*, from *nasci*, to be born). Grown together; congenitally united.

ad nauseam (L.). To the point of producing nausea.

adner·val (L. *ad*, to; *nervus*, nerve). Adjacent to a nerve.

adnex·a (L. *ad*, to; *nectere*, to bind). Adjunctive parts, e.g. the a. of the uterus. Hence **adnexal**, pertaining to adnexa.

adnexec·tomy. Removal by surgery of the adnexa.

adnexi·tis. Inflammation of both ovary and uterine tube.

adnexoge·nesis (L. *adnexa*; G. *genesis*, production). The development of the adnexa in the embryo.

adnex·opexy (L. *adnexa*; G. *pēxis*, fixation). The operation of raising the Fallopian tube and ovary and fixing them to the abdominal wall.

adole·scence (L. *adolescere*, to grow). The period between puberty and maturity.

adŏ·nidin. A hygroscopic glycoside, obtained from the *Adonis vernalis*. Used as a heart tonic and its action resembles that of digitalis. Has also been used in treatment of epilepsy, when it is combined with bromide.

Adonis. A genus of ranunculaceous plants, including the pheasant eye narcissus, found in Europe, Asia and Africa. (See adonidin.)

ador·al (L. *ad*, to; *os*, mouth). Situated near the mouth.

adosculā·tion (L. *ad*, to; *osculari*, to kiss). Impregnation by means of external contact, without intromission.

ad pond. om. (L. *ad pondus omnium*). To the weight of the whole.

adre·nal (L. *ad*, to; *renes*, kidneys). 1. The suprarenal gland. 2. Adjacent to the kidney.

adrenalec·tomize (L. *ad*, to; *renes*, kidneys; G. *ektomē*, excision). To remove the adrenal glands.

adrenalec·tomy. Surgical removal of the adrenal gland(s).

adre·naline. $C_6H_3(OH)_2.CHOH.CH_2NH.CH_3.-\alpha$ -3:4-dihydroxyphenyl-β-methylaminoethanol. The hormone produced by the adrenal medulla. It can be produced synthetically and when injected as the hydrochloride, acts as a powerful vasopressor. In contact with exposed tissues or mucous membranes, it acts as a vasoconstrictor.

adrenali·noscope (*adrenaline*; G. *skopein*, to look at). An instrument used to detect the presence of adrenaline in a liquid.

adre·nalinuria (*adrenaline*; G. *ouron*, urine). The presence of adrenaline in the urine.

adre·nalism. Adrenal malfunction.

adre·nalone. A ketone derived from the oxidation of an epinephrine derivative. It is capable of raising the blood pressure.

adrenalŏ·pathy (L. *ad.*, to; *renes*, kidneys; G. *pathos*, disease). Any state in which the function of the adrenals is disturbed.

adre·nals. The suprarenal glands.

adrener·gic (L. *ad*, to; *renes*, kidneys; G. *ergon*, work). Applied to those autonomic nerve fibres stimulation of which leads to the production of adrenaline or a related substance at the myoneural junction.

adre·nin. The internal secretion of the adrenal medulla.

adreni·tis. Inflammation of the adrenals.

adrenocor·tical (L. *ad*, to; *renes*, kidneys; *cortex*, outward part). Pertaining to the adrenal cortex or to its hormone.

adre·nocorticotrŏ·phic, adre·nocorticotrŏ·pic (L. *ad*, to; *renes*, kidneys; *cortex* outward part; G. *tropos*, way). Stimulating the hormonal activity of the adrenal cortex. A. hormone: see ACTH.

adrenodon·tia (*adrenal*; G. *odous*, tooth). Tooth form showing adrenal predominance, i.e. with usually large canines and teeth showing a brownish discoloration.

adre·nogě·nital syndrome (L. *ad*, to; *renes*, kidney; *gignere*, to produce; G. *sun*, with; *dromos*, course). A condition characterized by the development of secondary male characters in females, usually accompanied by amenorrhoea, or of secondary female characters in males; due to hyperplasia or an adenoma of the androgenic zone of the adrenal cortex.

adre·nomedullotrop·ic (L. *ad*, to; *renes*, kidneys; *medulla*, marrow; G. *tropos*, way). Stimulating hormonal activity of the adrenal medulla.

adre·notrope. A person with an endocrine constitution in which adrenal influences are predominant.

adrenotrŏp·ic. Stimulating hormonal activity of the adrenal glands.

adrenŏ·tropin. An anterior pituitary hormone acting upon the adrenal gland.

adrō·mia (G. *a*, neg.; *dromos*, course). Absence of conduction.

adru·e. *Cyperus articulatus*, a West Indies plant, the root of which has tonic and anthelmintic properties.

adsor·bate (L. *ad*, to; *sorbēre*, to suck). The substance being adsorbed.

adsor·bent (L. *ad*, to; *sorbēre*, to suck). A substance causing adsorption.

adsorp·tion. The concentration of a substance at the surface of a solid or liquid.

adster·nal (L. *ad*, to; *sternum*). Near the sternum.

adstrin·gent (L. *ad*, to; *stringere*, to draw tight). Any agent causing vascular constriction, thus lessening secretion from a mucous membrane.

adstringen·tia (L.). Drugs acting by local contraction of tissues and lessening of secretion.

ADT. Abbreviation used on placebo prescriptions, signifying A 'any', T 'thing', and D 'what you please'.

A.D.Te. Symbol for anodal duration tetanus.

adul·teration (L. *adulterare*, to pollute). The fraudulent admixture of less valuable substances with foodstuffs, medicaments, etc.

advancement. Surgical detachment of a part, e.g. a muscle, and its subsequent replacement at a further advanced position.

adventi·tia (L. *adventicius*, coming from elsewhere, from *advenire*). The outer layer of the wall of a blood-vessel.

adventi·tial. Pertaining to the adventitia.

adventi·tious. 1. Accidental. 2. Acquired. 3. Occurring out of the usual place.

adynā·mia (G. *a*, neg.; *dunamis*, power). Deficiency or loss of muscular power. Hence **adynă·mic**, characterized by adynamia.

A.E. German abbreviation for antitoxin unit.

Aeby's plane (Aeby, C. T., Swiss anatomist, 1835–85). A plane passing through the nasion and basion and running perpendicular to the median plane of the cranium.

Aedes (G. *aēdēs*, unpleasant). A genus of culicine mosquitoes. **A. aegypti** (syn. *Stegomyia fasciata*) is the vector of viruses causing yellow fever, dengue, etc.; several other species are the intermediate hosts of *Filaria bancrofti*. Other species of the genus are *A. albopictus*, *A. calopus*, *A. fuscus*, *A. sollicitans*, *A. sylvestris*, and *A. variegatus*.

aedŏeŏcĕ·phalus (G. *aidoia*, genitals; *kephalē*, head). A monster foetus with no mouth, a nose resembling a penis, and possessing only one orbit.

aedŏeŏ·logy (G. *aidoia*, genitals; *logos*, treatise). The study of the genitalia.

Aeg. Abbreviation for L. *aeger*, the patient.

aegagrŏ·pilus (G. *aigagros*, wild goat; *pīlos*, hair). A hairy tumour located in the stomach.

aegi·lops (G. *aigilōps*, an ulcer of the eye). Abscess at the inner canthus of the eye.

aegŏ·phony (G. *aix*, goat; *phōnē*, sound). The peculiar nasal, bleating character of the patient's voice heard on pectoral auscultation at the upper border of pleural effusions.

aeĭ·pathy (G. *aei*, always). Any inveterate or unyielding disease.

aeraē·mia (G. *aēr*, air; *haima*, blood). The presence of air in the bloodstream.

aerā·rium (L.). An arrangement for the provision of fresh-air supplies.

aerā·tion (G. *aēr*, air). 1. Charging with air or gas. 2. The state of being aerated.

aerendocar·dia (G. *aēr*, air; *endon*, in; *kardia*, heart). The presence of air in the heart.

aerial. Relating to the air.

aero-anaerō·bic (G. *aēr*, air; *an-*, neg.; *aēr*, air; *bios*, life). Term applied to organisms that are both aerobic and anaerobic.

Aerobac·ter. A genus of Bacteriaceae residing in the intestines of normal persons, and including *A. aerogenes* and *A. cloacae*.

aerobe (G. *aēr*, air; *bios*, life). One of the Aerobia.

Aerobia (G. *aēr*, air; *bios*, life). Organisms requiring air or available oxygen in order to maintain life. Facultative A.: micro-organisms capable of growing both in presence or absence of free oxygen. Obligate or Obligatory A.: organisms always requiring free oxygen to maintain life.

aerō·bic (G. *aēr*, air; *bios*, life). Requiring air or available oxygen to live or grow.

aerobiŏ·logy (G. *aēr*, air; *bios*, life; *logos*, word). The branch of biology dealing with the distribution of living organisms through air.

aerobi·oscope (G. *aēr*, air; *bios*, life; *skopein*, to view). Apparatus for collecting and filtering bacteria from the air.

aerobiō·sis (G. *aēr*, air; *bios*, life). Life requiring the presence of air or available oxygen. Hence aerobiŏ·tic, living through air.

aerocele (G. *aēr*, air; *kēlē*, tumour). A diverticulum of one of the upper respiratory organs (larynx, trachea or bronchus) or a swelling containing air in free connection with one of these organs.

aerocol·pos (G. *aēr*, air; *kolpos*, hollow). Distension of the vagina with air or gas.

aerŏ·coly (G. *aēr*, air; L. *colon*). Distension of the colon with air or gas.

aerocystŏ·graphy (G. *aer*, air; *kustis*, bladder; *graphein*, to write). Examination of the bladder, after its inflation with air, by means of x-rays.

aerodynă·mics (G. *aer*, air; *dunamis*, power). The science of air in motion.

aero-emphysē·ma (G.). Condition in which air bubbles collect in the body tissues at high altitudes.

aerogăst·ria (G.). The presence of air or gas in the stomach.

aerogen (G. *aēr*, air; *gennan*, produce). Any gas-producing micro-organism. Aerogenesis: gas production. Aerogenic: producing gas.

aerŏ·meter (G. *aēr*, air; *metron*, measure). Instrument for measuring the density of gases.

aeromicrobe (G.). Any aerobic micro-organism.

aeroneurō·sis (G.). Nervous disease found in aviators and characterized by gastric symptoms and emotional disturbance with increased motor activity.

aerŏ·pathy (G.). Disease caused by changes in atmospheric pressure.

aeroperitō·nia (G.). The presence of air or gas in the peritoneum.

aerŏ·phagy (G. *aēr*, air; *phagein*, to eat). The swallowing of air.

aerophyte (G.). A microbe or other plant organism that draws its sustenance from the air.

aeroscope (G.). An instrument for examination of air purity.

aerosīnusī·tis (L.). Inflammation of the sinuses in aviators.

aerō·sis. Production of air in the body tissues.

aerosol. (Called also aerosol mist.) A finely atomized bactericidal solution, used to sterilize the air of a sickroom or other confined place.

aerothē·rapy (G. *aer*, air; *therapeia*, treatment). The use of air for the treatment of disease.

aerotonŏ·meter (G. *aēr*, air; *tonos*, tone; *metron*, measure). Instrument for measuring tension of gases in the blood.

aerŏ·tropism (G. *aēr*, air; *trepein*, to turn). The growth of an organism either inclining to or turning away from the air.

aesculā·pian. Relating to Aesculapius, the god of medicine.

Aesculapius. Son of Apollo and Coronis, and the god of healing in Greek mythology.

Aesculus hippocastanum. The horse chestnut. The bark and seeds of the tree are anti-rheumatic.

aesthematŏ·logy (G. *aisthesis*, feeling; *logos*, treatise). Science of the senses.

aesthē·sia (G.). Feeling or sensation.

aesthē·sioblast (G. *aisthēsis*, feeling; *blastos*, germ). An embryonic cell of the spinal ganglia.

aesthesiomā·nia (G.). Insanity characterized by sense perversion.

aesthesiŏ·meter (G. *aisthēsis*, feeling; *metron*, measure). Instrument for measuring dermal sensibility.

aesthē·sioneure (G.). A sensory neuron.

aesthē·sioneurō·sis. Any malfunction or disorder of the sensory nerves.

aesthesiŏ·scopy (G.). The marking out on the skin of pain areas.

aesthě·tic. Relating to sensation.

aestī·val (L. *aestivus*, from *aestas*, summer). Relating to or occurring during the summer. A.-autumnal: relating to or occurring during summer and autumn. A.-a. fever: tropical malaria.

aet. Abbreviation for L. *aetas*, age.

aetiŏ·logy (G. *aitia*, cause; *logos*, discourse). 1. The cause of phenomena, e.g. of a disease. 2. The science of such causes. Hence, aetiolŏ·gical: pertaining to aetiology.

afeb·rile (G. *a*, neg.; L. *febris*, fever). Without fever.

affect (L. *afficere*, to influence). 1. A stimulus arousing emotion. 2. Emotion associated with ideas.

affection. 1. Synonym for disease. 2. A mental state.

affective. Relating to affect.

affectī·vity. The totality of emotions of an individual.

af·ferent (L. *afferens*, from *afferre*, to bring). Leading towards the centre; conveying sensory impulses from the periphery towards the central nervous system.

afferen·tia (L.). Any afferent vessels, whether of blood or lymph.

affi·liation (L. *ad*, to; *filius*, son). In forensic medicine, the act of affixing the paternity of a child so as to provide for its maintenance.

affi·nity (L. *affinis*, neighbouring). 1. Selective relationship. 2. Selective attraction. 3. The property of an element of electing to combine preferentially with a particular element.

aff·lux, afflux·ion (L. *affluere*, to flow). The flow of blood or other fluid to a part.

affu·sion (L. *affundere*, to pour). Pouring of water upon the body, e.g. to reduce fever.

afi·brinogenaē·mia. Lack of fibrinogen in the blood.

African coast fever. See Rhodesian fever.

African lethargy. See trypanosomiasis.

African pepper. Cayenne pepper.

African tick fever. See under relapsing fever.

after-birth. Popular term for the placenta, cord and membranes, sometimes termed the secundines.

after-care. Care and nursing of convalescents.

after-cataract (Syn. cataracta secundaria). Opacity of the lens capsule after operation for cataract; remains of the lens substance.

after-damp. Poisonous gases, such as carbon monoxide, found in coal-mines after an explosion.

after-hearing. Having the sensation of continuing to hear sounds when they have ceased to exist.

after-image. Retinal impressions persisting after the stimulus of light has ceased.

after-nŷstag·mus. Nystagmus occurring after the abrupt cessation of a rotation, due to persistence of movement of the labyrinthine fluid after the head has become stationary. Syn. secondary nystagmus.

after-pains. Pains felt after childbirth, and due to contraction of the uterus.

after-perception. Perception of a sensation after the stimulus which caused it has passed away.

after-sensation. A sensation prolonged beyond the stimulus which produces it.

after-sound. The hearing of a sound after the stimulus producing it has ceased to exist.

after-stain. A secondary stain used in order to obtain greater distinction of detail.

after-taste. Taste persisting after the stimulus producing it has disappeared.

after-treatment. The treatment of a convalescent patient.

afunction (G. *a*, neg.; L. *fungi*, to perform). Absence of function.

Ag. Chemical symbol for silver.

AgCl. Silver chloride.

AgCN. Silver cyanide.

agalac·tia (G. *a*, neg.; *gala*, milk). Absence of milk secretion.

ă·gamete (G. *a*, neg.; *gamos*, marriage). An amoeba developing without sexual union. Hence **agă·mic**, characterized by the absence of sexual union.

Agamofilaria. A genus of nematode parasites.

agamŏ·gony (G.). Reproduction without sexual connexion.

Agamomermis culicis. A genus of nematodes.

agar (Malay). A culture medium having agar-agar as solidifying agent.

agar-agar. A gelatinous substance obtained from certain seaweeds of the order Rhodophyceae. Used to solidify nutrient media for bacterial cultures.

agar·ic. 1. A mushroom of the species of Polyporus, especially the *P. officinalis*, used as a haemostatic, and the *P. igniarius*, used as tinder. 2. (Bot.) Any mushroom.

Agaricus. A genus of mushrooms.

agă·ster (G. *a*, neg.; *gastēr*, stomach). Without a stomach.

agă·stric. Applied to conditions due to complete or partial absence of the stomach. **A. anaemia:** see anaemia, a.

age. Time that has elapsed since birth (chronological age). **Mental a.:** stage of mental development reached by an individual as determined by intelligence testing.

agĕ·nesis (G. *a*, neg.; *genesis*, beginning). 1. Aplasia, *q.v.* 2. Impotence.

agenosŏ·mus (G. *a*, neg.; *gennan*, beget; *sōma*, body). A monster foetus without genitals, or having only rudimentary ones.

agent (L. *agere*, to do). Any natural force or substance which acts, whether curatively or otherwise, upon the organism.

agerā·sia (G. *a*, neg.; *geron*, old man). An appearance of youth in an elderly or old person.

ageū·sia, ageū·stia (G. *a*, neg.; *geusis*, taste). Absence or loss of the sense of taste.

agger (L. *agger*, mound). In anatomy, a pile or mound. **A. nasi:** an oblique ridge on the inner surface of the nasal process of the maxilla.

agglŏ·merate (L. *agglomerare*, to heap up). Cluster or heap.

agglutinā·tion (L. *agglutinare*, to fasten to). 1. A joining together. 2. Loss of mobility and clumping of micro-organisms when specific immune serum is added, or of red blood corpuscles when incompatible blood serum is added. **A., group:** a. of one or more members of a group of related micro-organisms by an agglutinin specific for one of these.

agglū·tinator (L.). An agglutinin.

agglū·tinin. An antibody, *q.v.*, which causes clumping of micro-organisms or other cells suspended in a fluid.

agglū·tinogen (L. *agglutinare*, to fasten to; G. *gennan*, beget). The antigenic substance in microbial or other cells stimulating the production of agglutinins. Hence **agglutinogen·ic**, relating to the production of agglutinin.

agglū·tinoid. An agglutinin which is no longer capable of agglutinating, but which still has the power to unite with its agglutinogen.

aggluti·noscope (L. *agglutinare*, to fasten to; G. *skopein*, to view). Instrument for estimating agglutination.

agglū·tinum. The part of a bacillus which is able to agglutinate.

agglutinŏ·meter (L. *agglutinare*, to fasten to; G. *metron*, measure). An instrument for carrying out the Gruber-Widal test without using a microscope.

aggred. feb. Abbreviation for L. *aggrediente febre*, while fever is approaching.

aggregate (L. *aggregatus*, added). To crowd together.

aggregā·tion. The crowding together of materials.

aggressin. A substance produced in the body by bacteria, causing a weakening of the normal protective substances in the body.

AgI. Silver iodide.

agit. vas. Abbreviation for L. *agitato vase*, the container having been shaken.

agitā·tion (L. *agitare*, to shake). Excessive restlessness.

agitogrā·phia (L. *agitare*, to drive; G. *graphein*, to write). Excessive speed in writing, with generally unconscious omission of words or parts of words.

agitolă·lia (L. *agitare*, to drive; G. *lalein*, to speak). Excessive rapidity of speech.

aglaucop·sia (G. *a*, neg.; *glaukos*, green; *opsis*, vision). Inability to distinguish green colours.

aglobū·lia (G. *a*, neg.; L. *globulus*, globule). Decrease in the blood of the proportion of red cells. Also called **aglobuliosis** and **aglobulism**.

aglos·sia (G. *a*, neg.; *glōssa*, tongue). Congenital absence of the tongue.

aglossostō·mia (G. *a*, neg.; *glōssa*, tongue; *stoma*, mouth). Congenital absence of the tongue and closure of the mouth.

aglutī·tion (G. *a*, neg.; L. *glutire*, to swallow). Inability to swallow.

aglycae·mia (G. *a*, neg.; *glukus*, sweet; *haima*, blood). Absence of sugar from the blood.

aglycosū·ric. Without glycosuria.

ag·men. An aggregation.

ag·nate. Under Scottish law the closest relative on the paternal side of a person adjudged insane and appointed guardian of the insane person.

agnā·thia (G. *a*, neg.; *gnathos*, jaw). Congenital absence or defective development of the jaws.

Agnew's splint (Agnew, D. H., American surgeon, 1818-1892). 1. A splint for a fractured patella. 2. A splint for a fracture of the metacarpus.

agmatŏ·logy (G. *agmos*, fracture; *logos*, discourse). The sum of knowledge of fractures.

AgNO₃. Silver nitrate.

agnoe·a (G. *agnoia*, ignorance.) Loss of perception powers owing to disease.

agnō·sia (G. *a*, neg.; *gnosis*, knowledge). Inability to recognize a sensory impression in the absence of a lesion of the particular sensory organ; due to a cerebral lesion. **A., auditory**: disturbance in recognition of speech, noise or musical sounds. Syn. word-deafness. See also aphasia, subcortical sensory. **A., finger**: see finger agnosia. **A., tactile**: disturbance in recognition of objects or forms by touch; usually associated with other sensory disturbances and due to a lesion in the superior parietal lobe. Syn. asterognosis. **A., visual**: disturbance in visual recognition of objects and colours; due to a lesion of the basal part of the occipital lobe.

Ag₂O. Silver oxide.

agō·nia₁ (G. *agōnia*, anguish). 1. Distress of mind; severe anguish. 2. The death struggle.

agō·nia₂ (G. *agŏnos*, barren). Barrenness; sterility.

agomphi·asis (G. *a*, neg.; *gomphios*, a grinder-tooth). Looseness of the teeth.

agom·phious. Having no teeth.

agō·nal. Relating to the death agony.

agō·nad (G. *a*, neg.; *gonē*, seed). A person without gonads. Hence **agon·adal**, without sex glands.

agony (G. *agonia*, struggle). 1. Extreme suffering. 2. The death struggle.

agoraphō·bia (G. *agora*, market place; *phobos*, fear). Neurotic fear of open places.

Agostini's test. A gold chloride and potassium hydroxide test for dextrose in urine.

agram·matism (G. *a*, neg.; *gramma*, a letter). Inability to form sentences grammatically, owing to a cerebral disorder; involuntary use of abbreviated forms of expression (telegram style).

agră·nulocyte. A non-granular leucocyte.

Ag₃PO₄. Silver orthophosphate.

agră·nulocytō·sis (G. *a*, neg.; L. *grānulum*, dim. of *grānum*, grain; G. *kutos*, a container). Disease characterized by leucopenia with extreme decrease of granulocytes, associated with ulcerative inflammation of the throat or vagina and a grave general condition, sometimes caused by the taking of a drug such as amidopyrine or sulphonamide against which an idiosyncrasy has developed.

agranuloplas·tic (G. *a*, neg.; L. *grānum*, grain; G. *plassein*, to form). Not forming granular cells.

agră·phia (G. *a*, neg.; *graphein*, to write). Inability to write, owing to a lesion near Broca's area.

agrăem·ia (G. *agra*, seizure; *haima*, blood). Condition of blood which obtains when gout is present.

ag·ria (G. *agrios*, wild). An unyielding pustular skin eruption.

Agrimonia eupatoria. A rosaceous plant, yielding a tonic known as agrimony.

agriothȳ·mia (G. *agrios*, wild; *thumos*, mind). Insane savagery.

agromā·nia (G. *agros*, field; *mania*, madness). Morbid desire for solitude.

agrȳp·nia (G. *agrupnos*, sleepless). Insomnia or sleeplessness. Hence **agrypnot·ic**, a drug that prevents sleep.

Ag₂S. Silver sulphide.

Ag₂SO₄. Silver sulphate.

ague (Old Fr. *ague*, from L. *acutus*, acute.) Malarial fever.

agȳ·ria (G. *a*, neg.; *guros*, round). Failure of gyral differentiation, especially of the outer cortical layers.

ah. Symbol for hypermetropic astigmatism.

a.h. (L. *alternis horis*). Every other hour.

Ahlfeld's sign (Ahlfeld, F., German obstetrician, 1843–1929). Irregular spasms in portions of the uterus to be noted after the third month of pregnancy.

ahȳp·nia (G. *a*, neg.; *hupnos*, sleep). Insomnia.

A.I. Abbreviation for 1. Axio-incisal. 2. Artificial insemination.

aichmophō·bia (G. *aikhmē*, spearpoint; *phobos*, fear). Neurotic fear of sharp points.

aidoioman·tia (G. *aidoia*, pudenda). Abnormal sexual desire.

ailment. Any disorder or disease of the body.

ailurophō·bia (G. *ailouros*, cat; *phobos*, fear). Neurotic fear of cats.

ain·hum (Negro word, to saw). Tropical disease characterized by the development of a furrow around the proximal part of a toe, followed by swelling, ulcer formation, and finally by the spontaneous amputation of the toe.

air (G. *aer*). The atmosphere. **A. conduction**: the normal way of transmission of sounds to the ear, via the external auditory meatus and middle ear. **A. embolism**: embolism due to entry of air into the circulatory system. **A. sickness**: condition similar to sea sickness caused by flying.

Airol (Syn. Airoform; Airogen). Proprietary preparation of bismuth oxyiodogallate, used externally in cases of gonorrhoea.

Aitken's operation (Aitken, J., Scottish surgeon, died 1790). Double hebotomy in cases of narrow pelvis. **A.'s saw**: a chain saw used in the decapitation of a foetus.

Aitken's pill (Aitken, Sir W., Scottish physician, 1825–92). A pill containing iron, quinine, strychnine and arsenic.

akatam·ah (Afric.). An endemic form of peripheral neuritis in Bantu negroes, believed not to be beri-beri.

Akerlund deformity (Akerlund, A., Swedish radiologist, born 1887). A deformity in the duodenal cap, resulting from a chronic ulcer.

Aker-tuba. Derris or tuba-root. A horticultural and agricultural insecticide of great value. Has also been used as a lotion in cases of scabies.

akinē·sia, akinē·sis (G. *a*, neg.; *kinēsis*, motion) Marked absence of movements; especially used in relation to absence of automatic movements as occurring in persons with lesions of the basal cerebral ganglia.

aknephascō·pia (G. *a*, neg.; *knephas*, twilight; *skopein*, to view). Twilight blindness.

akor·ia (G. *a*, neg.; *koros*, satiety). Insatiable appetite.

Al. Chemical symbol for aluminium.

ala (L.). 1. A wing. 2. Any wing-like process. 3. The arm or shoulder; in animals, the shoulder-blade. **A. cinerea**: a cerebral area situated lateral to the nucleus intercalatus.

alā·lia (G. *a*, neg; *lalein*, to speak). Inability to speak owing to a defect of the vocal organs. Hence **alal·ic**, relating to alalia.

alanine. CH₃CHNH₂. COOH. α-aminopropionic acid.

Alanson's amputation (Alanson, E., British surgeon, 1747–1823). A circular amputation, with the stump shaped like a circular cone.

ā·lar (L. *ala*, wing). 1. Winglike. 2. Relating to the shoulder or axilla.

alas·trim (Portug. *alastrar*). A mild form of smallpox, occurring especially in South Africa and South America. Syn. amaas; variola minor. Hence **alastrim·ic**, relating to alastrim.

alā·tus (L. *ala*, wing). Winged.

alba (L. *albus*, white). The white fibrous tissue of the brain and nerves.

Albarran's disease (Albarran, J., Cuban surgeon, 1860–1912). Colibacilluria. **A.'s test**: a test for renal inadequacy; also called polyuria test.

albe·do (L.). Whiteness. **A. unguis**: the lunula of the nail.

Albee's operation (Albee, F. H., U.S. surgeon, born 1876). 1. A plastic operation for ankylosis of the hip joint. 2. Spinal transplant in cases of tuberculous disease of the spine.

Albers-Schönberg's disease (Albers-Schönberg, H. E., German radiologist, 1865–1921). Osteopetrosis.

Albert's disease (Albert, E., Austrian surgeon, 1841–1900). Achillobursitis. **A.'s operation:** removal of the lower end of the femur and upper end of the tibia so as to obtain ankylosis of the knee joint. **A.'s suture:** a form of Czerny's suture, in which the first row of stitches is passed through the entire thickness of the intestine.

al·bicans (L. *albicare*, to whiten). 1. White; whitish. 2. One of the corpora albicantia of the brain.

albidūr·ia. Having pale urine.

al·bine. Diamidophosphide of egg yolk.

Albini's nodules (Albini, G., Italian physiologist, 1830–1911). Small greyish nodules sometimes appearing on the edges of the auriculoventricular valves of infants.

al·binism (L. *albus*, white). Congenital absence of pigment in skin, hair, iris, choroid and retinal epithelium, resulting in defective vision, nystagmus and photophobia. Hence **albin·ic,** relating to albinism.

albino. An albinic individual.

Albright's disease (Albright, F., U.S. physician, born 1900). Osteitis fibrosa cystica.

Albright's solution. A preparation, given by injection, for the treatment of first-degree piles.

Albucid. A brand of sulphacetamide.

albugī·nea (L. *albus*, white). 1. White or whitish. 2. Layer of white fibrous tissue investing an organ or part, e.g. albuginea or tunica a. testis. **A. oculi:** the sclerotic coat of the eye.

albugineŏ·tomy (*albuginea*; G. *tomē*, a cutting). Incision of the tunica albuginea of the testicle.

albū·min (L. *albus*, white). 1. Nutritive material in a vegetable seed. 2. One of a class of proteins present in the white of an egg and occurring in many animal and vegetable tissues; coagulable on heating and soluble in distilled water and salt solutions.

albū·minate. A compound of albumin with some other substance.

albuminī·ferous (L. *albus*, white; *ferre*, to bear). Yielding albumin.

albuminī·meter (*albumen*; G. *metron*, measure). An instrument for quantitative estimation of albumin in a fluid.

albuminip·arous (*albumen*; L. *parĕre*, to produce). Yielding albumin.

albū·minoid (*albumen*; G. *eidos*, form). 1. Resembling albumin. 2. Any of the scleroproteins, *q.v.*

albuminŏ·lysis. The splitting up of protein material.

albuminŏ·meter. See albuminimeter.

albuminorrhoē·a. Over excretion of albumin.

albū·minose. See albumose.

albuminŏ·sis. Abnormal increase of the albuminous elements in the blood.

albū·minous. Containing, or of the nature of, albumin.

albuminū·ria (*albumen*; G. *ouron*, urine). Excretion of albumin (generally serum albumin) in the urine. **A., cyclic:** small amounts of a. discharged at definite periods during the day. **A., lordotic:** albuminuria caused by lordosis, *q.v.* **A., orthostatic:** a. associated with assumption of erect position, occurring mainly in children and adolescents, characterized by the presence of the so-called acetic acid-body in the urine (a precipitate forming on addition of 10 per cent acetic acid to cold urine) indicating secretion of a globulin bound to chondroitin-sulphuric acid, due to effect of erect, especially lordotic, stance on renal blood-flow. The condition is of no significance in otherwise healthy subjects, but is sometimes found to co-exist with albuminuria of nephritic or nephrotic origin. **A., postural:** same as a., orthostatic.

albuminūr·ic (*albumen*; G. *ouron*, urine). Characterized by or due to albuminuria. **A. retinitis:** see neuroretinopathy.

al·bumose. The first cleavage product in enzymatic decomposition of albumin. It is not coagulable by heat, but is precipitated by ammonium sulphate.

albumosū·ria. The presence of albumose in the urine.

Alcaligenes (Arabic *al qalīy*; G. *gennan*, to produce). A group of bacteria, intermediate between the coli and brucella groups, found in the intestinal tracts of normal animals.

alcaptonū·ria. See alkaptonuria.

Alcock's canal (Alcock, T., English anatomist, 1801–1859). The fascial sheath of the internal pudic artery.

al·cohol (Arabic *al Koh'l*). 1. Ethyl alcohol. 2. Any one of a class of organic compounds in which a hydroxyl group (OH) is attached to an alkyl radical, classified as monohydric, dihydric, etc., according to the number of OH groups it contains and primary, secondary and tertiary according to the nature of the C atom to which it is attached, i.e., $-CH_2OH$, $-CHOH$, $-C.OH$, respectively.

al·coholase. A ferment capable of changing lactic acid into alcohol.

alcoholaē·mia. The presence of alcohol in the bloodstream.

alcohŏl·ic. 1. Containing or producing alcohol. 2. One addicted to the use of alcoholic liquors. **A. dementia:** the final stage of mental deterioration resulting from chronic alcoholism. **A. hallucinosis:** a hallucinosis resulting from chronic alcoholism. **A. psychosis:** a psychosis due to chronic alcoholism occurring in the form of delirium tremens, *q.v.*, Korsakow's syndrome, *q.v.*, or as more or less progressive change in character, mental power, and emotional depths.

al·coholism. 1. Addiction to the intake of alcohol. 2. The morbid results of prolonged or excessive use of alcoholic liquors.

alcoholŏ·meter. An instrument for discovering alcohol percentages present in any substance.

al·coholophi·lia. Neurotic or morbid desire for the consumption of alcohol.

alcoholū·ria. The presence of alcohol in urine.

al·dehyde (Abbreviation of L. *alcohol dehydrogenatum*). Substance obtained by oxidation of a primary alcohol, containing characteristically the -CHO group.

aldohex·ose (*aldehyde*, *q.v.*; G. *hex*, six). Any hexose containing the aldehyde group.

aldol. β-hydroxybutyric aldehyde $CH_3CHOH.CH_2.CHO$.

aldose. Mono- or di-saccharide which contains an aldehyde group.

ale. Liquor made from fermented malt and hops, containing about 3–7 per cent alcohol.

alĕ·cithal (G. *a*, neg.; *lekithos*, yolk). Applied to ova having little or no yolk.

Alectorobius talaje. A tick which is found in Central and South America. Its bite often sets up suppuration.

alem·bic. A primitive form of chemist's retort.

Aleppo boil. See Oriental sore.

alē·thia (G. *a*, neg.; *lēthē*, forgetfulness). Inability to forget.

alē·tocyte (G. *alētēs*, wanderer; *kutos*, cell). A wandering cell.

aleū·cocytō·sis (G. *a*, neg.; *leukos*, white, *kutos*, cell). Insufficient formation of white cells. Hence **aleucocyt·ic,** without leucocytes.

aleukaē·mia (G. *a*, neg.; *leukos*, white; *haima*, blood). Deficiency of leucocytes in the blood, especially when occurring in the course of leukaemia.

aleukia haemorrhagica (G. *a*, neg.; *leukos*, white; *haima*, blood; *rhegnunai*, to break). See anaemia, aplastic.

Aleurisma. A genus of fungi, of which some species are found in human skin lesions.

aleurŏ·meter (G. *aleuron*, flour; *metron*, measure). Instrument for determining the value of bread flours.

al·euron (G., flour). Protein granules in the endosperm of seeds.

aleū·ronoid (G. *aleuron*, flour; *eidos*, form). Like flour.

Alexan·derism (Alexander of Macedon, 350–323 B.C.). A condition in which the sufferer has the insane belief that he is a great conqueror.

Alexander's operation (Alexander, W., British surgeon, 1844–1919). 1. Ligation of vertebral arteries for the relief of epilepsy. 2. Shortening of the round ligaments for prolapse and retroflexion of the uterus. 3. Prostatectomy by means of suprapubic and perineal incisions.

Alexander-Adams operation (Alexander, W., British surgeon, 1844–1919; Adams, J. A., Scottish gynaecologist, 1849–99). Same as Alexander's operation No. 2.

alex·ia (G. *a*, neg.; *lexis*, speech). A form of subcortical sensory aphasia, *q.v.*, characterized by inability or difficulty in understanding written or printed characters. Syn. word blindness. **A.**, **musical**: amusia, sensory, *q.v.*

alex·in (G. *alexein*, to help). A thermolabile substance present in normal blood serum, with lytic properties on cells sensitized by the specific antibody (amboceptor). Identical with Ehrlich's complement.

alex·ocyte (G. *alexein*, to help; *kutos*, cell). A cell which secretes alexins.

A.L.G. Abbreviation for axiolinguogingival.

Algae. A group of cryptogamous plants, which includes seaweed and some fresh-water plants.

alganaesthē·sia (G. *algos*, pain; *anaesthesia*). Analgesia.

algedon·ic (G. *algos*, pain; *hēdonē*, pleasure). Relating to pleasure and pain.

algĕŏ·scopy (G. *algos*, pain; *skopein*, to examine). Examination by means of discovering whether pressure at certain points produces pain.

algē·sia (G. *algos*, pain). 1. Pain. 2. Hypersensitivity to painful stimuli. Hence, **algesic**, painful; **algesiogen·ic**, producing pain.

algē·simeter. See algometer.

al·gid (L. *algidus*, cold). Cold; chilly.

algin·ic acid. A polyuronic acid obtained from certain algae, chiefly *Laminaria cloustoni* which grows on the west coasts of Scotland and Ireland. It is used in the form of its sodium salt as an emulsifying and suspending agent.

alginurē·sis (G. *algos*, pain; *ouresis*, urination). Painful passing of urine.

algioglandul·ular. Relating to the action of glands in response to painful stimuli. Also **algiomuscular**, producing painful muscular movement, and **algiovascular**, producing vascular action in response to painful stimuli.

algolag·nia (G. *algos*, pain; *lagneia*, lust). Sexual pleasure found in giving or experiencing pain.

algŏ·meter (G. *algos*, pain; *metron*, measure). An instrument for measuring sensitiveness to pain.

algŏ·phily (G. *algos*, pain; *philia*, love). A form of sexual perversion accompanied by desire to suffer pain.

algophŏ·bia (G. *algos*, pain; *phobos*, fear). Fear of suffering pain.

al·gospasm (G. *algos*, pain; *spasmos*, spasm). Any painful spasm.

ALH. Abbreviation used for combined sex hormone of the anterior lobe of the hypophysis.

Alibert's disease (Alibert, J. L., French dermatologist, 1768–1837). Mycosis fungoides, *q.v.* **A.'s keloid:** a growth due to hypertrophy of a cicatrix and bearing resemblance to a true skin tumour, or keloid.

ă·lible (L. *alibilis*, nutritious). Capable of being assimilated as food.

ă·lices. The spots appearing before the formation of pustules in smallpox.

āl·ienā·tion (L. *alienare*, to estrange). 1. Mental derangement. 2. Disturbance of recognition in which familiar objects appear strange as in déjà vu phenomenon, *q.v.*

aliĕ·nia (G. *a*, neg.; L. *lien*, spleen). Having no spleen.

ā·lienism. The study of mental disorders.

ā·lienist. A psychiatrist; one skilled in the treatment of mental disorders.

ă·liform (L. *ala*, wing; *forma*, shape). Wing-shaped.

align·ment (Fr. *ligne*, line). The placing of three or more points in a straight line.

ă·liment (L. *alimentum*). Nourishment; food.

aliment·ary. Nourishing, pertaining to aliment. **A. canal:** digestive tube from the lips to the anus, also called the **a. tract. A. intoxication:** in paediatrics a syndrome characterized by dehydration and usually acidosis due to excessive loss of fluids and sodium by diarrhoea and vomiting.

alimentā·tion (L. *alimentum*). The act of supplying with food. **Forced a.:** the feeding of a person against his wish.

alimentŏ·logy (L. *alimentum*; G. *logos*, discourse). The science of nutrition.

alinā·sal (L. *ala*, wing; *nasus*, nose). Relating to the ala nasi, or wing of the nose.

aliphat·ic (G. *aleiphar*, oil). 1. Pertaining to a fat. 2. Belonging to the open-chain series of organic compounds. (See under chain.)

alipogenet·ic (G. *a*, neg.; *lipos*, fat; *gennan*, to produce). Not fat-forming.

alipoid·ic (G. *a*, neg.; *lipos*, fat; *eidos*, form). Not having lipoids.

ă·liquot (L.). One of any number of equal parts into which the whole can be divided without leaving a remainder.

alisphĕ·noid (L. *ala*, wing; G. *sphēn*, wedge; *eidos*, form). The bone which in adults forms the main portion of the greater wing of the sphenoid.

alizarin. A natural dyestuff, 1:2-dihydroxyanthraquinone, obtained from the leaves of the madder plant, now prepared synthetically. Used as an oxidation-reduction indicator, a dyestuff and for the identification of aluminium in analysis.

alizarine oil. The same as sodium sulphoricinate, the sodium salt of sulphonated castor oil. It is little used in pharmacy, but is occasionally employed in making soapless shampoos.

alkalaē·mia (Arab. *al qalīy*; G. *haima*, blood). Uncompensated alkalosis.

alkales·cence. Slight alkalinity; having a slight alkaline reaction.

alkales·cent. Slightly alkaline.

alkali (Arab. *al qalīy*). 1. Hydroxides, carbonates and bicarbonates of lithium, sodium, potassium, rubidium, caesium. 2. Ammonia, amines and related bases which yield hydroxyl ions on solution in water. **A. reserve:** the total amount of available buffer-alkalis in the body.

alkali·meter. Instrument for ascertaining the alkali contained in any substance.

al·kaline. Yielding hydroxyl ions in an aqueous solution. **A. earths:** oxides and hydrates of calcium, barium, magnesium or aluminium. **A. reaction:** term used to denote solutions having a *p*H greater than 7 (i.e. solutions containing an excess of hydroxyl ions).

alkali·nity. An excess of hydroxyl ions in an aqueous solution. **A., actual:** a. with reference to the amount of ionized hydroxyl ions (dissociated alkali) present. **A., total:** a. with reference to the amount of both dissociated and undissociated alkali present.

alkalinūr·ia (*Alkali*; G. *ouron*, urine). Alkalinity of the urine.

alkalipē·nia (*Alkali*; G. *penēs*, poor). Loss or poverty of the body's alkali reserves.

al·kalize. To make alkaline.

al·kalizer. Any medicine which produces alkalization in the body.

al·kaloid. Organic nitrogenous bases, usually of vegetable origin, but possibly synthetic, containing nitrogen as the component of a heterocyclic ring structure. They often have considerable physiological effect, e.g. morphine, cocaine, hyoscyamine and nicotine.

alkalō·sis. Disturbance of the acid-base equilibrium, characterized by the presence of abnormal amounts of alkali in the body, due to accumulation of these alkalis, overdosage of alkalis, or to loss of acids, e.g. of chlorides through sweating, vomiting or diarrhoea, or of carbon dioxide through hyperpnoea.

Alkanet root. The dried root of *Anchusa tinctoria*. It contains 3 per cent of red amorphous substance, alkannin, *q.v.*

alkannin. Dark red colouring matter obtained from alkanet.

alkaptonūr·ia. A congenital metabolic disturbance, characterized by urinary excretions of homogentisic acid, due to inability to oxidize the product of tyrosine cleavage.

al·kyl. Univalent hydrocarbon radical, C_nH_{2n+1}.

all or none laws. The principle relating to nerve fibres and muscle cells (e.g. the heart muscle) which react to an adequate stimulus either maximally or not at all, i.e. according to the condition of the cell only and irrespective of the intensity of the stimulus.

allachaesthē·sia (G. *allakhē*, elsewhere; *aisthēsis*, feeling). Wrong localization of tactile impressions.

allaitement mixte (Fr.). Nursing of infants by both mother's milk and artificial feeding.

allantō·ic (G. *allas*, sausage). Relating to the allantois.

allan·toid (G. *allas*, sausage; *eidos*, form). 1. Resembling a sausage. 2. Relating to the allantois.

allantoi·dean. Animal of which the embryo has an allantois.

allan·tōin. The diureide of glyoxylic acid, a product of oxidation of uric acid, normally present in traces in the urine; also found in allantoic fluid and in many plants. Used to stimulate epithelialisation of wounds; the basis of the maggot treatment of chronic suppurative conditions.

allan·tōinūr·ia. Having allantoin in the urine.

allan·tōis. A foetal membrane developing as a prolongation of the embryonic yolk sac, contributing to the formation of the umbilical cord and placenta.

allax·is (G. *allassein*, to change). Metamorphosis; transformation.

allē·lomorph (G. *allēlōn*, of one another; *morphē*, form). 1. One of a pair of alternative genetic characters; a genetic character different from that transmitted by the corresponding gene in the corresponding chromosome. 2. One of the isomera existing in a solution which will first separate or crystallize out. **A. multiple:** any of three or more alternative or contrasting genetic characters.

allelomor·phic. Relating to an allelomorph.

allelomor·phism. The transmission of allelomorphic characters.

allel·ōtrope (G. *allēlōn*, of one another; *tropē*, turn). Either of two isomeric substances in equilibrium with one another.

Allen's cement (Allen, J., U.S. dentist, 1810–92). A cement for attaching porcelain teeth to a dental plate.

Allen's paradoxic law (Allen, F. M., U.S. physician, born 1879). In normal individuals, the more sugar is given the more it is used; in diabetics the reverse is the case. **A.'s treatment:** a dietetic treatment for patients with diabetes. It consists of giving a restricted diet after certain days of fasting. It is also called starvation diet.

Allen's test (Allen, C. W., U.S. physician, 1854–1906). A Fehling solution test to discover the presence of glucose in the urine.

Allen-Doisy test (Allen, E., U.S. anatomist, 1892–1943; Doisy, E. A., U.S. biological chemist, born 1900). A test for oestrogenic substance in laboratory animals.

allen·thesis (G. *allos*, another; *en*, in; *thesis*, a placing). Introduction of a foreign substance into the body.

al·lergen (G. *allos*, other; *ergon*, work; *gennan*, to produce). Any substance capable of producing allergy.

aller·gic. Relating to, or affected by, allergy.

al·lergy (G. *allos*, other; *ergon*, work). 1. A modified sensitiveness or hypersensitiveness to a substance or substances of protein or non-protein character, introduction of which into the body may cause a variety of symptoms, such as bronchial asthma, urticaria, dermatitis. 2. A condition denoting a change in the reaction of an organism to chronic or recurring infection.

alliā·ceous (L. *allium*, garlic). Relating to garlic.

alloeō·sis (G. *alloioein*, to alter). Alteration in the characteristics of a disease or syndrome.

alligā·tion. Ascertaining the value of a mixture containing known quantities of materials, all being of known individual value.

alligator forceps. A tooth forceps one of the jaws of which works with a double lever.

Allingham's operation (1) (Allingham, H. W., English surgeon, 1862-1904). Inguinal colostomy by an incision parallel with Poupart's ligament. **A.'s ulcer:** fissure of the anus.

Allingham's operation (2) (Allingham, W., English surgeon, 1830-1908). Excision of the rectum from the perineum.

Allis's inhaler (Allis, O. H., U.S. surgeon, 1833-1921). An apparatus for giving ether, in which the drop method is used. **A.'s sign:** relaxation of the fascia between the crest of the ilium and the greater trochanter, showing that there is a fracture of the neck of the femur.

Allium (L. garlic). A genus of liliaceous plants, including garlic. The garlic clove produces a digestive stimulant.

allobar·bitone. 5:5-diallylbarbituric acid. A hypnotic similar to barbitone, more rapidly excreted and of less prolonged action.

Allobophora agricola. A parasitic worm, which is sometimes found in the human intestine.

allocen·tric (G. *allos* other; *kentron*, centre). The centreing of attention on others rather than on oneself.

allochei·ria (G. *allos*, other; *kheir*, hand). The localization of a sensation in the corresponding member of the other side.

allochē·zia (G. *allos*, other; *khezein*, to defaecate). The discharge of faecal matter through an abnormal passage.

allochrō·ic (G. *allos*, other; *khrōs*, colour). Changing colour.

allocortex (G. *allos*, other; L. *cortex*, skin). Type of cerebral cortex deviating even in early foetal stages from the six-layer prototype. Syn. heterogeneous cortex. See also isocortex.

allŏ·dromy (G. *allos*, another; *dromos*, a running). Uneven heart rhythm.

allo-erot·ism (G. *allos*, another; *erotism*, from *erōs*, love). Erotic desires directed to other people as opposed to oneself.

allŏ·gamy (G. *allos*, other; *gamos*, marriage). Cross-fertilization.

Allogro·mia. A genus of parasites found in protozoa.

al·loker·atoplasty (G. *allos*, other; *keras*, horn; *plassein*, to form). Corneal grafting with foreign matter.

allokinē·sis (G. *allos*, other *kinēsis*, movement). Passive or reflex movements.

allolă·lia (G. *allos*, other; *lalia*, speech). Impairment of the speech faculty.

allŏ·merism (G. *allos*, another; *merismos*, division). Changes in the chemical composition of crystalline substances, while the crystalline form is still retained.

allometrō·pia (G. *allos*, other; *metron*, measure; *ōpē*, sight). Ocular refraction in indirect vision.

allomor·phism (G. *allos*, other; *morphē*, form). Similarity in chemical composition while differing in crystalline form.

allomorphō·sis. Relation of parts of organisms at some definite age to wholes or parts of others also at some definite age, but of different groups (races, varieties, species, etc.).

Allonal. A proprietary preparation of allyl*iso*propyl-barbiturate of amidopyrine and acetophenetidin, used as a sedative or hypnotic.

allŏ·nomous (G. *allos*, another; *nomos*, law). Regulated by outside stimuli.

al·lopath, allŏ·pathist (G. *allos*, other; *pathos*, disease). One who practises allopathy.

allŏ·pathy (G. *allos*, another; *pathos*, disease). The Galenic treatment by drugs which produce phenomena different from those of the disease treated; opposed to homeopathy.

allŏ·phasis (G. *allos*, other; *phasis*, statement). Unclear or incoherent speech.

allophthal·mia (G. *allos*, other; *ophthalmos*, eye). The same as heterophthalmia, *q.v.*

allopla·sia. The same as heteroplasia, *q.v.*

alloplasmat·ic (G. *allos*, another; *plassein*, to form). Applied to cell elements capable of differentiation to perform special functions.

allopsȳ·chic (G. *allos*, other; *psukhe*, mind). Relating to the mind's contacts with the outside world.

allopsychō·sis (G. *allos*, other; *psukhe*, mind). A delusional state in which malicious intentions are attributed to others.

allorhȳth·mia (G. *allos*, another; *rhuthmos*, rhythm). Continuous irregularity of the cardiac rhythm.

ăl·losome (G. *allos*, another; *sōma*, body). A chromosome differing from entosomes in form, size or behaviour. Syn. heterochromosomes.

al·lotherm (G. *allos*, other; *thermē*, heat). An organism whose temperature depends upon its environment.

allotō·pia (G. *allos*, other; *topos*, place). Wrong position of an organ. Same as dystopia.

allotox·in (G. *allos*, other; *toxikon*, poison). Any substance originating from blood or tissues with antitoxic properties.

allotriodon·tia (G. *allotrios*, strange; *odous*, tooth). 1. Transplantation of teeth from one person to another. 2. The existence of teeth in abnormal situations, as in a dermoid cyst or tumour.

allotriogeū·stia (G. *allotrios*, strange; *geusis*, taste). 1. Perversion of the sense of taste; gustatory hallucination. 2. Abnormality of appetite.

allotriŏ·phagy (G. *allotrios*, strange; *phagein*, to eat). The eating of substances unfit for consumption, such as earth or chalk.

allotriū·ria (G. *allotrios*, strange; *ouron*, urine). Any unusual or perverted condition of the urine.

al·lotrope (G. *allos*, another; *tropos*, turn). One of the forms in which an allotropic element may appear.

allotrō·phic (G. *allos*, another; *trophē*, nourishment). Being made unfit for nutritional purposes by being digested.

allotrop·ic. Characterized by allotropism.

allŏ·tropism (G. *allos*, another; *tropos*, turn). Difference in the physical forms of a single chemical element, e.g. sulphur, phosphorus.

allotrȳl·ic (G. *allotrios*, strange; *hūlē*, matter). Caused by the presence of foreign bodies.

alloxan. Mesoxalyl urea.

alloxantin. Derivative of alloxan and dialuric acid.

alloxū·ric bodies (G. *allos,* another; *oxus*, sharp; *ouron*, urine). Purine bases. See under purine.

allspice. The dried fully grown unripe fruit of *Pimenta officinalis*. Syn. pimento; Jamaica pepper.

allyl (L. *allium*, garlic). Unsaturated hydrocarbon radical $CH_2=CH.CH_2—$.

allyl-*iso*-thiocyanate. The active constituent of volatile oil of mustard.

allylthiocarbamide. $H_2N.CS.NHCH_2CH=CH_2$. Allyl-thio-urea, used in the resolution of fibrous tissue of burn scars. Syn. thiosinamine.

Almeida's disease (Almeida, F. P. de, Brazilian physician, born 1898). Paracoccidioidal granuloma. See under granuloma.

Almén's test(s) (Almén, A. T., Swedish physiologist, 1833–1903). 1. For albumin in urine. 2. For blood or blood pigment. 3. For dextrose.

almoner. A person who performs the social service work connected with hospital patients.

Al₂O₃. Aluminium oxide.

alō·chia (G. *a*, neg.; *lokhia*, lochia). Absence of the lochia.

Alocol. A proprietary colloidal aluminium hydroxide supplied in powder or tablet form. Used for acidity.

Aloe. A genus of liliaceous plants. The juice of the plants yields a bitter purgative which is employed chiefly in combination with soap, iron or strychnine in the treatment of chronic constipation.

alō·gia (G. *a*, neg.; *logos*, word). Inability to speak owing to a lesion of the central nervous system.

aloin. A mixture of crystalline active principles obtained from aloes. Used as a purgative.

alopē·cia (G. *alopekia*, baldness). Baldness. **A. areata:** a disturbance of hair-growth characterized by more or less acutely appearing patches of baldness. **A. cicatrisata:** a. characterized by numerous small bald patches coalescing into cicatricial areas with serrated borders. Syn. pseudo-pelade.

alpha (G. A). 1. The first letter of the Greek alphabet. 2. In physics, α-particles or α-rays, electropositively charged helium nuclei emitted from radio-active substances. 3. In chemistry, applied to that substitution product of (a) a straight chain compound in which the substituting atom or radical is attached to the C-atom connected with the characteristic group; (b) a polycyclic compound in which the substituting atom or radical is attached to the C-atom closest to the one shared by both rings; (c) a heterocyclic compound in which the substituting atom or radical is attached to the C-atom closest to the heterocyclic atom. 4. Alpha cells: a cell type in the islands of Langerhans, containing acidophile granules and tending to be arranged towards the periphery. 5. Alpha-haemolytic streptococci: strains of streptococci producing greenish discoloration in the immediate vicinity of colonies of streptococcus viridans and pneumococcus, when these are grown on solid media containing blood. Syn. streptococcus viridans.

Alquié's operation (Alquié, A. J., French surgeon, 1812–65). Extra-peritoneal shortening of the round ligaments.

alt. dieb. Abbreviation of L. *alternis diebus,* every other day. Sometimes abbreviated *altern. dies.*

alterative (*alterativus,* from medieval L. *alterare,* from *alter,* the other). A medicine altering favourably the processes of nutrition and excretion.

alternans. See pulsus alternans.

Alternaria. A genus of fungi responsible for some plant diseases and also found in man in some skin infections.

alternating. Occurring by turns, or periodically. **A. current:** electric current in which the direction periodically reverses. **A. paralysis:** see paralysis, crossed. **A. psychosis:** see manic depressive psychosis.

altern. hor. Abbreviation for L. *alternis horis,* every other hour.

altern. q.q. hor (L. *alternus quibusque horis*). Same as altern. hor.

Altmann's fluid (Altmann, R., German histologist, 1852–1900). A fixing fluid used in histology. It is composed of equal parts of 2 per cent osmic acid solution and 5 per cent potassium dichromate solution. **A.'s granules:** Rounded masses seen in the glandular and lymphocytic cells of vertebrates after staining with acid fuchsin. **A.'s theory:** that protoplasm consists of bioblasts clustered together and enclosed in indifferent matter.

altofrequent. Characterized by high frequency.

alum. May be either potassium aluminium sulphate [$KAl.(SO_4)_2 12H_2O$, potash alum] or ammonium aluminium sulphate [$NH_4Al(SO_4)_2.12H_2O$, ammonium alum]. Colourless crystals or white powder with a sweetish astringent taste. Astringent and haemostatic for local application.

alum precipitated toxoid. A diphtheria prophylactic.

alūmina. Aluminium oxide; Al_2O_3.

alūminated. Charged with alum.

alumĭnium (L. *alumen,* alum). A silver-white metallic element of low specific gravity. Symbol Al.

aluminō·sis. A type of pneumoconiosis caused by the inhalation of aluminium dust.

alvearium (L. *alvearium,* from *alveus,* cavity). The external opening of the ear.

al·vĕŏlar (L. *alveolus,* dim. of *alveus,* cavity). Pertaining to an alveolus. **A. gland:** a gland possessing alveoli.

al·veolec·tomy (L. *alveolus,* small cavity; G. *ektomē,* excision). Operation for the excision of the whole or part of an alveolar process.

alveoli·tis. Inflammation of an alveolus.

al·vĕŏlus (L.). 1. A round or oval structure with a conspicuous free lumen lined by glandular cells. 2. An acinus. 3. An air-cell, one of the terminal dilatations of the bronchioles in the lung. 4. The bony socket of a tooth. 5. A small cell or cavity.

al·veus (L.). 1. A canal or tube. 2. A cavity.

al·vine. Relating to the alvus.

al·vus (L.). The belly and viscera contained in it.

alym·phia (G. *a,* neg.; L. *lympha,* water). Absence of lymph.

alymphocytō·sis (G. *a,* neg.; L. *lympha;* G. *kutos,* cell). Grave deficiency or complete absence of lymphocytes from the blood.

A.M. Abbreviation for L. *ante meridiem,* before noon.

ă·ma (L. *hama,* a water-bucket). Enlargement of a semicircular canal in the internal ear.

ā·maas. Alastrim, *q.v.*

amacrat·ic (G. *hama,* together; *kratos,* strength). Amasthenic, *q.v.*

ă·macrine (G. *a,* neg.; *makros,* long; *is,* fibre). Applied to a type of nerve cell, formerly thought to be devoid of axis cylinders, occurring in the inner nuclear layer of the retina, in the olfactory bulb and in the cerebellum. Hence **amă·crinal,** pertaining to or of the nature of an amacrine.

Amadou. A fungus prepared with alkali and nitre, and used as a haemostatic.

amal·gam (Medieval L. *amalgama,* probably from G. *malagma,* a plaster). 1. A combination of mercury with any other metal. 2. Any soft alloy. **Dental a.:** a combination of silver, tin and mercury used for the filling of caries in the teeth.

amal·gamable. Being able to combine with mercury in an amalgam.

amal·gamator. An apparatus used to amalgamate an alloy with mercury.

Amanita. A genus of fungi belonging to the Agaricaceae. *A. phalloides* is a deadly poisonous species, and *A. muscaria* and *A. verna* are also poisonous varieties. The *A. rubescens,* however, is supposed to be edible.

amă·nitine. A poisonous alkaloid, the active principle from various types of non-edible fungi.

amā·ra (L. *amarus,* bitter). Bitter drugs, gustatory stimulation by which causes reflex increase in gastric secretion.

amaranth. The sodium salt of 4-sulpho-*x*-naphthaleneazo-*β*-naphthol-3: 6-disulphonic acid. It is used as a colouring for medicines.

amarthrī·tis (G. *hama,* together; *arthron,* joint). Condition of inflammation in a number of joints at the same time.

amasē·sis (G. *a,* neg.; *masasthai,* to chew). Inability to masticate.

amasthē·nic (G. *hama,* together; *sthenos,* strength). Bringing chemical light rays into focus.

amă·stia (G. *a,* neg.; *mastos,* breast). Congenital absence of breasts or nipples.

ă·mative (L. *amare,* to love). Disposed to love.

amato bodies. Bodies found in the leucocytes of patients with scarlet fever.

amaurō·sis (G. *amaurosis,* darkening). Partial or total blindness, especially that without demonstrable ocular lesion.

amaurot·ic. Relating to or affected with amaurosis. **A. idiocy:** see under idiocy.

amā·zia (G. *a,* neg.; *māzos,* breast). Congenital absence of the mammary gland.

amber. Yellow translucent fossil resin, found chiefly on the southern Baltic coast. **A. oil:** an oil with a penetrating odour produced by the destructive distillation of resins. It is used in liniments for its rubefacient qualities, and can be given on sugar for the relief of asthma.

am·bergris. A waxlike material found in the intestines of sperm-whales. Used in the manufacture of perfumes, also sometimes as a stimulant.

Amberg's lateral sinus line (Amberg, E., U.S. surgeon, born 1868). A line halving the angle formed by the anterior edge of the mastoid process and the temporal line.

ambidex·trous (L. *ambo,* both; *dexter,* right-handed). Capable of using both hands equally well. **Ambidexterity:** ability to use both hands with equal skill.

ambilaē·vous (L. *ambo,* both; *laevus,* left-handed). Clumsy; having no skill with either hand.

ambilat·eral (L. *ambo,* both; *latus,* side). Relating to or affecting both sides.

ambiō·pia. See diplopia.

ambi·valence (L. *ambo,* both; *valere,* to be strong). The simultaneous existence of opposite emotions, e.g. love and hate, with regard to the same object or action. Hence **ambi·valent,** characterized by ambivalence.

ambiver·sion. A character which stands between introversion and extroversion.

amblyacū·sia (G. *amblus,* dull; *akousis,* a hearing). Dullness of hearing.

amblyă·phia (G. *amblus*, dull; *haphē*, touch). Dullness of the sense of touch.

amblygeu·stia (G. *amblus*, dull; *geusis*, taste). Impaired sense of taste.

amblyŏ·pia (G. *amblus*, dull; *ōps*, eye). Dimness of vision, not caused by a discoverable lesion of the eye. **A. alcoholica**: impairment of vision due to the immoderate use of alcohol. **A. ex anopsia**: a. from non-use or unilateral suppression of visual perception. **A., toxic**: a. due to the effect of some poison such as quinine, lead, ergot, thallium, alcohol, or tobacco, and characterized by bilateral impairment of central vision with the development of central-caecal scotoma, initially for red and green, and by absence of ophthalmoscopic changes. **A., tobacco**: toxic a. due to nicotine poisoning.

amblyopiă·trics (G. *amblus*, dull; *opē*, sight; *iatrikos*, medical). The treatment of amblyopia.

ăm·blyoscope (G. *amblus*, dull; *skopein*, to view). Apparatus for the treatment of amblyopic eyes by stereoscopic exercises.

Amblystoma. A genus of salamanders. Called also axolotl.

ambocep·tor (L. *ambo*, both, *capere*, to take). A thermostable lytic antibody present in small quantities in normal serum, and found in much greater amounts in immune serum. Ambocep·toid: an amboceptor that has lost its cytophilic properties.

ambocep·torgen. An antigen that procures amboceptors.

ambomal·leal. Relating to the incus and the malleus.

ambon. The margin of the sockets of the long bones.

ambosex·ual. Bisexual, *q.v.*

ambrin. A cholesterin-like substance, the main constituent of ambergris.

am·bulance (L. *ambulare*, to walk). 1. A vehicle for the transference of sick and wounded. 2. A portable military hospital and its equipment. 3. The surgical staff of an army on service.

am·bulant. Able to walk.

am·bulatory. Relating to treatment, or to a disease, in which the patient is not confined to bed.

ambŭ·stion (L. *amburere*, to scorch). A burn or scald.

amē·lia (G. *a*, neg.; *melos*, limb). Congenital absence of limbs.

amē·lioration (L. *melius*, better). Improvement of the condition of a patient.

amē·loblast (Anglo-Fr. *amayller*, from medieval L. *amaltum*, enamel; G. *blastos*, germ). An epithelial cell forming the enamel of the tooth. Syn. adamantoblast.

ă·melus (G. *a*, neg.; *melos*, limb). A monster having no limbs.

amenorrhŏē·a (G. *a*, neg.; *mēn*, month; *rhein* flow). Absence of menstruation. **A., primary**: condition when menstruation has never occurred. **A., secondary**: a. setting in after more or less regular menstruation has occurred for some time. Hence **amenorrhoeal**, relating to amenorrhoea.

ă·ment (G. *a*, neg.; L. *mens*, mind). 1. An idiot. 2. Suffering from amentia.

amen·tia (G. *a*, neg.; L. *mens*, mind). Feeble-mindedness, as distinct from dementia, *q.v.*

ameri·sia (G. *a*, neg.; *merizein*, to divide). Inability to speak or write words correctly.

Ametă·bola. A class of insects, which do not undergo metamorphosis. Hence **ametabolous**, not undergoing metamorphosis.

amē·thocaine hydrochlor·ide. $(CH_3)_2N.(CH_2)_2O.CO.C_6H_4NH(CH_2)_3CH_3$. The hydrochloride of β-dimethylaminoethyl-*p-n*-butylaminobenzoate. A local anaesthetic.

amē·tria (1) (G. *a*, neg.; *mētrā*, uterus). Congenital absence of the uterus.

amē·tria (2) (G. *a*, neg.; *metron*, measure). Immoderation; asymmetry.

ametrohāē·mia (G. *a*, neg.; *mētra*, womb; *haima*, blood). Absence or deficiency of blood supply to the uterus.

ametrŏ·meter (G. *a*, neg.; *metron*, measure). An instrument for measuring degrees of ametropia.

ametrŏ·pia (G. *a*, neg.; *metron*, measure; *ōps*, eye). Imperfect vision due to defective refractive power of the eye. Hence **ametropic**, pertaining to or affected by ametropia.

Amh. An abbreviation for astigmatism with myopia.

amiän·thinopsy (G. *a*, neg.; *ianthinos*, violet-coloured; *opsis*, vision). Violet-blindness.

amiän·thoid (G. *amiantos*, a greenish stone). Like asbestos.

amiánthŏ·sis. Asbestosis.

Amici's disc (Amici, G. B., Italian physicist, 1784–1863). Krause's membrane, *q.v.*

ă·micine. A substance contained in the posterior lobe of the hypophysis, which inhibits growth.

amicrŏ·bic. Not due to microbes.

amicroscŏp·ic. Too small to be perceived through a microscope.

ă·midase (Fr. *amidon*). See aminase.

amide. Organic radical -CONH₂ derived from the organic acid radical -COOH by extraction of an acid chloride or ester with ammonia.

amidone. $(C_6H_5)_2C.(COC_2H_5)CH_2CHN(CH_3)_2.CH_3$. dl-2-dimethylamino-4:4-diphenylheptane-5-one. A synthetic analgesic.

amidines. A class of organic antibacterial substances containing the amidine radical $H_2N.C=NH$.

amido-ă·cetal. A substance of a highly toxic nature, which paralyses the respiratory system.

ami·mia (G. *a*, neg.; *mimos*, mimic). Inability to express by gestures.

aminacrine hydrochloride. 5-aminoacridine hydrochloride, an active antibacterial substance, non-staining and of low toxicity. Valuable for surface application.

ă·minase. An enzyme decomposing amino-acids into ammonia and keto-acids.

ă·mine. Any one of a group of compounds derived from ammonia by the substitution of alkyl or aryl radicals for one or more of the hydrogen atoms.

aminoaceto-*p*-phenetidide hydrochloride. An antipyretic which is used in rheumatic fever, malaria, influenza, etc. $p-H_2N.CH_2CONHC_6H_4OC_2H_5HCl$.

amino-acid. An organic acid in which one or more of the hydrogen atoms is replaced by NH_2; any one of the end-products of hydrolytic protein decomposition in animal metabolism. They include *leucine*, glycine, tyrosine, glutamic acid, aspartic acid, alanine *phenylalanine*, *lysine*, *arginine*, *histidine*, cystine, *valine*, *tryptophane*, *isoleucine*, *methionine*, serine, *threonine*, hydroxyglutamic acid, norleucine, proline. Those in italics are indispensable to the growth of higher animals.

aminoazobenzene. An oil-soluble yellow dye.

p-aminobenzoic acid. $p-H_2NC_6H_4COOH$. Essential amino-acid present in numerous micro-organisms, the utilization of which is inhibited by sulphonamides.

aminoazotoluene. Non-staining scarlet medicinal dye, soluble in oils and fats and not soluble in water.

amino-*p*-phenetidide hydrochloride. $p-H_2N.CH_2CONHC_6H_4OC_2H_5HCl$.

aminop·terin. Amino-pteroyl glutamic acid. A folic acid antagonist.

p-aminosalicylic acid. 4-amino-2-hydroxybenzoic acid. Used in the treatment of tuberculosis.

aminŏ·sis. The production of amino-acids in the body.

aminosŭ·ria (*amine*; G. *ouron*, urine). Condition in which amines are found in the urine.

amitō·sis (G. *a*, neg.; *mitos*, thread). Direct division of nucleus and cell; cell division without formation of chromosomes or spindle figures; contrary to mitosis. Hence **amitotic**, characterized by amitosis.

am·meter. An instrument used for measuring the strength of electric current in ampères.

ammo·acidū·ria. Condition where ammonia and amino-acids are found in the urine.

ammon. Abbreviation for ammonium.

Ammon's fissure (Ammon, F. A. von, German ophthalmologist and pathologist, 1799–1861). A pear-shaped cleft in the sclera, apparent in early foetal life. **A.'s operation:** 1. Blepharoplasty; excision of cicatricial tissue from eyelid and replacement by a flap of skin from the cheek. 2. Excision of lacrymal sac. 3. For ectropion. 4. For symblepharon.

Ammon's horn (Ammon, ram-headed Egyptian god). See under hippocampus.

ammonia (From Ammon, or Jupiter, near whose temple at Siwah in the Libyan desert ammonium chloride was prepared). A colourless pungent gas (NH_3), soluble in water. Hence **ammoniated**, combined with ammonia.

ammoniated mercury. NH_2HgCl. Used in ointments for the treatment of skin infections.

ammonirrhœ·a (*Ammonia*; G. *rhoia*, a flux). The passing of ammonia in the urine.

ammonium. A hypothetic univalent alkaline radical (NH_4) existing only in combination. It acts like an alkaline metal and forms salts when combined with acids.

ammonŏ·lysis. A process resembling hydrolysis, with ammonia replacing water.

Ammospermophilus leucurus. A squirrel-like rodent, which harbours the plague-transmitting flea.

ammothē·rapy (G. *ammos*, sand; *therapeia*, treatment). The use of sand-baths to promote healing.

amnē·sia (G. *amnēsia*, forgetfulness). Inability to remember past experiences, especially those connected with some mental or cerebral trauma. **Broca's a.:** inability to remember words heard. **A., retrograde:** inability to remember happenings of a period immediately preceding a particular event, e.g., a cerebral trauma.

amnē·sic. Pertaining to amnesia. For a. aphasia, see aphasia, amnesic.

amnichor·ial (G. *amnion*, the inner membrane round the foetus; *khorion*, the outer membrane round the foetus). Pertaining both to the amnion and to the chorion.

amnioclep·sis (G. *amnion*, the inner membrane round the foetus; *klepsia*, theft). Gradual seeping away of the amniotic fluid.

amniogen·esis (G. *amnion*, the inner membrane round the foetus; *genesis*, formation). The growth of the amnion.

amniō·ma. A tumour arising from surviving fragments of the amnion.

am·nion (G. *amnion*, the inner membrane round the foetus). The innermost of the foetal membranes; it is connected with the foetus at the umbilicus, ensheaths the umbilical cord and forms a sac which contains the foetus and the amniotic fluid.

amnioni·tis. Inflammation of the amnion.

amniorrhœ·a (G. *amnion*, the inner membrane round the foetus; *rhoia*, a flux). Uterine discharge of the liquor amnii.

amniotic. Pertaining to the amnion.

am·niotome (G. *amnion*, the inner membrane round the foetus; *tomē*, a cutting). An instrument for opening up the foetal membranes.

Amœ·ba (G. *amoibe*, transformation). A member of the family Amoebidae.

Amœ·bidae. A family of unicellular micro-organisms, composed of simply constituted protoplasm, having the power to produce pseudopodia (*q.v.*) which are used as organs of motion and nutrition.

amœbī·asis. 1. Any disease caused by Amoebae. 2. The condition due to infection with the trophozoite forms of *Endamoeba histolytica*, e.g. dysentery, amoebic, *q.v.*

amœbic. Relating to or caused by Amoebae.

amœ·bicide (G. *amoibē*, transformation; L. *caedere*, to destroy). An agent which destroys Amoebae.

Amœ·bobacter. A genus of water bacteria.

amœ·boid (G. *amoibē*, transformation; *eidos*, form). Resembling an Amoeba either in form or in movement.

amœbū·ria (G. *amoibē*, transformation; *ouron*, urine). The presence of Amoebae in the urine.

amœnomā·nia (L. *amoenus*, pleasant; G. *mania*, madness). A psychotic condition characterized by pleasant delusions or hallucinations.

amok, amuck (Malay *amoq*). A psychotic condition as first observed among the Malays, in which the affected person attacks with a weapon any person or thing he may encounter.

amorā·lia. Moral idiocy.

amor·pha (G. *a*, neg.; *morphē*, form). Diseases showing no pathological condition.

amor·phism. The condition of being amorphous.

amor·phinism. Condition produced by depriving an addict of morphine.

amor·phous (G. *a*, neg.; *morphē*, form). Formless; non-crystalline.

amor·phus (G.). A formless monster foetus, having no heart.

Amoss's sign (Amoss, H. L., U.S. physician, born 1880). In cases with fixed spine, the patient will place his hands behind him in trying to raise himself to a sitting posture.

amō·tio rě·tinae (L.). Detachment of the retina.

amp. Abbreviation for ampere.

ampelother·apy (G. *ampelos*, vine, *therapy*). The use of grapes in therapeutics.

am·perage. The power of an electric current expressed in amperes.

am·pēre (Ampère, A. H., 1775–1836). Unit of measurement of the intensity of an electric current; the current produced by an electro-motive force of one volt in a circuit, having one ohm resistance; the intensity of current which induces precipitation of 1·118 mg. of silver within one minute while passing through an aqueous solution of silver nitrate.

am·pērmeter (*Ampere*; G. *metron*, measure). See ammeter.

amphamphō·terodiplō·pia (G. *amphi*, on both sides; *amphoteros*, both together; *diplopia*). Double vision, either with both eyes together, or with either eye separately.

amphē·merous (G. *amphi*, on both sides; *hēmera*, day). Occurring every day.

amphetamine. $C_6H_5CH_2CH(NH_2)CH_3$. β-amino-propylbenzene. 1. Used as a vasoconstrictor in cases of hay fever. 2. A mental stimulant.

am·phi (G.). A prefix meaning around or on both sides of.

amphïar·kyochrome (G. *amphi*, on both sides; *arkus*, net; *khroma*, colour). A nerve cell with nodal joints joined by an easily stainable network.

amphiarthrō·sis (G. *amphi*, on both sides; *arthron*, joint). An articulation in which the osseous surfaces are connected by fibrocartilaginous discs and connected by external ligaments so that only slight movements are possible, e.g., between vertebrae.

amphiä·ster (G. *amphi*, on both sides; *astēr*, star). The achromatic figure in mitosis, comprising two asters connected by a spindle.

Amphǐ·bia (G. *amphi*, on both sides; *bios*, life). Class of vertebrata capable of living both on land and in water. Hence **amphibious**, able to live in water and on land.

amphiblă·stula (G. *amphi*, about; *blastos*, germ). The mulberry mass or morula stage in the development of a holoblastic egg.

amphibol·ic (G. *amphibolia*, ambiguity). Uncertain, vacillating; pertaining to a stage in a febrile disease (e.g., typhoid fever) characterized by steep temperature curves.

amphicrā·nia (G. *amphi*, on both sides; *kranion*, skull). Pain affecting both sides of the head.

amphicrē·atine. A leucomaine from muscle, $C_9H_{19}N_7O_4$.

amphicreatinine. A poisonous leucomaine from muscle.

amphichrō·ic (G. *amphi*, on both sides; *khroiein*, to dye). Capable of turning red litmus blue and blue litmus red.

am·phicyte. The same as a capsule cell, *q.v.*

amphidiarthrō·sis (G. *amphi*, on both sides; *diarthrōsis*, articulation). A mixed gliding and hinge articulation.

amphǐ·gony (G. *amphi*, on both sides; *gonos*, procreation). Sexual reproduction.

amphikār·yon (G. *amphi*, on both sides; *karuon*, nut). A nucleus containing two haploid groups of chromosomes.

Amphǐ·merus. A genus of trematodes.

amphimicrō·bian (G. *amphi*, on both sides; *microbe*). Having aerobic and anaerobic properties.

amphimix·is (G. *amphi*, on both sides; *mixis*, a mingling). Union of germ plasm of two individuals in sexual reproduction.

amphinuclēo·lus (G. *amphi*, on both sides; L. *nucleolus*, dim. of *nucleus*, from *nucula*, dim. of *nux*, nut). A nucleolus containing a basophile and an oxyphile component.

Amphiŏ·xus. A primitive marine organism; the simplest of the vertebrates.

Amphistō·ma. A genus of parasitic trematode worms.

am·phitene (G. *amphi*, on both sides; *tainia*, a strip). The synaptic stage of meiosis.

am·phitheatre. A lecture-room or operating theatre, with tiers of seats for students.

amphithy·mia (G. *amphi*, on both sides; *thumos*, spirit). A psychotic mental condition, in which the patient feels both elated and depressed.

amphitri·cha (G. *amphi*, on both sides; *thrix*, hair). Bacteria having a flagellum at each pole.

amphǐ·trichous. Pertaining to bacteria possessing one flagellum at each pole.

am·phocyte. Any amphophilic cell.

amphodiplō·pia (G. *amphō*, both; *diploos*, double; *ōps*, eye). Double vision in both eyes.

ampho·philic, amphŏ·philous (G. *ampho*, both; *philein*, to love). Staining alike with acid or with basic dyes.

amphor·ic (L. *amphora*, from G. *amphoreus*, a jar). Pertaining to sounds of hollow, metallic character, resembling those produced by blowing across the mouth of a bottle or by percussing a bellied flask; obtained on percussing or auscultating a pulmonary cavity.

amphorŏ·phony. An amphoric voice sound.

amphotě·ric, amphŏ·terous (G. *amphoteroi*, both). Double-sided. **A. reaction:** The property whereby substances are capable of acting both as acids and bases.

amphō·terism (G. *amphoteroi*, both). Possessing both acid and basic qualities.

amplificā·tion (L. *amplificare*, to enlarge). 1. Enlargement. 2. In microscopy, an enlargement of the visual field.

am·plifier. A device for magnifying electric impulses.

am·plitude. 1. The difference between the extreme position of a vibratory body, e.g. pendulum, and its position at rest. 2. Maximum departure of a current from the average value. **A. of accommodation:** total accommodative power of the eye.

am·poule (L. *ampulla*, a flask). A sealed glass capsule, holding one dose of a sterile solution of a drug.

ampŭl·la (L. *ampulla*, a flask). A dilated end of a canal. Hence **ampullar**, relating to an ampulla. **A. recti**, the dilated part of the rectum over the perineal flexure. **A. of vas deferens:** the lower sacculated portion of the vas deferens. **A. of Vater:** the dilatation of the common bile duct and the pancreatic duct as they open by a papilla in the second part of the duodenum.

ampul·late. Shaped like a flask.

ampulli·tis. Inflammation of an ampulla.

ampŭl·lula (L. *dim.*). A small ampulla, e.g. like those found in lymphatic vessels.

amputā·tion (L. *amputare*, to lop off). The surgical removal of a limb or other part of the body, i.e. the breast or the penis. **A. neuroma,** regenerative painful proliferation of a nerve-end at the site of an a. stump.

Amsler's marker. A type of caliper compass used to mark the point of application of the cautery in the Gonin operation.

amū·sia (G. *a*, neg.; *mousa*, music). Inability to produce (**motor a.**) or to understand (**sensory a.**) musical sounds and melodies; the first being usually associated with disturbances in motor speech and the latter with auditory agnosia.

Amussat's operation (Amussat, J. Z., French surgeon, 1796–1856). Lumbar colostomy by means of an incision across the outer border of the quadratus lumborum. **A.'s probe:** a probe used in lithotrity. **A.'s valves:** the same as Heister's valves, *q.v.*

amyasthē·nia (G. *a*, neg.; *mus*, muscle; *sthenos*, strength). Muscular weakness; the same as amyosthenia.

amychophō·bia (G. *amukhe*, a scratch; *phobos*, fear). Morbid fear of suffering scratches, e.g., from a cat.

amŷc·tic. Caustic.

amydricaine hydrochloride. $C_2H_5.C.(OCOC_6H_5)$. $(CH_2.N(CH_3)_2)_2HCl$. White crystalline powder soluble in water and alcohol. Useful taken internally in post-operative vomiting, and used also for lumbar anaesthesia injections.

amylase. An enzyme splitting starch to the disaccharide maltose.

amyelencephā·lia, amyelencē·phaly (G. *a*, neg.; *muelos*, marrow; *egkephalos*, within the head). Congenital absence of the spinal cord and brain.

amylene hydrate. $CH_3CH_2C(OH)$ $(CH_3)_2$. Syn. for tertiary amyl alcohol. Hypnotic and used chiefly as a solvent for tribromethylalcohol.

amŷel·enceph·alus. A monster without a spinal cord or brain.

amyē·lia (G. *a*, neg.; *muelos*, marrow). Congenital absence of rudimentary development of the spinal cord.

amyĕlin·ic. Having no myelin.

amyelinū·ria (G. *a*, neg.; *muelos*, marrow; *neuron*, sinew). Paralysis of the spine.

amy·locaine hydrochloride. $C_6H_5COOC.(CH_3)(C_2H_5)CH_2N(CH_3)_2.HCl$. Methyl-d-ethyl-β-dimethylaminoethyl benzoate hydrochloride. A local anaesthetic.

amyelŏ·trophy (G. *a*, neg.; *muelos*, marrow; *trophē*, nourishment). Atrophy of the spinal cord.

amŷ·elus (G. *a*, neg.; *muelos*, marrow). A monster without a spinal cord.

amȳg·dala (G. *amugdalē*, almond). 1. The tonsil. 2. A small lobule on the lower surface of the cerebellar hemisphere, projecting into the fourth ventricle. 3. Almond.

amy̆g·dalotome (G. *amugdalē*, almond; *tomē*, section). An instrument for performing tonsillectomy.

amy̆g·dalo-ū·vular. Relating to the amygdala and the cerebellar uvula.

a·myl (G. *amulon*, starch). The univalent radical of amyl-alcohol, C_5H_{11}. **A. nitrite**: $(C_5H_{11}NO_2)$, a yellowish volatile liquid of penetrating odour. Acts by vascular dilatation; used by inhalation, especially in angina pectoris.

amylā·ceous. Starch-like; containing starch.

amylāē·mia. The presence of starch in the bloodstream.

ă·mylase (G. *amulon*, starch). An enzyme causing molecular disintegration (hydrolysis) of starch.

ă·mylism. Poisoning through amyl alcohol.

amylobac·ter (G. *amulon*, starch; *baktērion*, dim. of *baktron*, a staff). A genus of schizomycetes characterized by the property of containing starch during some period of development.

ă·myloclast (G. *amulon*, starch; *klaein*, to break). An enzyme capable of splitting starch.

amy̆·lodyspep·sia (G. *amulon*, starch; *dyspepsia*). Inability to assimilate starch foods.

ă·mylogen·esis. Starch formation.

ă·myloid (G. *amulon*, starch; *eidos*, form). 1. Starch-like. 2. Protein derivative present in animal tissues under certain morbid conditions, so-called because of its resemblance to starch in respect of staining reactions. **A. degeneration**: deposition of amyloid (2) in animal tissues, especially in the walls of the small arteries and arterioles, leading to increase in volume, transparent glassy appearance, and disturbance in function of organs involved (commonly kidney, liver, spleen, intestine); occurring mainly during the course of long-standing suppuration or infections such as tuberculosis and syphilis. Syn. waxy degeneration; lardaceous degeneration.

amyloidō·sis. Localized or generalized amyloid degeneration. **A., primary**: a. not due to long-standing infection.

amylŏ·lysis (G. *amulon*, starch; *lusis*, solution). Conversion of starch into glucose.

amylopec·tin (G. *amulon*, starch; *pēktos*, fixed). One of the two main constituents of starch. It is insoluble. (See amylose.)

amylophā·gia (G. *amulon*, starch; *phagein*, to eat). Abnormal desire for starch consumption.

amy·loplast (G. *amulon*, starch; *plassein*, to form). The starch-forming plastids of plant cells. Hence amyloplastic, starch forming.

amylop·sin (G. *amulon*, starch; *opsis*, appearance). A pancreatic enzyme hydrolysing starch.

amylorrhōē·a (G. *amulon*, starch; *rhein*, to flow). The passing of excessive quantities of starch in the faeces.

ă·mylose. One of the two main constituents of starch. It is soluble in water. (See amylopectin.)

amylō·sis. Albuminoid degeneration.

amylosū·ria. The presence of amylose in urine.

ă·mylum (G. *amulon*). Starch.

amyoaesthē·sia (G. *a*, neg.; *mus*, muscle; *aisthēsis*, feeling). Lack of muscle sense.

amyocar·dia (G. *a*, neg.; *mus*, muscle; *kardia*, heart). Weakness of the heart muscle.

amyostat·ic. See extra-pyramidal.

amyosthē·nia (G. *a*, neg.; *mus*, muscle; *sthenos*, strength). Muscular weakness.

amyotax·y. Muscle ataxia.

amyotō·nia congenita (G. *a*, neg.; *mus*, muscle; *tonos*, tone). See myatonia congenita. Syn. Oppenheim's disease.

amyotrō·phia (G. *a*, neg.; *mus*, muscle; *trophē*, nourishment). Muscular atrophy.

amyotrō·phic. Characterized by muscular disease due to progressive atrophy. **A. lateral sclerosis**: chronic disease due to degeneration of pyramidal tracts and anterior horns of spinal cord, characterized by spastic spinal paresis and progressive muscular atrophy.

amy̆·ous (G. *a*, neg.; *mus*, muscle). Having insufficient muscular tissue.

Amytal. A proprietary preparation of *iso*amylethylbarbituric acid, a white crystalline powder used as a sedative.

amy̆x·ia (G. *a*, neg.; *muxa*, mucus). Lacking in mucus. **amyxorrhoea**: absence of mucus secretion.

ana (G.). Usually written in prescriptions, etc., as āā, signifying so much of each.

anabasine. An insecticidal alkaloid from *Anabasis aphylla*.

ană·basis (G. *anabainein*, to ascend). The stage in which a disease increases in severity.

anabat·ic. Increasing in severity.

anabiō·sis (G. *anabiōsis*, a revival). Re-awakening to life after an apparent death. Hence, **anabiotic**, capable of being stimulated into life.

anabŏl·ic (G. *anaballein*, to throw up). Pertaining to anabolism.

ană·bolism. Assimilating metabolism; the formation of molecules of higher from those of lower energy content, and their incorporation into organized tissue; opposed to catabolism, *q.v.*

anabrō·sis (G. *ana*, up; *brōsis*, eating, from *bibrōskein*). Superficial types of ulceration.

anacamp·tic (G. *anakamptein*, to bend back). Reflected; pertaining to or causing a reflection, as of sound or light.

anacamp·tics. The study of reflection of sound or light.

anacamptŏ·meter (G. *anakamptein*, to bend back; *metron*, measure). An instrument for measuring reflexes.

Anacardium. A genus of tropical tree. *A. accidentale* yields the cashew nut, a gum, and cardol, *q.v.*

anacatadi·dymus (G. *ana*, up; *kata*, down; *didumos*, twin). A double monster, joined together near the middle.

anacathar·sis (G. *ana*, up; *katharsis*, cleansing). Vomiting.

anachlorhy̆·dria. Lack of hydrochloric acid in the gastric juices.

anachō·lea (G. *ana*, up; *chŏlē*, bile). Deficient secretion of bile.

anachorē·sis. The conveying of micro-organisms to tissue lesions.

anachromā·sis (G. *ana*, up; *khrōma*, colour). The totality of the prophasic transformations of the nucleus by which arise spireme threads and chromosomes.

ană·cid (G. *an*, neg.; L. *acidus*, sour, from *acere*, to be sour). Pertaining to anacidity.

anaci·dity. Lack of acidity; especially of free hydrochloric acid in the gastric juice.

anaclasi·meter (G. *anaklasis*, reflection; *metron*, measure). An apparatus used to measure eye refraction.

ană·clasis (G. *anaklasis*, reflection). 1. Reflection or refraction of light or sound. 2. Forcible flexion of the ankylosed joint.

anaclă·stic. Pertaining to refraction or to anaclasis.

anaco·bra. Cobra venom after treatment with formaldehyde.

anacroā·sia. (G. *an*, neg.; *akrŏāsis*, a hearing). Inability to understand the spoken word, although capable of understanding words read.

anacrot·ic (G. *ana*, up; *krotos*, knock). Relating to anacrotism.

anac·rotism. Notch-like elevations on the ascending limb of the pulse curve.

anaculture. Bacterial culture treated with formalin and then incubated.

anacū·sia, anacu·sis (G. *an*, neg.; *akouein*, to hear). Total deafness.

Anacyclus pyrethrum. See under pyrethrum.

anade·nia (G. *an*, neg.; *adēn*, gland). 1. Insufficiency of glandular function. 2. Syn. for achylia, *q.v.*

anadicrot·ic (G. *ana*, up; *dis*, twice; *krotos*, knock). Relating to anadicrotism.

anadi·crotism. Double indentation on the ascending limb of the pulse curve.

anadi·dymus (G. *ana*, up; *didumos*, twin). Double monster, separated above, but joined below.

anadip·sia (G. *ana*, up; *dipsa*, thirst). Intense thirst.

anadre·nalism, anadre·nia. Absent or indequate function of the adrenal glands.

anae·mia (G. *an*, neg.; *haima*, blood). Deficiency in the number of red corpuscles and/or haemoglobin. **A. achlorhydric, simple:** a. essential hypochromic, *q.v.* **A., achrestic:** severe hyperchromic a., characterized by megalocytosis, presence of megaloblasts in the bone marrow, of free hydrochloric acid in the gastric secretion, due to failure to utilize or to mobilize from tissue stores the antipernicious anaemia liver factor. **A., acute haemolytic:** ortho- or hyperchromic a. of unusually sudden onset with fever and sometimes intestinal symptoms, characterized by rapid decrease in red cells, reticulocytosis, normoblastosis, leucocytosis with presence of myelocytes and myeloblasts in the blood, hyperbilirubinaemia, with jaundice, increased excretion of urobilin and sometimes haemoglobinuria, some enlargement of the spleen, liver and lymph nodes, and usually normal fragility of the red cells. Syn. Lederer's anaemia. **A., agastric:** (of either iron deficiency or pernicious anaemia type) occurring after gastrectomy. **A., alimentary:** hypochromic a. due to iron deficiency in the food. **A., aplastic:** severe disease often characterized by progressive decrease of all cellular elements (red cells, white cells, platelets) in bone-marrow and blood, usually accompanied by multiple haemorrhages in skin, mucous membranes and viscera. **A., cow's milk:** a., alimentary, *q.v.* above. **A., erythroblastic:** chronic progressive a., characterized by normoblastosis, microcytosis, polychromasia, reticulocytosis and leucocytosis, osteoporosis of long and medullary thickening of flat bones, splenomegaly, mongoloid facies; affecting almost exclusively children of Syrian, Italian and Greek stock. Syn. Cooley's a.; Thalassaemia; Mediterranean a. **A., essential hypochromic:** hypochromic a. characterized by microcytosis due to iron deficiency, often associated with achlorhydria and sometimes with glossitis, dysphagia and koilonychia, affecting more often middle-aged women. Synonyms Paterson's syndrome; Plummer-Vinson's syndrome. **A., goat's milk:** see a. alimentary above. **A., haemolytic:** any a. due to excessive destruction of red blood cells. **A., hyperchromic:** any a. in which the haemoglobin content of the individual red blood corpuscles is above normal, i.e., with a colour index above 1. **A., hypochromic:** any a. in which the haemoglobin content of the red blood corpuscles is below normal, i.e., with a colour index below 1. **A., idiopathic hypochromic:** a., essential hypochromic, *q.v.* above. **A., infantum pseudoleukaemica:** an obsolete term covering conditions characterized by anaemia with normoblastosis, leucocytosis with immature white cells in the blood, enlargement of spleen and liver, occurring during the first three years of life and probably due to deficiency of one or more factors in the diet. **A., leuco-erythroblastic:** leuco-erythroblastosis, *q.v.* **A., macrocytic:** any a. characterized by the presence of macrocytes in the blood. **A., megaloblastic:** any a. characterized by the presence of megaloblasts in the blood and/or in the bone marrow. **A., megalocytic:** any a. characterized by the presence of megalocytes (*q.v.*) in bone marrow and blood. **A., microcytic:** any a. characterized by the presence of microcytes (*q.v.*) in the blood. **A., normoblastic:** any a. characterized by the presence of normoblasts (*q.v.*) in the blood. **A., osteosclerotic:** the same as leuco-erythroblastosis, *q.v.* above. **A., pernicious:** a hyperchromic a. characterized by megalocytosis, presence of megaloblasts in bone marrow and often in the blood, anisocytosis, poikilocytosis, polychromasia, leucopenia, by achlorhydria and glossitis, hyperbilirubinuria with straw-coloured discoloration of skin and mucous membranes and increased excretion of urobilin, slight enlargement of the spleen, retinal haemorrhages and commonly associated with subacute combined degeneration of the cord (*q.v.*), due to lack of intrinsic factor (*q.v.*) . Syn. Addison's a.; Biermer's a. **A., sickle cell:** a haemolytic a. of dominant inheritance, mainly characterized by the presence of sickle-shaped erythrocytes, occurring almost exclusively in negroes. **A., splenic:** a syndrome characterized by the association of (usually hypochromic) anaemia, leucopenia and splenomegaly due to Banti's disease or to chronic thrombotic or other obstruction of the splenic or the portal vein. **A., tropical megalocytic:** a hyperchromic a. characterized by megalocytosis, probably due to deficiency of Castle's intrinsic factor (*q.v.*) or some other factor in the diet.

anae·mic. Relating to anaemia. **A. infarct:** an infarct which, owing to relative lack of collateral circulation, remains pale and does not develop into a haemorrhagic infarct. **A. murmur:** cardiac or vascular murmur caused by anaemia.

anae·robe (G. *an*, neg.; *aer*, air; *bios*, life). A micro-organism capable of living without air or free oxygen. **A., facultative:** a micro-organism capable of growing in both presence and absence of free oxygen. **A. obligate** (or obligatory) micro-organism growing only in the absence of free oxygen.

anaero·bia, anae·robes. Pl. of anaerobe.

anaero·bic. Living in the absence of oxygen or air.

anaer·obiōsis. Life without free oxygen. Syn. anoxybiosis.

Anaeromyces bronchitica. A micro-organism found in cases of tropical bronchitis.

anaer·ophyte (G. *an*, neg.; *aer*, air; *phuton*, a plant). A vegetable anaerobic organism.

anaer·oplasty (G. *an*, neg.; *aer*, air; *plassein*, to form). The application of water to open wounds so as to exclude air.

anaero·sis (G. *an*, neg.; *aēr*, air). Interruption of the respiratory process.

anaesthe·sia (G. *an*, neg.; *aisthēsis*, feeling). A condition of total or partial insensibility, particularly to touch. **A., basal:** partial general a. produced by preliminary medication through a drug such as morphine, allowing reduction of the amount of an inhalation anaesthetic for producing a complete a. **A., block,** see a., field-block and a., nerve-block. **A., caudal:** a. produced by injection of an anaesthetic drug into the caudal portion of the spinal canal. **A., central:** a. due to a lesion of the central nervous system. **A., conduction:** see a. nerve-block. **A., crossed:** a. of one side of the body due to a lesion of the other side of the brain. **A., dissociated:** a. for pain and temperature without disturbance of the tactile sense. **A., dolorosa:** the association of pain and insensibility to touch in the same area. **A., field-block:** a. produced by encircling the operative field by subcutaneous injections of a local anaesthetic. **A., general:** a. affecting the whole body, with loss of consciousness. **A., girdle:** insensibility to touch, etc., in an area encircling a section of the body. **A., glove:** insensibility to touch, etc., of the hand from finger-tips to wrist. **A., intratracheal:** a. induced by administra-

c

tion of an inhalation anaesthetic by a tube into the trachea. **A., intravenous**: a. induced by intravenous administration of a general anaesthetic. **A., inhalation**: a. induced by inhaling the vapour of an anaesthetic. **A., local**: a. of a limited area. **A., nerve-block**: local a. induced by the injection of an anaesthetic into or at the sides of a sensory nerve. **A., parasacral**: regional a. induced by injection of an anaesthetic into the sacral nerves at their emergence from the sacral foramina. **A., paravertebral**: regional a. induced by the injection of an anaesthetic into the spinal nerves at their emergence from the spine. **A., rectal**: general anaesthesia induced by the rectal administration of an anaesthetic. **A., refrigeration**: the use of refrigeration (with ice packs) of limbs to induce anaesthesia prior to amputation. **A., regional**: nerve-block a. (q.v.). **A., saddleshaped**: insensibility to touch, etc., of a saddle-shaped area, including anus, perineum, posterior part of scrotum, upper medial part of the thighs, due to a lesion of the cauda equina. **A., segmental**: a. affecting a segment of the body, due to lesion of a posterior nerve root. **A., spinal**: a. of the lower half of the body induced by the injection of an anaesthetic into the subarachnoidal space of the cord. **A., splanchnic**: a. of the abdominal viscera induced by injection of an anaesthetic into the coeliac plexus. **A., thermal**: loss of heat sense due to a central nervous lesion.

anaesthesi·meter (G. *an*, neg.; *aisthesis*, feeling; *metron*, measure). 1. An instrument for measuring the amount of an anaesthetic administered. 2. aesthesiometer (*q.v.*)

anaesthet·ic (G. *an*, neg.; *aisthēsis*, feeling). 1. Insensible to touch, or pain. 2. A substance producing anaesthesia. **A., general**: a substance inducing anaesthesia of the whole body with loss of consciousness. **A., local**: a substance inducing anaesthesia of an area where it is locally applied.

anaes·thetist. One who administers an anaesthetic.

anaes·thetize. To bring under the action of an anaesthetic.

anage·nesis (G. *ana*, again; *genesis*, production). Reproduction of tissue. Hence **anagenetic**, relating to anagenesis.

anagnosasthe·nia (G. *anagnōsis*, a reading; *asthĕneia*, weakness). Neurasthenic condition, in which the patient is unable to read.

anagocyt·ic (G. *an*, neg.; *agein*, to bring; *kutos*, cell) Inhibiting cell growth.

anagotox·ic (G. *an*, neg.; *agein*, to bring; *toxikon*, poison). Against toxin.

anákhré (Afr.). See goundou.

anak·mēsis (G. *an*, neg.; *akmē*, prime of life). Arrest of growth.

anakusia. See Anacusia.

a·nal (L. *anus*). Pertaining to the anus. **A. character**: in psycho-analysis a character held to be determined by fixation to an early stage of development of the libido, comprising the following qualities: over-accentuated orderliness, parsimony or avarice, and obstinacy or defiance. **A. erotism**: In psychology, early phase in sexual development, in which sexual interest centres on the anal region **A. fissure**: a tear in the mucous membrane of the anus. **A. fistula**: a sinus leading from the rectum or anal canal into the perirectal tissue with or without breaking through the skin at some point near the anus.

analep·tic (G. *analēpsis*, restoration). A restorative medicine or agent.

anal·gecize (G. *an*, neg.; *algos*, pain). To render analgesic.

analge·sia (G.). Insensibility to pain.

analge·sic (G.). Relieving pain; remedy that relieves pain.

anal·gia (G.). Absence of pain.

analler·gic. The quality of being not allergic.

ana·logous (G. *analogos*, proportionate). Conforming to; corresponding in certain particulars.

a·nalogue (G. *analogos*, proportionate). Part or organ having the same function as another, but of a different structure; e.g., gills and lungs. Cf. homologue.

ana·logy (G. *analŏgia*). Similarity in structure, function, origin, or other particulars.

a·nalyser (G. *analuein*, to analyse). 1. In a polarimeter, the Nicol prism, which extinguishes light rays not swinging in one particular plane. 2. A receptor together with its central nervous connections by which sensitivity to stimuli is differentiated. 3. An indicator, *q.v.*

ana·lysis (G. *analusis*). The determination of the constituent parts of a compound body or of a total experience. Psychoanalysis, *q.v.* **A., colorimetric** quantitative determination of substances by means of the colour intensity of the reaction products. **A., diffusion**: determination of size of particles and molecular weight by diffusion. **A., elementary**: quantitative determination of constituents of an organic compound by combustion. **A., gasometric**: a. of gases by means of an eudiometer, *q.v.* **A., gravimetric**: quantitative determination of the elements of a substance by weighing its constituents directly or indirectly. **A., qualitative**: determination of the nature of the constituents of a substance. **A., quantitative**: determination of the proportionate amounts of the constituents of a substance. **A., spectral**: qualitative determination of elements by their characteristic radiation by means of a spectroscope. **A., volumetric**: quantitative determination of the constituents of a substance by titration with a standard solution.

a·nalyst (G. *analuein*, to analyse). Person who makes an analysis.

analyt·ic. Pertaining to analysis.

Anam boil. Syn. Annam ulcer; oriental sore.

anamnē·sis (G. *anamnēsis*, a recalling). Medical history; information in respect of past or present illnesses gained from the patient or other persons.

anamnes·tic. Relating to the anamnesis or medical history of the patient.

anamniŏt·ic (G. *an*, neg.; *amnion*). Without amnion.

anamorphŏ·sis (G. *ana*, up; *morphe*, form). An abnormal transformation, due either to degeneration or to change in the habits of a plant.

ananabā·sis (G. *an*, neg.; *ana*. up; *basis*, a going). Inability to go up to high places.

ana·naphylaxis (G. *an*, neg.; *ana*, against; *phulax*, protector). Anti-anaphylaxis.

anan·drious (G. *anandria*, want of manhood). Impotent.

anan·giŏplā·sia (G. *an*, neg.; *aggeion*, vessel; *plassein*, to form). Congenital shrinking of the lumen of arteries.

anapeirat·ic (G. *anapeirasthai*, to do again). Caused by excessive use.

anapep·sia. Absence of pepsin from the secretions of the stomach.

ana·naphase (G. *ana*, up; *phasis*, phase). The phase of mitosis characterized by the passage of the daughter chromosomes towards the poles.

ana·phia (G. *an*, neg.; *haphē*, touch). Having no sense of touch.

anaphorē·sis (G. *an*, neg.; *a*, neg.; *phorein*, to convey). Deficient perspiration.

anaphoret·ic (G. *an*, neg.; *a*, neg.; *phorein*, to convey). 1. Checking perspiration. 2. An agent checking perspiration.

anaphor·ia (G. *ana*, up; *phorein*, to convey). An upward tendency of the eyes and of the visual axes.

anaphrodĭ·sia (G. *an*, neg.; *Aphrodite*, Venus). Absence or impairment of the sexual libido.

anaphrodĭ·siac. 1. Relating to anaphrodisia. 2. An agent that allays the sexual desire.

anaphylac·tia (G. *ana*, against; *phulax*, protector). The condition resulting from anaphylaxis.

anaphylac·tic. Pertaining to anaphylaxis.

anaphylac·tin. A substance supposed to be part of the originally injected protein and to be responsible for induction of anaphylaxis.

anaphylac·togen (G. *ana*, against; *phulax*, protector; *gennan*, to produce). The antigen connected with the production of anaphylaxis.

anaphylac·toid (G. *ana*, against; *phulax*, protector; *eidos*, form). Resembling anaphylaxis. **A. purpura:** see purpura, a.

anaphylatox·in (G. *ana*, against; *phulax*, protector; *toxikon*, poison). The toxic protein fraction which produces the symptoms in anaphylaxis; supposed to be formed by anaphylactin and the newly injected protein.

anaphylax·is (G. *ana*, against; *phulax*, protector). Hypersensitiveness or susceptibility produced by inoculation of a soluble protein to further doses of the same protein when given after an interval of not less than 12-14 days.

anaphyl·odiagnō·sis (G. *anaphylaxis*; *dia*, through; *gnosis*, knowledge). The diagnosis of disease through the study of anaphylactic reactions.

anaplā·sia (G. *ana*, backward; *plassein*, to form). The reversion of certain tissues, especially tumour cells, to a less differentiated type.

Anaplasma. Sporozoan organisms found in red blood cells.

anaplā·stic (G. *ana*, backward; *plassein*, to form). 1. Relating to anaplasty. 2. Restoring a lost or defective part.

an·aplasty. Plastic surgery.

anap·nograph (G. *anapnoē*, respiration; *graphein*, to record). An apparatus for measuring the pressure of respired air.

anap·tic. Relating to anaphia.

anarax·ia. See under malocclusion.

anar·chic (G. *an*, neg.; *archē*, rule). Against the law.

anār·ic (G. *a*, neg.; L. *nāris*, nostril). Without a nose.

anarith·mia (G. *a*, neg.; *arithmein*, to number). Inability to reckon, owing to a central brain lesion.

anarrhēx·is (G. *ana*, again; *rhēxis*, fracture). The operation of re-breaking a bone.

anar·thria (G. *anarthros*, inarticulate). Defective speech powers. See also aphasia, subcortical motor.

anar·throus (G. *an*, neg.; *arthron*, joint). 1. Jointless. 2. Inarticulate.

anasar·ca (G. *ana*, throughout; *sarx*, flesh). Oedema of the subcutaneous tissues of the trunk.

anasar·cous. Affected with anasarca.

anascit·ic. Having no ascites.

anasō·mia (G. *ana*, against; *sōma*, body). A condition characterized by the abnormal adherence of the limbs to the body.

anaspā·dias (G. *ana*, up; *spān*, to tear). Condition in which the urethra opens on the upper surface of the penis.

anastal·tic (G. *ana*, upwards; *staltikos*, contractile). Astringent.

anastat·ic (G. *anastasis*, resurrection). Restorative.

anastigmat·ic (G. *an*, neg.; *a*, neg.; *stigma*, mark). Free from astigmatism.

anā·stole (G. *anastolē*, a drawing back). Retraction.

anas·tomose (G. *anastomoein*, to provide with a mouth). To produce anastomosis; to communicate by anastomosis.

anastomō·sis. 1. A communication between two vessels. 2. The development or establishment of a communication between two different hollow parts or organs.

anastomŏ·tic. 1. Pertaining to anastomosis. 2. A communicating blood vessel.

anat. Abbreviation for anatomical.

anatŏ·mical, anatŏ·mic (G. *ana*, apart; *temnein*, to cut). Pertaining to anatomy.

ană·tomist. An expert in anatomy.

ană·tomy (G. *anatōme*, dissection). The science of the form and structure of organisms and their organs. **A., artistic:** a. applied to painting and sculpture. **A., comparative:** comparison of the anatomical character of different animal species. **A., general:** a. applied to the body tissues in general, opposed to special a. **A., morbid:** pathological a. **A., pathological:** a. applied to diseased organs. **A., regional:** a. applied to a particular region or to certain related parts. **A., special:** a. applied to a particular organ. **A., surgical:** a. with reference to the structural interrelation of parts. **A., topographic:** surgical a.

anā·topism (G. *ana*, backward; *tŏpos*, place). A mental state in which the patient fails to act according to the usages of his particular sphere of society.

anatox·in (G. *ana*, backward; *toxikon*, poison). A toxin complex so modified that the toxophore group has more or less completely disappeared while the haptophore group is retained. Syn. toxoid. Hence, **anatoxic**, pertaining to anatoxin.

ă·natricrot·ic (G. *ana*, up; *trēis*, three; *krotos*, stroke). Making three indentations on the upward grade of a sphygmogram.

anatri·crotism. A pulse beat which produces an anatricrotic sphygmogram.

anatrip·sis (G. *anatripsis*, a rubbing). 1. Rubbing; friction. 2. A centripetal movement in massage. 3. A crushing, e.g., of calculi.

anatrō·phic. Correcting atrophy.

anatrō·pia. See under anaphoria.

anax·on, anaxone (G. *an*, neg.; *axōn*, axis). A neuron devoid of axis-cylinder processes.

anazot·ic (G. *an*, neg.; *azot*, nitrogen). Without azote or nitrogen.

anazotū·ria (G. *an*, neg.; *azot*, nitrogen; *ouron*, urine). Deficient excretions of nitrogen in the urine.

anchone (G. *agkhōnē*, a throttling). Throat spasm in cases of hysteria.

an·chorage (L. *ancŏra*, anchor). 1. The fixation of a floating or displaced viscus. 2. In dentistry, the points of fixation of a dental filling or bridge. 3. In orthodontia, the resistance from which force is applied.

anchu·sin. Red colouring matter derived from alkanet root.

ancĭ·pital (L. *anceps*, two-headed). Two-edged.

an·con (G. *agkōn*, elbow). Originally the olecranon process; applied to the elbow generally.

an·conad. Towards the elbow.

anconag·ra (G. *agkōn*, elbow; *agra*, seizure). Gout in the elbow.

an·conal. Relating to the elbow.

ancōn·eus. See under muscles.

anconi·tis. Inflammation of the elbow.

an·cyroid (G. *agkura*, anchor; *eidos*, form). Hook-shaped.

Andernach's ossicles (Andernach, J. W. von, German physician, 1478-1574). The wormian bones.

Anders's disease (Anders, J. M., U.S. physician, 1854-1936). Adiposis tuberosa simplex, a disorder in which fatty masses are deposited in the tissues.

Andersch's ganglion (Andersch, C. S., German anatomist, 1732-77). The same as the petrous ganglion. **A.'s nerve:** the tympanic nerve.

Anderson's pill (Anderson, P., seventeenth-century Scottish physician). The compound gamboge pill.

Andral's decubitus (Andral, G., French physician, 1797-1876). Decubitus, *q.v.* on the sound side; the position a patient takes up in the prodromal stage of pleurisy.

andrană·tomy (G. *anēr*, man; *anatomē*, dissection). Male anatomy.

Andrewes's test (Andrewes, C. M., British physician born 1896). A qualitative test for the presence of uraemia.

Andrews's operation (Andrews, E. W., U.S. surgeon, 1857–1927). 1. Radical cure of an inguinal hernia by overlapping sutures. 2. Radical cure of a vaginal hydrocele by eversion of the tunica vaginalis.

andriă·trics (G. *anēr*, man; *iātrikos*, healing). The science of men's diseases and their treatment.

an·drogen (G. *anēr*, man; *gennan*, to produce). 1. Having the function of or producing a male sex hormone. 2. Producing male sex characteristics. Hence, **androgenic**, producing masculine sex characteristics.

androgĕ·nesis (G. *anēr*, man; *gennan*, to produce). Ovular development with paternal chromosomes only.

andrŏ·genous. Giving birth to male children.

androglŏs·sia (G. *anēr*, man; *glōssa*, tongue). Male timbre or quality heard in some female voices.

andrŏ·gyna, an·drogyne (G. *anēr*, man; *gunē*, woman). 1. A hermaphrodite. 2. A female pseudo-hermaphrodite. 3. An androgynous plant.

andrŏ·gynism. Female hermaphroditism.

andrŏ·gynous. 1. Having the characteristics of both sexes; hermaphrodite. 2. Pseudo-hermaphroditic. 3. Having both stamens and pistils in the same flower cluster.

andrŏ·gynus. A male pseudo-hermaphrodite.

an·droid (G. *anēr*, man; *eidos*, shape). Like a man.

andromān·ia (G. *anēr*, man; *mania*, frenzy). Nymphomania.

androphŏ·bia (G. *anēr*, man; *phŏbos*, fear). A morbid antipathy towards the male sex.

an·drostene (G. *anēr*, *andros*, man; with the conventional ending -*ene* for unsaturated hydrocarbons containing one double bond, in official chemical nomenclature). An unsaturated polycyclic hydrocarbon, $C_{19}H_{30}$. A steroid.

androstē·nediol, androstēn·diol. A crystalline androgenic steroid, $C_{19}H_{30}O_2$.

andrŏ·sterone (G. *anēr*, man; *stereos*, solid). Male sex hormone, present in normal male urine.

anec·tasin (G. *an*, neg.; *ektăsis*, extension; from G. *ek* out and *tăsis*, verbal noun of *teinein* to stretch—a stretching out or distension). A substance produced by bacteria, having an effect on the vasomotor nerves opposite to that of ectasin (a substance having the properties of a vasomotor dilator).

anĕ·deous (G. *an*, neg.; *aidoion*, genitals). Without genitals.

Anel's operation (Anel, D., French surgeon, 1679–1730). 1. Proximal ligature of an artery in cases of aneurysm. 2. Instrumental dilatation of the lacrimal duct, followed by the injection of an astringent. A.'s **probe**: a special probe for the lacrimal canals.

anelec·tric (G. *an*, neg.; *elektron*, amber). Non-electric, or parting rapidly with electricity.

anelec·trode (G. *ana*, up; *elektron*, amber). The positive pole of a galvanic battery.

ă·nelectrŏ·tonous (G. *an*, up; *elektron*, amber; *tonos*, tension). The decrease in excitability in irritable tissue during the passage of electric current through it at the anode. See Pflüger's Law.

anemŏ·meter (G. *anemos*, wind; *metron*, measure). Instrument for measuring the velocity of air currents.

anemŏ·pathy (G. *anemos*, wind; *păthos*, affection). Therapy by means of inhalation.

anemophŏ·bia (G. *anemos*, wind; *phobos*, fear). Morbid fear of winds.

anencephā·lia, anencĕ·phaly. (G. *an*, neg.; *egkephalos*, brain). Congenital absence of the brain.

anencephal·ic. Pertaining to or characterized by anencephalia.

anencephalohāē·mia (G. *an*, neg.; *egkephalos*, brain; *haima*, blood). Inadequate supply of blood to the brain.

anencĕ·phalus (G). A monster characterized by absence of a brain.

anener·gia (G. *an*, neg.; *energeia*, action). Lack of vigour or power.

anen·terous (G. *an*, neg.; *enteron*, intestine). Having no intestine, as a tapeworm or a fluke.

aneosinophĭ·lia. Absence of the eosinophils in the bloodstream.

anĕ·pia (G. *an*, neg.; *ĕpos*, word). Having no power to speak.

anepiplŏ·ic (G. *an*, neg.; *epiploon*, the caul). Having no epiploon or omentum.

anergă·sia (G. *an*, neg.; *ergăsia*, work). Absence of functional activity.

aner·gia (G. *an*, neg.; *ergon*, work). Sluggishness; inactivity.

aner·gic. Pertaining to anergia.

ă·nergy (G. *an*, neg.; *ergon*, work). Absence of sensitivity to an antigen or the condition resulting from desensitization.

ă·neroid (G. *a*, neg.; *nēros*, liquid; *eidos*, form). Applied to a barometer containing no fluid.

aneryth·rocyte (G. *an*, neg.; *eruthros*, red; *kutos*, a container). A red blood cell without haemoglobin.

anerythroplā·sia (G. *an*, neg.; *eruthros*, red; *plassein*, to form). Impairment or absence of red blood cell formation.

anerythroplă·stic. Characterized by anerythroplasia.

anerythrop·sia (G. *an*, neg.; *eruthros*, red; *opsis*, sight). Impaired colour perception of red.

ă·nethol. An essential principle, $C_3H_5.C_6H_4.OCH_3$, of the oils of fennel and anise.

Anethum. A genus of plants, which includes fennel.

ă·netic (G. *anĕtos*, relaxed). Soothing; anodyne.

anetoder·mia (G. *anĕtos*, relaxed; *derma*, skin). Atrophic, lax skin.

ă·netus. Intermittent fever.

anēū·ria (G. *a*, neg.; *neuron*, nerve). Without nervous energy.

anēur·ic. Pertaining to aneuria.

aneurilem·mic (G. *a*, neg.; *neuron*, nerve; *lemma*, husk). Without a neurilemma.

ă·neurine (G. *an*, neg.; *neuron*, nerve). Vitamin B_1, a water-soluble compound containing the pyrimidine and thiazole ring systems, present in especially large amounts in the germ of cereals, in yeast and in the seed of pulses, and by absorption from plant foods in animal tissues rich in nuclear material; deficiency of aneurine in the diet causes beri-beri. Syn. thiamine.

ă·neurysm (G. *aneurusmos*, a widening). A circumscribed dilatation of the walls of an artery. A., **arterio-venous**: an abnormal communication between an artery and a vein. A., **cardiac**: a. of the heart, affecting usually the anterior wall of the left ventricle near the apex, due to an outward bulging of an area which has been weakened by ischaemic necrosis. A., **cirsoid**: a form of congenital arterio-venous a. occurring in the scalp, characterized by a mass of dilated tortuous vessels. A., **dissecting**: a condition characterized by a haemorrhage in the media of the aorta between the middle and outer thirds beginning at the base and spreading along the vessel for a variable distance, splitting the media into two layers, usually rupturing externally, originating from the passage of blood through atheromatous cracks in the interior to the rupture of vasa vasorum into a degenerated media; not causing a dilatation of the vessel and therefore not a true aneurysm. A., **false**: a haematoma due to a rupture of an arterial wall, having its walls formed by the surrounding tissues. **A., fusiform:** a dilatation of a segment of a vessel. **A., mycotic:** an a. caused by the effects of an infected embolus on the wall of a vessel. **A., sacculated, saccular:** a pouch-shaped dilatation of a vessel at one point. **A., spurious:** see false a. **A., true:** any a. in which the sac is formed by the vessel wall.

aneurȳs·mal. Of the nature of or pertaining to an aneurysm.

aneurysmat·ic. Affected with or of the nature of an aneurysm.

aneurysmec·tomy (G. *aneurusma*, aneurysm; *ektomē*, excision). Excision of the sac of an aneurysm.

aneurys·moplasty (G. *aneurusma*, aneurysm; *plassein*, to form). Restoration of the artery in an aneurysm.

aneurysmor·rhaphy (G. *aneurusma*, aneurysm; *raphē*, suture). The suturing of an aneurysm. (See also endoaneurysmorrhaphy).

aneurysmŏ·tomy (G. *aneurusma*, aneurysm; *tomē*, section). Incision into the sac of an aneurysm.

anfractŭŏ·sity (L. *anfractus*, bending). A cerebral sulcus.

anfrac·tuous. Convoluted.

angeī·tis (G. *aggeion*, vessel). Inflammation of a lymph vessel or a blood vessel.

angel's wing. A name given to a deformity characterized by abnormal prominence of both scapulae. Sometimes called winged scapulae.

angiăl·gia (G. *aggeion*, vessel; *algos*, pain). Pain felt in any blood vessel.

angiectă·sia (G. *aggeion*, vessel; *ektasis*, extension). Abnormal dilatation of a blood vessel.

angiectat·ic. Relating to or characterized by dilated blood vessels.

angiěc·tomy. The excision of a blood vessel.

angi·itis. Angeitis, *q.v.*

angi·na (G. *agkhein*, to throttle). Any disease associated with a sense of choking or suffocation. **A. abdominis:** condition characterized by severe abdominal pain due to transient or permanent occlusion of abdominal arteries. **A., follicular:** the same as follicular tonsillitis. **A., Ludovici:** phlegmonous inflammation of the floor of the mouth. Syn. Ludwig's angina. **A. lacunaris:** the same as lacunar tonsillitis. **A. pectoris:** a condition characterized by severe constricting pain in the chest, especially retrosternally, usually radiating to one or both shoulders and arm, and angor animi (*q.v.*) due to transient insufficiency of blood to the heart. **A. tonsillaris:** the same as tonsillitis, *q.v.*

an·ginoid (G. *agkhein*, to throttle, *eidos*, form). Resembling an angina.

an·ginose. Pertaining to angina; characterized by symptoms of suffocation.

an·gio-ată·xia (G. *aggeion*, vessel; *ataxis*, disorder). An irregularity in the tension of the blood vessels.

an·gioblast (G. *aggeion*, vessel; *blastos*, germ). Embryonic cell capable of development into vascular tissue.

angioblastō·ma. A blood vessel tumour.

angiocar·diogram (G. *aggeion*, vessel; *kardia*, heart; *gramma*, a picture). The radiological study of malformations of the heart and great vessels by the injection of radio-opaque substances.

angiocardī·tis (G. *aggeion*, vessel; *kardia*, heart). Inflammation of the main blood channels and the heart.

angiochei·loscope (G. *aggeion*, vessel; *kheilos*, lip; *skopein*, to view). An instrument for observing the blood circulation of the lips.

an·giocholecystī·tis (G. *aggeion*, vessel; *kholē*, bile; *kustis*, bladder). Inflammation of the gall-bladder and bile ducts.

an·gioclast (G. *aggeion*, vessel; *klaein*, to break). An instrument used to compress bleeding arteries.

Angiococcus. A genus of micro-organisms.

an·giodystrŏ·phia (G. *aggeion*, vessel; *dus-*, ill; *trophē*, nourishment). Impairment of the nutrition of the blood vessels.

an·giofibrō·ma (G. *aggeion*, vessel; L. *fibra*, fibre). A benign tumour composed of fibrous and angiomatous tissues.

angiogĕ·nesis (G. *aggeion*, vessel; *genesis*, formation). The development of the vessels.

angiogĕ·nic. Developing into blood vessels.

angiogliŏ·ma. A vascular form of glioma, *q.v.*

an·gioid (G. *aggeion*, vessel; *eidos*, form). Resembling a blood vessel. **A. streaks:** a sometimes recessively inherited affection characterized by a network of reddish or brown streaks situated between the retinal and choroidal vessels, radiating from a ring round the optic disc to the peripheral parts of the retina; probably due to rupture of Bruch's membrane.

an·giokeratō·ma (G. *aggeion*, vessel; *keras*, horn). A benign tumour characterized by small warty growths enclosing capillary telangiectases, affecting usually hands and feet.

an·giolipō·ma (G. *aggeion*, vessel; *lipos*, animal fat). A benign tumour composed of angiomatous and lipomatous tissue.

an·giolith (G. *aggeion*, vessel; *lithos*, stone). A calculus on the wall of a blood vessel. Also called phlebolith.

angiŏ·logy (G. *aggeion*, vessel; *logos*, treatise). The part of anatomy pertaining to the blood vessels and lymphatics.

angiolŭ·poid (G. *aggeion*, vessel; L. *lupus*, wolf; G. *eidos*, form). A form of sarcoidosis of Boeck, *q.v.*, in which the skin lesions are arranged in groups or plaques on the face, especially about the nose and eyes.

an·giolymphangiŏ·ma. An angioma in which both lymph and blood vessels are affected.

an·giolymphō·ma. A lymph vessel tumour.

angiŏ·ma (G. *aggeion*, vessel). A benign neoplasm derived from blood vessels. **A. serpiginosum:** a condition characterized by minute, gyrate-like arranged angiomata, spreading slowly and intermittently. **A., capillary:** an a. composed of new-formed capillaries affecting only one segment of a vessel. **A., cavernous:** an a. composed of large blood spaces lined by endothelium, occurring mainly in the liver.

angiomalā·cia (G. *aggeion*, vessel; *malakia*, softness). The softening of vessel walls in disease.

angiomatō·sis (G. *aggeion*, vessel). A condition characterized by multiple angiomata.

angiŏ·matous. Pertaining to an angioma.

an·giomĕ·galy (G. *aggeion*, vessel; *megas*, large). Enlargement of the blood vessels.

angiŏ·meter (G. *aggeion*, vessel; *metron*, measure). An instrument for measuring the tension of blood vessels.

an·giomyocar·diac (G. *aggeion*, vessel; *mus*, muscle; *kardia*, heart). Pertaining to or affecting the vessels and the heart muscle.

an·giomyŏ·ma (G. *aggeion*, vessel; *mus*, muscle). A benign tumour composed of angiomatous and myomatous tissue.

an·giomyoneurō·ma (G. *aggeion*, vessel; *mus*, muscle; *neuron*, sinew). Glomus tumour, *q.v.*

an·giomyŏ·pathy (G. *aggeion*, vessel; *mus*, muscle; *pathos*, disease). Blood vessel disturbances in which muscles are involved.

an·giomyosarcō·ma (G. *aggeion*, vessel; *mus*, muscle; *sarx*, flesh). A mixed tumour composed of angiomatous, myomatous and sarcomatous tissues.

an·gionecrō·sis (G. *aggeion*, vessel; *nekros*, dead). Necrosis of blood vessel walls.

an·gionē·oplasm. A blood vessel tumour.

angioneurec·tomy (G. *aggeion*, vessel; *neuron*, nerve; *ektomē*, excision). Excision of vessels and nerves.

an·gioneurō·sis (G. *aggeion*, vessel; *neuron*, nerve). Functional disorder of the vasomotor system.

angioneurotic oedema. Localized oedema of some parts (e.g., eyelid or lip) of acute onset and tending to recur, supposed to be due to vasomotor disturbance; considered by some authorities as an allergic symptom.

an·gioneurŏ·tomy (G. *aggeion*, vessel; *neuron*, nerve; *tomē*, a cutting). The division of the nerves and blood vessels of a part.

an·gionō·ma (G. *aggeion*, vessel). A blood vessel ulcer.

an·giopară·lysis (G. *aggeion*, vessel; *parĕsis*, paralysis). Paralysis of blood vessels.

an·giopă·rĕsis (G. *aggeion*, vessel; *parĕsis*, paralysis). Paralysis due to vasomotor defect.

an·giopathŏ·logy (G. *aggeion*, vessel; *pathos* (medical), affection; *logos*, discourse). Study of diseases of blood vessels.

angiŏ·pathy (G. *aggeion*, vessel; *pathos* (medical), affection). Any disease of the vascular system.

an·giophakomatō·sis. Lindau's disease, *q.v.*

an·gioplä·ny (G. *aggeion*, vessel; *planē*, a wandering). Any blood vessel of abnormal construction, or which takes an abnormal course.

an·gioplast (G. *aggeion*, vessel; *plassein*, to form). An embryo cell from which blood vessels develop.

an·gioplasty (G. *aggeion*, vessel; *plassein*, to form). Plastic surgery of blood vessels.

angiopoiē·sis (G. *aggeion*, vessel; *poiein*, to make). New formation of blood vessels. Hence, **angiopoietic**, forming new blood vessels.

an·giopressure. Method of controlling haemorrhage from a vessel by applying haemostatic forceps with pressure.

an·giorrhā·gia (G. *aggeion*, vessel; *rhēgnunai*, I break). Bleeding from a vessel.

angiŏr·rhaphy (G. *aggeion*, vessel; *rhaphē*, suture). Suture of a vessel.

angiorrhex·is (G. *aggeion*, vessel; *rhexis*, rupture). Rupture of a blood vessel.

angiorrhoē·a (G. *aggeion*, vessel; *rhein*, flow). Oozing of blood.

angiosarcō·ma (G. *aggeion*, vessel; *sarx*, flesh). A sarcoma composed of vascular tissues.

an·giosclerō·sis (G. *aggeion*, vessel; *sclerosis*). Hardening of blood vessel walls. Hence, **angiosclerotic**, relating to or characterized by angiosclerosis.

an·gioscope (G. *aggeion*, vessel; *skopein*, to view). An instrument used for the examination of blood vessels.

an·gioscotō·ma (G. *aggeion*, vessel; *skotos*, darkness). Defective vision caused by retinal blood vessel shadows.

an·gioscotŏ·metry (G. *aggeion*, vessel; *skotos*, darkness; *metron*, measure). Tracing of thin bands in the visual field, corresponding to the retinal vessels, of physiological blindness.

an·giosiali·tis (G. *aggeion*, vessel; *siălon*, saliva). Inflammation of a duct of a salivary gland.

an·giospasm (G. *aggeion*, vessel; *spasmos*, spasm). A vasomotor spasm.

angiospă·stic (G. *aggeion*, vessel; *spasmos*, spasm). Characterized by angiospasm.

an·giosperm (G. *aggeion*, vessel; *sperma*, seed). A plant giving its seeds within a closed vessel or ovary.

an·giostax·is (G. *aggeion*, vessel; *staxis*, a dripping). Haemorrhagic diathesis.

an·giostenō·sis (G. *aggeion*, vessel; *stenōsis*, a narrowing). Narrowing of a vessel.

an·giosteō·sis (G. *aggeion*, vessel; *osteon*, bone). Calcification of a blood vessel.

Angiostomidae. A family of Nematoda.

angiŏ·strophy (G. *aggeion*, vessel; *strephein*, to twist). Stoppage of a haemorrhage by twisting a blood vessel.

angioti·tis (G. *aggeion*, vessel; *ous*, ear). Inflammation of the blood vessels of the ear.

angiŏ·tomy (G. *aggeion*, vessel; *tomē*, a cutting). Incision into a vessel.

angiotō·nia (G. *aggeion*, vessel; *tŏnos*, tension). The tension of blood vessels.

an·giotribe (G. *aggeion*, vessel; *tribein*, to crush). A clamp with powerful jaws, used to occlude arteries.

an·giotripsy (G. *aggeion*, vessel; *tribein*, to crush). Vascular compression by means of the angiotribe.

an·giotrŏ·phic (G. *aggeion*, vessel; *trophē*, nutrition). Affecting or relating to vascular nutrition.

an·giotrŏ·pheneurō·sis (G. *aggeion*, vessel; *trophē*, nutrition; *neurosis*). Neurosis of the blood vessels characterized by trophic disorder.

angle (L. *angulus*). 1. A corner. 2. The degree of divergence of two lines or planes that meet each other; the space between two such lines. **A. of aperture:** a. at the focus of a lens between the two lines drawn from opposite sides of its periphery. **A., axial:** the a. formed by two surfaces of a body, the line of union of which is parallel with its axis. **A., biorbital:** the a. formed by the two optical axes. **A., carrying:** a. formed by the axes of the upper and lower arm when the latter is extended. **A., costal:** a. between the lower border of the false ribs and the sternal axis. **A., critical:** a. of incidence whose sine is equal to the refractive index. **A. of deviation:** the total amount of deviation between incident and emergent rays. **A. of incidence:** a. made by the incident ray with a line perpendicular to the surface of the refracting medium. **A. of jaw:** a. between lower border of mandibular body and the posterior border of the mandibular ramus. **A., optic:** a. between the two visual axes. **A. of polarization:** a. at which light is most completely polarized. **A. of reflection:** a. between the reflected ray and a line perpendicular to the surface of the medium. **A. of refraction:** a. between the ray leaving a refracting medium and a line perpendicular to the surface of the medium. **A., visual:** a. between the lines drawn from the periphery of an object seen at the nodal point. **Angle α:** a. formed at the nodal point between the optic and visual axes. **Angle γ:** a. between the optic and fixation axes. **Angle κ:** a. formed at the nodal point between the central pupillary line and the visual axis.

Angle's classification of malocclusion (Angle, E. H., U.S. orthodontist, 1855-1930). There are three classes of malocclusion. 1. Neutro-occlusion. 2. Disto-occlusion. 3. Mesio-occlusion. **A.'s splint:** a wire splint used in securing the teeth in fractures of the lower jaw.

Anglesey leg (Named after the Marquis of Anglesey, 1768-1854, for whom it was made). A wooden artificial leg, very little used to-day.

anglicus sudor (L.). English sweating fever. A contagious disease, often having a fatal outcome, which occurred in England during the fifteenth and sixteenth centuries. It was characterized by fever, much perspiration, rash and circulatory symptoms. Syn. ephemera maligna.

angor (L. a strangling). The same as angina. **A. animi:** a sense of imminent death. **A. pectoris:** the same as angina pectoris.

angostura. The bark of the *Calipea cusparia*, used as a febrifuge and tonic.

Angström unit. A°, 10^{-8} cm., unit used for measuring wavelengths.

Anguillula. Strongyloides, *q.v.* A genus of small nematode worms.

anguillulō·sis. The presence of strongyloides in the body.

Anguillulidae. A family of Nematoda.

Anguillulina putrefaciens. A nematode which has its normal habitat in onions, and is sometimes found in man.

an·gular. Sharp-cornered, or having angles.

angulā·tion. Formation of sharp angles.

angulus (L.). Angle.

anhaematō·sis (G. *an*, neg.; *haimatoein*, to make into blood). Defect of blood formation.

anhaemolyt·ic (G. *an*, neg.; *haima*, blood; *lusis*, a dissolving). Not haemolytic.

anhă·phia (G. *an*, neg.; *haphē*, touch). Absence or loss of the sense of touch.

anhelā·tion (L. *anhelāre*, to pant). Shortness of breath.

anhepā·tia (G. *an*, neg.; *hēpar*, liver). Loss of liver function.

anhepat·ic. Not arising from the liver.

anhidrō·sis (G. *an*, neg.; *hidrōs*, sweat). Diminution or absence of perspiration.

anhidrot·ic. Lessening perspiration.

anhormō·nia. Deficiency of hormones.

anhydrāe·mia (G. *an*, neg.; *hudōr*, water; *haima*, blood). Diminution of watery constituents in the blood.

anhydrā·tion (G. *an*, neg.; *hudōr*, water). The state of not being hydrated.

anhȳ·dride (G. *an*, neg.; *hudōr*, water). A compound usually derived from an acid by the abstraction of the elements of water.

anhydrochlor·ic. Characterized by absence or marked deficiency of hydrochloric acid.

an·hydromȳē·lia (G. *an*, neg.; *hudōr*, water; *muĕlos*, marrow). Absence or deficiency of spinal cord fluid.

anhȳ·drous (G. *an*, neg.; *hudōr*, water). Deprived of all water; applied especially to water of crystallization.

anhȳp·nia (G. *an*, neg.; *hupnos*, sleep). Sleeplessness; insomnia.

aniän·thinopsy (G. *an*, neg.; *ianthīnos*, violet-coloured; *opsis*, vision). Inability to perceive violet tints.

anictĕ·ric. Without icterus. (See jaundice.)

ani·dean. Relating to an anideus.

ani·deus (G. *an*, neg.; *eidos*, form). A double monster, in which the parasitic foetus is a shapeless mass. Hence, anidous, without form.

anidrō·sis (G. *an*, neg.; *hidrōs*, sweat). See anhidrosis.

ă·nile (L. *ănus*, old woman). Imbecile; like an old woman.

ă·nilide (Arab. *al-nil*, dark blue). A derivative of aniline formed by the substitution of acyl radicals for the H atoms of the NH₂ group.

ă·niline (Arab. *al-nil*, dark blue). $C_6H_5NH_2$. Phenylamine, obtained by the reduction of nitrobenzene. Parent substance of a group of dyestuffs, and also of a group of substances having antipyretic properties.

anili·nophile (Arab. *al-nil*, dark blue; G. *philein*, to love). Readily stained with aniline.

ă·nilism. Poisoning caused by the fumes from aniline dye manufacture.

ă·nima (L. *anima*, air). 1. The mind. 2. A current of air, breath. In the plural, *animae*, the swimming-bladders of herring.

ă·nimal. A living organism, endowed with life, sensation and voluntary motion.

animā·tion. The state of being alive.

an·ion. An electronegative ion.

aniri·dia (G. *an*, neg.; *iris*, iris). Absence or defect of the iris.

anischū·ria (G. *an*, neg.; *ischouria*, retention of the urine). The same as enuresis, *q.v.*

aniseed. Seed of anise, used as a carminative.

ani·sochromat·ic (G. *anĭsos*, unequal; *khrōma*, colour). Not having the same colour throughout.

anisochrō·mia (G. *anĭsos*, unequal; *khrōma*, colour). Heterochromia, *q.v.*

anisocŏr·ia (G. *anĭsos*, unequal; *kŏrē*, pupil). Inequality of the pupillary diameter.

anisocytō·sis (G. *anĭsos*, unequal; *kutos*, cell). Abnormal inequality in the size of the red blood corpuscles.

anisodăc·tylus (G. *anĭsos*, unequal; *daktulos*, digit). Having unequal digits.

anĭ·sodont (G. *anĭsos*, unequal; *ŏdous*, tooth). Having teeth of uneven lengths.

anisŏ·gamy (G. *anĭsos*, unequal; *gamos*, marriage). Fusion of two gametes of unequal form or size.

anisŏ·gnathus (G. *anĭsos*, unequal; *gnathos*, jaw). Having one jaw considerably wider than the other, especially in the molar region.

ani·soleucocytō·sis (G. *anĭsos*, unequal; *leukos*, white; *kutos*, cell). Inequality of the proportion of leucocytes in the blood.

anisomăs·tia (G. *anĭsos*, unequal; *mastos*, breast). Inequality of the size of the breasts.

anisomē·lia (G. *anĭsos*, unequal; *melos*, limb). Inequality between corresponding limbs.

anisomē·ria (G. *anĭsos*, unequal; *meros*, part). 1. The condition of having unequal organs. 2. The condition of not being isomeric.

ani·sometrō·pia (G. *anĭsos*, unequal; *metron*, measure; *ōps*, eye). A difference in the refraction of the two eyes.

anisosthĕn·ic (G. *anĭsos*, unequal; *sthenos*, power). Not of equal power, as of corresponding muscles.

anisotŏn·ic (G. *anĭsos*, unequal; *tonos*, tension). Exerting unequal osmotic pressure.

anisotrop·ic (G. *anĭsos*, unequal; *tropos*, direction). Doubly refractile, rotating the plane through which polarised light passes through the object.

anitrō·genous. Not nitrogenous.

ankle. The joint situated between the lower leg and the foot.

ankle clonus (G. *klonos*, turmoil). Abnormally increased ankle jerk in which the gastrocnemius muscle contracts rhythmically on sudden flexure of the foot.

ankle jerk. Reflex contraction of the gastrocnemius muscle, producing plantar flexion of the foot on sharp tapping of the Achilles tendon; mediated by the second sacral segment of the cord.

ankle, tailor's. A ganglion or synovial sac over the external malleolus in tailors, due to their posture when at work.

ankȳ·la, an·kyle (G. *agkulē*, flexure). 1. An angular part, particularly the elbow. 2. Ankylosis of a joint with flexion. 3. Abnormal adhesion of parts.

ankyloblĕ·pharon (G. *agkulē*, flexure; *blepharon*, eyelid). The adhesion of the ciliary edges of the eyelids. Syn. total symblepharon.

ankylochei·lia, ankylochī·lia (G. *agkulē*, flexure; *kheilos*, lip). Adhesion of the lips.

ankylocol·pos (G. *agkulē*, flexure; *kolpos*, womb). Adhesion between walls of, and hence atresia of the vagina.

an·kylodactȳl·ia (G. *agkulē*, flexure; *daktulos*, finger). Adhesion of fingers or toes to one another.

ankylodŏn·tia (G. *agkulē*, flexure; *odous*, tooth). Irregularity in the position of the teeth.

ankyloglŏs·sia, ankyloglŏs·sum (G. *agkulē*, flexure; *glōssa*, tongue). Tongue-tie.

ankylomĕ·lē (G. *agkulē*, flexure; *mĕlos*, limb). Abnormal adhesions between limbs, as between fingers or toes.

an·kylomele (G. *agkulē*, flexure; *mēlē*, probe). A curved probe.

ankylŏ·merism (G. *agkulē*, flexure; *meros*, part). Abnormal adhesion of parts to each other.

ankylophō·bia (G. *agkulē*, flexure; *phobos*, fear). Morbid fear of ankylosis.

ankylopoiĕt·ic (G. *agkulē*, flexure; *poiein*, to make). Causing ankylosis.

ankyloprŏc·tia (G. *agkulē*, flexure; *prōktos*, anus). Atresia of the anus.

ankylorrhĭ·nia (G. *agkulē*, flexure; *rhis*, nose). Abnormal adhesion between walls of a nostril.

an·kylose (G. *agkulē*, flexure). To be or to become firmly united or consolidated.

ankylŏ·sis (G. *agkulē*, flexure). Union of the bones forming an articulation, resulting in a stiff joint. A., false: non-bony union between two bones or two parts of a bone.

Ankylŏ·stoma (G. *agkulos*, crooked; *stŏma*, mouth). A genus of nematode parasites, the hookworms. A. canicum: the hookworm commonly found in dogs and cats. A. duodenale, a nematode worm inhabiting the small intestine.

ankylostomī·asis (G. *agkulē*, flexure; *stoma*, mouth). The morbid condition due to infestation with *A. duodenale*, characterized by anaemia, digestive upset, mental inertia. Syn. hookworm disease.

ankylō·tia (G. *agkulē*, flexure; *ous*, ear). Abnormal adhesions closing the external meatus of the ear.

ankylot·ic. Relating to or characterized by ankylosis.

ankў·lotome (G. *agkulē*, flexure; *tomē*, section). A knife for cutting adhesions.

ankylurē·thria (G. *agkulē*, flexure; *urethra*). A stricture of the urethra.

an·kyroid (G. *agkura*, a hook; *eidos*, form). Shaped like a hook.

anlage. (Ger. *Anlage*, predisposition). 1. The inherited organization of an individual or an organ, especially in early development, which forms the basis of later development. 2. The embryonic area in which traces of any particular part first appear.

Annam ulcer. See under Oriental sore.

Annandale's operation (Annandale, T., Scottish surgeon, 1838–1907). 1. For displaced semilunar cartilages; exposure of knee joint and stitching cartilages in their proper place. (Not used to-day.) 2. For genu valgum, partial excision of both condyles of femur. (Not used to-day.) These operations are only of historic interest.

anneal. To temper by heat.

annec·tant (L. *ad*, to; *nectare*, to join). Connecting.

Annelida. The phylum of segmented worms.

annuens (L.). The rectus capitis anticus minor muscle.

an·nular (L. *ānŭlus*, a ring). Ring-like.

annulor·rhaphy (L. *ānŭlus*, a ring; G. *raphē*, suture). Closure of a hernial ring or sac by suture.

an·nulus (L. *ānŭlus*, a ring). A circular opening.

An.O.C. Abbreviation for anodal opening contraction.

anochlē·sia (G.). 1. Calmness. 2. Catalepsy.

anoci-association (L. *a*, neg.; *nocēre*, to injure; *associare*, to associate). Exclusion of harmful associations by blocking sensory perceptions.

anococcў·geal (L. *ānus*, anus; G. *kokkux*, coccyx). Pertaining both to the anus and the coccyx.

anō·dal (G. *ana*, up; *hŏdos*, road). Relating to the anode; electro-positive. A. closure: the closure of an electric circuit with the anode placed on the muscle or nerve to be examined.

ă·node. The positive electrode, *q.v.*

anodĭ·nia (G. *an*, neg.; *ŏdûne*, pain). Absence of pains at labour.

anod·mia (G. *an*, neg.; *odmē*, smell). Absence of the sense of smell.

anodŏn·tia (G. *an*, neg.; *odous*, tooth). Absence of the teeth. Hence **anodontism**, the complete absence of dental organs.

an·odyne (G. *an*, neg.; *odunē*, pain). A medicine that relieves pain, e.g., morphine, atropine, etc.

anoes·trus (G. *an*, neg.; *oistros*, vehement desire). The period of sexual quiescence in females.

anomalō·pia (G. *anōmalos*, irregular; *ōpē*, sight). A type of colour blindness.

anō·maloscope (G. *anōmalos*, irregular; *skopein*, to view). An instrument used in examining the eye for colour perception.

anŏ·maly (G. *anōmalos*, irregular). Deviation from the normal. **Colour a.:** red-green colour blindness in varying degrees.

anō·mia (L. *a*, neg.; L. *nōmen*, name). Inability to name objects; loss of power to recall names.

anonў·chia (G. *an*, neg.; *onux*, nail). Absence of nail formation.

anō·nymous (G. *an*, neg.; *ŏnuma*, name). Nameless.

anŏŏp·sia (G. *anō*, up; *ops*, eye). Strabismus with the eye turned upwards.

ā·noperinē·al (L. *anus*, anus; G. *perineos*, perineum). Relating to anus and perineum.

Anŏ·pheles (G. *anŏphelēs*, hurtful). A subgenus of Anophelini (*q.v.*) comprising *A. maculipennis*, *A. bifurcatus* and other species transmitting malaria to man.

Anophelini. A tribe of the family Culicinae comprising various sub-genera of mosquitoes transmitting malarial plasmodia to man.

anŏ·phelism. The infestation of an area with Anopheles.

anophthal·mia, anophthal·mos (G. *an*, neg.; *ophthalmos*, eye). Congenital absence of the eyes; complete failure in the outgrowth of the primary optic vesicle.

anō·pia (G. *an*, neg.; *ops*, eye). Absence of sight, especially blindness due to a scotoma.

ā·noplasty. A plastic operation on the anus, to increase or decrease its size.

Anoplura. A sub-genus of the Hemiptera, *q.v.*

anor·chism (G. *an*, neg.; *orkhis*, a testicle). Absence of testicles.

ānorec·tal. Relating to the anus and the rectum.

anorec·tic, anorec·tous (G. *an*, neg.; *ŏrexis*, appetite). Without appetite.

anorex·ia. (G. *an*, neg.; *orexis*, appetite). Absence of appetite. A. nervosa: a neurotic affection, occurring mostly in young females, characterized by extreme aversion from food with corresponding loss of body-weight, cessation of menstruation and some loss of hair.

anorganic (G. *an*, neg.; *organon*, bodily organ). Not organic; derived from inanimate, mineral substances. A. chemistry: the chemistry of elements and their compounds with the exception of the compounds of carbon.

anorthō·pia (G. *an*, neg.; *orthos*, straight; *opsis*, vision). Distorted vision in which straight lines appear to be curved.

anor·thoscope (G. *an*, neg.; *orthos*, straight; *skopein*, to view). An instrument for combining two different objects or images into one visual image.

anorthō·sis (G. *an*, neg.; *orthōsis*, a making straight). Absence or defect of erectility.

ā·noscope (L. *anus*, anus; G. *skopein*, to view). Instrument for examining visually the rectum.

anos·mia (G. *an*, neg.; *osmē*, smell). Absence of the sense of smell.

anosodiaphor·ia (G. *a*, neg.; *nosos*, disease; *diaphora*, difference). A state of mind in which the patient is indifferent to his sickness.

anosognō·sia (G. *a*, neg.; *nŏsos*, disease; *gnōsis*, knowledge). A state of mind in which the patient has lost power to realize that he has any illness or defect.

anosphrā·sia (G. *an*, neg.; *osphrēsis*, smell). Absence of the sense of smell.

ānospī·nal. Relating to the anus and spine.

anosteoplă·sia (G. *an*, neg.; *osteon*, bone; *plăsis*, conformation). Defective formation of bone.

anō·tia (G. *an*, neg.; *ous*, ear). Congenital absence of the ears.

anotrŏ·pia (G. *anō*, upward; *trŏpē*, a turn). The same as hyperphoria, *q.v.*

anō·tus. A monster foetus having no ears.

anō·varism (G. *an*, neg.; L. *ovum*, egg). Congenital absence of the ovaries.

ānovēsi·cal (L. *anus*; *vēsica*, bladder). Relating to the anus and bladder.

anovulā·tion. Cessation of ovulation.

anoxāē·mia (G. *an*, neg.; *oxus*, keen; *haima*, blood). Deficiency of oxygen in the blood. **A., anaemic:** reduction in the volume of oxygen that can be furnished to the tissues by the blood, owing to deficiency of haemoglobin in anaemia or to presence of altered haemoglobin as in nitrite poisoning; or to displacement of O_2 by CO in carbon monoxide poisoning. **A., anoxic:** reduction in oxygen tension in the arterial blood, owing to 1. Reduced O_2 tension in inspired air. 2. Shallow respiration. 3. Inability of the lungs to take up O_2. **A., histotoxic:** a. due to disturbance of cellular capacity to utilize oxygen. **A., stagnant:** a. due to impeded circulation of the blood.

anox·ia (G. *an*, neg.; *oxus*, keen). Lack of oxygen.

anoxybiō·sis (G. *an*, neg.; *oxus*, keen; *bios*, life). Life without oxygen. The same as anaerobiosis.

an·sa (L.). A loop. **A. hypoglossi:** a loop formed by the descending ramus of the hypoglossal nerve. **A. lenticularis:** a bundle of nerve fibres passing from the optic thalamus to the globus pallidus. **A. peduncularis:** a bundle of nerve fibres passing from the optic thalamus to the insula and the temporal cortex.

an·serine (L. *anserinus*, from *anser*, goose). Silly; pertaining to or of the nature of a goose.

an·siform (L. *ansa*, loop; *forma*, shape). Loop-shaped.

Anstie's rule (Anstie, F. E., British physician, 1833–1874). A rule used in examination of patients for life insurance. The amount of absolute alcohol which can be taken daily without injury is 1½ ounces, i.e. about 3 oz. of whisky, brandy, etc., 4 glasses of sherry or port and 1 pint of champagne or light wine. **A.'s test:** a test for the presence of alcohol in blood, using potassium dichromate dissolved in concentrated sulphuric acid.

antā·cid (G. *anti*, against; L. *acidus*, acid). A substance binding or neutralizing an acid.

antă·gonism (G. *antagōnistēs*, an opponent). Opposition, contrariness.

antă·gonist. 1. An organ (e.g., a muscle, nerve or endocrine gland) that acts in opposition to another. 2. A drug neutralizing the effects of another.

antăl·kaline (G. *anti*, against; Arab. *al qalīy*, alkali). An agent that acts against alkalinity.

antaphrodĭ·siac (G. *anti*, against; *aphrodisia*, adjective formed from *Aphroditē* (Venus)). Lessening sexual desire.

ante (L.). Before.

ante cibum (L. *ante*, before; *cibus*, food). Before a meal.

antecū·bital. In front of the cubitus, or forearm.

antefeb·rile (L. *ante*, before; *febris*, fever). The period before a fever.

anteflect (L. *ante*, before; *flectere*, to bend). To bend forward.

anteflexion. A bending forward. **A, uterine:** normal position of the uterus in which the body of the uterus is bent forward.

antehypŏ·physis. The anterior lobe of the pituitary body, or hypophysis.

ante mortem (L.). Before death.

antenā·tal (L. *ante*, before; *natus*, birth). Before birth.

anten·na (L.). Feeler seen in pairs on the heads of arthropods.

ante partum (L. *ante*, before; *partus*, birth). Before delivery.

anteprandial (L.). Before the mid-day meal.

antēr·ior (L.). Before; in front of; relating to the ventral aspect of the body. **A. lobe:** the glandular part of the pituitary body. **A. rotation:** forward turning of the presenting part in labour.

antero- (L.). A prefix signifying before, or in advance of.

anterodor·sal (L. *anterior*, before; *dorsum*). Relating to the ventral aspect of the dorsum.

antero-external (L. *anterior*, before; *externus*, external). Relating to the front of the outer side.

an·terograde (L. *anterior*, before; *gradus*, a step). Extending forwards.

antero-inferior (L. *anterior*, before; *inferior*). Situated in front and below.

antero-interior (L. *anterior*, before; *interior*). Situated ventrally and internally.

antero-internal. In front and to the inner side.

an·tero-lă·teral (L. *anterior*, before; *latus*, side). In front and to one side.

anteromē·dian (L. *anterior*, before; *medius*, middle). In front and towards the middle.

an·teropostē·rior (L. *anterior*, before; *posterior*, rear). From before backward.

anterosupē·rior (L. *anterior*, before; *superior*). In front and above.

anterotā·tion (L. *ante*, before; *rotare*, revolve). A rotation forward.

antever·sion (L. *ante*, before; *vertere*, to turn). A turning or bending forward. **A. uteri:** normal position of the uterus in which the uterus is tilted forward. Hence **anteverted**, tipped forward.

an·thelix (G. *anthelix*, the interior curvature of the ear). The ridge surrounding the concha of the external ear posteriorly.

anthelmin·tic (G. *anti*, against; *helmins*, a worm). Remedy expelling or killing worms.

an·thema (G.). A rash.

Anthemis. A genus of flowering plants. **A. nobilis**, the common camomile.

anthiŏ·maline. Lithium antimony thiomalate. Used in the treatment of lymphogranuloma inguinale, schistosomiasis and leishmaniasis.

Anthyomyia canicularis. Small, black fly, of which the larvae are sometimes found in human intestines.

anthophō·bia (G. *anthos*, flower; *phobos*, fear). A morbid fear of flowers.

anthoris·ma (G. *anti*, against; *horisma*, boundary). A diffuse type of swelling.

an·thracene (G. *anthrax*, coal). A colourless, crystalline, polynuclear hydrocarbon, obtained from coal tar and used in the manufacture of certain dyes.

anthrā·cia (G. *anthrax*, carbuncle). An unhealthy state characterized by the presence of carbuncles.

an·thracoid (G. *anthrax*; *eidos*, form). Resembling anthrax.

anthracŏ·meter (G. *anthrax*, coal; *metron*, measure). An instrument for measuring the quantity of carbon dioxide in air.

an·thracosilicō·sis (G. *anthrax*, coal; L. *silex*, stone). See silicosis.

anthracŏ·sis (G. *anthrax*, coal). Carbon deposits in lungs, seen in city dwellers, especially in coal miners.

anthracot·ic. Relating to or affected with anthracosis.

anthraquinone (G. *anthrax*, coal; Peruv. *kina*). Oxidation product of the hydrocarbon compound anthracene. A number of drugs inducing peristalsis of the colon are derived from it.

an·thrax (G. *anthrax*, carbuncle). An acute infectious disease produced by the *Bacillus anthracis*. There are two main forms of the disease: **Skin a.** and **Pulmonary a.** Syn. wool-sorter's disease and malignant pustule.

an·thropobīo·logy (G. *anthrōpos*, man; *bios*, life; *logos*, discourse). Biological study of man and the anthropoid apes.

anthropogĕn·esis (G. *anthrōpos*, man; *gennan*, to produce). The evolution of man.

an·thropoid (G. *anthrōpos*, man; *eidos*, form). Man-like.

anthropŏ·logy (G. *anthrōpos*, man; *logos*, discourse). The science of man, or of the natural history of mankind.

anthropŏ·metry (G. *anthrōpos*, man; *metron*, measure). Measurement of the human body.

anthropomor·phic (G. *anthrōpos*, man; *morphē*, form). Pertaining to anthropomorphism.

anthropomor·phism (G. *anthrōpos*, man; *morphē*, form). Ascription of human characteristics to any non-human species or object.

anthropŏ·pathy (G. *anthrōpos*, man; *pathos*, emotion). The attribution to non-human subjects of human emotions.

anthropŏ·phagy (G. *anthrōpos*, man; *phagein*, to eat). Cannibalism.

anthropophō·bia (G. *anthrōpos*, man; *phobos*, fear). Fear of society; a form of neurosis.

anthropophu·ism (G. *anthrōpos*, man; *phuē*, nature). The ascription of human attributes to the gods.

anthropŏ·sophist (G. *anthrōpos*, man; *sophistēs*, a sage). One who possesses the wisdom of men.

anthropŏ·sophy (G. *anthrōpos*, man; *sophia*, wisdom). Knowledge of the nature of man.

anthropŏ·tomy (G. *anthrōpos*, man; *tomē*, section). Human anatomy.

anti- (G.). A prefix signifying against.

anti-abortus. An agent destructive to the *Brucella abortus.*

anti-agglutinin (G. *anti*, against; L. *glutinare*, to glue). An antibody neutralizing the corresponding agglutinin.

anti-aggressin (G. *anti*, against; L. *aggrediri*, to attack). An antibody neutralizing the corresponding aggressin.

anti-albumide. A product, parapeptone, of imperfect digestion of albumin.

anti-amboceptor (G. *anti*, against; L. *ambo*, both; *capere*, to take). A substance inhibiting the action of an amboceptor.

anti-anaphylax·is (G. *anti*, against; *ana*, upon; *phulax*, a guard). Insusceptibility to anaphylaxis, occurring probably when an excess of antibodies is present in the circulatory blood, preventing the antigen from reaching the cells. Syn. desensitization.

anti-antidote. A substance acting against an antidote.

antibactēr·ial (G. *anti*, against; *baktērion*, dim. of *baktron*, a stick). Acting against bacteria.

antibiō·sis (G. *anti*, against; *bios*, life). An association between two or more organisms which is injurious to one of them.

antibiŏ·tic (G. *anti*, against; *bios*, life). 1. Tending to destroy life. 2. Substance derived from living micro-organisms, especially fungi, which will destroy or inhibit the growth of other micro-organisms.

antibody. Specific constituent of the body-fluids which may be present normally (state of 'natural' immunity) or which may be developed by inoculation of antigens, such as antitoxins. Syn. immune body.

antibrā·chium (G. *anti*, against; *brakhiōn*, arm). The forearm.

antibrō·mic (G. *anti*, against; *brōmos*, a smell). Deodorant.

anticachec·tic (G. *anti*, against; *kakhexia*, from *kakos*, bad; *hexis*, condition). An agent preventing cachexia.

anticanit·ic (G. *anti*, against; L. *canities*, greyness). Acting against the greying of hair.

anticar·dium (G. *anti*, against; *kardia*, heart). The pit of the stomach.

anticatarrh·al. Relieving catarrh.

anti·cipate (L. *ante*, before; *capere*, to take). To occur before the expected time.

anticoă·gulant. A substance preventing the coagulation of blood.

anticom·plement (G. *anti*, against; L. *complementum*, complement). An antibody checking the action of a complement, *q.v.*

anticri·sis. Any circumstance which prevents the occurrence of a crisis.

anti·cus (L.). Anterior; in front of.

an·tidote (G. *anti*, against; *dotos*, granted). An agent preventing or counteracting the action of a poison. **Chemical a.:** an a. changing the chemical nature of a poison, rendering it harmless. **Mechanical a.:** an a. preventing absorption of a poison by making the body tissues impervious to it or by holding the poison in suspension. **Physiological a.:** a substance possessing properties antagonistic to the corresponding poison.

antidrōm·ic (G. *anti*, against; *drŏmos*, racecourse). Pertaining to impulses passing in the opposite direction to the normal.

anti-enzyme (G. *anti*, against; *en*, in; *zumē*, a leaven). A substance inhibiting the action of an enzyme.

anti-epileptic. Remedy counteracting epilepsy.

anti-epithē·lial. An agent destructive to epithelial cells.

antifĕ·brile (G. *anti*, against; L. *febris*, fever). Diminishing fever.

Antifeb·rin. Syn. for acetanilide.

antifer·ment (G. *anti*, against; L. *fermentum*, a ferment). 1. An agent preventing fermentation. 2. An anti-enzyme.

antiformin. A preparation containing in equal parts a 7·5 per cent solution of sodium or potassium hypochlorite and of sodium hydrate. It has powerful solvent action on certain organic substances and is used for rendering tubercle bacilli more easily visible in sputum-preparations.

antigalac·tic (G. *anti*, against; *gala*, milk). An agent inhibiting the secretion of milk.

an·tigen (G. *anti*, against; *gennan*, to form). Any substance which after inoculation into the body is capable of giving rise to antibodies in the animal body and thus inducing immunity.

antigenothē·rapy (G. *anti*, against; *gennan*, to produce; *therapeia*, treatment). The treatment of diseases by the injection of antigens to promote the formation in the body of antibodies.

antihaemŏ·lysin (G. *anti*, against; *haima*, blood; *luein*, to loosen). A substance produced in the blood serum by the injection of haemolysins.

antihaemorrhā·gic. Stopping haemorrhage.

antihor·mone (G. *anti*, against; *hormē*, an onset). An antibody inhibiting the activity of a hormone, produced in response to injection of that hormone.

anti-icter·ic. An agent which relieves jaundice.

antihĭ·stamine. Substance counteracting the liberation of histamine in the tissues. Some of the principal antihistamine drugs are Antergen, Neoantergen, now usually called Anthisan, Benadryl and its derivatives, Dramamine and Phenergan.

antiketogĕ·nesis (G. *anti*, against; L. *acetum*, vinegar; G. *gennan*, to form). Prevention of formation of acetone-bodies; reduction in the number of acetone-bodies.

antiketogenet·ic, antiketogen·ic. Inhibiting formation of acetone-bodies.

antilethar·gic (G. *anti*, against; *lethargia*, drowsiness). Preventing sleep.

antilī·poid. An antibody capable of reacting with a lipoid.

antilō·bium (G. *anti*, against; *lŏbus*, lobe). The tragus of the ear.

antilȳ·sin (G. *anti*, against; *luein*, loosen). An antibody opposing the activity of a lysin.

antilys·sic (G. *anti*, against; *lussa*, rabies). Acting against hydrophobia.

antimalā·rial. Preventing malaria.

an·timere (G. *anti*, against; *meros*, a part). 1. Any segment of the body bounded by planes at right angles to the long axis of the body. 2. One of the symmetrical parts of a bilateral organism.

antimetrō·pia (G. *anti*, against; *metron*, measure; *ops*, eye). Hypermetropia in one eye accompanied by myopia in the other.

antimicrō·bic. Acting against the growth of microbes.

anti·mony (L. *antimonium*). A metallic element with a bluish-white lustre. It has been used extensively in the past, notably by Paracelsus and his followers, and has now again come into use in modern medicine in the treatment of certain protozoic tropical diseases. Symbol Sb.

antimony and potassium tartrate. KOOC.CHOH. CHOH.COO(SbO), $\frac{1}{2}$ H$_2$O. Syn. tartar emetic.

antimycot·ic (G. *anti*, against; *mukēs*, mushroom). Destructive to fungi.

antimydriăt·ic (G. *anti*, against; *mudriasis*, an undue enlargement of the pupil). Pertaining to a drug acting against mydriasis.

antinarcot·ic (G. *anti*, against; *narkoein*, to benumb). Preventing narcotism.

antinephrit·ic (G. *anti*, against; *nephros*, kidney). Any agent useful in the treatment of kidney diseases.

antineural·gic. An agent that abates neuralgia.

anti·nion (G. *anti*, against; *inion*, occiput). The frontal pole of the cranium.

anti-op·sonin (G. *anti*, against; *opsōnion*, provisions). A substance opposing the action of an opsonin.

antiō·tomy (G. *antiotomia*). Surgical removal of the tonsils.

antiparalyt·ic. An agent which relieves the condition of paralysis.

antiparasit·ic. Destructive to parasites.

anti·pathy (G. *anti*, against; *pathos*, affection). A feeling of aversion; a quality of opposition.

antipellagra factor (G. *anti*, against; *pella*, skin; *agra*, seizure; L. *factor*, from *facere*). Vitamin B$_6$, see under vitamin.

antiperistal·sis (G. *anti*, against; *peristellein*, to wrap up). Reversed peristalsis, occurs in some cases of intestinal obstruction.

antiphlogis·tic (G. *anti*, against; *phlox*, a flame). Counteracting fever or inflammation.

Antiphlogistine. A proprietary cataplasm used in the treatment of inflammation and congestion.

antiphthis·ic. An agent relieving phthisis.

antiplas·tic (G. *anti*, against; *plassein*, to form). An agent unfavourable to the healing process.

antipneumocŏc·cal (G. *anti*, against; *pneumōn*, from *pnein*, to breathe; *kokkos*, a seed). Acting against pneumonia. **A. serum:** serum containing antibodies against pneumococci.

antiprō·teāse. A substance possessed by bacteria which hinders proteolytic action.

antiprothrom·bin (G. *anti*, against; *pro*, before; *thrombōsis*, a clot). A substance such as heparin, *q.v.*, holding prothrombin in combination and inhibiting thereby its combination with calcium.

antiprotozō·al. Destructive to protozoa.

antiprurit·ic (G. *anti*, against; L. *pruritus*, an itching). Relieving itching.

antipȳ·ic (G. *anti*, against; *puon*, pus). Preventing suppuration.

antipyogen·ic (G. *anti*, against; *puon*, pus; *gennan*, to form). Preventing the formation of pus.

an·tipyrē·sis (G. *anti*, against; *puretos*, fever). The use of antipyretics.

antipyret·ic (G. *anti*, against; *puretos*, fever). 1. Reducing temperature. 2. A febrifuge.

antipyrot·ic (G. *anti*, against; *purōsis*, a burning). An agent that is effective in the treatment of burns.

antirachĭt·ic (G. *anti*, against; *rakhitis*, rickets). Curative and preventive of rickets.

anti-Rh. See under Rh. factor.

antirheumat·ic. Relieving rheumatism.

Antirrhī·num. A genus of scrophulariaceous plants, which has homeopathic uses as a purgative and diuretic.

antiscarlatī·nal. Counteracting scarlet fever.

antiscorbū·tic (G. *anti*, against; L.L. *scorbutus*, scurvy). Acting against scurvy.

antisep·sis (G. *anti*, against; *sēpsis*, putrefaction). Prevention of sepsis by means of chemical substances (such as phenols, dyestuffs, antibiotics) which destroy or inhibit multiplication of pathogenic micro-organisms.

antisep·tic (G. *anti*, against; *sēpsis*, putrefaction). Destroying, or inhibiting the growth of, micro-organisms.

antisē·rum (G. *anti*, against; L. *serum*). Serum containing specific antibodies. Syn. immune serum.

antisiā·lic (G. *anti*, against; *sialon*, saliva). Checking the flow of saliva.

antisō·cial. Against the principles governing society.

antisō·cialism. The manifestation of antisocial characteristics in psychopathic personalities.

antispasmod·ic (G. *anti*, against; *spasmos*, spasm). Relieving spasm.

antispas·tic (G. *anti*, against; *spasmos*, spasm). 1. Antispasmodic. 2. Revulsive. 3. Counter-irritant.

antispirochāe·tal (G. *anti*, against; *speira*, coil; *khaitē*, hair). Effective against spirochaetes.

antistal·sis (G. *anti*, against; *stalsis*, from *stellein*, to repress). A reverse or backward movement of the contents of the bowels.

antistaphylococ·cal Effective against staphylococci.

antisteri·lity. Effective against sterility.

antistreptococ·cal. Effective against streptococci.

antisudor·al, antisudorif·ic (G. *anti*, against; L. *sudor* sweat). Diminishing perspiration.

antisyphilit·ic. Effective against syphilis.

antitabet·ic. Effective against tabes dorsalis.

antitetan·ic. Effective against tetanus.

anti·thĕnar (G. *anti*, against; *thĕnar*, palm or sole). Situated opposite to the palm or sole. See also hypothenar.

antither·mic (G. *anti*, against; *thermē*, heat). Cooling, antipyretic.

antithrom·bin (G. *anti*, against; *thrombos*, clot). 1. A substance neutralizing formed thrombin and preventing its action. 2. A substance inhibiting the formation of thrombin from its precursors.

antiton·ic. Diminishing tonicity.

antithȳ·roid. Effective against thyroid influences.

Antithyroidin 'Moebius'. Thyroidectomized sheep's serum, once used in the treatment of exophthalmic goitre.

antitox·ic (G. *anti*, against; *toxikon*, poison). 1. Counteracting poisons; antidotal. 2. Acting against a toxin. **A. serum:** a serum containing antitoxin.

antitox·igen (G. *anti*, against; *toxikon*, poison; *gennan*, to form). Any preparation or substance capable of forming an antitoxin in the body.

antitox·in (G. *anti*, against; *toxikon*, poison). A specific antibody produced in response to a toxin, capable of neutralizing that particular toxin.

antitoxinum. Latinized form of antitoxin.

anti·trăgus (G. *anti*, against; *trăgos*, goat). The process of the external ear opposite the tragus.

antitris·mus (G. *anti*, against; *trismos*, (1) a scream; (2) grinding of the teeth). A spasm which prevents the mouth from closing.

an·titrope (G. *anti*, against; *trepein*, to turn). The same as antimere (2).

antitryp·sia (G. *anti*, against; *tripsis*, friction). A substance inhibiting the action of trypsin.

antituber·culin. An antibody formed when tuberculin is injected into the system.

antity̆·phoid. Effective against typhoid.

antivaccina·tion. Opposed to the practice of vaccination.

antivĕ·nene, antivĕ·nin (G. *anti*, against; L. *venenum*, venom). Immune serum containing antibodies against snake poison.

antivi·ral. Effective against a virus.

antivivisec·tion (G. *anti*, against; L. *vivus*, living; *secare*, to cut). Opposed to experiments on living animals.

antizymot·ic (G. *anti*, against; *zumē*, leaven). Preventing any infectious disease.

antopognŏ·sia (G. *an*, neg.; *topos*, a place; *gnōsis*, knowledge). Inability of a patient to recognize the relationships of his own body.

an·tral (L. *antrum*, cavity). Relating or pertaining to an antrum.

antrec·tomy (L. *antrum*; G. *ektōmē*, excision). Excision of the walls of an antrum, especially the mastoid antrum.

antri·tis. Inflammation of the antrum.

antro-attico·tomy. The operation of opening the mastoid antrum and the attic of the tympanum.

an·trocele (L. *antrum*, cavity; G. *kēlē*, tumour). Accumulation of fluid in the maxillary antrum.

antrody̆·nia (L. *antrum*, cavity; G. *odunē*, pain). Any antral pain.

antronā·sal. Relating to the antrum and the nose.

an·troscope (L. *antrum*; G. *skopein*, to view). Instrument for visual examination of the mastoid antrum.

antrŏ·stomy (L. *antrum*; G. *stoma*, mouth). The operation of making an opening into the antrum of Highmore for drainage purposes.

an·trotome (L. *antrum*; G. *tomē*, a cutting). Instrument for opening up the mastoid antrum.

antrŏ·tomy (L. *antrum*; G. *tomē*, a cutting). Incision of an antrum, especially the surgical opening of the mastoid antrum (Schwartze's operation).

antrotympan·ic (L. *antrum*; G. *tumpanon*, a drum). Relating to the antrum and tympanic cavity.

antrotympani·tis (L. *antrum*; G. *tumpanon*, a drum). Inflammation of the mastoid antrum and the middle ear.

an·trum (L.). 1. A cavity, especially in bone, e.g., the mastoid a. or the antrum Highmori in the maxillary bone. 2. The prepyloric portion of the stomach.

anu·clear (G. *a*, neg.; L. *nucleus*, kernal). Without nuclei.

anurĕ·sis (G. *an*, neg.; *ouron*, urine). The same as anuria, *q.v.*

anuret·ic (G. *an*, neg.; *ouron*, urine). Affected with anuria.

anū·ria (G. *an*, neg.; *ouron*, urine). Absence of urinary secretion.

anū·rous (G. *an*, neg.; *oura*, a tail). Having no tail.

ā·nus (L.) The rectal exit. **Artificial a.:** opening of the bowel to the exterior at a point above the normal anus. **A., imperforate:** the same as atresia ani, *q.v.*

an·vil. See under incus.

anxī·ety. A feeling of fear or uncertainty.

anxiety-neurŏ·sis. A form of neurosis in which fear or apprehension is the main force controlling the ideas and behaviour of the patient.

any̆p·nia (G. *an*, neg.; *hupnos*, sleep). Insomnia.

A.O. Abbreviation for anodal opening.

A.O.C. Abbreviation of anodal opening contraction.

āor·ta (G. *aortē*). The main arterial trunk, arising from the left cardiac ventricle. (See also under artery.)

āortal·gia (G. *aortē*; *algos*, pain). Any pain felt in the aorta.

āortarc·tia (G. *aortē*; L. *artare*, to constrict). Narrowing of the aorta.

āortectā·sis (G. *aortē*; *ektăsis*, extension). Dilation of the aorta.

āor·tic (G. *aortē*). Pertaining to the aorta. **A. murmur:** a pathological mumur due to abnormal condition of the a. valves. **A. plexus:** the plexus of sympathetic nerves lying in front and on the sides of the aorta between the origins of the superior and inferior mesenteric arteries. **A. regurgitation (or A. insufficiency):** insufficient closure of the a. ostium, leading to regurgitation of blood from the aorta into the left cardiac ventricle. **A. sounds:** the heart sounds that can be normally heard over the second right intercostal space close to the sternal margin. **A. stenosis:** abnormal narrowing of the a. ostium, impeding thereby the passage of blood from the left ventricle into the aorta.

āorti·tis. Inflammation of the aorta.

āortoclā·sia (G. *aortē*; *klaein*, to break). Rupture of the aorta.

āor·tolith (G. *aortē; lithos*, a stone). An aortic calculus.

āortoclerō·sis (G. *aortē*; *skleros*, hard). Sclerosis of the aorta.

āortostenō·sis (G. *aortē*; *stĕnos*, narrow). Abnormal narrowing of the aorta.

āortŏ·tomy (G. *aortē*; *tomē*, a cutting). Incision of the aorta.

āŏs·mic (G. *a*, neg.; *osmē*, odour). Without odour.

A.P. Abbreviation for artificial pneumothorax. See under pneumothorax.

apan·dria (G. *apo*, from; *anēr*, man). Morbid dislike of the male sex.

apan·thropy (G. *apo*, from; *anthrōpos*, man). A type of melancholy characterized by morbid dislike of human companionship.

aparĕū·nia (G. *a*, neg.; *para*, beside; *eunē*, a bed). Impossibility of coitus.

apathet·ic (G. *a*, neg.; *pathētikos*, sensitive). Indifferent.

ape hand. A hand with outward rotated thumb which has become flat with the palm, as occurring in progressive muscular atrophy and in amyotrophic lateral sclerosis.

apel·lous (G. *a*, neg.; *pella*, skin). 1. Having no skin. 2. Without a prepuce.

Apenta water. An aperient mineral water from Hungary.

apep·sia (G. *a*, neg.; *pepsis*, digestion). Failure of the power to digest food.

apĕ·rient (L. *aperire*, to open). Laxative; opening.

ā·peristăl·sis (G. *a*, neg.; *peristellein*, to compress). Cessation of peristalsis.

apĕ·ritive. Stimulating to the appetite.

apertŏ·meter (L. *aperire*, to open; G. *metron*, measure). Apparatus used to measure the aperture angles of microscopic objects.

Apert's syndrome (Apert, E., French paediatrician, 1868–1940). See acrocephalosyndactylia.

apertū·ra (L. *apertura*, from *aperire* to open). An opening, e.g., **A. spinalis:** the vertebral foramen.

aperture. An opening or orifice.

ā·pex (L.). The summit or extremity of anything. **A. beat:** the impulse of the heart that can be felt or seen at a circumscribed area of the chest wall during systole.

aphă·gia (G. *a*, neg.; *phagein*, to eat). Inability to swallow.

apha·kia (G. *a*, neg.; *phăkos*, lentil). Absence of the crystalline lens of the eye.

apha·kic. Without a crystalline lens.

aphalan·gia (G. *a*, neg.; *phalagx*, finger). Congenital absence of fingers or toes.

aphă·nisis (G. disappearance). Morbid fear of losing sexual capabilities.

Aphanocap·sa, Aphanocap·ta. A genus of Schizomycetes.

Aphanozoa (G. *aphănēs*, invisible; *zŏŏn*, an animal). Ultramicroscopic organisms.

aphā·sia (G. *a*, neg.; *phăsis*, a saying). Partial or complete inability to speak in articulated manner and/or comprehend spoken words; differently interpreted by different authors, e.g., as disorder of symbolic formulation and expression (Head) or as disorder of a basal mental function to grasp the specific nature of a process or to differentiate a 'figure' from the surrounding 'ground' (Goldstein). Classified into Motor (cortical, subcortical, transcortical); Sensory (cortical, subcortical) and Conduction or Central a., or (Head) into Verbal, Syntactical, Nominal and Semantic a. **A., amnesic:** difficulty in finding words as names when words and phrases in certain uses can be evoked more easily; thought to be due to a diffuse cerebral lesion or to a focal lesion between temporal and frontal lobes. **A., central:** severe disturbance in speaking, repeating and reading with relatively slight limitations in understanding words; assumed to be due to a lesion between motor and sensory speech areas involving the island of Reil and the neighbouring parts of the temporal lobe, central convolutions and frontal lobe. **A., conduction:** same as A., central. **A., cortical motor:** a. predominantly characterized by difficulty in articulation, producing retarded scanty speech, usually associated with defects in writing and understanding and other processes not directly concerned with production of speech; due to a lesion in Broca's area (*q.v.*) of the left cerebral hemisphere. **A., cortical sensory:** a. characterized by difficulty in understanding of speech and written words, usually associated with paraphrasia, paragrammation, perseveration and/or defects of other mental processes; due to a lesion of the posterior part of the first temporal convolution and neighbouring parts of Henschl's convolution, the parietal lobe and the posterior part of the island of Reil. Syn. Wernicke's a.; true a. **A., expressive:** motor aphasia. **A., jargon:** severe literal paraphasia. **A., musical:** amusia, motor, *q.v.* **A., nominal:** disturbance in the use of words as names and of appreciating the nominal significance of words. **A., receptive:** sensory a. **A., semantic:** inability to recognize the ultimate significance and intention of words and phrases apart from their direct meaning, with loss of power to appreciate or to formulate the logical conclusion of thoughts or actions. **A., subcortical motor:** a. characterized by defect in use of lip, tongue and larynx muscles for production of speech (only), assumed to be due to a lesion cutting off Broca's area from deeper centres. Syn. pure motor a.; word-muteness; anarthria. **A., subcortical sensory:** a. characterized by difficulty in understanding speech or written words, assumed to be due to a lesion of an area below the middle part of the first temporal convolution. Syn. pure sensory a. See also alexia, word-blindness, word-deafness. **A., syntactical:** a. characterized by rapid speech, dropping of smaller words (articles, conjunctions, etc.) and lack of that perfect balance and rhythm necessary to make sounds uttered by the speaker easily understandable to the auditor; assumed to be due to a lesion in the upper convolution of the temporal lobe. **A., transcortical motor:** a. characterized by difficulty in spontaneous speech; sometimes a phase in recovery from cortical motor a., or possibly due to a minor lesion of the speech area. **A., verbal:** a. characterized by disturbance of power to form words in speech and writing, whether for 'external' or 'internal' use, without gross defect in understanding; assumed to be due to a lesion in the lower portion of the precentral and post-central convolution.

aphē·mia (G. *a*, neg.; *phēmē*, voice). Motor aphasia.

aphephō·bia (G. *haphē*, touch; *phobos*, fear). A morbid dread of being touched.

Aphiochǣ·ta ferrugĭ·nia. A genus of fly, found in India, which causes cutaneous myiasis in human beings.

aphō·nia (G. *a*, neg.; *phōnē*, a sound). Inability to speak, due to defect in the vocal apparatus; voicelessness.

aphō·nic. Characterized by aphonia.

aphonogĕ·lia (G. *a*, neg.; *phōnē*, a sound; *gĕlōs*, laughter). Inability to laugh aloud.

aphorē·sis (G. *a*, neg.; *phŏrein*, to bear). Inability to support pain.

aphosphorō·sis. A condition arising from deficiency of phosphorus.

aphrā·sia (G. *a*, neg.; *phrazein*, to tell). Inability to speak in connected phrases.

aphrodi·sia (G. *Aphroditē* (Venus)). Sexual desire.

aphrodi·siac. Stimulating or arousing sexual desire.

aphrodi·siomā·nia. Excessive sexual interest.

aphronē·sia (G. *a*, neg.; *phrŏnēsis*, prudence). Mental derangement; lunacy.

aphrŏ·nia (G. *a*, neg.; *phrŏnein*, to think). Defective mental powers.

aph·tha (G.). Stomatitis, with small white vesicles in the mouth, especially in children. Syn. aphthous stomatitis, thrush.

aphthae (Pl. of *aphtha*). **A., tropical:** tropical sprue.

aphthon·gia (G. *a*, neg.; *phthoggos*, sound). Aphasia caused by spasm of the muscles innervated by the hypoglossal and facial nerves.

aph·thous. Pertaining to aphthae.

ā·pical (L. *apex*). Relating to the apex. **A. murmur:** an abnormal sound heard over the apex of the heart.

apicec·tomy, apico·ectomy (L. *apex*; G. *ektomē*, excision). Excision of the apex or root-end of a tooth.

apicŏ·lysis (L. *apex*; G. *luein*, loosen). Pneumonolysis, *q.v.*, performed at the apical portion of the lung.

apilocā·tor (L. *apex*; *locus*, a place). Instrument for locating the apex of the root of a tooth.

Apiol. A volatile oil obtained by alcoholic extraction from the fruit of the common parsley. Has been used in cases of primary amenorrhoea and also in dysmenorrhoea.

ā·piother·apy (L. *apis*, bee; G. *therapeia*, treatment). Treatment of certain conditions, e.g., rheumatism, by means of bee stings.

apiphō·bia (L. *apis*, bee; G. *phobos*, fear). Morbid fear of bees.

Apis mellifica (L.). The honey bee.

Apium. A genus of umbelliferous plants, which includes celery and parsley.

aplacen·tal (G. *a*, neg.; L. *placenta*). Without a placenta.

aplana·sia (G. *a*, neg.; *plănān*, to wander). Entire or almost entire absence of spherical aberration.

aplanat·ic (G. *a*, neg.; *plănān*, to wander). Without spherical aberration; rectilinear.

aplā·sia (G. *a*, neg.; *plassein*, to form). Failure of an organ or tissue to develop. Syn. agenesis.

aplas·tic (G. *a*, neg.; *plassein*, to form). Structureless; formless. **A. Anaemia:** see anaemia.

Aplectana. A genus of parasitic nematodes.

apleu·ria (G. *a*, neg.; *pleura*, rib). Absence of ribs.

apnoe·a (G. *a*, neg.; *pnein*, to breathe). 1. Absence of respiration, e.g., in the foetus. 2. A transient cessation of respiration. 3. Asphyxia.

ap·neumato·sis (G. *a*, neg.; *pneumatosis*, inflation). Collapse of lung air cells.

apneu·mia (G. *a*, neg.; *pneumōn*, lung). Congenital absence of the lungs.

apobio·sis (G. *apo*, away; *bios*, life). Death of the physiological body.

apocamno·sis (G. *apokamnein*, to grow weary). Great fatigue.

apochromat·ic (G. *apo*, away; *khrōma*, colour). Free from chromatic and spherical aberration. A. lens: a lens in which rays of three or more colours are brought to the same focus.

ă·pocrine (G. *apo*, away; *krinein*, to separate). Denoting a form of sweat glands in which a portion of the cytoplasm leaves the cell together with the product of secretion; found mainly in axillary and pubic regions.

apo·dia (G. *a*, neg.; *pous*, foot). Congenital absence of the feet.

ă·pogee (G. *apogeios*, far from land). The climax or point of greatest severity in a disease.

apo·lar (G. *a*, neg.; *pŏlos*, pole (of an axis)). 1. Without a pole. 2. Applied to the ganglion cells lacking nerve processes.

Apollinaris water. Effervescent table waters from Remagen in Germany.

Apollonia. The patron saint of dentistry, martyred in A.D. 249.

apomorphine. A crystalline alkaloid derived from morphine, used as an emetic.

apomye·lin (G. *apo*, away; *mŭelos*, marrow). A substance derived from brain tissue.

aponeuro·sis (G. *apo*, away; *neuron*, tendon). A fibrous membranous expansion of a tendon giving attachment to or enclosing muscles.

aponeurosi·tis. Inflammation of an aponeurosis.

aponeurot·ic (G. *apo*, away; *neuron*, tendon). Pertaining to an aponeurosis.

apŏ·nia (G.). Absence of pain.

apon·ic. Relieving pain.

apophlegmat·ic (G. *apophlegmatizein*, to discharge phlegm). Expectorant.

apophylax·is (G. *apo*, away; *phylaxis*). Diminution of the blood's phylactic capabilities.

apophy·seal, apophy·sial (G. *apo*, away; *phusis*, growth). Relating to an apophysis.

apo·physis (G. *apo*, away; *phusis*, growth). A bony protuberance which was never during its development separated from the bone by cartilage.

apophysi·tis (G. *apo*, away; *phusis*, growth). Inflammation of an apophysis.

apoplec·tic (G. *apoplessein*, to disable). Pertaining to or affected with apoplexy.

apoplec·tiform. Resembling apoplexy.

apoplex·y (G. *apoplessein*, to disable). Sudden loss of cerebral function due to haemorrhage or thrombosis of a cerebral vessel. Term was formerly also used in regard to haemorrhages in other parts of the body.

Apoquinamine. $C_{19}H_{22}N_2O$, an alkaloid obtained from quinamine.

apŏ·sia (G. *a*, neg.; *posis*, a drink). Absence of thirst.

aposi·tia (G. *apo*, away; *sĭtos*, food). Distaste of food.

apŏ·stasis (G.). 1. An abcess. 2. A bony exfoliation. 3. The crisis of a disease.

apostē·ma (G.). An abscess.

Apostoli's treatment (Apostoli, G., French physician, 1847–1900). A form of electrical treatment sometimes used in uterine disease, the anode being placed in the cervical canal and the cathode applied externally.

apothanā·sia (G. *apo*, away; *thănătos*, death). Prolonging life.

apothecaries' weight (G. *apothēkē*, a storehouse). A system of weights and measures used in compounding medicines. The standard weight is the troy pound of 5,760 gr.; 1 lb. = 12 oz.; 1 oz. = 8 dr.; 1 dr. = 3 scr.; 1 scruple = 20 gr. Apothecaries' fluid or wine measure (U.S.) 1 gallon = 8 pints; 1 pint = 16 fluid oz.; 1 fl. oz. = 8 fl. drams; 1 fl. dr. = 60 minims.

apŏ·thecary (G. *apothēkē*). A druggist; a preparer and seller of drugs.

apŏ·thesis (G. *apothesis*). The reduction of a fracture or dislocation.

apotrip·sis (G. *apotrĭbein*, to rub off). The removal of an opacity in the cornea.

apparā·tus (L. from *apparare*, to prepare). 1. A mechanical appliance or an instrument composed of several parts. 2. A group of parts acting together in the performance of some particular function. A., auditory: the external and internal ear, the tympanum and the auditory tube. A. lacrimalis: the lacrimal apparatus.

appen·dage (L. *appendere*). That which is attached to an organ as part of it, e.g., *caecal a.*, the appendix vermiformis.

appendec·tomy (L. *appendix*; G. *ektomē*, excision). Excision of the vermiform appendix.

appendici·tis. Inflammation of the vermiform appendix, characterized, when acute, by sudden onset of abdominal pain, especially in the right iliac fossa, fever, tachycardia, vomiting and tenderness in the right iliac fossa, especially over McBurney's point.

appendicŏ·stomy (L. *appendix*; G. *stoma*, a mouth). Artificial fistula of the appendix vermiformis made in order to irrigate the colon.

appendi·cular. Relating to the vermiform appendix.

appen·dix. An appendage or adjunct, e.g., appendix vermiformis, the worm-like a. of the caecum. Appendices epiploicae: fatty projections of the serous coat of the colon.

appen·dotome. An instrument employed for the removal of the appendix vermiformis.

appercep·tion (L. *ad*, to; *percipere*, perceive). The conscious reception of a sensory impression.

ap·petite (L. *appetere*, to long for). 1. Desire for food. 2. Any natural desire.

applanat·ic, applanā·tion. Flattening.

applanŏ·meter (L. *ad*, to; *planus*, flat; G. *metron*, measure). Instrument for determining the amount of pressure required to flatten a given area of the surface of the eye. Syn. applanation tonometer.

apple. The fruit of the *Pyrus malus*.

apple jelly nodule. A soft, brownish-red translucent nodule situated in the corium, the most characteristic sign of lupus vulgaris.

applicā·tor. An instrument for applying medicine to a part. Radium a.: a metal plaque containing radium salt used in the treatment of superficial growths of the skin.

apposi·tion. 1. The act of fitting together. 2. The state of being fitted together. 3. Accretion.

aprac·tic. Characterized by apraxia.

aprax·ia (G. *a*, neg.; *prassein*, to do). Inability to manipulate common objects and to execute planned movements in the absence of motor or sensory defects, usually due to a lesion in the Sylvian region of the brain. A., ideational, A., ideatry: form of a. characterized by inability to appreciate the purpose of a voluntary action, with confusion as to the spatio-temporal relations in the movement-sequence, usually due to a lesion in the parietal lobe. A., ideokinetic, A., ideo-motor: form of a. characterized by loss of conception of motion. A., limb-kinetic, A., motor: form of a. characterized by inability to combine action of several muscle groups necessary for the execution of a particular skilled act.

aproc·tia (G. *a*, neg.; *prōktos*, anus). Absence of the anus.

Aprokta. A genus of filaria organisms.

apron (Old Fr. *naperon*). 1. A cloth or rubber covering to prevent clothing from becoming soiled. 2. The omentum. **A., hottentot**: abnormally or artificially elongated labia minora, as common in Hottentot women.

aprosex·ia (G. *aprosexia*, want of attention). Inability to fix the attention.

aprosō·pia (G. *a*, neg.; *prosōpon*, face). Partial or complete absence of the face.

apsithy·ria (G. *a*, neg.; *psithurîzein*, whisper). Hysterical aphonia, with inability to whisper.

apsȳ·chia (G. *a*, neg.; *psukhe*, spirit). A faint.

apsychō·sis (G. *a*, neg.; *psukhe*, mind). Loss of the power of thought.

A.P.T. Abbreviation for alum precipitated toxoid, *q.v.*

aptȳ·alia, aptȳ·alism (G. *a*, neg.; *ptualon*, spittle). Lack of saliva.

ā·pus (G. *a*, neg.; *pous*, foot). A monster without lower limbs, or without feet.

apyknomor·phous (G. *a*, neg.; *puknos*, compact; *morphē*, form). Applied to a cell either not staining systematically, or else staining feebly.

apyret·ic (G. *a*, neg.; *puretos*, fever). Without fever.

apyrex·ia (G. *a*, neg.; *puretos*, fever). Absence of fever.

A.Q. Abbreviation for achievement quotient.

Aq. (L. *aqua*). Water.

Aq. astr. (L. *aqua astricta*). Frozen water.

Aq. bull. (L. *aqua bulliens*). Boiling water.

Aq. cal. (L. *aqua calida*). Hot water.

Aq. dest. (L. *aqua destillata*). Distilled water.

Aq. pur. (L. *aqua pura*). Pure water.

Aq. tep. (L. *aqua tepida*). Tepid water.

aqua (L.). Water.

aquae (L. *aqua*). In pharmacy, medicated waters, e.g., *Aqua amygdalarum amararum*, bitter almond water.

ā·quapuncture (L. *aqua*, water; *punctura*, puncture). Perforation of the skin by water jets.

ā·queduct, aquaeduc·tus (L. *aqua*, water; *ductus*, from *ducere*, to lead). A canal. **A. Sylvii**: canal situated in the midbrain, leading from third to fourth ventricle.

aqueous. Watery; e.g., **a humour**, the fluid in the anterior chamber of the eye.

aquula externa (L.). The perilymph in the inner ear. **a. interna**, the endolymph.

arabin. Syn. for arabic acid, a carbohydrate derived from gum arabic.

arā·binose (G. *araps*, an Arab). A pentose, occurring as D-Arabinose in some bacteria and as L-Arabinose in various polysaccharides.

arabinosū·ria (G. *araps*, an Arab; *ouron*, urine). The presence of arabinose in the urine.

Arachis. The peanut.

arachnephō·bia (G. *arakhnē*, spider; *phobos*, fear). A morbid dread of spiders.

Arachnida. A genus of Arthropoda, which includes spiders.

arachnī·tis (G. *arakhnē*, spider). See under arachnoiditis.

arāch·nodaktȳ·ly (G. *arakhnē*, spider, *daktulos*, finger). Developmental anomaly, mostly congenital, characterized by abnormally long and slender bones of the extremities, especially at the distal parts ('spider fingers'), hypotonic muscles and poorness of subcutaneous fat tissue. Often associated with dolichocephaly, ectopy of the lens and congenital lesions of the heart. Syn. dolichostenomelia; Marfan's disease.

arach·noid (G. *arakhnē*, spider; *eidos*, form). 1. Resembling a web; e.g., arachnoid space, the space between a. and dura mater. 2. The a. membrane, the middle of the three coverings of the brain.

arachnoi·dal. Of or relating to the arachnoid.

arachnoidi·tis (G. *arakhnē*, spider). Inflammation of the arachnoidal membrane.

arachnō·pia (G. *arakhnē*, spider). The arachnoid and pia considered together.

Aran's green cancer (Aran, F. A., French physician, 1817–61). Invasion of the orbit by leukaemic masses. **A.'s law**: basal skull fractures are due to injury to the vault, the extension to the basis cranii taking place by irradiation along the line of the shortest circle.

Aran-Duchenne's disease (Aran, F. A., 1817–61; Duchenne, G. B. A., 1806–75, French physicians). Progressive muscular atrophy.

ar·bor (L.). Tree.

arbor vitae (L. tree of life). 1. Tree-like figure in a section of the cerebellum; the branched central mass of medullary substance surrounded on its outer surface by a narrow layer of grey matter. 2. The tree-like appearance of the internal folds of the cervix uteri.

arbores·cent (L. *arborescere*, to grow into a tree). Branching.

arborizā·tion (L. *arbor*, tree). 1. Branching of nerve cell processes. 2. More especially, the end-branches of the auriculo-ventricular bundle of His. **A. block**, impairment of conduction through the distal parts of the conduction system of the heart: usually caused by ischaemic necrosis of the heart muscle.

arbutin. A crystalline glycoside, $C_{12}U_{16}O_7,\frac{1}{2}H_2O$, obtained from the dried leaves of the *Arctostaphylos uva-ursi* (Ericaceae). It is diuretic, astringent and antiseptic, and is used in cases of urethritis, etc.

arc (L. *arcus*, bow). Part of the circumference of a circle. Also used to denote a more or less curved way. **A., reflex**: the pathway of a reflex along the afferent nerve to a centre and back to the periphery along the efferent nerve.

arcade (L. *arcus*, arch). Any anatomical feature which consists of a series of arches.

Arcella. A genus of amoebae.

arch (L. *arcus*). Term used for various curved portions of the body, e.g., **arch of the aorta**, the curved section of the aorta between its rising and descending parts. **A., deep femoral**: a thickening of the fascia transversalis as it passes downwards beneath the inguinal ligament to form the anterior wall of the femoral sheath. **A., jugular**: a transverse venous arch forming the anterior jugular veins in front of the trachea. **A., plantar**: an arterial arch in the foot made up of the termination of the external plantar artery. **A., superficial palmar**: the distal termination of the ulnar artery in the hand. **A., suprapubic**: a line joining the ischial tuberosities in front, it is bounded on each side by the ischiopubic ramus and above by their meeting to form the subpubic angle.

archā·ic (G. *arkhaios*, ancient). Very old; out of date.

archebiō·sis (G. *arkhe*, beginning; *bios*, life). Spontaneous generation.

archegō·nium (G. *arkhe*, beginning; *gŏnē*, offspring). The female reproductive organ of the higher cryptogams.

archĕ·gony (G. *arkhe*, beginning; *gŏne*, offspring). Spontaneous generation.

archencĕ·phalon (G. *arkhe*, beginning; *en*, in; *kephăle*, head). The primitive brain.

archen·teron (G. *arkhe*, beginning; *enteron*, intestine). Cavity formed by invagination of the blastodermic vesicle; the primitive enteron.

ar·cheocyte (G. *arkhaios*, ancient; *kutos*, cell). A wandering amoebic cell.

archespor·ium (G. *arkhe*, beginning; *spora*, seed). The layer of cells which gives rise to mother spore-cells.

ar·chetype (G. *arkhe*, beginning; *tupos*, type). A standard type; a prototype.

ar·chiblast (G. *arkhe*, beginning; *blastos*, germ). The formative part of the protoplasm of an ovum, as opposed to the nutritive portion.

archiblast·ic. Relating to the archiblast.

archiblastō·ma. A tumour deriving from archiblastic substance.

ar·chicyte (G. *arkhē*, beginning; *kutos*, cell). A fertilized egg in the pre-segmentation stage.

archicy̆·tula (L. dim. for archicyte). A fertilized egg in which the nucleus has become discernible.

ar·chigaster (G. *arkhe*, beginning; *gastēr*, belly). The embryonic alimentary canal.

archigŏ·nocyte (G. *arkhe*, beginning; *gŏnē*, offspring; *kutos*, cell). The primary germ cell, which is produced by the segmentation of the egg.

Archil, syn. **Orchil.** The word Archil, or more properly Orchil, was originally the name of the plant from which the dye, which goes under this name, is obtained. It appears that before the introduction of Orchil into this country a similar dye, obtained from certain lichens in Scotland, was in use under the name of 'Cork'. This is given in Miller's *Plant Names* as the name of the lichens yielding Archil. (Martindale.)

archineph·ron (G. *arkhe*, beginning; *nephros*, kidney). The primary renal apparatus; the Wolffian body.

archipal·lial. Relating to the archipallium.

archipal·lium (G. *arkhe*, beginning; L. *pallium*, cloak). The phylogenetically older portion of the cerebral cortex; the olfactory brain. Syn. rhinencephalon.

ar·chiplasm (G. *arkhe*, beginning; *plasma*, from *plassein*, to form). See archoplasm.

ar·chistome (G. *arkhe*, beginning; *stoma*, mouth). The blastophore, *q.v.*

ar·chocele (G. *arkhos*, rectum; *kēlē*, hernia). Rectal hernia.

ar·choplasm (G. *arkhe*, beginning; *plassein*, to form). Substance composing astral rays and spindle fibres.

archoptō·ma (G. *arkhos*, rectum; *ptōma*, a fall). Prolapse of the rectum.

archorrhā·gia (G. *arkhos*, rectum; *rhēgnunai*, to break). Haemorrhage of the rectum.

ar·chos (G. *arkhos*). The rectum.

archostegnō·sis (G. *arkhos*, rectum; *stĕgnōsis*, a stoppage). Stricture of the rectum.

ar·ciform (L. *arcus*, arc; *forma*, shape). Arcuate; bow-shaped.

arctā·tion. (Corrupt L. *arctatio*, narrowing). Constriction of the lumen of a canal.

Arctium. A genus of composite-flowering plants, which includes *A. lappa*, the burdock.

ar·cuate (L. *arcus*, arc). Arch-shaped; bow-shaped. **A. fibres**: association fibres connecting neighbouring regions in cerebral convolutions or in the cerebellum.

ar·cus (L.). A bow or arch, e.g., **arcus aortae**, arch of the aorta. **A. dentalis**: the dental arch. **A. juvenalis**: a white ring around the cornea occurring in young persons and resembling the arcus senilis. **A. parieto-occipitalis**: a curved gyrus in the occipital lobe of the brain. **A. senilis**: a greyish circle at the periphery of the cornea, occurring usually only in advanced age owing to simple senile degeneration of the cornea with deposition of cholesterol. **A. tendineus**: a thickened part of the pelvic fascia on the lateral pelvic wall commonly known as the *white line*. **A. volaris**: the palmar arch. **A. zygomaticus**: the zygomatic arch.

ar·dent (L. *ardēre*, to glow). 1. Eager. 2. Feverish.

ar·dour (L. *ardor*). Violent heat; burning.

area (L. *area*). Any delimited surface. **Audito-psychic a.**: a portion of the auditory cortex of the brain which includes part of the superior temporal gyrus. **Auricular a.**: an area on the sacropelvic surface of the hip bone which articulates with the auricular surface of the sacrum. **A., of broca**: the motor speech area; it occupies the triangular and opercular parts of the inferior frontal gyrus of the brain. **A. postrema**: a narrow strip of vascular nervous tissue in the medullary part of the fourth ventricle of the brain. **Premotor a.**: the anterior portion of the pre-central gyrus and the posterior extremities of the frontal gyri of the brain. **Sensory psychic A.**: a strip of sensory cortex of the brain including part of the postcentral gyrus and paracentral lobule and the anterior portions of the superior and inferior parietal lobules. **Visuo-psychic a.**: a portion of visual cortex of the brain including part of the cuneus and lingual gyrus and a large portion of the occipital lobe.

areā·tus (L. *area*). Circumscribed.

Areca. A genus of Asiatic palm trees, including the *A. catechu*, of which the fruit is anthelmintic.

areflex·ia (G. *a*, neg.; L. *reflectere*, to bend back). The absence of a reflex.

arenā·tion (L. *arena*, sand). Sand-bath; application of hot sand to the body.

areocar·dia (G. *araios*, thin; *kardia*, heart). The same as bradycardia, *q.v.*

arĕ·ola (L. *areola*, dim. of *area*, space). 1. Any interstice in a tissue. 2. The brownish ring around the nipple. 3. That section of the iris surrounding the pupil of the eye.

arĕ·olar. Relating to or characterized by areolae, e.g., **A. tissue**: intercellular tissue.

areoli·tis. Inflammation of the mammary areola.

areŏ·meter (G. *araios*, slight; *metron*, measure). Instrument for measuring the specific gravity of fluids.

arevare·va (Polynesian). A severe skin affection, believed by some authorities to be due to excessive use of kava, an alcoholic beverage distilled from the awa root.

arg. Abbreviation for (L.) *argentum*, silver.

Argas (G. *argēeis*, white, shining). A genus of ticks which includes the common fowl tick.

Argasidae (G. *argēeis*). A family of ticks.

Argein. A brand of silver proteinate.

ar·gema (G. *argēeis*, shining). Corneal ulcer.

argentaffine carcinoma. See carcinoid.

argentā·tion (L. *argentum*, silver). Staining with a preparation of silver.

argen·tum (L. silver). A metallic element, symbol Ag., of which various salts and preparations are used in medicine.

argillā·ceous (G. *argillos*, potter's earth). Made of clay.

ar·ginase (L. *argentum*, silver). An enzyme splitting arginine into ornithine and urea.

ar·ginine. $H_2N.C(=NH).CH_2CH_2CH(NH_2).COOH$. a-amino-δ-guanidino-n-valeric acid.

ar·gon (G. *argos*, inert). An inert gaseous element present in the air. Symb. Ar.

Argyll Robertson pupil (Argyll Robertson, D.M.C.L., Scottish physician, 1837–1909). A pupil which does not contract to light falling on it, but will contract with accommodation for near objects.

argy̆·ria (G. *arguros*, silver). A greyish-blue discoloration of organs due to prolonged administration of silver, leading to the deposition of silver granules in these organs.

argy̆·ric (G. *arguros*, silver). Relating to silver.

ar·gyrism (G. *arguros*, silver). Chronic silver poisoning

Argyrol. A brand of mild silver proteinate used in the treatment of conjunctivitis, etc.

argy·rophil (G. *arguros*, silver; *philein*, to love). Easily stained with silver.

argyrō·sis (G. *arguros*, silver). The same as argyria.

arhigō·sis (G. *a*, neg.; *rhīgos*, cold). Inability to perceive cold.

ariboflavinō·sis. A condition, characterized by skin eruptions around the mouth, nose and eyes, caused by a lack of riboflavin in the diet.

aristocar·dia (G. *aristos*, best; *kardia*, heart). Misplacement of the heart towards the right side of the body.

ă·rithmomā·nia (G. *arithmos*, number; *mania*, madness). Obsessional neurosis characterized by uncalled-for counting of objects or numbers.

ar·kyrochrome (G. *arkus*, net; *khrōma*, colour). Applied to Nissl's bodies, *q.v.*, arranged in network.

Arlt's operation (Arlt, C. F., Ritter von, Austrian physician, 1812–87). An operation on the eye for distichiasis. **A.'s sinus:** a small cavity which may occasionally be observed in the lower portion of the lacrimal sac. **A.'s trachoma:** granular conjunctivitis.

arm (L. *armus*, shoulder). The upper limb, from shoulder to wrist.

armamentār·ium (L. from *armare*, to arm). Outfit of medicines or instruments.

Armanni-Ebstein cells (Armanni, L., Italian pathologist, 1839–1903; Ebstein, W., German physician, 1836–1912). Small epithelial cells containing glycogen found in the terminal part of the first convoluted renal tubule; commonly found in cases of diabetes.

ar·mature (L. *armatura*, armour). A piece of soft iron placed across the poles of a horseshoe magnet to preserve its power.

Armenian bole. A red-coloured clay used in the manufacture of tooth powders.

Armigeres obturbans. A dengue-transmitting mosquito.

armorā·cia (L.). Horseradish.

armpit. Axilla, *q.v.*

Armstrong's disease. See choriomeningitis, lymphocytic.

Arndt's law (Arndt, R., German physician, 1835–1900). Physiological activity is stimulated by weak stimuli and inhibited or abolished by strong stimuli.

Arneth's formula (Arneth, J., German physician, born 1873). The polymorphonuclear leucocytes are classified into five groups, depending on the number of lobes (1 to 5) which they contain. The normal is 1 lobe 5 per cent; 2 lobes 35 per cent; 3 lobes 41 per cent; 4 lobes 17 per cent; 5 lobes 2 per cent.

Arnica. A genus of composite flowering plants, which includes *A. montana*, or leopard's bane, of which the flowers or root may be used as a cardiac stimulant. Is also used externally for bruises, sprains, etc.

Arnold's bodies (Arnold, J., German pathologist, 1835–1915). Erythrocyte segments seen in the blood.

Arnold's canal (Arnold, F., German anatomist, 1803–1890). The passage for the auricular branch of the pneumogastric nerve through the petrous portion of the temporal bone. **A.'s ganglion:** the otic ganglion. **A.'s operculum:** the operculum of the Island of Reil.

Arnold's test (Arnold, V., Austrian physician, born 1864). A para-amido-acetophenone test for acetoacetic acid in the urine.

Arnott's bed (Arnott, N., Scottish physician, 1788–1874). A water bed.

Arnoux's sign. A sign of twin pregnancy, being the rhythm of the foetal heart-beat produced by the presence of two hearts, the action of both being perceptible.

arō·ma (G. *arōma*, spice). Fragrance.

D

aromat·ic. 1. Property pertaining to certain plants containing essential oils of a fragrant odour or taste. 2. Term applied to carbon compounds originating from benzene or containing one or more carbon rings. **A. series:** carbocyclic or heterocyclic compounds containing fully conjugated systems of double bonds.

Aronson's serum (Aronson, H., German bacteriologist, 1865–1919). An anti-streptococcal serum.

arrector pili (L. *arrigere*, to erect, *pĭlus*, a hair). Smooth muscle fibres surrounding the hair follicles; on their contraction the follicles become erected, thus producing 'goose-flesh' (cutis anserina).

arrest (L. *ad*, to; *restare*, to remain). Stoppage, detention.

arrested head. The child's head in parturition which is hindered, but not impacted, in the pelvic cavity.

arrhě·noblastō·ma (G. *arrhēn*, male; *blastos*, germ). Neoplasm of the ovary which may give rise to Cushing's syndrome, *q.v.*

arrhenogen·ic (G. *arrhēn*, male, *gĕnos*, offspring). Having only male offspring.

arrhinencě·phaly, a(r)rinencephā·lia (G. *a*, neg.; *rhis*, nose; *egkephalos*, the brain). Partial or complete congenital absence of the olfactory bulb.

arrhi·nia (G. *a*, neg.; *rhis*, nose). Congenital absence of the nose.

arrhyth·mia (G. *a*, neg.; *rhuthmos*, rhythm). Without rhythm; irregular.

arrō·sion (L. *arrodere*, gnaw). Destruction of a part, e.g. a bone or vessel walls, by constant pressure or by ulcerative process.

arrowroot. Originally the starch derived from *Maranta arundinacea* (West Indies, etc.) but now used to designate starchy preparations from various other tropical plants.

Arsacetin. A brand of sodium acetylarsonilate.

Arsamin. A brand of sodium aminoarsonate.

ar·senate (G. *arsenikon*, yellow orpiment). Any salt of arsenic acid.

ar·senic (G. *arsenikon*, from Arab. *az-zernikh*, the orpiment). 1. An element (Symb. As.); brittle, of steel-grey colour. Used in medicine as an alterative, more especially in various skin diseases. 2. **A.** trioxide, or white arsenic.

arsen·ic. Pertaining to arsenic.

arsenic trioxide. As_2O_3. Arsenious oxide.

arsě·nical. Containing or pertaining to arsenic.

arsenicŏ·phagy (G. *arsenikon.* yellow orpiment; *phagein*, to eat). The habit of arsenic eating.

ar·senide (G. *arsenikon*, yellow orpiment; *eidos*, form). A compound of arsenic with another element.

ar·senism. Chronic arsenical poisoning.

ar·senite. Any salt of arsenous acid.

arsenizā·tion. Treatment with arsenic.

arseno-. A prefix. Arsenic combined in the form —As–As—, e.g., arsenobenzene: C_6H_5–As–As–C_6H_5.

Arsenobillon. A brand of arsphenamine.

ar·senous. A compound of trivalent arsenic.

arsenum (L.). Arsenic.

arsphen·amine. 3:3-diamino- 4:4-dihydroxyarsenobenzene. A bright yellow powder, used in the treatment of syphilis.

ar·tefact (L. *ars*, art; *facere*, to make). Any artificial product resulting from a physical or chemical agency.

Artemisia. A genus of composite flowering plants, including the southernwood, which has stimulant and anthelmintic properties.

artē·ria (G. *artēria*, artery). A hollow tube; an artery.

artē·rial. Pertaining to an artery.

arterializā·tion. 1. Oxygenation of venous blood, e.g., in the lungs. 2. Vascularization.

arteriā·sis. Degeneration of arterial walls.

arteriĕc·tomy (G. *artēria*, artery; *ektomē*, excision). Surgical removal of a part of an artery.

arteriĕctŏ·pia (G. *artēria*, artery; *ektopos*, out of place). Displacement of an artery.

arterii·tis. See under arteritis.

artē·rioăt·ony. Relaxation of arterial walls.

artēr·iocapi·llary (G. *artēria*, artery; L. *capillus*, hair). Pertaining to arteries and capillaries.

arteriŏ·graphy (G. *artēria*, artery; *graphein*, to write). 1. Radiological visualization of arteries by means of intravascular injection of some substance opaque to X-rays. 2. A description of the arteries. 3. A graphic representation of the pulse waves.

arteriŏ·lar. Relating to arterioles.

arteriole (G. *artēria*). A small artery. **Arteriolae rectae,** the straight arterioles of the kidney.

artēr·iolith (G. *artēria*, artery; *līthos*, stone). A chalky mass found in an artery.

arteriŏ·logy (G. *artēria*, artery; *logos*, discourse). That section of anatomy which relates to the arteries.

artēr·iomală·cia (G. *artēria*, artery; *malăkia*, softness). Softening of the arterial coats.

arteriŏ·meter (G. *artēria*, artery; *metron*, measure). Instrument for measuring the changes in arterial pulse beats.

artēr·ionecrŏ·sis (G. *artēria*, artery; *nekros*, dead). Necrosis of the arteries.

arteriŏ·pathy (G. *artēria*, artery; *pathos*, sickness). Any disease of the arteries.

artēr·ioplă·sty (G. *artēria*, artery; *plassein*, to form). Operation for aneurysm; making a new channel out of the sac walls.

artēr·iorē·nal (G. *artēria*, artery; L. *renes*, kidneys). Relating to the arteries of the kidneys.

artēr·iorrhā·gia (G. *artēria*, artery; *rhēgnunai*, to break). Arterial haemorrhage.

arteriŏr·rhaphy (G. *artēria*, artery; *rhaphē*, suture). Suture of an artery.

artēr·iorrhex·ia (G. *artēria*, artery; *rhēxis*, rupture). Rupture of an artery.

arteriosclerosis (G. *artēria*, artery; *sklēros*, hard). Chronic morbid condition of the arterial walls, especially of the intima; characterized by thickening and decrease of elasticity of the walls and narrowing of the lumen.

artēr·iosclerŏt·ic (G. *artēria*, artery; *sklēros*, hard). Pertaining to arteriosclerosis.

artēr·iospasm (G. *artēria*, artery; *spasma*, convulsion). Spasm of an artery.

artēr·iostenŏ·sis (G. *artēria*, artery; *stenos*, narrow). Contraction of the lumen of an artery.

artēr·iostŏ·sis (G. *artēria*, artery; *osteŏn*, bone). Ossification of an artery.

artēr·iotome (G. *artēria*, artery; *tomē*, section). A surgical instrument for the performance of arteriotomy.

arteriŏ·tomy (G. *artēria*, artery; *tomē*, section). Blood-letting from an artery.

artēr·iovē·nous (G. *artēria*, artery; L. *vena*, vein). Referring to both arteries and veins. **A.-V. anastomosis** (G. *anastomoein*, to furnish with a mouth), a direct connection between arterioles and veins through which blood may pass without traversing capillaries, such as is present in the skin of the distal parts, functioning under extreme degrees of cold or warmth. **A.-V. aneurysm:** aneurysm between an artery and a vein.

artēr·iover·sion (G. *artēria*, artery; L. *vertere*, to turn). Surgical eversion of the coats of a bleeding artery in order to stop a haemorrhage.

arterī·tis (G. *artēria*, artery). Inflammation of an artery or of the external coat of an artery. See also **endarteritis, peri-arteritis** and **thromboangeitis.**

ar·tery (G. *artēria*, from *ăēr*, air, and *tērein*, to keep. In ancient times it was believed that these vessels contained air). A vessel carrying blood from the heart towards the periphery. **Abdominal aorta:** continuation of thoracic aorta below diaphragm. Divides into left and right common iliac arteries. **Aberrant renal a.:** an uncommon artery arising from the phrenic, testicular, inferior mesenteric common or external iliac and supplying the lower pole of the kidney. **Accessory meningeal a.:** branch of maxillary a., entering the cranium through the foramen ovale. **Accessory renal a.:** arises from the aorta close to the main renal artery and usually above it and supplies the upper part of the kidney. **Acromio-thoracic a.:** branch of axillary artery. Divides into deltoid, acromial, clavicular and pectoral branches. **Alar thoracic a.:** a small branch of the axillary artery and it supplies the axillary glands. **Anterior caecal a.:** a branch of the ileocaecal artery and distributed to the front of the caecum. **Anterior carpal a.:** a small branch of the radial artery which goes to the structures on the front of the wrist. **Anterior cerebral a.:** arises from internal carotid. Lies in longitudinal fissure of brain and supplies cerebrum. **Anterior choroidal a.:** a branch of the intracranial portion of the internal carotid artery and terminates in the choroid plexus of the brain. **Anterior communicating a.:** small artery connecting anterior cerebral arteries on each side and completing circle of Willis anteriorly. **Anterior ethmoidal a.:** branch of ophthalmic artery to middle and anterior ethmoidal and frontal sinuses, and to meninges and nose. **Anterior inferior cerebellar a.:** arises from basilar artery. Supplies cerebellum. **Anterior interosseous a.:** branch of common interosseous artery. Runs down forearm on anterior aspect of interosseous ligament. **Anterior spinal a.:** branch of vertebral. Runs down whole length of spinal cord anteriorly. **Anterior tibial a.:** branch of popliteal artery. Passes forwards above interosseous ligament and runs down on latter to form dorsalis pedis artery at ankle. **Anterior tympanic a.:** branch of maxillary artery. Enters middle ear through squamotympanic fissure. **Anterior ulnar recurrent a.;** anterior branches of ulnar artery near elbow. Supply muscles and joint. **Appendicular a.:** branch of ileocolic artery. Enters meso-appendix to supply appendix. **Arcuate a.:** branch of dorsalis pedis. Crosses dorsum of foot and gives off second, third and fourth dorsal metatarsal arteries. **Ascending aorta:** arises from left ventricle and continues as arch of aorta. **Ascending cervical a.:** branch of inferior thyroid artery. Ascends on transverse processes of cervical vertebrae. **Ascending palatine a.:** branch of facial artery to soft palate and pharynx. **Ascending pharyngeal a.:** branch of external carotid artery to pharynx. **Axillary a.:** continuation of subclavian artery at outer border of first rib. Ends as brachial artery at lower border of teres major. **Azygos vaginal a.:** small branch of vaginal artery supplying the vagina and bladder. **Basilar a.:** arises from junction of two vertebral arteries. Lies on pons, and divides into two posterior cerebral arteries. **Brachial a.:** continuation of axillary artery at lower border of teres major. Divides at elbow into ulnar and radial arteries. **Buccal a.:** branch of maxillary artery to buccinator muscle. **Carotico-tympanic a.:** branch of internal carotid artery in the petrous bone and supplies the tympanic cavity. **Central a. of retina:** branch of ophthalmic artery to retina. Runs in optic nerve. **Charcot's a.:** a branch of lenticulostriate artery which supplies the internal capsule often called the artery of cerebral haemorrhage. **Circumflex fibular a.:** branch of anterior tibial artery and supplies muscles in the anterior compartment of the leg. **Circumflex scapular a.:** branch of subscapular artery to infraspinous fossa. **Cochlear a.:** a branch of the internal auditory

ARTERIES

1. FRONTAL BRANCH OF SUPERFICIAL TEMPORAL
2. SUPRA-ORBITAL
3. LATERAL NASAL
4. SUPERIOR LABIAL
5. INFERIOR LABIAL
6. SUBMENTAL
7. MENTAL
8. FACIAL
9. PARIETAL BRANCH OF SUPERFICIAL TEMPORAL
10. SUPERFICIAL TEMPORAL
11. OCCIPITAL
12. INTERNAL CAROTID
13. EXTERNAL CAROTID
14. SUPERIOR THYROID
15. COMMON CAROTID
16. SUBCLAVIAN
17. ACROMIOTHORACIC
18. LATERAL THORACIC
19. AXILLARY
20. SUBSCAPULAR
21. HUMERAL CIRCUMFLEX
22. BRACHIAL
23. PROFUNDA BRACHII
24. ULNAR COLLATERAL
25. SUPRATROCHLEAR
26. ULNAR RECURRENT
27. RADIAL RECURRENT
28. INTEROSSEOUS
29. ULNAR
30. RADIAL
31. DEEP PALMAR ARCH
32. SUPERFICIAL PALMAR ARCH
33. PALMAR INTEROSSEOUS
34. INNOMINATE
35. AORTA
36. INTERCOSTALS
37. GASTRIC (L.) ⎫ Coeliac
38. SPLENIC ⎬ axis
39. HEPATIC ⎭
40. SUPRARENAL
41. SUPERIOR MESENTERIC
42. RENAL
43. TESTICULAR
44. LUMBAR
45. INFERIOR MESENTERIC
46. MIDSACRAL
47. COMMON ILIAC
48. CIRCUMFLEX ILIAC (deep)
49. INTERNAL ILIAC
50. EXTERNAL ILIAC
51. INFERIOR EPIGASTRIC
52. INFERIOR PUDENDAL
53. FEMORAL
54. FEMORAL CIRCUMFLEX
55. DESCENDING BRANCH OF THE FEMORAL
56. PROFUNDA FEMORIS
57. DESCENDING GENICULAR
58. POPLITEAL
59. MEDIAL SUPERIOR GENICULAR
60. MEDIAL INFERIOR GENICULAR
61. ANTERIOR TIBIAL
62. POSTERIOR TIBIAL
63. PERONEAL
64. LATERAL TARSAL
65. DORSALIS PEDIS
66. MEDIAL PLANTAR
67. LATERAL PLANTAR
68. DORSAL METATARSAL
69. DIGITAL

artery and supplies the cochlea. **Coeliac a.:** short trunk arising from abdominal aorta between crura of diaphragm. Divides into left gastric, hepatic and splenic arteries. **Colic a.:** a branch of the superior mesenteric artery and supplies the ascending colon. **Common carotid a.:** branch of arch of aorta on left side, and of innominate artery on right side. Lies in anterior triangle of neck and divides into internal and external carotid arteries. **Common iliac a.:** terminal branch of abdominal aorta. Divides into external and internal iliac arteries. **Common interosseous a.:** short artery. Branch of ulnar artery at elbow. Divides into anterior and posterior interosseous arteries at upper border of interosseous ligament. **Coronary a.:** or left gastric artery: a branch of the coeliac artery and supplies the lesser curvature of the stomach. **Cremasteric a.:** branch of inferior epigastric artery and supplies the cremaster muscle and coverings of the spermatic cord. **Cricothyroid a.:** branch of superior thyroid artery and lies on cricothyroid ligament and anastomoses with its fellow of the opposite side. **Cystic a.:** branch of hepatic artery. Lies behind right hepatic duct and above cystic duct. Supplies gall bladder. **Deep auricular a.:** branch of maxillary artery to external auditory meatus and temporomandibular joint. **Deep cervical a.:** arises from costocervical trunk of subclavian artery. Ascends among muscles of back of neck. **Deep circumflex iliac a.:** branch of external iliac artery to muscles arising from crest of ilium. **Deep external pudendal a.:** branch of the common femoral artery and distributed to the skin of the scrotum and penis in the male and the labium majus in the female. **Deep femoral a.:** a large branch of the femoral artery and supplies the muscles on the back of the thigh. **Deep a. of penis:** branch of internal pudendal artery. Lies in corpus cavernosum. **Deep plantar a.:** branch of dorsalis pedis artery supplies muscles on the sole of the foot. **Deep temporal a.:** anterior and posterior branches of maxillary artery in temporal fossa. Supply temporalis muscle. **Descending aorta:** the continuation of the arch of the aorta. Divided into thoracic and abdominal portions. **Descending genicular a.:** branch of femoral artery. Takes part in anastomosis around knee. **Descending thoracic aorta:** part of aorta contained in posterior mediastinum. **Dorsal nasal a.:** terminal branch of ophthalmic artery to nose. **Dorsal a. of penis:** branch of internal pudendal artery to dorsum of penis or clitoris. **Dorsalis indicis a.:** branch of radial artery supplies the radial side of the index finger. **Dorsalis linguae a.:** branch of lingual artery and supplies the mucous membrane and substance of the tongue, the tonsil and the soft palate. **Dorsalis pedis a.:** continuation of anterior tibial artery at ankle. Gives rise to arcuate artery and anastomoses with plantar artery in first intermetatarsal space. **Dorsalis pollicis a.:** small branch of the radial artery distributed to both sides of the thumb. **Dorsalis scapulae a.:** branch of subscapular artery supplies muscles attached to scapula. **Duodenal a. or inferior pancreaticoduodenal a.:** a small branch of the superior mesenteric artery and supplies the duodenum and pancreas. **External carotid a.:** branch of common carotid artery. Lies in anterior triangle of neck and in parotid gland. **External iliac a.:** branch of common iliac artery. Continuous with femoral artery at inguinal ligament. **External mammary a.:** lateral thoracic branch of the second part of the axillary artery and supplies the breast. **Facial a.:** branch of external carotid artery to face. **Femoral a.:** continuation of external iliac artery beyond inguinal ligament. Becomes popliteal artery at opening in adductor magnus. **Frenulum linguae a.:** a small branch of the lingual artery supplying the frenum of

the tongue. **Frontal a.:** or supratrochlear artery, a small branch of the ophthalmic a. and is distributed to the structures over the frontal bone. **Gastroduodenal a.:** branch of hepatic artery. Passes behind pylorus and divides into right gastro-epiploic and superior pancreaticoduodenal arteries. **Greater palatine a.:** branch of maxillary artery. Descends in greater palatine canal to palate. **Hepatic a.:** branch of coeliac artery. Lies in lesser omentum and passes to porta hepatis, where it divides into right and left branches. **Humeral circumflex a., anterior and posterior:** branches of the axillary artery and forming a circle round the upper part of the humerus and supplying the muscles in that area. **Hyaloid a.:** a branch of the arteria centralis retinae supplying the lens in the foetus. **Hypogastric a. (umbilical a.):** branch of common iliac a. in the foetus. **Ileocaecal a.:** branch of ileocolic artery supplies the caecum and ileum. **Ileocolic a.:** terminal branch of superior mesenteric artery. Supplies terminal ileum and caecum. **Iliolumbar a.:** branch of internal iliac artery to iliac fossa. **Inferior dental a.:** branch of maxillary artery to lower jaw. Runs in mandibular canal to teeth. **Inferior epigastric a.:** branch of external iliac artery to lower part of anterior abdominal wall and rectus sheath. **Inferior gluteal a.:** branch of internal iliac artery. Leaves pelvis through greater sciatic notch below pyriformis muscle and supplies gluteus maximus. **Inferior haemorrhoidal a.:** see inferior rectal artery. **Inferior laryngeal a.:** branch of inferior thyroid artery. Accompanies recurrent laryngeal nerve to larynx. **Inferior mesenteric a.:** branch of abdominal aorta to left side of colon and rectum. **Inferior pancreaticoduodenal a.:** branch of superior mesenteric artery. Lies in groove between pancreas and duodenum. Anastomoses with superior pancreaticoduodenal artery. **Inferior profunda a.** (ulnar collateral artery): a branch of the brachial artery about the middle of the arm and supplies the muscles of that region. **Inferior rectal a.:** branch of internal pudendal artery supplies the external anal sphincter, levator ani muscles and anal canal. **Inferior thyroid a.:** branch of thyrocervical trunk of subclavian artery. Supplies lower pole of thyroid gland. Closely related to recurrent laryngeal nerve. **Inferior tympanic a.:** branch of ascending pharyngeal artery to middle ear. **Inferior ulnar collateral a.** (anastomotica magna): branch of the brachial artery just proximal to the elbow and takes part in the anastomosis around the elbow joint. **Inferior vesical a.:** branch of internal iliac artery to bladder. **Infrahyoid a.:** branch of superior thyroid artery. Lies in thyrohyoid membrane. **Infraorbital a.:** branch of maxillary artery. Runs along floor of orbit and appears on cheek. **Infundibular a.:** a small branch of the right coronary artery supplies the outer surface of the right ventricle of the heart. **Innominate a.:** branch of arch of aorta. Soon divides into right subclavian and right common carotid arteries. **Internal auditory a.:** branch of basilar artery. Enters internal auditory meatus and supplies internal ear. **Internal carotid a.:** branch of common carotid artery. **Internal iliac a.:** branch of common iliac artery. Passes into pelvis to supply branches to pelvic viscera. **Internal mammary a.:** branch of subclavian artery. Lies behind costal cartilages and forms superior epigastric and musculophrenic arteries. **Internal maxillary a.** (maxillary artery): larger of the two terminal branches of the external carotid supplies the pterygoid region, pharynx, and dura mater. **Internal pudendal a.:** branch of internal iliac artery. Runs into Alcock's canal to perineum. **Interventricular a.:** branch of right coronary artery and supplies the surface of the heart. **Jejunal a.:** branches of the superior mesenteric artery supplying the upper loops of small intestine. **Lacrimal a.:** branch of ophthalmic artery. Traverses lateral wall of orbit to lacrimal gland. **Lateral anterior malleolar a.:** branch of anterior tibial artery to lateral malleolus. **Lateral calcaneal a.:** branch of peroneal artery supplying the plantar surface of the heel. **Lateral femoral circumflex a.:** large branch of arteria profunda femoris artery supplies muscles on the outer side of the thigh and the hip joint. **Lateral plantar a.:** terminal branch of posterior tibial artery. Forms plantar arch with dorsalis pedis artery. Supplies adjacent muscles and toes. **Lateral sacral a.:** branch of internal iliac to posterior wall of pelvis. **Lateral thoracic a.:** branch of axillary artery. Passes to side of chest and supplies muscles. **Left gastric a.:** branch of coeliac artery. Passes into lesser omentum and supplies lesser curve of stomach. **Left gastro-epiploic a.:** branch of splenic artery to greater curve of stomach. **Lenticulostriate a.:** branch of middle cerebral artery supplying the internal capsule of the brain. **Lenticulothalamic a.:** branch of middle cerebral artery supplies the lentiform nucleus and the thalamus. **Lingual a.:** branch of external carotid artery to tongue. **Lumbar a.:** branches of abdominal aorta on body of each lumbar vertebra. Pass laterally to posterior abdominal wall. **Malleolar a.:** branch of peroneal artery supplies the skin over the internal malleolus. **Marginal a.:** branch of left coronary artery supplying the apex of the heart. **Masseteric a.:** branch of middle meningeal artery to masseteric muscle. **Mastoid a.:** branch of the posterior auricular artery distributed to tympanic cavity and the mastoid air cells. **Maxillary a.:** branch of external carotid artery to pterygoid fossa. **Medial anterior malleolar a.:** branch of anterior tibial artery to medial malleolus. **Medial calcaneal a.:** branch of peroneal artery supplying the plantar surface of the heel. **Medial femoral circumflex a.:** branch of profunda femoris artery. Passes backwards between pectineus and psoas, adductor brevis and obturator externus, adductor magnus and quadratus femoris, and so appears in gluteal region. **Medial plantar a.:** terminal branch of posterior tibial artery. Supplies muscles of medial side of foot and three superficial digital branches. **Median a.:** branch of anterior interosseous artery. Accompanies median nerve. **Median sacral a.:** branch of abdominal aorta at its bifurcation. Lies in midline of sacrum anteriorly. **Mental a.:** branch of inferior dental artery. Escapes from mental foramen and supplies chin. **Metatarsal a.** (arcuate artery): branch of dorsalis pedis artery and distributed to the intermetatarsal spaces of the foot. **Middle cerebral a.:** largest branch of internal carotid. Lies in Sylvian fissure and supplies cerebrum. **Middle colic a.:** branch of superior mesenteric artery. Enters transverse mesocolon and supplies transverse colon. **Middle haemorrhoidal a.:** see middle rectal artery. **Middle meningeal a.:** branch of maxillary artery. Enters cranium through foramen spinosum and supplies meninges. **Middle rectal a.:** branch of internal iliac artery to lower part of rectum. **Middle temporal a.:** branch of superficial temporal artery to temporalis muscle. **Middle vesical a.:** branch of inferior vesical artery supplies the base of the bladder and the vas deferens. **Musculophrenic a.:** terminal branch of internal mammary artery. Supplies upper lateral quadrant of abdomen and diaphragm. **Mylohyoid a.:** branch of inferior dental artery to chin. **Nasopalatine a.:** branch of maxillary artery supplies the nasal septum. **Obturator a.:** branch of internal iliac artery. Leaves pelvis through obturator canal and supplies obturator muscles. **Obturator abnormal a.:** branch of inferior epigastric artery in 30 per cent of cases passes over femoral ring to supply

muscles on inner side of thigh and hip joint. **Occipital a.:** branch of external carotid artery to occipital region of scalp. **A. of bulb:** branch of internal pudendal artery to bulb. **A. of cerebral haemorrhage:** lenticulostriate artery branch of middle cerebral. **A. of vas deferens:** branch of middle vesical artery and supplies the vas deferens. **Ophthalmic a.:** branch of internal carotid artery to orbit. **Ovarian a.:** branch of abdominal aorta. Enters broad ligament and supplies ovary. **Pancreatica magna a.:** branch of splenic artery supplying the pancreas. **Perforating peroneal a.:** branch of peroneal artery and supplies the foot. **Pericardiacophrenic a.:** branch of internal mammary. Accompanies phrenic nerve. **Peroneal a.:** branch of posterior tibial artery. Descends along medial crest of fibula to calcaneum. **Phrenic a.:** branch of abdominal aorta to under surface of diaphragm. **Popliteal a.:** continuation of femoral artery from opening in adductor magnus. Forms posterior tibial artery at lower border of popliteus muscle. **Posterior auricular a.:** branch of external carotid artery. Supplies occipital regions of scalp. **Posterior caecal a.:** branch of ileocolic artery supplies the posterior surface of caecum. **Posterior carpal a.:** branch of common interosseous artery and supplies structures on the back of the wrist joint. **Posterior cerebral a.:** branch of basilar artery. Supplies tentorial surface of cerebrum. **Posterior choroidal a.:** branch of the posterior cerebral artery supplies the choroid plexus. **Posterior communicating a.:** branch of internal carotid artery at base of brain. Anastomoses with posterior cerebral artery, a branch of basilar artery. Completes circle of Willis posteriorly. **Posterior ethmoidal a.:** branch of ophthalmic artery to posterior ethmoidal sinuses and meninges. **Posterior inferior cerebellar a.:** branch of vertebral. Passes laterally to supply cerebellum. **Posterior interosseous a.:** branch of common interosseous artery. Runs down forearm on posterior aspect of interosseous membrane. **Posterior interosseous recurrent a.:** branch of posterior interosseous artery supplies back of elbow. **Posterior meningeal a.:** branch of vertebral artery supplies the dura mater of the posterior cranial fossa. **Posterior scapular a.:** branch of thyroid axis (thyrocervical trunk) and supplies muscles in the lower part of the neck. **Posterior septal a.:** branch of third part of maxillary artery and supplies the nasal septum. **Posterior spinal a.:** branch of vertebral artery. Forms free anastomosis around posterior roots of spinal nerves. **Posterior superior dental aa.:** branches of maxillary artery to posterior part of maxilla. Supply molar and premolar teeth. **Posterior tibial a.:** terminal branch of popliteal artery. Passes down on tibialis posticus. Divides into medial and lateral plantar arteries. **Posterior tibial recurrent a.:** an inconstant branch of the anterior tibial artery and supplies structures around the knee joint. **Posterior ulnar recurrent aa.:** branches of ulnar artery near elbow. Supply muscles and joint. **Princeps pollicis a.:** branch of radial artery. Supplies palmar aspect of thumb. **Profunda femoris a.:** branch of femoral artery. Passes downwards behind femoral artery to supply muscles of back of thigh. **Profunda linguae a.:** the terminal portion of the lingual artery to the inferior portion of tip of tongue. **Profunda superior a.** (Profunda artery): branch of the brachial artery and supplies muscles of arm. **Prostatic a.:** branch of the anterior division of the internal iliac artery which supplies the prostate gland. **Pterygo-palatine a.:** branch of third part of maxillary artery which supplies the pharyngotympanic tube and sphenoidal sinus. **Pubic a.:** branch of inferior epigastric artery supplies structures in the region of the os pubis. **Pulmonary a.:**

arises from right ventricle. Divides into right and left branches. **Pyloric a.:** branch of hepatic artery and supplies the lesser curvature of the stomach and omentum. **Radial a.:** branch of brachial artery at elbow. Passes down among muscles of forearm to wrist, where it turns backwards and dives between two heads of first dorsal interosseous muscle to anastomose with deep palmar arch. **Radial recurrent a.:** branch of radial artery. Takes part in anastomosis around elbow. **Radialis indicis a.:** branch of deep palmar arch supplies the index finger. **Ranine a.:** a branch of the lingual artery and supplies the anterior part of the tongue. **Renal a.:** large trunk arising from abdominal aorta. Enters hilum of kidney. **Right colic a.:** branch of superior mesenteric artery to ascending colon. **Right gastric a.:** branch of hepatic artery. Supplies lesser curve of stomach. **Right gastro-epiploic a.:** branch of gastroduodenal artery. Supplies greater curve of stomach. **Sciatic a.** (inferior gluteal artery): branch of internal iliac artery and supplies pelvic structures. **Short gastric aa.:** branches of splenic artery to fundus of stomach. **Small meningeal a.:** branch of middle meningeal and supplies the dura mater of middle fossa. **Spermatic a.** (testicular artery): arises from aorta and supplies the spermatic cord and testicle. **Sphenopalatine a.:** terminal branch of maxillary artery. Enters nose through sphenopalatine foramen and supplies mucous membrane of nose. **Splenic a.:** branch of coeliac artery. Runs along upper border of pancreas to spleen. **Sternomastoid a.:** branch of superior thyroid artery and supplies the sternomastoid muscle. **Stylomastoid a.:** branch of posterior auricular artery. Enters stylomastoid foramen. **Subclavian a.:** branch of arch of aorta on left side and innominate artery on right side. Prolonged as axillary artery at first rib. **Subcostal a.:** branch of thoracic aorta. Runs laterally beneath twelfth rib. **Sublingual a.:** a branch of the lingual artery supplies the sublingual gland and adjacent muscles. **Submental a.:** branch of facial artery to chin. **Subscapular a.:** branch of axillary artery. Passes along axillary border of scapula. Ends in muscles. **Superficial cervical a.:** branch of transverse cervical artery. Ascends deep to trapezius. **Superior circumflex iliac a.:** branch of femoral artery to region of crest of ilium. **Superficial epigastric a.:** branch of femoral artery to abdominal wall. **Superficial external pudendal a.:** branch of the femoral artery and supplies the inguinal glands. **Superficial perineal a.:** branch of internal pudendal artery and supplies the scrotum. **Superficial temporal a.:** one of terminal branches of external carotid artery. Supplies temporal region of scalp. **Superior cerebellar a.:** branch of basilar. Supplies cerebellum. **Superior epigastric a.:** terminal branch of internal mammary artery. Enters rectus sheath and anastomoses with deep epigastric artery. **Superior gluteal a.:** branch of internal iliac artery. Leaves pelvis through greater sciatic notch above piriformis muscle. Supplies gluteal muscles. **Superior haemorrhoidal a.** (superior rectal): is the continuation of the inferior mesenteric artery. **Superior intercostal a.:** branch of costocervical trunk of subclavian artery. Descends in front of necks of first and second ribs. Gives off first and second posterior intercostal arteries. **Superior labial a.:** branch of facial artery to upper lip. **Superior laryngeal a.:** branch of superior thyroid artery. Runs with internal laryngeal nerve to larynx. **Superior mesenteric a.:** branch of abdominal aorta. Passes behind neck of pancreas and enters mesentery of small intestine. Supplies branches to small intestine and right half of large intestine. **Superior pancreaticoduodenal a.:** branch of gastroduodenal artery. Lies in groove between pancreas and duo-

denum. Anastomoses with inferior pancreatico-duodenal artery. **Superior rectal a.:** terminal branch of inferior mesenteric artery. Supplies rectum as far as anal canal. **Superior thoracic a.:** branch of axillary artery to pectoral muscles. **Superior thyroid a.:** branch of external carotid artery to upper pole of thyroid gland. **Superior vesical aa.:** branches of internal iliac arteries to bladder. **Suprahyoid a.:** branch of lingual artery. Runs along upper border of hyoid bone. **Supra-orbital a.:** branch of ophthalmic artery. Crosses orbit and turns up over eyebrow to forehead. **Suprarenal a.:** small artery which arises from the aorta and goes to the suprarenal gland. **Suprascapular a.:** branch of thyrocervical trunk of subclavian artery. Passes to suprascapular notch and supplies muscles in supra- and infraspinous fossae. **Suprasternal a.:** branch of suprascapular artery and supplies the structures over the sternum. **Supratrochlear a.:** branch of brachial artery to muscles around elbow. **Sural cutaneous a.:** branch of popliteal artery and supplies the skin of the upper and back part of the leg. **Tarsal a.:** branch of dorsalis pedis to dorsal joints. **Testicular a.:** branch of abdominal aorta. Leaves abdomen with vas deferens via inguinal canal. Supplies testicle. **Thyrocervical a.** (thyroid axis): a short artery arising from the subclavian artery. **Thyroidea ima a.:** an inconstant branch of the innominate artery and supplies the lower part of the thyroid gland. **Tonsillar a.:** branch of facial artery to tonsil. **Transverse cervical a.:** branch of thyrocervical trunk of subclavian artery. Passes laterally across neck. Divides into superficial cervical artery and descending scapular artery. **Transverse facial a.:** branch of superficial temporal artery. Runs along upper border of zygomatic arch. **Transverse perineal a.:** branch of internal pudendal artery. Supplies perineum. **Tympanic a.:** branch of the maxillary which supplies the tympanum. **Ulnar a.:** branch of brachial artery at elbow. Passes along medial border of forearm to wrist. Continued into palm as superficial palmar arch. **Ulnar collateral a.:** branch of brachial artery. Accompanies ulnar nerve. **Umbilical a.:** arises from internal iliac artery and passes along anterior abdominal wall to umbilicus. Only functional in foetus. **Uterine a.:** branch of internal iliac artery. Reaches side of uterus after traversing broad ligament and crossing ureter. Ascends along side of uterus and anastomoses with ovarian artery. **Vaginal a.:** branch of uterine artery to vagina. **Vertebral a.:** branch of subclavian artery. Runs up through foramina of lateral processes of cervical vertebrae. Enters cranium through foramen magnum and ends by joining vertebral artery of opposite side to form basilar artery. **Vesiculodeferential a.:** branch of internal iliac artery. Supplies bladder base and vas deferens. **Vestibular a.:** branch of internal auditory artery and supplies the utricle, saccule, and semicircular canals. **Vidian a.:** branch of the maxillary artery which supplies the pharynx and tympanum. **Zygomatic a.:** branch of superficial temporal artery supplying the skin over the face.

arthral·gia (G. *arthron*, joint; *algos*, pain). Pain in a joint.

arthral·gic. Pertaining to arthralgia.

arthrec·tomy (G. *arthron*, joint; *ektomē*, excision). Excision of a joint.

arthrit·ic. Relating to arthritis.

arthri·tis (G. *arthron*, joint). Inflammation of a joint. **A. deformans:** see osteo-arthritis. **A. fungosa:** form of tuberculous disease of a joint. **Rheumatoid a.:** subacute or chronic disease of joints with febrile stages, occurring more often in females between the ages of 35 and 45 years, affecting especially the small joints of the hands and feet.

arthri·tism (G. *arthron*, joint). Constitutional disposition (diathesis) to gout, formation of renal or biliary stones, diabetes, obesity, and to eczema or psoriasis.

ar·throbactēr·ium (G. *arthron*, joint; *baktērion*, a small stick). Any bacterium that multiplies by separation into arthrospores.

ar·throcele (G. *arthron*, joint; *kēlē*, tumour). Any swelling of the joint.

arthroclā·sia (G. *arthron*, joint; *klaein*, to break). Operation for breaking up an ankylosed joint to produce free movement.

arthrŏ·desis (G. *arthron*, joint; *dĕsis*, a binding). Surgical fixation of a joint by the artificial production of bony union.

arthrodia (G. *arthrōdia*, from *arthron*, joint; *eidos*, form). A joint with a kind of articulation in which surfaces are only slightly concave and convex. A joint with a gliding movement.

arthro-oedē·ma (G. *arthron*, joint; *oidema*, a swelling). Oedema affecting a joint.

arthro-empyē·sis (G. *arthron*, joint; *empuēsis*, suppuration). Suppuration in a joint.

Arthrographis langeroni. A genus of fungi. Is known to produce onychomycosis in human beings.

arthrŏ·graphy (G. *arthron*, joint; *graphein*, to write). 1. Radiological visualization of the cavity of a joint by means of an intra-articular injection of some substance opaque to X-rays. 2. A description of the joints.

ar·throgrypō·sis (G. *arthron*, joint; *grupōsis*, curvature). 1. Abnormal persistent flexure of a joint. 2. Obsolete term for tetany.

ar·throlith (G. *arthron*, joint; *lithos*, stone). Calculous deposit in a joint.

arthrŏ·logy (G. *arthron*, joint; *logos*, a discourse). The part of anatomy pertaining to joints.

arthrŏ·lysis (G. *arthron*, joint; *luein*, to loosen). Surgical freeing of an ankylosed joint by division or removal of adhesions, etc.

arthrŏ·meter (G. *arthron*, joint; *metron*, measure). An instrument for measuring joint movement angles.

arthropathŏ·logy. Joint pathology.

arthrŏ·pathy (G. *arthron*, joint; *pathos*, disease). 1. Any joint disease. 2. Charcot's disease, *q.v.*

ar·throphŷte (G. *arthron*, joint; *phuton*, a plant). An outgrowth or a free body in a joint.

ar·throplasty (G. *arthron*, joint; *plassein*, to form). 1. The making of an artificial joint. 2. Reconstruction of a new joint from an ankylosed joint.

Arthropoda (G. *arthron*, joint; *pous*, foot). A phylum of the animal series comprising crustacea, myriapoda, insecta and arachnida.

ar·throsclerō·sis (G. *arthron*, joint; *sklērōsis*, a hardening). Hardening of the joints.

arthrŏ·sis (G. *arthroein*, to articulate). 1. An articulation or joint. 2. Any degenerative disease of a joint. See osteo-arthritis.

ar·throspore (G. *arthron*, joint; *spŏra*, seed). A spore formed by simple division or fission.

ar·throsynovi·tis (G. *arthron*, joint; *sŭn*, together). Inflammation of the membranes of a joint.

ar·throtome (G. *arthron*, joint; *tomē*, section). A type of knife used in operations on joints.

arthrŏ·tomy (G. *arthron*, joint; *tomē*, section). Incision of a joint.

arthroty·phoid (G. *arthron*, joint; *tupōhdēs*, delirious). A kind of typhoid fever characterized by symptoms like those seen in rheumatic fever.

arthroxĕ·sis (G. *arthron*, joint; *xĕsis*, a scraping). Scraping of an articular surface of a joint.

ar·ticle. Any interarticular section.

arti·cular (L. *articularis* from *articulus*, dim. of *artus*, a joint). Pertaining to an articulation or joint.

arti·culate. 1. Divided into joints. 2. Distinct, clear.

articulatio (L.). Articulation.

articulā·tion. 1. A joint; a connection between two or more bones. 2. The enunciation of speech.

arti·culator. Instrument for supporting the casts of the jaws while arranging artificial teeth on the plates.

articulo mortis (L.). At the moment of death.

artifī·cial (L. *ars*, art; *facere*, to make). Something produced not spontaneously but by some art or device. **A. anus:** see anus, a. **A. eye:** an imitation of the front part of the eye made of glass, rubber or plastic, and worn as a substitute for a lost eye for cosmetic reasons. **A. feeding:** feeding of an infant with food other than mother's milk. **A. lung:** an apparatus inducing artificial respiration, used in cases of respiratory paralysis. See also Drinker's apparatus, Paul-Bragg's apparatus. Syn. iron lung. **A. respiration:** the inducing of respiration by manual or mechanical means in cases of present or impending asphyxiation. See also Schaefer's, Schultze's methods of a. respiration, and above, A. lung.

Arum. A genus of plants. **A. maculatum:** yields sago.

aryepiglŏt·tic (G. *arutaina*, a ladle or cup; *epi*, on, *glōttis*, glottis). The same as arytaeno-epiglottic, *q.v.*

aryl. Abbreviation for aromatic alkyl, C_6H_5, aromatic radical.

arytaeno·epiglot·tic (G. *arutaina*, ladle or cup; *epi*, on; *glōttis*, glottis). Connecting the arytaenoid cartilage and the epiglottis.

arytāē·noid (G. *arutaina*, ladle or cup; *eidos*, form). 1. Resembling the mouth of a pitcher. 2. Relating to the a. cartilage. **A. cartilage:** the pyramid-shaped cartilage at the back of the larynx.

arytaenoidec·tomy (G. *arutaina*, ladle or cup; *eidos*, form; *ektomē*, excision). Removal of an arytaenoid cartilage.

arytaenoidī·tis (G. *arutaina*, ladle or cup; *eidos*, form). Inflammation of the arytaenoid cartilage or muscles.

Arzberger's pear (Arzberger, F., Austrian physicist, 1833–1905). A hollow oval-shaped ball for insertion into the rectum where it is cooled by passing water through it.

As. 1. Symbol for arsenic. 2. Abbreviation for astigmatism.

As. H. Abbreviation for hypermetropic astigmatism.

As. M. Abbreviation for myopic astigmatism.

as·ab. A type of venereal disease found in Africa.

asā·cria. Congenital absence of the sacrum.

asafoē·tida (L. *foetidus*, foetid). A gum resin obtained from the root of the *Ferula foetida*. Of unpleasant taste and therefore formerly used in the treatment of hysteria.

asbes·tiform. Of fibrous structure.

asbes·tos (G. *asbestos*, quick lime). A silicate of magnesium. Used in the manufacture of fireproof fabrics.

asbestō·sis. Pneumoconiosis due to inhalation of dust containing asbestos fibre; characterized by fine and diffuse fibrosis of the lungs, pleural adhesions, especially at the basal parts, and by the presence of 'asbestos bodies', typically of dumbbell or club shape with an asbestos fibre lying centrally, in the lesions; often leading to the development of bronchiectasis or pulmonary cavities.

ascarī·asis (G. *askaris*, a maw-worm). The condition of harbouring ascaris worms within the body, sometimes resulting in appendicitis, cholangitis, peritonitis, or, if there are numerous worms, in mechanical intestinal obstruction.

Ască·ridae (G. *askaris*). A family of nematode worms, comprising the genera *Ascaris*, *Ascarid*, *Lagochilascaris* and *Toxocara*, parasitic to man and to domestic animals and inhabiting mainly the small intestine of the host.

ască·ricide (G. *askaris*, L. *caedere*, to kill). A medicine that kills ascarides.

ascaridi·asis. Ascariasis, *q.v.*

ascăr·idole. Terpenoid constituent of oil of chenopodium.

Ascaris (G. *askaris*). A genus of nematode worms. **A. lumbricoides,** the common round worm of man and pig. The ova are passed in the stools and reach the intestine of a new host by ingestion of food or liquids. There they hatch out and the larvae migrate at once through the portal circulation and thoracic duct, eventually returning to the intestine where they grow into mature worms. **A. mystax:** an intestinal worm found in dogs and cats and sometimes also in children. **A. trichiuris:** the whipworm.

ascending (L. *ascendere*, to go up). Taking an upward course; e.g., a. colon. **A. degeneration:** a degeneration of nerve fibres beginning at some peripheral and progressing towards the central part.

Ascherson's vesicles (Ascherson, F. M., German physician, 1798–1879). Minute fat globules formed by agitating oil and liquid albumin.

Aschheim-Zondek test (Aschheim, S., German gynaecologist, born 1878; Zondek, B., German gynaecologist, born 1891). A test for pregnancy, carried out by injecting the urine of pregnant women into immature female mice. This produces premature maturation of the animals' ovarian follicles.

Aschoff bodies (Aschoff, L., German pathologist 1866–1942). Submiliary collections of cells and leucocytes in the interstitial tissues of the heart in rheumatic myocarditis.

As₂(CH₃)₄O. Cacodyl oxide.

asci·tēs (G. *askitēs*, from *askos*, bag). An abnormal collection of serous fluid in the peritoneal cavity, due to systemic circulatory insufficiency, the obstruction of the portal circulation (as in cirrhosis of the liver) or to inflammation of the peritoneum.

ascit·ic (G. *askitēs* from *askos*, bag). Pertaining to or affected with ascites.

Asclē·pias. A genus of asclepidaceous plants.

Ascoli's reaction (Ascoli, A., Italian serologist, born 1877). The thermo-precipitation test.

As·comycē·tes. A group of fungi which includes Penicillium and Achorion. These fungi are characterized by the asexual formation of spores within the sacs (asci).

ascor·bic acid (G. *a*, neg.; L.L. *scorbutus*, scurvy).

$$CO-C(OH)=C(OH)-CH.CHOH.CH_2OH.$$

Ascorbic acid is the anolic form of 3-keto-*l*-gulofuranolactone. Vitamin C, a water-soluble substance present in germinating seeds, green leaves and ripening fruits; synthesized in the bodies of most animals, except man, monkey, and guinea-pig, who develop scurvy when fed on a diet deficient in this factor.

as·cospores (G. *askos*, bag; *spora*, seed). Sexual structures in ascomycetes.

as·cus (G. *askos*, bag). In hyphal fungi, the structure (sac) in which the ascospores are formed.

-ase. A suffix designating an enzyme. Usually attached to a root describing the substance on which the enzyme acts.

asē·cretory. Having no secretion.

Aselli's glands or **pancreas** (Aselli, G., Italian anatomist, 1581–1626). A group of lymphatic glands situated at the root of the mesentery.

asep·sis (G. *a*, neg.; *sēpein*, to corrupt). Absence of living pathogenic micro-organisms.

asep·tic. Free from living pathogenic micro-organisms. **A. surgery:** surgery in which every instrument, dressing, the hands of the surgeon, etc., are made germ free.

asex·ual (G. *a*, neg.; L. *sexus*, sex). Without sex; non-sexual.

ash. 1. The residue of any burning process. 2. A tree of the genus *Fraxinus*.

asiā·lia (G. *a*, neg.; *sialon*, saliva). Deficiency or absence of salivary secretion.

-asis. Abstract suffix indicating a state or condition.

asĭ·tia (G. *a*, neg.; *sitos*, food). The same as anorexia; a loathing of food.

askĕ·lia (G. *a*, neg.; *skelos*, the leg). Non-development of the legs.

asō·ma (G. *a*, neg.; *sōma*, body). Omphalositic monster with absence of trunk.

aspar·tic acid (G. *aspharagos*, asparagus). HOOC-CH₂.CH(NH₂).COOH, *a*-aminosuccinic acid. Syn. Asparaginic acid.

aspăs·tic (G. *a*, neg.; *spaein*, to pull). Non-spastic.

aspeci·fic. Non-specific.

as·pect (L. *aspectus*, from *aspicere*, to look at). The look or appearance. **Dorsal a.:** the aspect towards the back.

aspergil·lar. Relating to Aspergillus.

aspergillō·sis (L. *aspergere*, to sprinkle). Infection with some species of aspergillus, affecting either middle ear, an abraded cornea, or the lungs. **A. pulmonary:** condition due to infection of bronchi and lungs by **Aspergillus fumigatus** or, more rarely, **Aspergillus nidulans:** characterized by the development of nodular formations in the lungs resembling aggregated tubercles, which may result in lobular consolidation, fibrosis, bronchiectasis, cavity formation, or emphysema, usually accompanied by fever and general wasting.

Aspergillus (L. *aspergere*, to sprinkle). A genus of hyphal fungi, including the species of **A. fumigatus, A. nidulans, A. bouffardi, A. niger, A. flavescens** and others, many of which give rise to antibiotic substances.

aspermat·ic (G. *a*, neg.; *sperma*, seed). Relating to aspermatism.

asper·mia, asper·matism (G. *a*, neg.; *sperma*, seed). 1. Inability to produce semen. 2. Inability to ejaculate semen during coitus.

asphyx·ia (G. *a*, neg.; *sphuxis*, pulsation). Suffocation; the suspension of life due to deprivation of oxygen. **Local a.:** lack of tissue respiration. **A. neonatorum:** respiratory failure of the new-born. There are two forms, **A. livida** and **A. pallida:** in the first the child is cyanotic, in the second it is pale and cold. The latter form is the more dangerous.

asphyx·iant (G. *a*, neg.; *sphuxis*, pulsation). An agent or condition capable of producing asphyxia.

asphyx·iate (G. *a*, neg.; *sphuxis*, pulsation). To produce or cause asphyxia.

asphyxiā·tion. Suffocation.

aspi·dinol. A constituent of male fern, which is also formed by the decomposition of filicic acid.

aspirā·tion (L. *aspirare*, to breathe). 1. The act of sucking up or sucking in; imbibition. 2. The act of using an aspirator. 3. Withdrawing fluids or gases from a cavity by suction.

aspirā·tor (L. *aspirare*, to breathe). An apparatus for withdrawing fluids or gases from a cavity by suction.

Aspirin. The name Aspirin is free in Great Britain and Northern Ireland, but is proprietary in all other countries. It is used for brands of acetyl-salicylic acid and aspirin tablets are employed as analgesics and antipyretics.

asplē·nia (G. *a*, neg.; *splen*, spleen). Congenital absence of the spleen.

Asplenium. A genus of ferns.

asporogen·ic (G. *a*, neg.; *spŏra*, seed; *gennan*, to produce). Not reproduced by means of spores.

aspŏr·ous (G. *a*, neg.; *spŏra*, seed). Without spores.

assault (L. *assultare*, to attack). In forensic medicine, unlawful attack on a person. **Indecent a.**: the touching or the attempt to touch, on the part of a male, any of the sexual organs of a female against her will.

assay (Old Fr. *assay*, from L. *exagium*, from *exigere*, to examine). The testing or analysing of a drug or a metal in order to determine the proportions of its constituents. **Biological a.**: the quantitative testing of a drug on an experimental animal or on an isolated animal organ.

Assézat's triangle (Assézat, J., French anthropologist, 1832–76). A triangle bounded by lines uniting the alveolar and basal points and the nasion.

assi·milable (L. *ad*, to; *similis*, like). Capable of being assimilated.

assimilā·tion. Metabolism; the process of changing food into tissue.

assō·ciated (L. *associare*, to join to). Joined; attached. **A. movements:** coincident movements of muscles other than the leading one which are involuntarily connected with its action.

association (L. *associare*, to join to). 1. Connection between objects or states. 2. Connection between an object or state and a mental experience. **A. centres:** areas of the cerebral cortex in which various sensual perceptions are supposed to be integrated. **A. fibres** or **A. tracts:** fibres or tracts connecting certain cortical areas in the same cerebral hemisphere. **A., free:** a psychotherapeutic method based upon the assumption that an individual relieved from the necessity of logical thinking and reporting everything going through his mind necessarily reveals subconscious material.

astā·sia (G. *a*, neg.; *stăsis*, a standing). Hysterical inability to stand.

astat·ic (G. *a*, neg.; *stăsis*, a standing). 1. Not static. 2. Not tending to take a fixed position.

ă·steatō·sis (G. *a*, neg.; *stĕar*, tallow). Absence of sebaceous secretion.

aster (G. *astēr*, star). 1. The stellate structure surrounding the centrosome. 2. Formerly also the stellate group of chromosomes during mitosis.

astē·reognō·sis (G. *a*, neg.; *stereos*, solid; *gnōsis*, knowledge). See agnosia, tactile.

astē·rion (G. *astēr*, star). A point on the skull corresponding to the junction of the occipital, parietal and temporal bones.

aster·nal (G. *a*, neg.; *sternon*, chest). 1. Without a sternum. 2. Not connected with the sternum.

aster·nia (G. *a*, neg.; *sternon*, chest). Absence of the sternum.

ă·steroid (G. *astēr*, star; *eidos*, from). Stellate. **A. hyalitis:** inflammation of the vitreous humour when spherical or star-shaped bodies are found in the vitreous.

asthē·nia (G. *a*, neg.; *sthenos*, strength). 1. Absence of strength; more especially adynamia. 2. Congenital constitutional anomaly characterized by tall and slender build.

asthē·nic (G. *a*, neg.; *sthenos*, strength). Characterized by asthenia.

asthenō·pia (G. *a*, neg.; *sthenos*, strength; *ōps*, the eye). Weakness of the ocular muscles or of visual power, due to errors of refraction, heterophoria, etc.

asthenō·pic. Characterized by asthenopia.

asthma (G. *asthma*, panting). A paroxysmal attack of severe dyspnoea, with a feeling of constriction and suffocation. **A., bronchial:** a. caused by spasm of the smaller divisions of the bronchi, with bronchial swelling and increased secretion. Though this condition can be produced in experimental animals by sensitization with various substances (production of an allergic condition) its 'natural' occurrence in man seems partly conditioned by a psychological (neurotic) factor. **A., cardiac:** a. due to sudden decompensation of the left ventricle leading to engorgement of the lungs. **A., uraemic:** a. due to uraemia. **A. crystals:** acicular crystals present in the sputum of asthmatic patients. Syn. Charcot-Leyden's crystals. **A., hay:** see under hay fever.

asthmat·ic (G. *asthma*, panting). Pertaining to or affected with asthma.

astigmat·ic (G. *a*, neg.; *stigma*, a mark). Pertaining to or affected with astigmatism.

astig·matism (G. *a*, neg.; *stigma*, a mark). Refractive anomaly due to abnormality of the corneal curvature, or more rarely to imperfection of the lens or the ciliary muscles, owing to which rays of light from a point do not converge to a point on the retina.

astigmatō·meter (G. *a*, neg.; *stigma*, a mark; *metron*, measure). An instrument for measuring the degree of astigmatism.

astră·galectomy (G. *astragalos*; *ektomē*, excision). Excision of the astragalus.

astră·galus (G. *astragalos*). The ankle bone or talus, upon which the tibia rests.

astrin·gent (L. *astringere*, to bind). The same as adstringent, *q.v.* Substance which binds or draws together soft tissues, by causing vascular contraction.

as·troblast (G. *astron*, star; *blastos*, germ). A glial cell less differentiated than the astrocyte.

as·troblastō·ma (G. *astron*, star; *blastos*, germ). A neoplasm derived from astroblasts, occurring especially in childhood.

as·trocyte (G. *astron*, star; *kutos*, cell). A type of glial cell characterized by a small cell body with a very large number of long slender processes.

astrocytō·ma (G. *astron*, star; *kutos*, cell). A relatively benign neoplasm which may occur anywhere in the central nervous system, characterized by differentiation of its cells into more or less characteristic astrocytes.

astrog·lia (G. *astron*, star; *glia*, glue). The same as macroglia, *q.v.*

as·trosphere (G. *astron*, star; *sphaira*, sphere). The central area of the aster (1) exclusive of the rays. Syn. attraction sphere; centrosome (1).

A.-V. interval. The time interval between the beginning of auricular and ventricular systoles.

asȳ·lum (G. *asūlon*, sanctuary). An institution for the care of the insane.

asym·metry (G. *a*, neg.; *summetria*, symmetry). 1. Absence of symmetry; unlikeness of corresponding organs that are normally of the same size, etc. 2. The linkage of carbon atoms to four different univalent atoms or atom groups.

asymptomat·ic (G. *a*, neg.; *sun*, together; *ptōma*, from *piptein*, to fall). Having no symptoms.

asȳn·chronism (G. *a*, neg.; *sun*, with; *khronos*, time). Absence of synchronism.

asȳn·clitism (G. *a*, neg.; *sun*, with; *klisis*, a bending). The condition of obliquity of two or more objects to each other; e.g., the oblique presentation of the presenting foetal part in parturition.

asynē·chia (G. *a*, neg.; *sunekheia*, a continuity). Absence of continuity in structure.

asyner·gia, asȳn·ergy (G. *a*, neg.; *sunergia*, co-operation). Lack of synergy; inability to co-ordinate different muscle groups as would be necessary for carrying out complex movements.

asynŏd·ia (G. *a*, neg.; *sunŏdia*, a journeying together). Sexual incapacity.

asynō·via (G. *a*, neg.; *sun*, with; L. *ovum*, egg). Absence or deficiency of the synovial fluid.

asystemat·ic. Diffuse; not restricted to a particular system.

asys·tŏle, asystŏ·lia (G. *a*, neg.; *sustŏlē*, contraction). Failure of the heart, or of a heart chamber, to beat.

asystol·ic. Characterized by asystole.

atac·tic (G. *ataxia*, disorder). Pertaining to or affected with ataxia.

atacti·lia (G. *a*, neg.; L. *tactus*, from *tangere*, to touch). Inability to recognize tactile impressions.

ă·tavism (L. *ătăvus*, ancestor). An obsolescent term, formerly applied to various mental defects, but limited to conditions appearing nowadays in man which were at one time normal characters of (e.g., prehistoric) man or of his progenitors.

atavis·tic. Characterized by atavism.

atax·ia, atax·y (G. *ataxia*, lack of order from *taxis*, arrangement). Inco-ordination of muscular action, usually without loss of muscular power. **Friedreich's a.:** a form of hereditary ataxia beginning in early life and due to sclerosis of the posterior and lateral columns of the spinal cord. **Hereditary cerebellar a.:** form of ataxia associated with congenital cerebellar defects, usually starting in young adult life. **Locomotor a.:** syn. tabes dorsalis.

ataxi-amnesic (G. *ataxia*; *amnesia*, forgetfulness). Marked by both ataxia and amnesia.

atax·iaphā·sia (G. *ataxia*; *aphasia*, from *phasis*, speech). A condition characterized by both ataxia and aphasia.

atax·ic (G. *ataxia*, lack of order). Pertaining to or affected with ataxia.

Atebrin. A proprietary preparation of the dihydrochloride of 2-chloro-5-(ω-diethylamino-x-methyl-butylamino)-7-methoxy-acridine. It is used to combat malaria.

atelec·tasis (G. *atĕlēs*, imperfect; *ektasis*, extension). 1. Failure of lung to expand at birth. 2. Collapse of a lung which has previously expanded.

ateleiŏ·sis (G. *ateleia*, incompleteness). Simple nanism, a form of hereditary infantilism not associated with any detectable lesion or dysfunction of endocrine or other organs.

atelencephă·lia (G. *atĕlēs*, imperfect; *egkephalos*, the brain). Imperfect development of the brain.

athalpŏ·sis (G. *a*, neg.; *thalpŏs*, warmth). Inability to feel warmth.

athē·lia (G. *a*, neg.; *thēlē*, nipple). Absence of a nipple.

ather·mic (G. *a*, neg.; *thermē*, heat). 1. Without loss of heat energy. 2. Without fever.

atherŏ·ma (G. *athărē*, porridge). 1. A sebaceous retention cyst containing cheesy material. Syn. wen. 2. Fatty and hyaline degeneration of the intimal layer of the arteries.

atherŏ·matous. Affected with atheroma.

atherosclerŏ·sis, atherŏ·sis (G. *athărē*, porridge; *sklēros*, hard). Atheromatous degeneration. (See atheroma, 2.)

ath·etoid (G. *athetos*, not fixed; *eidos*, form). Affected with athetosis.

athetŏ·sis (G. *athetos*, not fixed). A condition characterized by involuntary, slow, more or less rhythmical movements of the limbs, especially of fingers, from position of supination, abduction and extension to pronation, adduction and flexion, due to cerebral disorder, especially to striatal lesions. **A., double:** bilateral a.

athrep·sia (G. *a*, neg.; *trephein*, to rear). 1. Defective nutrition, especially in infants. 2. Immunity to malignant tumour cells owing to absence of suitable nourishment for their growth.

athrom·bia (G. *a*, neg.; *thrombos*, a clot). Defective blood clotting

athȳrŏ·sis, athȳroid·ism (G. *a*, neg.; *thureos*, a shield). 1. Absence of the thyroid gland. 2. The state resulting therefrom.

at·īte. The substance contained in milk that reduces nitrate to nitrite.

atlan·tal (G. *atlas*). Relating to the atlas.

at·las (G.). The first cervical vertebra.

atlo·axoid (G. *atlas*, first cervical vertebra; *axōn*, the second cervical vertebra; *eidos*, form). Relating to the first and second cervical vertebrae.

atlŏ·dymous (G. *atlas*, cervical vertebra; *didumos*, twin). A monster with two heads on a single neck and body.

at·mograph (G. *atmos*, steam; *graphos*, to record). An instrument for recording respirations.

at·mosphere (G. *atmos*, steam; *sphaira*, sphere). 1. Any gaseous medium, especially the air surrounding the earth. 2. A unit of pressure; the pressure exerted by the air upon the earth at 760 mm. barometric pressure, 14·7 lb. to the square inch.

atmospher·ic. Relating to the atmosphere.

atŏ·cia (G. *a*, neg.; *tŏkos*, birth). Sterility in the female.

atom (G. *atomos*, indivisible). The smallest unit of an element which is not changed by any chemical re-action; composed of a positively charged nucleus (a closely packed group of protons and neutrons, some 2,000 times heavier than the electrons) and of electrons surrounding the nucleus and neutralizing the electro-positive charge of the nucleus; the electrons are arranged in a series of 'orbits' around the nucleus and their distribution over these 'orbits' determines the chemical properties of the atom. The nuclear charge determines the place of the atom in the periodic system of chemical elements.

atom·ic (G. *atomos*, indivisible). Relating to an atom. **A. number:** systematic placing of an element, determined by the number of extranuclear electrons surrounding the nucleus. **A. weight:** the weight of an atom of an element measured by an arbitrary scale based on an atomic weight of 16 for oxygen.

atomĭ·city (G. *atomos*, indivisible). Chemical valence.

a·tomizer (G. *atomos*, indivisible). A spraying instrument.

atŏ·nic (G. *a*, neg.; *tonos*, tone). Characterized by atony.

atonĭ·city (G. *a*, neg.; *tonos*, tone). Lack of tone.

a·tony (G. *a*, neg.; *tonos*, tone). Lack of tone.

a·topen (G. *a*, neg.; *topos*, place). The substance that causes atopy.

Atophan. A brand of cinchophen.

atop·ic (G. *a*, neg.; *topos*, place). 1. Displaced. 2. Pertaining to atopy or to an atopen.

a·topy (G. *a*, neg.; *topos*, place). Natural or inherited hypersensitiveness to some substances.

atox·ic (G. *a*, neg.; *toxikon*, poison). Not toxic.

Atoxyl. A brand of sodium aminoarsonate.

atrac·toid (G. *atraktos*, spindle; *eidos*, form). Spindle-shaped.

atrĕ·mia (G. *a*, neg.; *tremein*, tremble). Hysterical inability to stand and walk. Syn. abasia-astasia.

atrĕ·sia (G. *a*, neg.; *trēsis*, a boring). Imperforation of an opening or of a canal. **A. ani:** imperforate anus.

atrĕ·sic, atretic (G. *a*, neg.; *trēsis*, a boring). Characterized by atresia.

atretocĕ·phalus (G. *a*, neg.; *trēsis*, a boring; *kephalē*, head). A monster foetus with imperforate nose or mouth.

at·rial. Relating to an atrium.

Atricha (G. *a*, neg.; *thrix*, hair). A group of bacteria, having some forms without flagella.

atri·chia (G. *a*, neg.; *thrix*, hair). Absence of the hair; baldness.

at·rioventric·ular (L. *atrium*, hall; *ventriculus*, dim. of *venter*, belly). Auriculoventricular, *q.v.*

atrip·licism. A disease occurring in North China, characterized by local oedema, disturbances of sensibility, vasomotor and trophic disorders, due to poisoning with the plant *Atriplex littoralis*.

at·rium (L. *atrium*, hall). 1. The auricle of the heart. 2. The part of the tympanic cavity of the ear below the head of the malleus.

Atrŏpa (G. *atrŏpos*, undeviating). A genus of plants of the order Solanaceae. *A. belladonna*, the deadly nightshade.

atrŏ·phia (G.). See atrophy.

atroph·ic (G. *atrophia*, atrophy). Pertaining to or affected with atrophy.

atrophoder·ma (G. *atrophia*, atrophy; *derma*, skin). Atrophy of the skin.

at·rophy (G. *atrophia*). Diminution in volume or abnormal smallness of cells, tissues or organs, resulting from developmental or nutritional disturbance. **Acute yellow a. of the liver:** acute hepatitis, a disease characterized by a grave general condition, deep jaundice, diminution in size of liver, gravely disturbed metabolism, excretion of cystine and tyrosine crystals in the urine, and progressive coma. **Brown a.:** presence of brownish granules in atrophic cells, occurring especially in the heart muscle. **Infantile a.:** severely reduced state of nutrition in an infant due to inadequate diet or to factors preventing normal ingestion and absorption of the food. **Optic a.:** a. of the optic nerve. **Peroneal muscular a.:** (Charcot-Marie-Tooth), progressive chronic disease, probably affecting primarily peripheral nerves, starting usually in peroneal muscles, of familial character, usually beginning in early childhood. **Pigmented a.:** the same as brown a. **Progressive muscular a.:** chronic disease due to lesions of the anterior horns of the spinal cord, characterized by progressive a. of the distal parts of the extremities and fibrillary twitchings, beginning in middle life. **Senile a.:** the more or less physiological a. of old age.

at·ropine (G. *Atropos*, the undeviating; one of the Fates who cut off life's thread). Alkaloid formed by racemization of hyoscyamine, the active principle of *Atropa belladonna*; paralysing the parasympathetic system and therefore mydriatic, antispasmodic and inhibiting external secretion of glands innervated by the parasympathetic nerve.

at·ropinism, at·ropism (G. *atrŏpos*, undeviating). The condition produced by the prolonged use of atropine.

at·tar (Persian, essence). Any volatile oil of vegetable origin.

atten·tion (L. *attentio*, from *attendere*). The direction of conscious thought upon a particular object or to a particular sensation.

atten·uate (L. *attenuare*). To make thin.

atten·uated (L. *attenuare*). Wasted; weakened; thinned.

attenuā·tion (L. *attenuare*). A weakening or a thinning.

at·tic (G. *attikos*, of Attica). The portion of the tympanic cavity above the atrium. Syn. recessus epitympanicus.

atticŏ·tomy (G. *attikos*; *tomē*, section). Surgical opening of the tympanic cavity.

at·titude (L. *aptitudo*, fitness). Posture.

attrac·tion (L. *attrahere*, to draw to). The forces acting between particles tending to draw them together. **A. sphere:** central mass of the aster in mitosis.

at·trahens (L. *attrahere*). A muscle that draws forward.

attri·tion (L. *atterere*, to rub away). Wearing away by means of rubbing or friction.

atў·pia (G. *a*, neg.; *tupos*, type). Irregularity.

atў·pical, Not conforming to type.

A.U. Abbreviation for Angström unit.

Au. (L. *aurum*, gold). The symbol for gold.

Aubert's phenomenon (Aubert, H., German physiologist, 1826–92). An optical illusion by which, when the head is bent to one side, a vertical line appears oblique towards the opposite side.

au·diogram (L. *audire*, to hear; G. *gramma*, a writing). A graphic recording of an audiometer, showing the relation of audibility to the frequency of sound.

audiŏ·meter (L. *audire*, to hear; G. *metron*, measure). Instrument for measuring the perception of sound.

audiŏ·metry (L. *audire*, to hear; G. *metron*, measure). Measurement of the perception of sound.

au·diphone (L. *audire*, to hear; *phōnē*, voice). Instrument for assisting perception of sound.

au·ditory (L. *audire*, to hear). Relating to the act or organs of hearing. **A. amnesia:** mind-deafness, *q.v.* **A. aura:** an a. sensation immediately preceding an epileptic attack. **A. centre:** the cerebral area relating to hearing.

au·ditus (L. *auditus*, from *audire*). Hearing.

Auenbrugger's sign (Auenbrugger, L. J., Austrian physician, 1722–1809). Bulging of the epigastric region in cases of extensive pericardial effusion.

Auerbach's ganglia (Auerbach, L., German anatomist, 1828–97). The ganglionic nodes in A.'s plexus. **A.'s plexus:** plexus myentericus, a nerve plexus situated between the longitudinal and circular muscular layers of the stomach and intestine.

Aufrecht's sign (Aufrecht, E., German physician, 1844–1933). Short and feeble breathing heard just above the jugular fossa on placing the stethoscope over the trachea; noted in stenosis of trachea.

augment. To increase.

augnā·thus (G. *au*, besides; *gnathos*, jaw). A monster with two lower jaws.

au·la (G. *aulē*, hall). The anterior portion of the third ventricle.

aulatē·la (G. *aulē*, hall; L. *tela*, web). The membrane covering the aula.

au·lic (G. *aulē*, hall). Pertaining to the aula.

auliplex·us (G. *aulē*, hall; L. *plexus*). The portion of the choroid plexus within the aula.

au·lix (L. from G. *aulax*, furrow). The fissure of Monro.

au·ra (G. *aura*, air). A sensation immediately preceding an epileptic fit.

au·ral (L. *auris*, the ear). Relating to the ear. **A. vertigo:** vertigo due to some disturbance of the labyrinth. See Menière's syndrome.

Aureomycin. A powerful antibiotic derived from streptomyces aureofaciens. It possesses a wide range of antibacterial activity and has been found effective in amoebic infections.

au·ricle (L. *auricula*, dim. of *auris*, ear). 1. The external ear, the cartilaginous structure acting as a collector of sound. 2. One of the upper cavities of the heart.

auri·cular (L. *auricula*, dim. of *auris*, ear). Relating to the ear or to cardiac auricles. **A. extrasystole:** extrasystole arising in an auricle. **A. fibrillation:** a paroxysmal or chronic condition in which the muscle fibres of the auricle take on independent and incoordinate action, while the ventricle responds as best it can to the stimuli and beats with complete irregularity. **A. flutter:** a condition either paroxysmal or chronic in which the auricular muscle is in a state of continuous excitation and contracts at a very great pace. The ventricle also beats rapidly but is unable to follow the rhythm of the auricle. **A. node:** a complex of nerve cells in the lower part of the a. septum; the origin of the auriculoventricular bundle, *q.v.*, in mammals.

auri·culocrā·nial (L. *auricula*; G. *kranion*, skull). Relating to both the ear and the cranium.

auri·culotem·poral (L. *auricula*; *tempora*, pl. of *tempus*). Relating to both ear and temple.

auri·culoventric·ular (L. *auricula*; *ventriculus*, dim. of *venter*). Relating to both auricle and ventricle of the heart. Syn. atrioventricular. **A.-v. bundle:** a complex of nerve cells conducting stimuli from the auricular node to the cardiac ventricles. Syn. His's muscle bundle. See also complex, ventricular.

au·riform (L. *auris, forma*). Ear-shaped.

au·ris (L.). The ear.

au·riscope (L. *auris*; G. *skopein*, to see). Instrument for examining the ear. Syn. otoscope.

au·rist. A specialist in diseases of the ear.

aurococ·cus. The *Staphylococcus pyogenes aureus*.

aurothĕ·rapy (L. *aurum*, gold; G. *therapeia*, medical treatment). The use of gold in treatment.

aurum (L.). Gold. Symbol: Au.

auscult; aus·cultate (L. *auscultare*, to listen to). To examine by auscultation.

auscultā·tion (L. *auscultare*, to listen to). Method of examining an organ by listening, either directly with the ear or by means of a stethoscope, to the sounds produced in it.

auscul·tātory. Relating to auscultation.

Australian X disease. A severe type of encephalitis caused by a virus, first recognized in 1907 in certain parts of Australia.

au·tacoid (G. *autos*, self; *akos*, remedy). Endocrine.

autar·cesis (G. *autos*, self; *arkein*, to defend). Natural immunity brought about by action of the body cells and not by means of artificially introduced antibodies.

au·tism (G. *autos*, self). A mental attitude in which the individual concentrates excessively on himself and turns away from the realities of the external world. One of the main symptoms of schizophrenia.

autis·tic (G. *autos*, self). Relating to autism.

auto-agglutinā·tion (G. *autos*, self; L. *agglutinare*). Spontaneous agglutination.

auto-antitox·in (G. *autos*, self; *antitoxin*). Antitoxin produced within the body, protecting it from disease.

au·toblast (G. *autos*, self; *blastos*, germ). A micro-organism.

autoch·thonous (G. *autos*, self; *chthōn*, land). Formed in the place where it is found.

au·toclave (G. *autos*, self; L. *clāvis*, key). 1. Self-fastening; self-closing. 2. Apparatus for sterilizing by high-pressure steam.

autoconduc·tion (G. *autos*, self; L. *conducere*, to bring together). A method of treatment by high frequency currents, in which the patient is standing in a solenoid receiving the current by induction.

autocytŏ·lysin (G. *autos*, self; *kutos*, a cell; *luein*, to to loosen). Autolysin, *q.v.*

autocytŏ·lysis (G. *autos*, self; *kutos*, a cell; *luein*, to loosen). Autolysis, *q.v.*

autodiges·tion (G. *autos*, self; L. *digerere*, to digest). Digestion of an organ by its own secretions.

autoē·cious (G. *autos*, self; *oikos*, a house). Relating to parasites having only one host.

auto·erŏ·ticism (G. *autos*, self; *erōs*, love). Sexual gratification by means of activities directed towards oneself.

autŏ·gamy (G. *autos*, self; *gamos*, marriage). 1. Self-fertilization. 2. Conjugation of closely related cells or karyogamy within a single cell.

autogĕ·nesis (G. *autos*, self; *genesis*, production). Self-production; spontaneous generation.

autogenet·ic (G. *autos*, self; *genesis*, production). Self-produced.

autŏ·genous (G. *autos*, self; *gennan*, to produce). Relating to a process or product generated within the body. **A. vaccine**: vaccine produced from the particular strain of micro-organism harboured by the patient.

au·tograft. A graft taken from any part of the patient's body for transference to another part of it.

autohaemothĕ·rapy (G. *autos*, self; *haima*, blood; *therapeia*, treatment). Treatment of a patient by intramuscular injection of his own blood.

autohydrŏ·lysis. Spontaneous hydrolysis.

autohȳp·notism (G. *autos*, self; *hupnos*, sleep). Self-induced hypnotism.

auto-immunizā·tion (G. *autos*, self; L. *immunis*, exempt). Spontaneous immunization.

auto-infec·tion (G. *autos*, self; L. *inficere*, infect). Self-infection.

auto-inŏ·culable (G. *autos*, self; L. *inoculare*). Capable of being inoculated upon the person already infected.

auto-inoculā·tion (G. *autos*, self; *inoculare*). Spread of an infection or other process, which has already infected the individual, to some other part of the body by contact, blood or lymph stream, etc.

auto-intoxicā·tion (G. *autos*, self; *toxikon*, poison). 1. A morbid condition due to toxic substances elaborated within the body. 2. The condition believed to be due to excessive intestinal putrefaction with absorption of toxic products.

autokĕ·ratoplasty (G. *autos*, self; *keras*, horn; *plassein*, to form). The carrying out of a corneal graft with tissue removed from the patient's other eye.

autolē·sion (G. *autos*, self; *laedere*, to hurt). Self-injury.

autŏ·lysate (G. *autos*, self; *luein*, to loosen). Substance obtained by permitting bacteria to digest themselves by the enzymes they produce.

autŏ·lysin (G. *autos*, self; *luein*, to loosen). A lysin acting upon the cells of the organism in which it has been formed.

autŏ·lysis (G. *autos*, self; *luein*, to loosen). Digestion of cells or cell-products by enzymes which have originated within the cells themselves.

automat·ic (G. *automatizein*, to act of oneself). Self-acting; performed without voluntary action.

autŏ·matism (G. *automatizein*, to act of oneself). Performance of actions without independent consciousness or intention.

automysophō·bia (G. *autos*, self; *musos*, uncleanness; *phobos*, fear). Neurotic fear of personal uncleanliness.

autonom·ic, autŏ·nomous (G. *autos*, self; *nomos*, a law). 1. Having independent origin, action or function. 2. Self-governing. **A. nervous system**: that part of the nervous system by which efferent impulses pass to tissues other than multinuclear striated muscle; it comprises the parasympathetic and the sympathetic nervous systems; its function cannot be influenced at will.

autŏ·nomy (G. *autos*, self; *nomos*, law). Self-law; subject to its intrinsic laws only.

autŏ·pathy (G. *autos*, self; *pathos*, disease). A disease for which no external cause can be held to account.

autophō·bia (G. *autos*, self; *phobos*, fear). Neurotic fear of one's self or of solitude.

autŏ·phony (G. *autos*, self; *phōnē*, voice). Altered resonance of the individual's voice as heard by himself.

au·toplasty (G. *autos*, self; *plassein*, to form). Repair of a wound by grafting fresh parts removed from the patient's body.

autop·sy (G. *autos*, self; *opsis*, vision). A post-mortem examination.

autŏr·rhaphy (G. *autos*, self; *raphē*, suture). Suture of a wound by tissue taken from its flaps.

autosē·rum (G. *autos*, self; L. *sĕrum*). Serum derived from the patient for whose treatment it is used.

autosex·ualism (G. *autos*, self; L. *sexus*, sex). Narcissism, *q.v.*

au·tosite (G. *autos*, self; *sitos*, food). 1. A monster capable of independent existence after birth. 2. That portion of a double monster that nourishes the other.

au·tosome (G. *autos*, self; *sōma*, body). A chromosome other than an allosome. Syn. euchromosome.

autosuggestion (G. *autos*, self; L. *suggestio*, from *suggerere*, to suggest). Self-suggestion; the influencing of one's own judgment by responding to own suggestion.

autothĕ·rapy (G. *autos*, self; *therapeia*, treatment). 1. Spontaneous cure of disease. 2. Autohaemotherapy.

autŏ·tomy (G. *autos*, self; *tomē*, section). Self-dismemberment.

autotox·in (G. *autos*, self; *toxikon*, poison). Any poisonous substance produced in the body.

autotransfū·sion (G. *autos*, self; L. *transfusio* from *transfundere*, to pour through). Forcing blood to the vital centres by bandaging the limbs and lowering the upper part of the body.

au·totransplantā·tion (G. *autos*, self; L. *trans*, across; *plantare*, to plant). Transplantation of tissue from one site to another in the same individual.

autotrŏ·phic (G. *autos*, self; *trephein*, to rear). Applied to micro-organisms able to utilize CO_2 and ammonia or nitrites as sources of C and N, respectively, and synthesizing from these simple substances their characteristic cellular components.

autovaccinā·tion (G. *autos*, self; L. *vacca*, a cow). Vaccination by the micro-organisms developed in the patient's body.

auxano·logy (G. *auxanein*, to increase; *logos*, a treatise). The science of growth.

auxanŏ·meter (G. *auxanein*, to increase; *metron*, measure). Instrument for measuring the growth of micro-organisms.

auxē·sis (G.). Increase in size by cell expansion without cell division.

auxi·liary (L. *auxiliaris*, helping). Giving assistance.

auxo-action (G. *auxē*, increase; L. *agere*, to act). The stimulating action of any substance.

auxocar·dia (G. *auxē*, increase; *kardia*, heart). Normal increase of the heart-volume during diastole.

aux·ochrome, auxochrŏm·ic (G. *auxē*, increase; *khrōma*, colour). See under dye.

aux·ocyte (G. *auxē*, increase; *kutos*, cell). The primary spermatocyte during its early growth stages.

auxŏ·logy (G. *auxē*, increase; *logos*, treatise). The science of growth.

auxospi·reme (G. *auxē*, increase; *speira*, a coil). The spireme of an auxocyte.

aval·vular. Without valves.

A. V. node. Auriculoventricular node, *q.v.*

avariŏ·sis (Fr. *avarie*, harm). Syphilis, *q.v.*

avas·cular (G. *a*, neg.; L. *vasculum*, dim. of *vas*, vessel). Not vascular; bloodless.

avascularizā·tion. Rendering bloodless.

Avellis's symptom complex (Avellis, G., German laryngologist, 1864–1916). Paralysis of one-half of the soft palate, associated with a recurrent nerve paralysis on the same side.

Avena (L. oat). A genus of grasses.

average deviation. Average amount by which individual values differ from the arithmetic mean of a series.

Avertin. A proprietary preparation of tribromoethyl alcohol, used as a basal narcotic in general surgery and given *per rectum*.

aviator's disease. Hypobaropathy, characterized by vasomotor disturbances and headache.

avi·dity (L. *aviditas*, from *avere*, to crave). Power of attraction; in chemistry, the property of certain acids to supplant another acid in its salt-compound.

avi·rulent (G. *a*, neg.; L. *virus*, poison). Not virulent.

avitaminŏ·sis (G. *a*, neg.; L. *vita*, life). Disease due to lack of a vitamin or of several vitamins.

Avogadro's law (Avogadro, A., Italian physicist, 1776–1856). Equal volumes of gases, at like temperature and pressure, contain an equal number of molecules.

avoirdupois (Fr.). A system of weights in which 16 ounces make one pound, the latter being equivalent to 453·6 grammes.

avul·sion (L. *avulsio*, from *avellere*, to tear away). The wrenching away of a part.

axanthop·sis (G. *a*, neg.; *xanthos*, yellow; *opsis*, vision). Yellow-blindness.

ax·ial, ax·ile (L. *axis*). Pertaining to an axis.

axi·fugal (L. *axis*; *fugere*, to flee). Centrifugal.

axilem·ma (L. *axis*; G. *lemma*, a husk). The sheath of an axis-cylinder of medullated nerve fibre.

axil·la (L.). The armpit.

axil·lary. Pertaining to the axilla.

axio- (L. *axis*). A prefix used in dentistry and meaning 'pertaining to the long axis of a tooth', e.g., axiocervical, relating to the axial and cervical walls of a dental cavity.

ax·ion. The brain and spinal cord.

axi·petal (L. *axis*; *petere*, to seek). Centripetal; in a direction towards an axone.

ax·is (L.). An imaginary line through the centre of a body. 2. The second cervical vertebra. A. cylinder: an axon surrounded by a myelin sheath; the conducting part of a nerve. A., fixation: the line joining a point in the middle of the eye on the optic a. with the point of fixation. A., optic: the line upon which the refracting surfaces of the eye should be centred. A. traction: traction on the foetus in the pelvic axis to hasten delivery. A.-t. forceps: forceps to perform axis traction. A., visual: the line joining the point of fixation and the fovea and passing through the nodal point.

axolem·ma (G. *axōn*, axis; *lemma*, husk). A delicate membrane, perhaps an artificial product of fixation, found under certain conditions to enclose the axis-cylinder.

Axolotl. See under amblystoma.

axon, axone (G. *axōn*, axis). 1. A fibre projecting from the cell body of a neuron and conducting impulses towards the dendrites of the next neuron. 2. The body axis. A. cervix: the second portion of an axis. A. degeneration: disintegration of the axis-cylinder. A. hill: first portion of an axon, characterized by absence of Nissl bodies. A. hillock: the first portion of the axon, a conical, clear area consisting of delicate axon fibrils; syn. implantation cone. A.-reflex: a reflex originating without ganglion-cells by conduction from one branch of a nerve-fibre to another.

ax·onal. Relating to an axis.

axonŏ·meter (G. *axōn*, axis; *metron*, measure). Instrument for locating the axis of astigmatism.

ax·oplasm (G. *axōn*, axis; *plassein*, to form). The substance holding together the fibrillae of an axon.

axospon·gium (G. *axōn*, axis; *spoggos*, sponge). Reticular structure of the axis-cylinder.

Ayerza's disease (Ayerza, A., Argentinian physician, 1861–1918). A form of erythraemia, characterized by cyanosis, dyspepsia, and hyperplasia of the bone marrow and associated with sclerosis of the pulmonary artery.

azo-compound (G. *a*, neg.; *zōē*, life). Organic compounds of the form R-N = N-R, R being an aromatic radical.

azŏ·ic (G. *a*, neg.; *zōē*, life). Destitute of living organisms.

azo-itch. A type of pruritus seen in persons working with azo dyes.

azŏŏsper·mia (G. *a*, neg.; *zōon*, an animal; *sperma*, germ). Absence of living spermatozoa.

azotaē·mia (G. *a*, neg.; *zōē*, life; *haima*, blood). Presence of abnormally high amounts of nitrogenous waste products (urea, etc.) in the blood. A., extrarenal: a. not due to renal disease but, e.g., to loss of chlorides, as in prolonged vomiting or diarrhoea, profuse sweating, etc.

azotae·mic (G. *a*, neg.; *zōē*, life, *haima*, blood). Pertaining to or characterized by azotaemia.

ā·zote (G. *a*, neg.; *zōē*, life). Nitrogen.

Azotobacter (G. *a*, neg.; *zōē*, life; *baktērion*, dim. of *baktron*, a stick). See nitrobacteria.

azotŏ·meter. An instrument for measuring the quantities of nitrogen in solutions.

azotū·ria (G. *a*, neg.; *zōē*, life; *ouron*, urine). Increase of nitrogen, especially urea, in the urine.

Aztec type. See under idiot.

azure granules. Cytoplasmic granules in lymphocytes staining red with Leishman- or Giemsa-stain.

azū·rophil (Medieval L. *azura*, from Arab. *allazward*, from Pers. *lazhward*, azure blue; G. *philein*, to love). Staining readily with an azure dye.

azurophi·lia. A condition in which azurophil granulation cells are found in the blood.

az·ȳgos (G. *a*, neg.; *zugon*, yoke). Not paired, term applied to certain muscles and veins.

az·ȳgous (G. *a*, neg.; *zugon*, yoke). Single; not in pairs.

azym·ic (G. *a*, neg.; *zumē*, ferment). Not causing fermentation.

azȳ·mous (G. *a*, neg.; *zumē*, ferment). Unfermented, unleavened.

B

β. The second letter of the Greek alphabet. See Beta.

B. Abbreviation for bacillus.

Ba. Symbol of barium.

Babes-Ernst bodies (Babès, V., Rumanian bacteriologist, 1854–1926; Ernst, P., German pathologist, 1859–1937). Granules in bacteria, staining more deeply than the rest of the cytoplasm.

Babesia, Babesidae (Babès, V., Rumanian bacteriologist, 1854–1926). Piroplasma, *q.v.*

Babinski's phenomenon or reflex (Babinski, J. F. F., French physician, 1857–1932). Extension of big toe with flexion of other toes on exciting sole of foot. It indicates a lesion of the pyramidal tract and occurs in organic but not in hysterical hemiplegia. **B.'s sign:** Diminution or loss of Achilles tendon reflex occurs in true but not in hysterical sciatica.

baby. An infant.

Baccelli's sign (Bacelli, G., Italian physician, 1832–1916). Aphonic pectoriloquy. The whispered voice is transmitted through a serous, but not purulent, exudate. The sign is generally considered unreliable.

Bacillā·ceae (L. *bacillus*, dim. of *baculus*). One of the lower families of bacteria.

bacillae·mia (L. *bacillus*, dim. of *baculus*; G. *haima*, blood). The presence of bacilli in the blood, without evidence of active multiplication.

bacil·lary (L. *bacillus*). 1. Relating to bacilli. 2. Caused by bacilli.

bacil·liform (L. *bacillus*; *forma*, shape). Resembling a bacillus.

bacilli·parous (L. *bacillus*; *parere*, to produce). Producing bacilli.

bacillophō·bia (L. *bacillus*, G. *phŏbos*. fear). Neurotic fear of microbes.

bacillū·ria (L. *bacillus*; G. *ouron*, urine). The presence of bacilli in the urine.

bacil·lus (L. *bacillus*, dim. of *baculus*, rod). A straight rod-shaped bacterium. **B. anthracis:** the cause of anthrax. **B. coli:** see bacterium coli. **B. pyocyaneus:** see pseudomonas pyocyanea. **B. typhosus:** see salmonella typhi.

bacitrā·cin. An antibiotic derived from organisms of the Bacillus subtilis group.

back. The posterior aspect of the trunk.

BaCl₂. Barium chloride.

Bact. Abbreviation for Bacterium.

bacterae·mia (G. *baktērion*, dim. of *baktron*; *haima*, blood). Presence of bacteria in the blood.

bacte·ria (G. *baktērion*, dim. of *baktron*, rod). 1. Unicellular micro-organisms in size between 0·2 and 60 μ which grow without the aid of chlorophyll and reproduce themselves usually by transverse division, and under suitable conditions with considerable rapidity. They comprise the families Coccaceae, Bacteriaceae, Spirillaceae and Trichobacteria. Syn. Schizomycetes. 2. In a less strict sense, microbes. **B., higher:** a family of micro-organisms intermediate between lower bacteria (Eubacteria) and moulds, growing out into branching threads and developing certain portions of their substance into productive bodies from which the new individuals grow; comprising the genera of Actinobacillus, Leptotrichia, Actinomyces and Erysipelothrix.

Bacteriaceae (G. *baktērion*). One of the lower families of bacteria. These micro-organisms multiply by fission.

bactēr·ial (G. *baktērion*). Relating to or caused by bacteria.

bac·terichō·lia (G. *baktērion*; *kholē*, bile). The presence of bacteria in the bile ducts.

bactericī·dal (G. *baktērion*; L. *caedere*, to kill). Destroying bacteria.

bactĕ·ricīde. An agent capable of destroying bacteria.

bactĕ·riform (G. *baktērion*; L. *forma*, shape). Shaped like a bacterium.

bac·terin. A bacterial vaccine.

bacteriŏ·logist (G. *baktērion*; *logos*, a treatise). One versed in bacteriology.

bacteriŏ·logy (G. *baktērion*; *logos*, treatise). The science pertaining to micro-organisms.

bacteriŏ·lysis (G. *baktērion*; *luein*, to loosen). Disintegration of bacteria.

bacteriŏ·lysin (G. *baktērion*; *luein*, to loosen). A specific antibody developed in the blood by the action of any one bacterium and causing the disintegration of the same bacterium.

bacteriolyt·ic (G. *baktērion*; *luein*, to loosen). Pertaining to bacteriolysis.

bacteriopathology (G. *baktērion*; *pathos*, disease). The science of micro-organisms in relation to pathology.

bactĕ·riophage (G. *baktērion*; *phagein*, to eat). Term applied to a group of filter-passing bodies, *q.v.*, of 20–50 μ diameter with a bacteriolytic action, widely distributed in nature.

bacteriophō·bia (G. *baktērion*; *phŏbos*, fear). Neurotic dread of bacteria.

bacteriŏ·scopy (G. *baktērion*; *skopein*, to view). The examination of bacteria through a microscope.

bacteriŏ·sis. Any disease caused by bacteria.

bactĕ·rio-solvent (G. *baktērion*; L. *solvere*, to loosen). An agent capable of causing the solution of bacteria.

bacteriŏ·stasis (G. *baktērion*, bacterium; *stăsis*, a standing still). Preventing the growth of bacteria.

bactĕr·iostăt·ic. Pertaining to bacteriostasis.

bactĕr·iothĕ·rapy (G. *baktērion*; *therapeia*, treatment). Treating disease by means of introducing bacteria into the body.

bactĕr·iotoxae·mia (G. *baktērion*; *toxikon*, poison). A condition characterized by the existence of bacterial toxins in the system.

bactĕr·iotrope (G. *baktērion*, bacterium; *trŏpē*, a turn). Having affinity to bacteria.

bactĕr·iotrop·ic. Opsonic, *q.v.*

bacteriŏ·tropin. Opsonin, *q.v.*

bactĕr·ium (G. *baktērion*, dim. of *baktron*, rod). Any of the genus of bacteria or schizomycetes. They may be spherical (cocci); straight rods (bacilli); twisted rods (spirilla). Those requiring free oxygen are *aerobic*, those not requiring free oxygen are *anaerobic*. **B. coli:** occurs normally in the intestines but is pathogenic if it gains entrance to the urinary system.

bacteriū·ria (G. *baktērion*; *ouron*, urine). The presence of bacteria in the urine.

bac·teroid (G. *baktērion*; *eidos*, form). Like a bacterium.

Bacteroides. A genus of anaerobic intestinal bacteria, mainly non-pathogenic.

bacū·liform (L. *baculum*, rod; *forma*, shape). Shaped like a rod.

Badal's operation (Badal, A. J., French ophthalmologist, 1840–1939). Rupture of the infratrochlear nerve for the relief of pain in glaucoma.

Baelz's disease (Baelz, E. von, German physician, 1845–1913). Progressive ulceration and ultimate destruction of the mucous glands of the lips; myxadenitis labialis.

Baer's vesicle (Baer, E. von, Russian anatomist, 1792–1876). The ovule.

bag. Any sac or pouch.

bag of waters. Foetal membranes containing the liquor amnii.

bagă·sse (Fr.). Fibre left after extracting sugar from sugar cane.

bagassō·sis (Fr. *bagasse*, fibre). Form of pneumonoconiosis due to inhalation of bagasse, characterized by cough, dyspnoea, scanty and sometimes bloodstained sputum, mild fever and patchy consolidation of the lungs.

Bagdad sore. Oriental sore, *q.v.*

Baillarger's outer band, line or **layer** (Baillarger, F., French physician, 1806–91). A white band in the layer of large pyramidal cells of the cortex cerebri. **B.'s internal band** or **line**: a white band between the layer of large pyramidal cells and the polymorphous layers of the cortex. **B.'s sign**: difference in the size of the pupils in persons with paralytic dementia.

Bain-marie (Fr. bath). A vessel containing water in which test-tubes, etc., are placed to be warmed or to be kept at a particular temperature.

bake. To harden anything by subjecting it to considerable heat.

bakendjia (African). An infectious disease, prevalent in the Congo, resembling in symptoms dengue fever. Syn. red fever of the Congo.

Baker's cyst (Baker, W. M., English surgeon, 1839–1896). Hernial protrusions of synovial membrane through the capsule of joints, most commonly occurring about the knee joint.

bakers' itch. Dermatitis, caused by the handling of yeast.

bakers' leg. Knock knee or genu valgum.

bakers' stigmata. Corns on the fingers, caused by the kneading of dough.

B.A.L. British Anti-Lewisite, $CH_2SH.CHSH.CH_2$ OH, 2:3 dimercaptopropanol. See dimepacrol.

bă·lance (L. *bilanx*, a balance having two scales [plates]). 1. An instrument for weighing. 2. Equilibrium.

balan·ic (G. *balanos*, primarily, an acorn, the glans penis). Relating to the glans penis.

balani·tis. Inflammation of the glans penis.

bă·lanoblenorrhōē·a (G. *balanos*, acorn; *blenna*, a mucous discharge; *rhein*, to flow). Inflammation of the glans penis due to gonorrhoeal infection.

bă·lanoplasty (G. *balanos*, acorn; *plassein*, to form). Plastic surgery applied to the glans penis.

bă·lanoposthi·tis (G. *balanos*, acorn; *posthē*, prepuce). Inflammation of the glans penis and of the inner surface of the prepuce.

bă·lanopos·thomikō·sis (G. *balanos*, acorn; *posthē*, prepuce). Balanitis complicated by gangrene.

bă·lanoprepū·tial (G. *balanos*, acorn; L. *praeputium*, prepuce). Relating to the glans penis and prepuce.

Balanti·dium (G. *balantidion*, dim. of *balantion*, a bag). A genus of ciliata. **B. coli**: a protozoan parasite, harbouring in the large intestine and producing ulcerative lesions; the largest protozoon affecting man (60–100 μ: 40–70 μ).

bă·lanus (G. *balanos*, acorn). 1. The glans penis. 2. The glans clitoris.

Balbiani's body (Balbiani, E. G., French embryologist, 1823–99). The yolk-nucleus or idiosome, a small body observed near the nucleus of the oocyte.

Balfour's disease (Balfour, G. W., British physician, 1822–1903). Chloroma, a condition with leukaemic deposits in bone, found especially in children and young adults.

Balkan splint (or frame). An apparatus used for the treatment of fractures of the femur by extension.

ball and socket joint. A joint, such as that of the hip, in which motion is possible in all directions. Syn. enarthrosis.

ball thrombus. An unattached *ante-mortem* clot in the heart.

Ball's operation (Ball, Sir C. B., Irish surgeon, 1851–1916). 1. The radical cure of an inguinal hernia by the obliteration of the neck of the sac, which is partially dissected out and then twisted around its own axis; the fundus is then cut off and the stump secured in the ring. 2. A special method of iliac colostomy. 3. Section of the cutaneous nerves to the anus for the relief of pruritus ani.

Ballet's disease (Ballet, G., French neurologist, 1853–1916). Ophthalmoplegia externa, *q.v.* **B.'s sign**: loss of all voluntary movements of the eyeball with preservation of the automatic movements.

Ballingall's disease (Ballingall, Sir G., British surgeon, 1780–1885). See under mycetoma.

ballis·tic (G. *ballein*, to throw). Relating to projectiles.

ballis·tics (G. *ballein*, to throw). Science of the movement of projectiles.

ballis·tocār·diogram (G. *ballein*, to throw; *kardia*, heart; *gramma*, a writing). An apparatus used to record the velocity of blood leaving the heart at each single heartbeat.

ballooning. The distension of a cavity by air or a water-bag.

ballottement (Fr.). Term relating to the phenomenon that a body suspended in a fluid, such as the foetus in the amniotic fluid, falls back, when suddenly pushed, into its original position.

balm (G. *balsamon*, the balsam tree). A soothing application.

bal·neology (L. *balneum*, bath; G. *logos*, discourse). The science pertaining to baths and their effect on the human organism.

bal·neother·apy (L. *balneum*, bath; G. *therapeia*, treatment). The treatment of disease by baths.

balneum (L.). A bath.

balsam (G. *balsamon*). A mixture of resins and volatile oils obtained from certain plants.

balsam·ic (G. *balsamon*). Pertaining to or resembling balsam.

Balser's fat-necrosis (Balser, W., German physician). An acute disease of the pancreas with areas of fat-necrosis in the interlobular tissue of that organ, in the omentum and mesentery, and sometimes in the pericardial fat and bone marrow.

Bamberger's bulbar pulse (Bamberger, H. von, Austrian physician, 1822–88). Pulsation in the internal jugular vein in cases of tricuspid insufficiency. The pulsation is synchronous with the systole. **B.'s haematogenic albuminuria**: the presence of albumin in the urine in cases of very severe anaemia.

band. Any structure or appliance that binds or is used for binding.

band-kerati·tis (G. *keras*, horn). Band-shaped opacity of the cornea in the exposed part slightly below the pupillary centre, occurring rarely as primary condition in advanced age, more commonly associated with irido-cyclitis.

Bandl's ring (Bandl, L., German obstetrician, 1842–1892). Retraction ring, sometimes felt above the pubis during parturition.

bandy leg. Bowed leg.

banian. Indian fig tree, the *Ficus bengalensis*, the bark of which has tonic properties.

bant. To practise William Banting's method of reducing obesity.

Banti's disease (Banti, G., Italian pathologist, 1852–1925). Enlargement of the spleen with progressive anaemia, followed by cirrhosis of the liver and ascites.

Banting treatment (Banting, W., English undertaker, 1797–1878). A method, devised by Banting, for the reduction of corpulence by the withdrawal of carbohydrates and the use of a nitrogenous diet.

bar·aesthesiŏ·meter (G. *băros*, weight; *aisthēsis*, perception; *metron*, measure). An instrument used to measure weight or pressure sensitiveness.

baragnŏ·sis (G. *băros*, weight; *a*, neg.; *gnōsis*, knowledge). Inability to recognize weight.

Bárány's sign (Bárány, R., Hungarian otologist, 1876–1936). See past-pointing.

Barbados leg. See elephantiasis.

barbed-wire disease. Confinement neurosis of prisoners of war.

barbers' dermatitis. Dermatitis of the hands of barbers.

barbers' itch. See sycosis.

barbiers (E. Indian). A native form of beri-beri.

barbitone. Barbital. $(C_2H_5)_2.C.CO.NH.CO.NH.CO$ 5:5-diethylbarbituric acid, used in the treatment of insomnia.

barbi·turate. Any derivative of barbituric acid. Such compounds are used as hypnotics or sedatives.

barbituric acid. Malonyl-urea, $CH_2CONHCONHCO$. A compound with hypnotic effect.

Barcoo rot (Austral., Barcoo is a river in Queensland). See under desert sore.

Bard's sign (Bard, L., Swiss physician, 1857–1930). To differentiate between organic and congenital nystagmus; in organic nystagmus eyeball oscillations increase when the patient follows the physician's finger, moved before his eye alternately from right to left and from left to right. In congenital n. the oscillations disappear under these conditions.

Bardinet's ligament (Bardinet, B. A., French physician, 1819–74). The posterior fasciculus of the internal lateral ligament of the elbow-joint; it is attached above to the postero-inferior portion of the internal condyle, and below to the inner side of the olecranon process.

barium (G. *baros*, weight). A metal of the group of alkaline earths. Symbol Ba. **B. enema:** an enema containing Ba. salts; used for radiological examination of the lower part of the intestinal tract, Ba. being opaque to X-rays. **B. meal:** a paste-like or fluid mixture containing Ba. salts, used for radiological examination of the alimentary tract.

bark. The outer covering of tree trunks and branches.

Barkow's ligament (Barkow, H. L., German anatomist, 1798–1873). Ligamentous bundles lying in the fatty tissue of the olecranon fossa.

Barlow's disease (Barlow, Sir T., English physician 1845–1943). Infantile scurvy, a disease seen in children under two years of age, frequently associated with rickets. The bones are tender and there may be subperiosteal haemorrhages. There is often sponginess of the gums with haemorrhages. It is due to deficiency of vitamin C in the diet.

Barnes's bag or dilator (Barnes, R., English obstetrician, 1817–1907). A lyre-shaped rubber bag for dilating the cervix uteri. **B.'s cervical zone:** the lowest fourth of the internal surface of the uterus. **B.'s curve:** the segment of a circle, having at its centre the sacral promontory and its concavity backward.

barŏ·meter (G. *băros*, weight; *metron*, a measure). An instrument used to measure atmospheric pressure.

barren (Old Fr. *baraine*). Sterile; incapable of producing offspring.

Bartholin's duct (Bartholin, C., Danish anatomist, 1655–1738). The larger and longer of the sublingual ducts. **B.'s foramen:** the obturator foramen. **B.'s glands:** the vulvovaginal glands.

bartholinitis. Inflammation of Bartholin's glands.

Barton's bandage (Barton, J. R., American surgeon, 1794–1871). A bandage used in fractures of the mandible. **B.'s fracture:** a fracture of the articular surface of the lower end of the radius.

Bartonella bacilliformis. A blood parasite which produces Oroya fever. See also Carrion's disease.

Baruch's sign (Baruch, S., American physician, 1840–1921). A sign used in the diagnosis of typhoid fever. The rectal temperature does not rise if the patient is placed in a tepid bath (75° F.) for 15 minutes.

barū·ria (G. *băros*, weight; *ouron*, urine). Condition in which urine of high specific gravity is passed.

bă·ryenocephā·lia (G. *bărŭs*, heavy; *egkephălos*, brain). Dimness of intellect.

baryglos·sia (G. *bărŭs*, heavy; *glōssa*, tongue). Slow and thickened speech.

barythy·mia (G. *bărŭs*, heavy; *thumos*, mind). The same as melancholia.

bā·sal (G. *basis*). Pertaining to the base. **B. cell carcinoma:** see under carcinoma. **B. ganglia:** thalamus and corpus striatum. **B. metabolic rate:** the minimal production of heat after 12 hours' fasting and sleep and during absolute rest.

base (G. *basis*). 1. The lower part of an organ. 2. The chief substance of a mixture. 3. An element or radical with which an acid may unite to form a salt.

Basedow's disease (Basedow, C. A. von, German physician, 1799–1854). Exophthalmic goitre.

ba·si-arachnoidi·tis (G. *basis*, a base; *arakhnē*, spider). Arachnoiditis confined to the base of the skull.

bā·sic (G. *basis*, base). 1. Alkaline. 2. Basal or basilar.

basichrōmat·in (G. *basis*, base; *khrōma*, colour). The basophile part of a nucleus.

basichrō·miole (G. *basis*, base; *khrōma*, colour). Basophil particle composing the chromatin of the nucleus.

basicrā·nial (G. *basis*, base; *kranion*, skull). Relating to the base of the skull.

basi·dium (G. *basis*, base). Fructification cells, bearing spores, of certain of the higher fungi.

basihy·al (G. *basis*, base; *huoeidēs*, the hyoid bone). Applied to the bone of the hyoid arch.

bā·silar (G. *basis*, base). Pertaining to the base. **B. impression:** congenital or acquired (e.g., due to Paget's disease, tuberculosis, etc.) anomaly of the occipital bone and the upper cervical vertebrae, resulting in a stenosis of the foramen magnum and cephalic bulging of the clivus and neighbouring bony structures into the posterior cranial fossa. (Syn. platybasia). **B. membrane:** membrane of the internal ear, separating the scala tympani from the scala vestibuli and the cochlear duct; the basis of Corti's organ.

basilem·ma (G. *basis*, base; *lemma*, rind). The basement membrane.

basil·ic (G. *basilikos*, royal). Prominent.

basilicon ointment. Rosin cerate, consisting of rosin 35 gm.; yellow wax 15 gm.; lard 50 gm.

basilō·ma. Carcinoma characterized by basal cells.

bā·sin. The third ventricle of the brain.

bā·sioglos·sus (G. *basis*, base; *glōssa*, tongue). The hyoid portion of the hyoglossus muscle.

bā·sion (G. *basis*, base). The centre of the anterior margin of the foramen magnum.

bā·siotribe (G. *basis*, base; *tribein*, to crush). An instrument for crushing the foetal head.

bā·siotrip·sy (G. *basis*, base; *tribein*, to crush). The operation of crushing the foetal head.

basirrhi·nal (G. *basis*, base; *rhis*, nose). Relating to the base of the brain and the nose.

E

bā·sis (G. *basis*, base). Foundation or beginning, or the main ingredient of any compound. **B. cerebri:** the base of the brain. **B. cordis:** the base of the heart.

basisphē·noid (G. *basis*, base; *sphēn*, a wedge; *eidos*, shape). The base of the sphenoid bone.

basket cell. A nerve cell surrounded by a network of fibrils derived from the axis cylinder of another cell.

Basle nomenclature. See under B.N.A.

bā·socyte (G. *basis*, base; *kutos*, cell). A basophil cell.

bā·socytopē·nia (G. *basis*, base; *kutos*, cell; *penia*, poverty). Basophilic leucopenia.

bā·socytō·sis. Condition characterized by great increase in the number of basophil leucocytes in the blood.

bā·sophil, bā·sophile (G. *basis*, base; *philein*, to love). Applied to cells readily stained by basic dyes. **B. adenoma:** see Cushing's syndrome. **B. erythrocyte:** see basophilia. **B. leucocyte:** a leucocyte found normally in connective tissue and present to about 1 per cent of all the leucocytes in the peripheral blood. Syn. mast-cell.

basophi·lia (G. *basis*, base; *philein*, to love). 1. Abnormal amount of basophil leucocytes in the blood. 2. Condition characterized by the presence of intracellular basophil granules in the red blood cells, occurring, e.g., in lead poisoning.

basophil·ic (G. *basis*, base; *philein*, to love). Basophil, *q.v.*

basŏ·philism (G. *basis*, base; *philein*, to love). The same as Cushing's syndrome, *q.v.*

basophō·bia (G. *basis*, a step; *phŏbos*, fear). Neurotic inability to stand or walk.

Bassia. A genus of tropical trees, including *B. latifolia*, *B. longifolia* and *B. butyracea*, from the seeds of which is obtained a semi-solid yellow oil with an unpleasant odour and taste.

Bassini's operation (Bassini, L., Italian surgeon, 1844-1924). A method for the radical cure of inguinal hernia. The conjoined tendon of the internal oblique and transversalis muscles is sutured to Poupart's ligament behind the spermatic cord.

bassorin. An insoluble part of tragancanth and many other gums.

bas·tard. Born out of wedlock; illegitimate.

Bastian-Bruns law (Bastian, H. C., British neurologist, 1837-1915; Bruns, L., German neurologist, 1858-1916). In complete transverse lesions of the spinal cord above the lumbar enlargement, the tendon reflexes of the lower extremities are abolished.

Bateman's disease (Bateman, T., English physician, 1778-1821). Molluscum contagiosum. **B.'s drops:** tinctura pectoralis, a weak tincture of opium, camphor and catechu; a popular remedy for coughs.

bath. 1. A vessel or occasionally a room used for bathing. 2. Any medium in which the body is washed and immersed for cleansing or therapeutic reasons. **B., Aix:** the massage of a portion of the body over which a stream of hot water, either in one large jet or from innumerable small ones, is passing. Syn. Vichy douche. **B., hot:** water bath used in the treatment of rheumatism. Mud or peat baths used for a similar purpose. **B., hot air:** consists of a box or chamber with walls composed of felt or asbestos, and arranged so that the contained air can be heated to a required temperature by an oil or gas burner or by electricity. **B., radiant heat:** an enclosed cylinder in which electric incandescent lamps are used as heating agents. **B., Russian:** similar to Turkish b., but the air is full of vapour of steam. **B., Turkish:** consists in the exposure of the unclothed body to dry heat at varying temperatures (of 220° F., or more).

Baths:

1. **Water.** Variable factors:

(i) *Temperature*

very hot	104-110° F.	⎫
hot	98-108° F.	⎬ Analgesic, Sedative and
warm	90-104° F.	⎭ Diaphoretic.
tepid	85-95° F.	Sedative.
cool	32-70° F.	Stimulating.

The temperature may be maintained at a constant level throughout, gradually raised or lowered (Ziemssen) or rapidly alternated (contrast baths).

(ii) *Mode of Application*
still water,
running water,
shower, (Scottish douche),
douche, a stream of water being applied under pressure, either alone or under still water, hot, cold, or alternately 105° F. for six minutes, followed by 70° F. for four minutes (contrast douches),
sheet, the body is wrapped in a sheet soaked in cold water to reduce temperature.

2. **Alkaline:** Water containing potassium carbonate 1 oz, or sodium carbonate 2 oz., per 10 gallons hot water.

3. **Medicated:** Produced by addition of various medications, pine, sulphur, bran, etc., to thermal water.

4. **Sulphur:** Exposure to natural water containing sulphides or sulphuretted hydrogen, or artificially produced by addition of 4-8 oz. potassium sulphide or sublimed sulphur to 30 gallons water.

5. **Mustard:** Household mustard, $\frac{1}{2}$–1 oz. per gallon, is stirred into hot water until the lather is yellow in colour. Used formerly in emergency treatment of infant convulsions, and as a footbath.

6. **Seaweed:** Contains seaweed or a decoction thereof, and therefore contains chlorides and iodides in solution.

7. **Vichy:** The reclining patient is massaged under a thermal douche.

8. **Brine:** Baths of artificial or natural water, with a mineral content of 0·2-30 per cent, mainly sodium chloride, but also chlorides of other elements and traces of bromides and iodides. May be non-gaseous or aerated with carbon dioxide, administered cold, warm, or hot, producing respectively stimulation, sedation, or analgesia. The usual concentration of 3-9 per cent is produced by water dilution, or the addition of 'mutterlanges' (salt concentrates) to the natural water as appropriate.

9. **Aerated:**

(i) *Carbon Dioxide.* Many natural waters contain dissolved carbon dioxide whose bubbles collect on the skin of immersed limb, and moving along its surface, give rise to cutaneous nerve stimulation, producing a warm pricking sensation which enables the bath to be taken at a lower temperature than would otherwise be possible.

(ii) *Nauheim.* Natural bath of carbon dioxide aerated brine.

(iii) *Schwalbach.* Artificial bath containing ferrous carbonate and made effervescent by carbon dioxide.

(iv) *Hafussi.* Hot water bath artificially impregnated with carbon dioxide in which hands and feet are immersed.

(v) *Oxygen.* Bath made effervescent by impregnation with oxygen.

(vi) *Sulphuretted.* Natural waters aerated with sulphuretted hydrogen.

(vii) *Foam.* Produced by blowing air or oxygen through hot water containing a saponin. The whole body is immersed in foam and rapidly attains a high temperature.

10. **Vapour:** (Berthollet.) Exposure to steam, naturally or artificially generated, in the former instance possibly admixed with natural gases, such as sulphuretted hydrogen. Temperature 122° F., i.e. hotter than hottest water bath.

11. **Russian:** Vapour bath generated by throwing water on heated metal. Followed by a friction, and a plunge into cold water, usually a lake or river.

12. **Swedish:** As for Russian, steam generated by action of water on hot stone.

13. **Hot air:** Exposure of body to hot air, which has a diaphoretic effect.

14. **Turkish:** Hot-air bath in which bather is subjected to a graded increase in temperature, then rubbed down, and finally given a cold douche.

15. **Indian:** A process similar to the Turkish bath with the addition of massage.

16. **Egyptian:** A modification of the Turkish bath in which the temperature, having reached the upper limit, is then reduced by similar stages to the initial level.

17. **Mud:** A paste of mineral earth and mineral waters of varying composition is applied locally or generally, left for 15 minutes, and then washed off with warm saline. The initial temperature of 104° F. is increased as is the duration of application at subsequent baths. In natural mud baths the patient lies on a slab exposed to the sun which supplies the heat. Mud is so poor a conductor of heat that the layer in contact with the body surface rapidly attains body temperature and remains at this level, so that there is no risk of burning even at high temperature.

18. **Sand:** Heated dry sand used in the same manner as mud.

19. **Peat:** An organic earth used in the same manner as mud.

20. **Wax:** Paraffin wax, melting point 115° to 120° F. used at a temperature of 120° to 130° F. and usually thermostatically controlled. Low heat conductivity enables higher temperature to be used than in the case of water baths. Mainly used for the hands and feet.

21. **Electric:**

(i) *Radiant heat.* Carbon or special tungsten filament electric bulbs in a cradle or cabinet, the walls of which are of polished metal to reflect the heat rays on to the body. Used to expose a part or whole of the body to infra-red and visible radiant energy.

(ii) *Infra-red.* Similar to radiant heat except that the radiating elements are of metal or fire clay raised to a temperature just below dull red, thus eliminating the visible rays.

(iii) *Sinusoidal.* Alternating current of 25 to 60 cycles surged between maximum and minimum thirty times per minute. Used in arm and leg baths to stimulate the peripheral circulation.

(iv) *Galvanic.* Continuous or interrupted unidirectional currents. Used in arm and leg baths in the treatment of neuritis and paralysed muscles.

(v) *Faradic.* Damped oscillatory discharges produced by a modified induction coil and used in arm and leg baths to exercise skeletal muscles.

bathophō·bia (G. *bathos*, depth; *phŏbos*, fear). Neurotic dread of looking down from a high place.

bath·yanaesthē·sia (G. *bathus*, deep; *anaisthēsia*, insensibility). Absence of deep sensibility.

bathycar·dia (G. *bathus*, deep; *kardia*, heart). A non-pathological condition in which the heart is placed low, due to anatomical structure.

bathygǎst·ria (G. *bathus*, deep; *gastēr*, stomach). Gastroptosis, *q.v.*

bathypnoe·a (G. *bathus*, deep; *pnein*, to breathe). Deep respiration.

batonō·ma (G. *bǎton*, blackberry). A tumour thought to be due to vegetable organisms.

bat·rachoplasty (G. *batrakhos*, frog; *plassein*, to form). A surgical operation performed in cases of ranula.

bat·tarism. Stammering.

bat·tery. Set of connected cells for the provision of electric current.

Battey's operation (Battey, R., American surgeon, 1828–95). Removal of the ovaries to eliminate their physiological influence, and so produce the menopause.

Battle's incision (Battle, W. H., English surgeon, 1855–1936). An incision along the outer border of the right rectus muscle; the muscle is retracted inwards and the posterior sheath of the rectus incised. Used in removal of the appendix.

battledore placenta. A placenta with a marginal insertion of the cord.

Bauhin's valve (Bauhin, C., Swiss anatomist, 1560–1624). The ileocaecal valve, guarding the entrance to the caecum.

Bazin's disease. See erythema induratum.

B.B.B. Abbreviation for blood-brain barrier.

B.C.G. Bacille Calmette-Guérin (Calmette, A. L. C., French bacteriologist, 1863–1933; Guérin, C., French bacteriologist, born 1872). A vaccine in which tubercle bacilli are attenuated by special treatment with regard to virulence but not with regard to antigenic action. Used for inoculation against tuberculosis.

B.D. Abbreviation for buccodistal.

b.d. Abbreviation for L. *bis die* (twice each day).

bdella (G.). A leech.

bdellŏ·meter. An instrument used in place of a leech.

bdelÿg·mia (G.). Nausea.

Be. Symbol for beryllium.

beak (L.L. *beccus*). 1. Mandibular portion of forceps. 2. Lower end of calamus scriptorius. 3. The pad or splenium of the corpus callosum.

beaker. Wide-mouthed glass vessel.

Beard's disease (Beard, G. M., American physician, 1839–83). Nervous exhaustion; neurasthenia.

Beard-Valleix's points. See under Valleix's points douloureux.

beat. The pulsation of blood in the heart and vessels.

Beatty-Wright's friction sound. The sound produced by inflammation of the pleura.

Beau's disease (Beau, J. H. S., French physician, 1806–65). Asystole; cardiac insufficiency.

Beaumês's sign (Beaumês, L., French physician, born 1865). Retrosternal pain in angina pectoris.

Beauvais's disease. Chronic articular rheumatism.

Bechterew's accessory lemniscus (Bechterew, V. M., Russian neurologist, 1857–1927). Same as B.'s tract, *q.v.* below. **B.'s disease:** ankylosis of the vertebral column, usually associated with muscular atrophy and sensory symptoms. **B.'s layer:** the layer of fibres between and parallel to the tangential fibres and Baillarger's layer in the cerebral cortex. **B.'s nucleus:** the nucleus of the vestibular portion of the auditory nerve. **B.'s sign:** anaesthesia of the popliteal space in tabes dorsalis. **B.'s tract:** the central tract of the tegmentum lying between the mesial side of the superior olivary body and the fillet.

Becker's sign (Becker, O. H. E., German oculist, 1828–90). Increased pulsation of the retinal arteries in exophthalmic goitre.

Béclard's hernia (Béclard, P. A., French anatomist, 1785–1825). Hernia which presents at the saphenous opening in the thigh. **B.'s nucleus:** the bony nucleus which appears in the lower epiphysis of the femur at the end of the ninth month of foetal life.

Becquerel's rays (Becquerel, A. M., French physicist, 1852–1908). Radiations of electrified particles or ions projected from radioactive bodies such as uranium, radium, polonium, or their salts.

bedbug. The *Cimex lectularius.*

Bed·lam (=Bethlehem). Asylum for the insane (from the hospital of St. Mary of Bethlehem in London, used as an asylum for the insane from the beginning of the fifteenth century).

Bednar's aphthae (Bednar, A., Austrian physician, 1816–88). Small roundish ulcerative patches in symmetrical spots on both sides of the posterior portion of the hard palate in cachectic infants.

beeswax. The wax obtained from honeycomb of the bee, **Apis mellifica.** Natural wax is yellow, white when bleached. Used in the preparation of ointments.

Begbie's disease (Begbie, J., Scottish physician, 1798–1869). 1. Exophthalmic goitre, Graves' disease. 2. Localized rhythmic chorea.

beget. Procreate.

Beggiatoa. A group of bacteria containing large amounts of sulphur. They are found mainly in stagnant water.

behaviour. The totality of responses to stimuli.

behaviourism. A psychological method and theory based on the objective study of responses (*behaviour*) without reference to consciousness (*sensations, feeling,* etc.).

Béhier-Hardy's symptom (Béhier, L. H., French physician, 1813–75; Hardy, L. P. A., French physician, 1811–93). Aphonia, an early symptom in pulmonary gangrene.

Beigel's disease (Beigel, H., German physician, 1830–70). 1. Trichorrhexis nodosa. 2. A trichomycosis of false hair which is communicated to the natural hair in contact with it.

bel. The unit of a logarithmic scale expressing the difference in levels of intensity of sound; equal to 10 decibels, *q.v.*

belch. An eructation of wind from the stomach.

Bell's mania (Bell, L. V., American physician, 1806–62). Very intense delirium associated with high fever, but without physical signs of pneumonia or of any of the exanthemata.

Bell's muscle (Bell, J., Scottish anatomist, 1763–1820). The urethro-ureteric ridge in the trigone of the urinary bladder.

Bell's paralysis (Bell, Sir C., Scottish physiologist, 1774–1842). Peripheral paralysis of the facial nerve. **B.'s phenomenon:** an outward and upward rolling of the eyeball when an attempt is made to close the eye: it occurs on the affected side in peripheral facial paralysis.

belladonna. The *Atropa belladonna,* commonly known as deadly nightshade. The leaves and tops, and also the root, are used in medicine, yielding hyoscyamine. Used as a narcotic and anodyne and is an antispasmodic and mydriatic.

Bellini's ducts (Bellini, L., Italian anatomist, 1643–1704). The excretory ducts of the kidney. **B.'s ligament:** a ligamentous band extending from the capsule of the hip-joint to the greater trochanter of the femur. **B.'s tubes:** the straight uriniferous tubules.

Bellocq's cannula or sound (Bellocq, J. J., French surgeon, 1732–1807). A hollow sound containing a curved spring, used for passing a thread through the nostril and mouth to draw in a plug in acute epistaxis.

belly. The abdomen.

Benadryl $(C_6H_5)_2CHOCH_2CH_2N(CH_3)_2$. β-dimethyl-aminoethylbenzhydryl ether. An antihistaminic drug.

Bence-Jones's bodies (Bence-Jones, H., English physician, 1813–73). Peculiar protein substance found in the urine in certain bone-marrow affections, especially multiple myeloma. **B.-J.'s cylinders:** long cylindrical formations derived from the seminiferous tubules, sometimes seen in urine.

Benedict's test for glucose in urine. Take 5 cc. of Benedict's solution and add 10 drops of urine and boil in a test-tube. A green or orange brown precipitate indicates the presence of a reducing sugar.

Benedikt's syndrome (Benedikt, M., Austrian physician, 1835–1920). Paralysis of the oculo-motor nerve of one side and hemiplegia and clonic spasm or tremor on the other.

Benerva. A brand of aneurine hydrochloride.

Benger's food. A proprietary food containing trypsin and amylopsin.

benign, benig·nant (L. *benignus*). Not endangering health or life; mild; opposite to malignant.

Béniqué's sound (Béniqué, P. J., French physician, 1806–51). A urethral sound.

Bennet's corpuscles (Bennet, J. H., English obstetrician, 1816–91). Large epithelial cells filled with fatty detritus, found in the contents of some ovarian cysts.

Bennett's fracture (Bennett, E. H., Irish surgeon, 1837–1907). A longitudinal fracture of the first metacarpal bone, extending into the carpometacarpal joint and complicated by luxation.

Benson's disease (Benson, A. H., English ophthalmologist). Asteroid hyalitis, *q.v.*

bentonite. A native colloidal, hydrated aluminium silicate, the principal constituent being montmorillonite $Al_2O_3,4SiO_2$, H_2O. Absorbs water to form sols and gels which can be used as suspending and emulsifying agents.

benzaldehyde. The oil of bitter almonds, C_6H_5CHO.

benzamide. A white crystalline substance derived from bitter almonds, $C_6H_5CONH_2$.

benzamine. The lactate and hydrochloride of 2:2:6-trimethyl-4-benzoyloxy-piperidine. A local anaesthetic.

Benzedrine. A proprietary preparation of Beta-amino-propylbenzene, used as a vasoconstrictor by inhalation in cases of hay fever, etc. Syn. amphetamine.

benzene (Ult. from Arab. *lubān jāwi,* frank-incense of Java). A liquid volatile hydrocarbon from coal tar, C_6H_6.

benzidine. $H_2N.C_6H_4.C_6H_4NH_2$ 4:4'-diamino-diphenyl, a crystalline compound produced by the action of acid on hydrazo benzene.

benzidine test. A test for detecting minimal amounts of blood in excretions, especially in faeces.

benzin, benzine, benzinum. Petroleum ether.

benzoate. Salt or ester derived from benzoic acid.

benzocaine. $H_2NC_6H_4COOC_2H_5$.Ethyl-*p*-amino-benzoate. A local anaesthetic.

benzoic acid. C_6H_5COOH. A crystalline, white acid obtained from coal tar.

benzoin. 1. The resin obtained from the Asian tree, *Styrax benzoin.* It is used as an expectorant. 2. $C_6H_5CHOHCO.C_6H_5$. Substance obtained by the action of dilute potassium cyanide solution on benzaldehyde.

ben·zolism. Benzene poisoning.

benzothe·rapy. The treatment of disease with benzoates.

benzpyrin. A polynuclear, aromatic hydrocarbon $C_{20}H_{12}$, which has carcinogenic properties.

benzyl benzoate. $C_6H_5CH_2OCOC_6H_5$. Used in the treatment of scabies.

benzyl penicillin. Penicillin-G; an antibiotic obtained from a mould of the genus penicillium.

Béraneck's tuberculin (Béraneck, E., Swiss bacteriologist, 1859–1920). Tuberculin made from filtrates of tubercule bacilli; lime and phosphoric acid being used as extractives.

Bérard's aneurysm (Bérard, A., French surgeon, 1802–46). An arteriovenous aneurysm having its sac in the tissue immediately surrounding the affected vein.

Béraud's ligament (Béraud, B. J. J., French surgeon, 1823–65). The suspensory ligament of the pericardium attached to the third and fourth dorsal vertebrae. **B.'s valve:** a fold of mucous membrane occasionally found in the lacrimal sac, which it separates from the nasal duct.

Berberis. A genus of shrubs, of which many have medicinal properties.

bergamot. A fragrant oil derived from the *Citrus bergamia.*

Berger's paraesthesia (Berger, E., Austrian neurologist, 1844–85). Paraesthesia of one or both legs in young subjects, aetiology unknown. **B.'s sign:** irregular pupil seen sometimes in early cases of tabes dorsalis.

Bergeron's disease (Bergeron, E. J., French physician, 1817–1900). An affection characterized by abrupt lightning-like and involuntary muscular contractions, usually limited to the head and arms, sometimes involving the two extremities of one side. Also known as electric chorea.

Bergmann's fibres (or Bergmann-Deiters' fibres) (Bergmann, E. von, German surgeon, 1838–1907; Deiters, O.F.C., German neurologist, 1834–63). The fibres of neuroglial cells of the cerebellum which pass to the surface. **B.'s incision:** an oblique lumbar incision to expose the kidney.

beriberi (Singhalese). A deficiency disease, due to lack of vitamin B_1 in the diet; characterized by polyneuritis and cardiac insufficiency.

Berin. A brand of aneurine hydrochloride.

Berlin's disease (Berlin, R., German ophthalmologist, 1833–97). Commotio retinae; traumatic oedema of the retina.

Bernard's canal (Bernard, C., French physiologist, 1813–78). The accessory pancreatic duct.

Bernhardt's paraesthesia, Bernhardt-Roth's symptom-complex (Bernhardt, M., German neurologist, 1844–1915; Roth, V. K., Russian neurologist, 1848–1916). Paraesthesia limited to the distribution of the external cutaneous nerve of the thigh.

Bernheimer's fibres (Bernheimer, S., Austrian ophthalmologist, 1861–1918). A tract of nerve-fibres extending from the optic tract to Luys's body.

berry. Any small, round, juicy fruit.

Bertiella satyri. A genus of tapeworm.

Bertillonage (Bertillon, A., French criminologist, 1853–1914). A system of recording the anatomic measurements and peculiarities of criminals for the purpose of future identification.

Bertin's bones (Bertin, E. J., French anatomist, 1712–81). The sphenoid spongy (turbinal) bones. **B.'s columns:** the fibrovascular septa which lie between the Malpighian pyramids of the kidney. **B.'s ligament:** the iliofemoral ligament.

Bertrand's test (Bertrand, G., French chemist, born 1861). A Fehling solution test for dextrose.

beryllium. A metal: called also glucinum. Symbol Be.

Berzelius's test (Berzelius, J. J., Swedish chemist, 1779–1848). A metaphosphoric acid test for albumin.

Besnier's rheumatism (Besnier, E., French physician, 1831–1909). Simple chronic articular rheumatism; chronic arthrosynovitis.

Best's operation (Best, V., Scottish surgeon, 1836–75). Subcutaneous suture of the external abdominal ring in cases of inguinal hernia.

bestiā·lity. Sexual relations with an animal.

Bestucheff's mixture or tincture (Bestucheff, A. P., Russian general, 1693–1766). The ethereal tincture of iron chloride used in erysipelas.

Beta (G. β, *bēta*). 1. Second letter in the Greek alphabet. 2. In physics: β-particles or rays; electrons emitted from radio-active substances. 3. In chemistry, applied to that substitution-product of (*a*) a straight chain compound in which the substituting atom or radical is attached to the C-atom next but one to the characteristic group; (*b*) a dicyclic compound in which the substituting atom or radical is attached to the 2, 3, 6, or 7 C-atom. 4. Beta-cells; the cell-type making up the bulk of an island of Langerhans and producing insulin.

beta-brocaine. Benzamine borate. A local anaesthetic.

β-eucaine. A brand of benzamine hydrochloride.

β-haemolytic streptococci (G. *streptos,* curved; *kokkos,* a grain). Strains of streptococci producing a zone of complete haemolysis at the margins of their colonies on blood-containing media.

β-hydroxybutyric acid. $CH_3.CHOH.CH_2COOH.$ An intermediate product of fatty acid oxidation.

β-oxidation theory. The conception according to which oxidation of fatty acids in human metabolism begins at the carbon atom in the β position, with the subsequent splitting off of two carbon atoms and formation of CO_2 and H_2O. The fatty acid chains thus formed are smaller by two carbon atoms but always retain the original odd or even number.

bē·tacism (G. *bēta*). Over-use of the b-sound in speech.

bē·tanin. The red pigment of beetroot.

betaine hydrochloride. $\overset{+}{(N(CH_3)_3}. \overset{-}{CH_2COO)}HCl.$ Used in achlorhydria to supplement gastric hydrochloric acid.

between-brain. The diencephalon.

Betz's giant cells (or giant pyramids) (Betz, V., Russian anatomist, 1834–94). Large ganglion-cells in the deeper layers of the cortex, especially in the ascending frontal convolution and the paracentral lobule.

Bevan's incision (Bevan, A. D., American surgeon, 1861–1943). A vertical incision along the outer border of the right rectus muscle, to expose the gall-bladder.

bex·ia. Smallpox of Brazil.

Bezold's ganglion (Bezold, A. von, German physiologist, 1836–68). A ganglion in the interauricular septum of the frog's heart.

Bezold's mastoiditis (Bezold, F., German aurist, 1836–68). Destruction of the apex of the mastoid process, tending to the formation of an abcess in the neck. **B.'s symptom:** an inflammatory swelling a short distance below the apex of the mastoid process indicates mastoid suppuration.

bezoar (Pers. *pādzahr*). Any concretion formed in the gastro-intestinal tract.

Bi. Symbol for bismuth.

bi- (L). Prefix meaning two or twice.

Bial's test (Bial, M., German physician, 1870–1908). A hydrochloric acid, orcin and liquor ferri sesquichloratis test for pentose in the urine.

Bianchi's nodule (Bianchi, G. B., Italian anatomist, 1681–1761). The corpora arantii, *q.v.*

Bianchi's syndrome (Bianchi, L., Italian psychiatrist, 1848–1927). Sensory aphasia with apraxia and alexia which is seen in lesions of the left parietal lobe of the brain.

bibā·sic (L. *bis,* twice; G. *basis,* base). Having two hydrogen atoms replaceable by bases.

bib·liomā·nia (G. *biblion,* book; *mania,* madness). Abnormal desire to acquire books.

bib·ulous (L. *bibulus,* from *bibere,* to drink). Having absorbent properties.

bĭcap·sular (L. *bis*, twice; *capsula*, a small box). Possessing two capsules.

bĭcar·bonate (L. *bis*, twice; *carbo*, coal). Acid carbonate. Any salt of carbonic acid in which one of the hydrogen atoms has been replaced by a base.

bĭcĕl·lular (L. *bis*, twice; *cella*, cell). Composed of two cells.

bĭcĕ·phalus (L. *bis*, twice; G. *kephale*, the head). See under dicephalus.

bi·ceps (L. *bis*, twice; *caput*, head). Having two heads; term applied to various muscles.

Bichat's canal (Bichat, M. F. X., French anatomist, 1771–1802). A canal considered by B. to exist between the subarachnoid space and the third ventricle. **B.'s fat-ball**: the buccal fat-pad, a mass of fat lying in the space between the buccinator and the anterior border of the masseter; well developed in infants. **B.'s fissure**: the transverse curved fissure passing below the splenium, its extremities corresponding to the beginning of the Sylvian fissure. It affords passage to the pia, which forms within the hemispheres, the tela choroidea and the choroid plexus.

bĭcĭ·pital (L. *bis*, twice; *caput*, head). 1. Pertaining to the biceps muscle. 2. Double-headed.

bicon·cave (L. *bis*, twice; *concavus*, hollow). Concave on both surfaces.

bicon·vex (L. *bis*, twice; *convexus*, rounded). Convex on both surfaces.

bicor·nuate (L. *bis*, twice; *cornutus*, from *cornu*, horn). Having two horns.

bicor·poral, bicor·porate (L. *bis*, twice; *corpus*, body). Consisting of two bodies.

bicou·dé (Fr.). Bent twice.

bĭcrescen·tic (L. *bis*, twice; *crescere*, to grow). Applied to a tooth with two ridges in the shape of a double crescent.

bicŭs·pid (L. *bis*, twice; *cuspis*, point). Having two cusps or points, as the premolar teeth. **B. valve**: the mitral valve of the heart.

b.i.d. Abbreviation for L. *bis in die*, twice daily.

Bidder's ganglion (Bidder, H. F., German anatomist, 1810–94). An accumulation of ganglion cells in the interauricular septum and the auriculoventricular groove of the frog's heart.

biden·tal (L. *bis*, twice; *dens*, tooth). Having two teeth or tooth-like prominences.

bidermō·ma (L. *bis*, two; G. *derma*, skin). A growth comprising two germ layers.

bidet (Fr.). A basin for irrigating the vagina or for use as a sitzbath.

bi·duous (L. *bis*, twice; *dies*, day). For two days.

Biebrich scarlet red. A red dye soluble in oils and fats, but insoluble in water. It is used as an epithelial stimulant.

Bier's hyperaemia (Bier, A. V., German surgeon, 1861-1949). A method of treatment by artificially causing passive congestion in the diseased part. **B.'s local anaesthesia**: 1. Anaesthesia caused in a limb by intravenous injections of ½ per cent cocaine after the part has been rendered bloodless by being raised and constricted. 2. Anaesthesia of the lower part of the body caused by injection of an anaesthetic into the spinal membranes.

Biermer's anaemia (Biermer, A., German physician, 1827–92). See Addison's disease. **B.'s change of pitch**: in hydropneumothorax the tympanitic sound is lower in pitch when the patient is sitting than when he is lying down.

Biernacki's symptom (Biernacki, E., Polish physician, 1866–1911). Analgesia of the ulnar nerve at the elbow; observed in tabes dorsalis and paretic dementia.

Biesiadecki's fossa (Biesiadecki, A. von, Polish physician, 1839–88). The fossa iliaco-sub-fascialis; a peritoneal recess bounded in front by a more or less well-defined fold, the inner surface looking upward over the psoas towards the root of the mesentery, the outer extending to the crest of the ilium.

Biett's collar (Biett, L. T., French dermatologist, 1781–1840). A zone of lenticulopapular syphilide on the neck.

bi·fid (L. *bis*, twice; *findere*, to cleave). Cleft; divided into two; forked; e.g. b. spine, see under spina bifida.

bifō·cal (L. *bis*, twice; *focus*, hearth). With a double focus. Applied to a system of lenses with two different foci.

bifor·ate (L. *bis*, twice; *fōris*, a door). Having two apertures or pores (foramina).

bifurcā·tion (L. *bis*, twice; *furca*, a fork). Division into two branches.

bigas·ter (L. *bis*, twice; G. *gaster*, stomach). Having two bellies, as a muscle.

Bigelow's ligament (Bigelow, H. J., American surgeon, 1818–90). The Y-ligament of the hip-joint. **B.'s septum**: the calcar femorale, a nearly vertical spur of compact tissue in the neck of the femur, a little in front of the lesser trochanter.

bigĕ·minal (L. *bis*, twice; *geminus*, twin). Occurring in two pairs.

bigĕ·minum (L. *bis*, twice; *geminus*, twin). One of the corpora bigemina.

bigĕ·miny (L. *bis*, twice; *geminare*, to double). A form of allorhythmia in which every two pulse-beats are separated by an interval longer than the preceding one.

bi·labe (L. *bis*, twice; *labium*, lip). An instrument for removing foreign bodies from the bladder through the urethra.

bilammel·lar (L. *bis*, twice; *lamella*, dim. of *lamina*, a plate). Consisting of two lamellae.

bilǎ·minar (L. *bis*, twice; *lamina*, a plate). Consisting of two layers.

bilǎ·teral (L. *bis*, twice; *latus*, side). Relating to two sides; affecting both sides of the body.

bile (L. *bilis*). The external secretion of the liver; an alkaline fluid composed of b. acids, b. pigments, cholesterol, lecithin, soaps, fatty acids, calcium and magnesium phosphates and other inorganic salts. **B. pigments**, see bilirubin.

Bilharzia (Bilharz, T. M., German physician, 1825-62) A genus of trematode worms. Syn. Schistosoma.

bilharziō·sis, bilharzi·asis. See Schistosomiasis.

bi·liary (L. *bilis*, bile). Pertaining to or conveying bile. **B. cirrhosis**: hypertrophic cirrhosis of the liver, with jaundice, due to disease of extra- and intra-hepatic bile ducts.

bilige·nesis. The production of bile.

bi·lious (L. *biliosus*, from *bilis*, bile). 1. Pertaining to the bile. 2. Pertaining to biliousness.

bi·liousness (L. *biliosus*, from *bilis*, bile). A popular name for a variety of conditions marked by nausea and abdominal upsets.

bilirū·bin (L. *bilis*, bile; *ruber*, red). A compound of two pyrrole-methenes joined by a methylene group; the chief pigment of bile, derived from haemoglobin and formed in the reticulo-endothelial tissue.

bilirubinǣ·mia (L. *bilis*, bile; *ruber*, red; G. *haima*, blood). See under hyperbilirubinaemia.

bilirū·binate. A salt of bilirubin.

bilirubinū·ria (L. *bilis*, bile; *ruber*, red; G. *ouron*, urine). Presence of bilirubin in the urine.

biliver·din (L. *bilis*, bile; *viridis*, green). The oxidation product of bilirubin.

Billroth's disease (Billroth, T., Austrian surgeon, 1829–94). 1. Spurious meningocele, a chronic, localized, extracranial collection of cerebrospinal fluid which retains a permanent connection with the subdural space. 2. Malignant lymphoma. Syn. Hodgkin's disease.

bilōbed (L. *bis*, twice; G. *lobos*, lobe). Having two lobes.

bilŏ·cular (L. *bis*, twice; *loculus*, dim. of *locus*, place). Having two locules or compartments.

bĭl·tong. Dried meat of a buck, native in South Africa.

bīmă·culate (L. *bis*, twice; *macula*, a spot). Having two spots.

bīmă·nous (L. *bis*, twice; *manus*, hand). Having two hands.

bīmă·nual (L. *bis*, twice; *manus*, hand). With both hands; two-handed; ambidextrous.

bīmăs·toid (L. *bis*, twice; G. *mastos*, breast; *eidos*, shape). Relating to the two mastoid eminences.

bīmaxil·lary (L. *bis*, twice; *maxilla*, jaw). Relating to both jaws.

bimolĕ·cular. Relating to two molecules.

bi·nary (L. *binarius*, from *bini*, two by two). Composed of two elements. **B. colour:** any colour composed of two primary colours. **B. fission:** cell division into two equal parts.

binau·ral (L. *bini*, two by two; *auris*, the ear). 1. Having two ears. 2. Pertaining to both ears acting together. 3. Used for both ears.

binaurĭ·cular (L. *bini*, two by two; *auricula*, dim. of *auris*, ear). Relating to both auricles.

bin·der. An abdominal bandage.

Binet's test, Binet-Simon scale (Binet, A., French physiologist, 1857–1911; Simon, T., French physician, born 1873). A method of testing the mental capacity of children.

Bing's entotic test (Bing, A., German otologist, 1844–1922). Spoken words which are not audible through an ear trumpet, but may be heard when spoken into a trumpet joined to a catheter in the pharyngo-tympanic tube, indicates that there exists a lesion of the sound-conducting apparatus.

binŏ·cular (L. *bini*, two by two; *oculus*, eye). Relating to both eyes acting together. **B. vision:** vision with the two eyes, normally characterized by a single perception of the object fixed, although two images are formed in the two retinae.

binŏ·vular (L. *bini*, two by two; *ovum*, egg). Produced by two ova.

Binswanger's dementia (Binswanger, O., German neurologist, 1859–1929). A form of pre-senile dementia, characterized by impaired memory and dullness of intellect.

binū·clear, binū·cleate (L. *bini*, two by two; *nucleus*, dim. of *nux*, nut). Having two nuclei.

Binz's test (Binz, K., German pharmacologist, 1832–1913). An iodine-potassium iodide test for quinine in the urine.

bio- (G. *bios*, life). A prefix signifying life.

bi·oblast (G. *bios*, life; *blastos*, germ). A primitive formative cell.

biochĕ·mistry (G. *bios*, life; Arab. *al-kimia*). The chemistry of living tissues. Syn. physiological chemistry.

$(BiO)_2CO_3 + \frac{1}{2}H_2O$. Approximate formula for basic bismuth carbonate.

biocoenō·sis (G. *bios*, life; *koinos*, common). The relation between organisms living in association.

biodynam·ics (G. *bios*, life; *dunamis*, force). The dynamics of life.

bio-energet·ics (G. *bios*, life; *ergon*, work). Transformation of energy from one form to another in living organisms.

biogĕ·nesis (G. *bios*, life; *gennan*, to produce). The doctrine that living matter arises only from living matter.

biogenet·ic (G. *bios*, life; *gennan*, to produce). Relating to biogenesis. **B. law:** the principle according to which the development of an individual animal re-capitulates that of the ancestral series to which it belongs (phylogeny).

biokinet·ics (G. *bios*, life; *kinein*, to move). The science treating of the movements of living organisms.

Biol. Abbreviation for biology.

biolŏ·gical (G. *bios*, life; *logos*, treatise). Pertaining to biology. **B. assay:** see under assay, biological.

biŏ·logist (G. *bios*, life; *logos*, treatise). One versed in biology.

biŏ·logy (G. *bios*, life; *logos*, treatise). The science pertaining to living organisms.

biŏ·lysis (G. *bios*, life; *luein*, to loosen). Destruction of life.

biolyt·ic (G. *bios*, life; *luein*, to loosen). Pertaining to biolysis.

biŏ·metry (G. *bios*, life; *metron*, measure). Application of statistics to biology.

biomicrŏ·scopy (G. *bios*, life; *mikros*, small; *skopein*, to view). 1. Examination of vital processes by the microscope. 2. Examination of the living eye by the slit-lamp.

bionŏ·mics (G. *bios*, life; *nomos*, law). Oecology, *q.v.* A branch of natural history dealing with organisms and their environment.

biŏ·nomy (G. *bios*, life; *nomos*, law). Measurement of life phenomena.

biŏ·phagism (G. *bios*, life; *phagein*, to eat). Feeding on living organisms.

biŏ·phore (G. *bios*, life; *pherein*, to bear). See pangen.

bio·physics (G. *bios*, life; *phusis*, nature). Study of physical phenomena in living matter.

bi·oplasm (G. *bios*, life; *plasma*, anything moulded). Protoplasm; the active part of the cell-plasm.

bi·oplast (G. *bios*, life; *plassein*, to form). 1. A cell. 2. The bioplasm.

biŏp·sia, biŏp·sy (G. *bios*, life; *opsis*, vision). Microscopic examination of tissue excised from the living body.

biŏ·scopy (G. *bios*, life; *skopein*, to view). Inspection of the body to determine whether life is extinct.

biŏ·sis (G. *bios*, life). Vitality.

biostat·ics (G. *bios*, life; *statikos*, causing to stand). The science of organic structure in relation to function.

biostati·stics. The science dealing with the laws of mortality in human beings.

Biot's respiration (Biot, C., nineteenth-century French physician). Meningitic respiration; rapid, short breathing, with pauses lasting from several seconds to half a minute, sometimes observed in healthy subjects during sleep, but most frequently in meningitis, when it is an unfavourable prognostic sign.

biotax·is, bi·otaxy (G. *bios*, life; *taxis*, arrangement). Taxonomy, *q.v.*

biothĕ·rapy. Treatment by means of living organisms.

biŏt·ic (G. *bios*, life). Pertaining to life; vital.

biŏ·tomy (G. *bios*, life; *tomē*, a cutting). Vivisection, *q.v.*

biotox·in. A toxin obtained from living tissue.

bi·otype (G. *bios*, life; *tupos*, type). Transmitted character.

bi·para (L. *bis*, twice; *parere*, to bear). A woman who has had two children.

bi·parasit·ic (L. *bis*, twice; G. *parasitos*, parasite). Parasitic upon a parasite.

bi·parí·etal (L. *bis*, twice; *paries*, a wall). Relating to both parietal bones. **B. diameter:** the distance between the two parietal eminences.

bi·parous (L. *bis*, twice; *parere*, to bear). Giving birth to two offspring.

bipar·tite (L. *bis*, twice; *pars*, part). In biology, composed of two parts or divisions.

bi·ped (L. *bis*, twice; *pes*, foot). Having two feet.

biper·forate (L. *bis*, twice; *per*, through; *forare*, to pierce). Having two perforations.

bipō·lar (L. *bis*, twice; G. *pŏlos*, pole). 1. Having two poles. 2. Applied to a nerve-cell having two projecting fibres.

BIPP. An artificial name given by Rutherford Morison (English surgeon, 1853–1939) and applied to a wound dressing composed of bismuth subnitrate 1 part, iodoform 2 parts and liquid paraffin 1 part.

birch. A tree of the genus *Betula*. It produces oils that are used in medicine.

Bird's formula (Bird, G., English physician, 1815–54). The last two figures of the specific gravity of the urine roughly indicate the number of grains of solids to the ounce of urine.

Bird's sign (Bird, S. D. Australian physician, 1833–1904). A well-defined zone of dullness with absence of respiratory sound in hydatid cyst of the lung.

birefrāc·tive, birefrin·gent (L. *bis*, twice; *refringere*, to break up). Doubly refractive.

birhī·nia (L. *bis*, twice; G. *rhis*, nose). Developmental dysplasia characterized by the presence of a double nose.

Birkett's hernia (Birkett, J., English surgeon, 1815–1904). Intraperitoneal inguinal hernia; hernia into the vaginal process of the peritoneum.

birth. The delivery of a child; parturition. **B.-control:** regulation of number of offspring by preventing or controlling conception. **B.-mark:** naevus pigmentosus. **B.-palsy:** a paresis due to a trauma received at birth. **B., posthumous:** b. of a child after the death of its father. **B., precocious:** b. of a child after a shorter pregnancy than normal. **B., premature:** see under labour. **B.-rate:** the proportion of births per thousand of the total population. **B.-trauma:** 1. Injury to the child occurring in the course of the birth process. 2. In psycho-analysis the mental trauma to the child occurring in the course of its birth which, in later life, may be the source of neurotic anxiety.

bische. A form of dysentery occurring in Trinidad.

Bischoff's operation (Bischoff, J. J., German gynaecologist, 1841–92). Abdominal hysterectomy of the gravid uterus.

Bischoff's test (Bischoff, C. A., German chemist, 1855–1908). A sulphuric acid and cane sugar test for biliary acids.

bisec·tion (L. *bis*, twice; *secare*, to cut). The act of cutting in two.

bisex·ual (L. *bis*, twice; *sexus*, sex). Having the characteristics of both sexes; hermaphroditic. Also called ambosexual.

bisexŭā·lity (L. *bis*, twice; *sexus*, sex). 1. Hermaphroditism. 2. Sexual attraction to individuals of both sexes.

Bishop's sphygmoscope (Bishop, L. F., American physician, 1864–1941). An instrument for measuring blood pressure.

Biskra boil, B. button (from Biskra, an Algerian town). See under Oriental sore.

Bismarck brown. A brown basic azo-dye, used in histological and bacteriological work.

Bismarsen. A proprietary preparation of bismuth arsphenamine sulphonate. Used in the treatment of syphilis.

Bismosan. A proprietary suspension of bismuth salicylate in oil.

bis·muth (L. *bisemuthum*). A pinkish-white metal. Derivatives used as astringents, antiseptics and for radiological examination of the alimentary tract. Symbol Bi.

bismuthō·sis. Chronic bismuth poisoning.

bi·stoury (Fr. *bistouri*). A long, slender, straight or curved surgical knife.

bisul·phide. A sulphur compound containing two atoms of sulphur to one of the other element.

bite. 1. Coaptation of upper and lower teeth. 2. Corrosion of a substance with an acid.

bitem·poral (L. *bis*, twice; *tempora*, temples). Pertaining to the two temporal bones. **B. hemianopia:** see under hemianopia.

Bitot's spots (Bitot, P., French physician, 1822–88). Xerosis conjunctivae.

bitter. Having an unpalatable astringent taste.

bitters. Medicines characterized by a bitter taste; they increase gastric secretion by reflex action on gustatory stimulation.

Bittner milk factor. Carcinogenic factor occurring in breast tissue and milk of certain high cancer-bearing strains of mice. Milk from such animals is capable of increasing cancer incidence when fed to mice of low cancer strains.

bituminō·sis. Pneumoconiosis caused by the inhalation of dust from soft coal.

bi·uret (L. *bis*, twice; G. *ouron*, urine). A substance obtained from urea; amide of allophanic acid. **B. test:** a test for detecting protein or amino-acids which contain the CONH group, performed by adding one drop of copper sulphate and potassium hydroxide; a violet colour is formed when protein or a protein derivative is present.

bi·valence (L. *bis*, twice; *valere*, to be strong). Property of an element to combine with two univalent or one bivalent atom or radical.

bi·valent (L. *bis*, twice; *valere*, to be strong). 1. Having a double valence. 2. Pertaining to bivalence. 3. Applied to two coupling chromosomes.

bi·valve (L. *bis*, twice; *valva*, the leaf of a door). Having two valves.

bi·venter (L. *bis*, twice; *venter*, belly). A muscle with two bellies.

Bizzozero's blood-platelets (Bizzozero, G., Italian physician, 1846–1901). Small round or elliptical non-nucleated bodies in the blood of mammals, including man. **B.'s corpuscles:** see under Neumann's corpuscles. **B.'s crystals:** see under Charcot's crystals.

black. The colour resulting from total absorption of the light rays or that represented by total absence of light rays. **B. death:** plague, especially the epidemic of A.D. 1350. **B. eye:** ecchymosis of the tissues around the eye. **B. spit:** see miners' phthisis. **B. tongue:** 1. Hyperkeratosis of the tongue in which black patches occur, usually in front of the circumvallate papillae, with filiform projections resembling hairs; Syn. hairy tongue, melanoglossia. 2. Disease in dogs, characterized by necrosis of the tongue and buccal mucous membranes and bloody mucous diarrhoea, due to deficiency of vitamin B_2. **B. vomit:** haematemesis, especially that occurring in yellow fever.

blackhead. The same as comedo, *q.v.*

blackout. Momentary unconsciousness with failure of vision due to diminished circulation in the brain; a well-known risk among aviators who are subjected to centrifugal force.

blackwater fever. See under fever.

bladder. 1. A membranous sac containing fluid or gas. 2. The sac-like receptacle for the urine. **B., irritable:** frequency of micturition, not due to an intrinsic disease of the bladder. **B., trabeculated:** A b. with hypertrophied muscle trabeculae forming pouches between each other.

blain. A blister or pustule.

Blainville's ears (Blainville, H. M. D. de, French zoologist, 1778–1850). Congenital asymmetry of the auricles, in size or shape.

Blancard's pills (Blancard, S., Dutch physician, 1650–1702). Pills of iron iodide.

bland (L. *blandus*). Soothing.

Blandin's ganglion (Blandin, P. F., French surgeon, 1798–1849). The sublingual ganglion, a small gangliform enlargement situated between the lingual nerve and the sublingual gland. **B.'s gland**: a muciparous gland situated near the tip of the tongue in the median line: it opens by several ducts on the lower surface of the tongue.

Blasius's duct (Blasius, E., German surgeon, 1802–75). The duct of the parotid gland (Stenson's duct).

blast. 1. A disease in sheep. 2. The effect of an explosion, especially of shell or bomb. **Immersion b.**: the effect produced on the human body in the water from an underwater explosion.

blastē·ma (G. a sprout). Undifferentiated protoplasm.

blă·stid (G. *blastos*, germ). The small clear space in the fecundated ovum; the precursor of the nucleus.

blastocele. See under blastocoele.

blă·stochyle (G. *blastos*, germ; *khulos*, juice). The fluid in the blastocoele.

blă·stocoele (G. *blastos*, germ; *koilos*, hollow). The central, or cleavage, cavity of the blastula.

blă·stocyst (G. *blastos*, germ; *kustis*, pouch). The same as blastula, *q.v.*

Blastocystis hominis (G. *blastos*, germ; *kustis*, pouch; L. *homo*, man). A protozoan, found normally in the intestine in man.

Blastodendrion. A genus of fungi.

blă·stoderm (G. *blastos*, germ; *derma*, skin). Germinal membrane of an ovum; the layer of cells on the surface of the yolk from which the ovum develops.

blă·stogĕ·nesis (G. *blastos*, germ; *genesis*, production). Budding.

blastŏ·lysis (G. *blastos*, germ; *luein*, to loosen). Germ destruction.

blastō·ma (G. *blastos*, germ). Any tumour originating from embryonic cells.

blă·stomere (G. *blastos*, germ; *meros*, a part). Any one of the segments produced by the first cleavages of the fertilized ovum.

Blastomy·ces (G. *blastos*, germ; *mukēs*, mushroom). A genus of budding fungi. **B. dermatitidis**: the fungus causing American blastomycosis. Syn. Gilchristia dermatitidis.

Blastomycē·tes. Budding fungi; fungi reproducing themselves by abstriction of hernia-like protruding spores (buds).

blastomycet·ic, blastomycot·ic (G. *blastos*, germ; *mukēs*, mushroom). Pertaining to blastomycetes.

blastomycō·sis (G. *blastos*, germ; *mukēs*, mushroom; *ousia*, existence). Any disease caused by blastomycetes. **B., American**: a chronic disease, caused by B. dermatitidis, characterized by subacute development of cutaneous granulomata containing miliary abcesses, sometimes followed after a period of years by spread to lungs, testes, bone and other tissues. Syn. infectious granuloma; Gilchrist's disease. **B., European**: see under torulosis.

blă·stophore (G. *blastos*, germ; *pherein*, to bear). The portion of the sperm cell not forming a spermatozoon.

blă·stophthor·ia (G. *blastos*, germ; *phthora*, destruction). Degeneration of germ-plasm due to some chronic disease.

blă·stopore (G. *blastos*, germ; *poros*, passage). The orifice of the blastula. Also called archistome.

blă·stosphere (G. *blastos*, germ; *sphaira*, ball). Blastula, *q.v.*

blă·stula (G. *blastos*, germ). The stage in embryonal development, following the morula stage, in which the ovum consists of a hollow sphere surrounded by one-layered epithelium.

blastulă·tion (G. *blastos*, germ). Conversion of the morula into the blastula.

Blaud's pill (Blaud, P., French physician, 1774–1858). A pill containing equal parts of iron sulphate and potassium carbonate; given in anaemia, amenorrhoea, etc.

bleaching powder. Chlorinated lime, disinfectant owing to its content of free chlorine.

blear-eye. An eye affected with ulcerative blepharitis.

bleb. A small bubble or blister. See also under *bulla.*

bleeder. A person with haemophilia, *q.v.*

bleeding time. The period during which blood is flowing from a puncture in the skin when it is sucked away with blotting paper every 30 seconds. (Duke's test.)

blen·nadeni·tis (G. *blenna*, mucus; *adēn*, gland). Inflammation of the mucous glands.

blennĕm·ĕsis (G. *blenna*, mucus; *ĕmĕsis*, a vomiting). Vomiting mucus.

blen·noid. Like mucus.

blen·nophthal·mia (G. *blenna*, mucus; *ophthalmos*, eye). Inflammation of the conjunctiva.

blennorrhā·gia (G. *blenna*, mucus; *rhēgnunai*, to break). Blennorrhoea, *q.v.*

blennorrhō̄e·a (G. *blenna*, mucus; *rhoia*, flow). 1. Purulent conjunctivitis. 2. Purulent colpitis or urethritis, especially that caused by gonorrhoea.

blennostat·ic (G. *blenna*, mucus; *stasis*, a stopping). Counteracting too profuse secretion of mucus.

blennū·ria (G. *blenna*, mucus; *ouron*, urine). The presence of mucus in urine.

blĕ·pharadeni·tis (G. *blepharon*, eyelid; *adēn*, gland). Inflammation of the Meibomian glands.

blĕ·pharal (G. *blepharon*, eyelid). Relating to the eyelids.

blepharec·tomy (G. *blepharon*, eyelid; *ektomē*, excision). Surgical removal of an eyelid lesion.

blepharelō·sis (G. *blepharon*, eyelid; *heluein*, to roll). Ingrowing eyelashes.

blĕ·pharism (G. *blepharon*, eyelid). Rapid involuntary winking; spasm of the eyelids.

blephari·tis (G. *blepharon*, eyelid). Inflammation of the free margins of the eyelids.

blepharo-adenō·ma (G. *blepharon*, eyelid, *adēn*, gland). Adenoma of the margin of the eyelid.

blĕ·pharo-atherō·ma (G. *blepharon*, eyelid; *athērē*, gruel). Sebaceous cyst of the eyelid.

blĕ·pharocarcinō·ma (G. *blepharon*, eyelid; *karkinos*, ulcer). Carcinoma of the eyelid.

blĕ·pharochă·lasis (G. *blepharon*, eyelid; *khalasis*, a relaxing). 1. A usually bilateral condition of the eyelids, characterized by loss of elasticity and atrophy of the lids and subcutaneous tissue, leading to permanent bagginess of the lids. 2. Freeing of the skin of the eyelids, as done in the treatment of trachoma.

blĕ·pharoclō·nus (G. *blepharon*, eyelid; *klaein*, to break off). Spasm of the orbicularis palpebrarum muscle.

blĕ·pharodiă·stasis (G. *blepharon*, eyelid; *diastasis*, separation). Excessive separation of the eyelids.

blĕ·pharon (G.). The eyelid; palpebra.

blĕ·pharophimō·sis (G. *blepharon*, eyelid; *phimoun*, to muzzle). Abnormal narrowness of the palpebral opening.

blĕ·pharophthal·mia (G. *blepharon*, eyelid; *ophthalmos*, eye). Combined palpebral and ocular conjunctivitis.

blĕ·pharoplast (G. *blepharon*, eyelid; *plassein*, to form). The basal structure from which a cilium grows.

blĕ·pharoplasty (G. *blepharon*, eyelid; *plassein*, to form). A plastic operation on the eyelid.

blĕ·pharoplē·gia (G. *blepharon*, eyelid; *plēgē*, a stroke). Paralysis of the eyelid.

blĕ·pharoptō·sis (G. *blepharon*, eyelid; *ptosis*, a fall). Ptosis of the eyelid.

blepharŏr·rhaphy (G. *blepharon*, eyelid; *raphē*, a seam). Suturing of the eyelids.

blĕ·pharospasm (G. *blepharon*, eyelid; *spasmos*, spasm). Spasm of the orbicularis palpebrarum muscle.

blĕ·pharostenō·sis (G. *blepharon*, eyelid; *stenos*, narrow). Narrowing of the interpalpebral opening.

blĕ·pharosynech·ia (G. *blepharon*, eyelid; *sunekheia*, continuity). Adhesion between the upper and lower eyelids.

blepharŏ·tomy (G. *blepharon*, eyelid; *tomē*, a cutting). Incision into the eyelid.

Blessig's groove (Blessig, R., German physician, 1830–78). The slight groove in the embryonic eye which marks off the fundus of the optic cup from the zone encircling the periphery of the lens, and corresponds in position with the future ora serrata.

blind. Unable to see. B. spot: the entrance of the optic nerve in the retina, an area containing neither rods nor cones and being insensitive to light stimulation.

blindness. Absence of vision.

blinking. Involuntary winking.

blister. A vesicle between epidermis and true skin, resulting from the exudation of a serous fluid.

blistering. Producing a blister.

block. 1. To obstruct, e.g. the passage of neural impulses; to repress or to inhibit, e.g. the function of a tissue. 2. In dentistry, a mass of gold foil for filling teeth.

Blocq's disease (Blocq, P. O., French physician, 1860–96). Astasia abasia; hysteric ataxia.

blood. The fluid circulating in the arteries and veins. B.-brain barrier: a hypothetical barrier which separates the blood from the parenchyma of the central nervous system. B. corpuscles: the cellular particles of the b. See also erythrocyte and leucocyte. B.-count: a count of the absolute number of red and white b. cells in a given quantity of b. B.-count, differential: a count of the relative numbers of white b. cells in a given quantity of b. B.-group: term relating to the classification of b. into several groups according to the property of its serum to effect, or not to effect, agglutination and haemolysis of the red b. corpuscles of another individual. See Moss's blood grouping, and also Rhesus factor. B.-pigment: see haemoglobin. B.-plasma: the fluid part of the b. B.-platelet: circular bodies from $1-3\mu$ in diameter, normally present in b. (about 2–400,000 per c.mm.) derived from megakaryocytes; related to the process of coagulation and thrombus-formation. Syn. thrombocyte. B.-poisoning: the morbid condition due to the circulation of pathogenic bacteria or their products in the b. B.-pressure: the pressure of circulating b. on arterial walls. B.-serum: the fluid squeezed out during the process of coagulation; b.-plasma less fibrin. B.-sugar, B.-urea, B.-chlorides, etc.: the amount of these substances present in the b. B. typing: determination of the b.-group, *q.v.* B.-vessel: an artery or a vein.

bloodless. Anaemic.

blood-letting. Opening of a blood-vessel, usually of a vein, for the abstraction of blood.

blue. A primary colour.

blue eye. The condition caused by infestation with the nematode *Harbronema*, characterized by blue-coloured eyelids.

blue pill. A mercury pill containing 33% mercury.

blue sclerotics. A condition of usually dominant inheritance, characterized by uniformly light blue sclerae (owing to diminution in scleral opaqueness) usually in association with osteogenesis imperfecta and nerve deafness.

blue-yellow blindness. A very rare congenital, more often acquired, defect of colour vision. Syn. tritanopia.

Blumenau's nucleus (Blumenau, L., Russian neurologist, 1862-1932). The lateral nucleus of the cuneate nucleus.

Blumenbach's clivus (Blumenbach, J. F., German physiologist, 1752-1840). The inclined surface of the sphenoid bone situated behind the posterior clinoid processes; it is continuous with the basilar process of the occipital bone. B.'s process: the uncinate process of the ethmoid bone.

Blumenthal's disease (Blumenthal, F., German physician, born 1870). Erythroleukaemia.

blush. To become red in the face, due to shame or emotion.

B.M.R. Abbreviation for basal metabolic rate.

B.N.A. Abbreviation for Basle Nomina Anatomica; a system of anatomical nomenclature agreed at Basle in Switzerland in the year 1895.

Boas's sign (Boas, I., German physician, 1858-1938). The presence of lactic acid in the gastric contents indicates cancer of the stomach.

Boas-Oppler bacillus (Boas, I., German physician, 1858-1938; Oppler, B., German physician). The *Lactobacillus Boas-Oppleri*.

Bochdalek's canal (Bochdalek, V., Austrian anatomist, 1801-83). A very small duct which passes through the membrana tympani. B.'s ganglion: a small supramaxillary ganglion on the middle superior dental nerve.

Bock's pharyngeal nerve (Bock, A. C., German anatomist, 1782-1833). The posterior efferent (pterygopalatine) branch of the sphenopalatine ganglion.

Bockhart's impetigo (Bockhart, M., nineteenth-century German physician). Epidermic abscesses caused by pyogenic micrococci and involving the hair follicles.

Bodo. A genus of Bodonidae.

Bodonidae. A family of flagellates; occasionally found in human faeces.

body. 1. Mass of matter. 2. The animal structure. 3. The trunk, as opposed to the head and the limbs. 4. The important or the largest part of an organ. 5. Cadaver or corpse.

Boeck's disease (Boeck, C. P. M., Norwegian dermatologist, 1845–1917). See sarcoidosis.

Boeck's scabies (Boeck, C. W., Norwegian dermatologist, 1808–75). Scabies crustosa; Norwegian itch; a severe form of scabies said to be contracted by handling the skins of wolves containing the itch-mite.

Boedeker's test (Boedeker, C. H. D., German chemist, 1815–95). An acetic acid and potassium ferrocyanide test for albumin.

Boerhaave's glands (Boerhaave, H., Dutch physician, 1668–1738). The sudoriparous glands.

Boettcher's cells (Boettcher, A., German anatomist, 1831–89). Dark-coloured cells with a basally situated nucleus, found between Claudius's cells. B.'s crystals: crystals found in the spermatic fluid and probably identical with Charcot's crystals, though of a somewhat different system of crystallization.

Bogros's space (Bogros, A. J., French anatomist, 1786-1823). A retroperitoneal space in the iliac fossa which lodges the external iliac artery.

Bogrow's fibres. A tract of nerve fibres passing from the optic tract to the optic thalamus.

Böhler's splint (Böhler, L., Austrian surgeon, born 1885). A wooden splint, with a head rounded to fit into the axilla.

Böhme's Indol test. See Ehrlich's reagent.

Bohun upas. *Antiaris toxicaria*, a deadly poisonous tree found in Java.

boil. A furuncle; a localized abscess of the skin due to infection of a hair-follicle or sweat-gland, usually by staphylococci.

Bolognini's sign. On pressure with the tips of the fingers of both hands alternately upon right and left of the abdomen of a patient resting on his back with abdominal muscles relaxed by flexion of the thighs, a sensation of friction within the abdomen is perceived; this is observed in the early stages of measles.

bolŏ·meter (G. *bolē*, a throw; *metron*, measure). 1. An instrument used to measure the force of the heart beat. 2. An instrument for measuring radiant energy by registering the change in the conductivity of a black body.

bolus (L.). A pill-like mass of large size.

bone. 1. The hard tissue forming the skeleton of the higher vertebrates, composed of a dense form of connective tissue containing ossein and osseomucoid impregnated with mineral salts, especially calcium phosphate. 2. Any distinct piece of skeleton. **Cancellous b.:** b. consisting chiefly of cancellous or spongy tissue. **B. conduction:** the transmission of sound waves to the auditory nerve by way of the bones of the skull. **B., flat.:** a bone approximating in form to a plate, e.g. a rib. **B., long.:** a b. consisting of a long shaft and two expanded ends, e.g. the humerus. **B., rider's:** an ossification of the lower tendon of the adductor longus muscle, due to often repeated pressure. **Basi-occipital:** the compressed quadrilateral mass of the occipital bone which projects forwards and upwards in front of the foramen magnum. **Bertin's** or sphenoidal conchae are situated on the anterior and inferior surfaces of the body of the sphenoid, of which they form a large part. **Bregmatic:** a small ossicle which develops at times in the anterior fontanelle of the foetal skull. **Calcaneum** or os calcis, the heel bone and the largest bone of the tarsus. **Capitate** or os magnum, the largest bone of the carpus. **Cuboid:** a large tarsal bone situated on the outer side of the foot. **Cuneiform:** three bones situated in front of the scaphoid bone. Cuneiform bone of hand. Syn. triquetral. **Epipteric:** a small bone inconstant in size and shape situated at the pterion of the skull. **Ethmoid** is situated at the anterior part of the base of the skull, where it lies in the middle line in front of the sphenoid. A portion of it occupies the ethmoidal notch between the orbital plates of the frontal, whence the greater part of the bone projects downwards, to take part in the formation of the orbits and nasal fossae. **Exoccipital:** the condylar portions of the occipital bone which are placed on each side of the foramen magnum of the skull. **Femur:** thigh bone, and extends from the hip to the knee. **Fibula,** or peroneal bone, is situated on the lateral or postaxial side of the tibia. It is very slender for its length. **Frontal:** forms the forehead and greater part of the roof of each orbit, and lies in front of the parietal bones. **Hamate:** a carpal bone which is characterized by a hook-like process on its palmar surface. **Hip** (os coxae) or innominate bone forms the lateral, and one half of the ventral, wall of the pelvis. **Humerus:** a long bone which extends from the shoulder to the elbow. **Hyoid:** a small bone situated in the median line of the neck between the chin and the thyroid cartilage of the larynx. **Innominate:** see hip. **Intermaxillary:** a small portion of the maxilla which bears the central and lateral incisor teeth. It is an independent bone in many animals. **Interparietal:** the upper part of the tabular portion of the occipital bone which may remain separate throughout life. **Ischium:** forms the lower and back part of the hip bone. **Lacrimal:** a small bone situated at the anterior part of the inner wall of the orbit, where it lies behind the frontal process of the maxilla, and in front of the orbital plate of the ethmoid. **Lunate:** a carpal bone which is characterized by the crescentic concavity on its distal surface. **Malar:** see zygomatic bone. **Mandible** or lower jaw which supports the teeth, and articu-

lates on each side with the anterior part of the articular fossa of the temporal in a freely movable manner. **Maxilla** or upper jaw, it forms, with its fellow, a large part of the face, and, besides supporting the upper teeth of its own side, it enters into the formation of the orbit, nasal fossa, and hard palate. **Nasal:** a small bone, which articulates with its fellow by its medial border and forms with it the bridge of the nose. **Navicular pedis,** or scaphoid bone, so named from its fancied resemblance to a boat. It is situated on the medial side of the foot, where it is placed in front of the talus, and behind the three cuneiform bones. **Occipital** is so named because it occupies the posterior and inferior parts of the cranium. It is flat and curved, its long axis extending from above downwards and forwards. **Palatine:** enters into the formation of the hard palate, the outer wall of the nasal fossa, and the floor of the orbit. It consists of a horizontal and perpendicular plate, which meet at a right angle, and of four processes. **Parietal** are so named because they form a large part of the cranial wall. They lie between the frontal and occipital, and superiorly they articulate with each other by the sagittal or interparietal suture. Each bone is quadrilateral and curved, and presents two surfaces, four borders, and four angles. **Pisiform:** a small pea-shaped carpal bone placed in front of the triquetral bone. **Pubic** (os pubis): a part of the hip bone which lies in the ventral wall of the pelvis. **Radius** is the preaxial (lateral) bone of the forearm. It is parallel with, and shorter than, the ulna, and extends from the elbow to the wrist. **Scaphoid:** characterized by its boat-like shape is a carpal bone and lies with its long axis oblique, the broad end being directed proximally and medially. **Scaphoid pedis:** see navicular pedis. **Sphenoid** is so named from the wedge-like position which it occupies in the base of the skull, where it lies with its long axis placed transversely. It enters into the formation of the anterior, middle, and posterior fossae, of the base, the temporal and nasal fossae, and the orbits. **Talus,** or astragalus, is characterized by having a head, neck, and body. It is situated between the tibia proximally and the calcaneum distally, is grasped laterally by the tibial and fibular malleoli, and has the navicular in front. **Temporal** (ossa temporis) are so named because the hair over the temple is the first to become grey, thus indicating advance in life. Each bone is situated on the lateral aspect of the head below the parietal. **Tibia,** or shin bone, is the medial or foreaxial and larger of the two bones of the leg, and alone transmits the weight of the body to the foot. **Trapezium** is the lateral bone of the distal row of the carpus, and is characterized by a groove and ridge on its palmar surface, and a saddle-shaped facet on its distal surface. **Trapezoid:** a small carpal bone in the distal row of the carpus and somewhat resembles the trapezium but is destitute of a groove and tuberosity. **Triquetral:** a small bone in the proximal row of the carpus and is characterized by its resemblance to a wedge, or pyramid, and it lies obliquely with its base directed laterally and proximally. **Tympanic:** a circular disc of bone which forms the tympanic ring in the foetal skull. **Ulna** is the postaxial (medial) bone of the forearm. It is parallel with, and longer than, the radius, and extends from the elbow to the wrist. **Unciform:** syn. hamate. **Vomer** is situated in the median plane, and forms part of the septum of the nose. It presents two surfaces, four borders, and an anterior extremity. **Wormian:** name for any one of a number of small inconstant bones in the cranial sutures. **Zygomatic** or malar bone is situated between the zygomatic process of the frontal and zygoma of the temporal on the one hand, and the zygomatic process of the maxilla on the other, where it separates the orbit from the temporal fossa.

bone calibrator. An instrument designed to enable the surgeon to ascertain correctly the length of screw required to grip from cortex to cortex in the operation of bone screwing.

bonelet. A small bone.

bonesetter. One who manipulates fractured and displaced joint surfaces.

Bonfils's disease (Bonfils, E. A., French physician of the nineteenth century). See under Hodgkin's disease.

Bonnet's capsule (Bonnet, A., French surgeon, 1802–58). Tenon's capsule; the posterior portion of the sheath of the eyeball.

Bonnier's syndrome (Bonnier, P., French physician, 1861–1918). Clinical symptoms resulting from a lesion of Deiters's nucleus or vestibular tracts, causing vertigo and ocular disturbances.

bŏŏ·pia (G. *bous*, ox; *ŏps*, eye). The cowlike appearance seen in the eye of patients with hysteria.

boracic acid. See boric acid.

borage. A plant, *Borago officinalis*, used mainly as an aperient and diaphoretic.

bor·ate. A salt of boric acid.

borax. $Na_2B_4O_6.10H_2O$. Sodium pyroborate. A mild antiseptic.

borboryg·mus (G. *borborugmos*, a rumbling in the bowels). Intestinal rumbling due to movements of a mixture of fluid and gas.

Bordet-Gengou's phenomenon. See under complement, fixation of.

Bordier-Fraenkel's sign. See under Bell's phenomenon.

boric acid. H_3BO_3. A weakly monobasic acid which is used as a mild antiseptic. Syn. boracic acid.

Bornholm disease (Bornholm, a Danish island in the Baltic Sea). Epidemic pleurodynia.

boron (Arab. *buraq*, borax). A non-metallic element. Symbol B. Occurs in two allotropic forms—as a powder and as a crystalline substance.

Borrelia. A family of spirochaetes. Syn. Spironema.

Borsieri's line (Borsieri, G. B., French physician, 1725–85). In the early stages of scarlatina, a line drawn on the skin with the finger-nail leaves a white streak which quickly turns red and diminishes in size.

Borthen's operation (Borthen, J., contemporary Norwegian ophthalmologist). Iridotasis.

Bose's hooks (Bose, H., German surgeon, 1840–1900). Hooks for use in performing tracheotomy.

boss. An eminence.

bŏs·selated. Covered with bosses.

Botallo's or Botal's duct (Botallo L., Italian physician, born 1530). Ductus arteriosus Botalli, a short vessel in the foetus between the main pulmonary artery and the aorta. **B.'s foramen:** the foramen ovale in the interauricular septum of the foetal heart. **B.'s ligament:** the remains of B.'s duct.

bŏ·tany (G. *botanē*, herb). The science of plants.

Botelho's test (Botelho, French physician). A nitric acid and iodine test for cancer.

bothriocĕ·phalus (G. *bothrion*, a small pit; *kephalē*, the head). See under Diphylobothriinae worms. **B. latus:** Diphyllobothrium latum, *q.v.*

bot·ryoid (G. *botrūs*, bunch of grapes; *eidos*, form). Shaped like a bunch of grapes.

bot·rўomŷ·ces (G. *botrūs*, bunch of grapes; *mukēs*, mushroom). Obsolete term for fungi occurring in clusters.

bot·ryomycō·sis (G. *botrus*, bunch of grapes; *mukēs*, mushroom). See under granuloma pyogenicum.

Biotrytis. A genus of fungi.

bŏ·tulism (L. *botulus*, sausage). An acute and usually fatal disease due to poisoning with the exotoxins of *Bacillus botulini*, characterized by paralysis of cranial motor nerves and diaphragm and by disturbance of secretion in mouth and pharynx.

boubas (Brazilian). Yaws.

Bouchard's disease (Bouchard, C. J., French physician, 1837–1915). Dilatation of the stomach caused by imperfect functioning of the gastric muscular fibres. **B.'s nodosities:** enlargement of the second phalangeal joints of the fingers, associated with dilatation of the stomach.

Bouchardat's treatment (Bouchardat, A., French chemist, 1806–86). Treatment of diabetes mellitus by exclusion of carbohydrates from the diet.

Bouchut's tubes (Bouchut, J. A. E., French physician, 1818–91). A variety of tubes for intubation of the larynx.

Boudin's law (Boudin, J. C. M. F. J., French physician, 1806–67). Malaria and tuberculosis are antagonistic.

Bougard's paste (Bougard, J. J., French physician, 1815–84). A caustic paste containing mercury bichloride, zinc chloride, arsenic, cinnabar, starch and wheat flour.

bou·gie (Fr. *bougie*, from Arab. Bijiyah, town in Algeria, from which wax candles—bougies—were first imported into Europe). A slender cylindrical instrument for exploring or dilating the urethra or other canals.

Bouillaud's disease (Bouillaud, J. B., French physician, 1796–1881). Infective endocarditis. **B.'s metallic tinkling:** a peculiar clink sometimes heard to the right of the apex beat in cardiac hypertrophy.

bouillon (Fr. *bouillir*). 1. Broth made from meat. 2. A fluid medium for culturing micro-organisms, prepared from finely chopped meat.

Boulton's solution. A compound tincture of iodine, phenol, glycerol and distilled water, used for spraying in rhinitis.

Bourget's test (Bourget, L., Swiss physician, 1856–1913). A starch and ammonium persulphate solution test for iodides in the urine.

Bourneville's disease (Bourneville, D. M., French physician, 1840–1909). Tuberous sclerosis.

boutonnière (Fr.). 1. A buttonhole incision. 2. External urethrotomy.

Bouveret's disease (Bouveret, L., French physician, 1850–1929). Paroxysmal tachycardia. **B.'s sign in intestinal obstruction:** great distension of the caecum and a large elevation in the right iliac fossa (sign applicable only to the large intestine).

Boveri's test (Boveri, P., Italian neurologist, 1879–1932). A potassium permanganate test for excess of globulin in cerebrospinal fluid.

bŏ·vine (L. *bovinus*, from *bos*). Pertaining to or derived from the ox or cow. **B. tubercle bacilli:** strains of tubercle bacillus causing tuberculosis in cattle, but also pathogenic to man. **B. heart:** an extremely hypertrophied heart.

bowel (Late L. *botellus*, dim. of *botulus*, sausage). The intestine.

bow-leg. Genu varum.

Bowman's capsule (Bowman, Sir W., English surgeon, 1816–92). The expanded portion forming the beginning of a uriniferous tubule. **B.'s discs:** the products of a breaking up of muscle-fibres in the direction of the transverse striations. **B.'s glands:** slightly branched tubes, identical in structure with serous glands found in mucous membrane. **B.'s membrane:** the anterior elastic lamina of the cornea. **B.'s muscle:** the ciliary muscle. **B.'s probe:** a probe for dilating strictures of the lacrimal duct. **B.'s sarcous elements:** muscle-caskets; the small elongated prisms of contractile substance which produce the appearance of dark stripes in voluntary muscle. **B.'s tubes:** artificial tubes formed between the lamellae of the cornea by injection of air or coloured fluid.

Bowman-Müller's capsule. The same as Bowman's capsule, *q.v.*

Boyer's bursa (Boyer, A., French surgeon, 1757-1833). The subhyoid bursa. **B.'s cyst:** cystic enlargement of the subhyoid bursa.

Bozeman's catheter (Bozeman, N., American surgeon, 1825-1905). A double-current catheter.

Bozzi's foramen. Soemmering's yellow spot, the macula lutea of the retina.

Bozzolo's sign (Bozzolo, C., Italian physician, 1845-1920). Visible pulsation of the arteries of the nares, said to occur in some cases of aneurysm of the thoracic aorta.

Br. Symbol for bromine.

Brach-Romberg's sign. The same as Romberg's sign, *q.v.*

Brachet's mesolateral fold (Brachet, J. L., Belgian physiologist, 1789-1858). The right lamella of the primitive mesentery which passes to the dorsal aspect of the right lobe of the liver. Its free edge bounds the foramen of Winslow.

brā·chia (G. *brakhiōn*, arm). Plural of brachium, *q.v.* **B. quadrigemina:** bundles of fibres passing from anterior and posterior to optic thalamus and corpus geniculatum mediale.

brā·chial (G. *brakhiōn*, arm). Pertaining to the arm.

brachiăl·gia (G. *brakhiōn*, arm; *algos*, pain). Pain in the arm.

brachiā·lis (G. *brakhiōn*, arm). A muscle of the upper arm.

brā·chiocephal·ic (G. *brakhiōn*, arm; *kephalē*, head). Pertaining to both the arm and head.

brā·chiocrū·ral (G. *brakhiōn*, arm; L. *crus*, leg). Pertaining to both arm and leg.

brā·chiocū·bital (G. *brakhiōn*, arm; L. *cubitus*, the elbow). Pertaining to both the arm and the fore-arm.

brā·chiofā·cial (G. *brakhiōn*, arm; L. *facies*, face). Pertaining to both arm and face.

brā·chioradiā·lis. The supinator longus muscle.

brachiŏ·tomy (G. *brakhiōn*, arm; *tomē*, a cutting). Amputation of a foetal arm during delivery.

brā·chium (G. *brakhiōn*, arm). 1. The arm, especially the part between the shoulder and elbow. 2. Any arm-like structure. **B. conjunctivum:** the superior cerebellar peduncle, *q.v.* **B. pontis:** the middle cerebellar peduncle, *q.v.*

Bracht-Wächter bodies (Bracht, E. F. E., German pathologist, born 1882). Small necrotic areas seen in the myocardium in cases of bacterial endocarditis.

brăchycephal·ic (G. *brakhus*, short; *kephalē*, head). Having a skull with a transverse diameter more than 80 per cent of the long diameter.

brā·chycĕ·phaly (G. *brakhus*, short; *kephalē*, head). The condition of being brachycephalic.

brā·chydac·tyly (G. *brakhus*, short; *daktulos*, finger). Having abnormally short fingers.

brachygnă·thism (G. *brakhus*, short; *gnathos*, jaw). Abnormal shortness of jaw.

brachygnă·thous (G. *brakhus*, short; *gnathos*, jaw). Having short jaws.

brady-aesthē·sia (G. *bradus*, slow; *aisthēsis*, feeling). Dullness of perception.

brady-ar·thria (G. *bradus*, slow; *arthroein*, to articulate). Slow articulation of words.

bradycar·dia (G. *bradus*, slow; *kardia*, heart). Abnormal infrequency of pulse; slowness of the heart-beat.

bradyĕcoi·a (G. *bradus*, slow; *akouein*, to hear). Subnormal acuteness of hearing; hardness of hearing.

bradylă·lia (G. *bradus*, slow; *lalein*, to talk). Slowness of speech.

bradyphā·sia (G. *bradus*, slow; *phasis*, statement). Abnormal slowness of speech, due to cerebral disorder.

bradyphrā·sia (G. *bradus*, slow; *phrasis*, speech). The same as bradyphasia, *q.v.*

bradypnōē·a (G. *bradus*, slow; *pnein*, to breathe). Abnormal infrequency of breathing.

brady-uria (G. *bradus*, slow; *ouron*, urine). Abnormally slow passing of urine.

braille (Braille, L., blind French teacher, 1809-1852). A tangible system of printing, used by the blind.

Brailsford-Morquio's disease. See chondro-osteo-dystrophy.

brain. That part of the central nervous system that is contained in the skull of vertebrates, and consisting of the cerebrum, the cerebellum, the pons and the medulla, together with the pituitary body.

brain-sand. Carbonate and phosphate of calcium and organic matter in the epithalamus. Syn. acervulus cerebri.

branch. Offshoot of blood-vessels, nerves or lymphatics from the trunk or main stem.

bran·chia (G. *bragkhia*, gills). 1. The gills of fish. 2. Analogous structure of clefts in the human embryo.

bran·chial (G. *bragkhia*, gills). Relating to the branchia.

branchiŏ·genous (G. *bragkhia*, gills; *gennan*, to produce). Derived from a branchial cleft.

branchiŏ·ma (G. *bragkhia*, gills). Any tumour derived from remains of the branchial clefts.

bran·chiomere (G. *bragkhia*, gills; *mĕros*, part). The segment of the lateral mesoderm between each two branchial clefts.

Brand's method (Brand, E., German physician, 1827-97). A system of baths used in treatment of typhoid fever.

Brande's test (Brande, W. T., English chemist, 1788-1866). A chlorine water and ammonia test for quinine.

Brandt's method (Brandt, R., Swedish physician, 1819-95). Treatment of affections of the uterine tubes by massage in an endeavour to force out their contents into the uterus.

brandy. A spirit distilled from wine. (Spiritus vini gallici.)

brash. Pyrosis.

Brassica. A genus of plants which includes the cabbage.

Braun's canal (Braun, M., German anatomist, 1850-1930). The neurenteric canal.

Braun's hook (Braun, G. von, Austrian gynaecologist, 1829-1911). An instrument, shaped like a hook, and used for decapitation of the foetus.

Braun's test (Braun, C. H., German physician, 1847-1911). A sodium hydroxide and trinitrophenol test for dextrose in urine.

Braune's canal (Braune, C. W., German anatomist, 1831-92). The continuous passage formed by the uterine cavity and the vagina during labour, after full dilatation of the os. **B.'s muscle:** the musculus pubo-rectalis. **B.'s valvule:** the fold that marks the cardiac sphincter between the oesophagus and the stomach.

Bravais-Jackson's epilepsy. The same as Jackson's epilepsy, *q.v.*

Braxton-Hicks's sign (Braxton-Hicks, J., English gynaecologist, 1825-97). The small intermittent contractions of the uterus which commence at the end of the third month of pregnancy.

bread. Flour, moistened with water, kneaded and baked. Most kinds of bread are leavened by addition of yeast.

breakbone fever. See dengue.

breast. 1. The chest. 2. The mamma. **Chicken b.:** deformity of the chest characterized by prominence of the sternum and the sternal parts of the ribs. **Funnel b.:** a deformity of the chest, characterized by a depression of the wall at the sternal part.

breath. The air exhaled from the lungs. **B. sounds:** the sounds heard on auscultation during respiration.

breathing. Taking air into the lungs and expelling it. **B., abdominal:** b. in which the walls of the abdomen move more than those of the chest; more common in men than in women. **B., amphoric:** a form of cavernous b. characterized by a hollow metallic sound. **B., bronchial:** the blowing high-pitched respiratory sound heard on auscultation over areas of consolidated lung tissue; expiration being as long as inspiration and separated from it by a distinct pause. **B., broncho-vesicular:** a form of respiratory sound intermediate between bronchial and vesicular b. **B., cavernous:** a form of bronchial b. characterized by a hollow character of both inspiratory and expiratory sounds, the latter being hollower and more prolonged than the former; as heard over pulmonary cavities. **B., cog-wheel:** a respiratory sound heard on auscultation of the lungs in cases of jerky (neurotic) breathing resembling that of cogwheels. **B., mouth:** habitual b. through the mouth instead of through the nose. **B., puerile:** a form of harsh vesicular breathing, as heard normally in children and in some forms of emphysema. **B., thoracic:** b. in which the chest walls move more extensively than the walls of the abdomen. **B., tubular:** a form of high-pitched bronchial breathing of whiffing character heard over areas of consolidated or collapsed lung tissue. **B., vesicular:** the normal respiratory faint rustling sound heard on auscultation during inspiration and expiration, the former phase being two or three times as long as the latter. **B., vesiculo-bronchial:** a form of respiratory sound intermediate between vesicular and bronchial breathing.

Brecht's cartilages. The ossa suprasternalia, two small cartilaginous or bony nodules near each sternoclavicular joint, above the sternum; regarded as rudiments of the episternal bone, well developed in some animals.

Breda's disease (Breda, A., Italian dermatologist, 1850-1933). The same as yaws, *q.v.*

breech. The buttocks. **B. presentation:** that uterine position of the foetus during labour in which the foetal buttocks present at the uterine orifice.

breg·ma (G.). The junction of the coronal and sagittal sutures.

Brehmer's method (Brehmer, H., German physician, 1826-89). A method of treating tuberculosis by physical and dietetic means.

Brenner's formula (Brenner, R., German physician, 1821-84). Given the same electrical current, the cathodal closing contraction is four times stronger than the cathodal opening contraction.

Breschet's canals or veins (Breschet (or Brechet), G., French anatomist, 1784-1845). The canals and veins of the diploe. **B.'s bones:** the ossa suprasternalia. **B.'s helicotrema:** the helicotrema, the foramen of communication between the scala vestibuli and the scala tympani. **B.'s sinus:** the sphenoparietal sinus.

Bretonneau's diphtheria (Bretonneau, P., French physician, 1778-1862). Diphtheria of the pharynx. **B.'s method:** the administration of quinine in a single large dose after the paroxysm in malaria.

breviduc·tor. The adductor brevis muscle of the thigh.

breviflex·or. Any short flexor muscle.

brevissimus oculi (L.). The obliquus inferior muscle, the shortest muscle of the eye.

brickdust deposit. Urinary sediment consisting of urates.

bricklayers' itch. Dermatitis caused by irritation due to the handling of mortar.

bridge. 1. A narrow band of tissue. 2. The upper ridge of the nose. 3. In electricity, an apparatus for measuring the resistance of a conductor. **B. corpuscle:** see desmosome.

Bright's blindness (Bright, R., English physician, 1789-1858). Partial or complete blindness in cases of uraemia. **B.'s disease:** a term used to denote acute or chronic nephritis. **B.'s disease (acute):** acute nephritis. **B.'s disease (chronic):** chronic nephritis.

brilliant green. An antiseptic dyestuff of the triphenylmethane series.

Brinton's disease (Brinton, W., English physician, 1823-67). 1. Linitis plastica; hypertrophy and sclerosis of the submucous connective tissue of the stomach. 2. Infantile scurvy.

Briquet's ataxia (Briquet, P., French physician, 1796-1881). Hysterical ataxia; astasia abasia. **B.'s syndrome:** shortness of breath and aphonia in hysterical paralysis of the diaphragm.

Brissaud's bundle (Brissaud, E., French physician. 1852-1909). 'Psychic or intellectual' bundle in the inferior cerebellar peduncle. **B.'s convolution:** gyrus parietalis transversus.

Brissaud-Marie's syndrome (Brissaud, E.; Marie, P., French neurologist, 1853-1940). Hysterical unilateral spasm of the tongue and lips.

Britannia metal. An alloy of tin, antimony, copper and bismuth.

British-Anti-Lewisite. See B.A.L.

Broadbent's sign (Broadbent, Sir W. H., English physician, 1835-1907). In cases of adherent pericardium there is a visible retraction on the left side in the region of the 11th and 12th ribs.

Broca's aphasia (Broca, P. P., French anatomist, 1824-80). Cortical motor aphasia. **B.'s area:** the medial portion of the anterior olfactory lobe; area parolfactoria; gyrus olfactorius medialis. **B.'s centre:** the posterior part of the left third frontal convolution, the centre for speech. **B.'s convolution:** the third frontal convolution of the left hemisphere. **B.'s olfactory area:** the posterior end of the gyrus rectus, lying anteriorly to the mesial root of the olfactory tract; trigonum olfactorium. **B.'s point:** the centre of the external auditory meatus. **B.'s pouch:** a pear-shaped sac lying in the tissues of the labia majora. It is analogous in structure to the dartos, but contains no muscular fibres.

Brodie's abscess (Brodie, Sir B. C., English surgeon, 1783-1862). Chronic pyogenic abscess of bone, usually situated in the head of the tibia. **B.'s bursa:** the semimembranosus-gastrocnemius bursa. **B.'s disease:** pulpy disease of a joint, especially the knee-joint. **B.'s joint:** hysterical arthroneuralgia. **B.'s pain:** the pain caused by lifting a fold of skin in the neighbourhood of a joint in articular neuralgia.

Brodmann's areas (Brodmann, K., German psychiatrist, 1868-1918). Cortical areas distinguished by the structure and disposition of cellular layers.

Broesike's fossa (Broesike, G., German surgeon, born 1853). The parajejunal fossa, a recess in the peritoneal cavity situated in the first part of the mesojejunum and behind the superior mesenteric artery.

Brokaw's ring (Brokaw, A. V. L., U.S. surgeon, 1853-1907). A ring of rubber tubing threaded with catgut, used in intestinal anastomosis.

bromhidrō·sis (G. *brōmos*, stench; *hidrōs*, sweat). Foul perspiration.

brō·mide (G. *brōmos*, stench). A salt of hydrobromic acid.

brō·midrosiphō·bia (G. *brōmos*, stench; *hidrōs*, sweat; *phobos*, fear). Neurotic fear of bodily odours.

bromidrō·sis (G. *brōmos*, stench; *hidrōs*, sweat). Offensive-smelling perspiration.

brō·mine (G. *brōmos*, stench). A reddish-brown fuming liquid element of the halogen group. Symbol Br.

bromism (G. *brōmos*, stench). Poisoning by bromides.

bromoder·ma. A dermatitis caused by the use of bromides.

bromo-ï·odism (G. *brŏmos*, stench; *iŏdēs*, violet or rust-coloured). Poisoning with iodine and bromide.

bromvaletone. H₂N.CONHCOCHBr.CH(CH₃)₂. α-bromo-*iso*-valerylcarbamide. Sedative and hypnotic.

bronch·adeni·tis (G. *brogkhos*, windpipe; *adēn*, gland). Inflammation of the bronchial glands.

bron·chi (G. *brogkhos*, windpipe). The plural of bronchus, *q.v.*

bron·chia (G. *brogkhos*, windpipe). The bronchial tubes smaller than the main bronchi.

bron·chial. Pertaining to the bronchi.

bronchiĕc·tasis (G. *brogkhos*, windpipe; *ektasis*, extension). Congenital or acquired dilatation of a bronchus or of bronchi; a condition characterized at later stages by paroxysmal cough with expectoration of large amounts of foetid sputum, by clubbing fingers, haemoptyses, and impairment of general condition.

bron·chiectat·ic. Pertaining to or affected with bronchiectasis.

bronchi·loquy (G. *brogkhos*, windpipe; L. *loqui*, to speak). Bronchophony.

bronchiocele. See under bronchocele.

bron·chiogen·ic (G. *brogkhos*, windpipe; *gennan*, to produce). Arising from a bronchus.

bron·chiole. A minute end-branch of a bronchus.

bron·chiolec·tasis (G. *brogkhos*, windpipe; *ektasis*, extension). Dilatation of the bronchioles.

bron·chiolith (G. *brogkhos*, windpipe; *lithos*, a stone). See under broncholith.

bron·chioli·tis. Inflammation of the bronchioles. Syn. capillary bronchitis. **B. fibrosa obliterans:** a condition characterized by obstruction of the lumen of the bronchioles by desquamated epithelial cells and fibrous overgrowth, leading to intense dyspnoea and cyanosis.

bron·chiospäs·mus (G. *brogkhos*, windpipe; *spasmos*, spasm). Spasm of a bronchus or of the bronchi.

bron·chiostenŏ·sis (G. *brogkhos*, windpipe; *stenos*, narrow). Stenosis of a bronchus.

bronchit·ic. Affected with bronchitis.

bronchi·tis (G. *brogkhos*, windpipe). Inflammation of the bronchial tubes. **Capillary b.:** bronchiolitis. **Croupous b.** or **Fibrinous b.:** b. with formation and expectoration of fibrinous casts of the bronchial tubes.

broncho-aegophony (G. *brogkhos*, windpipe; *aix*, goat; *phŏnē*, voice). Bronchophony with aegophony.

bron·chocele (G. *brogkhos*, windpipe; *kēlē*, tumour). A diverticulum of a bronchus.

bron·choconstric·tor (G. *brogkhos*, windpipe; L. *constringere*, constrict). An agent constricting the calibre of the bronchial tubes.

bron·chodilatā·tion (G. *brogkhos*, windpipe; L. *dilatare*, to dilate). Dilatation of a bronchus; bronchiectasis.

bron·chodilā·tor (G. *brogkhos*, windpipe; L. *dilatare*, to dilate). An agent dilating the calibre of the bronchial tubes.

bron·cho-oesophagŏ·scopy (G. *brogkhos*, windpipe; *oisophagos*, oesophagus; *skopein*, to view). Endoscopic inspection of the oesophagus and bronchi.

bron·cholith (G. *brogkhos*, windpipe; *lithos*, stone). A calculus or concretion formed in a bronchial tube.

bron·chiolithi·asis (G. *brogkhos*, windpipe; *lithos*, stone). The formation of bronchial calculi.

bron·chomycŏ·sis (G. *brogkhos*, windpipe; *mukēs*, mushroom). Mycotic infection of the bronchi.

bronchŏ·pathy (G. *brogkhos*, windpipe; *pathos*, disease). Any disease of the bronchi.

bronchŏ·phony (G. *brogkhos*, windpipe; *phŏnē*, voice). 1. The resonance of the voice of a subject as heard when auscultating the main bronchi. 2. The pathological phenomenon that the voice is heard as under (1) when lung-parts other than the main bronchi are auscultated, a sign of consolidation of the lungs,

consolidated lung tissue being a better conductor of sound than air-containing lung-tissue.

bron·choplasty (G. *brogkhos*, windpipe; *plassein*, to form). The operation of closing a bronchial fistula.

bron·chopneumŏ·nia (G. *brogkhos*, windpipe; *pneumŏn*, the lungs). Focal, often lobular, inflammation of the lungs commencing in the bronchi.

bron·chopul·monary (G. *brogkhos*, windpipe; L. *pulmo*, a lung). Relating to the bronchi and the lungs.

bronchorrhā·gia (G. *brogkhos*, windpipe; *rhēgnunai*, to break out). Haemorrhage from the bronchi.

bronchorrhoē·a (G. *brogkhos*, windpipe; *rheein*, to flow). Profuse bronchial discharge.

bron·choscope (G. *brogkhos*, windpipe; *skopein*, to view). An instrument for examining the bronchi.

bronchŏ·scopy (G. *brogkhos*, windpipe; *skopein*, to view). Instrumental inspection of the interior of a bronchus.

bron·chospirochetŏ·sis Haemorrhagic bronchitis, due to infection by the spirochaeta bronchialis.

bronchostenŏ·sis. See under bronchiostenosis.

bron·chotome. A surgical instrument used in carrying out bronchotomy.

bronchŏ·tomy (G. *brogkhos*, windpipe; *tomē*, a cutting). Incision into a bronchus.

bron·chotrachē·al (G. *brogkhos*, windpipe; *tracheia*, rough). Relating to the bronchi and trachea.

bron·chovesï·cular (G. *brogkhos*, windpipe; L. *vesicula*, dim. of *vesica*, bladder). Both bronchial and vesicular.

bron·chus (G. *brogkhos*, windpipe). One of the main branches of the trachea.

bronze (It. *bronzo*, from L. *(aes) Brundisium*). 1. An alloy of copper and tin. 2. Of a bronze colour. **B. diabetes:** haemochromatosis with diabetes mellitus.

Brooke's disease (Brooke, H. A. G., English dermatologist, 1854–1919). Keratosis follicularis, also known as Darier's disease.

Brossard's type of progressive muscular atrophy. Femoral type with claw-like appearance of the toes. See also Eichhorst's type.

broth. The same as bouillon, *q.v.*

brow. The forehead; the superciliary ridge; the eyebrow. **B. presentation:** that uterine position of the foetus during labour in which the foetal brows present at the uterine orifice.

brown induration (L. *indurare*, to harden). Induration of the lung caused by chronic congestion of the lung in heart-disease and stasis of blood, characterized by decreased size of alveoli and increase in connective tissue and pigment derived from haemoglobin.

Brown's phenomenon (Brown, R., Scottish botanist, 1773–1858). Brownian molecular movement; the spontaneous movements of inorganic particles and micro-organisms in a fluid medium; pedesis.

Brown-Séquard's paralysis (Brown-Séquard, C. E., French physiologist, 1818–94). Paralysis and hyperaesthesia of one side and anaesthesia of the other side of the body.

Browne (Crichton). See Crichton-Browne.

Bruce's septicaemia (Bruce, Sir D., English surgeon, 1855–1931). Malta fever.

Bruce and Muir, septomarginal tract of (Bruce, A., Scottish neurologist, 1854–1911; Muir, J. C., contemporary Scottish neurologist). A part of the descending posteromedial tract of the spinal cord.

Brucella. A genus of bacteria. **B. abortus:** the bacterium causing abortus fever, *q.v.*, in man and contagious abortion in cows. **B. melitensis:** the bacterium causing Malta or Mediterranean fever, *q.v.*

brucel·lar. Relating to Brucella.

brucellŏ·sis. Any disease caused by an organism of the Brucella group.

Bruch's glands (Bruch, K. W. L., German anatomist, 1819–84). Lymph-follicles found in the conjunctiva about the inner canthus of ruminants. **B.'s layer or membrane**: the lamina basalis which forms the inner boundary of the choroid.

brucine. An alkaloid from various species of *Strychnos*.

Bruck's disease (Bruck, A., German physician, born 1865). A syndrome consisting of multiple fractures and marked by deformity of bones, ankylosis of most of the joints, and muscular atrophy.

Bruecke's lines (Bruecke, E. W., Ritter von, German physiologist, 1819-92). The broad bands which alternate with Krause's membranes in the fibrils of striated muscles. **B.'s muscle**: 1. See Bowman's muscle. 2. The muscularis mucosae of the small and large intestines. **B.'s tunica nervea**: the layers of the retina, exclusive of the rods and cones.

Bruggiser's hernia. The same as Krönlein's hernia, *q.v.*

bruit (Fr.). An abnormal sound heard during auscultation; see also murmur. **B. de diable**: a rushing sound heard in the veins of the neck in anaemia. **B. de galop**: see gallop rhythm. **B. de pot felé**: a cracked pot sound, heard over pulmonary cavities.

Brunn's cell-nests (or **epithelial nests**) (Brunn, A. von, German anatomist, 1849-72). Branched or solid groups of flat epithelial cells occurring in all normal bladders. **Brunn's glands**: see Brunner's glands.

Brunner's glands (Brunner, J. K., German anatomist, 1653-1727). The racemose glands found in the wall of the duodenum.

Brunonian theory (Brown, J., Scottish physician, 1735-88). Brownism; the doctrine that both physiological and pathological phenomena are due to variations in a natural stimulus, its excess causing sthenic and its deficiency asthenic diseases.

Bryobia practiosa. A small red spider, irritating to man and usually found in clover fields.

Bryonia. A genus of plants, some of which have roots with cathartic properties.

Bryant's ampulla (Bryant, T., English surgeon, 1828-1914). The apparent distension of an artery immediately above a ligature, due to the contraction of the vessel above the ampulla, where it is not completely filled by the clot. **B.'s iliofemoral triangle**: the triangle formed by a vertical line dropped from the anterior superior iliac spine to the horizontal plane of the body; by a second line drawn from the anterior superior iliac spine to the tip of the trochanter; and by a third, the test-line, which joins the two at a right angle to the vertical line. Shortening of the neck of the femur will be indicated by a shortening of the test line. **B.'s line**: the base of B.'s iliofemoral triangle towards which the trochanter moves in fracture of the neck of the femur.

Bryson's sign (Bryson, A., English physician, 1802-60). Diminished power of expansion of the thorax during inspiration, occasionally observed in exophthalmic goitre and neurasthenia.

bubo (G. *boubōn*, the groin). An inflammation and swelling of a lymph node, particularly of the groin, especially when due to a venereal disease or to plague.

bubon d'emblée (Fr.). Bubo of venereal origin, without any visible primary lesion.

bubon·ic (G. *boubōn*). Pertaining to a bubo. **B. plague**: see under plague.

bubŏ·nocele (G. *boubōn*, groin; *kēlē*, tumour). An incomplete indirect inguinal hernia the sac of which is retained in the inguinal canal.

bucca (L.). 1. The cheek; the hollow part of the cheek. 2. The mouth.

buc·cal (L. *bucca*). Pertaining to the bucca or cheek.

buccodi·stal (L. *bucca*, check; *distarc*, to be distant). Pertaining to th ɛ buccal and distal walls of a cavity.

buccolā·bial (L. *bucca*, cheek; *labium*, lip). Pertaining to the cheek and lip.

buccoling·ual (L. *bucca*, cheek; *lingua*, tongue). Pertaining to the cheek and tongue.

buccopharyngē·al (L. *bucca*, mouth; G. *pharugx*, pharynx). Pertaining to the mouth and pharynx.

Buchner's albuminoid bodies (Buchner, H., German bacteriologist, 1850-92). Defensive proteins, i.e., those existing in the blood and rendering the system immune to infectious diseases.

Buchwald's atrophy. Idiopathic progressive diffuse atrophy of the skin.

Buck's extension (Buck, G., American surgeon, 1807-77). An apparatus consisting of a weight and pulley for applying extension to a limb. **B.'s fascia**: the sheath of the corpora cavernosa and the corpus spongiosum, which arises from the symphysis pubis by the suspensory ligament of the penis and is continuous with the deep layer of the superficial perineal fascia.

bud. Any small part bearing some resemblance to plant buds.

Budd's cirrhosis (Budd, G., English physician, 1808-82). Hepatic cirrhosis due to auto-intoxication from the gastro-intestinal tract. **B.'s jaundice**: acute yellow atrophy of the liver; Rokitansky's disease.

budding. A form of reproduction or cell-division; gemmation. **B. fungi**: blastomycetes.

Budge's centres (Budge, J. L., German anatomist, 1811-84). 1. The ciliospinal centre in the cervical spinal cord. 2. The genitospinal centre in the lumbar spinal cord.

Budin's obstetrical joint (Budin, P. C., French gynaecologist, 1846-1907). Articulation between the ex- and supra-occipital bones in the foetal and infantile skull.

Buehlmann's fibres. Certain lines on decayed teeth.

Buengner's bands (Buengner, O. von, German surgeon, 1858-1905). Protoplasmic bands within which the neurofibrillar cell processes travel in regenerating nerves.

Buerger's disease (Buerger, L., American physician, 1879-1943). The same as thrombo-angiitis obliterans, *q.v.*

Buetschli's nuclear spindle (Buetschli, O., German zoologist, 1848-1920). The spindle-shaped figure observed during karyokinesis.

buffer. Any substance preventing changes in the pH of a solution by combining with and thus nullifying the effect of any acid or alkali that may be added. **B. solution**: a solution to which an acid or an alkali may be added without producing a significant change in its pH.

bufonin (L. *bufo*, toad). A poisonous principle found in skin secretions of toads and lizards. Related to the steroids.

bufother·apy. Therapeutic application of toad toxins.

bug. An insect belonging to the Hemiptera family.

buggery. Sodomy; sexual intercourse through the anus.

Buhl's desquamative pneumonia (Buhl, L. von, German pathologist, 1816-80). Caseous pneumonia in which the exudate consists chiefly of desquamated alveolar epithelium. **B.'s disease**: acute fatty degeneration of the viscera of the newborn, with haemorrhages in various parts of the body.

bulb (L. *bulbus*). 1. Any globular or fusiform structure, e.g., a fusiform expansion of a canal or vessel. 2. The medulla oblongata.

bulbar (L. *bulbus*, bulb). 1. Bulbous. 2. Pertaining to the medulla. **B. paralysis**: paralysis of the tongue, lips, pharynx and larynx, due to a degenerative lesion of the motor nuclei of cranial nerves in the medulla oblongata.

bul·boid. Shaped like a bulb.

bulbonū·clear (L. *bulbus*, bulb; *nucleus*, from *nucula*, dim. of *nux*, nut). Pertaining to the medulla nuclei.

bulbopon·tine (L. *bulbus*, bulb; *pons*, a bridge). Relating to both cerebral pons and medulla oblongata.

bulbo-urē·thral (L. *bulbus*, bulb; G. *ourēthra*, urethra). Relating to the bulb of the urethra.

bulbous (L. *bulbus*, bulb). Terminating in a bulb, or having bulbs.

bulbus (L.). A bulb, *q.v.*

buli·mia (G. *bous*, ox; *limos*, hunger). Excessive hunger.

bulla (L., a bubble). 1. A bulging structure. 2. A bleb; a unilocular elevation of the epidermis containing serous fluid. **B. ethmoidalis:** the bulging region of the inner wall of the ethmoidal labyrinth in the middle nasal meatus.

Buller's shield (Buller, F., Canadian ophthalmologist, 1844–1905). A watch-glass in a frame of adhesive plaster or rubber worn before a sound eye to protect it from an infected eye.

bul·lous (L. *bulla*, a bubble). Marked by the presence of bullae.

bundle. A collection or group of fibres; a fasciculus. **B. branch block:** that form of heart-block in which nervous conduction is impaired in one of the main branches of the auriculoventricular bundle.

Bunge's amputation (Bunge, R., German surgeon, born 1870). Aperiosteal amputation.

bū·ninoid (G. *bounos*, hill; *eidos*, form). Having a rounded shape.

bū·nion. A swelling or a bursa of the foot, especially on the metatarso-phalangeal joint of the great toe.

Bunsen burner (Bunsen, R. W. E. von, German chemist, 1811–99). A gas burner for laboratory use.

buphthal·mia, buphthal·mos (G. *bous*, ox; *ophthalmos*, eye). Enlargement of the whole globe of the eye with enlarged, globular and thinned cornea and abnormally deep anterior chamber, due to congenital obstruction of drainage of the intra-ocular fluid resulting in congenital glaucoma.

Burckhardt's corpuscles. Peculiar roundish or angular bodies of a yellowish colour, found in the secretion of trachoma.

Burdach's column (Burdach, C. F., German physiologist, 1776–1847). The postero-external column of the spinal cord. **B.'s fissure:** a small fissure between the island of Reil and the operculum. **B.'s nucleus:** the cuneate nucleus, a small nucleus of grey matter in the funiculus cuneatus of the medulla oblongata, forming the termination of the long fibres of B.'s column. **B.'s operculum:** see Arnold's operculum.

burette, buret. A long cylindrical glass vessel, graduated and fitted with a stopcock at the lower end; used for delivering measured volumes of liquid.

burn. 1. To sear or scorch. 2. An injury due to dry heat. 3. In chemistry, to oxygenize. 4. In surgery, to cauterize. 5. To become inflamed.

Burnett's disinfecting fluid (Burnett, Sir W., English surgeon, 1779–1861). A strong solution of zinc chloride with a little iron chloride.

Burns' amaurosis (Burns, J., Scottish physician, 1774–1880). Post-marital amblyopia; impaired vision caused by sexual excess.

Burns's ligament (Burns, A., Scottish anatomist, 1781–1813). See under Hey's ligament. **B.'s space:** the fascial space at the suprasternal notch.

Burow's vein (Burow, K. A. von, German anatomist, 1809–74). A non-constant venous trunk formed by branches of the inferior epigastric veins and joining the umbilical vein.

burr. A dental instrument used for excavating.

bursa (G. *byrsa*, a hide). A small sac containing viscid fluid interposed between moving parts, as between bony prominences and tendons. **B. omentalis:** the lesser peritoneal sac covering the posterior surface of the stomach, quadrate and caudate lobes of the liver, upper surface of the pancreas, part of the spleen and transverse colon, communicating with the general peritoneal cavity through the foramen epiploicum.

bur·sal (G. *byrsa*). Pertaining to a bursa or sac.

Bursata. A group of Nematoda.

bursec·tomy (G. *byrsa*, a hide; *ektomē*, excision). Surgical removal of a bursa.

bursī·tis (G. *byrsa*, a hide). Inflammation of a bursa. See also Baker's cyst.

bur·solith (G. *byrsa*, a hide; *lithos*, stone). A calculus contained in a bursa.

bur·sula (L. dim. of *bursa*). Any small sac.

Burton's line (Burton, H., English physician, 1799–1849). A blue line along the margins of the gums in chronic lead poisoning.

Busk's fluke. *Fasciolopsis buskii*, a fluke occurring in the small intestine in inhabitants of India.

butacaine sulphate. $[p\text{-}NH_5C_6H_4COO(CH_2)_3.N(CH_2CH_2CH_2CH_3)_2]_2H_2SO_4$. The sulphate of di-*n*-butylaminopropyl-*p*-aminobenzoate. A local anaesthetic.

butter. An oily substance made from cream by means of churning.

buttermilk. Milk from which the milk fat has been extracted.

buttocks. The nates, or gluteal region.

button anastomō·sis (G. *anastomoein*, to open out). Intestinal anastomosis by means of a Murphy button, *q.v.*

buttonhole incision. Any small straight incision.

butylchloral hydrate. $CH_3CHCl.CCl_2CH(OH)_2$. 2:2-dichloro-3-chlorobutane-1:1-diol. A weak hypnotic.

butyl (G. *bouturon*, butter). An alkyl radical, C_4H_9.

butyrā·ceous (G. *bouturon*, butter). With butter-like consistency.

butyrate (G. *bouturon*, butter). A salt or ester of butyric acid.

butyric acid (G. *bouturon*, butter). $CH_3CH_2CH_2COOH$. A constituent of butter.

butyrŏ·meter (G. *bouturon*, butter; *metron*, measure). Instrument for estimating the amount of fat in milk.

byssinō·sis (G. *bussos*, cotton). The form of pneumonokoniosis caused by the inhalation of cotton-dust.

byssophthī·sis. Phthisis caused by the inhalation of cotton-dust.

bys·sus (G.). Lint or cotton.

bў·thus (G. *bythos*, depth). The base of the abdomen.

F

C

C. 1. Symbol of carbon. 2. Abbreviation for Centigrade.

C. substance. A specific substance of carbohydrate character, one of the major antigenic constituents in group A haemolytic streptococci.

Ca. Symbol of calcium.

cabbage. A green vegetable, *Brassica oleracea*, which contains the A, B, and C vitamins.

Cabot's ring bodies (Cabot, R. C., American physician, 1868–1939). Intracellular and extracellular bodies having the general shape of a ring, found in the red blood cells in severe anaemia.

cacaesthen·ic (G. *kakos*, bad; *aisthesis*, perception). Having impaired or defective organs of sense.

cacaesthē·sia. A sensibility disorder.

cacanthrax (G. *kakos*, bad; *anthrax*, charcoal). Contagious anthrax.

cachec·tic (G. *kakos*, bad; *hexis*, condition). Characterized by cachexia.

cachet (Fr. *cacher*, to hide). Flat capsule for enclosing a drug of disagreeable taste.

cachex·ia (G. *kakos*, bad; *hexis*, condition). A very severely lowered state caused by some systemic disease, and especially by carcinoma. **C., pituitary:** see under Simmond's disease. **C. strumipriva** or **C. thyreopriva:** myxoedema occurring after thyroidectomy, caused by removal of too much of the gland. **C., urinary:** the state found in patients with chronic kidney disease when suppuration is present. **C., verminous:** the debility seen when there is infestation with worms.

cachinnā·tion (L. *cachinnare*, to laugh). Hysterical laughter.

cacidrō·sis (G. *kakos*, bad; *hidrōs*, sweat). Excessive and offensive perspiration.

cacochȳ·lia (G. *kakos*, bad; *chulos*, juice). Abnormal condition of the gastric juices.

că·codyl (G. *kakōdēs*, evil-smelling; *hule*, matter). Dimethylarsine, an organic compound of arsenic.

cacō·dylate (G. *kakōdēs*, evil-smelling; *hule*, matter). A salt of cacodylic acid.

cacodylic acid. Dimethylarsinic acid.

cacoë·thic (G. *kakos*, bad; *ēthos*, disposition). Malignant.

cacogě·nesis (G. *kakos*, bad; *genesis*, formation). Abnormal development.

cacogēu·sia (G. *kakos*, bad; *geusis*, taste). An unpleasant taste.

Caconema. A genus of nematodes.

cacŏ·trophy (G. *kakos*, bad; *trophe*, nourishment). Malnutrition.

Cactus. A genus of plants, some of which yield cardiac and other stimulants.

cacu·men (L.). The top of any organ.

cadă·ver (L.). A dead body; a corpse.

cadaver·ic. Relating to a cadaver.

cadă·verine. A putrefactive intermediate product of proteolysis, $H_2N.(CH_2)_5NH_2$ pentamethylenediamine.

cadă·verous. Pertaining to or resembling a dead body.

cad·mium (G. *kadmia*). A bluish-white metallic element resembling zinc. Symbol Cd.

Cadū·ceus (G.). The wand of Mercury. Symbol of the medical profession.

cāe·cal (L. *caecus*, blind). Relating to the caecum.

cāecŏ·stomy (L. *caecus*, blind; G. *stŏma*, mouth). The surgical establishment of an artificial anus leading into the caecum.

cāe·cum (L. *caecus*, blind). The blind pouch at the beginning of the large intestine.

Caesarean section (Julius Caesar is believed to have been delivered at birth by this method). Extraction of the foetus by abdominal incision.

caffeine. A purine base, $C_8H_{10}O_2N_4$, which has uses as a stimulant and as a cardiac tonic.

caisson disease (Fr. *caisse*, from L. *capsa*, box). Condition occurring in persons working under high atmospheric pressure (c. workers, divers, tunnel workers) on too rapid return to normal pressure. Under high atmospheric pressure nitrogen is absorbed by the tissues from the blood and unless return to normal pressure is slow enough for reabsorption of nitrogen by the blood to take place, nitrogen bubbles form in the tissues or in the blood, giving rise to gaseous emboli; spinal cord and brain are usually mainly affected and sensory and/or motor pareses may result.

Cajal's cells (Cajal, S. Ramon y, Spanish neurologist, 1852–1934). The multipolar nerve cells of the cerebral cortex.

calamine. A basic zinc carbonate. It is used in the making of various soothing lotions and unguents and as a dusting powder.

calamus scriptorius (L. *calamus*, a reed-pen; *scribere*, to write). A groove on the dorsal surface of the medulla oblongata at its caudal end.

calcā·neal (L. *calx*, heel). Relating to the calcaneum.

calcaneo-apophysitis (L. *calx*, heel; G. *apophusis*, bone process). A chronic disease affecting the epiphysis of the calcaneum; causing fragmentation of the disc of bone.

calcā·neo-astră·galoid (L. *calx*, heel; G. *astragalos*, knuckle). Relating to the calcaneum and the astragalus.

calcā·neo-cā·vus (L. *calx*, heel; *cavus*, hollow). See under talipes cavus.

calcā·neum, calcā·neus (L. *calx*, heel). The heel-bone or os calcis.

cal·car (L. *calcar*, from *calx*, heel). 1. Any spur or spur-like point. 2. The calcaneum. **C. avis:** pes hippocampi minoris. **C. pedis:** the heel.

calca·rea (L. *calx*, lime). Lime; calx. **C. usta:** quicklime, calcium oxide.

calca·reous (L. *calx*, lime). Containing calcium.

cal·carine (L. *calcar*, from *calx*, heel). 1. Spur-shaped. 2. Relating to the hippocampus minor. **C. fissure:** fissure on the mesial surface of the occipital lobe.

calcariū·ria (L. *calx*, lime; G. *ouron*, urine). Urinary excretion of calcium salts.

calci·ferol (L. *calx*, lime; *ferre*, to bear, *oleum*, oil). Vitamin D., a fat-soluble substance derived from ergosterol by photo-chemical changes, found in relatively large amounts in the livers of certain fish (cod, halibut), also present in egg-yolk, yeasts, fungi and, immediately after exposure to sunlight only, in green vegetables; deficiency in this substance in the diet of infants is a cause of rickets.

calcificā·tion (L. *calx*, lime; *facere*, to make). The deposition of calcium salts (about 9 parts of calcium carbonate to 1 part of calcium phosphate) in the tissues. **C., metastatic:** deposition of calcium salts in living tissues other than bone, preceded by its removal from bone.

calci·meter (L. *calx*, lime; G. *metron*, measure). An instrument used to estimate the quantity of calcium in any part of the body or in the blood.

calcinā·tion (Mediaeval L. *calcinare*, from *calx*, lime). Roasting or expelling volatile constituents of a substance by heat.

calcinō·sis (L. *calx*, lime). A condition characterized by abnormal deposition of calcium salts in the soft tissues, either localized (usually in older people) or generalized (often affecting younger individuals). See also calcification, metastatic.

cal·ciorrhă·chia (L. *calx*, lime; G. *rhakhis*, spine). A condition in which calcium is present in the spinal fluid.

calcipē·nia (L. *calx*, lime; G. *penia*, poverty). Absence or deficiency of calcium in the system.

calcium (L. *calx*, lime). A bivalent element of the magnesium group, widely distributed in nature; the basic element of limestone; essential to life; daily requirement in man about 0·7 grm.; symbol Ca. **C. carbonate:** $CaCO_3$, one of the salts occurring in bone. **C. phosphate, C. metaphosphate** $(Ca(PO_3)_2)$, dicalcium phosphate $(CaHPO_4)$, calcium pyrophosphate $(Ca_2P_2O_7)$ or tricalcium phosphate $(Ca(PO_4)_2)$, the last being the main mineral salt of bone.

cal·culous (L. *calculus*, pebble, dim. of *calx*, lime). Of the nature of a calculus.

calculus (L.). An abnormal stone-like concretion (usually containing calcium salts) in the body, e.g., in the gall-bladder, salivary glands, bile ducts or urinary system.

Caldani's ligament (Caldani, L. M. A., Italian anatomist, 1725–1813). A small fibrotic band which extends from the inner border of the coracoid process to the lower border of the clavicle.

calefā·cient (L. *calidus*, warm; *facere*, to make). Creating warmth.

calf. The fleshy part of the leg below the knee at the back. It is formed by the gastrocnemius muscles.

ca·libre (Fr.). The inner diameter of a tube or canal.

ca·librate (Fr. *calibre*). To graduate a measuring instrument from a given standard.

cali·go (L.). Poorness of vision.

ca·lipers (Fr. *calibre*). Compasses with curved legs; instrument for measuring a diameter.

Callaway's test (Callaway, T., English physician, 1791–1848). A measurement test for dislocation of the humerus. The axillary line is longer on the injured side.

Calleja's olfactory islets (Calleja y Sanchez, C., Spanish anatomist, died 1913). Nests of large stellate cells interspersed with small nests of minute pyramidal cells, found in the cortex of the hippocampal gyrus.

Calliphora. A genus of flies which includes the *C. vomitoria*, or bluebottle.

callomā·nia (G. *kallos*, beauty; *mania*, madness). A mental condition in which the patient suffers from delusions of personal good looks.

callō·sal (L. *callus*, hard skin or flesh). Relating to the corpus callosum.

callō·sity (L. *callus*, hard skin or flesh). A localized thickening of the epidermis on parts exposed to pressure, differing from a corn in the absence of the peg.

callō·so-mar·ginal (L. *callus*, hard skin or flesh; *margo*, margin). Relating to the callosal and marginal gyri of the brain.

callō·sum (L. *callus*, hard skin or flesh). See under corpus callosum.

cal·lous (L. *callus*, hard skin or flesh). Hard; indurated.

cal·lus (L.). 1. A callosity. 2. The reparative growth of osseous tissue around a fracture.

calomel (G. *kalos*, beautiful; *melas*, black). Mercurous chloride, Hg_2Cl_2; used as a purgative.

Calori's bursa (Calori, L., Italian anatomist, 1807–96). The bursa interposed between the trachea and the arch of the aorta.

calor·ic (L. *calor*, heat). Relating to calory or to heat or heat-production. **C. test:** a test for labyrinthine function depending on the fact that douching of the external auditory meatus with warm or cold water induces convection currents in the endolymph, causing nystagmus to (warm) or away from (cold) the stimulated side.

ca·lorie (L. *calor*, heat). A heat unit; the amount of heat required to raise the temperature of 1 g. of water through 1° Centigrade. Kilo-calorie=1,000 calories.

ca·lorifā·cient (L. *calor*, heat; *facere*, to make). Heat-producing.

calori·fic (L. *calor*, heat; *facere*, to make). Heat-producing.

calori·meter (L. *calor*, heat; G. *metron*, measure). Apparatus for direct estimation of the caloric energy produced by an organism or by an organic substance by measuring the rise in temperature of a known quantity of water or air surrounding a ventilated compartment in which the organism is placed or the substance burned.

calori·metry (L. *calor*, heat; *metron*, measure). Estimation of caloric value of energy. **C., direct:** c. by means of a calorimeter, *q.v.* **C., indirect:** c. by measuring the amount of oxygen used, and/or the amount of CO_2 given off, by respiration or by the burning of an organic substance.

calva·ria, calva·rium (L. *calvaria*, skull, from *calvus*, bald). The skullcap.

calvi·tiēs (L. *calvus*, bald). Baldness.

calx (L.). 1. The heel. 2. Calcium oxide.

calў·ciform (G. *kalux*, flower-cup; L. *forma*, shape). Cup-shaped.

cā·lyx (G. *kalux*, flower-cup). A cup-shaped structure, e.g., one of the funnel-shaped structures surrounding the renal pyramids.

Campbell's area (Campbell, A. W., English pathologist, 1868–1937). The precentral area of the cortex cerebri.

Campbell's ligament (Campbell, W. F., American surgeon, 1867–1926). The suspensory ligament of the axilla.

Camper's angle (Camper, P., Dutch anatomist, 1722–89). The angle formed by Camper's line and a line joining the acanthion and the auricular point. **C.'s chiasma:** the interlacing of the fibres of the tendons of the flexor digitorum sublimis. **C.'s fascia:** the subcutaneous layer of the superficial fascia of the upper part of the thigh. **C.'s ligament:** the triangular ligament. **C.'s line:** a line passing from the external auditory meatus to just below the nasal spine.

cam·phor. A white crystalline substance from the *Cinnamomum camphora* (growing in Japan and Formosa) or synthetically produced from turpentine. It has a variety of medical uses, is sedative, carminative, anti-spasmodic, diaphoretic and anti-pyretic.

cam·phorism. Camphor poisoning.

campi·meter (L. *campus*, field; G. *metron*, measure). A screen over the surface of which test-objects are moved.

campi·metry (L. *campus*, field; G. *metron*, measure). Examination of vision of the central area of the retina by a campimeter.

camp·todacty̆·lia, camp·todac·tyly (G. *kamptos*, flexible; *daktulos*, finger). Congenital or acquired permanent flexion of one or more fingers.

campylorrhi·nus (G. *kampulos*, curved; *rhis*, nose). Monster with nasal deformity.

canal (L. *canalis*). A tubular channel or passage. C., alimentary: the digestive tube from the mouth to the anus. C., auditory: the meatus acousticus externus. C., blastophoric: opening marking the remains of the notochordal canal. C., ciliary: tubular ring in the sclera around the iridal margin. C., cranio-pharyngeal: a foetal structure between pharynx and anterior lobe of pituitary body. C., neural: see neural canal. C., neurenteric: passage between posterior part of neural tube to enteron; also called c. notochordal. C. semicircular: canals in the inner ear which act as receptor organs on which static sense depends.

canali·cular (L. *canaliculus*, dim. of *canalis*). Relating to a canaliculus.

canali·culus (L.). A small channel or groove.

căn·aliză·tion. 1. The making of channels. 2. Surgical wound drainage without the use of tubes.

cancel·late, can·cellated, can·cellous (L. *cancelli*, lattice). Resembling lattice work; especially applied to the spongy portion of bone.

cancel·lus (L., lattice). 1. Space or unit of structure in cancellous bone. 2. Spongy lattice textures of bone.

can·cer (L., crab). 1. Carcinoma, *q.v.* 2. Sometimes loosely used to denote any malignant neoplasm. C. à deux: cancer occurring in husband and wife. C. en cuirasse: metastatic carcinomatosis of the skin of the chest, usually due to carcinoma of the breast. Adenoid c.: the same as adenocarcinoma, *q.v.* Colloid c.: a cancer the tissue of which has undergone 'colloid degeneration', *q.v.* Contact c.: a cancerous metastasis on the surface of a part which is in contact with the surface of another part affected with c. C. juice: the milky juice yielded on scraping the cut surface of carcinomatous tissue.

can·ceroci·dal (L. *cancer*; *caldere*, to kill). Destroying cancer cells.

cancerogen·ic (L. *cancer*, G. *gennan*, to produce). Causing cancer.

Canceromy̆·ces (L. *cancer*; G. *mukēs*, mushroom). A fungus thought by some to be the causal agent in cancer.

can·cerophō·bia (L. *cancer*; G. *phobos*, fear). Neurotic fear of acquiring or of being affected by cancer.

can·cerous (L. *cancer*). Of the nature of cancer.

can·criform (L. *cancer*; *forma*, shape). Resembling cancer.

can·croid (L. *cancer*; G. *eidos*, form). Like a cancer.

cancrum (L.). Canker. C. oris: see under noma.

canes·cent (L. *canus*, grey). Of a greyish colour.

cane sugar. Sucrose. Syn. saccharose.

că·nine (L. *canis*, dog). Resembling or relating to a dog, or the sharp tearing teeth of a dog. C. tooth: the tooth lateral to the incisor teeth. Syn. cuspid tooth.

caninus muscle (L. *canis*, dog). The muscle which raises the angle of the mouth.

cani·tiēs (L.). Greyness of the hair.

canker. Ulceration.

cannabinol. A constituent of the oil obtained from Indian hemp.

cannabis (L.). Hemp.

can·nula (L. dim., of *canna*, reed). A tube for insertion into a part, usually fitted with a trocar.

Canquoin's paste (Canquoin, A., French physician, 1795–1881). Zinc chloride mixed with flour and water.

can·thal (G. *kanthos*, corner of the eye). Relating to a canthus.

canthari·asis (G. *kantharos*, beetle). The presence of beetle larvae in the system.

Canthă·ridēs (pl. of L. *Cantharis*, *q.v.*). Spanish flies.

canthă·ridin. A blistering agent obtained from the Spanish fly.

canthă·ridism. A morbid condition produced by excessive use of cantharides.

Can·tharis. 1. A genus of beetles. 2. The Spanish fly. C. (Meloe) vesicatoria. Cantharides are used externally for blistering. Although large doses taken internally are poisonous, small doses are sometimes used as diuretics.

canthec·tomy (G. *kanthos*, corner of the eye; *ektomē*, excision). Excision of a canthus.

canthi·tis (G. *kanthos*, corner of the eye). Inflammation of a canthus.

canthŏ·lysis (G. *kanthos*, corner of the eye; *luein*, to loosen). Canthectomy, with a section of the external canthal ligament.

can·thoplasty (G. *kanthos*, corner of the eye; *plassein*, to form). 1. Any operation for restoration of the canthus. 2. An operation for increasing the length of the palpebral fissure by slitting the outer canthus.

canthor·rhaphy (G. *kanthos*, corner of the eye; *haphē*, suture). Suturing of the canthus.

canthŏ·tomy (G. *kanthos*, corner of the eye; *tomē*, a cutting). Slitting of the canthus.

canthus (G. *kanthos*). The angle formed by the junction of the eyelids.

canula. The same as cannula, *q.v.*

CaO. Calcium oxide.

Ca(OH)$_2$. Calcium hydroxide.

caoutchouc (Fr.). Gum elastic.

capă·city (L. *capacitas*). 1. Containing or holding power. 2. Volume. Thermal c.: the amount of calories required to raise the temperature of a body 1° Centigrade. Vital c.: the amount of air that can be expelled by forcible expiration after forcible inspiration.

cap·illarectă·sia (L. *capillaris*, of the hair; G. *ektăsis*, extension). Dilatation of capillaries.

capillari·tis. Inflammation of the capillaries.

capillă·rity (L. *capillus*, hair). The physical phenomena relating to the rise of fluids in capillary tubes.

capil·lary (L. *capillus*). 1. One of the minute vessels forming the capillary system intermediate between the arteries and veins. 2. A minute lymph vessel. 3. Pertaining to the capillaries. 4. Hair-like. C. attraction: the phenomenon that in a c. tube a fluid rises to a level higher than in a communicating vessel of larger bore owing to the adhesive force between the fluid and the capillary wall. C. bronchitis: bronchiolitis. C. pulse: pulsation of c. blood vessels.

capil·lus (L.). A hair.

capital (L. *caput*, head). Of vital importance.

că·pitate (L. *caput*, head). Shaped like a head.

capitation fee. The fee in respect of each insured person per annum received by a general practitioner under the National Health Service Act.

capita·tum. The os magnum of the carpus.

capitel·lum (L. *caput*, head). 1. The bulb of a hair. 2. A small rounded prominence of a bone. 3. The rounded eminence at the lower end of the humerus.

capi·tular. Relating to the head of a bone.

capi·tulum (L. *caput*, head). A small head-like structure.

cap·rate. Salt or ester of capric acid.

capric acid. A monobasic fatty acid $CH_3(CH_2)_8COOH$.

cap·rŏate. Salt or ester of caproic acid.

capro·ic acid. A monobasic fatty acid, $CH_3(CH_2)_4COOH$.

cap·sicism. Addiction to capsicum.

Capsicum. A genus of solanaceous plants, including Cayenne or red pepper. From the dried fruit of C. *frutescens* a strong local stimulant is obtained, which is used in neuralgia and similar complaints. It is sometimes given internally in cases of malaria.

capsī·tis. Inflammation of the crystalline lens capsule.

capsula (L.). The internal capsule in the brain.

cap·sular (L. capsula). Relating to a capsule.

cap·sule (L. capsula, dim. of capsa, box). 1. A membrane, sheath or other structure enclosing a part or an organism, e.g., many, if not all, bacteria in which it consists of a carbohydrate compound containing, in some instances, nitrogen. 2. A soluble shell for enclosing drugs. C. cell: or cell capsule, the lining or cell-wall to any cell. C. externa: a thin layer of white fibres surrounding the corpus striatum. C., interna: a bundle of white fibres separating the optic thalamus and the caudate nucleus from the lenticular nucleus.

capsulec·tomy (L. capsula, a small box; ektomē, excision). Excision of a capsule.

capsuli·tis. Inflammation of a capsule.

cap·sulo-lenti·cular (L. capsula, a small box; lens, a lentil). Relating to the crystalline lens and its capsule.

capsulō·ma. A tumour of the renal capsule.

capsulor·rhaphy (L. capsula, dim. of capsa, box; G. rhaphē, suture). Suture of a capsule, especially in the sense of reducing it.

capsū·lotome (L. capsula; G. tomē, a cutting). Instrument for performing capsulotomy.

capsulŏ·tomy (L. capsula, small box; tomē, a cutting). Incision of the capsule of the ocular lens.

Capuron's cardinal points (Capuron, J., French physician, 1767–1850). Four fixed points of the pelvic inlet, the two iliopectineal eminences anteriorly and the two sacro-iliac joints posteriorly.

caput (L., head). 1. The head. 2. The chief part or beginning of an organ. C. medusae: that relatively rare form of collateral circulation established in cases of portal obstruction with the systemic circulation in which the epigastric veins of the abdominal wall which communicate with the veins at the hilus of the liver by way of the round ligament become dilated, forming a figure of rays converging to the umbilicus. C. natiforme: see C. quadratum below. C. obstipum: see under torticollis. C. quadratum: deformity of the cranial vault due to rickets, characterized by square shape, division into four mounds corresponding to the two frontal and the two parietal bones by abnormal depression of the anterior fontanelle and the sagittal and coronal sutures, and bossing of the frontal and parietal tubera owing to periosteal new bone formation. Syn. C. natiforme. C. succedaneum: an oedematous swelling of the soft parts of the cranium on the presenting part of a foetus, due to pressure upon the presenting part by the cervix of the maternal uterus.

Carabelli's tubercle (Carabelli, G., Austrian dentist, 1787–1842). An occasional fifth tubercle lingual to the antero-internal cusp of the first upper molar tooth.

carat. A measure of the excellence of gold, pure gold being 24 carats.

că·raway. Dried ripe fruits of Carum carvi (Umbelliferae). Used as a carminative.

car·bachol. $(H_2N.COOCH_2CH_2N(CH_2)_3) + Cl−$. Carbamylcholine chloride. Action similar to acetylcholine, but more stable.

car·bamide. $H_2N.CO.NH_2$. Syn. for urea. It has a diuretic action when administered orally.

carbarsone. Para-carbaminophenylarsonic acid, used in the treatment of intestinal amoebiasis.

carbhaēmoglŏ·bin (L. carbo, coal; G. haima, blood; L. globus, globe). An easily dissociable compound of carbon dioxide and haemoglobin.

car·binol. Methyl alcohol.

car·bo (L., coal). Charcoal. C. animalis: animal charcoal. C. ligni: wood charcoal.

carbocyc·lic (L. carbo, coal; G. kuklos, circle). Applied to cyclic compounds, q.v., in which the ring is composed of carbon atoms.

carbogă·seous (L. carbo, coal; G. khaŏs, chaos). Charged with carbon dioxide gas.

carbohaē·mia (L. carbo, coal; G. haima, blood). Impaired oxidation of the blood.

car·bohaemoglŏ·bin. Haemoglobin united with carbon dioxide.

carbohȳ·drase (L. carbo, coal; G. hŭdor, water). Any enzyme hydrolyzing a carbohydrate.

carbohȳ·drate (L. carbo, coal; G. hŭdor, water). Name applied to a group of substances which usually have the general formula $C_n(H_2O)_n$ or to de-oxidation products. They are classified, according to complexity of structure (value of n), into mono- or di-saccharides which are crystalline, and polysaccharides which are amorphous.

car·bolate. Salts of carbolic acid (phenol).

car·bolfuchs·in. A mixture of one part of fuchsin with 90 parts of 5 per cent carbolic acid dissolved in 10 parts of alcohol; used for staining.

carbŏ·lic (L. carbo, coal; oleum, oil). Containing or derived from coal tar.

carbolic acid. Phenol, C_6H_5OH, derived from coal tar. Parent member of a group of antiseptics.

car·bolism. Carbolic acid poisoning.

car·bolize. To impregnate with carbolic acid.

carbolū·ria (L. carbo, coal; G. ouron, urine). A condition in which carbolic acid is present in the urine.

car·bon (L. carbo, coal). A non-metallic element occurring as diamond, graphite and coal, in carbon dioxide, carbonates, and in all vegetable and animal tissues. Symbol C.

carbon dioxide (CO_2). A colourless gas of pungent smell. Present at 0·03 per cent in the atmospheric air. CO_2 combining power: the capacity of the blood to bring dissolved carbon dioxide (H_2CO_3; a weak acid) into its combined condition (mainly as Na HCO_3, a weak base). CO_2 snow: the snow-like substance produced by the solidification of fluid CO_2.

carbon monoxide (CO). A colourless, non-odorous poisonous gas, originating during incomplete combustion of coal.

car·bonate. Any salt of carbonic acid containing the CO_3 radical.

car·bonated. 1. Containing carbon dioxide. 2. Changed into a carbonate.

carbon·ic acid. H_2CO_3. An unstable acid found only in solution by the dissolution of CO_2 in water. It reacts with bases, e.g., sodium and potassium, to form carbonates and bicarbonates.

car·bonize. To convert into charcoal; to char.

carbonū·ria (L. carbo, coal; G. ouron, urine). The presence of carbon compounds in the urine.

car·bonyl (L. carbo, coal; G. hulē, matter). The CO radical.

Carboxydomonas. Bacteria which are capable of growing in the absence of organic matter. They obtain their energy from the oxidation of carbon monoxide to carbon dioxide.

carbox·yhaemoglŏ·bin (L. carbo, coal; G. oxus, sharp; haima, blood; L. glŏbus, globe). The reversible combination of carbon monoxide and haemoglobin formed in the blood on inhalation of carbon monoxide; diminishing or abolishing the oxygen-carrying power of the blood.

carbox·yhaemoglobinaē·mia. Carbon monoxide poisoning.

carbox·yl (L. carbo, coal; G. oxus, sharp; hulē, matter). The CO.OH group, characteristic of the organic salts.

carbox·ylase (L. carbo, coal; G. oxus, sharp; hulē, matter). An enzyme acting on the carboxyl group, splitting off carbon dioxide.

carbromal. a-Bromo-a-ethylbutyrylcarbamide. A hypnotic that is valuable in cases of insomnia due to worry, etc., but not so efficient in the allaying of pain. It is free from after-effects.

car·buncle (L. *carbunculus*, dim. of *carbo*). A staphylococcal infection of hair follicles or sweat glands and the surrounding subcutaneous tissue, discharging on the surface by several openings.

carbunc·ular. Like a carbuncle.

Carcassone's ligament (Carcassone, M., French surgeon, born 1728). The deep layer of the perineal fascia. Syn. Colles's fascia.

carcinec·tomy (G. *karkinos*, crab or cancer; *ektomē*, excision). The surgical removal of a carcinoma.

car·cinelcō·sis (G. *karkinos*, cancer; *helkōsis*, ulceration). Cancerous ulceration.

car·cinogen (G. *karkinos*, cancer; *gennan*, to produce). Any cancer forming agent.

car·cinogĕ·nesis (G. *karkinos*, cancer; *gennan*, to produce). Development of cancer.

carcinogen·ic (G. *karkinos*, cancer; *gennan*, to produce). Applied to agents inducing cancer.

car·cinoid (G. *karkinos*, cancer; *eidos*, form). A benign tumour occurring usually in the vermiform appendix, but occasionally also in the small intestine, resembling carcinoma microscopically, but scarcely giving rise to any symptoms, composed of lipoid containing cells derived from the Kultschitzky cells of the intestinal mucosa which belong to the chromaffine system and are intensely stained by silver impregnation. Syn. argentaffine carcinoma; Kultschitzky-cell carcinoma.

carcinŏ·lysis (G. *karkinos*, cancer; *luein*, to dissolve). Destruction of cancer cells.

carcinō·ma (G. *karkinoma*, cancer). A malignant epithelial tumour, tending to invade the lymph spaces of the surrounding connective tissue and spreading primarily by lymphatic permeation and embolism but also by the blood-stream to form metastasis, both tending to ulcerate and causing by its growth destruction of the invaded tissue and general cachexia. **Adeno-c:** carcinoma formed of columnar epithelium in imperfect glandular form. **C., basal-celled:** an invasive, non-metastasizing neoplasm of the skin, probably derived from cells of the basal layer of the epidermis, characterized by slow growth and failure to spread by metastases, occurring especially at the upper part of the face about the nose, eyelid, cheek or ear. Syn. rodent ulcer. **Chimney-sweep c.:** c. of the scrotum occurring in chimney-sweeps and due to the action of soot. **Colloid c.,** c. with mucoid degeneration of the stroma; an undesirable term. **Cylindrical c.:** c. derived from cylindrical or columnar-shaped cells. **Fibrous c.:** the same as scirrhous c. **Medullary c.** or **Encephaloid c.:** a c. almost entirely composed of cells, having very little fibrous stroma. **Scirrhous c.:** a c. of hard consistency due to the dense fibrous stroma. **Simple c.:** a c. in which cells are arranged in solid cords. **Squamous c.:** c. derived from squamous epithelial cells. Syn. epithelioma.

carcinō·matophō·bia (G. *karkinoma*, cancer; *phobos*, fear). Neurotic dread of cancer.

carcinomatō·sis (G. *karkinoma*, cancer). More or less extensive spread of carcinomatous metastases.

carcinŏ·matous (G. *karkinoma*, cancer). Relating to or of the nature of carcinoma.

carcinō·sis. The same as carcinomatosis, *q.v.*

Cardarelli's symptom (Cardarelli, A., Italian physician, 1831-1926). Tracheal tugging.

car·dia (G. *kardia*). 1. The heart. 2. The oesophageal orifice of the stomach.

car·diac (G. *kardia*, heart). 1. Relating to the heart. 2. Relating to the cardia of the stomach. 3. A drug acting especially on the heart. **C. asthma:** see under asthma. **C. cycle:** the succession of auricular and ventricular systole and diastole. **C. decompensation:** congestive circulatory failure. **C. failure:** inability to maintain an efficient circulation of the blood. **C. index:** see under index.

cardiăg·ra (G. *kardia*, heart; *agra*, seizure). Severe pain in the heart.

cardial·gia (G. *kardia*, heart; *algos*, pain). Heartburn.

cardiă·meter (G. *kardia*, heart; *metron*, measure). An instrument used for finding the position of the cardia.

car·diamor·phia (G. *kardia*, heart; *a* neg.; *morphē*, form). Heart deformity.

cardianaesthē·sia (G. *kardia*, heart; *anaisthēsia*, insensibility). Absence of feeling in the heart.

car·diant. Any heart stimulant.

cardi·azol. Preparations of leptazol, used as heart stimulants.

cardiĕctă·sis (G. *kardia*, heart; *ektasis*, extension). Dilatation of the heart.

cardiĕc·tomy (G. *kardia*, heart; *ektomē*, excision). Excision of the cardiac end of the stomach.

car·dinal (L. *cardo*, hinge). Chief or principal. **C. movements:** movements of the eye around the transverse and vertical axes of Listing's plane. *q.v.*

cardio-accĕ·lerator (G. *kardia*, heart; L. *accelerare*, from *celer*, swift). Hastening the action of the heart.

cardio-augmen·tor (G. *kardia*, heart; L. *augēre*, to increase). Increasing the force of the heart's action.

car·diocele (G. *kardia*, heart; *kēlē*, hernia). Hernia of the heart. **C. abdominalis:** hernia of heart into the abdominal cavity.

car·diocentē·sis (G. *kardia*, heart; *kentēsis*, puncture). Puncture of one of the chambers of the heart.

cardiŏ·clasis (G. *kardia*, heart; *klăsis*, a fracture). A rupture of the heart.

car·diōdiō·sis (G. *kardia*, heart; *diosis*, a pushing off). The operation in which the cardiac end of the stomach is dilated.

car·diodynă·mics (G. *kardia*, heart; *dunamis*, power). The science of the forces relating to the action of the heart.

car·diodỹ·nia (G. *kardia*, heart; *ŏdŭnē*, pain). Pain of the heart.

car·diogĕ·nesis (G. *kardia*, heart; *gennan*, to produce). The growth of the foetal heart.

car·diogen·ic (G. *kardia*, heart; *gennan*, to produce). Originating in the heart.

car·diogram (G. *kardia*, heart; *gramma*, a picture). A recording of the heart's pulsation, taken through the chest wall.

car·diograph (G. *kardia*, heart; *graphein*, to write). Instrument for recording the heart's pulsation graphically.

cardiŏ·graphy (G. *kardia*, heart; *graphein*, to write). Examination by means of the cardiograph.

car·dioid (G. *kardia*, heart; *eidos*, form). Heart-shaped.

cardio-inhĭ·bitory (G. *kardia*, heart; L. *inhibēre*, prevent). Inhibiting the action of the heart.

car·diolith (G. *kardia*, heart; *lithos*, stone). A calculus in the heart.

cardiŏ·logist (G. *kardia*, heart; *logos*, treatise). A specialist in heart diseases.

cardiŏ·logy (G. *kardia*, heart; *logos*, treatise). That part of the science of medicine pertaining to the heart.

cardiŏ·lysis (G. *kardia*, heart; *lusis*, loosening). Resection of the ribs and sternum over the pericardium, as performed for severing adhesions between the pericardium and the external surrounding parts, which prevent proper diastolic stretching of the heart.

car·diomalā·cia (G. *kardia*, heart; *mălăkia*, softness). Softening of the heart muscles.

car·diomĕ·galy (G. *kardia*, heart; *megas*, large). General enlargement of the heart.

cardĭŏ·meter (G. *kardia*, heart; *metron*, measure). An apparatus for estimating the changes in the systolic and diastolic sizes of the cardiac ventricles.

car·diomoti·lity (G. *kardia*, heart; L. *mŏvēre*, to move). The heart's movements.

car·diomyolipō·sis (G. *kardia*, heart; *mus*, muscle; *lipos*, fat). Fatty degeneration of the muscles of the heart.

car·dionecrō·sis (G. *kardia*, heart; *nekrōsis*, deadness). Necrosis of the heart.

car·dioneph·ric (G. *kardia*, heart; *nephros*, kidney). Relating to the heart and the kidney.

car·dioneurō·sis (G. *kardia*, heart; *neuron*, nerve). A nervous disorder, characterized by malfunctioning of the heart.

car·dio-omen·topexy (G. *kardia*, heart; L. *omentum*, adipose membrane; G. *pēxis*, a fixing). Suturing of an area of the omentum to the heart to provide it with an additional blood supply.

car·diopath (G. *kardia*, heart; *pathos*, disease). A sufferer from heart disease.

car·diopath·ic. Relating to disease of the heart.

cardĭŏ·pathy (G. *kardia*, heart; *pathos*, suffering). Any disease of the heart.

car·diopericardī·tis (G. *kardia*, heart; *peri*, around; *kardia*, heart). Inflammation of the heart tissues and the pericardium.

cardiophŏ·bia (G. *kardia*, heart; *phobos*, fear). Neurotic dread of heart disease.

cardioplē·gia (G. *kardia*, heart; *plēgē*, a stroke). 1. Any injury done to the heart. 2. Paralysis of the heart.

car·diopneumat·ic (G. *kardia*, heart; *pneuma*, breath). The same as cardio-respiratory, *q.v.*

car·diopneumopex·y (G. *kardia*, heart; *pneumōn*, lung; *pēxis*, a fixing). Suturing of an area of the lung to provide the heart with an additional blood supply.

car·diopul·monary, car·diopulmon·ic (G. *kardia*, heart; L. *pulmo*, lung). Relating to both heart and lungs.

cardiopunc·ture (G. *kardia*, heart; L. *punctura*, from *pungere*, to puncture). The same as cardiocentesis, *q.v.*

car·diores·piratory (G. *kardia*, heart; L. *spirare*, to breathe). Relating to both heart and respiration.

cardiopylor·ic (G. *kardia*, heart; *pulōros*, the pylorus). Relating both to the heart and the pylorus.

car·diorē·nal (G. *kardia*, heart; L. *rēnes*, the kidneys). Relating to the heart and the kidney.

car·dĭŏr·rhaphy (G. *kardia*, heart; *rhaphē*, suture). Suturing of the heart.

car·diorrhex·is (G. *kardia*, heart; *rhēxis*, rupture). Rupture of the heart.

car·diosclerō·sis (G. *kardia*, heart; *sklēros*, hard). Fibrous induration of the tissues of the heart.

car·dioscope (G. *kardia*, heart; *skopein*, to view). An instrument for examining the interior of the heart.

car·diospasm (G. *kardia*, heart; *spasmos*, spasm). Spasm of the cardiac sphincter of the stomach, preventing the proper passage of food from the oesophagus to the stomach. See also achalasia.

cardiosphyg·mograph (G. *kardia*, heart; *sphugmos*, pulsation; *graphein*, to write). Instrument for recording graphically the apex beat, the radial and the venous pulse.

car·diotachŏ·meter (G. *kardia*, heart; *tachos*, speed; *metron*, measure). An apparatus for recording the number of heartbeats in a given period.

car·diothy·rotoxicō·sis (G. *kardia*, heart; *thureoeidēs; toxikon*, poison). Hyperthyroidism with severe involvement of the heart.

cardĭŏ·tomy (G. *kardia*, heart; *tomē*, a cutting). 1. Incision of the cardiac end of the stomach. 2. Incision of the heart.

car·dioton·ic (G. *kardia* heart; *tonos*, tone). Having a stimulating effect on the heart.

car·diotox·ic (G. *kardia*, heart; *toxikon*, poison). Having a poisonous effect upon the heart.

car·diovas·cular (G. *kardia*, heart; L. *vasculum*, dim. of *vas*, vessel). Relating to both heart and blood vessels.

cardi·tis (G. *kardia*, heart). Inflammation of the endocardium, myocardium and pericardium.

car·divalvuli·tis (G. *kardia*, heart; *valvula*, dim. of *valva*). Inflammation of the valves of the heart.

car·dol. An irritant oil from cashew nuts.

Cardophyllin. A brand of theophyllene and ethylenediamine.

cā·rīēs (L., decay). 1. Inflammatory destruction of bone. 2. Dental decay affecting the enamel, dentine and cementum with secondary infection of the pulp.

cari·na (L., keel). 1. Any keel-like structure. 2. Mesial ridge on the lower surface of the fornix cerebri.

că·rinate, carinā·tion (L. *carina*, keel). Keeled; resembling a keel.

cā·rious (L. *caries*, decay). Relating to caries.

car·minative (L. *carminare*, to card (wool, etc.)). A drug promoting absorption or expulsion of intestinal gases.

carmine (Sanskrit, *krimi*, a worm). Red colouring matter derived from cochineal by precipitation with alum.

carmi·nophil (Sanskrit, *krimi*, a worm; G. *philein*, to love). Easily stained with carmine.

car·neous (L. *caro*, flesh). Fleshy.

car·nificā·tion (L. *caro*, flesh; *facere*, to make). Inflammatory consolidation of the lungs by which their appearance becomes flesh-like.

carni·vorous (L. *caro*, flesh; *vorare*, to eat). Flesh-eating.

carnophŏ·bia (L. *caro*, flesh; G. *phobos*, fear). Abnormal dislike of meat-eating.

car·nose (L. *caro*, flesh). Resembling or relating to flesh.

Carnot's solution (Carnot, P., French physician, born 1869). A solution of gelatin, 5 per cent to 10 per cent, in normal saline; a local haemostatic.

că·rotene (L. *carota*, carrot). A yellow pigment occurring in certain plants; a precursor of Vitamin A, to which it is converted in the animal body.

carŏ·tid (G. *karoein*, to stupefy). 1. The carotid artery, the principal large artery on each side of the neck. 2. Of or relating to the c. artery. **C. body** or **C. gland:** a structure belonging to the chromaffine system, *q.v.*, lying at the bifurcation of the common c. artery: Syn. glomus caroticum. **C. sinus:** the bifurcation of the carotid artery. **C. sinus reflex:** reflex vasomotor and cardio-inhibitory phenomena originating from the nerve-plexus at the c. sinus.

car·otinaē·mia (L. *carota*, carrot; G. *haima*, blood). Presence of carotene in the blood in an abnormally large amount, resulting in yellowish discolouration of the skin, especially of naso-labial folds and the palms of the hands.

car·pal (G. *karpos*, wrist). Relating to the carpus or wrist.

carpec·tomy (G. *karpos*, wrist; *ektomē*, excision). Excision of one or more of the carpal bones.

carphŏ·logy (G. *karphos*, a dry stalk; *legein*, to collect). Picking and fumbling at bedclothes, as occurring in patients delirious from grave illness.

Carpoglȳ·phus passulā·rum. A mite which is found sometimes in dried fruit, and which may cause skin disorders in human beings handling infested fruit.

car·pometacar·pal (G. *karpos*, wrist; *meta*, after; *karpos*, wrist). Relating to the carpus and metacarpus.

carpopĕ·dal spasm (G. *karpos*, wrist; L. *pes*, foot; G. *spasmos*, spasm). Tonic intermittent cramps affecting the hands and feet.

car·pophalan·geal (G. *karpos*, wrist; *phalanx*, the bone between two joints of the fingers and toes). Relating to both carpus and phalanges.

car·pus (G. *karpos*, wrist). The wrist; the eight wrist-bones.

carrefour sensitif (Fr.). The back part of the posterior limb of the internal capsule of the cerebrum, crossed by sensory nerve tracts.

Carrel-Dakin fluid. See under Dakin's solution.

car·rier. Person harbouring and spreading pathogenic micro-organisms to which he is or has become immune.

Carrión's disease (Carrión, D. A., Peruvian student, 1850-86). An infectious fever caused by the *Bartonella bacilliformis*, and transmitted by the sandfly, *Phlebotomus verrucarum*.

carrot. The plant *Daucus carota*, the seed of which is used as a diuretic and as a stimulant.

Carswell's grapes (Carswell, Sir R., English physician, 1793-1857). A racemose arrangement of tuberculous infiltration about the bronchioles in pulmonary tuberculosis.

Carthamus. A genus of plants, the flowers of which are diuretic and aperient.

car·tilage (L. *cartilago*). Gristle; a tissue forming the main part of the embryonic skeleton in vertebrates, becoming in nearly all vertebrates converted into bone and hyaline c., which consists of an avascular intercellular tissue with c. cells interspersed; chemically mainly composed of chondromucoid (*q.v*), chondro-albumin (*q.v.*) and collagen (*q.v.*). **Intermediary c.:** 1. c. in process of transformation into bone. 2. c. lying between epiphysis and diaphysis of a bone. **Reticular c.:** c. in which the cells are surrounded by elastic fibres. **Temporary c.:** c. which is ultimately replaced by osseous tissue.

car·tilagï·nifica·tion (L. *cartilago*, cartilage; *facere*, to make). Conversion into cartilage.

cartilagï·niform (L. *cartilago*, cartilage; *forma*, shape). Resembling cartilage.

cartilä·ginous (L. *cartilago*, cartilage). Of the nature of cartilage.

cä·runcle (L. *carunculus*, dim. of *caro*, flesh). 1. A small reddish structure at the base of the plica semilunaris of the eyelid. 2. A small, red, tender polypoidal tumour arising from the opening of the female urethra and projecting into the vestibule, composed of angiomatous tissue covered by squamous epithelium.

Carus's curve (Carus, K. G., German obstetrician, 1789-1869). The longitudinal axis of the pelvic canal, which forms a curved line, having the symphysis pubis as its centre.

car·vacrol. A phenolic substance isomeric with thymol, present in oil of thyme.

carvone. A terpene ketone, principal constituent of oil of caraway.

casca·ra (Sp., bark). C. sagrada, a laxative prepared from the bark of the *Rhamnus purshiana*, a shrub growing in the Pacific states of U.S.A.

case. An instance of any disease.

ca·seäse (L. *caseus*, cheese). A ferment acting upon casein.

caseä·tion (L. *caseus*, cheese). 1. Form of necrosis characteristic of tuberculosis and syphilis, characterized by transformation of tissue into a structureless cheesy mass by the combination of coagulation necrosis and fatty degeneration. 2. Precipitation of casein as a calcium paracaseinate.

ca·sein (L. *caseus*, cheese). The protein of milk. **C. hydrolysate:** see Casydrol.

caseïn·ic. $C_{12}H_{24}N_2O_5$, an acid present in casein.

caseï·nogen (L. *caseus*, cheese; G. *gennan*, to produce). A protein of milk yielding casein when acted upon by rennin.

cä·seöse (L. *caseus*, cheese). A proteose produced during digestion of casein.

cä·seous (L. *caseus*, cheese). Resembling cheese. **C. degeneration:** the same as caseation, *q.v.*

cashew nut. The kidney-shaped fruit of the Indian tree, *Anarcardium occidentale*.

CaSO₄. Calcium sulphate.

Cassava (Sp. *casabe*). The *Manihot utilissima* and *M. aipi*, from the starchy roots of which tapioca is produced.

Casserio's fontanelle (Casserio, G., Italian anatomist, 1556-1616). The fontanelle formed by the temporal, occipital and parietal bones. **C.'s muscle:** 1. Ligamentous fibres attached to the malleus. 2. The coraco-brachialis. **C.'s perforating nerve:** the external cutaneous nerve of the arm.

Cassia. A genus of leguminous plants which yield senna.

cast. A structure possessing the form of the cavity in which it has been moulded: e.g., bronchial c. **C., urinary:** a cylindrical structure formed in the renal tubules under certain morbid conditions.

Castellanella. A genus of trypanosomes, including the *C. castellani* which is the agent causing a serious type of sleeping sickness.

Castle's factors (Castle, W. B., American physician, born, 1897). 1. Intrinsic factor contained in gastric juices which, together with 2., the extrinsic factor, contained in certain foods, provides 3., the anti-anaemic factor stored in the liver, from where it is released to promote maturation of red blood corpuscles.

castor oil. A vegetable oil expressed from the seeds of *Ricinis communis*, used as a purgative.

casträ·tion (L. *castrare*). Removal of the sex-glands. **C. cells:** see under cell. **C. complex:** the unconscious thoughts pertaining to the idea of having been deprived, or the expectation of being deprived, of the (male) genitals.

cä·sualty (L. *casus*, accident). An accidental injury or the person thus injured.

Casydrol. A proprietary mixture of amino-acids and simple peptides prepared from casein and meat proteins by enzymic digestion. It is used in cases of gastro-intestinal carcinoma, intestinal obstruction, pyloric stenosis, peptic ulcer, etc.

catabä·sial (G. *kata*, down; *basis*, base). Relating to a skull in which the basion is lower than the opisthion.

catä·basis (G. *kata*, down; *bainein*, to go). The abating stage of any disorder.

catabol·ic (G. *kata*, down; *ballein*, to throw). Relating to catabolism.

catä·bolite (G. *kata*, down; *ballein*, to throw). Any product of catabolism.

catä·bolism (G. *kata*, down; *ballein*, to throw). Destructive metabolism; the breakdown of large molecules with the release of energy in the living organism.

catacau·sis (G. *kata*, down; *kausis*, a burning). Spontaneous combustion.

catacrot·ic (G. *kata*, down; *krotos*, beat). Denoting elevation of the descending line of a sphygmogram or the pulse-undulation causing this elevation.

catä·crotism (G. *kata*, down; *krotos*, beat). The occurrence of a minor pulsatory expansion of the artery after the main beat.

catadicrot·ic (G. *kata*, down; *dis*, twice; *krotos*, beat). Denoting two elevations in the descending line of a sphygmogram or the pulse undulations causing these elevations.

catadï·crotism (G. *kata*, down; *dis*, twice; *krotos*, beat). The occurrence of two minor pulsatory expansions of the artery after the main beat.

catadï·dymus (G. *kata*, down; *didumos*, twin). A twin monster fused into one in the upper and in some of the lower parts.

catadiŏp·tric (G. *kata*, down; *dia*, through; *optos*, visible). Relating to both reflection and refraction of light rays.

catagĕ·nesis (G. *kata*, down; *gennan*, to produce). Retrogression.

catagenet·ic. Relating to catagenesis.

catagmat·ic (G. *katagma*, fracture). Having the capacity to consolidate fractured bone.

că·talase (G. *kata*, down; *luein*, to dissolve). An enzyme with the property of splitting off active oxygen from peroxides; widely distributed in animal and vegetable matter.

că·talepsy (G. *kata*, down; *lēpsis*, a seizing). Abnormally long retention of positions in which limbs are passively placed, as occurring especially in catatonia or hypnosis.

catalep·tic (G. *kata*, down; *lēpsis*, a seizing). Relating to or affected with catalepsy.

catalep·tiform (G. *kata*, down; *lēpsis*, a seizing; L. *forma*, shape). Resembling catalepsy.

catalep·toid (G. *kata*, down; *lēpsis*, a seizing; *eidos*, shape). Resembling catalepsy.

cată·lysis (G. *kata*, down; *luein*, dissolve). A chemical reaction effected by a small quantity of a third substance which does not appear in the end-products of the reaction.

că·talyst (G. *kata*, down; *luein*, dissolve). A substance effecting catalysis.

catalyt·ic (G. *kata*, down; *luein*, dissolve). Relating to or produced by catalysis.

că·talyzer (G. *kata*, down; *luein*, dissolve). A substance effecting catalysis.

catamē·nia (G. *kata*, down; *mēn*, month). The menses.

catamē·nial (G. *kata*, down; *mēn*, month). Pertaining to the catamenia.

cataphā·sis (G. *kata*, down; *phasis*, statement). Perpetual repetition of the same answer to a question.

cată·phora (G. *kataphora*, an attack of lethargy). Coma somnolentium, a coma punctuated by brief periods of half consciousness.

cataphorē·sis (G. *kata*, down; *pherein*, to bear). 1. Movement of suspended particles under the influence of an electric current. 2. Diffusion of electrically charged drugs through the skin or a mucous membrane.

cataphoret·ic (G. *kata*, down; *pherein*, to bear). Relating to cataphoresis.

cataphor·ia (G. *kata*, down; *phoros*, a bearing). Hypophoria of both eyes.

cataplā·sia (G. *kata*, down; *plassein*, to form). Reversionary metamorphosis; a form of atrophy in which the cells revert to earlier and more embryonic types.

că·taplasm (G. *kata*, down; *plasma*, a thing moulded). A poultice, a soft pasty preparation for application to the body surface.

că·taract (G. *katarrhaktēs*, a waterfall). Opacity of the crystalline lens or its capsule. **C., after-:** remnants of the lens left behind after extra-capsular extraction, or destruction, of the lens. **C., aridosiliquose:** over-ripe c. with thickened capsule. **C., black:** a form of senile c. occupying nearly the entire tissue of the lens, the dark colour being due to deposition of pigment from products of slow decomposition of lenticular proteins. **C., blue-dot:** the same as c., punctiform, *q.v.* **C. brunescens:** the same as c., black, *q.v.* **C., cachectic:** bilateral cortical c., as sequel to acute toxic illness. **C. calcarea:** impregnation of lenticular opacities with calcium salts, occurring especially in later stages of complicated c. **C., capsular:** capsular opacity. **C., capsulo-lenticular:** c. of the lens and its capsule. **C., chalky:** the same as c. aridosiliquose, *q.v.* **C., choroidal:** c. following inflammatory or degenerative processes in the posterior segment of the eye. **C., coerulea:** the same as c., punctiform, *q.v.* **C., complicated:** c. due to intra-ocular diseases, usually involving the anterior and posterior portions of the cortex and characterized by rosette-like arrangement and polychromatic lustre in the early stages. **C., concussion:** c. due to contusion of the eye. **C., coronary:** a form of punctate c., developing just after the age of puberty, characterized by crown-like arrangement. **C., cortical:** c. involving the lenticular cortex only. **C., cuneiform:** a form of cortical c., developing in the peripheral parts of the deep cortex, forming radiating spikes pointing towards the centre; the typical form of senile c. **C., cupuliform:** a form of cortical c. involving only the posterior cortical layer, usually associated with nuclear sclerosis and obstructing vision early owing to its proximity to the nodal point of the dioptric system. **C., dermatogenous:** c. associated with certain skin diseases, such as sclerodermia or neurodermatitis. **C., diabetic:** c. associated with diabetes mellitus, either of widespread subcapsular or of senile type, involving usually both eyes, arising relatively early in life, and of rather acute development. **C., dilacerated:** congenital c. involving in infants the superficial, and in adults the deep, zone of the nucleus, characterized by opacities of very fine and thin shape. **C., dust-like:** the same as c., perinuclear punctate, *q.v.* **C., endocrine:** c. characterized by discrete punctate cortical opacities, early onset and bilateral occurrence, associated with certain endocrine diseases such as tetany and cretinism, also with myotonic dystrophia. **C., fusiform:** a form of congenital c.; syn. spindle-shaped, axial or coralliform c. **C., gypseous:** the same as c. calcarea, *q.v.* **C., hard:** the same as c. nuclear, *q.v.* **C., heterochromic:** c. associated with chronic uveitis. **C., hypermature:** c. owing to which the lens has become inspissated and shrunken. **C., immature:** c. leaving the lenticular cortex still clear. **C. intumescens:** c. in the stage of development characterized by swelling of the lens. **C. lactea:** an opacity consisting of a milky-white fluid. **C., lamellar:** a form of c. in young individuals characterized by localized opacities which are enclosed by new clear fibres. **C., mature:** c. extending right up to the capsule. **C., morgagnian:** c. which has resulted in liquefaction of the cortex. **C. nigra:** the same as c., black, *q.v.* **C., nuclear:** an intensification of lenticular sclerosis beginning normally about the fifth decade. **C. ossea:** formation of true bone in the lens, occurring after rupture or disintegration of the capsule. **C., perinuclear punctate:** form of cortical c. characterized by thickening of the anterior and posterior bands of the adult nucleus. **C. polaris:** opacity of one of the lenticular poles (anterior or posterior). **C., posterior saucer-shaped:** the same as c. cupuliform, *q.v.* **C., punctiform:** a condition characterized by punctiform opacities of bluish appearance scattered in the lenticular nucleus and cortex, not interfering with vision, the blue colour being due to the dispersion of light by the minute particles in the opalescent medium. **C., pyramidal:** an anterior capsular c., protruding conically owing to the dragging upon adhesions of the lens to the cornea when the anterior chamber is re-formed. **C., radiational:** c. due to radiant energy. **C., secondary:** 1. After-c. 2. Complicated c. **C., senile:** c. becoming manifest in old age, but usually of congenital character. **C., snowflake:** a typical form of diabetic c. **C., soft:** cortical c. **C., subcapsular:** congenital or acquired c. involving the subcapsular epithelium. **C., total:** opacity of the entire lens. **C., zonular:** the same as c. lamellar, *q.v.*

cataract-extraction. Surgical removal of the cataractous lens.

catarac·tous (G. *katarrhaktēs*, cataract). Pertaining to or affected with cataract.

catarrh (G. *katarrhein*, to flow down). Mild inflammation of a mucous membrane.

catar·rhal (G. *katarrhein*, to flow down). Of the nature of catarrh. **C. jaundice:** see under jaundice.

catatō·nia, cată·tony (G. *kata*, down; *tonos*, tension). A symptom of schizophrenia in which the body or limbs retain any posture in which they are placed by the observer. Syn. flexibilitas cerea.

cataton·ic. Relating to catatonia.

că·techu. A powerful astringent. A dried aqueous extract from the leaves and young shoots of *Uncaria gambier.*

că·telectrŏ·tonus (G. *kata*, down; *ēlektron*, amber; *tonos*, tension). Increase in excitability in irritable tissue during the passage of electric current through it at the cathode.

că·tenating (L. *catenare*, from *catena*, chain). Connecting; linking.

că·tenoid. Chain-like.

catgut. A ligature substance made from the intestines of sheep and other animals.

cathar·mos (G. *kathairein*, to cleanse). An incantation to prevent or cure disease.

cathar·sis (G. *kathairein*). 1. Purgation. 2. Emotional purification. 3. In psycho-analysis, elimination of a complex by bringing it to consciousness.

cathar·tic. 1. Relating to catharsis. 2. A drug promoting intestinal peristalsis.

că·theter (G. *kathĕtēr*). A hollow tube for introduction through a narrow canal, especially through the urethra for draining the bladder or through the pharyngotympanic tube for abolishing an occlusion of this canal.

că·theterism (G. *kathĕtēr*). Repeated use of a catheter.

că·theterizā·tion (G. *kathĕtēr*). The passing of a catheter.

cathex·is (G. *kathexis*, retention). The accumulation or concentration of psychic energy on a particular idea or object. **C. of the ego:** libido directed towards the self; ego libido; narcissism. **C., object:** libido directed towards some object; also called object libido.

cathŏ·dal (G. *kata*, down; *hodos*, road). Relating to the cathode.

că·thode (G. *kata*, down; *hodos*, road). The negative electrode, *q.v.* **C. rays:** negative electrons emanating from the cathode, normally travelling in straight lines, usually produced in tubes containing a gas under low pressure, causing many substances struck by them to fluoresce; the point of impact of high-speed cathode rays is the source of X-rays.

cathod·ic (G. *kata*, down; *hodos*, road). 1. Cathodal. 2. Efferent or centrifugal.

că·tholyte. That part of an electrolyte that adjoins the cathode.

că·tion (G. *kation*, descending). An electro-positive ion.

cat·ling. A long, straight amputation knife with a sharp point.

catop·trics (G. *katoptron*, a mirror). The phenomena related to the reflection of light rays.

catoptrophō·bia (G. *katoptron*, mirror; *phobos*, fear). A neurotic fear of mirrors.

cauda (L.). A tail; a termination. **C. equina:** the nerve roots of the lumbar and sacral plexus, from their resemblance to a horse's tail.

cau·dal (L. *cauda*, tail). 1. Relating to a cauda. 2. Relating to the lower or tail end of the long axis of the body.

cau·date (L. *cauda*, tail). Having or resembling a tail. **C. lobe:** tail-like process of the liver. **C. nucleus:** a portion of the corpus striatum, forming part of the outer wall of the lateral ventricle.

cau·dex (L.). A stalk, or any part resembling a stalk.

caul. 1. A piece of the foetal membranes which sometimes envelop a child's head during birth. 2. The great omentum.

Cau·lobacter vibrĭoides. An organism from water.

Caulobacteriā·lēs. A genus of aquatic Schizomycetes.

cau·sal. Relating to a cause.

causal·gia (G. *kausos*, heat; *algos*, pain). A condition characterized by intense burning pain referred to a sensory nerve segment which is also over-reactive to an effective stimulus (the intensely painful sensation radiating far beyond the area stimulated and persisting abnormally long), due to an association of incomplete lesion of a sensory (usually the median or posterior tibial) nerve with disorder in the mechanism of sensation at higher (cerebral) levels.

cause (L. *causa*). The circumstance or agent which brings about a condition or has an effect.

caus·tic (G. *kaustikos*, from *kaiein*, to burn). An escharotic.

cau·terant (G. *kautēr*, from *kaiein*, to burn). A caustic.

cau·terizā·tion (G. *kaiein*, to burn). The application of a cautery.

cau·terize (G. *kaiein*, to burn). To burn with a cautery or a caustic.

cau·tery (G. *kautēr*, from *kaiein*, to burn). An instrument for destroying tissue by burning. **Actual c.:** the white-hot iron (*ferrum candens*). **Galvanic c.:** an electrically heated platinum wire. (See also Paquelin's c., thermocautery.)

cava (L. *cavus*, hollow). 1. A cavity. 2. Either of the large veins opening directly into the right auricle.

ca·val (L. *cavus*, hollow). 1. Hollow. 2. Pertaining to a cavity.

că·vascope (L. *cavus*, hollow; G. *skopein*, to view). An apparatus for examining a cavity.

cavern (L. *caverna*, from *cavus*, hollow). A cavity of pathologic origin.

cavernī·tis (L. *caverna*, from *cavus*, hollow). Inflammation of the cavernous tissue of the penis (corpora cavernosa).

cavernō·ma (L. *caverna*, from *cavus*, hollow). A cavernous angioma.

că·vernous (L. *caverna*, from *cavus*, hollow). 1. Having hollow spaces. 2. Relating to the corpora cavernosa. 3. Relating to the venous sinus at the side of the body of the sphenoid bone.

cavil·la (L. dim. of *cavus*, hollow). The sphenoid bone.

că·vitary (L. *cavus*, hollow). 1. Hollow. 2. Having a body-cavity or an intestinal tract; applied to nematode worms.

cavitas glenoidalis (L.). The glenoid cavity.

cavitā·tion (L. *cavus*, hollow). Formation of cavities.

cavī·tis. Inflammation of a vena cava.

că·vity (L. *cavus*, hollow). 1. A hollow, e.g., the abdominal c. 2. A space in the lung, either hollow or filled with purulent matter, formed by liquefaction of caseous areas and expectoration of the resulting debris.

cavoval·gus (L. *cavus*, hollow; *valgus*, bow-legged). Cavus combined with valgus; see also talipes cavovalgus.

că·vum (L. *cavus*, hollow). A cavity.

că·vus (L.). Talipes cavus, *q.v.*

Cayenne pepper. See under Capsicum.

Cazenave's disease (Cazenave, P.L.A., French physican, 1795–1877). 1. Lupus erythematosus. 2. Pemphigus foliaceus. **C.'s vitiligo:** see Celsus's area.

Cb. Symbol of columbium.

cc. Abbreviation for cubic centimetre.

CCl₄. Carbon tetrachloride. Anthelmintic solvent.

CCl₃CHO. Chloral.

CCl₃CH(OH)₂. Chloral hydrate.

Cd. Symbol of Cadmium.

cĕăs·mic (G. *keazein*, to cleave). A condition characterized by the continuation after birth of embryonic fissures.

cē·bocephā·lia (G. *kēbos*, monkey; *kephalē*, head). A cyclocephalic monster with rudimentary nose and palate.

Cel. Abbreviation for Celsius.

cel. A velocity unit of 1 cm. per second.

celectome (G. *kele*, tumour; *ektomē*, excision). A surgical instrument used for detaching a portion of tissue from a tumour.

cell (L. *cella*, closet). 1. Ultimate unit of animal and plant structure, consisting of cytoplasm, nucleus and central nucleoli. 2. Galvanic element. **Cs., alpha:** see under Alpha. **C., basket:** 1. A cell of the cerebellar cortex the axon of which gives off fibrils forming a network around the body of a Purkinje cell. 2. Spindle-shaped element between the basement membrane and glandular cells in certain glands. **C., beta:** see under Beta. **C., castration:** applied to any one of enlarged basophile cells of the anterior pituitary gland, filled with one or more large globules of a colloid-like substance, which are found in gonadectomized rats. **C., caudate:** a glia c., characterized by tail-like prolongations. **C.-cones:** cancer nests of a squamous carcinoma. **C., daughter:** any one of the cells formed by the division of a mother c. **C., foam:** 1. A cell of foam-like appearance which is due to the presence of lipoid substances, as seen in tissues affected by Niemann-Pick's disease, xanthoma, etc. 2. A vacuolated connective tissue c. in rhinoscleroma; syn. Mikulicz's c. **C., giant:** see under giant. **C., heart-failure:** see under heart-failure. **Cs., islet:** cells of the islets of Langerhans, in the pancreas, secreting insulin. **C., mossy:** a glia c. characterized by a large body and numerous short processes. **C., mother:** any c. giving rise by division to daughter cells. **C., motor:** the neuron of a motor nerve fibre. **C.-nest:** any mass of epithelial cells surrounded by connective tissue. **C., pavement:** see under pavement epithelium. **C.-plate:** a membrane originating from thickenings of the spindle fibres in the equatorial plate; splitting in the following stage of mitosis into layers between which the new partition wall is formed. **C.-sap:** enchylema, *q.v.* **C., spindle:** a spindle-shaped c. **C., squamous:** a flattened, scale-like c. (See also squamous epithelum.) **C., stab** or **C., staff:** a juvenile polymorphonuclear leucocyte whose nucleus is not yet segmented. **C., stem:** any primitive c. giving rise in foetal or post-foetal development to more specialized cells.

cella (L., closet). 1. A cell. 2. The central portion of the paracele.

Cellfalcicula. A race of soil bacteria capable of oxidizing cellulose.

celli·ferous. Cell-bearing.

cel·liform. Resembling a cell.

cellobi·ase (L. *cellula*, dim. of *cella*; G. *bios*, life). An enzyme hydrolyzing cellobiose to glucose.

cellobi·ose (L. *cella*, cell; G. *bios*, life). A disaccharide produced from cellulose by acid or enzymic hydrolysis.

cel·lophane (L. *cella*; G. *phainein*, to appear). A product of cellulose which is transparent.

cel·lular. Composed of cells.

cel·lulase (L. *cellula*, dim. of *cella*). An enzyme hydrolyzing cellulose to cellobiose, present in certain bacteria, protozoa and snails.

cel·lule (L. *cellula*, dim. of *cella*, cell). A minute cavity or cell.

cellulici·dal (L. *cella*, cell; *caedere*, to kill). Destructive of cells.

celluli·fugal (L. *cellula*, cellule; *fugere*, to flee). Relating to the transmission of impulses from a nerve cell.

celluli·petal (L. *cellula*, cellule; *petere*, to seek). Relating to the transmission of impulses towards a nerve cell.

celluli·tis. Diffuse inflammation of the areolar tissue.

cel·luloid. 1. Resembling cells. 2. A substance, resembling ivory, and mainly composed of camphor and pyroxylin.

Cellumonas. A genus of Bacteriaceae capable of digesting cellulose.

cel·lulose (L. *cellula*, cellule). A polysaccharide forming cell walls in plants; chemically one of the most resistant substances elaborated by living cells.

cē·loscope (G. *koilos*, hollow; *skopein*, to view). An instrument for examining a cavity.

celosō·mia (G. *kēlē*, hernia; *sōma*, body). Congenital defect of the thoracic or abdominal wall with protrusion of the viscera.

celosō·mus (G. *kēlē*, hernia; *sōma*, body). A monster with defect of the sternum and protrusion of the thoracic or abdominal organs.

Celsius's thermometer (Celsius, A., Swedish astronomer, 1701–44). Also called Centigrade thermometer. One which has 100 degrees between ice melting point and the boiling point of water, the former being zero on the scale and the latter 100°.

Celsus's area (Celsus, A. C., Roman physician, 1st century A.D.). Alopecia areata. **C.'s chancre:** chancroid. **C.'s kerion:** inflamed and suppurating ringworm. **C.'s papulae:** lichen agrius, a form of acute papular eczema.

cement (L. *caementum*, quarry-stone). 1. A plastic material that hardens when dried, used in dentistry. 2. Cementum, *q.v.*

cementi·tis. Inflammation of the cementum.

cemen·toblast (L. *caementum*, quarry-stone; G. *blastos*, germ). A cell depositing cementum upon the dentine of the tooth root.

cementoclā·sia (L. *caementum*, quarry-stone; G. *klaein*, to break). Destruction of the cementum of a tooth root.

cementogĕ·nesis (L. *caementum*, quarry-stone; G. *gennan*, to produce). Formation of cementum.

cementō·ma (L. *caementum*, quarry-stone). A tumour derived from dental cementum.

cemen·tum (L. *caementum*, quarry-stone). The thin layer of bony tissue covering the root of a tooth. Syn. dental cement; crusta petrosa.

cenadel·phus (G. *koinos*, common; *adelphos*, brother). A double monster foetus, with both parts equally developed.

centē·simal (L. *centesimus*, from *centum*, hundred). In the proportion of one to one hundred.

centē·sis (G. *kentēsis*, a puncture). Puncture; perforation.

cen·tigrade (L. *centum*, hundred; *gradus*, step). Having a hundred degrees. (See also under Celsius.)

centigramme (L. *centum*, hundred; G. *gramma*, a small weight). The one-hundredth part of a gramme.

centilitre (L. *centum*, a hundred; G. *litra*, a pound). One-hundredth part of a litre.

centimetre (L. *centum*, hundred; G. *metron*, measure). The one-hundredth part of a metre.

centinor·mal (L. *centum*, hundred; *norma*, a rule). $\left(\frac{n}{100}\right)$ A solution of one-hundredth strength of a normal solution. *q.v.*

centipede (L. *centum*, hundred; *pes*, foot). An arthropod distinguished by possessing a pair of legs for each segment of its body.

cen·trad (G. *kentron*, centre). Towards the centre.

cen·tral (G. *kentron*, centre). Situated at the centre. **C. bodies:** the structure at the centre of the aster during mitosis, comprising the centrosome and the centriole. **C. spindle:** the primary spindle connecting the c. bodies.

centre (L. *centrum*, from G. *kentron*). 1. The middle point of any surface or of a body. 2. Any part of the central nervous system which is supposed to regulate or control a particular function.

cen·tric. Relating to a centre.

centri·ciput (L. *centrum*, centre; *caput*, head). The mid-head; the second cranial segment between the sinciput and the occiput.

centri·fugal (L. *centrum*, centre; *fugere*, to flee). Receding from the centre. **C. force:** tendency of a body moving in a curve around another body to leave its axis of motion.

cen·trifugaliza·tion (L. *centrum*, centre; *fugere*, to flee). Separation of a substance by means of a centrifuge.

cen·trifuge (L. *centrum*, centre; *fugere*, to flee). 1. An apparatus for separating substances by centrifugal force. 2. To submit to the action of a centrifuge.

cen·triole (L. *centrum*, centre). A minute structure in the centrosome, at the centre of the aster.

centri·petal (L. *centrum*, centre; *petere*, to seek). Travelling towards the centre.

cen·trocine·sia (G. *kentron*, centre; *kinēsis*, movement). Movement derived from the stimulation of a centre.

centrodes·mus (L. *centrum*, centre; *desmos*, a bond). The structure primarily connecting the centrioles and thought to give rise to the central spindle.

centrolĕ·cithal (L. *centrum*, centre; G. *lekithos*, yolk). Applied to ova having the yolk mainly in the central region.

cen·tromere (L. *centrum*, centre; G. *meros*, part). The part of the sperm containing the central bodies.

centrophor·ium (L. *centrum*, centre; G. *phorios*, secret). A form of the Golgi apparatus, *q.v.*, in the membrane of Descemet, with the form of a hollow sphere.

cen·troplasm (L. *centrum*, centre; G. *plassein*, to form). The substance of the centrosome.

cen·trosome (L. *centrum*, centre; G. *sōma*, body). The larger of the central bodies, *q.v.*, composed of centroplasm and containing the centriole.

cen·trosphere (L. *centrum*, centre; G. *sphaira*, sphere). The granular area surrounding the centrosome from which the astral rays radiate.

cen·trum (L., centre). 1. A central or middle part. 2. The body of a vertebra. **C. ovale:** the central area of white matter of the brain.

ce·phalad (G. *kephalē*, head). Towards the head.

cephală·gra (G. *kephalē*, head; *agra*, seizure). Gouty pain in the head.

cephalal·gia (G. *kephalē*, head; *algos*, pain). Pain in the head; headache.

ce·phalhaēmat·ocele (G. *kephalē*, head; *haima*, blood; *kēlē*, tumour). A haematocele beneath the scalp and communicating with a dural sinus.

ce·phalhaēmatō·ma (G. *kephalē*, head; *haima*, blood). A collection of blood beneath the pericranium in the new-born, not limited by suture lines.

cephalhŷ·drocele (G. *kephalē*, head; *hudōr*, water; *kēlē*, tumour). A collection of cerebrospinal fluid beneath the scalp in cases of skull fracture.

cephal·ic (G. *kephalē*, head). Relating to the head.

ce·phalin (G. *kephalē*, head). A generic type of phospholipid composed of two molecules of fatty acid, one of phosphoric acid, one of glycerol, and one of the base amino-ethyl alcohol; present in animal tissues. Syn. kephalin.

cephaliza·tion (G. *kephalē*, head). Concentration of parts towards the brain.

cephă·locele (G. *kephalē*, head; *kēlē*, hernia). Hernia of the brain.

ce·phalocentē·sis (G. *kephalē*, head; *kentēsis*, puncture). Surgical puncture of the head.

ce·phaloedē·ma (G. *kephalē*, head; *oidēma*, a swelling). Oedema of the head.

ce·phalogas·ter (G. *kephalē*, head; *gastēr*, belly). The anterior division of the enteric canal.

ce·phaloid (G. *kephalē*, head; *eidos*, form). Resembling a head.

cephalō·ma (G. *kephalē*, head). A soft cancer.

cephalŏ·melus (G. *kephalē*, head; *melos*, limb). A monster with a supernumerary limb attached to the head.

ce·phalomeningī·tis (G. *kephalē*, head; *mēnigx*, a membrane). Inflammation of the brain membranes.

cephalŏ·meter (G. *kephalē*, head; *metron*, measure). Craniometer, *q.v.*

cephalŏ·metry (G. *kephalē*, head; *metron*, measure). Craniometry, *q.v.*

ce·phalone. An idiot with an abnormally large head.

cephalŏ·pagus (G. *kephalē*, head; *pēgnunai*, to fix). Double monster with heads united at the top.

ce·phaloplē·gia (G. *kephalē*, head; *plēgē*, a stroke). Paralysis of head and face muscles.

ce·phalorrhachī·dian (G. *kephalē*, head; *rhakhis*, spine). Relating to the head and spine; cerebro-spinal.

ce·phalothoracŏ·pagus (G. *kephalē*, head; *thōrax*, thorax; *pēgnunai*, to fix). A double-headed monster with united thoraces and necks.

cephalothor·ax (G. *kephalē*, head; *thōrax*, thorax). Head and thorax fused into a single organ; one of the chief characteristics of Arachnida.

ce·phalotome (G. *kephalē*, head; *tomē*, a cutting). Craniotome, *q.v.*

cephalŏ·tomy (G. *kephalē*, head; *tomē*, a cutting). The same as craniotomy, *q.v.*

ce·phalotribe (G. *kephalē*, head; *tribein*, to crush). Instrument for performing cephalotripsy.

ce·phalotripsy (G. *kephalē*, head; *tribein*, to crush). Instrumental crushing of the foetal head in labour.

ce·ra (L., wax). Beeswax.

cerā·ceous (L. *cera*, wax). Waxy; resembling wax.

ce·rate (L. *cera*, wax). In pharmacy, an ointment-like preparation with a basis of wax, which does not melt when applied to the skin.

cercā·ria (G. *kerkos*, tail). A trematode in its tailed stage of larval life.

Cercomonas. A genus of flagellate protozoa.

ce·real (L. *ceres*). Any edible grain.

cerebel·lar (L. *cerebellum*, dim. of *cerebrum*, brain). Relating to the cerebellum.

ce·rebellī·tis. Inflammation of the cerebellum.

ce·rebello-pon·tine (L. *cerebellum*; *pons*, a bridge). Relating to both cerebellum and pons cerebri or to the angle formed by these structures.

ce·rebello-rubral (L. *cerebellum*; *ruber*, red). Relating to a nervous pathway extending from the cerebellum to the nucleus ruber.

ce·rebello-spinal (L. *cerebellum*; *spina*, spine). Relating to the cerebellum and the spinal cord.

cerebel·lum (L. *cerebellum*, dim. of *cerebrum*, brain). The inferior part of the brain, lying below the cerebrum and above the pons and medulla oblongata; having mainly the function of controlling postural reactions (anterior lobe with its spino-cerebellar afferents and rubro-spinal efferents), of participating in the integration of volitional movements (neocerebellar portion) and of equilibrium (lingula and and flocculonodular lobe).

ce·rebral (L. *cerebrum*, brain). Relating to the brain.

cerebra·tion (L. *cerebrum*, brain). Cerebral activity.

cerebri·fugal (L. *cerebrum*, brain; *fugere*, to flee). Conducting impulses from the brain.

cerebri·petal (L. *cerebrum*, brain; *petere*, to seek). Conducting impulses towards the brain.

cerebri·tis. Inflammation of the cerebrum.

cĕ·rebrocar·diac (L. *cerebrum*, brain; G. *kardia*, heart). Relating to both the brain and the heart.

cĕ·rebrol. An oil-like substance obtained from the brain.

cerebrŏ·logy (L. *cerebrum*, brain; G. *logos*, word). Knowledge or study of the brain.

cĕ·rebron (L. *cerebrum*, brain). The same as phrenosin, *q.v.*

cerebrŏ·pathy (L. *cerebrum*, brain; G. *pathos*, disease). Disorder of the brain.

cĕ·rebropon·tile (L. *cerebrum*, brain; *pons*, a bridge). Relating to both cerebrum and pons.

cĕ·rebroret·inal syndromes (L. *cerebrum*, brain; *rētē*, a net; G. *sun*, together; *dromos*, a running). Applied to various heredo-degenerative conditions characterized by the association of retinal lesions with mental defect. Cf. idiocy, amaurotic. (See also epiloia.)

cĕ·rebroside (L. *cerebrum*, brain). A glucoside containing galactose, the base sphingosine and a fatty acid. Five cerebrosides have been isolated (phrenosin, kerasin, nervon, oxynervon, sulfosin); they differ from each other only in the fatty acid they contain. They occur in the brain and nerves, making up a considerable portion of the myelin sheaths and in relatively small amounts in other organs, especially liver, spleen and heart. Abnormal accumulation of the c., kerasin, in various organs is one of the basic factors in Gaucher's disease, *q.v.*

cĕ·rebrospi·nal (L. *cerebrum*, brain; *spina*, spine). Relating to the brain and spinal cord. C. fever: see under fever. C. fluid: the fluid occupying the space between the arachnoid membrane and the pia mater; formed by the choroid plexuses of the cerebral ventricles; serving as a fluid buffer for the central nervous system, as a reservoir for regulating the contents of the cranium and as a mechanism for the exchange of gases and nutrients of the nervous system. C. meningitis: the same as c. fever, *q.v.*, under fever.

cĕ·rebrum (L., brain). All the structures of the brain taken collectively, with the exception of the cerebellum, pons and medulla.

cerevi·siae fermen·tum (L.). Brewers' yeast.

ce·rium (L.). One of the rarer metals. Symbol Ce.

ceroli·poid (L. *cera*, wax; G. *lipos*, fat; *eidos*, form). A wax-like material from plants.

cerŏ·ma (G. *kērōma*, a wax-like mass). A tissue tumour with waxy degeneration.

cer·tifiable. Capable of being certified. Said of persons so mentally deranged that they must be placed in institutions.

cerū·men (L. *cera*, wax). The waxy secretion of the glands of the external auditory meatus.

cerū·minal. Relating to cerumen.

cerū·minŏ·sis. Excessive secretion of cerumen.

cerū·minous. Pertaining to cerumen.

cĕ·ruse (L. *cērussa*, white lead). White lead.

cervi·cal (L. from *cervix*, neck). Relating to (1) the neck, (2) the cervix uteri, or (3) the first part of the spinal cord. C. rib: see under rib.

cervicā·lis (L. *cervix*, neck). Cervical.

cervicec·tomy (L. *cervix*, neck; G. *ektomē*, excision). Excision of the cervix uteri.

cervici·tis (L. *cervix*, neck). Inflammation of the cervix uteri.

cer·vico-axil·lary (L. *cervix*, neck; *axilla*). Relating to the neck and the axilla.

cervicobrǎ·chial (L. *cervix*, neck; G. *brakhion*, arm). Relating to the neck and the arm.

cer·vicodor·sal (L. *cervix*, neck; *dorsum*, back). Relating to the neck and the back.

cer·vicofā·cial (L. *cervix*, neck; *facies*, face). Relating to the neck and the face.

cer·vico-hū·meral (L. *cervix*, neck; *humerus*, shoulder). Relating to the neck and the upper arm.

cer·vico-occi·pital (L. *cervix*, neck; *caput*, head). Relating to the neck and the back of the head.

cer·vicoplasty (L. *cervix*, neck; G. *plassein*, to form). Plastic surgery of the neck.

cer·vicoscǎ·pular (L. *cervix*, neck; *scapulae*, the shoulder-blades). Relating to the neck and the scapula.

cer·vicothorǎ·cic (L. *cervix*, neck; G. *thorax*). Relating to the neck and the thorax.

cer·vicovagi·nal (L. *cervix*, neck; *vagina*). Relating to the cervix uteri and the vagina.

cervi·meter (L. *cervix*, neck; G. *metron*, measure). An instrument used for measuring the cervix uteri.

cer·vix (L.). 1. The neck. 2. Any neck-like structure. C. uteri: the cylindrical part of the uterus between the internal and external orifices.

Cestoda (G. *kestos*, girdle; *eidos*, form). The true tapeworms, a sub-class of Cestoidea, having a definite scolex or pseudoscolex and an onchosphere with six hooks.

cestoid. Like a tapeworm.

Cestoidea (G. *kestos*, girdle; *eidos*, form). A class of endoparasitic flat worms, commonly known as tapeworms; found in the adult stage almost exclusively in the alimentary tract of vertebrates, although the larval form may inhabit various tissues of both vertebrates and invertebrates. Syn. Platyhelminthes.

cetrimide. A cationic detergent and antiseptic consisting mainly of cetyltrimethylammonium bromide.

cetylpyridi·nium chloride. A substance similar to CTAB.

Ceylon moss. *Gracilaria lichenoides*, a seaweed yielding agar.

CG. Abbreviation for phosgene.

C_H. The symbol for hydrogen ion concentration.

$(CH_2)_2$. Ethylene.

C_2H_2. Acetylene.

C_6H_6. Benzene.

Chabert's disease (Chabert, P., French veterinary surgeon, 1737-1814). Symptomatic anthrax.

Chagas's disease (Chagas, C., Brazilian physician, 1879-1934). A kind of trypanosomiasis which is found in Brazil.

Chagasia. A genus of anopheline mosquitoes found in the South American states.

chain (L. *catena*, chain). 1. A series of connected links of metal, e.g., chain saw, a surgeon's saw with teeth linked like a chain. 2. A series of connected substances or events. 3. In organic chemistry, a series of atoms linked together by one or more bonds. 4. Micro-organismal growth characterized by end-to-end arrangement of the individual cells.

chalǎ·zion (G. *khalaza*, hailstone). A retention cyst of the Meibomian glands in the eyelid.

chalci·tis (G. *khalkos*, copper). Inflammation of the eyes due to brass dust-particles.

chalcō·sis (G. *khalkos*, copper). A deposit of copper particles in the tissues.

chalicō·sis (G. *khalix*, gravel). The same as silicosis.

chalk (L. *calx*, lime). Carbonate of lime.

chǎ·maecephal·ic (G. *khamai*, on the earth; *kephalē*, head). Having a cephalic height index below 70°. (See under index.)

chǎ·maeprosop·ic (G. *khamai*, on the earth; *prosōpon*, face). Having a facial index below 51°.

chamber (L. *camera*, from G. *kamara*, a vaulted enclosure). A cavity or space. Anterior c.: the space between the cornea and iris. **Posterior c.:** the space between iris and lens.

champagne. French sparkling wine with up to 13 per cent of alcohol.

chan·cre (Fr. *chancre*, from L. *cancer*, crab). The primary lesion in syphilis, a small papule quickly enlarging to a round or oval sore of about 1 cm. diameter, the centre of which soon ulcerates while the surrounding tissue becomes indurated.

chan·criform (Fr. *chancre*; L. *forma*, shape). Like a chancre.

chan·croid (Fr. *chancre*; G. *eidos*, form). A soft venereal sore of non-syphilitic origin. Syn. ulcus molle.

chancroi·dal. Relating to chancroid.

chan·crous. Chancre-like; of the nature of chancre.

change of life. The menopause.

channel. A groove through which anything may flow.

Chaoul's therapy and tube (Chaoul, H., German radiologist, born 1887). Low voltage X-ray therapy.

chap. A small fissure of the skin.

chappa. A yaw-like disease found in the western part of Africa.

chă·racter. In natural history and heredity the collective peculiarities and traits of animal and plant life.

charbon (Fr., coal). Anthrax.

charcoal. The carbon residue of charred organic material.

Charcot's artery (Charcot, J. M., French neurologist, 1825–93). The artery of cerebral haemorrhage (middle cerebral artery). **C.'s cirrhosis:** biliary cirrhosis (also called Hanot's disease). **C.'s crystals:** octahedral crystals of the phosphate of Schreiner's base (spermin) found in the sputum of asthma, in seminal fluid, leukaemic blood and faeces. **C.'s disease:** 1. Amyotrophic lateral sclerosis. 2. Tabetic arthropathy. 3. Multiple cerebrospinal sclerosis. **C.'s fever:** fever occurring in jaundice, due to impacted gallstones. **C.'s gait:** the gait of Friedreich's ataxia. **C.'s joints:** enlarged joints found in C.'s disease and generally associated with tabes dorsalis. **C.'s pain:** hysterical pain in the ovarian region. **C.'s posterior root-zone:** see under Burdach's column. **C.'s sensory crossway:** the posterior third of the posterior limb of the internal capsule. **C.'s sign:** in facial paralysis the eyebrow is raised; in facial contracture it is lowered. **C.'s syndrome:** intermittent claudication, an affection connected with arteriosclerosis of the lower extremities. **C.'s triad:** nystagmus, intention tremor and scanning speech; an early sign of disseminated sclerosis. **C.'s zones:** the hysterogenic zones.

Charcot-Guinon's disease (Charcot, J. M.; Guinon, G., French physician, 1859–1929). Dementia complicating some cases of progressive muscular atrophy.

Charcot-Leyden's crystals. The same as Charcot's crystals, *q.v.*

Charcot-Marie's symptom (Charcot, J. M.; Marie, P., French neurologist, 1853–1940). The same as Marie's symptom, *q.v.* **C.-M.'s type of progressive muscular atrophy:** the neurotic type of p.m.a., progressive neural m.a., commencing in the muscles of the feet and legs. **C.-M.-Tooth's type of P.M.A.:** the same as C.-M.'s type, above mentioned.

Charcot-Neumann's crystals. The same as Charcot's crystals, *q.v.*

Charcot-Vigouroux's sign. The same as Vigouroux's sign, *q.v.*

charlatan (Fr.). A quack; a person claiming medical skill but not qualified as a practitioner.

chart. A record of temperature fluctuation, etc., recorded on graph paper.

char·ta (L. *charta*, from G. *khartēs*). Medicated paper; wrapper for powders.

Chassaignac's muscle (Chassaignac, C. M. E., French surgeon, 1805–79). A non-constant muscle extending across the axilla from the lower border of the latissimus dorsi to that of the pectoralis minor or to the brachial fascia. **C.'s tubercle:** the carotid tubercle on the transverse process of the 6th cervical vertebra.

chaudepisse (Fr.). The painful urination of the acute stage of gonorrhoea.

chaulmoo·gric acid. Found with hydnocarpic acid as a glyceride in chaulmoogra oil. Used in the treatment of leprosy.

Chaussier's areola (Chaussier, F., French physician, 1746–1828). The areola of inflammatory induration of a malignant pustule. **C.'s line:** the raphe of the corpus callosum.

C_2H_5Br. Ethyl bromide.

$CHCl_3$. Chloroform.

C_2H_5Cl. Ethyl chloride.

$CCl_3CH(OH)_2$. Chloral hydrate.

CH_3COOH. Acetic acid.

Cheadle's disease (Cheadle, W. B., English paediatrician, 1835–1910). Infantile scurvy.

cheek. The side of the face.

cheek bone. The malar bone.

cheese (L. *caseus*). A food made of pressed curds.

chee·sy. Caseous; like cheese.

cheilec·tomy (G. *kheilos*, lip; *ektomē*, excision). The operation of chiselling off the excessive bony edges of a joint cavity caused by osteo-arthritis.

cheilectrŏ·pion (G. *kheilos*, lip; *ektrepein*, to turn aside). Eversion of the lip.

cheili·tis (G. *kheilos*, lip). Inflammation of the lip. **C., exfoliative:** a condition characterized by swelling and tenderness of a lip, usually the lower, with formation of a loosely adherent crust, recurring after removal. **C. glandularis:** a condition usually affecting the lower lip only, characterized by swelling and hemp-seed-sized nodules about the orifices of the mucous glands, discharging mucopurulent matter.

chei·locarcinō·ma (G. *kheilos*, lip; *karkinos*, cancer). Cancer of the lip.

chei·lognā·thopalatŏ·schisis (G. *kheilos*, lip; *gnathos*, jaw; L. *palatum*, palate; G. *skhizein*, to cleave). Congenital fissure of upper lip, alveolar process and palate; hare-lip and cleft palate.

cheilŏ·gnathus (G. *kheilos*, lip; *gnathos*, jaw). Congenital fissure of the upper lip; hare-lip.

cheilon·cus (G. *kheilos*, lip; *ogkos*, tumour). A tumour of the lip.

cheilophā·gia (G. *kheilos*, lip; *phagein*, to eat). Biting the lips.

chei·loplasty (G. *kheilos*, lip; *plassein*, to form). Plastic operation on the lip.

cheilor·rhaphy (G. *kheilos*, lip; *rhaphē*, suture). Suturing the lip.

cheilŏ·schisis (G. *kheilos*, lip; *skhizein*, to cleave). Hare-lip.

cheilō·sis (G. *kheilos*, lip). A condition caused by riboflavin deficiency and affecting the lips and angles of the mouth.

chei·lostomat·oplasty (G. *kheilos*, lip; *stoma*, mouth; *plassein*, to form). Cheiloplasty, including restoration of the mouth.

cheilŏ·tomy (G. *kheilos*, lip; *tomē*, a cutting). Excision of part of the lip.

cheir·agre (G. *kheir*, hand; *agra*, seizure). Gout of the hand.

cheiromĕ·galy. A type of acromegaly in which the swelling occurs in the hands and feet.

cheiropom·pholyx (G. *kheir*, hand; *pompholux*, a water bubble). Skin diseases characterized by acute eruption of multiple vesicles in the stratum mucosum in hands and feet with a burning and itching sensation, often associated with, if not due to, epidermophytosis. Syn. dysidrosis.

chei·rospasm (G. *kheir*, hand; *spasmos*, spasm). Writers' cramp.

chē·loid (G. *khēlē*, claw; *eidos*, form). See keloid.

chelō·nian (G. *khělōnē*, tortoise). Relating to a tortoise.

chem·ic, chem·ical (Arab. (*al*) *kimia*). Relating to chemistry.

chě·micocau·tery. Cauterization by some chemical method.

chě·milumines·cence (Arab. (*al*) *kimia*; L. *lumen*, a light). Fluorescence initiated by a chemical reaction.

cheminō·sis. A disease produced by chemical means.

chě·miotax·is (Arab. (*al*) *kimia*; G. *tassein*, to arrange). See chemotaxis.

chě·mism. Chemical action.

chě·mist. One versed in chemistry; wrongly applied to an apothecary.

chě·mistry (Arab. (*al*) *kimia*). The science dealing with the composition and transformation of substances. **C., inorganic:** the c. of compounds not containing carbon. **C., organic:** the c. of compounds containing carbon. **C., physical:** the science dealing with the relations of the physical and chemical properties of substances. **C. physiological:** see under biochemistry.

chemorecep·tor (Arab. (*al*) *kimia*; L. *recĭpěre*, to receive). Applied to cells responding to minute chemical changes in the condition of their environment.

chemorē·flex. A reflex caused by chemical action.

chemo·sis (G. *khēmōsis*, swelling of the cornea). Oedema of the bulbar conjunctiva.

chemotac·tic (Arab. (*al*) *kimia*; G. *tassein*, to arrange). Relating to chemotaxis.

chemotax·is (Arab. (*al*) *kimia*; G. *tassein*, to arrange). Positional response (attraction or repulsion) of living cells to chemical stimuli.

chemothě·rapy (Arab. (*al*) *kimia*; G. *therapeuein*, to attend). The prevention or treatment of disease by chemical substances which, while effective against the pathogenic organism, have no harmful effects on the patient.

chemot·ic (G. *khēmōsis*, swelling of the cornea). Affected with chemosis.

chemō·tropism. See chemotaxis.

Chenopodium (G. *khēn*, goose; *pous*, foot). A genus of plants which produce anthelmintics effective against round worms and hookworm.

Cherchevsky's disease (Cherchevsky, M., contemporary Russian physician). Nervous ileus, an affection simulating intestinal obstruction; sometimes seen in neurasthenia.

cheromā·nia (G. *khairein*, to rejoice; *mania*, madness). A mental disorder characterized by cheerfulness.

cherophō·bia (G. *khairein*, to rejoice; *phobos*, fear). A neurotic fear of rejoicing.

Chervin's treatment (Chervin, C., French schoolmaster, 1824–96). A method of treating stammering.

chest. The thorax.

Cheyne's nystagmus (Cheyne, J., Scottish physician, 1777–1836). Nystagmus with rhythmic variation similar to that of Cheyne-Stokes respiration.

Cheyne-Stokes asthma (Cheyne, J., Scottish physician, 1777–1836; Stokes, W., Irish physician, 1804–78). Dyspnoea due to pulmonary congestion in advanced chronic myocarditis. **C.-S. respiration:** rhythmical breathing of a periodic type occurring in certain grave conditions of the central nervous system, heart and lungs, and in intoxications.

CHI₃. Iodoform.

C₂H₅I. Ethyl iodide.

Chiari's disease (Chiari, H., German pathologist, 1851–1916). Endophlebitis obliterans hepatica.

chi·asm (G. *khiasmos*, a diagonal arrangement). A crossing. **C., optic:** the junction of the optic nerves at which, in man, the nerve fibres from the nasal half of each retina cross and join the optic nerve of the opposite side.

chias·ma. The same as chiasm, *q.v.*

chias·mic. Like a chiasm; crosswise.

chichism. A pellagra-like disease found in the central American states.

chickenpox. See varicella.

chigger, chigoe (W. Indies). *Turga penetrans*, a sand flea occurring in tropical countries. **C. disease:** the condition due to infestation, mostly of the feet, with the pregnant female of the *Turga penetrans*, which attaches herself to the skin of man and higher animals, becoming almost entirely enclosed by the resultant swelling; after discharging her eggs through an aperture of the swelling, the flea dies, but the swelling often becomes secondarily infected.

chil·blain. A localized congestion and swelling of the skin, especially at the peripheral parts, sometimes followed by ulceration; due to a circulatory disorder influenced by cold. Syn. pernio; erythema pernio.

childbed. Labour; confinement.

childhood. The period of life between infancy and puberty.

chill. Cold sensation; feverish shivering.

Chilomastix mesnili (G. *kheilos*, lip; *mastix*, whip). A species of flagellates which may be transmitted to man, in whom they inhabit the intestine.

chilomastixi·asis. Infestation with *Chilomastix mesnili*.

chimpanzee. An anthropoid ape, which is frequently used for experimental purposes.

chin. The anterior prominence of the lower jaw.

Chinacrin. A preparation of mepacrine hydrochloride, which is used in combating malaria.

Chiniofon. A compound containing hydroxyquinoline, sulphonic acid and sodium bicarbonate. It is used in the treatment of amoebic dysentery.

chirā·gra (G. *kheir*, hand; *agra*, seizure). Any pain of the hand.

chi·roplasty (G. *kheir*, hand; *plassein*, to form). Plastic operation on the hand.

chirŏ·podist (G. *kheir*, hand; *pous*, foot). One who treats hands and feet, particularly for corns, bunions and affections of the nails.

chiroprac·tic (G. *kheir*, hand; *prassein*, to do). System of treatment based on the idea that disease is due to lesions of the central nervous system and can be cured by spinal manipulation.

chi·rospasm (G. *kheir*, hand; *spasmos*, spasm). Writers' cramp.

chirur·gia (G. *kheirourgia*, from *kheir*, hand; *ergon*, work). Surgery, *q.v.*

chirur·gical (G. *kheirourgia*, surgery). Surgical.

chi·tin (G. *khitōn*, tunic). A polysaccharide forming the basis of the hard shells of crustaceans and insects.

chlamydozoa (G. *khlamus*, cloak; *zōon*, animal). S. J. M. von Prowazek's (German zoologist, 1876–1915) term for inclusion bodies (*q.v.*) which he believed to be protozoa surrounded by material produced by the invaded cell.

chlōas·ma (G. *khloazein*, to be green). Patchy hyperpigmentation of the skin. **C. uterinum:** c. occurring during pregnancy or associated with ovarian dysfunction.

chloral (G. *khlōros*, green). 1. A pungent colourless mobile liquid, trichloracetaldehyde, $Cl_3C.CHO$, prepared by the mutual action of alcohol and chlorine. 2. Chloral hydrate, a deliquescent, crystalline substance; anodyne, hypnotic and antispasmodic. $CCl_3.CH(OH)_2$.

chlor·alism. Addiction to the use of chloral.

chlor·alose. A substance obtained by heating chlora with glucose: a hypnotic and sedative.

chloram·phĕ·nicol. An antibiotic, originally isolated from a streptomyces but now prepared synthetically. Syn. chloromycetin.

chlor·ate (G. *khlōros*, green). A compound of chloric acid and a base.

chlor·butol. Trichloro-tert.-butyl alcohol. A mild sedative and analgesic.

chlor·ide (G. *khlōros*, green). A binary compound containing chlorine.

chloridū·ria (G. *khlōros*, green; *ouron*, urine). Condition where there is an excess of chlorine in the urine.

chlor·inated (G. *khlōros*, green). Treated with chlorine.

chlorinā·tion (G. *khlōros*, green). Saturation with chlorine, or introduction of chlorine into a compound.

chlor·ine (G. *khlōros*, green). A non-metallic gaseous element of the group of halogens; occurring as chlorides in many minerals and in vegetable and animal tissues. Symbol Cl.

chlor·ite (G. *khlōros*, green). Any one of the salts of chlorous acid.

chloro·anaemia. See under chlorosis.

chloroā·zidin. A substance which slowly liberates chlorine and is thus used to produce a prolonged bactericidal action.

Chlorodyne. An analgesic containing chloroform, ether, alcohol, morphine hydrochloride and dilute hydrocyanic acid.

chlŏr·oform (G. *khlōros*, green; L. *formica*, ant). Trichlormethane; a heavy, colourless liquid which acts, when inhaled, as a general anaesthetic.

chlŏr·oformism. Addiction to the use of chloroform as a narcotic.

chlorō·ma (G. *khlōros*, green). A condition, mainly affecting children and adolescents, characterized by the association of myeloid leukaemia with tumours of greenish tint in the flat bones, especially of face and skull, probably arising from bone-marrow cells, but on section seen to be situated subperiosteally, composed of myeloid, usually oxydase-positive cells, invading the surrounding tissues and often leading, for mechanical reasons, to exophthalmia and blindness; the greenish colour is probably due to a porphyrin.

chloromycĕ·tin. See chloramphenicol.

chloropĕ·nic (G. *khlōros*, green; *penia*, poverty). Lacking in chlorine.

chloroper·cha. A solution of gutta-percha in chloroform, used in dental surgery for filling root canals.

chlorophenyl*iso*propylbiguanide. The chemical name of Paludrine.

chlor·ophyll (G. *khlōros*, green; *phullon*, leaf). The green pigment of plants, having the structure of a porphyrin nucleus with a centrally bound magnesium atom; the substance effecting photosynthesis in plants, i.e., assimilation of CO_2 under the influence of light and subsequent fixation of carbon.

chlorō·pia, chlorop·sia (G. *khlōros*, green; *opsis*, vision). Vision in which all objects appear green.

chlor·oplast, chloroplas·tid (G. *khlōros*, green; *plassein*, to form). A cell containing chlorophyll, freely moving in the tissue fluids of plants in response to light.

chlor·oquine. A synthetic antimalarial drug of the quinoline family.

chlorō·sis (G. *khlōros*, green). A form of anaemia formerly common in women about or after puberty, but now relatively rare. It is characterized by hypochromic anaemia and a greenish tint of the skin and is often associated with gastric and menstrual dysfunction.

chlorot·ic (G. *khlōros*, green). Relating to or affected with chlorosis.

chlorox·ylenol. A powerful and non-irritant bactericide. Syn. *para*chloro*meta*xylenol.

chlorurāe·mia. The presence of urinary chlorides in the blood.

chō·ana (G. *khoanē*, funnel). 1. A funnel-like opening. 2. Any of the posterior nasal openings.

chŏ·colate (Sp. *chocolate*, from Mexican *chocolatl* (*choco*=cocoa, *latl*=water)). Hardened paste of the cacao seed, sweetened with sugar. C_2H_5OH. Ethyl alcohol.

choke. To suffocate; to prevent access of air to the lungs by compression of the trachea or by its obstruction.

choked disc (G. *diskos*, quoit). Papilloedema, *q.v.*

choking. Partial or complete suffocation by the lodgment of a foreign body in the upper respiratory tract or by the inhalation of any irrespirable gas or vapour.

cholāe·mia (G. *khŏlē*, bile; *haima*, blood). 1. The presence of bile in the blood. 2. Condition of acute hepatic insufficiency, as in acute yellow atrophy or in final stages of cirrhosis of the liver, characterized by (1) and by jaundice, a peculiar oral foetor resembling the smell of raw liver, and by more or less severe impairment of consciousness.

cholāe·mic (G. *khŏlē*, bile; *haima*, blood). Relating to cholaemia.

chō·lagogue (G. *khŏlē*, bile; *agōgos*, leading). Promoting the flow of bile.

cho·langiectā·sia, cho·langiectā·sis (G. *khŏlē*, bile; *aggeion*, vessel; *ektasis*, extension). Dilatation of biliary ducts.

cholangiō·ma (G. *khŏlē*, bile; *aggeion*, vessel). Tumour arising from bile-duct cells.

cholangi·tis (G. *khŏlē*, bile; *aggeion*, vessel). Inflammation of a bile-duct.

cholas·cos (G. *khŏlē*, bile; *askos*, bag). The entry of bile into the peritoneal cavity.

chō·late (G. *khŏte*, bile). Any salt of cholic acid.

chō·lecyst (G. *khŏlē*, bile; *kustis*, bladder). The gall-bladder.

chō·lecystectā·sia (G. *khŏlē*, bile; *kustis*, bladder; *ektasis*, extension). Dilatation of the gall-bladder.

chō·lecystec·tomy (G. *khŏlē*, bile; *kustis*, bladder; *ektomē*, excision). Excision of the gall-bladder.

chō·lecystenterŏ·stomy (G. *khŏlē*, bile; *kustis*, bladder; *enteron*, bowel; *stoma*, mouth). Surgical establishment of a direct communication between gall-bladder and small intestine.

cholecysti·tis (G. *khŏlē*, bile; *kustis*, bladder). Inflammation of the gall-bladder.

chō·lecystocolŏ·stomy (G. *khŏlē*, bile; *kustis*, bladder; *kŏlon*, colon; *stoma*, mouth). Surgical establishment of a direct communication between gall-bladder and colon.

chō·lecystocolŏ·tomy (G. *khŏlē*, bile; *kustis*, bladder; *kŏlon*, colon; *tomē*, a cutting). An incision into gall-bladder and colon.

chō·lecys·toduodenŏ·stomy (G. *khŏlē*, bile; *kustis*, bladder; L. *duodeni*, twelve each; G. *stoma*, mouth). Surgical establishment of a direct communication between gall-bladder and duodenum.

cholecys·togastrŏ·stomy (G. *khŏlē*, bile; *kustis*, bladder; *gastēr*, stomach; *stoma*, mouth). Surgical establishment of a direct communication between gall-bladder and stomach.

cholecys·togram (G. *khŏlē*, bile; *kustis*, bladder; *gramma*, picture). An X-ray film of the gall-bladder obtained by cholecystography.

cholecystŏ·graphy (G. *khŏlē*, bile; *kustis*, bladder; *graphein*, to write). Visualization of the gall-bladder by X-rays after it has been made opaque to X-rays by ingestion of a suitable substance which, after absorption from the gastro-intestinal tract, is secreted from the liver into the gall-bladder.

cholecys·tolithi·asis (G. *khŏlē*, bile; *kustis*, bladder; *lithos*, stone). The presence of one or more gall-stones in the gall-bladder.

cholecys·toli·thotripsy (G. *khŏlē*, bile; *kustis*, bladder; *lithos*, stone; *tribein*, to crush). The crushing of gall-stones in the gall-bladder.

cholecystŏ·pathy (G. *khŏlē*, bile; *kustis*, bladder; *pathos*, disease). Any disease of the gall-bladder.

cholecys·topexy (G. *khŏlē*, bile; *kustis*, bladder; *pēxis*, fixation). Suturing the gall-bladder to the abdominal wall.

cholecystŏ·stomy (G. *khŏlē*, bile; *kustis*, bladder; *stoma*, mouth). Surgical establishment of a fistula between gall-bladder and abdominal wall.

cholecystŏ·tomy (G. *khŏlē*, bile; *kustis*, bladder; *tomē*, a cutting). Incision into the gall-bladder.

choledochec·tomy (G. *khŏlē*, bile; *dekhesthai*, to receive; *ektomē*, excision). Excision of part of the common bile duct.

choledochi·tis (G. *khŏlē*, bile; *dekhesthai*, to receive). Inflammation of the common bile duct.

cholĕ·dochoduodenŏ·stomy (G. *khŏlē*, bile; *dekhesthai*, to receive; L. *duodeni*, twelve each; G. *stoma*, mouth). Surgical establishment of an artificial communication between common bile duct and duodenum.

cholĕ·docho-enterŏ·stomy (G. *khŏlē*, bile; *dekhesthai*, to receive; *enteron*, intestine; *stoma*, mouth). Surgical establishment of a direct communication between common bile duct and small intestine.

choledŏ·cholith (G. *khŏlē*, bile; *dekhesthai*, to receive; *lithos*, stone). Stone in the common bile duct.

cholĕ·docholithŏ·tomy (G. *khŏlē*, bile; *dekhesthai*, to receive; *lithos*, stone; *tomē*, a cutting). Incision of the common bile duct for the removal of gall-stones.

cholĕ·docholith·otripsy (G. *khŏlē*, bile; *dekhesthai*, to receive; *lithos*, stone; *tribein*, to crush). The crushing of gall-stones in the common bile duct, without opening the duct.

chŏ·ledochŏ·stomy (G. *khŏlē*, bile; *dekhesthai*, to receive; *stoma*, mouth). Surgical establishment of a fistula between the common bile duct and the abdominal wall.

chŏ·ledochŏ·tomy (G. *khŏlē*, bile; *dekhesthai*, to receive; *tomē*, a cutting). An incision into the common bile duct.

chŏ·lithŏ·tomy (G. *khŏlē*, bile; *lithos*, stone; *tomē*, a cutting). Incision into the gall-bladder or a bile duct for the removal of gall-stones.

cholĕ·ic. Relating to the bile.

chŏ·lelith (G. *khŏlē*, bile; *lithos*, stone). A gall-stone.

chŏ·lelithi·asis (G. *khŏlē*, bile; *lithos*, stone). The presence of one or more calculi in the gall-bladder.

cholelith·ic (G. *khŏlē*, bile; *lithos*, stone). Relating to gall-stones.

chŏ·lelithŏ·trity (G. *khŏlē*, bile; *lithos*, stone; L. *terere*, to rub). Crushing of a gall-stone.

cholĕ·mesis (G. *khŏlē*, bile; *emĕein*, to vomit). Vomiting of bile.

chŏ·lera (G. *khŏlera*). An acute infectious disease caused by the *Vibrio cholerae*, characterized by fever or sub-normal temperature, vomiting and profuse diarrhoea producing dehydration of the body and hypochloraemia, peripheral circulatory insufficiency and cramp-like pains in leg muscles. Syn. Asiatic c. **C. infantum:** term applied to the more severe forms of infantile gastro-enteritis. **C. nostras:** gastro- enter-itis, resembling true (Asiatic) c., usually caused by bacilli of the paratyphoid or coli group. **C. sicca:** a form of c. characterized by death from circulatory collapse before onset of gastro-intestinal symptoms.

cholerā·ic (G. *kholera*). Relating to cholera.

cholerĕ·sis (G. *khŏlē*, bile). Secretion of bile.

choleret·ic (G. *khŏlē*, bile). Pertaining to or inducing choleresis.

chŏ·leric (G. *khŏlē*, bile). Relating to a temperament characterized by hyper-excitability.

cholĕ·riform (G. *kholera*, cholera; L. *forma*, shape). Resembling cholera.

chŏ·lerine (G. *kholera*, cholera). A form of Asiatic cholera, characterized by sudden onset and rapid recovery.

chŏ·lerophŏ·bia (G. *kholera*, cholera; *phobos*, fear). An abnormal dread of cholera.

cholestā·sis (G. *khŏlē*, bile; *stăsis*, a standing still). Arrestation of the flow of bile.

chŏ·lestĕătŏ·ma (G. *khŏlē*, bile; *stear*, fat). 1. A cere-bral tumour of congenital-developmental origin, arising from epithelial implantations, usually under the pia mater, composed of horny cholesterol-con-taining bodies which are derived from stratified epithelium. 2. A structure resembling microscopic-ally the cerebral cholesteatoma, occurring in the middle ear in chronic middle ear infections, due to ingrowing epithelium of the external meatus into the middle ear, where it becomes desquamated.

cholĕ·stenone. A ketone formed by oxidation of cholesterol.

cholĕ·sterol (G. *khŏlē*, bile; *stear*, fat). A complex unsaturated secondary alcohol containing a nucleus of four reduced rings. It occurs in various animal tissues in the free state and also as an ester with various fatty acids. Nervous tissue contains large amounts as do gall-stones. **C., blood:** the amount of c. present in the blood, normally up to 200 mgm. per 100 c.c. of blood.

cholĕ·sterolŏ·sis (G. *khŏlē*, bile; *stear*, fat). Deposition of masses of cholesterol ester in the gall-bladder mucosa, probably due to hyper-cholesterolaemia when accompanied by chronic catarrhal inflamma-tion of the gall-bladder. Syn. strawberry gall-bladder.

cholĕu·ria (G. *khŏlē*, bile; *ouron*, urine). The presence of bile in the urine.

chŏ·lic (G. *khŏlē*, bile). Relating to bile. **C. acid:** tri-hydroxy saturated acid, present in bile.

choline. Trimethyl-hydroxyethylammonium hydrox-ide; a substance occurring in all living cells and formed by hydrolysis of lecithin. See also acetylcho-line.

choliner·gic (G. *khŏlē*, bile; *ergon*, work). Applied to autonomic nerve fibres the stimulation of which causes liberation of acetylcholine at their myoneural junction.

chŏ·linĕ·sterase (G. *khŏlē*, bile; *stear*, fat). An enzyme hydrolyzing acetylcholine present in all body tissues and blood; inhibited by physostigmine and prostig-mine.

chŏ·lochrome (G. *khŏlē*, bile; *khrōma*, colour). Any bile pigment.

chologenet·ic (G. *khŏlē*, bile; *gennan*, to produce). Producing bile.

chŏ·lolith (G. *khŏlē*, bile; *lithos*, stone). A gall-stone.

cholorrhŏe·a (G. *khŏlē*, bile; *rheein*, to flow). Excessive secretion of bile.

cholu·ria (G. *khŏlē*, bile; *ouron*, urine). Urinary excretion of bile pigments.

chon·dral (G. *khondros*, cartilage). Relating to carti-lage; cartilaginous.

chondral·gia (G. *khondros*, cartilage; *algos*, pain). Pain in a cartilage.

chondrec·tomy (G. *khondros*, cartilage; *ektomē*, ex-cision). Excision of a cartilage.

chon·dric (G. *khondros*, cartilage). Pertaining to cartilage.

chon·drificā·tion (G. *khondros*, cartilage; L. *facere*, to make). Conversion into cartilage.

chon·drigen (G. *khondros*, cartilage; *gennan*, to pro-duce). The collagenous substance of hyaline cartilage.

G

chon·drin (G. *khondros*, cartilage). A gelatin-like protein from cartilage.

chon·driocont (G. *khondros*, cartilage; *kontos*, a pole). A rod-shaped or fibrillar chondriosome.

chon·driomere (G. *khondros*, cartilage; *meros*, part). Plastomere, *q.v.*

chon·driomite (G. *khondros*, cartilage; *mitos*, a thread). A chondriosome arranged as a linear series of granules.

chon·driosome (G. *khondros*, cartilage; *sōma*, body). 1. A general term comprising all forms of mitochondria, chondrioconts, chondriomites and other cytoplasmic bodies of similar function. 2. Granular type of mitochondria, as occurring in the sexual cells of vertebrates and in undifferentiated cells generally.

chondri·tis (G. *khondros*, cartilage). Inflammation of a cartilage.

chon·driosphere (G. *khondros*, cartilage; *sphaira*, sphere). A spherical chondriosome.

chon·dro-adenō·ma (G. *khondros*, cartilage; *adēn*, a gland). An adenoma containing cartilaginous substance.

chon·drōăl·bumin (G. *khondros*, cartilage; L. *albumen*, white of egg). One of the main constituents of cartilage; resembling in some respects elastin and keratin.

chon·droblast (G. *khondros*, cartilage; *blastos*, germ). An embryonic cell-forming cartilage.

chon·droclast (G. *khondros*, cartilage; *klaein*, to break). A cell-absorbing cartilage.

chondrocos·tal (G. *khondros*, cartilage; L. *costa*, rib). Relating to the ribs and costal cartilages.

chondrocrā·nium (G. *khondros*, cartilage; *kranion*, skull). The cartilaginous cranium, as that of the embryo.

chon·drocyte (G. *khondros*, cartilage; *kutos*, a container). A cartilage cell.

chon·drodystrō·phia (G. *khondros*, cartilage; *dus-*, inseparable pejorative prefix=Eng. un— or mis—; *trophē*, nourishment). The same as achondroplasia, *q.v.*

chon·drofibrō·ma (G. *khondros*, cartilage; L. *fibra*, fibre). A tumour composed of cartilaginous and fibromatous elements.

chondrogen·esis (G. *khondros*, cartilage; *gennan*, to form). The formation of cartilage.

chondroglos·sus (G. *khondros*, cartilage; *glossa*, tongue). A muscle passing from the hyoid bone to the tongue.

chon·droid (G. *khondros*, cartilage; *eidos*, form). Resembling cartilage.

chondröit·ic acid (G. *khondros*, cartilage). An acid derived from cartilage, found in traces in urine.

chondrō·itin (G. *khondros*, cartilage). A hyaline substance present as chondroitin sulphuric acid in the hydrolysis products of cartilage. A combination of sulphuric acid, acetic acid, glucuronic acid and galactosamine.

chon·drolipō·ma (G. *khondros*, cartilage; *lipos*, fat). A cartilaginous and fatty tumour.

chondrō·logy (G. *khondros*, cartilage; *logos*, discourse). Knowledge of cartilages.

chondrō·lysis (G. *khondros*, cartilage; *luein*, to loosen). Removal of costal cartilages so that the chest wall is more mobile.

chondrō·ma (G. *khondros*, cartilage). A tumour originating from cartilaginous cells.

chon·dromalā·cia (G. *khondros*, cartilage; *malakia*, softness). A morbid softening of the cartilages.

chondrō·matous (G. *khondros*, cartilage). Pertaining to or of the nature of a chondroma.

chondromū·coid (G. *khondros*, cartilage; L. *mucus*; G. *eidos*, form). A substance composed of a protein and chondroitin-sulphuric acid; one of the main constituents of cartilage.

Chondromȳ·ces (G. *khondros*, cartilage; *mukēs*, mushroom). A genus of bacteria.

chon·dromyō·ma (G. *khondros*, cartilage; *mus*, muscle). A tumour composed of cartilaginous and myomatous tissue.

chon·dromyxō·ma (G. *khondros*, cartilage; *muxa*, mucus). A tumour composed of cartilaginous and myxomatous tissue.

chon·dro-os·teodys·trophy (G. *khondros*, cartilage; *osteon*, bone; *dus-*, inseparable pejorative prefix; *trophē*, nourishment). A frequently familial, congenital disease characterized by multiple disturbances in the epiphyses, the occurrence of pseudo-epiphyses and supernumerary ossification centres, and absence of various osseous nuclei, leading to disturbance of height and growth. Syn. Brailsford-Morquio's disease.

chondrō·pathy (G. *khondros*, cartilage; *pathos*, disease). Any cartilaginous disease.

chon·droplasty (G. *khondros*, cartilage; *plassein*, to form). A plastic operation for the repair of a cartilage.

chon·droporō·sis (G. *khondros*, cartilage; *poros*, a passage). The thinning of cartilage by the formation of spaces; occurring during the process of ossification.

chon·drosarcō·ma (G. *khondros*, cartilage; *sarx*, flesh). Sarcoma arising from a chondroma.

chondrosă·mine (G. *khondros*, cartilage; *ammoniakon*, sal-ammoniac). A galactosamine derived from chondrosin.

chondrō·sin (G. *khondros*, cartilage). A substance derived from chondroitin; decomposed by hydrolysis into chondrosamine, and glucuronic acid.

chondrō·sis (G. *khondros*, cartilage). Formation of cartilage.

chon·drotome (G. *khondros*, cartilage; *tomē*, a cutting). An instrument for cutting cartilage.

chondrō·tomy (G. *khondros*, cartilage; *tomē*, a cutting). Division of a cartilage.

chondroxi·phoid (G. *khondros*, cartilage; *xiphos*, a sword; *eidos*, form). Relating to the costal cartilages and the ensiform cartilage.

Chondrus. A genus of seaweeds, some of which have properties useful in the treatment of bronchial and renal diseases.

Chopart's joint (Chopart, F., French surgeon, 1743–95). The mediotarsal articulation; the line of articulation which separates the astragalus and os calcis from the remaining tarsal bones.

chor·da (G. *khordē*, a chord). 1. A chord, tendon or nerve filament. 2. That part of a vertebrate embryo which gives rise to the vertebral column. **Chordae tendineae:** fibrous bands from papillary muscles to auriculoventricular valves. **Chorda tympani:** a branch of the facial nerve joining the lingual branch of the trigeminal nerve supplying the submaxillary and sublingual glands. **Chordae willisii:** fibrous bands crossing the cavity of the dural sinuses.

chor·dal (G. *khordē*, a chord). Relating to a chorda, especially to the notochord, *q.v.*

chordec·tomy (G. *khordē*, a chord; *ektomē*, excision). Surgical removal of a chord.

chordee (G. *khordē*, a chord). Painful, curved erection of the penis with concavity downwards, due to inflammatory periurethral infiltration.

chordi·tis (G. *khordē*, chord). Inflammation of the vocal cords.

chordō·ma (G. *khordē*, chord). A tumour of low malignancy arising from remnants of the notochord, occurring at the upper and lower ends of the vertebral column between the foramen magnum and the pituitary body (spheno-occipital synchondrosis) or in the sacro-coccygeal region (intervertebral discs) respectively, composed of chordal cells distended with mucinous material closely packed together without any intercellular substance.

chordo-skeleton (G. *khordē*, chord; *skeleton*, a mummy). The portion of the skeleton surrounding the notochord.

chordŏ·tomy (G. *khordē*, chord; *tomē*, a cutting). Division of an antero-lateral column of the spinal cord.

chorē·a (G. *khoreia*, a dance). A disease of the nervous system related to, if not a form of, rheumatic fever, more common in females, occurring mainly during childhood, adolescence or pregnancy, liable to recur, and characterized by involuntary, purposeless movements, incoordination of voluntary movements, muscular weakness or flaccid paresis and some degree of psychic disturbance. Syn. Sydenham's c.; C. minor; St. Vitus's dance. **C., electric:** 1. A form of c. minor, characterized by violent movements. See Bergeron's disease. 2. An epidemic disease, possibly related to epidemic encephalitis, prevalent in Northern Italy about 1846. **C., hereditary:** a chronic disease inherited by dominant transmission, becoming manifest during the 3rd or 4th decade of life, characterized by involuntary movements, muscular incoordination and paresis, ataxy, slurring articulation and progressive mental failure, and, pathologically, by degenerative changes in the cerebral cortex and the basal ganglia. Syn. Huntington's chorea; C. major. **C. mollis:** a form of Sydenham's c. characterized by a relatively severe degree of temporary paresis affecting the whole musculature. Syn. Limp c.

chorē·iform (G. *khoreia*, a dance; L. *forma*, shape). Resembling chorea.

chorē·al, chorē·ic (G. *khoreia*, a dance). Relating to chorea.

choreo-ă·thetoid (G. *khoreia*, a dance; *athetos*, without position; *eidos*, form). Relating to choreo-athetosis.

choreo-athetō·sis (G. *khoreia*, a dance; *athetos*, without position). Combination of chorea minor and athetosis.

chŏ·reoid (G. *khoreia*, a dance; *eidos*, form). Resembling chorea.

chŏ·rio-adenō·ma destruens (G. *khorion*, the afterbirth; *adēn*, gland; L. *destruere*, to destroy). Destructive placental mole; a condition sometimes following hydatid mole, occurring especially in multiparae over forty years of age; rarely giving rise to metastases, but if so, only in the pelvic region; histologically characterized by overgrowth of all the elements of the chorionic villi (connective tissue, Langhans's cells and syncytium).

chor·ioblastō·sis (G. *khorion*, the afterbirth; *blastanein*, to grow). Overgrowth of chorionic villi.

chor·iocapillă·ris (G. *khorion*, the afterbirth; L. *capillus*, hair). The capillary layer over the inner portion of the choroid coat of the eye.

chŏ·riocele (G. *khorion*, membrane; *kelē*, hernia). A hernia of the choroid coat of the eye.

chŏ·rioi·dal (G. *khorion*, membrane; *eidos*, form). Pertaining to the chorion.

chorio-epitheliō·ma (G. *khorion*, membrane; *epi*, upon; *thēlē*, nipple). See under chorionepithelioma.

chŏ·rioid (G. *khorion*, membrane; *eidos*, form). 1. Choroid. 2. Choroid plexus. 3. Resembling chorion. 4. Resembling corium.

chŏ·rioi·dal (G. *khorion*, membrane; *eidos*, form). Pertaining to the chorion.

chŏ·rioidi·tis (G. *khorion*, membrane; *eidos*, form). The same as choroiditis, *q.v.*

chŏ·rio-iri·tis (G. *khorion*, membrane; *iris*, rainbow). Inflammation of both choroid and iris.

choriō·ma (G. *khorion*, membrane). Any neoplasm originating from elements of the chorion.

chŏ·riomeningī·tis (G. *khorion*, membrane; *mēnigx*, membrane of the brain). **C., lymphocytic:** a form of acute, aseptic, benign meningitis caused by a virus, often transmitted to man by mice, characterized by fever, symptoms of meningeal irritation, a clear or slightly turbid cerebrospinal fluid with an increased cell content (1,500–3,000 cells per cmm. of c.s.f.) consisting almost entirely of lymphocytes, and pathologically (proven at least in intracerebrally inoculated monkeys and mice) by lymphocytic infiltration of pia mater and choroid plexus, sometimes with an exudate into the cerebral ventricles and by some perivascular glial and lymphocytic infiltration. A meningo-encephalomyelitic form and an influenza-like condition not involving the nervous system may also be caused by the same virus. (Syn. Armstrong's disease.)

chŏ·rion (G. *khorion*, membrane). The outermost of the foetal membranes formed from the trophoblast. **C. frondosum:** the villi-bearing part of the c. in its late developmental stages. **C. laeve:** the part of the c. from which villi have disappeared. **C. primitivum:** the c. in its first developmental stage when its entire surface is covered by villi.

chŏ·rionepitheliō·ma (G. *khorion*, membrane; *epi*, upon; *thēlē*, nipple). 1. A highly malignant tumour derived from epithelial cells of the chorionic villi left in the uterus after parturition or abortion, often preceded by a hydatid mole, *q.v.* (Syn. malignant deciduoma.) 2. A malignant teratoma occurring in the testicle or extremely rarely in the mediastinum, in which foetal membranes have been formed, the chorionic epithelium giving rise to the tumour, the other structures of the tumour being usually destroyed by the malignant growth; producing gynaecomastia and effecting a positive Aschheim-Zondek test.

chorion·ic (G. *khorion*, membrane). Relating to the chorion. **C. gonadotrophin.** Gonadotrophic hormone, from pregnancy urine: as pregnyl, gonon, etc.

chŏr·ioni·tis (G. *khorion*, membrane). Inflammation of the chorion.

chŏr·ioretini·tis (G. *khorion*, membrane; Mediaeval L. *retina*, from *rete*, net). Inflammation of both choroid and retina.

chŏ·roid (G. *khorion*, membrane; *eidos*, form). 1. The middle or vascular coat of the eye. 2. Pertaining to the choroid. **C., gyrate atrophy of:** progressive, frequently familial, disease characterized by atrophy of the c., the pigment epithelium and the retina, usually involving ultimately the greater part of the fundus. **C. plexus:** a highly vascular tissue, derived from ependymal cells, projecting fringe-like into the cavities of all the cerebral ventricles; forming the cerebrospinal fluid.

choroi·dal (G. *khorion*, membrane; *eidos*, form). Pertaining to the choroid. **C. sclerosis:** a condition of the c. coat characterized by primary degenerative vascular changes, usually leading to secondary depigmentation and degeneration of the retina.

chŏ·roiderē·mia (G. *khorion*, membrane; *eidos*, form; *erēmia*, a desert). Absence of both choroid and the epithelial pigment of the retina, except in the macular region; affecting practically only males and occurring bilaterally; causing night blindness, extreme contraction of the usual fields and limitation of colour-perception to the fixation point.

choroidi·tis (G. *khorion*, membrane; *eidos*, form). Inflammation of the choroid; classified as suppurative, exudative, or specific infective c.; as disseminate, diffuse, and circumscribed exudative c.; or as deep and superficial types. **C., Doyne's honeycomb:** see drusen.

choroido-iritis. The same as chorio-iritis, *q.v.*

choroidoretinitis. The same as chorioretinitis, *q.v.*

christŏ·pathy. Christian science: religious movement of American origin. The basic belief is in the unreality of pain and illness.

chromaesthē·sia (G. *khrōma*, colour; *aisthēsis*, perception). Chromato-aesthesia, *q.v.*

chromaf·fine (G. *khrōma*, colour; L. *affinis*, related to). Staining readily with chromium salts, as the cells of the c. system. **C. bodies:** see under paraganglion. **C. tumour:** a tumour composed of chromaffin tissue. Syn. chromaffinoma. See also phaeochromocytoma. **C. system:** applied to c. cells derived from embryonal sympathetic neurons, which are the essential constituent of the paraganglia (*q.v.*) and the carotid body (*q.v.*); the term usually includes also the cells of the adrenal medulla.

chrō·mate (G. *khroma*, skin). A salt of chromic acid.

chrō·matelop·sia (G. *khroma*, colour; *atelēs*, imperfect; *opsis*, vision). Imperfect vision for colours.

chromat·ic (G. *khroma*, colour). Relating to or possessing colour.

Chromatieae. A genus of Rhodobacteriaceae.

chrō·matid (G. *khrōma*, colour). Any one of the chromosomes composing a meiotic tetrad.

chrō·matin (G. *khrōma*, colour). The portion of the cell-nucleus that stains readily with basic dyes.

Chromatium. A genus of aquatic bacteria.

chrō·mato-aesthē·sia (G. *khrōma*, colour; *aisthēsis*, perception). Association of a specific colour with a non-visual sensation.

chrō·matoblast (G. *khrōma*, colour; *blastos*, germ). Melanoblast, *q.v.*

chromatŏ·genous (G. *khrōma*, colour; *gennan*, to produce). Forming colour.

chromatŏ·lysis (G. *khrōma*, colour; *luein*, to loosen). 1. Disintegration of the nuclear chromatin and thereby of the nucleus. Syn. karyolysis. 2. Disintegration of the Nissl bodies from nerve cells. Syn. Nissl's degeneration.

chromatŏ·meter (G. *khrōma*, colour; *metron*, measure). 1. A chart for measuring the intensity of colours. 2. An instrument for measuring colour perception.

chromă·tophane (G. *khrōma*, colour; *phainein*, to show). Coloured globules in the retinal cones of amphibia, reptiles and birds.

chromă·tophile. The same as chromophile, *q.v.*

chrō·matophŏ·bia (G. *khrōma*, colour; *phŏbos*, fear). Discomfort on looking at colours.

chromă·tophore (G. *khrōma*, colour; *phoros*, from *pherein*, to bear). Any cell containing pigmented granules.

chromatop·sia (G. *khrōma*, colour; *opsis*, vision). Abnormal sensation of colour, e.g., xanthopsia, *q.v.*, or vision in which colourless objects appear coloured.

chrō·matoptŏ·meter (G. *khrōma*, colour; *optos*, visible; *metron*, measure). An instrument for measuring the response to colour stimuli.

chromă·toscope (G. *khrōma*, colour; *skopein*, to view). Instrument for estimating the refractive index of coloured light.

chromatŏ·sis (G. *khrōma*, colour). Abnormal pigmentation of the skin.

chromi·dium (G. *khrōma*, colour). Chromatin particles outside the cell nucleus.

chromidrŏ·sis (G. *khrōma*, colour; *hidrōs*, sweat). Secretion of coloured sweat.

chrō·miole (G. *khrōma*, colour). 1. Nuclear granule. 2. More especially, the smallest visible organized part of a chromosome.

chrō·mium (G. *khrōma*, colour). A hard, grey, metallic element, one of the elements of the iron group. Symbol Cr. **C. trioxide:** a caustic agent CrO_3. Syn. chromic acid; chromic anhydride.

Chrō·mobactē·rīae (G. *khrōma*, colour; *baktērion*, dim. of *baktron*, a stick). The first tribe of the family bacteriaceae (including e.g., pyocyaneus) characterized by containing pigment as an integral part of the protoplasm.

chrō·moblast (G. *khrōma*, colour; *blastos*, germ). Embryonic precursor of a pigment cell.

chrō·moblastomycŏ·sis (G. *khrōma*, colour; *blastos*, germ; *mukēs*, mushroom). A disease caused by *Hormodendrum pedrosoi*, characterized by widespread warty granulomatous lesions of the legs.

chrō·mogen (G. *khrōma*, colour; *gennan*, to produce). Applied to any organic substance or organism capable of forming colouring matter.

chromogen·ic (G. *khrōma*, colour; *gennan*, to produce). 1. Producing pigment. 2. Relating to chromogen.

chromō·ma (G. *khrōma*, colour). A malignant tumour, reputedly deriving from chromatophore cells.

chrō·momere (G. *khrōma*, colour; *meros*, part). Any one of the linearly arranged granules of the spireme threads of a chromosome.

chromō·meter (G. *khrōma*, colour; *metron*, measure). 1. A chromomatometer. 2. A colorimeter.

chrō·momycō·sis (G. *khrōma*, colour; *mukēs*, mushroom). Chromoblastomycosis, *q.v.*

chromonē·ma (G. *khrōma*, colour; *nēma*, thread). The basichromatic thread giving rise to the spiremethread.

chrō·mophane (G. *khrōma*, colour; *phainein*, to show). Chromatophane, *q.v.*

chrō·mophile (G. *khrōma*, colour; *philein*, to love). 1. Staining readily. 2. Chromaffine, *q.v.*

chrō·mophobe (G. *khrōma*, colour; *phobos*, fear). Not, or not readily, stainable. **C. adenoma:** the commonest form of pituitary tumour, arising from the c. pituitary cells, overgrowth of which does not give rise by itself to endocrine symptoms but may produce symptoms of pituitary insufficiency through compression of pituitary tissue with endocrine activity.

chrō·mophore (G. *khrōma*, colour; *pherein*, to bear). 1. Carrying colour. 2. The atomic arrangement of a coloured body. 3. Applied to bacteria of the genus Chromobacterieae, *q.v.*

chromoplasm (G. *khrōma*, colour; *plasma*, something formed). The network of a nucleus, so called because it readily stains.

chrō·moplast (G. *khrōma*, colour; *plassein*, to form). 1. Plastids containing or producing pigment, other than the chloroplasts. 2. The large basichromatic nucleolus of the presynaptic nuclei.

chromoprō·tein (G. *khrōma*, colour; *prōteios*, from *prōtos*, first). Conjugated protein, the prosthetic group of which is coloured.

chromop·sia (G. *khrōma*, colour; *opsis*, vision). Chromatopsia, *q.v.*

chrō·moscope (G. *khrōma*, colour; *skopein*, to view). Chromatoscope, *q.v.*

chrō·mosome (G. *khrōma*, colour; *sōma*, body). Any one of the dark-staining bodies produced in mitosis by transverse fission of the spireme, which form characteristic figures, occur in every species in a constant number and transmit the genes of hereditary characters. **C., accessory:** the product of fusion of the unequal sex cs. **C., daughter:** the separated moiety of a c., produced by longitudinal chromosomal splitting during metaphase. **C., sex:** a c. carrying the sex-determining gene. **C., X-:** the larger of the pair of sex cs.; a zygote containing two X-cs. develops into a female individual. **C., Y-:** the smaller of the pair of sex cs.; a zygote containing one Y-c. develops into a male individual.

chronax·y,·ie (G. *khronos*, time; *axia*, value). The minimal duration of a constant current of twice rheobasic (*q.v.*) strength necessary to stimulate an excitable tissue.

chron·ic (G. *khronos*, time). Of long duration; opposite of acute.

chrŏ·nograph (G. *khronos*, time; *graphein*, to write). Instrument for recording intervals of time.

chronotrop·ic (G. *khronos*, time; *trepein*, turn). Applied to phenomena influencing the heart rate.

chrysarŏ·bin. A mixture of substances obtained by benzene extraction of araroba found in *Andira araroba aguiar*. Used as a parasiticide and in psoriasis and ringworm of the scalp.

Chrysomỹ·ia (G. *khrusos*, gold; *muia*, a fly). A genus of flies, certain species of which, found in Australia and in India, cause myiasis in man.

chrysothĕ·rapy (G. *khrusos*, gold; *therapeia*, treatment). Treatment by gold.

Chvostek's symptom (Chvostek, F., Austrian surgeon, 1835–84). Increase in the mechanical irritability of the motor nerves, especially the facial, in postoperative tetany. See also Weiss's sign.

chyle (G. *khulos*, juice). The fluid in the intestinal lymph-vessels during absorption, having a white colour owing to its abundant content of fat globules.

chylifac·tion (G. *khulos*, juice; L. *facere*, to make). Chylopoiesis, q.v.

chyli·ferous (G. *khulos*, juice; L. *ferre*, to bear). Transmitting chyle.

chylificā·tion (G. *khulos*, juice; L. *facere*, to make). Chylopoiesis, q.v.

chy·locele (G. *khulos*, juice; *kēlē*, tumour). An effusion of chylous fluid into the cavity of the tunica vaginalis testis.

chỹ·lopericar·dium (G. *khulos*, juice; *peri*, around; *kardia*, heart). Presence of chyle within the pericardium.

chỹ·loperitonĕ·um (G. *khulos*, juice; *peri*, around; *teinein*, to stretch). Presence of chyle within the peritoneal cavity.

chylopoiē·sis (G. *khulos*, juice; *poiein*, to make). Formation of chyle.

chỹ·lopoiĕt·ic (G. *khulos*, juice; *poiein*, to make). Chyle-forming.

chỹlorrhoē·a (G. *khulos*, juice; *rhein*, to flow). Excessive flow of chyle.

chylothor·ax (G. *khulos*, juice; *thōrax*, chest). Presence of chyle in the pleural cavity, usually due to rupture of the thoracic duct.

chỹ·lous (G. *khulos*, juice). Pertaining to or containing chyle.

chylū·ria (G. *khulos*, juice; *ouron*, urine). Presence of chyle in the urine, due to an opening of lymph vessels into some part of the urinary tract, as occurring, e.g., in filariasis.

chyme (G. *khumos*, juice). Food that has undergone gastric digestion but not intestinal digestion.

chymificā·tion (G. *khumos*, juice; L. *facere*, to make). Transformation of food into chyme by the digestive process.

chymŏ·trichy (G. *khumos*, juice; *thrix*, hair). Wavy hair.

C.I. Abbreviation of Colour Index.

Ciaccio's glands (Ciaccio, G. V., Italian anatomist, 1824–1901). The conjunctival glands.

Ciaglinski's tract (Ciaglinski, A., Polish histologist, work published 1891). A tract of ascending fibres in the posterior grey commissure of the thoracic part of the spinal cord.

cicatri·cial (L. *cicatrix*, scar). Relating to a scar.

cicatricŏ·tomy (L. *cicatrix*, scar; G. *tomē*, a cutting). Surgical removal of a scar.

ci·catrix (L. *cicatrix*, scar). Scar; the connective tissue replacing a localized loss of substance.

ci·catrizā·tion (L. *cicatrix*, scar). The process of wound-healing.

ci·catrize (L. *cicatrix*, scar). To heal by scar-formation.

ci·lia (L. *cilium*, eyelid). 1. The eyelashes. 2. The hair-like processes of infusoria. 3. The hair-like process of epithelial cells in some of the organs of the upper respiratory tract.

ci·liary (L. *cilium*, eyelid). 1. Relating to the c. body. **C. body:** an annular structure just behind the corneo-scleral margin, containing the c. muscle and bearing the c. processes. **C. muscle:** the unstriped muscle innervated by parasympathetic fibres of the oculomotor nerve, supporting and adjusting the shape of the lens.

Ciliā·ta (L. *cilium*, eyelid). A sub-class of infusoria characterized by having cilia (2) in both young and adult stages.

ciliā·ted (L. *cilium*, eyelid). Possessing cilia.

ci·liospi·nal reflex (L. *cilium*, eyelid; *spina*, spine; *reflectere*, to bend back). Pupillary dilatation on homolateral stimulation of the skin of the neck.

ci·lium (L.). One of the cilia.

cillŏ·sis (L. *cilium*, eyelid). Spasmodic twitching of the eyelid.

cim·bia (Ital. *cimbia*, a fillet). The band of white matter lying upon the ventral surface of the crus cerebri.

Cimex lectularius. The common bed-bug.

cin·chocaine. The β-diethylaminoethylamide of α-butyloxycinchoninic acid. A local anaesthetic.

Cinchona. Genus of evergreen trees, some of which yield quinine.

cin·chonism (Countess of Chinchon, supposed introducer of the drug in Spain, 1639). Quinine poisoning.

cin·chophen. 2-phenylquinoline-4-carboxylic acid. Possesses an antipyretic action and assists the excretion of uric acid.

cinē·rea (L. *cinereus*, from *cinis*, ashes). The grey matter of the brain, spinal cord and ganglia.

cin·gulum (L.). 1. A girdle or zone. 2. The waist. 3. Herpes zoster (shingles). 4. The association bundle in the gyrus fornicatus of the brain, connecting the areas of the limbic lobe and this lobe with other parts of the rhinencephalon. Syn. fasciculus areatus.

cin·nabar (L. *cinnabaris*, dragon's blood dye). Vermilion.

cinnamic acid. $C_9H_8O_2$; occurs in tolu balsams and some benzoin resins.

cin·namon (G. *kinnamōmon*). The dried inner bark of the C. *saigonicum*. It is used as spice and is carminative and astringent.

cion (G. *kiōn*, pillar). The uvula.

cionec·tomy (G. *kiōn*, pillar; *ektomē*, excision). Excision of the uvula.

cioni·tis (*kiōn*, uvula). Inflammation of the uvula.

cir·cinate (L. *circinare*, from G. *kirkinos*, a circle). Ring-shaped.

circle (L. *circulus*). A ring. **C. of diffusion:** the imperfect image formed by incomplete focalization.

circuit (L. *circuitus*). The path of an electric current.

cir·cular (L. *circulus*, circle). 1. Relating to a circle; ring-shaped. **C. amputation:** amputation with an incision surrounding. 2. Characterized by alternation; cyclic, q.v.

circulā·tion (L. *circulatio*, ult. from *circus*). Passage in a circle, as the c. of the blood. **Foetal c.:** blood c. of the foetus, placenta and umbilical cord. **Portal c.:** the blood flow through the intestinal, mesenteric and splenic vein and its end branches in the liver. **Pulmonary c.:** the c. of blood through the pulmonary arteries, the lungs and the pulmonary veins. **Systemic c.:** the c. of blood through the body, excepting the pulmonary c.

circulā·tory. Relating to the circulation.

cir·culus (L.). A circle. **C. arteriosus Willisii:** a vascular ring at the base of the brain, formed by anterior communicating, right and left anterior cerebral, posterior communicating and right and left posterior cerebral arteries.

circumci·sion (L. *circum*, round; *caedere*, to cut). Removal or excision of a circular portion of the prepuce.

circumclū·sion (L. *circum*, round; *claudere*, to shut). Arterial compression by means of a wire and a pin.

circumduc·tion (L. *circum*, round; *ducere*, to lead). Circular movement, as of a limb.

cir·cumflex (L. *circum*, round; *flectere*, to bend). Surrounding, as a vessel or nerve; winding around.

circumgem·mal (L. *circum*, round; *gemma*, a bud). Applied to various nerve fibrils at the surface of the taste buds.

cir·cumpolarizā·tion (L. *circum*, round; G. *polos*, axis of the sphere). The rotation of a ray of polarized light.

cir·cumscribed (L. *circum*, round; *scribere*, to write). Clearly defined or limited.

circumval·late (L. *circum*, round; *vallum*, a wall). Surrounded by a wall; e.g., circumvallate papillae.

circus (L.). **C. movement:** 1. Persisting circulatory movement of an excitatory or contraction wave in the cardiac auricle, caused by abnormal slowing of conduction rate and shortening of refractory period, leading to auricular flutter. 2. Forced movement of an individual in a circle, due to cerebral disorder.

cirrhō·sis (G. *kirrhos*, orange coloured). A term properly applied only to c. of the liver, in which the liver usually presents a yellowish discoloration. Owing to a confusion between *kirrhos* (orange coloured) and *skirrhos* (hard), the term is sometimes also applied to morbid changes in organs other than the liver which are characterized by fibrous overgrowth and parenchymatous destruction, but which do not manifest any yellowish discoloration. **C. of the liver:** a chronic, progressive disease characterized by destruction and irregular regeneration of the parenchymatous tissue of the liver with overgrowth of connective tissue, resulting in jaundice, enlargement of the spleen and portal obstruction, the last leading to ascites, new formation of collateral veins between portal and systemic circulation, and development of lower oesophageal and rectal varices. Syn. Laënnec's c.; portal c., multilobular c., atrophic c.; alcoholic c. **Alcoholic c.:** c. of the liver due to chronic alcoholism. **Atrophic c.:** the stage in the development of c. in which the liver is diminished in size. **Biliary c.:** c. of the liver due to inflammatory or non-inflammatory obstruction of the extra-hepatic and/or intra-hepatic bile ducts. **Cardiac c.:** cirrhose cardiaque, atrophy of liver cells in the central area of each lobule with fibrous overgrowth owing to pressure from the congested central vein as occurring in chronic congestion of the systemic circulation. **Hanot's c.:** see under Hanot. **Hypertrophic c.:** the stage in the development of c. in which the liver is increased in size. **Multilobular c.:** c. of the liver microscopically characterized by nodules of irregularly arranged liver cells and occupying an area of several liver lobules; the arrangement is, however, not truly lobular, as the normal relation of the central vein is lost. **Pigmentary c.:** see haemochromatosis. **Portal c.:** Laënnec's c.: or **Unilobular c.:** c. of the liver characterized by relatively intact arrangement of the liver lobules, especially of the central parts of the lobules.

cirrhot·ic (G. *kirrhos*, orange coloured). Relating to or affected with cirrhosis.

cir·soid (G. *kirsos*, varicocele; *eidos*, like). Resembling a varix.

cistern (L. *cisterna*, a tank). 1. A dilatation. 2. Any one of the large subarachnoidal spaces at the base of the brain.

citrate (L. *citrus*, the citrus-tree). Any salt of citric acid.

citrā·ted (L. *citrus*, citrus-tree). Applied to blood the coagulation of which has been prevented by the addition of one part of a 3·8 per cent solution of sodium citrate to 9 parts of blood.

citric acid. A crystalline acid obtained from citrous fruits (lemons, limes, etc.).

Citrus. A genus of rutaceous trees, including the lemon, orange and lime.

Civinini's spine (Civinini, F., Italian anatomist, 1805–44). A small spine on the outer border of the external pterygoid plate, giving attachment to the pterygospinous ligament.

Cl. Symbol of chlorine.

Clado's ligament (Clado, S., French gynaecologist, 1856–1905). The appendiculo-ovarian ligament. **C.'s anastomosis:** situated between the appendicular and ovarian arteries in the ligament.

Cladothrix (G. *klados*, branch; *thrix*, hair). A group of higher bacteria capable of separating ferric oxide from water containing iron.

clamp. An instrument for holding parts together or for compressing a structure such as a blood vessel. There are many varieties such as Blalock's clamps, used in heart surgery, Doyen's broad ligament clamp, used in gynaecological operations, and Lane's stomach clamp and Payr's clamp, both used in gastrotomy.

clapotage, clapotement (Fr. *clapoter*, splash). A splashing sound.

Clapton's line. Greenish discoloration of the gums and teeth, especially the incisors, in chronic copper poisoning.

clarificā·tion (L. *clarus*, clear; *facere*, make). Clearing; removing of turbidity from a liquid.

Clark's sign (Clark, A., American physician, 1807–87). A tympanic sound over the hepatic region in tympanites due to perforative peritoneal inflammation.

Clarke's column (Clarke, J. L., English anatomist, 1817–80). The nucleus dorsalis of the spinal cord. **C.'s cells:** pigmented cells of the nucleus dorsalis.

Clarke's corroding ulcer (Clarke, Sir C. M., English physician, 1782–1857). Progressive ulcer of the cervix uteri. **C.'s tongue:** the hard, fissured and nodular tongue of syphilitic glossitis sclerosa.

clasmā·tocyte (G. *klasma*, fragment; *kutos*, cell). A large proliferating connective tissue cell with phagocytic capacity.

claudicā·tion (L. *claudicare*, to limp). Lameness. **C., intermittent:** intermittent occurrence of limping due to impairment in the arterial circulation in a limb.

Claudius's cells (Claudius, F. M., Austrian anatomist, 1822–69). Polyhedral or conoidal cells lining the outer angle of the scala media of the cochlea. **C.'s fossa:** the ovarian fossa, a triangular space containing the ovary.

claustrophō·bia (L. *claustrum*, enclosure; G. *phŏbos*, fear). A form of obsessional neurosis characterized by fear of staying in a closed room.

clau·strum (L.). 1. A barrier. 2. A layer of grey matter between the island of Reil and the putamen.

clā·va (L. *clava*, club). Enlargement of the funiculus gracilis at the inferior angle of the rhomboid fossa.

clā·vate (L. *clava*, club). Club-shaped.

Claviceps (L. *clava*, club; *caput*, head). A genus of fungi. **C. purpurea:** the fungus from which ergot is derived.

clā·vicle (L. *clavicula*, dim. of *clavis*, key). The collar-bone.

clavi·cular. Relating to the clavicle.

clavi·culus (L. *claviculus*, dim. of *clavus*, a nail). One of Sharpey's fibres in bone.

clā·vus (L. *clavus*, a nail). A corn; a horny growth of the epidermis.

claw-foot. A form of talipes due to atrophy of the interossei and lumbricales muscles, characterized by depression of the heads of the metatarsal bones, overextension of the first and flexion of the last phalanges.

claw-hand. A condition of the hand caused by atrophy of the interossei muscles, characterized by overextension of the first and flexion of the other phalanges. Syn. *main en griffe.*

clear. To remove turbidity or cloudiness by means of a clearing substance.

clea·vage. 1. Segmentation; division. 2. Cell-division. 3. The splitting of a molecule into simpler molecules. **C. lines:** the linear clefts in the skin, indicating the direction of the connective tissue fibres. **C. nucleus:** the primary nucleus of the fecundated ovum.

cleft. 1. A fissure; a crevice. 2. Divided. **C. hand:** a congenital deformity in which the fingers are abnormally separated from each other. **C. palate:** a congenital developmental deformity characterized by persistence of fissures at one or both sides of the vomer in the hard palate and in the middle of the soft palate. Syn. palatoschisis.

cleidarthri·tis (G. *kleis,* clavicle; *arthron,* joint). Inflammation of the sternoclavicular joint.

cleidocos·tal (G. *kleis,* clavicle; L. *costa,* rib). Relating to both clavicle and ribs.

cleidocrā·nial (G. *kleis,* clavicle; *kranion,* cranium). Relating to both clavicle and cranium. **C. dysostosis:** see dysostosis, c.

cleidŏ·tomy (G. *kleis,* clavicle; *tomē,* a cutting). Operative division of the clavicles in cases of difficult labour due to a discrepancy in size between the foetal shoulders and the maternal pelvis.

cleithrophō·bia (G. *kleithron,* door bolt; *phŏbos,* fear). Morbid fear of being confined in an enclosed space.

Cleland's cutaneous ligaments (Cleland, J., Scottish anatomist, 1835–1925). Ligaments of the digits.

clē·oid (G. *kleis,* hook; *eidos,* form). A dental excavating instrument.

cleptomā·nia. See kleptomania.

Clevenger's fissure (Clevenger, S. V., American neurologist, 1843–1920). The inferior occipital fissure; the sulcus temporalis inferior.

climactĕ·ric (G. *klimaktēr,* from *klimax,* a ladder). Menopause.

cli·mate (G. *klima,* a region). The sum of meteorological conditions in a region, especially as regards their influence on health.

climat·ic (G. *klima,* a region). Pertaining to climate. **C. bubo:** lymphogranuloma inguinale, *q.v.*

climatŏ·logy (G. *klima,* a region; *logos,* treatise). The science dealing with climatic phenomena and conditions.

cli·matothĕ·rapy (G. *klima,* a region; *therapeia,* treatment). Use of climate as a therapeutic agent.

climax (G. *klimax,* ladder). The peak period in the course of any disease.

clin·ic (G. *klinē,* a couch). 1. An institution for the treatment of patients. 2. Medical instruction given in the presence of a patient.

cli·nical (G. *klinē,* a couch). 1. Relating to a clinic. 2. Relating to the signs of a disease as observed by the physician. **C. pathology:** see under pathology.

clini·cian (G. *kline,* a couch). A physician who examines and treats patients at the bedside.

clinocĕ·phalism (G. *klinein,* to bend; *kephalē,* head). Saddle-head: dolichocephalus with saddle-shaped depression of the skull due to early synostosis between sphenoid and parietal bones.

clinodac·tyly (G. *klinein,* to bend; *daktulos,* finger). Permanent phalangeal curvature in the longitudinal axis, congenital or acquired.

cli·noid (G. *klinē,* bed; *eidos,* form). Resembling a bed; applied to various bony structures, e.g., the

processes of the body and lesser wing of the sphenoid bone.

clitoridec·tomy (G. *kleitoris*; *ectomē,* excision). Removal of the clitoris.

clitorĭdi·tis (G. *kleitoris,* clitoris). Inflammation of the clitoris.

clitoridŏ·tomy (G. *kleitoris*; *tomē,* a cutting). Circumcision in the female as practised by some tribes.

cli·toris (G. *kleitoris*). A structure at the anterior end of the labia minora, the homologue of the penis in the female.

cli·vus (L.). A slope. **C. of Blumenbach:** the structure formed by the basilar part of the occipital bone and posterior surface of the dorsum sellae turcicae.

clŏā·ca (L. *cloaca,* a drain). 1. A common canal into which open the intestine, the reproductive and urinary ducts. It is found during a transient stage in the development of most mammals. 2. A sinus from a diseased bone.

clŏā·cal. Relating to the cloaca.

clŏ·nic (G. *klonos,* turmoil). Relating to clonus.

clonorchiŏ·sis (G. *klŏn,* a twig; *orkhis,* a testicle). Invasion of the bile ducts by *Clonorchis endimicus* or *Clonorchis sinensis.*

Clonorchis (G. *klŏn,* a twig; *orkhis,* a testicle). A genus of liver flukes, belonging to the sub-class of digenetic trematodes.

clŏ·nus (G. *klonos,* turmoil). Involuntary, rapid alternate contraction and relaxation of antagonistic pairs of muscles.

Clopton Havers's glands. The same as Havers's glands, *q.v.*

Cloquet's canal (Cloquet, J. G., French anatomist, 1790–1883). Hyaloid canal in the foetal vitreous body. **C.'s fascia:** the crural septum. **C.'s ganglion:** swelling of the nasopalatine nerve. **C.'s hernia:** femoral hernia.

Clostri·dium (G. *klōster,* spindle). The genus of large spore-bearing anaerobic bacilli, including *Cl. tetani, Cl. botulinum, Cl. chauvoei,* and the gas gangrene group.

clot. The solid coagulum of blood, serum, or milk.

cloudy swelling. A form of cellular degeneration, also constituting an early stage of parenchymatous inflammation, characterized by swelling of cells, loss of translucency, and formation of cytoplasmic granules; occurring mainly in kidney, liver and heart muscle. Syn. degeneration, albuminous.

clownism. Hysterical display of contortions and poses.

clubbed fingers. Club-shaped deformity of the end phalanges of fingers or toes, due to chronic pulmonary or cardiac disorder.

club-foot. See talipes.

club-hand. A congenital deformity of the wrist resulting in supination of the hand, often associated with absence of the radius.

clumping. See under agglutination.

clū·nis (L.). The buttocks.

cm. Abbreviation for centimetre.

cne·mial (G. *knēmē,* shin). Relating to the shin.

cne·mis (G. *knēmē,* shin). The shin or tibia.

C.N.S. Abbreviation for central nervous system.

CO. Carbon monoxide.

CO₂. Carbon dioxide.

cŏā·gulant (L. *coagulum,* from *cogere,* to collect). Causing coagulation.

cŏā·gulate. 1. To produce coagulation. 2. To undergo coagulation.

cŏā·gulation (L. *coagulum,* from *cogere,* to collect). Clotting; the process of becoming jelly-like; precipitation of proteins or conversion of a colloid from a sol into a gel state. **C.-necrosis:** a form of necrosis characterized by c. of intra- and extra-cellular protein and exudation of fibrin. **C. time**: the interval between withdrawal of blood and its conversion into a gel state.

coă·gulum (L. *coalescere*, to unite). The union of previously separate parts.

coarctā·tion (L. *coartare*, to compress). The narrowing of the lumen of a vessel or a canal. **C. of the aorta**: narrowing of the aorta where it is joined by the ductus arteriosus; leading to the establishment of collateral circulation (subscapular and internal mammaries with intercostal and epigastric arteries respectively) and arterial hypertension in the upper part of the body.

coat. Membrane covering a part; a tunic.

COC. Abbreviation for cathodal opening contraction.

cocaine (Peruv. *coca*). An alkaloid from coca leaves; a powerful local anaesthetic used in aqueous media in the form of its hydrochloride. $CH_3.N:C_6H_9(CO.O.CH_3).—CH.O.$

cocain·ism (Peruv. *coca*). Addiction to cocaine.

cocarbox·ylase. Aneurin pyrophosphate, a substance essential for the activity of carboxylase; present in yeast.

Coccā·ceae (G. *kokkos*, berry). One of the lower families of bacteria at the moment of their complete development of spherical form; in the process of multiplication lancet-shaped or flattened, dividing in one (e.g. streptococci), two (e.g. tetrads), three (e.g. sarcinae) or in any axis (e.g. staphylococci).

coc·cal. Relating to cocci.

cocci (G. *kokkos*, berry). Coccaceae, *q.v.*

Coccidiida (G. *kokkos*, berry). An order of sporozoa, comprising Eimeria, Isospora, Haemogregarina, etc.

coccidioi·dal granulō·ma, coccidiō·sis (G. *kokkos*, berry). One of the diseases caused by *Coccidioides immitis*, or *Paracoccidioides brasilensis tenuis* or *Paracoccidioides brasilensis cerebriformis*; characterized by cutaneous, pulmonary or oral granulomata, sometimes metastasizing into other parts.

Coc·cidiomor·pha (G. *kokkos*, berry; *morphē*, shape). A sub-class of sporozoa, comprising the order of Coccidiida.

Cocci·dium (G. *kokkos*, berry). The same as Coccidiida, *q.v.*

Coccobacillus. A rod-like bacillus found in putrefying liquid.

coccobactē·ria (G. *kokkos*, berry; *baktērion*, dim. of *baktron*, a staff). Coccaceae, *q.v.*

coc·cus, pl. **cocci** (G. *kokkos*, berry). 1. A member of the family of Coccaceae, *q.v.* 2. A genus of insects.

coccy̆·geal (G. *kokkus*, coccyx). Relating to the coccyx.

coccygec·tomy (G. *kokkux*; *ektomē*, excision). Excision of the coccyx.

coccy̆·geus. A muscle in the lower part of the pelvis (see muscles).

coc·cygody̆·nia (G. *kokkux*, coccyx; *odunē*, pain). Pain in the coccygeal region, usually marked on sitting.

coc·cyx (G. *kokkux*). The os coccygis; the most caudal bone of the spinal column.

cochineal. The dried bodies of a species of Mexican insects, found on cactus plants, and used in the production of scarlet dye.

cŏch·lea (G. *kokhlos*, a snail). A spiral canal resembling a snail-shell in the anterior part of the bony labyrinth, containing the receptors for auditory stimuli.

coch·lear (G. *kokhlos*, a snail). 1. Relating to the cochlea. 2. A spoon.

cochlei·tis. Inflammation of the cochlea.

Cock's peculiar tumour (Cock, E., English surgeon, 1805–92). Extensive septic ulceration of the scalp, resembling an epithelioma and developed from a neglected sebaceous cyst.

COCl. Abbreviation for cathodal opening clonus.

codeine (G. *kōdeia*, poppy-head). An opium alkaloid used to allay coughing, normally met with as codeine phosphate.

Codex Medicamentarius. The French Pharmacopoeia.

coefficient (L. *cum*, with; *efficere*, to effect). A numerical factor expressing the quantitative change of a value under certain conditions. **C. of correlation**: a number indicating the degree of correlation between two variables, the quotient of the average product of the deviations of the values of the variables divided by the product of the corresponding standard deviations of the variables. **C. of variation**: in statistics, the ratio of standard variation in a series to the arithmetic mean of the series.

coelen·teron (G. *koilos*, hollow; *enteron*, the gut). The primary embryonic alimentary canal.

coe·liac (G. *koilia*, from *koilos*, hollow). Relating to the belly; abdominal. **C. disease**: chronic disease of childhood, characterized by marked impairment of intestinal absorption of fat and calcium and to some degree of carbohydrates, resulting in the production of bulky, greyish stools, containing abnormally large amounts of split fat, by high faecal excretion of calcium, hypocalcaemia; causing general wasting, abdominal prominence, osteoporosis and retardation of growth. Syn. Gee's disease; Heuber-Herter's disease; intestinal infantilism.

coeliadel·phus (G. *koilia*, from *koilos*, hollow; *adelphos*, brother). A double monster united at the belly.

coe·lom, coelō·ma (G. *koilōma*, a cavity). The embryonic body-cavity.

coelosō·ma (G. *koilos*, hollow; *sōma*, body). Single autositic monsters, characterized by body-cleft and eventration.

Coe·nocyte (G. *koinos*, common; *kutos*, a container). A syncytial body in lower plants.

coe·nogă·mete (G. *koinos*, common; *gamein*, to marry). A multinuclear gamete.

Coenu·rus cerebra·lis (G. *koinos*, common; *oura*, tail). The cystic stage of a canine tapeworm, *Taenia multiceps*, found in the brain of sheep and other ruminants.

co-enzyme (L. *cum*, with; G. *en*, in; *zumē*, leaven). Term applied to substances necessary for the activity of a particular enzyme. **Co-enzyme I**: a dinucleotide (probably), containing the radicals of nicotinamide and adenine, acting as hydrogen-carrier in certain oxido-reduction reactions. **Co-enzyme II**: a substance similar to but not interchangeable with co-enzyme I, possessing an additional phosphate radical.

coeur. French for heart.

co-ferment. Co-enzyme, *q.v.*

coffee-ground vomit. Vomited matter containing partly digested blood mixed with other gastric contents.

coffin-lid crystals. Ammonio-magnesium phosphate crystals in urine.

cognac. French brandy.

cogwheel breathing. See under breathing.

cohabitation (L. *cum*, with; *habitare*, to dwell). 1. Living together of a man and woman. 2. Sexual intercourse.

cohere (L. *cohaerere*, to cling together). 1. To stick together. 2. To be consistent.

cohe·sion (L. *cohaerere*, to cling together). Attractive force between the molecules of a body.

cohe·sive (L. *cohaerere*, to cling together). 1. Cohering. 2. Producing cohesion.

Cohnheim's areas (Cohnheim, J. F., German anatomist, 1839–84). (Also called **C.'s fields**). Small polygonal fields visible on optic section of a sarcous element prism. **C.'s end-arteries**: the short arteries supplying the basal ganglia of the cerebrum. **C.'s frog**: a frog from which all blood has been removed and replaced by saline solution. **C.'s theory:** that all true tumours arise from cell-rests or embryonic cells left over after development of the foetus and its organs. **C.'s tumour germs:** small aberrant or heterotopic masses of embryonic tissue from which new growths may originate.

co·itus (L. *coire*, to meet). Sexual intercourse. **C. interruptus, C. reservatus:** c. in which seminal ejaculation into the vagina is prevented by withdrawal of the penis.

colā·tion (L. *colare*, to filter). The process of straining a liquid.

colchicine. An alkaloid, $C_{22}H_{25}O_6N$, made from colchicum. It is used to give relief in gout and experimentally for its effect on mitosis.

col·chicum. The corm and seeds of the meadow saffron, *Colchicum autumnale*, useful in cases of gout. The active principle is alkaloid colchicine.

cold. Popular term for coryza or catarrh of the upper respiratory tract.

colec·tomy (G. *kolon*, colon; *ektomē*, excision). Excision of a portion of the colon.

Coley's mixture (Coley, W. B., American surgeon, 1862-1936). A combination of the toxins of *Streptococcus erysipelatis* and *Bacillus prodigiosus*; has been used in the treatment of inoperable cases of cancer.

coli (G. *kolon*, colon). Of the colon. **Bacterium c.:** predominant micro-organism of the large intestine, a frequent pathogen elsewhere, e.g. in the urinary tract.

col·ic (G. *kolon*, colon). 1. Relating to the colon. 2. Spasmodic pain in the abdomen. **Biliary c.:** c. due to a morbid condition of the gall-bladder or its ducts, especially to the passage or incarceration of a gallstone. **Lead c.:** c. due to lead poisoning. **Renal c.:** c. due to the passage or incarceration of a stone in kidney or ureter.

colicysti·tis (G. *kolon*, colon; *kustis*, bladder). Cystitis due to infection with a member of the *Bacterium coli* group.

co·liform. Resembling *Bacterium coli*.

coli·tis (G. *kolon*, colon). Inflammation of the colon. **C., mucous:** a condition characterized by abdominal pains and the discharge of band- or tube-shaped pseudo-membranes *per rectum*, occurring usually in neuropathic subjects. **C., ulcerative:** a chronic disease with acute exacerbations, characterized by more or less extensive ulcerative inflammation of the colon and rectum with loss of haustrations; causing fluid motions containing blood, pus and mucus, leading to general wasting and anaemia.

col·lagen (G. *kolla*, glue; *gennan*, to produce). A protein constituent of fibrous tissue yielding gelatin on boiling.

collä·ginous (G. *kolla*, glue; *gennan*, to produce). Pertaining to or containing collagen.

collapse (L. *collapsus*, from *collabi*, to fall). 1. Shock, *q.v.* 2. Abnormal retraction of an organ. **C., massive:** c. of one or more lobes of the lung, occurring usually as result of chest wounds or abdominal operations; characterized by sudden onset of pain in the chest, severe dyspnoea, cyanosis, viscid sputum, tachycardia, fever, diminished movements of the affected side of the chest, dullness of percussion-note, tubular breathing, increased vocal fremitus, bronchophony and displacement of heart and mediastinum towards the affected side. **C. of the lungs:** 1. Absence of air from lung tissue previously expanded, due to bronchial obstruction from increased bronchial secretion and inhibition of cough reflex or from intrathoracic neoplasm or lymph node enlargement compressing the bronchus. 2. Congenital atelectasis.

collarette (L. *collare*, from *collum*, neck). Line of junction between the peripheral ciliary and the central pupillary zones of the iris. Syn. iris frill.

collä·teral (L. *cum*, with; *lateralis*, from *latus*, side). 1. Accompanying. 2. Accessory. 3. Applied to branches of an axis-cylinder passing at a right angle. **C. circulation:** blood circulation through anastomosing vessels.

Colles's fascia (Colles, A., Irish surgeon, 1773-1843). The deep layer of the urogenital fascia. **C.'s fracture:** fracture of the lower extremity of the radius. **C.'s ligament:** see triangular fascia.

colli·culus (L. *collis*, hill). A small eminence.

Collier's pontospinal tract. The tegmental portion of the fasciculus longitudinalis medialis.

colliquā·tion (L. *cum*, with; *liquare*, to liquefy). Liquefaction.

colli·quative (L. *cum*, with; *liquare*, to liquefy). Pertaining to colliquation.

col·located (L. *collocare*, to place with). Placed or arranged with something else, especially side by side.

collō·dion. A flexible cellulose plastic varnish.

collō·tion. A dressing made by dissolving gun-cotton in ether and alcohol.

col·loid (G. *kolla*, glue; *eidos*, form). 1. That state in which a solid, liquid or gaseous substance composed of particles of 1-100 mμ size (dispersed phase) is uniformly distributed in another solid, liquid or gaseous substance (dispersion medium or continuous phase). Two main classes are distinguished: suspensoid, or hydrophobic, or lyophobic c. and emulsoid, hydrophilic, or lyophilic c., the former being characterized by a dispersed phase consisting of particles of an insoluble substance suspended in a solid, fluid or gaseous dispersion medium, and in the latter the dispersed phase consists of a water-absorbing organic substance which is suspended in a liquid medium. 2. The jelly-like secretion of the thyroid gland. **C. degeneration:** condition of the tissues characterized by the presence in them of a jelly-like or mucoid, yellowish, translucent substance. **C. goitre:** a goitre characterized by accumulation of c. (2) matter in the distended acini of the gland, probably due to iodine deficiency in food and water. **C. milium:** a skin disease, mainly affecting the face, characterized by small, yellowish, translucent cyst-like structures containing gelatinous matter.

colloi·dal (G. *kolla*, glue; *eidos*, form). Having the properties of a colloid.

collō·ma (G. *kolla*, glue). A colloid cancer.

col·lum (L.). 1. The neck, particularly its anterior portion. 2. The neck-like part of an organ, e.g., collum femoris.

collunā·rium (L. *colluere*, to rinse; *naris*, nose). A nasal douche.

collutor·ium (L. *colluere*, to rinse; *os* mouth). A mouth-wash; a gargle.

colly·rium (G. *kollurion*, eye-salve). A medicinal lotion for the eye.

colobō·ma (G. *kolobos*, mutilated). Congenital absence of a portion of a structure of the eye, especially of the choroid, retina or iris, usually in the region of the foetal fissure and due to disturbance of the mechanism of its closure, probably initiated in the region of the optic cusp.

cō·locolō·stomy (G. *kolon*, colon; *stoma*, mouth). Surgical anastomosis of two portions of the colon.

cō·locynth. The dried pulp of *Citrullus colocynthis*, an ingredient of various purgatives.

cō·lofixā·tion. An operation for fixing the colon. (See colopexy.)

cō·lohĕ·patopexy (G. *kolon*, colon; *hēpar*, liver; *pēxis*, fixation). Surgical fixation of the colon to the liver.

cō·lon (G. *kolon*). 1. The part of the large intestine from the caecum to the end of the sigmoid flexure.

colon·ic (G. *kolon*, colon). Relating to the colon.

colonŏ·meter (L. *colonia*, colony; G. *metron*, measure). An apparatus used for estimating the number of bacteria on a culture-plate.

colony (L. *colonia*). An assemblage, as of micro-organisms in a culture.

colopex·ia, cŏ·lopexy (G. *kolon*, colon; *pēxis*, fixation). Suturing of a portion of the colon to the abdominal wall.

colopexŏ·tomy (G. *kolon*, colon; *pēxis*, fixation; *tomē*, section). Incision into a portion of the colon which has previously been sutured to the abdominal wall.

colŏ·phony. The residue left after removal of oil of turpentine from the exudate of various species of *Pinus*. Syn. resin.

coloptō·sis (G. *kolon*, colon; *ptōsis*, a fall). Downward displacement of the colon.

colori·meter (L. *color*, colour; G. *metron*, measure). An instrument for performing colorimetry.

colori·metry (L. *color*, colour; G. *metron*, measure). 1. Measurement of colour. 2. Estimation of the proportion of a substance in a liquid by determining the amount of water which has to be added to obtain a colour intensity equal to that of a liquid containing a known concentration of the substance or its equivalent.

colŏ·stomy (G. *kolon*, colon; *stoma*, mouth). Establishment of an artificial anus by making an opening into the colon.

colos·trum (L.). The first milk secreted by the breasts; it contains more protein, less fat and much less sugar than the true milk. C.-corpuscles: fatty, degenerated, yellowish-brown epithelial cells of the mammary glands.

colŏ·tomy (G. *kolon*, colon; *tomē*, section). Incision into the colon.

colour (L. *color*). Light rays emitted, reflected or refracted by an object and the visual sensations caused by it. C., basic: any one of the three colours red, yellow and blue. C.-blindness: imperfect perception of colour. C., complementary: a primary colour which added to another produces white. C., impure: c. containing light of more than one wave-length. C.-index: an index of the amount of haemoglobin in the red blood corpuscles; estimated by dividing the percentage of haemoglobin by the percentage of red cells, 5,000,000 per c.mm. being regarded as 100 per cent. C., primary: any one of the seven colours of the solar spectrum (red, orange, yellow, green, blue, indigo and violet). C., pure: the same as c., primary, *q.v.*

col·peurynter (G. *kolpos*, a hollow; *eurunein*, dilate). An inflatable bag for dilating the vagina.

colpeu·rysis (G. *kolpos*, a hollow; *eurunein*, dilate). Vaginal dilatation.

colpi·tis (G. *kolpos*, a hollow). Inflammation of the vagina.

col·pocele (G. *kolpos*, a hollow; *kēlē*, hernia). A hernia protruding into the vagina.

colpocy·stocele (G. *kolpos*, a hollow; *kustis*, bladder; *kēlē*, hernia). A protrusion of the bladder into the vagina with prolapse of the anterior vaginal wall.

col·pocystŏ·tomy (G. *kolpos*, a hollow; *kustis*, bladder; *tomē*, section). Incision into the bladder through the vaginal wall.

colpocy·sto-urĕ·terocystŏ·tomy (G. *kolpos*, a hollow; *kustis*, bladder; *oureteron*, ureter; *tomē*, a cutting). Operation for the exposure of the ureteric orifices by incision of the bladder and vagina.

col·podesmor·rhaphy (G. *kolpos*, a hollow; *desmos*, band; *rhaphē*, suture). Suturing of the vaginal sphincter.

colpoedē·ma (G. *kolpos*, a hollow; *oidema*, a swelling). Oedema of the vagina.

col·pohyperplā·sia (G. *kolpos*, a hollow; *hyper*, over; *plassein*, to form). Hyperplasia of the vagina.

col·pohysterec·tomy (G. *kolpos*, a hollow; *hustera*, uterus; *ektomē*, excision). Removal of the uterus through the vagina; transvaginal hysterectomy.

col·pohy·steropexy (G. *kolpos*, a hollow; *hustera*, uterus; *pēxis*, fixation). 2. Vaginal fixation of the uterus.

col·pohysteror·rhaphy (G. *kolpos*, a hollow; *hustera*, uterus; *rhaphē*, suture). Colpohysteropexy.

col·pohysterŏ·tomy (G. *kolpos*, a hollow; *hustera*, uterus; *tomē*, section). Incision into the uterus through the vagina; transvaginal hysterotomy.

col·pomyomec·tomy (G. *kolpos*, a hollow; *mus*, muscle; *ektomē*, excision). Myomectomy through the vagina.

colpŏ·pathy (G. *kolpos*, a hollow; *pathos*, disease). A vague term for any disease of the vagina.

col·poperinē·oplasty (G. *kolpos*, a hollow; *perinaion*, perineum; *plassein*, to form). Plastic surgery of the vagina and perineum; repair of a rupture involving perineum and vagina.

col·poperinĕŏr·rhaphy (G. *kolpos*, a hollow; *perinaion*, perineum; *rhaphē*, suture). The suturing of vagina and perineum.

col·popexy (G. *kolpos*, a hollow; *pēxis*, fixation). An operation for fixation of the vagina.

col·poplasty (G. *kolpos*, a hollow; *plassein*, to form). Plastic operation on the vagina.

colpoptō·sis (G. *kolpos*, a hollow; *ptōsis*, a fall). Prolapse of the vaginal walls.

colporrhā·gia (G. *kolpos*, a hollow; *rhēgnunai*, to burst forth). Vaginal haemorrhage.

col·por·rhaphy (G. *kolpos*, a hollow; *rhaphē*, suture). Operation for narrowing the vagina.

colporrhex·is (G. *kolpos*, a hollow; *rhēxis*, rupture). Rupture or laceration of the vagina.

col·poscope (G. *kolpos*, a hollow; *skopein*, to view). Instrument for visual examination of the vagina.

col·pospasm (G. *kolpos*, a hollow; *spusmos*, spasm). Spasm of the vagina.

col·postenō·sis (G. *kolpos*, a hollow; *stenōsis*, stricture). Constriction of the vagina.

colpŏ·tomy (G. *kolpos*, a hollow; *tomē*, section). Incision of the vagina.

col·po-urĕ·terocystŏ·tomy (G. *kolpos*, a hollow; *ourētēr*, ureter; *kustis*, bladder; *tomē*, section). Operation for exposure of the ureteral orifices by cutting through the vagina and bladder.

col·po-urĕ·terŏ·tomy (G. *kolpos*, a hollow; *ourētēr*, ureter; *tomē*, section). Incision of the lower end of the ureter through the vagina.

col·poxerō·sis (G. *kolpos*, a hollow; *xeros*, dry). A pathological dryness of the vagina.

columel·la (L., dim. of *columna*, column). 1. A small column. 2. The cochlear modiolus.

column (L. *columna*). 1. Applied to pillar-shaped parts; (2) more especially to any of the grey tracts of the spinal cord.

colum·nar (L. *columna*, column). Column-shaped.

coma (G. *kōma*). A state of absolute unconsciousness, as judged by the absence of any psychologically understandable response to external stimuli or internal need. C., diabetic: a condition occurring in severe, uncontrolled diabetes mellitus, characterized by coma, considerable hyperglycaemia, ketosis with decrease of alkali reserve, air-hunger (slow deep respiration), flaccidity, dehydration of tissues with softness of eyeballs and peripheral circulatory insufficiency.

cō·matose (G. *kōma*). In a state of coma.

combined degeneration of cord. See under cord, subacute combined degeneration.

combŭ·stion (L. *comburere*, to burn). 1. Process of burning. 2. Any chemical process accompanied by liberation of heat and sometimes of light and sound.

comē·do, comedones (plural) (L.). Plug or horny epithelial cell detritus and sebaceous matter in the duct of a sebaceous gland. Syn. blackhead.

co·mēs (L. *comes*, comrade). A companion, as a vein to an artery.

comma bacillus (G. *komma*, a segment; L. *bacillus*, dim. of *baculus*). *Vibrio cholerae*.

comma tract (G. *komma*, segment; L. *tractus*, extent, from *trahere*, to drag). A comma-shaped tract in the postero-lateral column of the spinal cord.

commen·sal (L. *cum*, with; *mensa*, a table). An organism living in or on an organism of another species without thereby injuring the host.

commen·salism (L. *cum*, with; *mensa*, a table). An association between two organisms of different species in which one partner is benefited whereas the other is neither injured nor benefited.

com·minuted (L. *comminuere*, to diminish). Broken into more than two pieces.

comminū·tion (L. *comminuere*, to diminish). Process of breaking into pieces.

commissū·ral (L. *commissura*, connection). Pertaining to a commissure. C. fibres: intercerebral fibres connecting corresponding areas of the two cerebral hemispheres.

com·missure (L. *commissura*, connection). A connection between two parts. C., anterior: a fascicle of medullary fibres in the ventral angle of the septum pellucidum. C., hippocampal: a triangular lamina of transverse medullary fibres connecting the two fornices. C., inferior: a strand of fibres in the optic chiasm. See Gudden's commissure. C., optic: callosal fibres passing from the medullary optic lamina to the splenium; perhaps associated with the bilateral cortical representation of the macula. C., posterior: a band of medullary fibres above the dorsal portion of the cephalic orifice of the Sylvian aqueduct. C., superior: a strand of fibres in the optic chiasm. Syn. Meynert's commissure.

com·missurŏ·tomy (L. *commissura*, connection; G. *tome*, cutting). Incision of a fibrous band, especially of cuspa of mitral valve for mitral stenosis.

commō·tio, commotion (L. *commotio*, disturbance). Concussion, *q.v.* C. retinae: see Berlin's disease.

commū·nicable (L. *communicare*). Transmissible.

commū·nicans (L. *communicare*). Communicating; connecting.

commū·nis (L.). Common; relating to more than one.

com·mutator (L. *commutare*, to change). An instrument for interrupting or reversing electric currents.

compatibil·ity (Mediaeval L. *compatibilis*, from L. *cum*, with; *pati*, to suffer). Of two or more drugs, the property of not undergoing an undesired chemical reaction when mixed.

compensā·tion (L. *compensare*, to balance). 1. Counterbalance of a structural or functional defect by hypertrophy or hyperfunction of unimpaired parts of the same organ or another organ. 2. In psychology the counterbalancing of an actual or supposed bodily or psychical defect by exhibiting a more or less highly estimated trait in an especially high degree.

compensā·tory (L. *compensare*, to balance). Effecting a compensation. C. hypertrophy: a hypertrophy counterbalancing a structural or functional defect of an organ. C. pause: a pause immediately succeeding a premature beat of the heart and compensating by its length for the prematurity of the beat.

com·plement (L. *complementum*). A thermolabile substance present in normal blood serum, with lytic properties on cells sensitized by the specific antibody (amboceptor). Syn. alexin. C., deviation of: the phenomenon observed when more antibody (amboceptor) is present in a mixture than can be taken up by the bacteria present in the mixture, that complement becomes bound to the excess antibody but not to the antibody which became attached to the bacterial cells. Syn. Neisser-Wechsberg's phenomenon. C., fixation of: the fixation of a c. by both an antigen and the corresponding specific antibody (amboceptor) whereby the complement becomes unavailable for effecting haemolysis in a second antigen-antibody system consisting of inactivated haemolytic serum and red blood corpuscles. Syn. Bordet-Gengou's phenomenon.

complemen·tal, complemen·tary (L. *complementum*). Supplying a deficiency. C. colours: any two colours of the spectrum which, when combined, produce white, e.g., blue and yellow. C. space: the lowest part of the pleural space which becomes filled out by the lungs on deep inspiration only.

complemen·toid (L. *complementum*, complement; G. *eidos*, form). A complement that has lost the property to cause lysis but still retains that of fixation.

complex (L. *complexus*, from *complecti*, to fold together). 1. Composite; complicated. 2. Any group of emotionally charged ideas which have been banished from consciousness but are active in the unconscious stratum of mental life. C., auricular: the P-wave in an electrocardiogram. C., ventricular: the Q R S T-waves in an electrocardiogram. C., Oedipus: unconscious sexual desire for the parent of the opposite sex.

complexion. The colour of the skin, especially the face.

complexus. A muscle in the back of the neck (see muscles).

complicā·tion. (L. *complicatio*, a multiplication). Condition adding to the severity of an existing disease: either a new manifestation of that disease or the supervention of a new disease.

compō·nent (L. *componere*, to unite). Constituent part or ingredient of a mixture.

compos mentis (L.). Of sound mind.

com·pound (L. *componere*, to unite). 1. To mix. 2. Composed of several parts. C. fracture: see under fracture.

comprehen·sion (L. *comprehendere*, to understand). Capacity to integrate diverse precepts and/or ideas and to understand the relation between them and one's own experience.

compress (L. *compressus*, from *comprimere*, to compress). 1. To force together. 2. (com·press) Folded cloth for local application or pressure.

compres·sion (L. *comprimere*, to compress). 1. Forcing together. 2. The state of being compressed.

compres·sor (L. *comprimere*, to compress). 1. Instrument for compressing a vessel. 2. Applied to muscles with a constricting function.

Concato's disease (Concato, L. M., Italian physician, 1825–82). Tuberculosis affecting successively various serous membranes, usually ending in pulmonary tuberculosis.

con·cave (L. *concavus*). With outline or surface curved like interior of circle.

concă·vity (L. *concavus*). A depression or fossa.

concă·vo-con·cave (L. *concavus*). Concave on both surfaces. Syn. biconcave.

concă·vo-con·vex (L. *concavus*; *convexus*). Having one side concave, the other convex.

concentrā·tion (L. *cum*, with; *centrare*, from G. *kentron*, centre). 1. The proportion between the amount of a dissolved substance and the solvent. 2. The act of increasing the proportionate amount of one or more constituents of a fluid, e.g. by evaporation. 3. The state of fixed attention. C. test: test for examining the renal function of excreting a urine of high specific gravity; in a patient having no manifest or latent oedema urine excreted after 24-hours' dry diet reaches normally a c. corresponding to 1030-1035 specific gravity.

concen·tric (L. *cum*, with; *centrum*, from G. *kentron*, centre). Having a common centre.

concep·tion (L. *concipere*, to conceive). 1. Sexual fecundation. 2. An idea; the formation of an idea.

con·cha (G. *kogkhē*, a shell). 1. The central part of the external ear. 2. The turbinate bone. 3. Applied to parts of shell-like appearance.

conchi·tis (G. *kogkhē*, a shell). Inflammation of the concha.

con·choscope (G. *kogkhē*, a shell; *skopein*, to view). A special instrument for examining the nasal cavity.

con·chotome (G. *kogkhē*, a shell; *tomē*, a cutting). An instrument for removal of part of the inferior turbinate bone of the nose.

conchŏ·tomy (G. *kogkhē*, a shell; *tomē*, a cutting). An operation for removal of turbinate bone.

concoc·tion (L. *concoquere*, to boil together). The boiling of two substances together.

concŏ·mitant (L. *concomitari*, to accompany). Accompanying.

concres·cence (L. *concrescere*, to grow together). 1. Growing together. 2. Union of roots of a tooth, or of adjacent teeth, by cemental proliferation.

concrē·tion (L. *concrescere*, to grow together). 1. A calculus. 2. Abnormal union of adjoining parts of membranes.

concu·bitus (L. *concumbere*, to lie with). Copulation.

concus·sion (L. *concussio*, from *concutere*, to shake). 1. Sudden application of mechanical force to the skull. 2. A state of unconsciousness, or impaired consciousness, however fleeting, suddenly produced by mechanical force applied to the skull, usually followed by amnesia.

concus·sor. An instrument used in applying massage.

condensā·tion (L. *condensare*, to thicken). 1. The passing of a gaseous substance into a liquid, or of a liquid into a solid state. 2. The act of making denser. 3. Fusion of events, pictures or elements of speech. 4. The process by which an idea may appropriate the whole cathexis, *q.v.*, of several other ideas, e.g. in dreams.

conden·ser (L. *condensare*, to thicken). 1. A system of lenses used for concentrating the rays of an illuminating source, e.g. in the microscope. 2. Apparatus for the accumulation of electricity.

condi·ment (L. *condimentum*, spice). A relish.

conditioned reflex (Mediaeval L. *conditionare*, from L. *condicere*, to proclaim). A reflex action artificially produced by association of ideas.

con·dom (L. *condomare*, to check or curb). A rubber sheath for the penis to prevent conception or infection during copulation.

conduc·tance (L. *conducere*, to bring together). 1. Capability to conduct. 2. Art of conducting. 3. The ratio between electric current flowing through a unit conductor and the difference of potentials at its ends; the reciprocal of resistance.

conduc·tion (L. *conducere*, to bring together). 1. The transmission of energy from one particle of matter to the next. 2. The transmission of excitation through living tissue, as through a nerve or specialized heart muscle fibres. **C. current:** movement of electricity in a conductor along the conductor, or in a vacuum, due to differences in potential.

conducti·vity (L. *conducere*, to bring together). Capacity for conduction of some form of energy (electricity, heat, light, sound or nervous impulse).

conduc·tor (L. *conducere*, to bring together). 1. Any agent for transmitting electricity, heat, nervous impulses, etc. 2. An individual transmitting to his offspring a genetical character which is not manifest in himself.

condū·plicate (L. *cum*, with; *duplicare*, to double). Folded lengthwise.

conduplicatio corporis. The folded up position of the foetus in transverse presentation.

Condy's fluid (Condy, H. B., English physician of the nineteenth century). A solution of sodium permanganate: used for purposes of disinfection.

con·dylar(G.*kondulos*, a knuckle). Relating to a condyle.

con·dylarthrō·sis (G. *kondulos*, a knuckle; *arthron*, joint). A joint consisting of a condyle and an elliptoid cavity.

con·dyle (G. *kondulos*, knuckle). A rounded articular eminence.

condylec·tomy (G. *kondulos*, knuckle; *ektomē*, excision). Excision of a condyle.

con·dyloid (G. *kondulos*, knuckle; *eidos*, form). Resembling or pertaining to a condyle.

condylō·ma (G. *kondulos*, knuckle). A papule or papilloma about the anus or the external genitalia. **C. acuminatum:** pointed papilloma at the external genital organs. **C. latum:** flat, broad, moist papule at the anus in secondary syphilis.

condylŏ·tomy (G. *kondulos*, knuckle; *tomē*, section). Division of a condyle; extra-articular osteotomy.

con·dylus (L.). Condyle.

cone (G. *kōnos*). 1. A pointed structure with a circular base. **Retinal c.:** one of the two elements of the bacillary or rod-and-cone layer of the retina, which constitute the specific receptors for vision, having less cytoplasm and a less deeply staining nucleus than a rod, not possessing visual purple and transverse striation; there are about 7,000,000 cones in the human retina. 2. The mechanical element of the tooth-crown. See also conus.

confabulā·tion (L. *cum*, with; *fabula*, talk). The ready narration of fictitious occurrences which the patient believes that he has experienced, and which are not hallucinations but are produced to fill gaps of defective memory, especially in respect of the immediate past; one of the main signs of Korsakow's syndrome, *q.v.*

confec·tion (L. *cum*, with; *facere*, to make). In pharmacy, a sweet excipient used with a prescribed medicinal substance.

confine·ment (L. *cum*, with; *finis*, border). The period of parturition.

confirm·atory (L. *confirmare*, to establish). Confirming.

conflict (L. *conflictio*, collision). Opposition between contradictory desires which may produce emotional tension leading to repression of one or other of the ideas.

con·fluens sin·uum (L. *confluere*, to flow together; *sinus*, a hollow). The place where the cranial sinuses unite; the torcular Herophili.

con·fluent (L. *confluere*, to flow together). Coalescing; running together, as of pustules in smallpox.

confu·sion (L. *confundere*, to mix). Disturbance of consciousness, characterized by impaired capacity to think clearly and with customary rapidity and to perceive, respond to and remember current stimuli, and by some degree of disorientation.

congelā·tion (L. *congelatio*, a freezing). 1. Freezing. 2. Frostbite.

congen·ital (L. *congenitus*, born with). Actually or potentially present at birth.

congĕ·sted (L. *congerere*, to collect). Hyperaemic; in a state of congestion.

congĕ·stion (L. *congerere*, to collect). Hyperaemia of an organ or part, as of the lungs or the liver.

conglobā·tion (L. *conglobare*, to make into a ball). Forming a rounded mass.

conglŏ·merate (L. *conglomerare*, to heap together). 1. Massed together, as of glands. 2. A mass of units without order.

conglū·tinated (L. *conglutinare*, to cement). Cemented; agglutinated.

conglutinā·tion (L. *conglutinare*, to cement). Adhering together; agglutination, *q.v.*

Congo red. An azo dye used as indicator, for detecting amyloidosis (by failure of normal urinary excretion of the dye owing to storage in amyloid-containing organs) and for detecting free mineral acids in the presence of organic acids, e.g. free hydrochloric acid in gastric juice. C. r. paper: filter paper stained with c. r., used especially for examining gastric juice for the presence of free acid, by which it is turned blue.

CO(NH₂)₂. Urea.

coni vasculosi. Small tubules which form the globus major of the epididymis.

cŏ·nic, cŏ·nical (G. *kōnos*, cone). Cone-shaped.

conĭ·diophore (G. *konia*, dust; *pherein*, to bear). The short stalk in hyphal fungi bearing the conidium.

coni·dium (G. *konia*, dust). The non-sexual spore in certain hyphal fungi.

Conium. Hemlock.

con·jugal (L. *conjugalis*, from *conjux*, spouse from *conjungere*, to join). Relating to marriage; affecting both husband and wife.

conjugata spuria (L. *conjugare*, to unite; *spurius*, illegitimate or wrong). Conjugate, external, *q.v.* conjugata vera: conjugate, true, *q.v.*

con·jugate (L. *conjugare*, to unite). Coupled. C. deviation: deviation of both eyes to the same direction and to the same extent, as in certain unilateral lesions of the cerebrum (towards the side of the lesion) or the pons (towards the contralateral side). C. diameter: the antero-posterior diameter of the brim of the pelvis. C., external: distance between the middle upper border of the symphysis pubis and the depression between the 5th lumbar vertebra and the sacral spine. C. proteins: proteins containing a prosthetic group. C., true: distance between upper posterior border of the symphysis pubis and promontorium.

conjugā·tion (L. *conjugare*, to unite). 1. Union of two unicellular organisms with exchange of nuclear material, in micro-organisms the common form of sexual reproduction. 2. Union of two sexual cells with nuclear division and union of chromosomes. 3. Combining of large molecules.

conjuncti·va (L. *conjunctivus*, from *conjungere*, to join). The mucous membrane covering the anterior portion of the globe of the eye, except the cornea.

conjunctī·val (L. *conjunctivus*, connective). C. folliculosis: a condition affecting children, characterized by the formation of discrete lymph follicles, mainly in the lower fornix, unaccompanied by c. inflammation. C. reflex: closing of eyelids on touching the conjunctiva.

conjunctivi·tis (L. *conjunctivus*, connective). Inflammation of the conjunctiva. C., follicular: any form of c. which is accompanied by the development of lymph follicles in the conjunctiva. C. phlyctenular: conjunctivitis with vesicles or ulcers surrounded by an inflamed area; arising during the course of a systemic tuberculous infection.

connate (L. *cum*, with; *natus*, birth). 1. Congenital. 2. United.

connec·tive (L. *connectere*, to fasten). Binding; connecting. C. tissue: a tissue of mesodermal origin, present in every organ, binding together and supporting the other elements of an organ; composed mainly of intercellular substance with collaginous or white, elastic or yellow fibres, or with reticular fibres, arranged in bundles or lattice-like patterns, respectively, any of which may predominate in a given area so as to determine the particular type of the tissue; its cellular elements include fibroblasts, undifferentiated cells, histiocytes, macrophages, fat cells, etc.

co·noid, conoid·al (G. *kōnos*, cone; *eidos*, shape). Conical.

Conolly's system (Conolly, J., English psychiatrist, 1795–1866). Means of treating the insane without the use of harsh restraints.

Conradi's line (Conradi, A. C., Norwegian physician, 1809–1869). A line drawn from the base of the xiphoid process to the point of the apex beat, indicating, under normal conditions, the upper limit of percussion-dullness of the left lobe of the liver.

consanguin·eous (L. *consanguineus*, from *cum*, with *sanguis*, blood). Of the same blood; descended from the same ancestor.

consangui·nity. Blood relationship; state of being descended from the same ancestor.

con·sciousness (L. *cum*, with; *scire*, to know). 1. State of being aware of personal existence and sensory impressions. 2. The 'upper stratum' of mental life of which the individual is aware at any given time.

consen·sual (L. *consensus*, from *cum*, with; *sentire*, to feel). Applied to a reflex induced in one organ by stimulation of another organ, e.g. the reflex narrowing of a pupil on illumination of the other eye.

conservā·tion (L. *conservare*, to preserve). Preservation without loss. C. of Energy, Law of: the principle that conversion of one form of energy into another proceeds without loss or gain of energy.

conser·vative (L. *conservare*, to preserve). Aiming at the preservation of bodily integrity.

consis·tence, consis·tency (L. *consistere*, to become hard). Degree of density or hardness.

consŏ·lidating (L. *consolidare*, to make firm). The healing of fractures or wounds.

consolidā·tion (L. *consolidare*, to make firm). State of becoming solid, as of a lung in pneumonia. See also hepatization.

con·stant (L. *constare*, to abide). Fixed; not changing; e.g. constant current.

constipā·tion (L. *constipare*, to crowd). Sluggishness or inaction of the bowels.

constitū·tion (L. *constituere*, to arrange). 1. The total of inherited (and, according to some authors, acquired) properties of characters and diatheses. 2. In chemistry, the arrangement of atoms in a molecule. Syn. structure. 3. Composition.

constrict (L. *constringere*, to bind). To draw together in one part; to compress or to contract.

constric·tor (L. *constringere*, to bind). A contracting or compressing muscle.

consul·tant (L. *consultare*, to take counsel). A specialist called in by the physician attending the patient to give advice.

consultā·tion (L. *consultatio*, from *consultare*, to take counsel). 1. The giving of medical advice. 2. Deliberation between two or more doctors with regard to a patient.

consump·tion (L. *consumptio*, from *consumere*, to waste). A progressive wasting away, used as a synonym for progressive tuberculosis.

consump·tive. 1. Pertaining to consumption. 2. A person suffering from tuberculosis of the lungs.

con·tact (L. *contactus*, from *contingere*, to touch). 1. A touching. 2. One who has been exposed to a contagious or infectious disease. C. lens: a glass lens worn directly upon the cornea.

contā·gion (L. *contagio*, from *cum*, with; *tangere*, to touch). 1. Transmission of a disease, either by direct contact or by an intermediate agent. 2. Transmission of a disease by direct transference from one host to another. 3. Contagium, *q.v.*

contā·gious (L. *contagio*, contact). Transmissible by contact, as of a communicable disease.

contā·gium (L.). Any micro-organism, virus or infectious matter producing or transmitting a disease.

contigū·ity (L. *contiguus*, from *contingere*, to touch). State of being contiguous.

conti·guous (L. *contiguus*, from *contingere*, to touch). In actual contact; neighbouring.

con·tinence (L. *continēre*, to hold). 1. Self-restraint. 2. Ability of a hollow organ to hold its contents.

conti·nued (L. *continuare*, to make or be continuous). Persisting, uninterrupted.

continū·ity (L. *continuitas*, from *continere*, to hold together). Uninterrupted connection.

contor·tion (L. *contortio*). A twisting.

con·tour (Fr. *contourner*). A boundary or outline.

contra-aperture (L. *contra*, against; *apertura*, opening). Counter-opening.

contracep·tion (L. *contra*, against; *concipere*, to conceive). The prevention of conception.

contracep·tive (L. *contra*, against; *concipere*, to conceive). An agent which prevents conception.

contract (L. *contrahere*, to draw together). 1. To draw together; to shrink. 2. To acquire by contagion.

contracted pelvis. A pelvis abnormally short in one or more diameters.

contrac·tile (L. *contrahere*, to draw together). Possessing the property of contracting.

contracti·lity (L. *contrahere*, to draw together). The property of contracting or shortening.

contractio praevia (L.). A narrowing of the lower uterine segment.

contrac·tion (L. *contractio*, from *contrahere*, to draw together). Decrease of volume; approximation of the walls of an organ. **C., anodal closing; C., anodal opening:** muscular c. occurring on closure or opening, respectively, of an electric circuit when the anode is placed on the muscle. **C., cathodal closing; C., cathodal opening:** muscular c. occurring on closure or opening, respectively, when the cathode is placed on the muscle. **C., Dupuytren's:** see under Dupuytren. **C., hourglass:** c. of the middle part of the stomach.

contrac·ture (L. *contrahere*, to draw together). 1. Involuntary permanent contraction of a muscle. 2. Permanent shortening of any of the other soft parts of the body (tendon, skin, etc). 3. Deformity of a joint due to 1 or 2.

contra-indicā·tion (L. *contra*, against; *indicare*, to show). Anything forbidding a particular method of treatment.

con·trală·teral (L. *contra*, against; *latus*, side). Opposite; especially opposite to the site of a lesion.

con·trast (L. *contra*, against; *stare*, to stand). **C. staining:** staining by means of two dyes which are differently taken up by the various tissue or cell elements.

con·travoli·tional (L. *contra*, against; *volo*, I am willing). Involuntary.

contre-coup (Fr.). Injury by transmitted force opposite to or remote from the point of contact.

control (Fr. *contrôler*, from Old Fr. *contreroller*, to check). Anything used as a standard for checking observations. **C. analysis:** the checking of psycho-analytic treatment by a more experienced analyst. **C. animal:** an animal used in a c. experiment. **C. experiment:** an experiment varying in a single factor from another experiment which it is meant to check.

contuse (L. *contundere*, to bruise). To bruise.

contū·sion (L. *contusio*, from *contundere*, bruise). A bruise from a blow by a blunt object, inflicted without breaking the integument.

cō·nus (G. *kōnos*, cone). 1. A cone. 2. A crescent of atrophic choroid tissue, usually at the temporal side of the optic papilla in myopia. 3. The conus medullaris, the cone-like termination of the enlargement of the lumbar spinal cord.

convalĕ·scence (L. *convalescere*, to recover). Period of recovery after an illness or lesion.

convalĕ·scent (L. *convalescere*, to recover). 1. One recovering from illness. 2. Recovering from illness.

convec·tion (L. *convehere*, to bring together). 1. Process of conveying. 2. Transmission of energy by the movement of energy-absorbing particles of the surrounding liquid or gaseous medium. **C. current:** the motion of electrically charged particles.

conver·gence (L. *convergere*, to incline together). Meeting, or tending to meet, at a point, as the co-ordinated movement of the two eyes on fixation upon a near object. **C.-reaction:** narrowing of the pupils on c. of the eyes. **C., relative:** that amount of c. which can be exerted or relaxed if accommodation is kept constant.

conver·gent (L. *convergere*, to incline together). Pertaining to convergence.

conver·sion (L. *convertere*, to change). The symbolic expression by means of physical manifestations of both repressed wishes and the defence set up against them, e.g. in a hysterical paresis. See also, neurosis, conversion.

con·vex (L. *convexus*). Curved outward on the exterior surface.

convexo-convex (L. *convexus*). Convex on both surfaces. Syn. biconvex.

con·voluted (L. *convolvere*, to roll together). Coiled; folded upon itself.

convolū·tion (L. *convolvere*, to roll together). A folding of any organ upon itself; especially any one of the rounded folds of the cortical surfaces of the brain. (Syn. gyrus.)

Convolvulus (L.). A genus of twining plants; the bindweed. Some species produce a laxative substance.

convul·sant (L. *convellere*, to wrench). A drug causing spasms.

convul·sion (L. *convulsio*, from *convellere*, to wrench). A violent involuntary contraction of an extensive group of muscles due to disturbance of cerebral function; a fit.

convul·sive (L. *convulsio*, from *convellere*, to wrench). Of the nature of a convulsion.

Cooper's fascia (Cooper, Sir A. P., English surgeon, 1768–1841). The fascia transversalis. **C.'s hernia:** encysted hernia of the tunica vaginalis. **C.'s irritable breast:** neuralgia of the mammary gland. **C.'s irritable testicle:** neuralgia of the testicle. **C.'s ligament:** the pectineal ligament. **C.'s suspensory ligaments:** fibrous bands which pass from the breast to the skin.

co-ordination (L. *cum*, with; *ordinare*, to dispose). Harmonious action, as of muscles.

copper (L. *cuprum*, from *aes cyprium*, copper). A metallic element. Symbol Cu. **C. wire arteries:** retinal arteries showing as early signs of sclerosis, increase in brightness of reflex assuming a burnished metallic appearance with a broader and softer reflex, resembling copper wire.

coprolā·lia (L. *kopros*, dung; *lalia*, chatter). An obsession for the utterance of obscene words.

cop·rolith (G. *kopros*, dung; *lithos*, stone). A mass of hardened faeces in the bowel.

coprŏ·phagy (G. *kopros*, dung; *phagein*, to eat). The eating of faeces.

coprophi·lia (G. *kopros*, dung; *philein*, to love). 1. The tendency to be attracted to faeces. 2. The property of growing on faecal matter.

coprophŏ·bia (G. *kopros*, dung; *phŏbos*, fear). Obsessional repugnance to faeces.

co propor·phyrin (G. *kopros*, dung; *porphureos*, purple). Four isomeric compounds derived from protoporphyrin 9 by substitution of the two vinyl groups by two propionyl groups. Two types are known, 1 and III, the former being usually present in small amounts in urine and faeces.

cop·roporphyrinū·ria (G. *kopros*, dung; *porphureos*, purple; *ouron*, urine). Urinary excretion of coproporphyrin.

coprostā·sis (G. *kopros*, dung; *stasis*, a standing). Accumulation of faeces in the bowel.

coprostĕ·rol (G. *kopros*, dung; *stear*, tallow). A sterol present in faeces.

cŏ·pula (L.). 1. A connecting structure. 2. Amboceptor, *q.v.* 3. Sexual intercourse.

copulā·tion (L. *copulare*, to unite). 1. The sexual union of the male and female. 2. In infusoria, conjugation between two cells which do not fuse after fertilization.

Coq. Abbreviation for the L. *coquere*, to boil.

cor (L.). The heart.

cor·aco-acrō·mial (G. *korax*, a hook (lit. crow's beak); *akron*, highest point; *ōmos*, shoulder). Relating to both coracoid process and acromion.

cor·acobrachiā·lis (G. *korax*, hook; *brakhiŏn*, arm). A muscle of the upper arm. (See muscles.)

cor·acoid (G. *korax*, a crow; *eidos*, form). Shaped like a crow's beak. 2. The c. process of the scapula.

Coramine. A proprietary preparation of pyridine β-carboxylic acid diethylamide, injected as a stimulant. Syn. nikethamide.

cord (G. *khordē*, a string). 1. A tendon; any string-like body. 2. Spinal c., *q.v.* 3. Umbilical c., *q.v.* 4. Vocal c., *q.v.* **Presentation of the c.:** in parturition, the descent of the umbilical c. between the presenting part and the membranes. **Prolapse of the c.:** in parturition, the descent of the umbilical c. after rupture of the amnion into or beyond the vagina. **C., subacute combined degeneration of the:** degenerative changes of both lateral and posterior columns of the spinal c., leading to objective and subjective disturbance of sensibility and proprioceptive reflexes, usually associated with, but sometimes preceding, pernicious anaemia.

cor·date (L. *cor*, heart). Heart-shaped.

cordec·tomy (G. *khordē*, a string; *ektomē*, excision). The surgical removal of a cord.

cor·dial (L. *cor*, heart). A heart stimulant.

core (L. *cor*, heart). 1. Any central part; a kernel. 2. The central slough of a boil. 3. A bare iron or a bundle of soft iron used as a magnet in a transformer or induction coil.

co·rē (G. *korē*). The pupil of the eye.

corectō·pia (G. *korē*, pupil of eye; *ektopos*, out of place). Displacement of the pupil, usually associated with ectopy of the lens. Syn. ectopia pupillae.

corĕ·mium (G. *korēma*, sweepings). A form of mycelium characterized by bundles of parallel hyphae.

corĕŏ·meter (G. *korē*, pupil of eye; *metron*, measure). Instrument for measuring the width of the pupil.

cor·eplasty (G. *korē*, pupil of eye; *plassein*, to form). Any operation for forming an artificial pupil.

corĕ·tomy (G. *korē*, pupil of eye; *tome*, section). Any cutting operation performed on the iris, see iridectomy; iridotomy.

coriăn·der. An aromatic and carminative principle from the dried fruits of *Coriandrum sativum*.

cor·ium (L.). The true skin; the layer of the skin between the epidermis and the subcutaneous tissue.

corn (L. *cornu*, horn). A local thickening and induration of the skin, as on the feet and toes, with a central horny peg projecting upon the papillary layer of the corium.

cor·nea (L. *corneus*, from *cornu*, horn). The transparent anterior portion of the eyeball. **C. guttata:** endothelial dystrophy of the c., usually affecting both eyes; starting as endothelial degeneration whereby the intra-ocular fluid gains access into the c., followed by dystrophic changes in the corneal epithelium and finally in the substantia propria.

cor·neal (L. *corneus*, from *cornu*, horn). Relating to the cornea. **C. dystrophy, familial:** congenital-developmental anomaly of the cornea, becoming manifest about the time of puberty, affecting both eyes and progressing slowly; characterized by the development of deposits of hyaline-like material in the superficial layers of the substantia propria in the axial region of the cornea; classified as nodular, reticular or lattice-like and ring-shaped types. **C. reflex:** reflex closing of the eyelids on touching the cornea.

corneo-irī·tis (L. *corneus*, horny; G. *iris*, rainbow). Inflammation of the cornea and the iris.

cor·neous (G. *corneus*, from *cornu*, horn). Horny, or horn-like.

cor·neum (L. *corneus*, from *cornu*, horn). The stratum corneum or horny layer of the skin.

cornflour. Flour derived from maize.

cornificā·tion (L. *cornu*, horn; *facere*, to make). The process of becoming horny; keratinization.

cor·nu (L. *cornu*, horn). A horn-shaped structure. **C. ammonis:** the hippocampus major. **C. cutaneum:** a horny excrescence resembling the horns of animals.

cor·nual. Relating to a cornu.

cornuco·pia (L. *cornu copiae*, horn of plenty). Part of the choroid plexus in the 4th ventricle of the brain.

corō·na (L. *corona*, crown). Any structure resembling a crown. **C. dentis:** the crown of a tooth. **C. mortis:** arterial circle which in case of an abnormal course of the obturator artery at the neck of a femoral hernia may easily be severed during herniotomy. **C. radiata:** a series of radiating fibres connecting cortical areas with the internal capsule. **C. veneris:** papular or pustular eruption on the upper part of the forehead in the secondary stage of syphilis.

corō·nal (L. *corona*, crown). Relating to a crown or to the top of the head. **C. suture:** the transverse suture between the frontal and parietal bones.

coronaria ventriculi (L.). The coronary or left gastric artery.

cŏ·ronary (L. *corona*, crown). Encircling; said of a vessel or nerve (e.g., c. artery) that encircles an organ. **C. occlusion:** partial or complete occlusion of a c. artery of the heart causing ischaemia of the related cardiac area and characterized by sudden onset of severe pain behind the sternum or referred to shoulder, arm or abdomen, by severe dyspnoea and fall in blood-pressure and followed usually within 36 hours by moderate fever and leucocytosis. **C. sclerosis:** 1. Arteriosclerosis of the coronary arteries. 2. The clinical syndrome due to (1). See also angina pectoris, c. occlusion. **C. thrombosis:** thrombosis of a coronary artery of the heart.

cŏ·roner (L. *corona*, crown). An officer who holds inquests on persons supposed to have died from an unnatural cause (such as violence or accident).

cŏ·ronoid (G. *korōnē*, crow; *eidos*, form). Curved like a crow's beak; applied to processes of bones thus curved.

cor·pora (Pl. of L. *corpus*, body). Bodies; especially applied to spherical or ovoid bodies. **C. amylacea:** small spheroid hyaline bodies, probably representing degenerated microglial or oligodendroglial cells, found in large numbers in the nervous system in old age. **C. arantii:** small tubercles found in the semilunar valves of the aorta and pulmonary arteries. **C. arenacea:** laminated structures found in the dura, in meningeal tumours and in degenerated nervous tissue. **C. bigemina:** the foetal c. quadrigemina. **C. geniculate:** (lateral and medial), cerebral structures beneath the pulvinar at the dorsal end of the thalamus, present in higher animals from amphibia onwards; relay stations for visual and auditory pathways, respectively. **C. libera:** free bodies within a cavity, especially that of a joint, e.g. pieces of normal or diseased articular tissue which have become severed from their place of attachment. **C. mamillaria:** the most caudal part of the interbrain in both hemispheres. **C. quadrigemina:** the four rounded structures above the Sylvian aqueduct and behind the third ventricle. See also corpus.

corpse (L. *corpus*, body). A cadaver; a dead body.

cor·pulence, cor·pulency (L. *corpulentus*, from *corpus*, body). Obesity.

cor·pulent (L. *corpulentus*). Obese.

cor·pus (L. *corpus*, body; pl. *corpora*). 1. A body; the human body. 2. The main shaft of a bone or other structure. **C. albicans:** the fibrous scar following final degeneration of a c. luteum. Syn. c. candicans. **C. callosum:** a band of fibres beneath the superior longitudinal fissure, connecting the two hemispheres. **C. candicans:** c. albicans, *q.v.* **C. haemorrhagicum:** the forming c. luteum of menstruation. **C. highmorianum:** the mediastinum testis, the connective tissue corresponding to a testicular hilus. **C. luteum:** the structure formed after rupture of a Graafian follicle, characterized by large ovoid or polyhedral cells having a clear, finely granulated cytoplasm and a yellow colour due to the pigment lutein or progesterone, *q.v.* **C. luysii:** a part of the nucleus ruber. **C. restiforme:** a bundle of nerve fibres on either side of the medulla oblongata passing to the cerebellum. **C. striatum:** basal ganglion in the mid-brain lateral to the optic thalamus, consisting of lenticular and caudate nuclei. See also corpora.

cor·puscle (L. *corpusculum*, dim. of *corpus*, body). 1. A minute body or particle. 2. A blood cell. **C., lamellar:** Vater corpuscle. **C., renal:** the Malpighian body. **C., thymic:** Hassall's corpuscles.

corpus·cular (L. *corpusculum*, dim. of *corpus*, body). Relating to or of the nature of a corpuscle.

correc·tant, correc·tive (L. *corrigere*, to set right). 1. Modifying favourably. 2. A substance improving taste, smell or colour of a drug.

correlā·tion (L. *cum*, with; *relatum*, pp. of *referre*, to restore). A reciprocal relation; a relation between two objects or attributes of such a character that the value assumed by the one determines the value of the other. **C. coefficient:** see coefficient of correlation.

Corrigan's cautery (Corrigan, Sir D. J., Irish physician, 1802–80). A primitive actual cautery with a wooden handle and a button-shaped iron end. **C.'s line:** purple line seen on the gum margins in copper-poisoning. **C.'s pulse:** the 'water-hammer pulse' of aortic insufficiency. **C.'s respiration:** slow respiration of the cerebral type. **C.'s sign:** abdominal pulsation felt in cases of aneurysm of the abdominal aorta.

corrode (L. *corrodere*, to gnaw). To wear gradually away, especially by a chemical process.

corrō·sion (L. *corrodere*, to gnaw). 1. The process of corroding. 2. The condition of being corroded.

corrō·sive (L. *corrodere*, to gnaw). Eating away or corroding.

cor·rugator (L. *corrugare*, to wrinkle). A muscle that contracts the skin into wrinkles.

cor·set (Fr. *corset*, ult. from L. *corpus*, body). A close-fitting support for the abdomen or chest, or both.

cor·tex (L., rind). 1. The bark of a tree or plant. 2. The outer layer of an organ beneath its capsule or membrane, such as the cerebral c., or the renal c.

Corti's arch (Corti, A., Italian anatomist, 1822–76). The arch formed in the organ of C. by the two files of rods, C.'s rods or fibres. **C.'s canal:** the canal formed by the basilar membrane and the arch of C. **C.'s cells:** the hair cells of C.'s organ. **C.'s fibres:** see C.'s rods. **C.'s ganglion:** the ganglion spirale, an aggregation of ganglion cells in the spiral canals of the cochlea. **C.'s membrane:** the membrane tectoria. **Organ of C.:** the spiral organ in which the branches of the cochlear part of the auditory nerve end. **C.'s rods:** the pillars of the arch of the organ of C. **C.'s teeth:** the auditory teeth; the tooth-like projections at the edge of the limbus laminae spiralis of the ear. **C.'s tunnel:** the same as C.'s canal, *q.v.*, above.

cor·tical (L. *cortex*, rind). Relating to the cortex. **C., cataract:** see under cataract c. **C. epilepsy:** epilepsy due to physical or chemical irritation of a c. motor focus, characterized by convulsions beginning in a certain small group of muscles on the side opposite to the c. lesion and spreading successively up or down from the originally affected part to further parts of the same side, or in severe seizures also finally to the other side. Syn. Jacksonian epilepsy. **C. necrosis of the kidney:** a condition characterized by bilateral necrosis of the renal cortex leading to uraemia; occurring as sequel to eclampsia or the most severe types of accidental haemorrhage (*q.v.*) or rarely to scarlet fever, diphtheria or acute pulmonary tuberculosis.

cortici·fugal (L. *cortex*, rind; *fugere*, to flee). Cortico-efferent, or departing from the cortex.

cortici·petal (L. *cortex*, rind; *petere*, to seek). Cortico-afferent, or approaching the cortex.

cortico-afferent (L. *cortex*, rind; *afferre*, to bring to). Conducting impulses from the periphery or from the lower centres to the cortex cerebri.

cortico-efferent (L. *cortex*, rind; *efferre*, to bring out). Conducting impulses from the cortex cerebri to the periphery or the lower centres.

cor·ticospi·nal (L. *cortex*, rind; *spina*, spine). Relating to the cortex cerebri and to the spinal cord.

corticostĕ·rone (L. *cortex*, cortex; Gr. *stereos*, solid). The hormone, or one of the hormones, of the adrenal cortex.

cor·tisone. One of the hormones of the adrenal cortex used in the treatment of rheumatoid arthritis.

Corvisart's disease (Corvisart des Marest, J. N., French physician, 1755–1821). Idiopathic cardiac hypertrophy. **C.'s facies:** the facies of cardiac insufficiency.

Corȳ·nebacte·ria (G. *korunē*, club; *baktērion*, dim. of *baktron*, stick). A genus of club-shaped and gram-positive bacilli, comprising the diphtheria and the diphtheroid bacilli.

corȳ·za (G. *koruza*, a running at the nose). Catarrhal inflammation of the nasal passages. Syn. rhinitis; 'Cold in the head'.

cosmet·ic (G. *kosmein*, from *kosmos*, order). 1. Beautifying. 2. A remedy for beautifying the skin, etc. **C. operation:** an operation for improving the appearance of a mutilated or unsightly part.

cos·ta (L.). A rib. **C. decima fluctuans:** floating 10th rib; defect in formation of costal cartilage normally joining the 10th rib to the costal arch, usually found in asthenic subjects. **C. spuria:** false rib; a rib of which the cartilage is either not directly or not at all connected with the sternum. **C. vera:** true rib; a rib directly connected with the sternum.

cos·tal (L. *costa*, rib). Relating to the ribs. **C. breathing or respiration:** respiration chiefly carried on by the chest muscles.

cos·tive (L. *constipare*, to crowd). Constipated.

cos·tiveness (L. *constipare*, to crowd). Constipation.

costochon·dral (L. *costa*, rib; G. *khondros*, cartilage). Relating to the ribs and their cartilages.

cos·toclavi·cular (L. *costa*, rib; *clavicula*, dim. of *clavis*, key). Relating to the ribs and the clavicle.

cos·tocŏ·racoid (L. *costa*, rib; G. *korax*, crow; *eidos*, form). Relating to the ribs and coracoid process.

cos·totome (L. *costa*, rib; G. *tomē*, section). A surgeon's knife used in performing costotomy.

costŏ·tomy (L. *costa*, rib; G. *tomē*, section). Resection of a portion of a rib.

cos·totrans·verse (L. *costa*, rib; *transvertere*, to turn across). Relating to the ribs and transverse vertebral processes.

cos·totransvertec·tomy (L. *costa*, rib; *transvertere*, to turn across; G. *ektomē*, excision). An operation for excision of the transverse process in the thoracic vertebra; and the adjoining part of the rib.

costover·tebral (L. *costa*, rib; *vertebra*, a spinal joint, from *vertere*, to turn). Relating to the ribs and vertebrae.

Cotard's syndrome (Cotard, J., French neurologist, 1840–87). A form of paranoia characterized by delusions of negation, with sensory disturbances and a suicidal impulse.

cotton. A textile obtained from the seeds of various varieties of the *Gossypium herbaceum.*

Cotunnius's canal (Cotugno, D., Italian anatomist, 1736–1822). The aquaeductus vestibuli. **C.'s disease:** sciatica. **C.'s liquor:** the perilymph of the osseous labyrinth of the ear. **C.'s nerve:** the nasopalatine nerve. **C.'s space:** the saccus endolymphaticus of the internal ear.

cotylē·don (G. *kotulēdōn*, from *kotulē*, anything hollow). 1. Any one of the enlarged vascular villi of the chorion, projecting into depressions of the decidua vera. 2. Any one of the lobular portions of the uterine surface of the placenta. 3. The seed-leaf in higher plants.

cŏ·tyloid (G. *kotulē*, cup; *eidos*, form). Cup-shaped; e.g., c. cavity, the acetabulum.

cough. 1. To expel suddenly air from the lungs accompanied by an explosive noise due to opening of the glottis. 2. The act of coughing.

coulomb (Coulomb, C. A. de, French physicist, 1736–1806). Unit of electric charge; the quantity of electricity transferred by a current of one ampere flowing against one ohm of resistance with a force of one volt.

counter-extension (L. *contra*, against; *extendere*, to stretch out). Traction upon the proximal extremity of a fractured limb opposing traction in the opposite direction, made to hold or bring the ends into their proper place.

counter-irritant (L. *contra*, against; *irritare*, to irritate). An agent producing counter-irritation.

counter-irritā·tion (L. *contra*, against; *irritare*, to irritate). The irritation of a superficial part of the body effected to relieve existing irritation in a deep-seated part.

counter-opening. An incision of an abscess opposite another opening to effect drainage.

counter-poison (L. *contra*, against; *potio*, a drink). A poison contracting another.

counter-puncture (L. *contra*, against; *punctura*, a pricking). A puncture made opposite to another puncture.

counter-stain. Contrast-staining, *q.v.*

counter-transference (L. *contra*, against; *transferre*, to carry across). In psycho-analytic treatment, phenomenon in which the analyst unconsciously tranfers his suppressed desires to the patient.

courses (L. *cursus*, from *currere*, to run). Menses, *q.v.*

couveuse (Fr. *couver*, from L. *cubare*, to recline). An incubator for new-born, especially prematurely born, infants.

cover-glass. A thin glass plate fixed over the object on a microscopic slide.

Cowper's glands (Cowper, W., English surgeon, 1666–1709). The bulbo-urethral, two compound tubular glands situated between the two layers of the triangular ligament, anteriorly to the prostate gland and corresponding to Bartholin's glands in the female. **C.'s ligament:** that portion of the fascia lata which is attached to the pubic crest.

Cowperian cyst (Cowper, W., English surgeon, 1666–1709). A retention cyst formed in one of C.'s glands.

Cowperitis. Inflammation of C.'s glands, usually gonorrhoeal in origin.

cowpox. Vaccinia, *q.v.*

cox·a (L.) The hip-joint. **C. plana:** see Perthes's disease. **C. valga:** a condition characterized by an increase of the angle between the neck and shaft of the femur. **C. vara:** the congenital or acquired condition where the angle between neck and shaft of the femur is smaller than normal, the neck being bent downwards, and sometimes also towards the posterior side. The position of the trochanter is higher than normal, the leg therefore shorter, usually rotated externally and impaired in abduction movements.

coxal·gia (L. *coxa*, the hip; G. *algos*, pain). Pain in the hip; disease of the hip-joint.

coxi·tis (L. *coxa*, the hip). Inflammation of the hip-joint.

coxofē·moral (L. *coxa*, the hip; *femur*, thigh). Relating to both hip and femur.

Cr. Symbol for chromium.

crab louse. The *Phthirus pubis.*

cracked pot sound. A peculiar sound elicited on percussion by which air is expelled from a cavity into a small bronchus. Syn. *bruit de pot felé.*

cradle. A frame for keeping the weight of bed-clothing from an injured part of the body.

cramp. Painful contraction of a group of muscles.

Crampton's muscle (Crampton, Sir P., Irish surgeon, 1777–1858). A bundle of striated muscle fibres extending from the annular ligament to the sclera.

crā·nial (G. *kranion*, skull). 1. Relating to the cranium. 2. Denoting a position relatively near the cranium. **C. nerve:** any of the nerves (in mammals, birds and reptiles, 12) originating within the cranium or from the medulla oblongata and passing to the peripheral parts through a foramen of the skull.

craniĕc·tomy (G. *kranion*, skull; *ektomē*, excision). Excision of a cranial bone.

crā·niocele (G. *kranion*, skull; *kēlē*, tumour). Encephalocele, *q.v.*

cranio-cĕ·rebral (G. *kranion*, skull; L. *cerebrum*, brain). Relating to both cranium and cerebrum.

crā·nioclast (G. *kranion*, skull; *klaein*, to break). Instrument for performing cranioclasty.

crā·nioclasty (G. *kranion*, skull; *klaein*, to break). Crushing of the foetal skull in labour with the cranioclast.

cranioclei·dal (G. *kranion*, skull; *kleis*, clavicle). Relating to both cranium and clavicle. **C. dysostosis:** see under dysostosis.

craniofā·cial (G. *kranion*, skull; L. *facies*, face). Relating to both cranium and face. **C. dysostosis:** see under dysostosis.

craniŏ·logy (G. *kranion*, skull; *logos*, treatise). The study of skulls.

craniŏ·meter (G. *kranion*, skull; *metron*, measure). Instrument for the measurement of skulls. Also called cephalometer.

craniomet·ric, craniomet·rical (Gr. *kranion*, skull; *metron*, measure). Relating to craniometry.

craniŏ·metry (G. *kranion*, skull; *metron*, measure). Measurement of skulls.

craniŏ·pagus (G. *kranion*, skull; *pēgnunai*, to fix). Double monster with fusion of the heads.

craniŏ·pathy (G. *kranion*, skull; *pathos*, disease). Any disease affecting the skull.

crā·niopharyngiŏ·ma (G. *kranion*, skull; *pharugx*, throat). A tumour arising from remnants of the embryonic craniopharyngeal duct, from which the

H

anterior pituitary lobe is derived, situated usually above the sella, developing in early life and frequently producing Fröhlich's syndrome by compression of the pituitary body.

crã·nioplasty (G. *kranion*, skull; *plassein*, to form). Plastic operations on the skull.

crã·niorrhachi·schisis (G. *kranion*, skull; *rhakhis*, spine; *skhisis*, cleavage). Congenital fissure of the skull and the spine.

craniŏ·schisis (G. *kranion*, skull; *skhisis*, cleavage). Congenital fissure of the cranium due to failure of closure of the cranial part of the neural groove.

crã·niostenŏ·sis (G. *kranion*, skull; *stenōsis*, narrowing). Premature ossification of the sutures of the skull.

crã·niostŏ·sis (G. *kranion*, skull; *osteon*, bone). Premature ossification of the cranial sutures.

crã·niotã·bēs (G. *kranion*, skull; L. *tabes*, a wasting away). 1. A condition characterized by areas, not sharply delimited and about the size of a shilling piece, of thinning in the cranial vault which when pressed with the finger indent and spring back with a crackle as of parchment; occurring in infants in rickets, affecting nearly always the posterior half of the skull, especially the occipital and parietal eminences and protuberance; due to increased destruction on the inner side of the cranial vault and failure in compensatory bone-formation. 2. A similar condition involving also the anterior half of the skull, due to osteogenesis imperfecta.

crã·niotome (G. *kranion*, skull; *tomē*, section). A cutting instrument for performing craniotomy.

craniŏ·tomy (G. *kranion*, skull; *tomē*, section). 1. Surgical opening of the skull. 2. Perforation of the foetal skull in labour, preliminary to cranioclasty.

crã·nium (G. *kranion*). 1. The skull of a vertebrate animal. 2. The part of the skull enclosing the brain.

crã·sis (G. *krasis*, a blend). Obsolete term denoting a normal admixture of the body fluids, as opposed to dyscrasia; also synonymous with constitution, temperament.

craw-craw. A form of filariasis, occurring especially on the West Coast of Africa, characterized by the formation of papules or pustules.

cream. The fatty content of milk, from which butter is prepared.

crease. A line produced by folding, e.g., ileofemoral c., the lower boundary of the buttock.

crē·atine (G. *kreas*, flesh). Methyl-guanidine-acetic acid; a product of protein metabolism, occurring mainly in muscle, partly as a phosphoric acid ester (phosphocreatine, q.v.); not excreted by the normal male adult in man.

creã·tinine (G. *kreas*, flesh). Anhydride of, and probably derived from, creatine. Normal constituent of urine in man.

creatinū·ria (G. *kreas*, flesh; *ouron*, urine). Excretion of creatine in the urine.

creatorrhŏē·a (G. *kreas*, flesh; *rhoia*, flow). Faecal excretion of undigested muscle fibres.

Credé's method (Credé, K. S. F., German gynaecologist, 1819–92). 1. A prophylactic measure against ophthalmia neonatorum by instillation into the eyes of newborn children of a few drops of a 1 per cent or 2 per cent solution of silver nitrate. 2. Manual expression of the placenta by grasping the uterus firmly through the abdominal walls, kneading it to excite contraction and then pressing downward towards the sacrum.

creeping disease, creeping eruption. The condition characterized by thin red lines of eruption gradually fading at one and extending at the other end, due to the burrowing into the skin of larvae of a species of certain flies (*Gastrophilus, Hypoderma bovis*, etc.). Syn. Myiasis linearis; Larva migrans.

cremaster muscle (G. *kreman*, to suspend). A muscle which extends the length of the spermatic cord and by its contraction draws up the testicle.

cremastē·ric (G. *kreman*, to suspend). Relating to the cremaster muscle. **C. reflex:** reflex retraction of the testis effected by the cremaster muscle on stimulation of the skin of the upper medial part of the thigh of the homolateral side, mediated by the 1st and 2nd lumbar segments of the spinal cord.

cremã·tion (L. *crematio*, a burning). The burning of dead bodies.

crē·mor (L., pap). Cream; any thick substance formed on the surface of a liquid.

crē·na (It.). A cleft or notch.

crē·nate, crē·nated (It. *crena*, cleft). Notched.

crenã·tion (It. *crena*, cleft). The condition of being notched.

crē·nocyte (It. *crena*, cleft; G. *kutos*, cell). A notched erythrocyte.

crenother·apy (G. *krēnē*, fountain; *therapeia*, treatment). Treatment of disease by means of waters from mineral springs.

Crenothrix (G. *krēnē*, fountain; *thrix*, hair). A genus of Schizomycetes.

crē·osote (G. *kreas*, meat; *sōzō*, I save). A colourless oily fluid obtained by distillation from wood tar. It is a powerful antiseptic.

crē·pitant (L. *crepitare*, to rattle). Crackling; see also crepitation.

crepitã·tio, crepitã·tion, crē·pitus (L. *crepitare*, to crackle). 1. The grating or crackling sound produced by the friction of two rough surfaces, such as the free ends of a fractured bone, in an osteo-arthritic joint, or in dry pleurisy (as heard during inspiration). 2. The fine crackling sounds heard on auscultation, mainly during inspiration in the first (c. indux) and resolving (c. redux) stages of pneumonia or bronchopneumonia, and in pulmonary collapse and oedema. 3. The sound produced by pressing an emphysematous tissue.

crē·scent (L. *crescere*, to grow). 1. Shaped like the crescent moon; e.g., myopic c., white crescent, usually on the temporal side of the optic disc in myopia, due to a separation of choroid and retina from the optic disc. 2. A sporont of *Plasmodium falciparum*.

crescen·tic (L. *crescere*, to grow). Crescent.

crē·sol. A mixture of phenolic bodies derived from coal tar. It has a similar action to phenol.

crest (L. *crista*, a crest). A ridge or linear prominence, especially of bone; the surmounting part of an organ or process, e.g. iliac crest.

crē·ta (L.). Chalk; native calcium carbonate.

cretin (Fr. *crétin*). One affected with cretinism.

crē·tinism (Fr. *crétin*). A congenital condition now almost generally assumed to be related to iodine deficiency in the soil and therefore in the drinking water; characterized by goitrous degeneration of the thyroid gland, causing dwarfism, failure of mental and sexual development, coarseness of features, broadness and plumpness of tongue and the various symptoms of myxoedema; occurring endemically in districts where goitre without c. is prevalent, but also in sporadic form in non-goitrous regions. See also myxoedema, congenital.

crē·tinoid (Fr. *crétin*; G. *eidos*, form). Resembling a cretin.

crē·tinous (Fr. *crétin*). Relating to cretinism.

crib·riform (L. *cribrum*, sieve; *forma*, shape). Perforated like a sieve, e.g., c. plate.

Crichton-Browne's sign (Crichton-Browne, Sir J., English physician, 1842–1938). Tremor of the labial commisures and outer angles of the eyes in the early stage of paralytic dementia.

cri·co-aryte·noid (G. *krikos*, a ring; *arutaina*, a ladle; *eidos*, form). Relating to the cricoid and arytenoid cartilages.

cri·coid (G. *krikos*, a ring; *eidos*, form). Ring-like. **C. cartilage**: the ring-like cartilage forming the inferior and posterior part of the larynx.

cricoidec·tomy (G. *krikos*, a ring; *eidos*, shape; *ektome*, excision). Excision of the cricoid cartilage.

cricothy·roid (G. *krikos*, a ring; *thureos*, from *thura*, a door; *eidos*, shape). Relating to the cricoid and thyroid cartilages.

cri·cotracheo·tomy (G. *krikos*, a ring; *trakhus*, rugged; *tome*, section). Tracheotomy through the cricoid cartilage.

crimino·logy (L. *crimen*, accusation; G. *logos*, a treatise). The study of crime.

cri·nis (L. *crinis*, hair). Hair. **C. capitis**: hair of the head. **C. pubis**: pubic hair.

cri·sis (G. *krisis*). 1. The turning-point in a disease, such as the sudden and permanent fall of febrile temperature or the sudden appearance of regenerative signs in a blood disease. 2. Paroxysmal pains, especially gastric, etc., c. in tabes dorsalis.

cris·ta (L.). A crest, e.g. **C. iliaca**: the crest of the ilium.

Crithi·dia (G. *krithidion*, dim. of *krithe*, barley). A genus of flagellata (trypanosomidae) characterized by elongated body and central kinetoplast; parasitic in invertebrates.

cri·tical (G. *kritikos*, critical, from *krites*, a judge). Relating to a crisis in disease, or a period of life. **C. pressure**: the premature saturation of a gas having c. temperature. **C. temperature**: the temperature above which a gas cannot be liquefied by any increase in pressure.

Crohn's disease. See ileitis, regional.

Crookes's tube (Crookes, Sir W., English physicist, 1832–1919). A highly exhausted vacuum tube with two electrodes, used in producing X-rays.

cross (L. *crux*). The result of c.-fertilization. **C.-birth**: shoulder-presentation. **C.-fertilization**: fertilization of plants or animals by the fertilizing substance of another species.

crossed. 1. Cross-shaped. 2. Affecting alternate sides of the body. **C. paralysis**: (1) Paralysis affecting the face on one side and the extremities on the other. (2) Paralysis affecting the arm on one side and the leg on the other. **C. reflex**: A reflex induced by stimulation of a part on the contralateral side.

crossing-over. A term applied to the breaking up of a linkage, q.v., between two genetic characters due to interchange of parts between two homologous chromosomes or linkage groups.

Crotalidae. A genus of snakes, which includes the rattlesnake.

crot·chet (Fr. *crochet*, dim. of *croc*, hook). A hook for extracting a foetus after the performance of craniotomy.

cro·tin (G. *kroton*, castor-berry shrub). The toxin from the seed of the tree, *Croton tiglii*, having characteristics similar to a microbial exotoxin.

croup. 1. A condition characterized by the formation of a fibrinous pseudo-membrane on the surface of a mucous membrane without development of extensive necrosis. 2. More especially, acute fibrinous inflammation of the larynx, usually caused by the *Bacillus diphtheriae*, and sometimes of the trachea and bronchi, causing a peculiar, harsh cough and, owing to the narrowing of the affected parts, dyspnoea and danger of suffocation. 3. An inflammatory process with fibrin-exudation, e.g. croupous pneumonia.

croup·ous. Relating to croup.

Crouzon's disease. See dysostosis, craniofacial.

crown (L. *corona*). See corona. **C. of a tooth**: the part of the tooth above the gum.

crowning (L. *corona*, crown). The appearance of the foetal head at the vulva during labour.

cru·cial (L. *crux*, cross). 1. Resembling a cross, as in c. incision. 2. Decisive; critical.

cru·ciform (L. *crux*, cross; *forma*, shape). Shaped like a cross.

crude (L. *crudus*, raw). In the natural form; raw.

cru·or (L.). 1. Coagulated blood. 2. Defibrinated blood.

cru·ra (L. pl. of *crus*, leg). Applied to parts resembling limbs. See also crus. **C. cerebelli**: see peduncles, cerebellar.

cru·reus (L. *crus*, leg). A muscle of the thigh.

cru·ral (L. *crus*, leg). 1. Pertaining to the thigh or to the leg. 2. Relating to the crura cerebelli or crura cerebri.

crus (L.). 1. The leg. 2. A limblike structure. **C. cerebri**: one of the two symmetrical tracts between medulla oblongata and cerebral hemispheres, forming the ventricular part of the mid-brain.

crust, crusta (L.). A mass produced by the drying of exudate on the skin. **Crusta lactea**: mild form of eczema on the scalp and face of milk-fed infants. **C. petrosa cementum**: the cement of a tooth.

crutch. A staff reaching from the armpit to the ground, used as a support in cases of leg injury or amputation. **C. paralysis**: see under paralysis, crutch.

Cruveilhier's atrophy (Cruveilhier, J., French pathologist, 1791–1874). Aran-Duchenne's disease, progressive muscular atrophy. **C.'s fascia**: the superficial layer of the perineal fascia. **C.'s plexus**: 1. A plexus of the posterior cervical region, derived from the great occipital nerve and the 1st and 2nd cervical nerves. 2. The plexus of varicose veins in one of the varieties of angioma. **C.'s ulcer**: ulcer of the stomach.

cry. An inarticulate vocal sound.

cryo·scopy (G. *kruos*, cold; *skopein*, to view). Determination of the freezing points of liquids, such as blood or urine, for estimating their molecular concentration.

crypt (G. *kruptein*, to hide). 1. A small sac or follicle. 2. A glandular cavity, e.g. Lieberkühn's crypts.

cryp·tic (G. *kruptein*, to hide). Concealed.

cryptoce·phalus (G. *kruptein*, to hide; *kephale*, head). A monster with a rudimentary head, only fragments of which are visible externally.

Cryptococcus (G. *kruptein*, to hide; *kokkos*, berry). A genus of yeast-like organisms having no asci and forming, in cultures, buds but no mycelium. **C. hominis**: the micro-organism causing torulosis. Syn. Torula histolytica.

cryptodi·dymus (G. *kruptein*, to hide; *didumos*, twin). A double monster in which one foetus is concealed in another.

cryp·togam (G. *kruptein*, to hide; *gamein*, to marry). Any lower plant having no true flowers but propagating by spores.

cryptogenet·ic, cryptogen·ic (G. *kruptein*, to hide; *gennan*, to produce). Obscure in origin.

cryptophthal·mos, cryptothal·mus (G. *kruptein*, to hide, *ophthalmos*, eye). Congenital union of the upper and lower eyelids, generally associated with developmental anomalies of the eyes.

cryptor·chism (G. *kruptein*, to hide; *orkhis*, testis). Failure of descent of the testicles from the abdomen or inguinal canal into the scrotum.

cryptorhet·ic (G. *kruptein*, to hide; *rhein*, to flow). Relating to internal secretion.

crys·tal (G. *krustallos*, ice). Any structure bounded by a plane, geometrically arranged surfaces and having a symmetrical internal structure. **Coffin-lid c.**: See under coffin-lid. **Charcot's, Leyden's, Teichmann's c.**, see under proper names.

crystal violet. A member of the Triphenylmethane dye family. Selective action against gram-positive bacteria.

crystäl·lin (G. *krustallos*, ice). A protein of the crystalline lens.

cry·stalline (G. *krustallos*, ice). Pertaining to or resembling a crystal. **C. lens:** the transparent lens of the eye. α-**C.**, β-**C.**: pseudo-globulins in the ocular lens. γ-**C.**: an albumin in the ocular lens.

crystalli·tis. Inflammation of the crystalline lens.

crystallizä·tion (G. *krustallos*, ice). Process of crystallizing; that form of conversion from a gaseous or liquid to a solid state in which the molecules of a substance become arranged in geometric forms.

crȳ·stallize (G. *krustallos*, ice). To be converted into crystalline structure.

crȳ·stalloid (G. *krustallos*, ice; *eidos*, form). Formerly applied to any of those substances which may pass through a semi-permeable membrane.

crystallū·ria (G. *krustallos*, ice; *ouron*, urine). The presence of crystals in the urine.

C.S.F. Abbreviation for cerebrospinal fluid.

C.S.M. Abbreviation for cerebrospinal meningitis.

CTAB. A proprietary preparation of cetyltrimethylammonium bromide, used as a wound and skin disinfectant.

Ctenocephalides. A species of flea. **Ct. canis:** the common dog flea.

Cu. Symbol for copper.

cubeba (L.). The dried unripe fruit of the Javanese plant *Piper cubeba.* An expectorant.

Cubebic acid. $C_{13}H_{14}O_7$, a white waxy material obtained from cubeb berries.

cū·bicle (L. *cubiculus*, dim. of *cubile*, bed). A single-bed ward, separated from the general ward by means of partitions.

cū·bital (L. *cubitum*, the elbow). Relating to the elbow.

cū·bitus (L. *cubitum*, elbow). **C. valgus:** a deformity of the elbow in which an exteriorly open angle is formed between upper arm and forearm. **C. varus:** a deformity of the elbow in which upper arm and forearm form an interiorly open angle.

cū·boid (G. *kubos*, cube; *eidos*, form). Like a cube. **C. bone:** one of the tarsal bones.

cuboi·dēs (G.). The cuboid bone.

cuirass (Fr. *cuirasse*, breastplate, from L. *coriaceus*, from *corium*, leather). A close-fitting bandage of the chest.

cul-de-sac (Fr.). Any cavity of which one end is closed.

Culex (L. *culex*, gnat). A genus of culicine mosquitoes transmitting filarial worms and avian malaria.

Culi·cidae (L. *culex*, gnat). A family of insects, order Diptera, comprising the culicinae and other species resembling mosquitoes but not blood-sucking in habit.

cū·licide (L. *culex*, gnat; *caedere*, to destroy). Any agent capable of destroying mosquitoes.

Culi·cinae (L. *culex*, gnat). A sub-family of Culicidae; the true mosquitoes.

Culicini (L. *culex*, gnat). A tribe of the Culicinae, comprising the Culex, Aedes and other groups of mosquitoes.

cul·men (L., a ridge). A part of the cerebellum near the vermis.

cul·tural (L. *cultura*, from *colere*, to cultivate). Relating to cultures, as of bacteria or tissues.

culture (L. *cultura*, from *colere*, to cultivate). Growth of micro-organisms or tissues in suitable media. **C. medium:** a substance used for the growth of micro-organisms. **Plate c.:** a culture of micro-organisms spread upon a flat surface of a medium. **Pure c.:** c. of a single strain of a micro-organism. **Slant c.:** a c. of micro-organisms made on the slanting surface of a medium. **Stab c.:** a c. of micro-organisms made by inoculating the medium by inserting deeply into it a needle bearing the micro-organisms.

cu. mm. Abbreviation for cubic millimetre.

cū·mulative (L. *cumulare*, to heap). Increasing; adding to; e.g., c. action of a drug, the summative effect produced by repeated administration of doses at intervals not long enough for the drug to be entirely excreted or detoxicated.

cū·neate (L. *cuneus*, wedge). Wedge-shaped. **C. fasciculus:** lateral part of the posterior white column in the upper thoracic and cervical regions ending in the c. nuclei at the lower part of the fourth ventricle.

cū·neiform (L. *cuneus*, wedge; *forma*, shape). Wedge-shaped. **C. bone:** any of the three distal tarsal bones.

cuneo-cuboid (L. *cuneus*, wedge; G. *kubos*, cube; *eidos*, form). Relating to both cuneiform and cuboid bones.

cū·neus (L. *cuneus*, wedge). The wedge-shaped lobe on the inner surface of the posterior part of the cerebral hemisphere.

cuni·culus (L. *cuniculus*, rabbit). The furrow of an itch-insect in the skin.

cunnilin·gus (L. *cunnus*, vulva; *lingere*, to lick). Licking the female external genitalia.

cunnus (L.). The vulva.

cup. A cupping-glass.

cū·pola (It. dim. of L. *cupa*, cask). The dome-shaped apex of the cochlea.

cupping. 1. Abstraction of blood by means of cupping-glasses. 2. The formation of a cuplike depression. **C. glass:** a glass cup in which a partial vacuum is produced in cupping.

cuprae·mia (L. *cuprum*, copper; G. *haima*, blood). The presence of copper in the blood.

cupres·sin. An oil obtained from cypresses.

cupric citrate. $Cu_2C_6H_4O_7.2H_2O$. An astringent.

cupric sulphate. $CuSO_4.5H_2O$. An astringent.

cu·prum (L.). Copper, *q.v.*

curare. A vegetable extract obtained from *Paullinia curare.* Its alkaloid is **curarine.** First known as a South American Indian arrow-poison, now used to promote muscular relaxation in anaesthesia.

cū·rative (L. *curare*, to heal). Having a healing effect.

curcū·min. Chemical indicator and dye. An alkaloid of *Curcuma longa*, the rhizome of which is called turmeric.

curd. The coagulum of milk, as formed after the addition of an acid.

cure (L. *cura*, care). The re-establishment of health; the successful treatment of disease.

curettage (Fr. *curer*, to cleanse). The removal of vegetations, necrotic tissue, retained placenta, etc., by means of a curette.

curette, curet (Fr. *curer*, to cleanse). A spoon-shaped instrument for scraping away tissue. There are many varieties such as the aural, eye, uterine and Volkmann's curette used to remove sequestrum.

curettement (Fr. *curer*, to cleanse). See under curettage.

curie (Curie, M. S., Polish physicist, 1867–1934; and Curie, P., French physicist, 1859–1906). Unit of measurement of radium emanations or of radioactive substances. **C.-therapy:** treatment by radium.

Curling's ulcer (Curling, T. B., English physician, 1811–81). A duodenal ulcer produced by extensive burns of the skin.

current (L. *currere*, to run). Transmission of electric force along a conductor. **C., alternating:** electric c. changing its direction at regular intervals. **C., direct:** electric c. flowing always in the same direction. **C., high-frequency:** alternating c. changing its direction 10,000 times or more per second.

Curschmann's spirals (Curschmann, H., German physician, 1846–1910). Spiral conglomerates of mucin with a light-coloured central thread, sometimes found in the sputum of bronchial asthma.

cur·vature (L. *curvare*, to curve). A bending or curving.

curve. A bending or flexure.

Cusco's speculum (Cusco, E. G., French surgeon, 1819–94). A vaginal speculum.

Cushing's law (Cushing, Harvey, American surgeon, 1869–1939). Increased intracranial tension raises the blood pressure above the pressure exerted against the vital centres in the medulla of the brain. **C.'s reaction:** a test for hypopituitarism. If 2 c.c. of an extract of the anterior lobe of the pituitary gland of an ox are injected subcutaneously, a rise of temperature indicates hypopituitarism. **C.'s suture:** a form of continuous Lembert suture. **C.'s syndrome:** (dystrophia adiposogenitalis) seen in lesions of the pituitary gland in which there is adiposity, atrophy of the external genitalia and changes in the secondary sexual characters.

cushion. A fatty mass in which is incorporated some elastic tissue which acts by relieving pressure on structures lying beneath.

cusp (L. *cuspis*, a point). One of the pointed parts of the crown of a tooth.

cuspid, cuspidate. Having a sharp point. **Cuspid teeth:** the four teeth having conical crowns. Syn. canine teeth.

cută·neous (L. *cutis*, skin). Relating to the skin. **C. reflex:** a reflex elicited by stimulation of the skin.

cu·ticle (L. *cuticula*, dim. of *cutis*, skin). 1. A pellicle. 2. The epidermis. 3. Thin layer of skin covering the nail at its base and sides. 4. The enamel covering a recently erupted tooth. 5. A thin skin on the surface of a liquid.

cuti·cula (L. *cuticula*, dim. of *cutis*, skin). Cuticle.

cuti·cular (L. *cuticula*, dim. of *cutis*, skin). Pertaining to a cuticle.

cu·tis (L., skin). The derma or true skin. **C. anserina:** gooseskin. **C. laxa:** see dermatolysis. **C. verticis gyrata:** a developmental deformity of the scalp, especially about the vertex, characterized by unusual laxness and movability, forming irregular folds, with cellular infiltration of the corium and absence of elastic fibres.

Cuvier's canals (Cuvier, G.L.C.F.D., French anatomist, 1769–1832). Two short vessels (in the embryo) opening into the common trunk of the omphalo-mesenteric veins, each being formed by the union of two veins, the anterior cardinal (or jugular) and the posterior cardinal. The right one becomes the superior vena cava; the left one disappears. **C.'s duct:** junctional termination of cardinal veins in the embryo.

cwt. Abbreviation for hundredweight.

Cy. Abbreviation for cyanogen, *q.v.*

cyanhidrŏ·sis (G. *kuanos*, blue; *hidrōs*, sweat). Secretion of bluish-coloured sweat, due to bacterial action.

cyanogen. A gas, with chemical formula, CN, for the radical and CN.CN, for dicyanogen, a highly poisonous gas. **C. bromide:** tear gas, BrCN. **C. chloride:** gas used to fumigate houses, etc. Its chemical formula is ClCN.

cyanŏ·pia (G. *kuanos*, blue; *ōps*, eye). Vision in which all objects appear blue, occurring occasionally in digitalis poisoning, retinal or choroidal diseases, or shortly after extraction of the lens.

cy·anosed (G. *kuanos*, blue). Affected with cyanosis.

cyanose tardif (G. *kuanos*, blue; Fr. *tardif*, delayed). Cyanosis from congenital heart disease beginning to appear only in later childhood or adolescence.

cyanŏ·sis (G. *kuanos*, blue). Bluish discoloration of the skin, mucous membranes or other tissues due to the presence of abnormally increased quantities or reduced haemoglobin (owing to insufficient aeration of the blood) or to presence of sulphaemoglobin or methaemoglobin in the blood.

cyanot·ic (G. *kuanos*, blue). Relating to or affected with cyanosis.

cȳ·athus (G. *kuathos*, a cup). A cup or glass.

cycle (G. *kuklos*, circle). A succession of events or symptoms.

cyclencĕ·phalus (G. *kuklos*, circle; *egkephalos*, the brain). A monster having both cerebral hemispheres joined into one.

cyclic (G. *kuklos*, circle). Pertaining to or occurring in cycles. **C. albuminuria:** see albuminuria, c. **C. compound:** any organic compound belonging to the ring or closed-chain series. **C. insanity:** see cyclothymia. **C. vomiting:** recurrent attacks of vomiting in children, associated with ketosis.

cycli·tis (G. *kuklos*, circle). Inflammation of the ciliary body, mostly associated with inflammation of the iris (iridocyclitis) or choroid (choriocyclitis).

cyclobar·bitone. Ethylcyclohexenylbarbituric acid. A short-acting barbiturate of mild effect.

cyclocephalus (G. *kuklos*, circle; *kephalē*, head). See Cyclopean brain.

cyclodiă·lysis (G. *kuklos*, circle; *dia*, through; *luein*, to loosen). Detachment of the ciliary body from the sclera.

cyclŏ·pean (G. *kuklos*, circle; *ōps*, eye). Pertaining to cyclops. **C. brain:** the result of incomplete development of the end-brain, characterized by defect of the eyes and optic tracts and absence of olfactory tracts.

cyclophor·ia (G. *kuklos*, circle; *pherein*, to bear). Tendency of one eye to rotate round the anteroposterior axis more than the other.

cycloplē·gia (G. *kuklos*, circle; *plēgē*, a stroke). Paralysis of the ciliary muscles of the eye, resulting in loss of power of accommodation.

cyclopropane. A gaseous anaesthetic, $CH_2CH_2CH_2$.

cyclops (G. *kuklos*, circle; *ōps*, eye). 1. A monster with the eyes fused into a single organ. 2. A genus of minute, free-swimming crustaceans.

cyclothȳ·mia (G. *kuklos*, circle; *thumos*, mind). A condition characterized by alternate periods of depression and exuberance, with absence of definite psychotic symptoms.

cyclotome (G. *kuklos*, circle; *tomē*, section). An instrument used for the performance of cyclotomy.

cyclŏ·tomy (G. *kuklos*, circle; *tomē*, section). Incision through the ciliary body.

cyc·lotron (G. *kuklos*, circle; *ēlektron*, amber). A machine for imparting extremely high velocities up to 100,000 miles (sec.) to atomic particles by means of electrical impulses; the charged atoms whirling in ever-widening circles in a chamber mounted between the poles of an immense magnet sped faster and faster by alternate changes of the electric field from negative to positive and vice versa; they finally shoot out through an opening to smash against a target, by impact on which the atoms are to be cracked.

cyematocar·dia (G. *kuēma*, embryo; *kardia*, heart). Foetal rhythm of the heart sounds.

cyemŏ·logy (G. *kuēma*, embryo; *logos*, treatise). The science of embryology.

cyē·sis (G. *kuēsis*, conception). Pregnancy.

cyē·tic (G. *kuēsis*, conception). Relating to pregnancy.

cȳ·linder (G. *kulindros*). 1. See cast, urinary. 2. A lens with one or both surfaces curved as a cylinder.

cylin·drical. Relating to or shaped like a cylinder.

cylin·droid (G. *kulindros*, cylinder; *eidos*, form). 1. Resembling a cylinder. 2. A mucous cast in urine, a pseudo-cylinder.

cylindrŏ·ma (G. *kulindros*, cylinder). A term sometimes applied to tumours having a stroma of elongated, thickened, twisted cords of hyaline material, e.g. as sometimes seen in basal cell carcinoma or in carcinoma of the salivary glands.

cylin·drosarcō·ma (G. *kulindros*, cylinder; *sarx*, flesh). A sarcoma containing cylindromatous elements.

cylindrū·ria (G. *kulindros*, cylinder; *ouron*, urine). Presence of casts in the urine.

cyllō·sis (G. *kullos*, crippled). Club foot.

cyst (G. *kustis*, bladder). A membranous sac containing fluid; a bladder. C., **allantoic:** a circumscribed dilatation of the urachus. C., **atheromatous:** an epidermoid, dermoid or retention c., of a hair follicle gland, developing during adult life, occurring on scalp, scrotum, etc. C., **branchial:** a c. resulting from incomplete closure of a branchial cleft. C., **compound:** a c. containing daughter cc. C., **daughter:** a c. developed from the wall of a primary or mother c. C., **dentigerous:** a cystic odontoma containing one or more imperfectly formed teeth, originating from a tooth follicle. C., **dermoid:** a teratoma composed essentially of structures derived from the ectoderm. C., **epidermoid:** a simple teratoma, occurring on the scalp, lined with stratified epithelium which after desquamation forms a soft putty-like substance. Syn. wen. C., **hydatid:** the larval or cysticercus stage of the *Taenia echinococcus*, developing in the host's liver, brain or other part. C., **implantation:** a c. originating from a piece of skin implanted into a deeper tissue, usually as the result of a trauma with a pointed instrument. C., **inclusion:** implantation c., *q.v.* C., **mother:** a primary c. enclosing secondary or daughter cc. C., **multilocular:** a c. containing numerous cavities separated by membranous septa. C., **parent:** mother c., *q.v.* C., **proliferation, proliferous:** a c. producing numerous daughter cc. C., **retention:** a structure due to obstruction of the excretory duct of a gland. C., **sebaceous:** retention c. of a sebaceous gland. C., **secondary:** daughter c., *q.v.* C., **sequestration:** a dermoid c. resulting from displacement of a portion of skin during embryonic development. C., **thyroglossal:** a c. resulting from imperfect closure of the thyroglossal duct. C., **unilocular:** a c. containing a single cavity.

cystă·denocarcinō·ma (G. *kustis*, bladder; *adēn*, gland; *karkinos*, cancer). A variety of mammary cancer, arising in mammary cysts or large ducts, of relatively slow growth.

cyst·adenō·ma (G. *kustis*, bladder; *adēn*, gland). An adenoma containing cysts.

cystal·gia (G. *kustis*, bladder; *algos*, pain). Any bladder pain.

cyst·auchenŏ·tomy (G. *kustis*, bladder; *aukhēn*, neck; *tomē*, section). An operation in which an incision is made into the neck of the urinary bladder.

cystectă·sia (G. *kustis*, bladder; *ektasis*, extension). Dilatation of the bladder.

cystec·tomy (G. *kustis*, bladder; *ektomē*, excision). 1. Excision of the cystic duct. 2. Excision of the gallbladder or part of the urinary bladder. 3. Removal of a cyst.

cyste·ine (G. *kustis*, bladder). α-amino-β-thiol-propionic acid, a reduction product of cystine, *q.v.*; activating oxidation-reduction reactions.

cystencĕ·phalus (G. *kustis*, bladder; *egkephalos*, brain). A monster with an undeveloped brain and hydrocephaly.

cysten·desis (G. *kustis*, bladder; *endĕsis*, a binding on). Suture of a wound in the gall bladder.

cystic (G. *kustis*, bladder). 1. Relating to a cyst. 2. Relating to the urinary bladder or to the gall-bladder. C. **degeneration:** degeneration of tissue with formation of cysts.

cysticercō·sis (G. *kustis*, bladder; *kerkos*, tail). Infestation with cysticerci.

Cysticercus (G. *kustis*, bladder; *kerkos*, tail). The larval stage of certain species of tapeworms, consisting of a head and neck which are attached to a cyst-like structure filled with fluid; living in tissues of animals serving as intermediate host until swallowed by an animal of a species serving as definitive host of the tapeworm in the intestine of which it develops into the adult tapeworm. See also, hydatid. C. **bovis:** the larval stage of the *Taenia saginata*, living in cattle. C. **cellulosae:** the larval stage of the *Taenia solium*, living in the pig and sometimes in man.

cysticō·tomy (G. *kustis*, bladder; *tomē*, section). Incision into the bile duct.

cys·tidotrachelō·tomy (G. *kustis*, bladder; *eidos*, form; *trakhelos*, neck; *tomē*, section). See cystauchenotomy.

cystināē·mia (Cystine, G. *haima*, blood). Condition in which cystine is present in the blood.

cys·tine (G. *kustis*, bladder). The disulphide corresponding to cysteine, *q.v.*, and of importance with the latter in biological oxidation/reduction mechanisms.

cystinū·ria (G. *kustis*, bladder; *ouron*, urine). Metabolic disturbance characterized by, usually permanent, urinary excretion of cystine.

cystistax·is (G. *kustis*, bladder; *staxis*, a dripping). The escape of blood into the bladder.

cysti·tis (G. *kustis*, bladder). Inflammation of the bladder.

cystitome (G. *kustis*, bladder; *tomē*, section). A special knife used in cataract operations.

cysti·tomy (G. *kustis*, bladder; *tomē*, section). Incision into the bladder.

cys·tobubŏ·nocele (G. *kustis*, bladder; *boubōn*, the groin; *kēlē*, hernia). Incomplete indirect inguinal hernia involving the bladder.

cys·tocele (G. *kustis*, bladder; *kēlē*, hernia). Protrusion of the bladder into the vagina; an early stage in genital prolapse.

cys·tocolŏ·stomy (G. *kustis*, bladder; *kolos*, colon; *stoma*, mouth). An anastomosis between the gallbladder and the colon.

cysto-enterocele (G. *kustis*, bladder; *enteron*, intestine; *kēlē*, hernia). A hernia which contains a part of the intestine.

cysto-epitheliō·ma (G. *kustis*, bladder; *epithelion*, skin). A squamous celled carcinoma containing cysts.

cys·tofibrō·ma (G. *kustis*, bladder; L. *fibra*, fibre). Cystic fibroma.

cys·toid (G. *kustis*, bladder; *eidos*, form) .Resembling a cyst.

cystolithec·tomy (G. *kustis*, bladder; *lithos*, stone; *ektomē*, excision). Removal of a stone from the gallbladder or the urinary bladder.

cys·tolithī·asis (G. *kustis*, bladder; *lithos*, stone). Formation of a stone in the bladder.

cystolū·tein (G. *kustis*, bladder; L. *luteus*, yellow). The yellow colouring matter found in cysts.

cystō·ma (G. *kustis*, bladder). A tumour composed of one or more cysts.

cystomēr·ocele (G. *kustis*, bladder; *mēros*, thigh; *kēlē*, hernia). Hernia of the bladder through the femoral ring.

cys·tomyxō·ma (G. *kustis*, bladder; *muxa*, mucus). A cystoma with myxomatous contents.

cys·topară·lysis (G. *kustis*, bladder; *paralusis*, paralysis). Paralysis of the bladder.

cystopex·ia (G. *kustis*, bladder; *pēxis*, fixation). Surgical fixation of the bladder.

cystophthī·sis (G. *kustis*, bladder; *phthisis*, decay). Bladder tuberculosis.

cys·toplasty (G. *kustis*, bladder; *plassein*, to form). Any plastic operation on the bladder.

cystoptō·sis (G. *kustis*, bladder; *ptōsis*, a falling). Prolapse of the vesical mucous membrane into the urethra.

cys·topyeli·tis (G. *kustis*, bladder; *puelos*, a trough). Inflammation of both urinary bladder and pelvis of the kidney.

cys·torecto·stomy (G. *kustis*, bladder; L. *rectus*, straight; G. *stoma*, mouth). The formation of a fistula between the rectum and the bladder.

cystorrhā·gia (G. *kustis*, bladder; *rhegnusthai*, to burst out). Haemorrhage from the bladder.

cystor·rhaphy (G. *kustis*, bladder; *rhaphē*, suture). Suture of the bladder.

cystŏ·schisis (G. *kustis*, bladder; *skhisis*, cleavage). A congenital fissure of the urinary bladder.

cystoscir·rhus (G. *kustis*, bladder; *skiros*, a hard covering). Carcinoma of the urinary bladder.

cys·toscope (G. *kustis*, bladder; *skopein*, to inspect). Instrument for inspecting the interior of the bladder.

cystŏ·scopy (G. *kustis*, bladder; *skopein*, to inspect). Examination of the interior of the bladder by the cystoscope.

cys·tospasm (G. *kustis*, bladder; *spasmos*, spasm). Spasm of the bladder.

cys·tospermi·tis (G. *kustis*, bladder; *sperma*, semen). Inflammation of the seminal vesicles.

cystŏ·stomy (G. *kustis*, bladder; *stoma*, mouth). The formation of a fistulous opening in the bladder wall.

cys·totome (G. *kustis*, bladder; *tomē*, section). 1. Knife used in cystotomy. 2. Knife used in rupturing the capsule of the lens in cataract operations.

cystŏ·tomy (G. *kustis*, bladder; *tomē*, section). 1. An incision into the bladder. 2. Surgical division of the anterior capsule of the lens.

cysto-urē·throscope (G. *kustis*, bladder; *ourēthra*, urethra; *skopein*, to view). Instrument for inspecting the bladder and urethra.

cȳ·taster (G. *kutos*, cell; *astēr*, star). 1. Aster, *q.v.* 2. An accessory aster, an aster not associated with chromosomes.

cȳ·toblast (G. *kutos*, cell; *blastos*, germ). 1. The nucleus of a cell. 2. Cytotrophoblast.

cytoche·mistry. The chemistry of cells.

cytochro·matin (G. *kutos*, cell; *khrōma*, colour). The chromophilic substance of a nerve cell. Syn. Nissl's bodies; tigroid substance.

cȳ·tochrome (G. *kutos*, cell; *khroma*, colour). A pigment, related to haemoglobin, widely distributed in cells of aerobic organisms, acting as oxidizing enzyme and as carrier of hydrogen.

cȳ·tochylē·ma (G. *kutos*, cell; *khulos*, juice). Cellsap.

cȳ·tocide (G. *kutos*, cell; L. *caedere*, to destroy). An agent capable of destroying cells.

cȳ·tode (G. *kutos*, cell; *eidos*, form). 1. A supposedly anuclear cell. 2. The simplest form of nuclear cell.

cytoden·drite (G. *kutos*, cell; *dendron*, tree). Collateral fibril of a nerve cell.

cytodes·ma (G. *kutos*, cell; *desmos*, band). Intercellular connections or bridges.

cȳ·todiagnō·sis (G. *kutos*, cell; *dia*, through; *gnōsis*, knowledge). The microscopical study of the cellular elements in fluids as an aid to diagnosis.

cytogĕ·nesis (G. *kutos*, cell; *gennan*, to produce). Cell-formation.

cytŏ·genous (G. *kutos*, cell; *gennan*, to produce). Producing cells.

cytoid (G. *kutos*, cell; *eidos*, form). Resembling a cell. C. **bodies**: transient structures observed in a phase of degeneration of the optic nerve, originating from enlarged non-medullated fibres.

cytokinē·sis (G. *kutos*, cell; *kinein*, to move). The changes of the cytoplasm during mitosis, meiosis and fertilization.

cytŏ·logy (G. *kutos*, cell; *logos*, a treatise). The branch of biology pertaining to the formation and function of cells.

cȳ·tolymph (G. *kutos*, cell; L. *lympha*, water). The ground-substance of the cytoplasm. Syn. cell-sap; enchylema.

cytŏlȳ·sin (G. *kutos*, cell; *luein*, to loosen). A specific antibody developed in the body by the injection of foreign cells of any kind and causing the disintegration of these foreign cells when they are again introduced.

cytŏ·lysis (G. *kutos*, cell; *luein*, to loosen). Cell-disintegration or dissolution.

cytō·ma (G. *kutos*, cell). A sarcoma.

cȳ·tomere (G. *kutos*, cell; *meros*, part). The cytoplasmic part of a spermatocyte, especially the flagella.

cytŏ·meter (G. *kutos*, cell; *metron*, measure). Instrument for counting or measuring cells.

cytomī·crosome (G. *kutos*, cell; *mikros*, small; *sōma*, body). A cytoplasmic microsome.

cytomitō·ma (G. *kutos*, cell; *mitos*, thread). The network of the cell-body.

cytomorphō·sis (G. *kutos*, cell; *morphōsis*, from *morphē*, shape). The developmental changes undergone by cells.

cyton (G. *kutos*, cell). A cell.

cȳ·tophil (G. *kutos*, cell; *philein*, to love). Having an affinity for cells.

cytophylax·is (G. *kutos*, cell; *phulassein*, to protect). Cell protection.

cȳ·toplasm (G. *kutos*, cell; *plassein*, to form). 1. Protoplasm as distinguished from the nucleus of the cell-body. 2. Formerly = protoplasm.

cytopoiē·sis (G. *kutos*, cell; *poiēsis*, fabrication). Cell-production.

cytŏ·scopy (G. *kutos*, cell; *skopein*, to inspect). The examination of cells.

cȳ·tosome (G. *kutos*, cell; *sōma*, body). The cell-body as distinguished from the nucleus.

cȳ·tostome (G. *kutos*, cell; *stoma*, mouth). The mouth of a protozoan.

cytotax·is (G. *kutos*, cell; *taxis*, arrangement). The directive influence which determines the arrangement of cells.

cytotox·in (G. *kutos*, cell; *toxikon*, poison). Cytolysin, *q.v.*

cȳ·totrŏ·phoblast (G. *kutos*, cell; *trephein*, to nourish; *blastos*, germ). One of the layers of the chorionic villi.

cȳ·tozyme (G. *kutos*, cell; *zumē*, a leaven). A tissue extract which activates prothrombin; of lipoid character, resembling cephalin.

Czermak's spaces (Czermak, J. N., Austrian physician, 1828–73). Gaps in the continuity of dentine.

D

Δ, δ. The fourth letter of the Greek alphabet. See under Delta.

D. (G. *dosis*). Abbreviation for dose and deuterium.

D. to N. ratio. Abbreviation for dextrose-nitrogen ratio.

dac·ryadenăl·gia (G. *dakruon*, tear; *adēn*, gland; *algos*, pain). Pain in lacrimal gland.

dac·ryadeni·tis (G. *dakruon*, tear; *adēn*, gland). See under dacryo-adenitis.

dac·ryadenoscir·rhus (G. *dakruon*, tear; *adēn*, gland; *skiros*, hard covering). A hard indurated tumour of the lacrimal gland.

dac·ryagogatrē·sia (G. *dakruon*, tear; *agōgos*, leading; *a*, neg.; *trēsis*, boring). Obstruction to the lacrimal duct.

dac·ryo-adeni·tis (G. *dakruon*, tear; *adēn*, gland). Inflammation of a lacrimal gland.

dac·ryoblennorrhōē·a (G. *dakruon*, tear; *blennos*, slime; *rhoia*, a flux). Dacryocystoblennorrhoea, *q.v.*

dac·ryocele (G. *dakruon*, tear; *kēlē*, hernia). See dacryocystocele.

dac·ryocyst (G. *dakruon*, tear; *kustis*, bladder). The lacrimal sac.

dac·ryocystal·gia (G. *dakruon*, tear; *kustis*, bladder; *algos*, pain). Pain in lacrimal sac.

dac·ryocysti·tis (G. *dakruon*, tear; *kustis*, bladder). Inflammation of the lacrimal sac.

dac·ryocys·toblennorrhōe·a (G. *dakruon*, tear; *kustis*, bladder; *blennos*, slime; *rhoia*, a flux). Chronic dacryocystitis with a muco-purulent discharge.

dac·ryocys·tocele (G. *dakruon*, tear; *kustis*, bladder; *kēlē*, hernia). Protrusion of a lacrimal sac.

dac·ryocys·torhinŏ·stomy (G. *dakruon*, tear; *kustis*, bladder; *rhis*, nose; *stoma*, mouth). The making of a permanent opening between lacrimal sac and nose.

dac·ryocys·totome (G. *dakruon*, tear; *kustis*, bladder; *tomē*, section). An instrument for operating on the lacrimal sac.

dac·ryocystŏ·tomy (G. *dakruon*, tear; *kustis*, bladder; *tomē*, section). Surgical puncture of the lacrimal sac.

dac·ryohaemorrhōe·a (G. *dakruon*, tear; *haima*, blood; *rhoia*, flow). The weeping of bloody tears.

dac·ryolith (G. *dakruon*, tear; *lithos*, stone). A calculus in the lacrimal passages.

dac·ryon (G. *dakruon*, tear). 1. A tear. 2. The point of junction of the frontal, lacrimal and superior maxillary bones.

dac·ryops (G. *dakruon*, tear; *ōps*, eye). Retention cyst of the lacrimal gland or duct.

dac·ryorrhōe·a (G. *dakruon*, tear; *rhoia*, flow). An excessive flow of tears.

dac·ryosō·len (G. *dakruon*, tear; *sōlen*, channel). A lacrimal duct, or canal. Hence dacryosolenitis, inflammation of a lacrimal duct.

dacryū·ria (G. *dakruon*, tear; *ouron*, urine). The voiding of urine which occurs with lacrimation in cases of hysteria.

dac·tyl (G. *daktulos*, finger). A digit of the hand or foot.

dac·tylar, dactyl·ic (G. *daktulos*, finger). Relating to a finger or toe.

dac·tylate (G. *daktulos*, finger). Resembling a finger.

dac·tylī·tis (G. *daktulos*, finger). Inflammation of a metacarpal or a phalanx of a finger or toe, usually due to tuberculosis or congenital syphilis, character-ized by diffuse infiltration of the bone-marrow with expansion or erosion of the medullary cavity and formation of new periosteal bone on the surface, the affected phalanx presenting a spindle-shaped swelling. (See also spina ventosa.)

dac·tylogrypō·sis (G. *daktulos*, finger; *grupos*, curved). Abnormal curvature of the fingers or toes.

dac·tyloid (G. *daktulos*, finger; *eidos*, form). Resembling a finger.

dactylŏ·logy (G. *daktulos*, finger; *logos*, discourse). Communication by signs made with the fingers, as by the manual alphabet of deaf-mutes.

dactylŏ·lysis (G. *daktulos*, finger; *luein*, to loosen). The falling off of a finger or toe. **D. spontanea:** ainhum, *q.v.*

dac·tylomĕ·galy (G. *daktulos*, finger; *megas*, large). A condition in which one finger or toe is larger than the rest.

dac·tylospasm (G. *daktulos*, finger; *spasmos*, seizure). Spasm of a finger.

dac·tylosym·physis (G. *daktulos*, finger; *sun*, together; *phusis*, from *phuein*, to grow). Syndactylism.

dac·tylus (G. *daktulos*). A finger or a toe.

D.A.H. Abbreviation for disordered action of the heart; see effort syndrome.

Dakin's solution (Dakin, H. D., American chemist, born 1880). Bicarbonate of soda 200 gm.; chlorinated lime 140 gm.; water 10 litres; mix, filter through cotton and add 40 gm. boric acid.

dak·ryon (G. *dakruon*, tear). See under dacryon.

Dalton's Law (Dalton, J., English chemist and physicist, 1766–1844). (The law of partial pressures.) The pressure exerted by a gaseous mixture is equal to the sum of the pressures which the constituents would exert if each occupied separately the volume of the mixture.

Daltonism (Dalton, J., English chemist and physicist, 1766–1844). Congenital colour blindness.

Damman's bacillus (Damman, K., German veterinary surgeon, 1839–1914). *Actinomyces necrophorus.*

Damoisseau's curve (Damoisseau, L. H. C., French physician, 1815–90). See under Ellis's line.

Dance's sign (Dance, J. B. H., French physician, 1797–1832). A slight depression about the right flank or iliac fossa, considered by D. to indicate invagination of the caecum in cases of intussusception.

dandruff, dandriff. Scurf on the head, coming off in small scales.

dandy fever (Corrupted form of dengue). Dengue, *q.v.*

Darier's disease (Darier, J., French dermatologist, 1856–1938). Keratosis follicularis; psorospermosis follicularis vegetans.

dark field or dark ground illumination. Microscopical method in which, by means of a mirror-condenser and by illuminating the object not from below but from the sides, a bright image is obtained from the object on a dark ground.

Darkshevich fibres (Darkshevich, L., Russian neurologist, 1858–1925). A tract of nerve fibres passing from the optic tract to the habenular ganglion. **D.'s nucleus:** a nucleus of nerve cells on each side of the upper part of the Sylvian aqueduct.

dartoid (G. *dartos*, flayed; *eidos*, form). Like the dartos.

dartos (G., flayed). The contractile layer beneath the skin of the scrotum.

Darwinian ear (Darwin, C. R., English naturalist, 1809–82). Congenital deformity of the human ear. **D.'s tubercle:** the auricular tubercle on the anterior surface of the helix.

Daubenton's angle and line (Daubenton, L. J. M., French physician, 1716–1800). The occipital angle and line; anthropometric indices on the skull. **D.'s plane:** a line passing through the opisthion and the inferior borders of the orbits.

Davai·nea (Davaine, C. J., French physician, 1812–82). A family of tapeworms.

Davidoff's cells (Davidoff, M. von, German histologist, died 1904). 'Cellules comprimées.' The cells of Paneth in the mucosa of the small intestine.

Davidsohn's sign (Davidsohn, H., German physician, 1842–1911). The illumination obtained on placing an electric light in the mouth will be absent, or less marked, on the side on which there is a tumour or empyema of the antrum of Highmore.

day-blindness. Impaired acuity and discomfort of vision on more or less intense illumination, probably due to a deficiency in the cones. Syn. hemeralopia.

D.C. Abbreviation for direct current.

D.Cc. Abbreviation for double concave.

D.Cx. Abbreviation for double convex.

D.D.S. Abbreviation for Doctor of Dental Surgery.

D.D.T. pp′-dichlorodiphenyltrichloroethane; a synthetic insecticide.

de-acǐ·dification. The neutralization of acid.

de-acetylā·tion (L. *de*, from; *acetum*, vinegar; G. *hulē*, matter). Removal of acetyl groups from a substance.

dead. Without life.

dead hand. A clinical condition marked by vascular disturbances of the fingers, arising in rotary tool cutters.

deaf. Lacking the sense of hearing. **Deaf-mutism:** the condition of being deaf and dumb.

deafness. The condition of being deaf; loss of power of hearing. **Cortical d.:** d. due to a lesion of the areas of the cerebral cortex associated with auditory function. **Mind-d.** agnosia, auditory d. **Word-d.:** agnosia, auditory d.

deǎ·midase. An enzyme hydrolyzing amides.

deamidā·tion. The hydrolysis of an amide to the parent carboxylic acid.

deǎ·minase (L. *de*, from; G. *ammoniakon*, salammoniac). An enzyme hydrolyzing amines.

deaminā·tion (L. *de*, from; G. *ammoniakon*, salammoniac). The hydrolysis of amines with the removal of the amino-group.

death. The cessation of life. **D.-instinct:** in psychoanalysis, the tendency to re-establish a state of things which was disturbed by the emergence of life, believed to be composed of regressive, self destroying and aggressive impulses. **D.-rate:** the mortality per 1,000 individuals in a given group during a given period, e.g. a year.

Deaver's windows (Deaver, J. B., American anatomist, 1855–1931). The fat-free portions of the mesentery framed by intestinal vascular arcades adjacent to the attached margin of the gut.

debi·litate (L. *debilitare*, from *debilis*, weak). To weaken.

debi·lity (L. *debilitas*, from *debilis*, weak). Weakness.

Débové's membrane or layer (Débové, G. M., French pathologist, 1845–1920). The basement membrane of the mucosa of the trachea, bronchi and intestinal tract.

débridement (F. *débrider*, to open up a wound). Cutting away damaged or infected tissue from a wound.

debris (F. *débris*). Rubbish; the remainder of a disintegrated substance.

decalcificā·tion (L. *de*, from; *calx*, lime; *facere*, to make). Removal or loss of calcium salts, from bone.

decal·cified (L. *de*, from; *calx*, lime; *facere*, to make). Freed from calcium salts.

decamethonium bromide, d. iodide. Muscle relaxing drugs whose properties resemble curare. They are used to abolish muscle tone during anaesthesia and to lower blood pressure.

decannulā·tion (L. *de*, from; *cannula*, dim. of *canna*, a reed). The removal of a cannula.

decantā·tion (Late L. *decanthare*, from G. *kanthos*, the corner of the eye). The removal of supernatant fluid from a liquid or solid sediment.

decapitā·tion (Late L. *decapitare*, from *de*, from; *caput*, head). Cutting off the head, e.g. of a foetus during labour.

decapsulā·tion (L. *de*, from; *capsula*, from *capsa*, a box). The stripping off of a capsule, e.g. of the renal capsule.

decarbonā·tion (L. *de*, from; *carbo*, coal). Removal of carbon dioxide from a substance.

decarbonizā·tion (L. *de*, from; *carbo*, coal). Removal of carbon from a substance.

decarbox·ylation, decarboxylizā·tion (L. *de*, from; *carbo*, coal; G. *oxus*, sharp; *hulé*, matter). Removal of one or more carboxyl groups, involving the decomposition of an organic acid to carbon dioxide.

decay. 1. Decline, as of life or health. 2. Aerobic proteolysis of compounds without production of foul odour.

decě·rebrate (L. *de*, from; *cerebrum*, brain). 1. To section the brain stem above the vestibular nucleus. 2. To remove the brain. 3. Having the brain removed. **D. rigidity:** the state after decerebration, characterized by increase in postural tonus, due to postural reflexes.

decerebrā·tion (L. *de*, from; *cerebrum*, brain). 1. Removal of the brain. 2. Section through the lower part of the mesencephalon.

decě·rebrize (L. *de*, from; *cerebrum*, brain). To decerebrate.

dechloridation. A diet without salt.

dechloruration. Producing a decreased excretion of chlorides in the urine.

decibel (L. *decimus*, from *decem*, ten). One-tenth of a bel, *q.v.*; unit for measurement of sound intensity on a logarithmic scale.

decǐ·dua (L. *decidere*, to fall away). The mucous membrane of the pregnant uterus. **D. basalis:** the part of the d. on which the ovum is lying. **D. capsularis:** the part of the d. which envelops the ovum. **D. parietalis (vera):** the part of the d. not in contact with the ovum. **D. serotina:** syn: decidua basalis.

decǐ·dual (L. *decidere*, to fall away). Relating to the decidua.

deciduī·tis (L. *decidere*, to fall away). Inflammation of the decidual endometrium. Syn. decidual endometritis.

decǐ·duoma (L. *decidere*, to fall away). An intrauterine tumour containing decidual remains. **D. malignum:** a variety of uterine sarcoma.

decǐ·duosarcō·ma (L. *decidere*, to fall away; G. *sarx*, flesh). See deciduoma malignum.

decǐ·duous (L. *decidere*, to fall away). Shedding periodically, or at certain seasons.

decinor·mal (L. *decimus*, from *decem*, ten; *norma*). **D. solution:** a solution one-tenth of normal solution strength.

decipa·ra (L. *decimus*, from *decem*, ten; *parere*, to produce). A woman pregnant for the tenth time.

dě·clinator. An instrument for retracting the dura mater when opening the skull.

decline. A wasting away of the strength of the body. A popular lay term for pulmonary tuberculosis.

declive (L. *declivis*, declivity). A sloping part.

declivis cerebelli (L.). The sloping posterior part of the monticulus of the cerebellar vermis.

decoc·tion (L. *decoquere*, to boil). A liquid preparation obtained by boiling a vegetable substance in water.

decollā·tion (L. *decollare*, to behead). Decapitation, *q.v.*

decollator. An instrument for foetal decapitation.

decolorā·tion (L. *de*, from; *color*, colour). Removal of colour.

decompensā·tion (L. *de*, from; *compensare*, to balance). 1. Failure of compensation. 2. Loss of sufficiency of function, as cardiac or circulatory d.

decomposi·tion (L. *de*, from; *componere*, to unite). 1. The separation of the component elements of a body. 2. Putrefaction.

decompres·sion (L. *de*, from; *comprimere*, to compress). The removal of pressure or compression, as the gradual release of atmospheric pressure practised on the return of caisson workers to the surface. **D. operation:** any operation for the relief of abnormal pressure, as the excision of a portion of a cranial bone in cases of abnormal cerebral pressure such as is caused by a cerebral tumour.

decontaminā·tion (L. *de*, from; *contaminatio*, a mixing). The removal of the clothes and cleansing of the skin of persons exposed to poisonous gases (e.g., mustard gas).

decorticā·tion (L. *de*, from; *cortex*, bark). 1. Removal of the cortex of an organ, especially of the kidney or of the cerebrum. 2. Decapsulation.

dec·rement (L. *decrementum*, decrease). Decline; decrease.

decrĕ·pit (L. *decrepitus*, worn out). Worn out; infirm.

decrĕ·pitude (L. *decrepitus*, worn out). Senile weakness.

decrudes·cence (L. *de*, from; *crudus*, raw). Decline in the severity of a disease.

decrustā·tion (L. *de*, from; *crusta*, crust). The removal of a crust.

decū·bital (L. *decumbere*, to lie). Relating to decubitus.

decū·bitus (L. *decumbere*, to lie). 1. The recumbent or horizontal posture. (2) A bedsore.

decursus fibrarum cerebralium (L.). The descent of the cerebral fibres.

decus·sate (L. *decussare*, from *decussis*, the number ten (X)). To intersect; to interlace.

decussā·tio (L. *decussare*, to divide crosswise, in the form of X). A decussation.

decussā·tion (L. *decussare*, to divide crosswise, in the form of X). An x-shaped crossing; an interlacing or crossing of symmetrical parts, as the crossing of the efferent fibres in the pyramids of the medulla.

dedenti·tion (L. *de*, from; *dens*, tooth). The shedding of teeth.

de d. in d. Abbreviation for L. *de die in diem*, from day to day.

deep. Far inside; away from the surface.

deep X-ray therapy. Irradiation of deep-lying tissues with X-rays.

Deetjen's bodies (Deetjen, N., German physician, 1867–1915). The blood platelets.

defaecā·tion (L. *defaecere*, to purify). The evacuation of the bowels.

defect (L. *deficere*, to fail). An imperfection; absence of a structure or function. Hence defective, imperfect.

defeminā·tion (L. *de*, from; *femina*, female). Loss of female and assumption of male characteristics.

dĕ·ferent (L. *deferens*, from *deferre*, to carry away). Carrying away or down.

dĕ·ferentec·tomy (L. *deferre*, to carry away; *ektomē*, exision). Excision of the vas deferens.

deferenti·tis. Inflammation of the vas deferens.

deferred (L. *differre*, to delay). Delayed. **D. shock:** late onset of shock.

deferves·cence (L. *de*, from; *fervescere*, to grow hot). Abatement of a febrile process.

defibrillā·tion (L. *de*, from; *fibrilla*, dim. of *fibra*). Blunt dissection as in dissection of the brain.

defī·brinate (L. *de*, from; *fibra*, a fibre). To remove fibrin, as in freshly voided blood by stirring.

defibrinā·tion (L. *de*, from; *fibra*, fibre). The removal of fibrin.

deficiency disease. Any condition caused by deficiency of certain food elements, such as vitamins, minerals or protein, in the diet.

defini·tion (L. *definire*, to define). Distinctness, as of an image given by a lens.

defi·nitive (L. *definitivus*, from *definire*, to define). Final; fully developed.

deflagration (L. *de*, from; *flagrare*, to burn). A sudden sparkling combustion.

deflec·tion (L. *de*, from; *flectere*, to bend). A turning aside.

deflorā·tion (L. *de*, from; *florare*, from *flos*, flower). The act of depriving of the state of virginity.

deflū·vium capillor·um (L. *de*, from; *fluere*, to flow; *capillus*, hair). Alopecia.

deform·ing (L. *de*, from; *formare*, from *forma*, shape). Disfiguring.

defor·mity (L. *deformitas*, deformity). Malformation or distortion of a body or of an organ.

defurfurā·tion (L. *de*, from; *furfur*, bran). Desquamation.

degang·lionate. The removal of a ganglion, or ganglia.

degas·sing. Resuscitation of persons overcome by toxic gases.

degĕ·neration (L. *degenerare*). 1. Deterioration, as of a species. 2. Conversion of cells, tissues or organs into structures with inferior function. **Albuminous d.:** cloudy swelling, *q.v.* **Amyloid d.:** wax-like d. caused by the deposition of amyloid within the walls of arterioles, and later within the parenchymatous tissue of certain organs. **Ascending d.:** afferent d. of nerve-fibres. **Calcareous d.:** calcification, *q.v.* **Caseous d.:** caseation, *q.v.* **Cheesy d.:** caseation, *q.v.* **Colloid d.:** an undesirable term for mucoid d. **Cystic d.:** d. with cyst-formation. **Descending d.:** efferent d. of nerve-fibres. **Fatty d.:** cell d. characterized by the appearance of droplets of neutral fat in the cytoplasm occurring under conditions of disturbed cellular oxygen metabolism. See also d., lipoidal; infiltration. **Fibrous d.:** Conversion of specific into fibrous tissue. **Grey d.:** d. of nervous tissue with loss of myelin-sheath and axis-cylinder. **Hyaline d.:** a form of d. affecting chiefly collagenous connective tissue and the fibrous tissue in the walls of blood-vessels, as in arteriosclerosis, characterized by homogeneous swelling of collagen. **Hydropic d.:** distension of epithelial cells with clear fluid, as in acute inflammation of surface epithelium (blisters, smallpox, etc.) due to alteration of the osmotic pressure of the cytoplasm. **Lardaceous d.:** amyloid d. **Lipoidal d.:** cell d. characterized by the appearance of droplets of lipoid substances, mainly cholesterol or cholesterol ester, in the cytoplasm, as in caseous tissue, atheroma, dermoid cysts, xanthoma, etc. **Mucoid d.:** cell d. with excessive secretion of mucin. **Nissl's d.:** see Nissl's d. **Parenchymatous d.:** see cloudy swelling. **Pigmentary d.:** d. with deposition of pigment. **Primary neuronal d.:** d. of a nerve resulting from injury to the nerve cell itself. **Secondary neuronal d.:** d. of the distal part of nervous tissue that has been separated from its cell, characterized by disintegration of the axons and medullary sheath and conversion of the cells of Schwann's sheath into phagocytes removing the remnants of the medullary sheath and axone. Syn. Wallerian d. **Senile d.:** d. due to old age. **Wallerian d.:** see d., secondary neuronal. **Zenker's d.:** see Zenker's d.

degluti·tion (L. *de*, from; *glutire*, to swallow). The act of swallowing.

degradā·tion (L. *de*, from; *gradus*, a step). Degeneration, retrograde metamorphosis.

degrease. Removal of fat, as from the bones when preparing a skeleton.

degree (L. *de*, from; *gradus*, a step). 1. Position in a graded series. 2. A division or interval in a scale, as on a thermometer. 3. A rank conferred by a college or university.

degustā·tion (L. *degustare*, to taste). The act of tasting.

dehis·cence (L. *dehiscere*, to gape). 1. A bursting; an opening. 2. The developmental formation of an opening, e.g., along a suture.

dehū·maniza·tion. The loss of human qualities; brutalization.

dehydrā·tion (L. *de*, from; G. *hudōr*, water). The removal of water from a substance.

dehȳ·drocholic acid. An oxidation product of the naturally occurring cholic acid. Used to increase the volume of bile (hydrocholeretic action).

dehydrō·genase (L. *de*, from; G. *hudōr*, water; *gennan*, to produce). An enzyme widely distributed in animal and vegetable tissues, catalyzing oxidation-reduction reactions by activating hydrogen atoms in a molecule so that these atoms can be 'accepted' by an appropriate substance, the original molecule becoming thereby oxidized and the 'acceptor' reduced.

dehydrogenā·tion (L. *de*, from; G. *hudōr*, water; *gennan* to produce). Oxidation by the action of a dehydrogenase, *q.v.*

dehȳp·notize (L. *de*, from; G. *hupnos*, sleep). To arouse from a hypnotic trance.

Deiter's cells (Deiters, O. F. K., German anatomist, 1834–63). 1. Supporting cells in the organ of Corti attached to the basilar membrane and receiving between their free extremities the hair-cells or cells of Corti of the outer row. 2. Astrocytes or spider-cells of the neuroglia. 3. Nerve-cells of the first type, the neuraxons of which become the axis-cylinders of nerve-fibres. **D.'s formation:** formatio reticularis. **D.'s nucleus:** a large nucleus situated in the oblongata between the inner portion of the cerebral peduncles and the restiform body. **D.'s phalanges:** the phalangeal processes of D.'s cells in the organ of Corti. **D.'s process:** the axis-cylinder process of a nerve-cell; the neuraxon.

déjà vu (F. *déjà*, already; *voir*, to see). Applied to a transitory illusion characterized by a feeling of familiarity on experiencing something new, supposed to be due to forgotten or repressed daydreams that dealt with a similar situation.

dejec·ta (L. *dejicere*, to throw down). Excreted matter, especially the faeces.

dejec·tion (L. *dejicere*, to throw down). 1. A discharge of excretions, especially of faeces. 2. Melancholy.

Déjérine's disease (Déjérine, J. J., French neurologist, 1849–1917). Interstitial neuritis of infancy, producing muscular atrophy.

delactā·tion (L. *de*, from; *lactare*, to give milk). The process of weaning.

delaminā·tion (L. *de*, from; *lamina*, plate). A splitting into layers.

deletēr·ious (G. *dēlētērios*, noxious). Harmful.

Delhi boil. Syn. Oriental sore. *q.v.*

deligā·tion (L. *de*, from; *ligare*, to tie). The application of a ligature.

delimitā·tion (L. *de*, from; *limitare*, to enclose). Determination of limits.

delinquency (L. *delinquentia*, a crime). Antisocial or criminal behaviour, especially in children.

deliques·cence (L. *deliquescere*, to dissolve). Liquefaction of hygroscopic substances by absorption of water from the atmosphere.

deliques·cent (L. *deliquescere*, to dissolve). Liquefying from absorption of atmospheric water.

delī·riant (L. *delirare*, to rave). Causing delirium.

delī·rious (L. *delirare*, to rave). Relating to or suffering from delirium.

delī·rium (L. *delirare*, to rave). A state of confusion (*q.v.*) with motor restlessness, transient hallucinations, disorientation and sometimes delusions. **D. tremens:** acute psychosis due to chronic alcoholism, characterized by disorientation with regard to time and space, visual, haptic and auditory hallucinations, extreme suggestibility, great restlessness, insomnia, fear and a coarse tremor especially of fingers, tongue, facial muscles; usually lasting 3–6 days, and sometimes followed by development of the Korsakow syndrome, *q.v.*

delī·ver (L. *de*, from; *liberare*, to liberate). To free; to remove; to d. a woman of a child or of the afterbirth.

delī·very (L. *de*. from; *liberare*, to liberate). The act of release from something; parturition; childbirth.

delomor·phous (G. *dēlos*, evident; *morphē*, form). Having a definite form; especially applied to the parietal cells of the tubular glands of the stomach.

delta (*delta*, Δ, δ, 4th letter of the Greek alphabet). 1. Any triangular space. 2. Denoting the 4th carbon atom in a chain.

del·toid (G. *delta; eidos*, form). 1. Delta-shaped. 2. A muscle of the shoulder.

deltoi·deus. Deltoid muscle.

delū·sion (L. *de*, from; *ludere*, to play). A false opinion, due to mental disease, the falsity of which cannot be made intelligible to the patient by arguments. **D., expansive; D. de grandeur:** d. in which the patient ascribes to himself eminent qualities, excessive wealth, etc.; occurring especially in general paralysis of the insane.

delū·sional (L. *de*, from; *ludere*, to play). Characterized by delusions.

demag·netize. To remove magnetic qualities.

demarcā·tion (Sp. *demarcar*, to mark out). Delimitation. **Line of d.:** red line forming at the limit of gangrenous area.

Demarquay's symptom (Demarquay, J. N., French surgeon, 1811–75). Immobility or lowering of the larynx during deglutition and phonation; said to indicate syphilitic induration of the trachea.

Dematium. A genus of fungi, of which some varieties have been found in lesions in man.

d'emblée (Fr.). At first onset; applied, e.g., to a mode of nervous discharge in which the number of motor neurons entering the reaction never exceeds that engaged initially.

demedicā·tion (L. *de*, from; *medicari*, to heal). To free the system from drugs.

dement (L. *dementare*, to drive mad). One affected by dementia.

demen·ted (L. *dementare*, to drive mad). Insane; of unsound mind.

demen·tia (L. *de*, from; *mens*, mind). Insanity characterized by marked loss of mental faculties. **D., paralytic:** general paralysis of the insane, *q.v.* **D. paranoides:** a form of schizophrenia, mainly characterized by paranoid delusions. **D. praecox:** schizophrenia, *q.v.* **D., senile:** d. due to organic cerebral changes of old age, characterized by impairment of intellectual functions and loss of interest in the environment. **D., traumatic:** progressive mental impairment, predominantly of the intellectual functions, resulting from structural damage to the brain.

Demerol. Syn. for Pethidine.

demi-bain (Fr.). Sitzbath.

demifacet. One half of an articulation surface adapted to articulate with two bones; e.g., a rib articulating with two thoracic vertebrae.

demi-gauntlet. A special form of bandage used for the hand and fingers.

demi-monstrosity. A variety of congenital deformity which does not prevent the exercise of its function.

dĕ·mineralizā·tion (L. *de*, from; Mediaeval L. *mineralis*, mineral). Abnormal loss of mineral salts.

Dĕ·modex (G. *dēmōs*, fat; *dēx*, worm). A genus of parasitic mites. **D. folliculorum**: a parasite found in sebaceous glands and hair follicles. Hence, **demodec·tic**, relating to Demodex.

demŏ·graphy (G. *dēmos*, people; *graphein*, to write). The statistical study of physical and social conditions of populations.

demonomā·nia (G. *daimōn*, spirit; *mania*, madness). A form of dementia in which the person imagines that he or she is possessed of a devil.

demonophŏ·bia (G. *daimōn*, spirit; *phobein*, to fear). A fear of devils or demons.

dĕ·monstrator (L. *de*, from; *monstrare*, to teach). A teacher for demonstrating dissections or experiments.

De Morgan's spots (De Morgan, C., English physician, 1811–76). Small red spots (capillary telangiectases) in the skin, formerly believed to appear on the skin of patients with cancer.

Demours's membrane (Demours, P., French ophthalmologist, 1702–95). The lamina basalis posterior of the cornea.

demucosā·tion. The removing of mucous membranes.

demul·cent (L. *de*, from; *mulcere*, to stroke). 1. Soothing; allaying irritation of surfaces, especially mucous membranes. 2. A drug, such as a mucilaginous liquid, with d. (1) properties.

De Mussey's point or symptom (de Mussey, N. F. O. G., French physician, 1813–85). A painful spot in cases of diaphragmatic pleurisy. The point is the intersection of a line along the left border of the sternum with another continuous with the 10th rib.

demȳ·elinated (L. *de*, from; G. *muelos*, marrow). Applied to nerve fibres which have lost their myelin sheaths.

demȳelinā·tion (L. *de*, from; G. *muelos*, marrow). Destruction of the myelin sheaths of nerve fibres.

dēnā·ture (L. *de*, from; *natura*, nature). To remove natural or original properties. **Denatured alcohol**: ethyl alcohol, rendered unfit for consumption.

dēnā·turize (L. *de*, from; *natura*, nature). Denature, *q.v.*

den·dric (G. *dendron*, tree). Having dendrites.

den·driform (G. *dendron*, tree; L. *forma*, shape). Branched.

den·drite (G. *dendron*, a tree). A protoplasmic branching process of a nerve-cell body.

dendrit·ic (G. *dendron*, a tree). 1. Branching like a tree. 2. Pertaining to a dendrite. **D. calculus**: a calculus filling and therefore having the shape of renal calyces and pelvis.

den·droid (G. *dendron*, a tree; *eidos*, form). Arborescent; dendritic (1).

dendron (G., a tree). Dendrite, *q.v.*

Deneke's spirillum (Deneke, T., German bacteriologist, born 1860). *Vibrio tyrogenus.*

dener·vated (L. *de*, from; *nervus*, a nerve). Deprived of nerve supply.

dengue (Swahili *kidinga popo*, corrupted to Sp. *dengue*, affectation, prudery, w. ref. to stiff neck). An acute epidemic virus disease of tropical and sub-tropical countries, transmitted by *Aedes aegypti*, *q.v.*, and *Aedes albopictus*, characterized by fever, severe pains in head, eyes, muscles and joints and sometimes a polymorph rash, lasting a few days, recurring after two to three days' interval in usually milder form, and usually followed by protracted convalescence.

denidā·tion (L. *de*, from; *nidus*, nest). The disintegration and shedding of the superficial portion of the uterus, as during menstruation.

Denigès's test (Denigès, G., French chemist, 1859–1935) for formaldehyde in milk. A solution of fuchsin and sodium bisulphite if added to milk containing formaldehyde will give a violet colour when pure hydrochloric acid is added to this mixture.

Denman's evolution, or version (Denman, T., English obstetrician, 1733–1815). A form of version used in cases of shoulder presentation.

Denonvilliers's fascia (Denonvilliers, C. P., French surgeon, 1808–72). The retrovesical fascia between the prostate gland and the rectum.

dens (L.). 1. A tooth. 2. Any tooth-shaped structure, e.g. the tooth-like process of the body of the second cervical vertebra. **D. lacteus**: a milk or temporary tooth. **D. serotinus; D. sapiens**: a wisdom tooth, or third molar tooth.

densĭ·meter (L. *densus*, thick; G. *metron*, measure). An instrument for measuring densities.

den·sity (L. *densitas*, from *densus*, thick). 1. Compactness; the mass of something per unit of volume. 2. The amount of electricity accumulated per unit of surface or volume. See also, gravity, specific. **D., absolute**: ratio between mass and volume of a body. **D., relative**: ratio between mass of a body of a given volume and (1) the weight of the same volume of water, or (2) that of a standard measured under the same conditions.

den·tal (L. *dens*, tooth). Pertaining to the teeth.

den·tate (L. *dentatus*, from *dens*, tooth). Toothed; notched. **d. nucleus**: a large group of nerve cells in the cerebellum.

dentā·tion (L. *dentatus*, from *dens*, tooth). A tooth-shaped projection.

dentā·tum (L. *dentatus*, from *dens*, tooth). The nucleus dentatus cerebelli.

dentia praecox (L.). A condition in which an infant is born with teeth.

dentibuc·cal (L. *dens*, tooth; *bucca*, cheek). Relating to the teeth and the cheek.

denti·culate. Having tooth-shaped projections or dentations.

den·ticule (L. *denticulus*, dim. of *dens*, tooth). A small tooth-like projection.

dentificā·tion (L. *dens*, tooth; *facere*, to make). Formation of teeth.

den·tiform (L. *dens*, tooth; *forma*, shape). Tooth-shaped.

den·tifrice (L. *dens*, tooth; *fricare*, to rub). A substance for cleaning the teeth.

denti·gerous (L. *dens*, tooth; *gerere*, to carry). Containing or bearing teeth.

dentiling·ual (L. *dens*, tooth; *lingua*, tongue). Relating to the teeth and the tongue.

den·tinal (L. *dens*, tooth). Pertaining to or composed of dentine.

den·tine (L. *dens*, tooth). The calcareous structure of the teeth, formed by odontoblasts, surrounding the entire pulp of the cavity except at the opening of the root canal.

dentin·ificā·tion (L. *dens*, tooth; *facere*, to make). Formation of dentine.

dentinī·tis (L. *dens*, tooth). Inflammation of the dentinal tubules.

den·tinoblast (L. *dens*, tooth; G. *blastos*, germ). A dentine-forming cell.

den·tinoid (L. *dens*, tooth; G. *eidos*, form). 1. Resembling dentine. 2. Relating to an odontoma.

dentinō·ma (L. *dens*, tooth). Odontoma, *q.v.*

den·tist (L. *dens*, tooth). A practitioner of dentistry.

den·tistry (L. *dens*, tooth). The science pertaining to the teeth.

denti·tion (L. *dentitio*, from *dentire*, from *dens*, tooth). The development and cutting of the teeth.

den·toid (L. *dens*, tooth; G. *eidos*, form). Resembling a tooth; tooth-shaped.

den·ture (L. *dens*, tooth). 1. The entire set of teeth. 2. A set of artificial teeth.

Denucé's ligament (Denucé, J. H. M., French surgeon, 1859–1924). A short and broad fibrous band in the wrist joint, connecting the radius with the ulna.

denū·cleated (L. *de*, from; *nucula*, dim. of *nux*, nut). Deprived of the nucleus.

denudā·tion (L. *de*, from; *nudare*, from *nudus*, bare). A laying bare or stripping; state of being made bare.

denutri·tion (L. *de*, from; *nutrire*, nourish). 1. A want of nutrition. 2. Atrophy and degeneration of tissue due to malnutrition.

de·odar. The *Cedrus deodara*, a Himalayan tree yielding a medical turpentine.

deō·dorant (L. *de*, from; *odor*, odour). An agent correcting offensive odours.

deō·dorize (L. *de*, from; *odor*, odour). To free from odour.

de-ossificā·tion (L. *de*, from; *os*, bone; *facere*, to make). Absorption of bone.

de-oxidā·tion, de-oxidizā·tion (L. *de*, from; G. *oxus*, sharp). Removal of oxygen.

de-ox·idize (L. *de*, from; G. *oxus*, sharp). To deprive of oxygen.

deoxycor·ticostĕ·rone. See desoxycorticosterone.

de-ox·ygenate (L. *de*, from; *oxus*, sharp; *gennan*, to produce). To deprive of oxygen.

de-oxygenā·tion (L. *de*, from; G. *oxus*, sharp; *gennan*, to produce). Removal or deprivation of oxygen.

depan·creatize (L. *de*, from; *pancreas*). Removal of the pancreas.

deper·sonalizā·tion (L. *de*, from; *persona*). Loss of feeling of personal existence or bodily integrity.

depigmentā·tion (L. *de*, from; *pigmentum*, from *pingere* to paint). Loss or removal of pigment.

dĕ·pilate (L. *depilare*, to pull out hair). To remove hair.

depilā·tion (L. *depilare*, to pull out hair). Removal or loss of hair.

depi·latory (L. *depilare*, to pull out hair). 1. An agent capable of removing hair. 2. Pertaining to such agent.

dĕ·pilous (L. *de*, from; *pilosus*, from *pilus*, hair). Without hair.

deplē·tion (L. *deplere*, to empty). 1. Exhaustion. 2. Loss of any body-material. 3. Loss of a fluid of the body, as the blood. 4. The state resulting from considerable loss of some body-fluid.

deplumā·tion (L. *de*, from; *pluma*, feather). The falling out of the eyelashes.

depolarizā·tion (L. *de*, from; G. *polos*, the axis of the sphere). 1. Prevention or neutralization of polarity. 2. Freeing from polarization.

depō·larize (L. *de*, from; G. *polos*, the axis of the sphere). To deprive of polarity.

depō·larizer (L. *de*, from; G. *polos*, the axis of the sphere). A device affecting, or a substance preventing polarization.

depō·sit (L. *depositum*, from *de*, from; *ponere*, to place). A sediment.

depravā·tion (L. *depravare*, to make crooked). 1. Deterioration. 2. Perversion.

depraved (L. *depravare*). Deteriorated; perverted; vitiated.

depres·sant (L. *deprimere*, to press down). 1. Lowering. 2. A drug lowering functional activity.

depressed. 1. Lowered. 2. Flattened from above. 3. Suffering from depression. **D. fracture:** a fracture in which one fragment is lying below the normal surface.

depres·sion (L. *depressio*, from *de*, from; *premere*, to press). 1. A hollow. 2. Inward or downward displacement. 3. Lowering of functional activity. 4. Emotional derangement resulting in a feeling of dejection and in general inactivity. **D., agitated:** d. or melancholia associated with great restlessness. **D., reactive:** d. conditioned by some environmental or external factor.

depres·somotor. Causing diminished motion.

depres·sor (L. *deprimere*, to press down). A muscle or an instrument that depresses or lowers anything. **D. nerve:** a branch of the vagus nerve, transmitting circulatory and respiratory impulses from the aorta to the medullary centres, resulting in lowering of the blood-pressure or in maintaining its height when other factors tend to elevate it.

deprimens (L. *deprimere*, to press down). Depressing. **D. oculi:** the rectus inferior muscle.

dĕ·purant (L. *de*, from; *purare*, from *purus*, clean). 1. Purifying. 2. A purifying agent or drug.

dĕ·purate (L. *de*, from; *purare*, to purify). To purify.

depū·rative. Depurant, *q.v.*

dĕ·purator. A depurant (2), *q.v.*

deradel·phus (G. *derē*, neck; *adelphos*, brother). A double monster fused in head and chest.

derangement (Fr. *déranger*). Disorder, especially mental disorder.

Dercum's disease (Dercum F. X., American physician, 1856–1931). Adiposis dolorosa.

derencĕ·phalocele (G. *derē*, neck; *egkephalos*, the brain; *kēlē*, tumour). Encephalocele, *q.v.*, through a fissure in the cervical vertebrae.

derencĕ·phalus (G. *derē*, neck; *egkephalos*, the brain). A monster with a rudimentary brain which is enclosed by the upper cervical vertebrae.

dĕ·rivant (L. *derivare*, to divert, from *de*, from; *rivus*, a stream). Derivative; a derivative drug.

derivā·tion (L. *derivare*, to divert). Counter-irritation, *q.v.*

deri·vative (L. *derivare*, to divert). 1. Derived from something primitive or original. 2. Producing derivation.

derma (G.). The true skin or cutis vera, the corium, consisting of the papillary and reticular layers and lying between the epidermis and subcutaneous tissue.

Dermacen·tor (G. *derma*, skin; *kentein*, prick). A genus of ticks. **D. Andersonii:** a tick of the family Ixodidae, transmitting Rocky Mountain fever. **D. variabilis:** the common wood tick, transmitting a mild form of Rocky Mountain spotted fever prevalent in the eastern part of North America.

der·mal (G. *derma*, skin). Pertaining to the skin.

dermă·noplasty (G. *derma*, skin; *ana*, up; *plassein*, to form). Skin-grafting.

dermatatrō·phia (G. *derma*, skin; *atrophia*, from *a*, neg.; *trophein*, to nourish). Atrophy of the skin.

dermatergō·sis (G. *derma*, skin; *ergon*, work). Any occupational skin disease.

dermati·tis (G. *derma*, skin). Inflammation of the skin. **D. artefacta:** 1. D. autophytica, *q.v.* 2. Skin lesions produced by the external action of foreign substances. **D. autophytica:** self-inflicted lesions of the skin. **D., berlock:** d. with subsequent pigmentation caused by application to the skin of perfume containing bergamot oil followed by exposure to sunlight. **D. exfoliativa infantum:** d. with profuse scaly desquamation of the horny layer of the epidermis, leaving moist denuded areas; occurring mainly in infants between the 2nd and 5th week of life. **D. factitia:** d. artefacta, *q.v.* **D. herpetiformis, Duhring:** chronic relapsing d. characterized by the development of intensely itching vesicles, pustules, erythematous and/or various other lesions tending to be grouped in clusters, and eosinophilia. **D. papillaris capillitii:**

chronic disease affecting the neck and adjacent parts of the hairy scalp, characterized by papulo-pustular perifolliculitis followed by keloid-like cicatricial changes with destruction of the smaller pilosebaceous follicles. Syn, sycosis nuchae. **D. pigmentée en forme de coulee:** d. berlock, *q.v.* **D. seborrhoica:** 1. An acute or subacute d., characterized by rounded or irregular reddish patches covered with yellow greasy scales, affecting mainly scalp, face and chest; believed to be caused by pityrosporon of Malassez. 2. D. seborrhoides, *q.v.* **D. seborrhoides:** a form of infantile eczema characterized by epidermal dyskeratosis (associated with a constitutional abnormality of epidermal metabolism) with secondary dermatitis. Syn. eczema seborrhoicum. **D. venenata:** d. due to local irritants of vegetable or mineral origin.

dermato-autoplasty (G. *derma*, skin; *autos*, self; *plassein*, to form). Transplantation of skin taken from the patient's own body.

Dermatobia. A genus of fly. **D. hominis:** a bot-fly of Central America, which deposits its eggs on the body of some arthropod which visits animals or man; the larvae are found in the skin of man or, more frequently, of cattle.

der·matocellulī·tis (G. *derma*, skin; L. *cellula*, dim. of *cella*, a cell). Inflammation of skin and subcutaneous cellular tissue.

der·matoconiō·sis (G. *derma*, skin; *kŏnis*, dust). Any skin disease resulting from contact with dust.

der·matocyst (G. *derma*, skin; *kustis*, bladder). Any skin cyst.

dermatŏ·graphy (G. *derma*, skin; *graphein*, to write). See dermographia.

der·matohĕ·teroplasty (G. *derma*, skin; *heteros*, other; *plassein*, to form). Skin-grafting by means of skin taken from another individual.

der·matoid (G. *derma*, skin; *eidos*, form). See dermoid.

dermatŏ·logist. An expert in the diseases of the skin.

dermatŏ·logy (G. *derma*, skin; *logos*, a treatise). The science of the skin and its diseases.

dermatŏ·lysis (G. *derma*, skin; *luein*, to loosen). A congenital condition characterized by hypertrophy of the skin, which is also loosely attached to the underlying structure, hanging in baggy folds. Syn. cutis laxa.

dermatŏ·ma (G. *derma*, skin). A tumour of the skin.

der·matome (G. *derma*, skin; *tome*, cutting). 1. Area of skin innervated by a single spinal nerve, dermatomere. 2. Instrument for cutting a skin graft.

der·matomere (G. *derma*, skin; *mĕros*, a part). 1. Dorsal portion of mesenchymal somites upon either side of the neural tube. 2. Any segment of skin innervated by one of the spinal nerves.

der·matomycō·sis (G. *derma*, skin; *mukēs*, mushroom). A skin disease caused by a fungus.

dermatomyŏ·ma (G. *derma*, skin; *mus*, muscle). Myoma originating from the non-striped muscle of hair, dermal glands or vessels, occurring especially in the buttocks and extremities, at embryonic fissures, and in the scrotum and labia.

der·matomyosī·tis (G. *derma*, skin; *mus*, muscle). A more or less chronic condition characterized by degenerative rather than inflammatory changes in blood-vessels, skin and muscles, resulting in muscular atrophy and corresponding weakness, sometimes also involving the heart muscle, by marked creatinuria, and sometimes by decalcification of the bones and/or calcinosis; probably closely allied to progressive symmetrical scleroderma.

der·matoneurō·sis (G. *derma*, skin; *neuron*, sinew). Any skin neurosis.

dermatophō·bia (G. *derma*, skin; *phobos*, fear). Fear of contracting a skin disease.

der·matophone (G. *derma*, skin; *phonē*, voice). An instrument used for hearing the blood current in the skin.

der·matophyte (G. *derma*, skin; *phuton*, plant). A group of fungi growing upon skin and mucous membranes, and not invading deeper structures, including the genera Microsporum, Achorion, Trichophyton and Epidermophyton.

dermatŏ·phytid (G. *derma*, skin; *phuton*, plant). Term applied to skin lesions caused by allergy to fungi.

dermatoplă·sty (G. *derma*, skin; *plassein*, to form). Plastic surgery of the skin; replacement of destroyed skin by skin-grafts.

dermatŏ·sis (G. *derma*, skin). Any disease of the skin.

der·matozō·on (G. *derma*, skin; *zōon*, animal). Any animal parasite of the skin.

dermatrō·phia (G. *derma*, skin; *atrophia*, atrophy). Dermatatrophia, *q.v.*

der·mic (G. *derma*, skin). Pertaining to the skin, or formed of skin.

der·mis (G. *derma*, skin). The true skin, the corium.

der·moblast (G. *derma*, skin; *blastos*, germ). The part of the mesoblast from which the corium is formed.

dermocȳ·ma (G. *derma*, skin; *kuma*, foetus). A foetal monster containing another one inside it.

dermogră·phia, dermŏ·graphy, dermogră·phism (G. *derma*, skin; *graphein*, to draw). The development of erythematous streaks or wheals on the skin from tracings made with a blunt instrument.

dermohāē·mia (G. *derma*, skin; *haima*, blood). Hyperaemia of the skin.

dermoid (G. *derma*, skin; *eidos*, form). 1. Resembling skin. 2. A congenital, usually cystic, tumour, derived from an inclusion of dermal tissue along the line of an embryonic fissure, e.g., in the middle line of the chest (mediastinal d.) or abdomen, in the skull (line of attachment of dura mater to tentorium cerebelli, in the line of the thyroglossal or of the craniopharyngeal duct, or of a branchial cleft; characterized by a lining of stratified squamous epithelium and the presence of elements of skin and its accessory structures, including sebaceous glands and hairs, and sometimes nails, bone, cartilage, striated muscle, etc. 3. A usually cystic tumour derived from the implantation of a small piece of skin in the deeper tissues, usually as a result of trauma with a pointed instrument. Syn. implantation cyst, implantation d. **Dermoid cyst:** d. (2) and (3) *q.v.* **D. process:** the nipple-shaped process, covered by stratified epithelium, in the wall of a d. cyst, representing the original d. tumour from which all the other solid elements are derived.

der·moplasty (G. *derma*, skin; *plassein*, to form). See dermatoplasty.

der·mosynovī·tis (G. *derma*, skin; *sun*, with; L. *ovum*, egg). Inflammation of a subcutaneous bursa, together with the adjacent skin.

derodī·dymus (G. *derē*, neck; *didumos*, twin). A double monster with two heads and spines and one trunk.

derris. The dried rhizome and roots of various species of *Derris* found in Burma, Siam, East Indies. From these an insecticide is produced, the most important constituent being rotenone.

desaturā·tion (L. *de*, from; *saturare*, from *satur*, filled). Conversion from a saturated into an unsaturated compound.

Desault's apparatus or bandage (Desault, P. J., French surgeon, 1744–95). A bandage for the arm in fracture of the clavicle, consisting of an axillary pad held by tapes about the neck, a sling for the hand, and two single-headed rollers. **D.'s splint:** one used in fracture of the thigh.

Descartes's body (Descartes, R., French philosopher. 1596–1650). The pineal body or gland.

Descemet's membrane (Descemet, J., French anatomist 1732–1810). The posterior elastic lamina of the cornea.

descemeti·tis. Inflammation of Descemet's membrane.

descemĕ·tocele. Protrusion of Descemet's membrane through a gap in the substantia propria of the cornea.

descen·dens (L.). Having a downward direction.

descending (L. *descendere*, descend). Having a downward direction, e.g., d. current, d. degeneration.

descen·sus (L. *descendere*, descend). Descent; prolapse. **D. testis:** descent of testicle into the scrotum.

Deschamp's needle (Deschamps, L., French surgeon, 1740–1824). A needle on a long handle used when inserting deep sutures.

desensitizā·tion (L. *de*, priv., *sentire*, to perceive). The production of insensitivity to an agent to which the individual has previously been sensitive or hypersensitive; the production of a condition in which antigens injected are neutralized in the blood by circulating antibodies. Syn. anti-anaphylaxis.

desen·sitize (L. *de*, priv.; *sentire*, to perceive). 1. To effect desensitization. 2. To deprive of sensation.

desert sore. Tropical ulcer which appears on the face, back of hands and lower extremities. It is also called veldt sore and Barcoo rot.

dĕ·siccant (L. *desiccare*, to dry up). 1. Causing desiccation. 2. A drying agent.

dĕ·siccate (L. *desiccare*, to dry up). To dry; to become dry.

desiccā·tion (L. *desiccare*, to dry up). The process of drying.

dĕ·siccative (L. *desiccare*, to dry up). Desiccant.

desmectā·sia (G. *desmos*, a ligature; *ekteinein*, to stretch). The stretching of a ligament.

desmī·tis (G. *desmos*, ligature). Inflammation of a ligament.

Desmobacteria. A group of bacteria corresponding to the genus Bacilli.

des·mocyte (G. *desmos*, ligature; *kutos*, a container). Fibroblast. *q.v.*

desmŏ·graphy (G. *desmos*, ligature; *graphein*, to write) A description of the ligaments.

desmoid (G. *desmos*, ligature; *eidos*, form). Resembling a ligament; fibroid. **D. tumour:** 1. Fibroma originating from fascia or tendon, especially from the sheath of the abdominal rectus muscle, tending to infiltrate the muscle, occurring mostly in women who have borne children. 2. A hard, sharply defined, slowly developing nodular fibroma, occurring singly or in small numbers, on trunk or extremities of either sex at any age.

desmŏ·logy (G. *desmos*, ligature; *logos*, treatise). Anatomy of the ligaments.

desmoplas·tic (G. *desmos*, ligature; *plassein*, to form). Promoting the growth of new connective tissue; especially applied to the marked proliferation of connective tissue in cancerous tissue.

desmorrhex·is (G. *desmos*, ligature; *rhēxis*, rupture). The rupture of a ligament.

desmŏ·sis (G. *desmos*, ligature). Any disease of the connective tissue in the body.

des·mosome (G. *desmos*, ligature; *soma*, body). The small central thickening of the intercellular bridges in epithelial tissues. Syn. bridge corpuscle.

desmŏ·tomy (G. *desmos*, ligature; *temnein*, to cut). The dissection of ligaments; the cutting of a ligament.

desoxycorticos·terone. One of the active hormones of the adrenal cortex concerned with life maintenance and electrolyte and water metabolism. It is used in cases of Addison's disease. Syn. DOCA; Deoxycorticosterone.

desoxyhex·ose (G. *oxus*, sharp; *hex*, six). A hexose in which the CHOH group is substituted by a CH_2 group; derived from glycosides, e.g. digitalis and strophanthus.

d'Espine's sign (d'Espine, J. H. A., French physician, 1844–1931). 1. Pectoriloquy heard in the adult below the bifurcation of the trachea and, in the child, below the 7th cervical vertebra; indicates enlargement of hilar lymph glands. 2. Bronchophony over the spinous processes is heard at lower level in pulmonary tuberculosis than in health.

desquamā·tion (L. *desquamare*, from *squama*, a scale). Shedding of the superficial epithelium.

Desvoidea obturbans. A dengue-transmitting mosquito.

deter·gent (L. *detergere*, to wipe away). 1. Cleansing. 2. A remedy used for the removal of crusts, scales, etc., from a surface.

deteriorā·tion (L. *deterior*, worse). The condition of becoming worse.

dethȳ·roidism. A condition arising from the absence of the thyroid gland, or the suppression of its function.

detor·sion (L. *detorquere*, to twist aside). Correction of abnormal curvature; the restoration of a deformed part to its proper position.

detoxicā·tion (L. *de*, priv.; G. *toxicon*, poison). The removal of toxic properties or effects.

detri·tion (L. *deterere*, to wear out). The wearing away by friction or use.

detrī·tus (L. *deterere*, to wear out). Any disintegrated substance.

detrū·sion (L. *detrudere*, to drive out). Displacement; ejection.

detrū·sor (L. *detrudere*, to drive out). 1. Any expelling agent. 2. A muscle serving to expel something. **D. urinæ:** a muscle in front of the pubis which, when it contracts, compresses the bladder.

Dettol. A proprietary disinfectant, whose active constituent is chloroxylenol.

detubā·tion. The removal of a tube.

detumes·cence (L. *detumescere*, to subside). The subsidence of a swelling.

deuteranŏ·pia (G. *deuteros*, second; *an*, priv.; *ops*, eye). Green-blindness, a defect in a factor essential for full colour-vision.

deute·rium (G. *deuteros*, second). A heavy isotope of hydrogen; hydrogen of atomic weight 2. Symbol H^2 or D.

deu·teroplasm (G. *deuteros*, second; *plassein*, to form). The inert nutritional constituents of protoplasm.

deu·teropor·phorin (G. *deuteros*, second; *porphuros*, purple). A compound derived from protoporphyrin by substitution of the two vinyl groups by two H-atoms.

development (Fr. *développer*). Process of maturing.

Deventer's diameter (Deventer, H. van, Dutch obstetrician, 1651–1724). The oblique diameter of the pelvic brim. **D.'s pelvis:** a simple non-rachitic pelvis, with shortened anteroposterior diameter.

Devergie's attitude de combat (Devergie, M. G., French physician, 1798–1879). A posture of a dead body characterized by flexion of the elbows and knees, with closure of the fingers and extension of the ankles. **D.'s disease:** pityriasis rubra pilaris.

deviā·tion (L. *deviare*, to turn aside). Turning aside from the ordinary or normal course or position. **D., average or mean:** in statistics, the arithmetic mean of the deviations of the empirical values from the mean value, added irrespective of their sign. **D., primary:** the d. of the axis of the squinting eye when the sound eye fixes. **D., secondary:** the d. of the axis of the sound eye when the squinting eye fixes. **D., standard:** in statistics, the square root of the mean of the sum of the squares of all deviations from the arithmetic mean of the observations. Syn. root mean square deviation. **D. conjugée:** see conjugated d. **D. of complement:** see complement, d. of.

deviŏ·meter. Instrument for measuring squint deviations.

desviscerā·tion (L. *de*, from; *viscerare*, from *viscus*, bowels). Removal of the viscera.

devī·talizā·tion (L. *de*, from; *vita*, life). Depriving of, or loosing, properties necessary to life.

devolū·tion (L. *devolvere*, to roll down). 1. Retrograde evolution. 2. Degeneration.

dew-point. The temperature at which air is saturated with water-vapour, or more generally at which a vapour begins to be converted into the liquid state.

dexter (L., right). Right; upon the right side.

dextrad (L. *dexter*, right; *ad*, to). Toward the right side.

dextral. Pertaining to the right side.

dex·trase. An enzyme which converts dextrose into lactic acid.

dextrau·ral (L. *dexter*, right; *auris*, ear). 1. Right-eared. 2. Pertaining to the right ear.

dextrin. A polyhexose formed by hydrolysis of starch; $(C_6H_{10}O_5)n$.

dextrocar·dia (L. *dexter*, right; G. *kardia*, heart). Congenital transposition of the heart to the right side of the thorax.

dex·trocar·diogram (L. *dexter*, right; G. *kardia*, heart; *gramma*, letter). That part of a cardiogram showing the action of the right ventricle.

dextrocĕ·rebral (L. *dexter*, right; *cerebrum*, brain). 1. Located in the right cerebral hemisphere. 2. Arising or dependent from the right side of the brain.

dextrŏ·cular (L. *dexter*, right; *oculus*, eye). 1. Right-eyed. 2. Pertaining to the right eye.

dextrorŏ·tatory (L. *dexter*, right; *rotare*, to rotate). Turning the plane of polarization to the right.

dextrose (L. *dexter*, right). Dextroglucose. See glucose.

dex·trosinī·stral (L. *dexter*, right; *sinister*, left). Extending from right to left.

dextrosū·ria (L. *dexter*, right; *ouron*, urine). The presence of dextrose in the urine.

dextrover·sion (L. *dexter*, right; *vertere*, to turn). A turning to the right.

dg. Abbreviation for decigram.

d'Herelle phenomenon (d' Herelle, F. H., French bacteriologist, born 1873). Syn. Twort-d'Herelle phenomenon. See bacteriophage.

dhobie itch (Hind. *dhobie*, laundryman). A term for tinea cruris, *q.v.*, in tropical countries.

di-. Latin prefix meaning twice.

diabē·tes (G. *dia*, through; *bainein*, to go). A disease characterized by polyuria. Employed without qualification, the term indicates d. mellitus. **D., bronzed:** haemochromatosis, *q.v.*, with d. mellitus. **D., experimental:** d. mellitus produced in animals by pancreatectomy or by administration of phlorhizin. **D., innocent:** see glycosuria. **D. insipidus, renal:** a disease characterized by chronic polyuria, polydipsia, and inability to form concentrated urine, caused by a lesion of the posterior part, or of the stem, of the pituitary gland, or of the tuber cinereum. **D. mellitus:** a chronic, often inherited, disease characterized (as now believed by most authorities) by an increased rate of gluconeogenesis, *q.v.*, accompanied by a normal rate of sugar utilization by the tissues, resulting in hyperglycaemia and glycosuria (and therefore polyuria, polydipsia, increased feeling of hunger, and loss of body weight) with or without abnormal ketosis, *q.v.*, due to insufficient secretion of insulin, *q.v.*, or excessive production of an anterior pituitary hormone.

diabet·ic (G. *dia*, through; *bainein*, to go). 1. Pertaining to diabetes. 2. One affected with diabetes.

diabetogen·ic (G. *dia*, through; *bainein*, to go; *gennan*, to produce). Producing diabetes.

diabrot·ic (G. *dia*, through; *bibrōskein*, to eat). 1. Corrosive. 2. A corrosive sublimate.

diacetae·mia (G. *dis*, twice; L. *acetum*, acid; G. *haima*, blood). The presence of diacetic acid in the blood.

diä·cetate (G. *dis*, twice; L. *acetum*, acid). A salt of aceto-acetic acid.

diacet·ic acid (G. *dis*, twice; L. *acetum*, acid). Aceto-acetic acid, *q.v.*

diacetū·ria (G. *dis*, twice; L. *acetum*, acid; G. *ouron*, urine). Urinary excretion of aceto-acetic acid.

diä·chylon (G. *dia*, through; *khulos*, juice). Lead plaster.

diä·cid (G. *dis*, twice; L. *acidus*, sour). Having two acidic groups.

diä·clasis (G. *dia*, through; *klaein*, to break). Breaking a bone over a wedge. Used in cases of rickets where the bone is bent or deformed.

di·ad (G. *dis*, twice). A bivalent radical.

diä·dochokinē·sia (G. *diadokhos*, successor; *kinein*, to move). The normal ability to perform alternative movements in rapid succession, as pronation and supination, or flexion and extension.

dī·agnose. To make a diagnosis, *q.v.*

diagnō·sis (G. *dia*, through; *gnōsis*, knowledge). The recognition of a disease from its signs and symptoms, and the determination of its character.

diagnos·tic (G. *dia*, through; *gnōsis*, knowledge). Serving to make a diagnosis.

dī·agnosti·cian (G. *dia*, through; *gnōsis*, knowledge). One skilled in diagnosing.

diagnŏ·stics (G. *dia*, through; *gnōsis*, knowledge). The science and art of recognising correctly morbid conditions.

dī·agram (G. *diagramma*, a geometrical figure). A sketch giving the essential features of an object.

diagrammat·ic (G. *diagramma*, a geometrical figure). Of the nature of a diagram.

diakinē·sis (G. *dia*, through; *kinein*, to move). The later prophase in the auxocyte.

Dial. Trade name of a preparation of diallylbarbituric acid, used as a hypnotic.

diäl·urate. Any salt of dialuric acid.

dialū·ric acid. Tartronyl urea; a crystalline acid, $C_4H_4N_2O_4$, obtainable from alloxan.

diäl·ysate (G. *dia*, through; *luein*, to loosen). That portion of a substance which has filtered through a semi-permeable membrane.

dīa·lysis (G. *dia*, through; *luein*, to loosen). Filtration through a semi-permeable membrane.

dī·alyzer (G. *dia*, through; *luein*, to loosen). An instrument for performing dialysis.

diä·meter (G. *diametros*). 1. Any straight line passing through the centre of a body or figure. 2. A unit of magnification, equal to the number of times the linear dimensions of an object are increased. **D., biparietal:** line joining the parietal eminences. **D., bitemporal:** line joining the extremities of the coronal suture. **D., fronto-occipital:** line joining the glabella and the protuberantia occipitalis externa. **D., mento-occipital:** line joining the chin and the external occipital protuberance. **D., trachelo-bregmatic:** line joining the centre of the anterior fontanelle and the junction of neck and floor of the mouth. **Diameters, pelvic:—** anteroposterior (of pelvic inlet); line joining the promontorium and the symphysis. Anteroposterior (of the pelvic outlet): line joining the coccygeal tip and the subpubic ligament. See also: conjugate, true; conjugate, external. Transverse (of pelvic inlet): line joining the two most widely separated parts of the pelvic inlet. Transverse (of pelvic outlet): line joining the ischial tuberosities.

dī·amide (G. *dis*, twice; G. *ammoniakon*, sal-ammoniac). A compound containing two –CO NH_2 groups.

diamino-acid. An acid having two amino NH_2 groups.

diamor·phine hydrochlor·ide. Diacetylmorphine hydrochloride. An analgesic similar in action to morphine though it possesses greater addiction properties. Syn. heroin hydrochloride.

di·apedē·sis (G. *dia*, through; *pēdan*, to leap). The passage of blood-corpuscles through unruptured walls of capillaries and venules.

diă·mine (G. *dis*, twice; *ammoniakon*, sal-ammoniac). A compound containing two –NH₂ groups.

di·aphane (G. *dia*, through; *phainein*, to show). A transparent membrane of an organ or cell.

diaphanŏ·meter (G. *dia*, through; *phainein*, to show; *metron*, measure). An instrument for estimating the transparency of fluids.

diaphă·noscope (G. *dia*, through; *phainein*, to show; *skopein*, to view). The illuminating instrument used in diaphanoscopy.

diaphanŏ·scopy (G. *dia*, through; *phainein*, to show; *skopein*, to view). Transillumination of body cavities by an electric light for diagnostic purposes.

diă·phanous (G. *dia*, through; *phainein*, to show). Transparent; transmitting light.

di·aphorē·sis (G. *dia*, through; *phorein*, to carry). Perspiration.

diaphoret·ic (G. *dia*, through; *phorein*, to carry). 1. Causing increased diaphoresis. 2. An agent producing increased diaphoresis.

di·aphragm (G. *diaphragma*, a partition-wall). 1. The muscular wall between the thorax and the abdomen. 2. A thin partitioning membrane or septum. 3. A device for regulating the illumination of an object, as in the microscope by regulating the aperture of the optical system.

diaphragma sellae (G. *diaphragma*, wall; L. *sella*, chair). The dural fold roofing the pituitary fossa.

di·aphragmal·gia (G. *diaphragma*, wall; *algos*, pain). Any diaphragmatic pain.

di·aphragmat·ic (G. *diaphragma*, wall). Pertaining to a diaphragm.

di·aphragmă·tocele (G. *diaphragma*, wall; *kēlē*, hernia). Hernia of a viscus through the diaphragm.

diă·physis (G. *dia*, through; *phuesthai*, to grow). The shaft of a long bone.

diaphysi·tis (G. *dia*, through; *phuesthai*, to grow). Inflammation of a diaphysis.

di·aplex, diaplex·us (G. *dia*, through; L. *plexus*, braid). The choroid plexus of the third cerebral ventricle.

diapŏ·physis (G. *dia*, through; *apo*, from; *phusia*, from *phuēsthai*, to grow). 1. The transverse process of a vertebra. 2. The articular part of a transverse process of a vertebra.

di·arch (G. *dis*, twice; *arkhon*, leader). A type of anastral bipolar spindle in higher plants.

diarrhōe·a (G. *dia*, through; *rheein*; to flow). Frequent evacuation of more or less fluid faeces. **Summer d.:** due to gastro-enteritis or entero-colitis, as occurring in the summer months.

diarthrŏ·sis (G. *dia*, through; *arthroein*, to articulate). A freely movable joint.

diă·schisis (G. *diaskhizein*, to sever). Functional disturbance of a cerebral area due to a lesion of part of it.

diă·schistic (G. *diaskhizein*, to sever). 1. Pertaining to diaschisis. 2. Undergoing both transverse and longitudinal division in meiosis.

Diă·sone. The disodium sulphoxylate derivative of 4:4-diaminodiphenylsulphone.

diastal·sis (G. *dia*, through; *stellein*, to set). The downward moving wave of contraction in the small intestine, preceded by a wave of inhibition.

di·astase (G. *diastasis*, separation). An enzyme found in the secretions of the salivary glands and the pancreas; also present in the germinating seeds of various grains; converting starch into dextrose and maltose. **D.-test:** quantitative estimation of d. in the urine, diagnostic for disturbances in the external secretion of the pancreas as occurring in acute affections of this gland.

diă·stasis (G. *diastasis*, separation). 1. A separation of bones without fracture, as of the pubic bones at the symphysis. 2. An incomplete dislocation, *q.v.*, in which the separation occurs only in a plane perpendicular to that of the articular surface. 3. A gap between the inner borders of the musculi recti abdominis.

di·astem, diastē·ma (G. *disatēma*, an interval). 1. A modified cytoplasm in the equatorial plane through which the cytosome divides in mitosis. 2. A vacant space or gap, as between teeth.

diastem·atocrā·nia (G. *diastēma*, interval; *kranion*, skull). Congenital longitudinal fissure of the cranium.

diastem·atomyē·lia (G. *diastēma*, interval; *muelos*, marrow.) Congenital splitting of part or all of the spinal cord, a minor degree of diplomyelia, *q.v.*

di·aster (G. *dis*, twice; *astēr*, star). The structure formed by the daughter chromosomes grouped near the poles of the spindle, during the later stages of the anaphase in mitosis. Syn. amphiaster.

diă·stolē (G., a drawing asunder). The period of dilatation of the heart-chambers following the systole.

diastol·ic (G. *diastolē*, a drawing asunder). Pertaining to or occurring during the diastole of the heart.

diather·mal, diather·mic, diather·matous (G. *dia*, through; *thermē*, heat). 1. Applied to bodies through which radiant heat can pass without becoming absorbed. 2. Pertaining to diathermy.

di·athermy (G. *dia*, through; *thermē*, heat). The method of increasing the temperature of the tissues beneath the skin by applying to the surface high-frequency currents, part of the electric energy of which is converted into heat by the resistance offered to the current by the body tissues.

diă·thesis (G. *dia*, through; *tithenai*, to put). A constitutional predisposition to a particular disease.

diathet·ic. Pertaining to diathesis.

diătomē·a (G. *dis*, twice; *atomos*, atom). A class of unicellular algae.

diatom·ic (G. *dis*, twice; *atomos*, atom). Consisting of two atoms. 2. Having two replaceable atoms or radicals.

diă·zo compounds (G. *dis*, twice; *a*, neg.; *zoe*, life). Organic compounds having a group of two N atoms, formed by the action of nitrous acid upon salts of certain aromatic amines.

diazotizā·tion. The process of converting into a diazo compound.

dibă·sic (G. *dis*, twice; *basis*, a base). 1. Doubly basic; of a salt, having two atoms of a monobasic element or radical; of an acid, having two hydrogen atoms replaceable by basic atoms or radicals; of a base, having two hydroxyl groups.

dibla·stula (G. *dis*, twice; *blastos*, germ). Gastrula, *q.v.*

Dibŏth·riocě·phalus latus (G. *dis*, twice; *bothros*, a pit; *kephalē*, head; L. *latus*, broad). Diphyllobothrium latum, *q.v.*

dibrō·mide (G. *dis*, twice; *brōmos*, a foetid odour). A compound containing two atoms of bromine combined with an element or radical.

dibū·tyl phthă·late. The dibutyl ester of phthalic acid. Used as an insect repellant.

dicarbox·ylic (G. *dis*, twice; L. *carbo*, coal; G. *oxus*, sharp). Having two carboxyl groups.

dicě·phalus (G. *dis*, twice; *kephalē*, head). A double-headed monster.

dichlor·ide (L. *dis*, twice; *khlōros*, pale green). A compound containing two atoms of chlorine combined with an element or radical.

dichŏ·tomy (G. *dikha*, asunder; *tomē*, section). 1. Division into two equivalent parts or branches. 2. The unethical practice of fee-splitting between the consultant and the practitioner who referred the patient to him.

I

dichrō·ic (G. *dis*, twice; *khrōma*, colour). Exhibiting or referring to dichroism.

di·chroism (G. *dis*, twice; *khrōs*, colour). 1. The phenomenon of bodies presenting different colours by transmitted light when viewed in two different directions. 2. The phenomenon of presenting different colours according to the degree of concentration or thickness of the layer through which light is transmitted.

dichrō·mate. Any salt of dichromic acid.

dichromat·ic (G. *dis*, twice; *khrōma*, colour). 1. Having two colours. 2. Dichroic. 3. Applied to the colour-sensations of one affected by dichromatopsia.

dichrō·matism (G. *dis*, twice; *khrōma*, colour). 1. Condition of being dichromatic. 2. Dichromatopsia, *q.v.* 3. Dichroism, *q.v.*

dichromatop·sia (G. *dis*, twice; *khrōma*, colour; *opsis*, vision). Form of colour-blindness in which not more than two of the primary colours (red, green or blue) can be recognized.

Dick test (Dick, G. F., born 1881, and Dick, Gladys H., born 1881, American physicians). A test for cases susceptible to scarlet fever. An intracutaneous injection of a filtrate of a culture of haemolytic streptococci produces a circular erythematous area after four to six hours in positive cases.

Dickey's fibres or suspensory ligament (Dickey, J. S., Irish anatomist, 1882–1912). The fibres derived from the tendon of the scalenus anterior that pass to the cervical pleura.

diclidī·tis (G. *diklis*, folding-door). Inflammation of any valve.

diclidostō·sis (G. *diklis*, folding-door; *osteon*, bone). Ossification in the valves of veins.

diclidŏ·tomy (G. *diklis*, folding-door; *tomē*, section). Incision into a valve.

dicor·ia (G. *dis*, double; *kŏrē*, pupil of the eyes). Double pupil.

dicou·marol. Methylene-bis-4-hydroxycoumarin, a substance producing prolongation of the prothrombin and coagulation times of the blood.

dicrot·ic (G. *dis*, twice; *krotos*, a beat). Pertaining to dicrotism.

dǐ·crotism (G. *dis*, twice; *krotos*, a beat). The condition of the pulse in which two beats can be felt after each cardiac systole; normally a second wave can be traced in the sphygmogram, but it is too small to be felt by the palpating finger.

dic·tyocyte (G. *diktuon*, a net; *kutos*, a container). A polygonal mesenchymal cell, with numerous short projections, non-granular, neutrophil or faintly basophil cytoplasm, a round or oval nucleus with a large nucleolus, producing reticulin and always found in close association with active reticulin formation.

dictyŏ·ma. Diktyoma, *q.v.*

dic·tyosomes (G. *diktuon*, net; *sōma*, body). The fragments collecting around the poles of the spindle during the final meiotic division, originating from the Golgi body.

didac·tylism (G. *dis*, twice; *daktulos*, finger). The presence of but two digits on a hand or foot, especially when congenital.

didel·phic (G. *dis*, twice; *delphus*, uterus). Having a double uterus and double vagina.

didymī·tis (G. *didumos*, twin). Inflammation of the testicle.

dǐ·dymus, dǐ·dymous (G. *didumos*, twin). 1. Twin. 2. Twin-monster. 3. Testicle.

dieb. alt. Abbreviation for L. *diebus alternis*, on alternate days.

Dieffenbach's operation (Dieffenbach, J. F., German surgeon, 1792–1842). An early operation for amputation at the hip joint. An elastic ligature was placed round the upper part of the thigh and a circular incision was made below this.

di-elec·tric (G. *dia*, through; *ēlektron*, amber). Any insulator in an electric field, so called because the field-lines pass through it. **D. constant:** a factor in the formula expressing the force between two electric charges separated by an insulator.

diencĕ·phalon (G. *dia*, through; *egkephalos*, brain). The interbrain, comprising thalamus, subthalamus, hypothalamus, epithalamus and metathalamus.

dienōē·strol. An artificial oestrogen.

diet (G. *diaita*, diet). The food-intake of an individual.

di·etary. 1. A special method of nutrition. 2. Pertaining to diet.

dietet·ic. Pertaining to diet.

dietet·ics. The science of nutrition.

dī·etist, dietǐ·cian, dietǐ·tian. An expert in matters relating to diet.

diĕ·thylstil·boestrol. U.S.P. name for stilboestrol.

Dietl's crises (Dietl, J., Austrian physician, 1804–78). Paroxysms of gastric distress and severe lumbar abdominal pain occurring in nephroptosis.

Dieudonné's medium (Dieudonné, A., German physician, born 1864). An alkaline medium for bacterial cultures.

Dieulafoy's aspirator (Dieulafoy, G., French physician, 1839–1911). A special glass syringe with a two-way cock, used for aspirating fluid from the chest. **D.'s triad:** muscular rigidity, tenderness and hyperaesthesia over the appendix area in cases of appendicitis.

difference of potential. A difference of electric potential, *q.v.* of two points in an electric field or circuit, measured in volts.

differen·tial (L. *differentia*, from *differre*, to differ). Relating to difference or differentiation. **D. blood count:** the count of the relative numbers of each of the various types of white blood corpuscles. **D. diagnosis:** a diagnosis based on the distinction between the characteristics of similar diseases or syndromes.

differentiā·tion (L. *differre*, to differ). 1. Distinguishing or differentiating. 2. A specialized development of structures or functions.

diffrac·tion (L. *diffringere*, to shatter). The departure from linear propagation of light or other wave phenomena when passing an obstacle of any character, e.g. when striking the edge of a narrow opening.

diffuse (L. *diffundere*, to scatter). Scattered; not localized, e.g., d. inflammation. **D. sclerosis:** a term covering various both sporadic and familial diseases, often of early manifestation, characterized by widespread demyelination of the white matter of the cerebral hemispheres, resulting in visual failure, mental deterioration and spastic paralysis, *q.v.* Syn. Schilder's disease, Pelizaeus-Merzbacher's disease, leucodystrophia cerebri progressiva.

diffū·sible (L. *diffundere*, to scatter). 1. Capable of diffusing. 2. Capable of being diffused.

diffusiŏ·meter (L. *diffundere*, to scatter; G. *metron*, measure). An instrument used for measuring diffusion speeds.

diffū·sion (L. *diffundere*, to scatter). A spreading or scattering out; propagation. **D. circle:** the imperfect image formed by incomplete focalization. **D. constant:** the number of cc. of a substance passing a membrane per mm. pressure difference.

digamet·ic (G. *dis*, twice; *gamein*, to marry). Having or producing two kinds of gametes, especially male-producing and female-producing gametes.

digas·tric (G. *dis*, twice; *gastēr*, belly). 1. Having two bellies, as the d. muscle. 2. Relation to the d. muscle.

digas·tricus (G. *dis*, twice; *gastēr*, stomach). The digastric muscle (see muscles).

Digĕ·nea (G. *dis*, twice; *gennan*, to produce). A sub-class of endoparasitic trematodes; developing through a coupled series of stages involving alternation of hosts, one of which is always a mollusc, and alternation of generations.

digĕ·nesis (G. *dis*, twice; *gennan*, to produce). Reproduction by alternation of sexual and asexual generation.

digenet·ic. 1. Relating to digenesis. 2. Relating to Digenea.

di·gerent. Digestant, *q.v.*

digest (L. *digerere*, to digest). 1. To convert into absorbable condition. 2. In pharmacy, the extraction of soluble substances in a hot medium.

digĕ·stant (L. *digerere*, to digest). Any substance promoting digestion.

digĕ·stion (L. *digerere*, to digest). 1. The change of food in the organism prior to absorption; the dissolution of food and its disintegration into simpler compounds. 2. The processes leading to 1.

digĕ·stive (L. *digerere*, to digest). Pertaining to or promoting digestion. **D. tract:** the alimentary canal, from the mouth to the anus.

digĭ·lanide. The glycoside derived from *Digitalis lanata*.

digit (L. *digitus*). A finger or toe.

di·gital (L. *digitus*, digit). Pertaining to the fingers or toes.

digitā·lin. A cardiac glycoside from the seeds of *Digitalis purpurea*.

digitā·lis. Foxglove leaves from the plant *Digitalis purpurea*. The leaves are 15 to 30 centimetres long and up to 15 centimetres broad. Odour faint. Taste very bitter, unpleasant. **Tincture of d.:** digitalis leaves in 70 per cent. alcohol. Dose 5 to 15 minims. This drug is given in cases of cardiac disorder. (Name derived from finger-like flowers.)

digitalizā·tion. To bring under the influence of digitalis.

di·gitate (L. *digitatus*, from *digitus*, finger). Having finger-like branches or processes.

digitā·tion. 1. State of being digitate. 2. A finger-like process.

di·gitus (L.). A finger or toe.

diglos·sia (G. *dis*, twice; *glōssa*, tongue). The state of having a bifid tongue.

dignā·thus (G. *dis*, twice; *gnathos*, jaw). A monster with two lower jaws.

dīhÿ·drate (G. *dis*, twice, *hudōr*, water). 1. A compound containing two molecules of water. 2. Sometimes also applied to a compound containing two hydroxyl groups.

dihÿ·dromor·phinone hydrochlor·ide. An analgesic allied to morphine. Syn. dilaudid hydrochloride.

dihÿ·drotachystĕ·rol. A reduction product of tachysterol, an intermediate irradiation product of ergosterol. It increases serum calcium and urinary excretion of phosphates. Used in idiopathic and hypoparathyroid tetany; it has no antirachitic activity. Syn. A.T.10.

dihÿstĕ·ria (G. *dis*, twice; *hustera*, uterus). Dimetria, *q.v.*

di-iodide (G. *dis*, twice; *iōdēs*, from *ion*, a violet). A compound containing two atoms of iodine combined with an element or radical.

diktÿō·ma (G. *diktuon*, net). Epithelial tumour growing from the ciliary body, having the structure of the embryonic retina, occurring in young children.

dil (L. *diluere*). Abbreviation for *dilutus*, diluted.

dī·lacerā·tion (L. *dilaceratio*, from *dis*, asunder; *lacerare*, from *lacer*, torn). 1. A tearing apart. 2. Discission, *q.v.*, of a membranous cataract by tearing the membranes apart. 3. Distortion of a tooth due to any injury during its development which did not interfere with its subsequent calcification.

dilatā·tion (L. *dilatare*, to widen). Expansion, enlargement, especially of a cavity or a canal.

dilate. To enlarge, to expand, to spread apart.

dilā·tor. 1. An instrument for enlarging a part such as lacrimal, oesophageal or uterine dilator. 2. A dilating muscle.

dilaudid hydrochloride. See dihydromorphinone hydrochloride.

di·luent (L. *diluere*, to dilute). Diluting; effecting dilution.

dilū·tion (L. *diluere*, to dilute). 1. The lowering of the strength of a solution, e.g. by addition of water. 2. A diluted liquid.

dī·merous (G. *dis*, twice; *meros*, part). Composed of two parts. Syn. bipartite.

dimepac·rol. 2:3-dimercaptopropanol, used in acute poisoning due to arsenic, mercury and gold. Syn. British Anti-Lewisite (B.A.L.).

dimĕ·thyl (G. *dis*, twice; *mĕta*, with; *hulē*, wood). 1. Ethane. 2. Any compound containing two methyl groups. **D. phthǎlate:** The same action and uses as dibutyl phthalate, *q.v.*

dimĕ·tria (G. *dis*, twice; *mētra*, womb). The state of having a double uterus.

diminū·tion (L. *diminuere*, to lessen). 1. Reduction in amount or degree. 2. Elimination of part of the nucleus, as in the formation of the primordial germ-cells.

dimor·phic. Dimorphous, *q.v.*

dimor·phism (G. *dis*, twice; *morphē*, form). 1. Difference in form. 2. Occurrence under two different forms.

dimor·phous (G. *dis*, twice; *morphē*, form). Pertaining to or characterized by dimorphism.

dimple. A small depression.

dinēur·ic (G. *dis*, twice; *neuron*, sinew). Having two axons.

dī·odone. The diethanolamine salt of 3:5-diiodo-4-pyridone-N-acetic acid, an X-ray contrast medium for examination of the urinary tract.

diō·doquin. 5:7-diiodo-8-hydroxyquinoline; used in the treatment of amoebiasis.

diōe·strum, diōe·strus (G. *dis*, twice; *oistros*, a sting). A short quiescent interval between two oestral periods within the oestrous cycle.

dioptō·meter (G. *diopsesthai*, to see through; *metron*, measure). An instrument for determining ocular refraction.

dioptō·scopy (G. *diopsesthai*, to see through; *skopein*, to view). A method of estimating refraction by means of the ophthalmoscope.

diop·tral (G. *dioptra*, an optical measuring instrument). Relating to a dioptre; expressed in dioptrics.

diop·tre (G. *dioptrikos*, from *dioptra*, an optical measuring instrument). The unit of measurement of refractive power of a lens with a focal distance of one metre.

diop·tric (G. *dioptrikos*, from *dioptra*, an optical measuring instrument). 1. Pertaining to dioptrics. 2. Pertaining to a dioptre.

diop·trics (G. *dioptrikos*, from *dioptra*, an optical measuring instrument). Branch of optics dealing with refraction.

diop·try. See dioptre.

dī·ose (G. *dis*, twice; mod. suffix -ose from words formed as glucose, from *glukus*, sweet). A monosaccharide with two carbon atoms in the chain.

diox·ide (G. *dis*, twice; *oxus*, sharp). Any oxide containing two atoms of oxygen.

di·phallus (G. *dis*, twice; *phallos*, membrum virile). A monster having a double penis.

diphā·sic (G. *dis*, twice; *phasis*, from *phainein*, to show). Occurring in two phases.

diphenan. *p*-benzylphenylcarbonate. An anthelmintic used especially against threadworms.

diphthē·ria (G. *diphthera*, membrane). An acute infectious disease caused by corynebacterium diphtheriae and characterized by fever, formation of pseudo-membranes on mucous membranes, especially of the upper respiratory tract, and sometimes by pareses.

diphther·ic, diphtherit·ic (G. *diphthera*, membrane). Pertaining to diphtheria.

diph·theroids (G. *diphthera*, membrane; *eidos*, form). A group of usually non-pathogenic bacilli, differing also from diphtheria bacillus in their fermentative reactions on carbohydrates and in not producing exotoxin.

diphthon·gia. Diplophonia, *q.v.*

Di·phyllobothrī·inae (G. *dis*, twice; *phullon*, a leaf; *bothros*, a pit). A group of tapeworms of the order Pseudo-phyllidea.

Diphyllobothrium latum (G. *dis*, twice; *phullon*, leaf; *bothros*, a pit; L. *lātus*, broad). A tapeworm of the group Diphyllobothriinae, requiring two intermediate hosts for its development, a fresh-water crustacean and a fresh-water fish (e.g. the pike). In the adult stage it is a parasite of man, dog, cat, pig and fox; it is one of the largest of the tapeworms, attaining commonly a length of 30 feet; in a small percentage of persons harbouring the parasite it gives rise to an anaemia indistinguishable from pernicious anaemia, curable by the expulsion of the worm. Syn. Dibothriocephalus latus; Bothriocephalus latus.

dǐ·phyodont (G. *di*, two; *phuein*, to produce; *odous*, tooth). Having a first dentition, which is shed, followed by a second, permanent one.

diplacū·sis (G. *diploos*, double; *akousis*, a hearing). Double hearing; the hearing of one sound as two, probably due to a lesion of the organ of Corti. **D. binauralis dysharmonica**: the hearing of the same sound at a different pitch by each ear. **D. b. echotica**: the hearing of a sound a fraction of a second later by one ear than by the other. **D. monauralis dysharmonica**: the hearing of a pure tone by one ear as a double tone of two different pitches.

diplē·gia (G. *dis*, twice; *plēgē*, stroke). Paralysis of symmetrical parts. **D., cerebral**: a condition characterized by spastic paralysis, frequently limited to the lower limbs, often associated with attacks of generalized convulsions and/or mental deficiency, due to primary neuronal degeneration in more or less symmetrical regions of the brain beginning during foetal or early post-foetal life. Syn. Little's disease.

diplobacil·lus (G. *diploos*, double; L. *bacillus*, dim. of *baculus*, a stick). A bacillus which is found in pairs.

diplobactē·rium (G. *diploos*, double; *baktērion*, dim. of *baktron*, a stick). Two bacteria adhering to each other to form a paired organism.

diploblast·ic (G. *diploos*, double; *blastos*, germ). Having two germinal layers.

diplocē·phalus (G. *diploos*, double; *kephalē*, head). A monster with two heads.

Dip·lococcus (G. *diploos*, double; *kokkos*, berry). Any one of those cocci which divide in one direction only and remain attached in pairs.

diplocōr·ia (G. *diploos*, double; *korē*, pupil of the eye). Double pupil.

dip·loē (G. *diploē*, fold). The spongious bony tissue between the cranial tables.

diplogě·nesis (G. *diploos*, double; *gennan*, to produce). The development of two parts instead of one, as in a double monster.

diplō·ic (G. *diploē*, fold). Relating to the diploe. **D. veins**: the veins between the two tables of the skull, a system of venous spaces freely communicating with one another.

dip·loid (G. *diploos*, double; *eidos*, form). 1. Doubly arranged. 2. Having the haploid or genetic number of chromosomes doubled, as in somatic cells.

diplō·ma (G., a folded paper). A document of graduation from an authorized body or council.

diplomyē·lia (G. *diploos*, double; *muelos*, marrow). Congenital doubling of part of the spinal cord.

diplonē·ma (G. *diploos*, double; *nēma*, thread). The auxocyte-spireme in the diplotene, *q.v.*, stage of meiosis.

dip·lophase (G. *diploos*, double; *phasis*, phase). The phase in which the nuclei are diploid, as in the sporophyte.

diplophō·nia (G. *diploos*, double; *phōnē*, voice). The synchronous production of two notes in the larynx, caused, e.g., by unilateral paresis of the vocal cords. Syn. diphthongia.

diplō·pia (G. *diploos*, double; *opsis*, vision). Double vision; the vision of one object as two.

diploscope (G. *diploos*, double; *skopein*, to view). An instrument for the investigation of binocular vision.

dip·losome (G. *diploos*, double; *sōma*, body). 1. Any small double body cell, as a pair of centrioles in which the auxocytespireme is longitudinally double. 2. Any one of the two structures into which, in animal cells, the centrosome divides during the prophase in mitosis.

dip·lotene (G. *diploos*, double; *tainia*, a riband). Applied to that stage in meiosis following the pachytene stage.

Dippel's animal oil (Dippel, J. K., German physician, 1673–1734). Oleum cornu cervi. Obtained by distilling bone and deer's horn.

diprosō·pic (G. *dis*, twice; *prosōpon*, face). Doubling of the face.

diprosō·pus (G. *dis*, twice; *prosōpon*, face). A monster with complete or partial doubling of the face.

dipsē·sis (G. *dipsa*, thirst). Extreme thirst.

dipsomā·nia (G. *dipsa*, thirst; *mania*, madness). Periodic alcoholism.

Dip·tera (G. *dis*, twice; *pteron*, wing). An order of insects including the flies and mosquitoes.

dip·terous (G. *dis*, twice; *pteron*, wing). 1. Possessing two wings or winglike processes. 2. Pertaining to the diptera.

dipȳ·gus (G. *dis*, twice; *pugē*, rump). A monster with doubling of the lower part of the trunk.

direct (L. *directus*, from *dirigere*, to straighten). Immediate; in a straight line. **D. current**: see current, d. **D. vision**: vision with the macula lutea, i.e. upon fixation of the subject.

direc·tor (L. *dirigere*, to straighten). A grooved instrument to direct a knife.

direc·toscope (L. *directus*; G. *skopein*, to view). An instrument used for the examination of the larynx.

disăc·charide (G. *dis*, twice; *sakkhar*, sugar). Any carbohydrate composed of two monosaccharide molecules less the elements of one molecule of water; of the formula $C_n (H_2O)_{n-1}$.

disarticulā·tion (L. *dis-*, apart; *articulus*, dim of *artus*, joint). Amputation of a limb at the joint.

disassimilā·tion (L. *dis-*, away; *assimilare*, to make like). Catabolism, *q.v.*

disc (G. *diskos*, quoit). 1. A circular plate or surface. 2. The optic papilla, the section of the optic nerve at its entrance into the eyeball as seen with the ophthalmoscope. 3. A small tablet for ocular medication. **D., accessory**: in skeletal muscle, a stripe bisecting the portion of the intermediate d., *q.v.*, between the telophragma and the succeeding anisotropic d. **D., intercalated**: straight, step-like or serrated lines extending across muscle fibre peripheral to the axial sarcoplasm, found in the heart of all animals down to and including teleost fish, probably produced irreversibly by the rhythmic contraction of the muscle. **D., intermediate**: the lighter or isotrope d. of a muscle fibre. **D., intervertebral**: the fibro-cartilaginous layer between the vertebrae. **D., theminal:** the median portion of the intermediate d., *q.v.* **D., transverse:** the dark or anisotropic d. in a muscle fibre.

discharge. 1. A morbid secretion. 2. The flowing of such a secretion. 3. The giving off of energy, e.g. of electricity.

dis·ciform (G. *diskos*, quoit; L. *forma*, shape). Disc-shaped.

discis·sion (L. *dis*, apart; *scindere*, to cleave). Incision into the capsule of the crystalline lens or into the lens itself in the operation for soft or membraneous cataract; allowing thus the aqueous humour to enter and to cause swelling, disintegration and eventually absorption of the lenticular fibres.

disci·tis (G. *diskos*, quoit). Inflammation of a disc.

discoid, discoi·dal (G. *diskos*, quoit; *eidos*, form). Disc-shaped. **D. cleavage:** cell division occurring only at the surface of a large yolk-mass.

dis·coplacen·ta (G. *diskos*, quoit; L. *placenta*, a cake). A disc-shaped placenta, as in man, apes and rodents.

discrete (L. *discretus*, from *discernere*, to separate). Separate; not confluent.

discus (L.) A disc.

discū·tient (L. *discutere*, dissipate). Scattering.

disdī·aclast (G. *dis*, twice; *dia*, through; *klaein*, to break). Any one of the doubly refractive elements of the contractile substance of muscular fibres.

disease (Old Fr. *desaise*, sickness). A process disturbing structure and/or function of the body, systemically or locally.

disengage·ment (L. *dis-*, apart; Fr. *engager*, engage). Emergence from a confined condition, as of the foetal head from the vaginal canal in parturition.

disinfect (L. *dis-*, apart; *inficere*, to taint). To destroy pathogenic organisms.

disinfec·tant (L. *dis-*, apart; *inficere*, to taint). An agent destroying pathogenic organisms.

disinfec·tion (L. *dis-*, apart; *inficere*, to taint). The destruction of all organisms and their products which are capable of producing disease. **Concurrent d.:** the regular d. of infective material throughout the course of a disease. **Terminal d.:** d. of material and rooms after the termination of an infective disease.

disinfestā·tion (L. *dis-*, apart; *infestare*, to attack). 1. Making free from insect or animal parasites. 2. Delousing.

disinvā·gination (L. *dis-*, apart; *in-*, into; *vagina*, a sheath). The undoing of an invagination.

disjoint. Disarticulate.

disjunc·tive (L. *disjungere*). Disjoining; applied to movements of the eyes when the fixation lines are moved out of parallelism, as in convergence or divergence.

disk. See disc.

disloca·tion (L. *dis-*, apart; *locare*, from *locus*, place). Displacement of one or more bones of a joint, or of an organ, from its normal position. **D., central:** d. of the femur in which the head has penetrated the fractured acetabulum. **D., complete:** d. in which contact between the articular surfaces has been lost. **D., complicated:** d. associated with injury to adjacent tissues. **D., compound:** d. in which a communication between the joint and the external air has been produced by injury to the soft parts. **D., double:** d. involving both ends of a bone. **D., iliac:** d. of the femur in which the head lies on the iliac bone. **D., infra-acromialis:** d. of the lateral clavicular end below the acromion. **D., infraglenoid:** anterior d. of the humerus head. **D., obturator:** d. of the femur in which the head lies at the obturator foramen on the external obturator muscle. **D., perineal:** d. of the femur in which the head lies in the perineum. **D., pubic:** d. of the femur in which the femur head lies on the superior ramus of the pubic bone against the ileopec-

tineal eminence. **D., sciatic:** d. of the femur in which the head lies on the sciatic notch. **D., subclavicular:** d. of the humerus in which the head is displaced below the clavicle, usually associated with fracture of the great tuberosity or the coracoid process and tearing the muscles attached to it. **D., subcoracoid:** d. of the humerus in which the head rests below the coracoid process upon the neck of the scapula. **D., subglenoid:** d. of the humerus in which the head is displaced on the axillary border of the scapula below the glenoid cavity, usually associated with compression of the axillary vessels. **D., subspinous:** 1. D. of the humerus in which the head rests on the posterior surface of the neck of the scapula. 2. D. of the femur in which the head rests below the anterior inferior iliac spine. **D., subtalar:** d. between the talus, calcaneus and naviculare in which the talus retains its normal relationship with the malleoli. **D. supraclavicular:** d. of the outer end of the clavicle above the acromion. **D., supracoracoid:** d. of the humerus in which the head rests above the coracoid process, usually accompanied by fracture of the acromion. **D., suprapubic:** d., pubic, *q.v.*

disordered action of the heart. See effort syndrome.

disorganizā·tion (L. *dis-*, apart; G. *organon*, instrument). Loss or absence of structural integrity.

disor·ientā·tion (L. *dis-*, apart; *oriens*, east, from *oriri*, to arise). Loss of the ability to locate oneself with regard to space and/or time.

dis·par (L.) Unequal.

dis·parate (L. *disparare*, to separate). Unequal; not indentical; not corresponding. **D. points:** non-corresponding points of the two retinae.

dispā·rity (L. *dispar*). Inequality; difference.

dispen·sary (L. *dispensare*, to weigh out). 1. Out-patients' clinic. 2. Any place where medicines are dispensed.

dispen·sing (L. *dispensare*, to weigh out). The preparing and issuing of drugs ordered in a prescription.

di·sperme (G. *dis*, twice; *sperma*, seed). The entrance of two spermatozoa into an egg.

disperse (L. *dispergere*, from *dis-*, apart; *spargere*, to scatter). Scattered. **D. phase:** see colloid. **D. system:** any substance containing at least one d. phase.

dispersidŏ·logy (L. *dispergere*, to disperse; G. *logos*, discourse). The chemistry of colloids.

disper·sion (L. *dispergere*, to disperse). Scattering. **D. of light:** the separation of light into its unicoloured components, arising from their difference in refraction or diffraction.

dispī·rem, dispī·reme (L. *dis-*, apart; G. *speira*, coil). The two spiremes in mitosis formed from the dividing nucleus.

displace·ment. 1. A position other than the normal. 2. The act of displacing. 3. In psychoanalysis, a process by which one idea may surrender to another the whole volume of its cathexis, *q.v.* (as observed especially in obsessional neuroses), or a replacement in the affective life of one idea by another which is more satisfactory and acceptable, or the shifting of sexual energy from one pathway to another (as in exhibitionism).

disposi·tion (L. *disponere*, to arrange). Susceptibility in respect of certain diseases or reactions. Syn. diathesis.

disrup·tive (L. *disrumpere*, to burst). Bursting.

dissect (L. *dissecare*, to cut up). To separate; to make a dissection.

dissecting (L. *dissecare*, to cut up). Separating. **D. aneurysm:** see aneurysm, d.

dissec·tion (L. *dissecare*, to cut up). Cutting of the parts of the body along natural lines of cleavage.

dissĕ·minated (L. *dis-*, apart; *seminare*, to sow). Scattered; spread over a large area. **D. sclerosis:** a chronic disease characterized by widespread occurrence of focal demyelination, *q.v.*, in the central nervous system, followed by gliosis, *q.v.*, progressing with remissions and relapses. While owing to the scattered arrangement of the lesions a great variety of syndromes may result, the most frequent clinical features include nystagmus, dysarthria ('staccato-speech'), intention tremor, spastic paraplegia and absence of abdominal reflexes. Syn. multiple sclerosis; insular sclerosis.

disseminā·tion (L. *dis-*, apart; *seminare*, to sow). A scattering; a spreading.

dissimilā·tion (L. *dis-*, apart; *similis*, like). Catabolism, *q.v.*

dissociā·tion (L. *dissociare*, to disunite). 1. Disintegration of molecules or ions of a compound into simpler molecules, as caused by heat, electrolysis, hydrolysis. 2. Separation of parts of a function; loosening, or loss, of a connection. 3. Disturbance of association.

dissolū·tion (L. *dissolvere*, to loosen). Separation of a body or compound into its parts; decomposition.

dissolve (L. *dissolvere*, to loosen). 1. To separate into component parts. 2. To make a solution of.

dissol·vent (L. *dissolvere*, to loosen). A solvent.

dis·sonance (L. *dis*, apart ; *sonus*, sound). Discord.

dis·tad (L. *distare*, to be distant; *ad*, to). Towards the distal part.

dis·tal (L. *distare*, to be distant). Peripheral; of two points of a body, the one which is more distant from the centre.

distance. The space between two points.

distensibil·ity. Capacity of being distended.

disten·tion. Enlargement.

distichi·asis (G. *dis*, twice; *stikhos*, a row). Having a double row of eyelashes, the lower one directed towards the eyeball.

dis·tillate (L. *destillare*, to drop down). The substance obtained by distillation.

distillā·tion (L. *destillare*, to drop down). Vaporization of a substance by heat and conversion of the vapour into the fluid state by cooling.

Distomata (G. *dis*, twice; *stoma*, mouth). A sub-order of the digenetic trematodes comprising the families Fasciolidae, Opisthorchiidae, Dicrocoeliidae, Plagiorchiidae, Echinostomatidae, Heterophydae and Troglotrematidae, all the members of which have two suckers.

distomi·asis (G. *dis*, twice; *stoma*, mouth). Any disease due to infestation with Distomata.

districhi·asis (G. *dis*, twice; *thrix*, hair). The growth of two hairs from a single follicle.

dis·trix (G. *dis*, twice; *thrix*, hair). A splitting of the hair ends.

dithī·o. Chemical name for the -S-S- group.

dithrǎ·nol. 1:8 dihydroxyanthranol, the chief active ingredient of chrysarobin.

ditō·cia (G. *dis*, twice; *tokos*, parturition). Giving birth to two offspring at a time.

Dittel's falciform fold (Dittel, L. von, Austrian anatomist, 1815–98). A thickening of the superficial fascia of the neck, bounding the orifice through which the external jugular vein penetrates the fascia behind the sternomastoid muscle. **D.'s operation:** removal of the lateral lobes of the prostate gland through an external incision.

Dittrich's plugs (Dittrich, F., German pathologist, 1815–59). Dirty white or greyish masses, consisting chiefly of fatty detritus, micro-organisms and crystals of margarine, found in the sputum of putrid bronchitis and pulmonary gangrene. **D.'s stenosis:** stenosis of the conus arteriosus.

diurē·sis (G. *dia*, through; *ouron*, urine). The increased secretion of urine.

diuret·ic (G. *dia*, through; *ouron*, urine). Promoting the secretion of urine.

diū·ria (L. *dies*, day; G. *ouron*, urine). Frequency of urination during the daytime.

diur·nal (L. *dies*, day). 1. Daily. 2. Occurring or active during daytime.

diutur·nal (L. *diuturnus*, lasting, from *diu*, long (time)). Lasting; of long duration.

dī·valent (G. *dis*, twice; L. *valere*, to be strong). Bivalent, *q.v.*

diver·gence (L. *dis*, asunder; *vergere*, to incline). A progressive separation from each other in moving from a common point.

diver·gent (L. *dis-*, asunder; *vergere*, to incline). Extending in different directions from a common point.

divers' paresis. See caisson disease.

divertic·ular (L. *divertere*, to turn aside). Pertaining to or caused by diverticulum.

diverticuli·tis (L. *diverticulum*). Inflammation of a diverticulum.

diverticulō·sis (L. *diverticulum*). The presence of many diverticula of the intestine.

divertī·culum (pl. **diverticula**) (L. *diverticulum*, from *divertere*, to turn aside). A small blind pouch arising from the wall of a hollow organ, such as the intestine or urinary bladder. **D., pulsion:** d. of the oesophagus, caused by pressure from within. **D., traction:** d. of the oesophagus, caused by traction from without the organ.

divul·sion (L. *divulsio*, a plucking apart). A tearing away; a forcible separation.

diz·ziness. Giddiness; vertigo.

D:N ratio. The ratio of glucose to nitrogen excreted in the urine.

D₂O. The symbol for deuterium oxide.

Dobell's solution (Dobell, H. B., English physician, 1828–1917). A solution of borax, sodium bicarbonate and phenol in glycerol and water; used as a spray for nasal and throat troubles.

Dobie's globule (Dobie, W. H., English physician, 1826–1915). A small round body rendered visible by staining methods in the centre of the transparent disc of a muscular fibril. **D.'s layer, or line:** see Krause's membrane.

DOCA. Syn. desoxycorticosterone acetate.

Dochez's antitoxin or serum (Dochez, A. R., American physician, born 1882). A scarlet fever antitoxic serum derived from horses which have been immunized with scarlet fever streptococcus.

doctor (L. *doctor*, teacher). A practitioner of medicine.

Doederlein's bacillus (Doederlein, A., German obstetrician, 1860–1941). A bacillus normally present in the secretions of the vagina.

Doehle's inclusion bodies (Doehle, P., German pathologist, 1855–1928). Bodies found in the leucocytes in scarlet fever.

Dogiel's end-bulbs, nerve-endings (Dogiel, H. S., Russian neurologist, 1852–1922). The sensory nerve endings, especially those of the 'end-bulb' type.

doisynol·ic acid. An artificial oestrogen containing part of the oestrone nucleus. It is extremely active when administered orally.

Dolan·tin. Syn. for pethidine.

dŏ·lichocephā·lia (G. *dolikhos*, long; *kephalē*, head). See dolichocephaly.

dŏ·lichocephal·ic (G. *dolikhos*, long; *kephalē*, head). Characterized by dolichocephaly.

dŏ·lichocě·phalus (G. *dolikhos*, long; *kephalē*, head). A skull having a breadth less than 75 per cent. of its length.

dŏ·lichocě·phaly (G. *dolikhos*, long; *kephalē*, head). The condition of having a dolichocephalus.

dolichofā·cial (G. *dolikhos*, long; L. *facies*, face). Dolichoprosopic, *q.v.*

dŏ·lichomor·phic (G. *dolikhos*, long; *morphē*, form). Inclining to height and slenderness.

dŏ·lichoprosop·ic (G. *dolikhos*, long; *prosōpon*, face). Having an abnormally long face.

Döllinger's tendinous ring (Döllinger, J. I. J., German physiologist, 1775–1841). A thickening of Descemet's membrane.

dŏ·lor (L). Pain.

dolori·fic (L. *dolor*, pain; *facere*, to make). Producing pain.

dolorŏ·sus (L. *dolor*, pain). Painful.

dŏ·matophō·bia (G. *dōma*, house; *phŏbos*, fear). Abnormal fear of being inside a house.

dŏ·minant (L. *dominari*, from *dominus*, a lord). Prevailing. See also inheritance, d.

Donders' glaucoma (Donders, F. C., Dutch physician, 1818–89). Simple atrophic glaucoma. **D.s' rings:** rainbow-coloured rings seen by patients in glaucoma and by normal and cataractous eyes when the pupil is dilated; supposed to be due to diffraction of light by the cortex of the crystalline lens.

Donné's corpuscles (Donné, A., French physician, 1801–78). 1. Leucocytes containing fat-drops, found in colostrum corpuscles. 2. See Bizzozero's blood platelets.

donor (L. *donare*, to give). One who gives his blood for transfusion to another person.

Donovan's solution (Donovan, E., English pharmacist, 1789–1837). A solution of mercuric and arsenic iodides, 1 per cent. of each.

dopa. Abbreviation of dihydroxyphenylalanine. **D.reaction:** the staining of the cytoplasm of melanoblastic cells with a 1:1000 solution of d., due to the reaction of the solution with an intracellular oxydase which produces a substance closely allied to melanin.

dope (Dutch *doop*). Slang term for any drug, especially a narcotic drug.

doraphō·bia (G. *dŏra*, hide; *phŏbos*, fear). Morbid dislike of animal fur or skin.

dor·mancy (L. *dormīre*, to sleep). The condition of being dormant.

dor·mant (L. *dormīre*, to sleep). Quiescent; inactive.

doromā·nia (G. *dōron*, gift; *mania*, madness). A morbid desire to make gifts.

dor·sad (L. *dorsum*, back; *ad*, to). Towards the back.

dor·sal (L. *dorsualis*, from *dorsum*, back). Pertaining to the dorsum or to the posterior part of an organ.

dorsal·gia (L. *dorsum*, back; G. *algos*, pain). Any back pain.

dorsalis (L. *dorsum*, back). Relating to the back.

dorsiflex·ion (L. *dorsum*, back; *flectere*, to bend). Bending in a dorsal direction.

dorsi·meson (L. *dorsum*, back; G. *mesos*, middle). The dorsal median line of the body.

dorsispi·nal. Relating to the back and the vertebrae.

dorso-anterior (L. *dorsum* back; *ante*, before.) Pertaining to the dorsal surface and the anterior part of a body.

dorsocĕ·phalad (L. *dorsum*, back; G. *kephalē*, head; L. *ad*, to). Towards the back of the head.

dorsolă·teral (L. *dorsum*, back; *lateralis*, from *latus*, side). Pertaining to the dorsal surface and the lateral part of a body.

dorsolum·bar. Relating to the back and to the lumbar region.

dorsopostē·rior (L. *dorsum*, back; *post*, after). Pertaining to the dorsal surface and the posterior part of a body.

dorsoven·trad (L. *dorsum*, back; *venter*, belly; *ad*, to). In a direction from back to front.

dorsum (L). The back; the posterior part of any organ.

Doryl. Trade name for carbaminoylcholine chloride. It slows the heart in cases of paroxysmal tachycardia and causes contraction of the musculature of the intestine and bladder.

dosage (G. *dosis*, a giving). The regulation of the doses of drugs or intensity and duration of current or rays to be applied.

dose (G. *dosis*, a giving). The measured quantity of a drug to be taken at one time.

dosim·eter (G. *dosis*, a giving; *metron*, measure). An apparatus for measuring doses.

dosimet·ric (G. *dosis*, a giving; *metron*, measure). Relating to dosimetry.

dosi·metry (G. *dosis*, a giving; *metron*, measure). The measurement of doses, especially of X-rays.

dot. A small speck.

dŏ·tage. Senility.

double. Twofold; in pairs. **D. hearing:** see diplacusis. **D. refraction:** the refraction of light in two different directions, a phenomenon produced by all crystals except those of the isometric system and by isotropic bodies when under mechanical strain or when in an electrical field. The ray which is refracted according to ordinary refraction is called ordinary ray and the other ray is called extraordinary ray; both rays are plane polarized in planes at right angles to one another; doubly refracting bodies with one optic axis are called uni-axial, those with two axes, bi-axial. **D. refraction, negative:** D. r. by a body in which (except along the optic axis) the extraordinary ray has a greater velocity than the ordinary ray. **D. r., positive:** d. r. by a body in which the extraordinary ray is more refracted than the ordinary ray so that the velocity of the former is less than that of the latter. **D. vision:** see diplopia.

douche (Fr.). 1. A stream of water or steam directed against a part, or into a cavity. 2. An apparatus for directing a jet of fluid or steam against or into a part.

Douglas's crescentic fold (Douglas, J., Scottish anatomist, 1675–1742). The lower border of the posterior sheath of the rectus abdominis. **D.'s cul-de-sac, or pouch of Douglas:** the pouch formed by the recto-uterine folds of the peritoneum. **D.'s line:** the curved lower edge of the internal layer of the aponeurosis of the internal oblique muscle of the abdomen. **D.'s septum:** in the foetus, the septum formed by the union of Rathke's folds, transforming the rectum into a complete canal.

dourine (Pers. from Arab. *darin*, filthy). A venereal disease of horses, characterized by oedema of the genital organs followed by anaemia and paralysis due to infection with *Trypanosoma equiperdum*.

Dover's powder (Dover, T., English physician, 1660–1742). A powder containing 10 per cent each of opium and ipecacuanha.

Doyère's hillock or imminence (Doyère, L., French physiologist, 1811–63). The slight prominence formed by the motor end-plates on a muscle fibre.

dr. Abbreviation for drachm.

drachm (G. *drakhmē*, a drachm). A weight of 60 grains; the eighth part of the apothecaries' ounce; the sixteenth part of the avoirdupois ounce. **Fluid d.:** the eighth part of a fluid ounce.

draconti·asis (G. *drakōn*, a snake). The disease caused by *Dracunculus medinensis*, q.v.

Dracun·culus medinen·sis. A species of threadworms belonging to the order Filaroidae, widely distributed and a common parasite of man in Africa, Arabia, India and the Dutch East Indies, the adult female of which harbours most frequently in the subcutaneous tissues, especially of arm, leg and shoulders, producing in the host anaphylactic symptoms (urticaria, vomiting, dyspnoea, diarrhoea) when she comes to the surface of the body; the larvae are discharged in a milky fluid through a lesion in the skin at parts coming in contact with water and undergo a further development in the body cavity of several species of Cyclops by which they are hunted and ingested; infection in susceptible hosts results from swallowing infected Cyclops in drinking water.

dragée (Fr.). A sugar-coated pill.

Dragendorff's test (Dragendorff, J. G. N., German physician, 1836–98). For bile pigments. If on to a film of urine on a porcelain tile a few drops of nitric acid are added a ring of colours is produced if bile is present.

drain. 1. To cause to flow off gradually; to draw off. 2. An open tube or other appliance used for drainage, q.v.

drainage. 1. A gradual flowing off. 2. The gradual removal, or a device for such removal, of excess fluids or of wound secretions.

dram. Drachm, q.v.

Drasch's cells (Drasch, O., Austrian histoloist, 1849–1911). The cuneiform cells of the mucous membrane of the trachea.

dras·tic (G. drastikos, effective). 1. Powerful. 2. A powerful purgative.

draught. A quantity of fluid medicine to be taken at one time.

draw. 1. To cause discharge, as from a poultice. 2. To extract a tooth. 3. To catheterize.

dream. A series of images and thoughts exhibited during sleep, a primitive method of psychic activity. **D.-state, epileptic:** a form of epileptic aura or an epileptic equivalent. **D. work:** the process by which latent d. thoughts are unconsciously converted into the manifest content of the d.

Drechsel's test for bile acids (Drechsel, E., Swiss chemist, 1843–97). The production of a red colour if bile acids are present in a substance treated with a little cane-sugar and a few drops of a mixture of phosphoric acid and water.

dre̅·panocyte (G. drepanon, a scythe; kutos, a container). Sickle cell, q.v.

dresser. A medical student whose special duty it is to dress wounds, etc.

dressing. 1. Application of some material to, or the bandaging of, a wound. 2. The material so applied.

Dressler's disease (Dressler, a German physician). Paroxysmal haemoglobinuria.

drill. An instrument used for boring into hard substances, such as bones or teeth.

Drinker's apparatus (Drinker, P., American public health engineer, born 1893). An artificial mechanical respirator, in which the body of a patient is enclosed in cases of respiratory paralysis, i.e. infantile paralysis.

drip, intravenous. The slow administration of intravenous saline, plasma, or blood.

drivel, drivelling. 1. Involuntary flow of saliva, as in infancy. 2. Childish or senile talk; decay of mental efficiency.

dro̅·mograph (G. dromein, to run; graphein, to write). An instrument for recording the velocity of the blood current.

dromomā·nia (G. dromos, a running; mania, madness). Vagabondage; a neurotic or psychotic desire to wander.

dromotrop·ic (G. dromos, a running; trepein, to turn). Affecting the conductivity of the heart muscle.

drop. A globule of liquid. 2. To let fall in drops. 3. The falling of a part, as from paralysis, e.g. wrist-drop. **D.-clysma; D.-enema:** enema running into the rectum at the rate of about 20–100 drops per minute. **D.-infusion:** intravenous or subcutaneous infusion, running in at the rate of about 20–60 drops a minute.

dropper. A bottle or pipette fitted to emit a fluid by drops.

droplet. A minute drop.

dropsical (G. hudrōps, from hudōr, water). Affected with or pertaining to dropsy.

dropsy (G. hudrōps, from hudōr, water). Abnormal accumulation of serous fluid in the cellular tissues or in a body cavity. Syn. oedema, q.v., D., wet: beri-beri, q.v.

Drosŏ·phila (G. drŏsos, dew; philein, to love). A genus of flies breeding mainly in decaying fruit.

drug (Fr. drogue). Any substance used as a medicine. **d. addiction:** habitual excess of the use of a drug.

drum. The tympanic membrane.

Drummond's sign (Drummond, Sir D., English physician, 1852–1932). The 'oral whiff' heard when the mouth is closed, disappearing on compression of the nostrils; synchronous with the cardiac systole and observed in certain cases of aneurysm of the thoracic aorta.

drusen (Germ. for glands). 1. Deposition of hyaline material in the cuticular layers of Bruch's membrane in the retina, usually associated with degenerative changes in the pigmentary epithelium, occurring in old age, in areas of retinal or choroid lesions, or in young adults as inherited primary degeneration. Syn. of the latter type: Doyne's honeycomb choroiditis. Syn. colloid bodies. 2. Concentric laminations of hyaline matter upon the optic disc, sometimes associated with retinitis pigmentosa or other retinopathies. Syn. hyaline bodies.

dry. Free from moisture, e.g. d. gangrene. **D. labour:** labour in which there is only a slight discharge of liquor amnii, e.g. because of premature rupture of the amnion. **D. pleurisy:** pleurisy without effusion.

Dubini's disease (Dubini, A., Italian physician, 1813–1902). Rapid rhythmic contractions of one or more groups of muscles, beginning in an extremity or a half of the face, and extending over the greater part or the whole of the body; electric chorea. Usually fatal; cases occur chiefly in Italy.

Dublin method (Rotunda Hospital, Dublin, Eire). Expulsion of the placenta by stimulating uterine contraction by kneading the uterus through the abdominal wall and then pressing it down to the sacrum.

Dubois's disease (Dubois, P., French obstetrician, 1795–1871). 1. The presence of multiple necrotic foci in the thymus glands of infants with congenital syphilis. 2. A cyst of the thymus caused by the growth of thymic tissue into Hassall's corpuscles.

Duchenne's attitude (Duchenne, G. B. A., French neurologist, 1806–75). In paralysis of the trapezius the shoulder droops; the shoulder-blade moves so that its internal edge, instead of being parallel to the vertebral column, becomes oblique from top to bottom and from without inwards. **D.'s disease:** 1. Tabes dorsalis. 2. Bulbar paralysis. **D.'s paralysis:** progressive muscular dystrophy with pseudo-hypertrophy. **D.'s sign:** falling in of the epigastrium during inspiration in cases of marked hydropericardium or impaired movement of the diaphragm from pressure or paralysis. **D.'s syndrome:** subacute or chronic anterior spinal paralysis with multiple neuritis.

Duchenne-Aran's disease. See under Aran-Duchenne.

Duchenne-Erb's paralysis. See under Erb.

Duchenne-Landouzy's type of progressive muscular atrophy. See under Landouzy-Déjérine.

Duckworth's syndrome (Duckworth, Sir D., English physician, 1840–1928). Complete cessation of respiration several hours before stoppage of the heart in certain cerebral diseases attended by intracranial pressure.

Ducrey's bacillus (Ducrey, A., Italian dermatologist, 1860–1940). A small oval streptobacillus, described as the pathogenic agent in chancroid.

duct (L. *ductus*, from *ducere*, to lead). A tube or channel, especially one for carrying off glandular secretion. **D. carcinoma:** a carcinoma of relatively low malignancy originating from the epithelium of a mammary d., usually near the nipple. **D. papilloma:** a papilloma originating from the epithelium of a mammary d., usually near the nipple. Syn. mammary adenocystoma, papillary cystoma.

ductile. Capable of being drawn out.

ductless gland. See endocrine gland.

ductule. A small duct.

ductuli, d. aberrantes (L.). Blind tubules between testis and epididymis opening into the epididymis below the globus major and at the globus minor, remnants of the mesonephric tubules. **D. efferentes:** the end branches of the tubules of the rete testis between mediastinum testis and globus major epididymis.

ductus (L.). A duct. **D. deferens:** the portion of the excretory duct of the testis beyond the epididymis. Syn. vas deferens.

Duddel's membrane (Duddel, B., 18th century English physician). The membrane of Descemet or of Demours.

Duhring's disease (Duhring, L. A., American dermatologist, 1845–1913). Dermatitis herpetiformis. **D.'s pruritus:** pruritus hiemalis.

Dukes's disease (Dukes, C., English physician, 1845–1925). Fourth disease, an affection resembling scarlet fever and measles.

Duke's test. See bleeding time.

dull. 1. Not resonant. 2. Blunt.

dullness. 1. Bluntness. 2. Lack of resonance, as on percussion of the lungs over an area of diminished content of air.

dumb. Unable to speak.

dum-dum (Dum Dum, town in India). A fever. Kalaazar, *q.v.*

dumping syndrome. Gastric discomfort, palpitations and cold sweats sometimes occurring after gastrectomy.

Duncan's folds (Duncan, J. M., British gynaecologist, 1826–90). The folds on the loose peritoneal surface of the uterus, seen immediately after delivery. **D.'s position of the placenta:** the marginal position generally assumed by the placenta on presenting itself at the os uteri for expulsion. **D.'s ventricle:** sinus Duncanii, the fifth ventricle; cavum septi pellucidi.

duodĕ·nal (L. *duodeni*, twelve each). Pertaining to the duodenum.

duodenec·tomy (L. *duodeni*, twelve each; G. *ektomē*, excision). Excision of part or all of the duodenum.

duodeni·tis (L. *duodeni*, twelve each). Inflammation of the duodenum.

duodeni·tis. Inflammation of the duodenum.

duodĕ·nochŏ·lecystŏ·tomy (L. *duodeni*, twelve each; G. *khŏlē*, gall; *kustis*, bladder; *tomē*, section). Formation of an artificial fistula between the duodenum and the gall-bladder.

duodeno-enterŏ·stomy (L. *duodeni*, twelve each; G. *enteron*, intestine; *stoma*, mouth). The formation of an artificial fistula between the duodenum and the small intestine.

duodĕ·nojejū·nal (L. *duodeni*, twelve each; *jejunus*, dry). Pertaining both to the duodenum and the jejunum.

duodenŏ·stomy (L. *duodeni*, twelve each; G. *stoma*, mouth). The formation of an artificial opening through the abdominal wall into the duodenum.

duodenŏ·tomy (L. *duodeni*, twelve each; G. *tomē*, section). An incision into the duodenum.

duodĕ·num (L. *duodeni*, twelve each). The first part of the small intestine, beginning at the pylorus.

Duplay's bursitis (Duplay, S., French surgeon, 1836–1924). Subdeltoid bursitis. **D.'s operation:** for epispadias.

dū·plicature (L. *duplicare*, to double). A doubling; a folding of a membrane upon itself.

dupli·city (L. *duplicitas*, from *duplex*, double). The condition of being double.

Dupré's bursitis (Dupré, E., French physician, 1862–1921). Inflammation of the bursa outside the capsule of the shoulder joint.

Dupré's muscle (Dupré, French anatomist at Hôtel Dieu of Paris. Work published in 1699). The subcrureus, in the thigh.

Dupuytren's contraction (Dupuytren, G., French surgeon, 1778–1835). Contraction of the palmar fascia. **D.'s egg-shell symptom:** the crackling sensation (egg-shell crackling) imparted on slight pressure in certain cases of sarcoma of the long bones. **D.'s finger:** see D.'s contraction. **D.'s fracture:** fracture of the lower end of the fibula, with displacement of the foot outwards and backwards. **D.'s hydrocele:** bilocular hydrocele of the tunica vaginalis testis, in which the sac fills the scrotum and extends into the abdominal cavity beneath the peritoneum.

dura, dura mater (L. *durus*, hard; *mater*, mother). The outermost of the three membranes of the brain and spinal cord.

dural. Relating to the dura.

duralumin. An aluminium and copper alloy.

Duret's nuclear arteries (Duret, H., French surgeon, 1849–1921). The arteries to the nuclei of cranial nerves. **D.'s rivers:** the subarachnoid canals.

Duroziez's disease (Duroziez, P. J., French physician, 1826–97). Congenital mitral stenosis. **D.'s murmur:** a double murmur heard over the femoral artery on light pressure with the stethoscope in cases of aortic insufficiency, mitral stenosis, lead poisoning and contracted kidney.

Duval's nucleus (Duval, M. M., French anatomist, 1844–1915). An aggregation of large multi-polar ganglion-cells situated ventrolaterally to the hypoglossal nucleus.

Duverney's foramen (Duverney, G. J., French anatomist, 1648–1730). See Winslow's foramen. **D.'s gland:** see Bartholin's glands.

dwarf. An individual of stunted growth.

dwarfism. The condition of abnormally small height or length. See also nanosomia, ateleiosis and microsomia.

dȳ·ad (G. *duas*, the number two). 1. A bivalent element or radical; bivalent. 2. A double chromosome, or one of a group of chromosomes as formed by the division of a tetrad.

dyaster. See diaster.

dye. An organic compound containing benzene rings with chromophoric and auxochromic groups attached, of which the former gives to the dye its colour property and the latter the property of conferring colour upon another substance. **D., acid:** any d. colouring acidophil constituents of protoplasm, such as most cytoplasmic granules. **D., basic:** any dye colouring basophil constituents of protoplasm, as nuclear tissue and chromatin of cells and bacteria.

dynă·mic (G. *dunamis*, power). 1. Relating to or characterized by energy. 2. Relating to or characterized by forces causing movement. 3. Relating to changes.

dynă·mics (G. *dunamis*, power). Branch of physics dealing with the action of forces or of motions.

dȳ·namo (G. *dunamis*, power). A machine for transforming mechanical into electrical energy by electromagnetic induction.

dynă·mograph (G. *dunamis*, power; *graphein*, to write). An instrument for recording muscular strength.

dynamŏ·meter (G. *dunamis*, power; *metron*, measure). 1. Instrument for measuring muscular power. 2.

Instrument for measuring the magnifying power of lenses.

dyne (G. *dunamis*, power). The unit of force; a force which gives to a mass of one gramme an increase in velocity of one centimetre per second.

dysacou·sia, dysacū·sis (G. *dus-*, bad; *akouein*, to hear). Discomfort in the hearing of ordinary sounds.

dysar·thria (G. *dus-*, bad; *arthron*, a joint). Impairment of articulated speech, due to an organic nervous lesion.

dysarthrō·sis (G. *dus-*, bad; *arthron*, joint). 1. A deformed joint. 2. A false joint.

dysbā·sia (G. *dus-*, bad; *basis*, step). Difficulty in walking. **D. intermittens:** Claudicatio intermittens, *q.v.*

dysbū·lia (G. *dus-*, bad; *boulē*, will). Impairment of will-power.

dyschĕ·zia (G. *dus-*, bad; *khězein*, to defaecate). Rectal constipation; difficulty in the final evacuation of faeces from the rectum.

dyschondroplā·sia (G. *dus-*, bad; *khondros*, cartilage; *plasis*, a forming). A congenitally developed dysplastic condition affecting the growing ends of long bones (including the metacarpal and phalangeal bones) characterized by the retention of areas of unossified cartilage at the diaphyses of long bones, resulting in dwarfism of the affected tissue; usually limited to one or two extremities. Syn. Ollier's disease; pseudochrondromata.

dys·chromatop·sia (G. *dus-*, bad; *khrōma*, colour; *opsis*, vision). Impairment of colour vision.

dyscor·ia (G. *dus-*, bad; *korē*, pupil of the eye). An abnormal form of the pupil.

dyscrā·sia (G. *dus-*, bad; *krasis*, mixture). Obsolescent term meaning a condition of morbid composition of body fluids, especially of the blood.

dys·diadŏ·chokinē·sia (G. *dus-*, bad; *diadokhos*, successor; *kinein*, to move). Impairment of diadochokinesia, *q.v.*

dysenter·ic (G. *dus-*, bad; *enteron*, intestine). Pertaining to or affected with dysentery.

dy̆·sentery (G. *dus-*, bad; *enteron*, intestine). One of a group of infectious diseases, characterized by, usually ulcerative, inflammation of the colon, the passage of frequent blood-containing stools, and tenesmus. **D., amoebic:** d. caused by the protozoon *Entamoeba histolytica*. **D., bacillary:** d. caused by the *Bacillus dysenteriae Shiga*, by *Bacillus paradysenteriae Flexner*, by Sonne's bacillus, or by related organisms.

dysfunc·tion (G. *dus-*, bad; L. *functio*, a performance). Impaired function, especially qualitatively abnormal function.

dys·galac·tia (G. *dus-*, bad; *gala*, milk). Disorder of milk secretion.

dysgen·ic (G. *dus-*, bad; *gennan*, to produce). Tending to deterioration of the race; the opposite of eugenic.

dysgĕ·nesis (G. *dus-*, bad; *gennan*, to produce). Sterility, especially of hybrid organisms among themselves.

dysgerminō·ma (G. *dus-*, bad; L. *germen*, an offshoot). A tumour arising from cells of germinal epithelial origin, containing remnants of an asexual foetus.

dysgeū·sia (G. *dus-*, bad; *geusis*, taste). Impairment or alteration of the sense of taste.

dysgrā·phia (G. *dus-*, bad; *graphein*, to write). Impairment of the ability to write, due to a central nervous lesion. See also agrammatism.

dyshaematopoiē·sis (G. *dus*, bad; *haima*, blood; *poiein*, to make). Conditions in which blood formation is defective.

dyshidrō·sis, dysidrō·sis (G. *dus-*, bad; *hidrōs*, sweat). Cheiro-pompholyx, *q.v.*

dyskeratō·sis (G. *dus-*, bad; *keras*, horn). Any skin disease characterized by abnormal keratinization of the epidermis.

dyskinē·sia (G. *dus-*, bad; *kinesis*, motion). 1. Impairment of voluntary movement. 2. Impairment of excretion, especially from the gall-bladder, due to hypertonicity of the peripheral sphincter, i.e., the sphincter of Oddi.

dyskoimē·sis (G. *dus-*, bad; *koimēsis*, a lying down to sleep). Difficulty in falling asleep.

dyslă·lia (G. *dus-*, bad; *lalein*, to talk). Impairment of articulation, due to a disturbance of the organs of speech or their motor nerves.

dyslex·ia (G. *dus-*, bad; *lexis*, from *legein*, to speak). Impairment of the ability to read, due to a central nervous lesion. See also alexia.

dyslō·gia (G. *dus-*, bad; *logos*, word). Difficulty in expressing ideas by speech, as in certain psychoses.

dysmasē·sis (G. *dus-*, bad; *māsēsis*, mastication). Difficulty in mastication.

dysmenorrhōē·a (G. *dus-*, bad; *men*, month; *rheein*, to flow). Painful menstruation.

dysmē·tria (G. *dus-*, bad; *metron*, measure). 1. Misjudgment of distances in the execution of motor acts, due to a central nervous, usually cerebellar, lesion. 2. Impairment of ability to compare weights placed in both hands, due to a central nervous, usually cerebellar, lesion.

dysmi·nia (G. *dus-*, bad; *mimeisthai*, to imitate). Impairment of the ability to make gestures.

dysō·pia, dysop·sia (G. *dus-*, bad; *opsis*, vision). Defective vision.

dysorex·ia (G. *dus-*, bad; *orexis*, appetite). A depraved or unnatural appetite.

dysos·mia (G. *dus-*, bad; *osmē*, smell). Impairment of the sense of smell.

dysostō·sis (G. *dus-*, bad; *osteon*, bone). Congenital malformation of bone. **D., cleidocranial or D. craniocleidal:** d. of cranial and clavicular bones, characterized by increased breadth of the skull, open fontanelles, prognathism, malformation of the palatal arch, and absence or malformation of the clavicles. **D., craniofacial:** d. of cranial and facial bones, due to premature synostosis in the base of the skull, characterized by striking prominence of the frontal region, digital markings of the cranial vault, shallowness of the orbits (causing exophthalmos and secondary changes of the optic nerve and other parts of the eye), poor development of the upper jaw and relative prognathism, and abnormal width between the orbits. Syn. Crouzon's disease.

dyspareu·nia (G. *duspareunos*, ill-mated). Painful sexual intercourse, commonly relating to the female partner.

dyspep·sia (G. *dus-*, bad; *peptein*, to digest). Impaired digestion; indigestion.

dyspep·tic (G. *dus-*, bad; *peptein*, to digest). Related to or suffering from indigestion.

dysphā·gia (G. *dus-*, bad; *phagein*, to devour). Difficulty in swallowing.

dysphā·sia (G. *dus-*, bad; *phasis*, a statement). Impairment of speech due to a central nervous lesion. See also aphasia.

dysphō·nia (G. *dus-*, bad; *phōnē*, voice). Impairment of phonation.

dysphor·ia (G. *dus-*, bad; *pherein*, to bear). Feeling of unease.

dysphrā·sia (G. *dus-*, bad; *phrasis*, speech). Impairment of speech due to impairment of mental power.

dyspitū·itarism (G. *dus-*, bad; L. *pituita*, phlegm). Any condition due to qualitative disordered function of the pituitary gland.

dysplā·sia (G. *dus-*, bad; *plassein*, to form). Abnormal tissue formation.

dysplas·tic (G. *dus-*, bad; *plassein*, to form). 1. Characterized by dysplasia. 2. Applied to all forms of constitutional physique which differ from the asthenic, pyknic and athletic types.

dyspnœ·a (G. *dus-*, bad; *pnein*, to breathe). Difficult breathing; shortness of breath. **D., cardiac:** due to heart disease. **D., renal:** due to renal disease. **D., Traube's:** dyspnoea with slow respiratory movements, noted in diabetes mellitus.

dyspnœ·ic (G. *dus-*, bad; *pnein*, to breathe). Pertaining to or affected with dyspnoea.

dysprâ·gia (G. *dus-*, bad; *prassein*, to do, to perform). Painful performance of any function.

dysprax·ia (G. *dus-*, bad; *prassein*, to perform). Impairment of purposeful performance.

dysrâ·phia (G. *dus-*, bad; *rhaphē*, seam). Imperfect closure of the primitive neural tube, resulting in cleft formation of the central parts of the spinal cord with distension or incomplete closure of the spinal canal. Syn. status dysraphicus.

dysrhyth·mia (G. *dus-*, bad; *rhuthmos*, rhythm). Disturbance or abnormality of rhythm.

dysteleŏ·logy (G. *dus-*, bad; *telos*, an end; *logos*, word). The doctrine of purposelessness in nature.

dysthy·mia (G. *dus-*, bad; *thumos*, mind). Mental perversion.

dysthy·roidism (G. *dus-*, bad; *thureos*, a shield; *eidos*, form). 1. Qualitative disorder of thyroid function. 2. The bodily condition resulting therefrom.

dysti·thia (G. *dus-*, bad; *tithēnos*, nursing). Difficulty in breast-feeding.

dystō·cia (G. *dus-*, bad; *tokos*, birth). Difficult parturition.

dystō·nia (G. *dus-*, bad; *tonos*, tone). Impaired tissue tonicity. **D., muscular:** see torsion spasm.

dystō·pia (G. *dus-*, bad; *topos*, place). Displacement of an organ.

dystō·sis. Dysostosis, *q.v.*

dystrō·phia (G. *dus-*, bad; *trophē*, from *trephein*, to nourish). Dystrophy, *q.v.* **D. adiposa corneae:** primary fatty degeneration of the cornea, peripheral or central, usually beginning in the deeper parenchymatous layers. **D. adiposogenitalis:** a condition characterized by obesity of the female type, hypogenitalism, with or without diabetes insipidus, due to hypofunction of the pituitary gland, which may itself be due to encroachment on pituitary tissue by a pituitary or craniopharyngeal tumour. Syn. Fröhlich's syndrome. **D. calcarea corneae:** deposition of calcium salts in the cornea. **D. myotonic:** heredo-degenerative disease characterized by muscular atrophy (especially of the distal parts of the extremities, of the face and sterno-mastoid muscle), myotonic reaction (especially of the hands after fist-closure), juvenile cataract, testicular atrophy, dysarthria, sensory changes, and usually some degree of mental debility. See also myotonia congenita. **D. urica corneae:** bilateral crystalline deposition of urea and sodium ureate in the cornea, not associated with gout.

dystroph·ic. Characterized by dystrophy. **D. myotonia:** Dystrophia, myotonic, *q.v.*

dystrophy (G. *dus-*, bad; *trophē*, from *trephein*, to nourish). Faulty nutrition. **D., progressive muscular:** heredo-degenerative disease of muscles, characterized by gradual onset in childhood or early adolescence, flaccidity and atrophy of the muscles of the trunk and especially of the proximal parts of the limbs with loss of deep reflexes and electrical reaction degeneration, and sometimes by pseudo-hypertrophy of muscles, especially those of the calves. The following types are distinguished: (1) Pseudo-hypertrophic type. (2) Erb's juvenile type. (3) Facio-scapulo-humeral type (Landouzy-Déjérine). (4) Distal type (Gower's). (5) Congenital or infantile myopathy. (6) Limited, transitory and late forms.

dysū·ria (G. *dus-*, bad; *ouron*, urine). Difficulty in micturition.

E

e. Abbreviation for electron.

ead. Abbreviation for L. *eadem*, the same (feminine).

Eales's disease (Eales, H., English physician, 1852–1913). A condition marked by repeated haemorrhages into the retina and vitreous.

ear. The organ of hearing, consisting of the external ear, the middle ear and the internal ear. **E., external:** the auricle and the external auditory meatus. **E., middle:** the cavity between the tympanic membrane and the osseous wall of the inner ear, containing the auditory ossicles. Syn. tympanum. **E., internal:** the bony labyrinth containing the membranous labyrinth (saccule, utricle, semicircular canals and cochlea) with the terminal fibres of the accoustic nerve.

ear drum. The tympanum.

ear wax. See cerumen.

Easton's syrup (Easton, J. E. A., English physician, 1807–65). A syrup of the phosphates of quinine, iron and strychnine.

ebb. A slow decline.

Eberstaller's sulcus (Eberstaller, O., contemporary Austrian anatomist). The sulcus intermedius secundus of the parietal cortex.

Eberth's bacillus (Eberth, K. J., German pathologist, 1835–1926). *Bacillus typhi abdominalis.* **E.'s lines:** Lineae scarlariformes; dark broken lines between the cardiac muscular cells, seen when stained with silver nitrate.

Eberthella. A genus of bacteria of the Salmonelleae family. **E. typhosa:** the organism causing typhoid fever.

Ebner's germ reticulum (Ebner, V., Austrian histologist, 1842–1925). A network of nucleated cells in the seminiferous tubules. **E.'s glands:** the acinous glands situated in the region of the circumvallate papillae of the tongue.

ébranlement (F.). The removal of a polypus by twisting it on its pedicle and avulsing it.

ē·briĕtas (L.). Drunkenness.

Ebstein's lesion (Ebstein, W., German physician, 1836–1912). Hyaline degeneration and insular necrosis of the epithelial cells of the renal tubules in diabetes mellitus.

eburnā·tion (L. *ebur*, ivory). Increase in the density of bone or cartilage. Seen in joints affected with osteoarthritis.

ebur·neous (L. *ebur*, ivory). Ivory-like, in consistency and/or colour.

E-C mixture. Mixture of ether and chloroform for inhalation anaesthesia.

ecau·date (L. *e*, out of; *cauda*, tail). Tailless.

Ecballium. A genus of plants including the *E. elaterium*, from which elaterium is obtained.

ecbol·ic (G. *ek*, out of; *bolē*, a throw, from *ballein*, to throw). Promoting expulsion from the uterus.

eccen·tric (G. *ek*, out of; *kentron*, centre). 1. Not having the same centre. 2. Situated away from the centre. 3. Peculiar in behaviour. 4. Directed outside the self.

eccen·tro-os·teochon·drodysplā·sia (G. *ek*, away; *kentron*, centre; *osteon*, bone; *khondros*, cartilage; *dys-*, bad; *plassein*, to form). Morquio's disease; a rare type of ossification characterized by multiple discrete centres of ossification. It is a familial condition.

eccen·tropiĕ·sis (G. *ek*, away; *kentron*, centre; *piesis*, pressure). Pressure from within.

ecchondrō·ma (G. *ek.* away; *khondros*, cartilage). Chondroma, *q.v.*

ecchondrō·sis (G. *ek*, away; *khondros*, cartilage). A cartilaginous outgrowth due to simple hyperplasia.

ecchon·drotome (G. *ek*, away; *khondros*, cartilage; *tomē*, a cutting). A surgical knife used in the excision of cartilage.

ecchordō·sis (G. *ek*, away; *khordē*, string). A tumour arising from remnants of the embryonic chorda dorsalis at the base of the skull, beneath the dura mater of the olivus Blumenbachii. See also chordoma.

ecchymō·sis (G. *ek*, away; *khumos*, juice). A macular haematoma, somewhat larger than petechia.

ecchymot·ic (G. *ek*, away; *khumos*, juice). Relating to or resembling an ecchymosis.

ec·crine (G. *ek*, away; *krinein*, to separate). Applied to a type of sweat gland, distributed generally over the surface of the body, excreting a dilute solution of sodium chloride, urea and lactate.

ec·crisis (G. *ek*, away; *krisis*, separation). The excretion of waste products.

eccyē·sis (G. *ek*, out; *kuēsis*, conception). Extrauterine gestation.

ec·deron (G. *ek*, out; *deros*, poetic form of *derma*, skin). The epithelial layer of skin or mucous membrane.

ecg. Abbreviation for electrocardiogram.

echid·nin (G. *ekhidna*, viper). Serpent venom.

echinococ·cus (G. *ekhinos*, hedgehog; *kokkos*, berry). The larval form of *Taenia echinococcus*, forming the hydatid cyst in various tissues (especially liver, lung, brain) of cattle, swine, man, etc., the adult form developing only in the dog.

echo. A reverberated sound.

echokinē·sia, echokinē·sis (G. *ekhō*, echo; *kinein*, to move). Unmotivated imitation of movements, as in psychotics.

echolā·lia (G. *ekhō*, echo; *lalia*, speech). 1. Unmotivated repetition of words. 2. A form of aphasia in which the patient can repeat words spoken to him, but cannot find words by himself.

echoprax·y (G. *ekhō*, echo; *praxis*, action). Echokinesia, *q.v.*

Eck's fistula (Eck, N. V., Russian physiologist, born 1847). An artificial anastomosis between the portal vein and the inferior vena cava.

Ecker's gyrus (Ecker, A., German physiologist, 1816–87). The gyrus descendens, the most posterior of the occipital convolutions. **E.'s sulcus:** the anterior or transverse occipital sulcus, usually joined to the horizontal part of the interparietal sulcus.

eclā·bium (G. *ek*, away; L. *labium*, lip). An eversion of the lip.

eclamp·sia (G. *eklampein*, to flash). A condition occurring in women with hypertensive toxaemia of pregnancy either in the last stage of pregnancy, during labour, or in early puerperium, characterized by epileptiform seizures followed by coma due to acute cerebral oedema, by rising blood pressure, and sometimes also other signs of hypertensive encephalopathy and renal insufficiency.

eclamp·tic (G. *eklampein*, to flash). Relating to or affected with eclampsia.

eclec·ticism (G. *ek*, away; *legein*, to select). The attempt to harmonize one or more divergent views by selecting from each such features as can be fused into a consistent whole.

ecmnē·sia (G. *ek*, away; *mnasthai*, to remember). A form of amnesia.

ecochlĕā·tion. Surgical removal of the cochlea.

ecŏ·logy. See oecology.

Economo's disease (von Economo, C., Austrian neurologist, 1876–1931). Encephalitis lethargica.

ecos·tate (L. *e*, out of; *costa*, rib). Without ribs.

écouvillon (F.). A stiff brush or swab used in the removal of débris from the uterus. Hence, *écouvillonage*, the operation of cleansing the inside of the uterus by means of a brush or swab.

écraseur (Fr. *écraser*, to crush). An instrument for removing a projecting part by gradually tightening a chain or wire loop around it.

ec·tad (G. *ektos*, outside; L. *ad*, to). On or towards the outer part.

ec·tal (G. *ektos*, outside). Outer; external.

ectā·sia, ec·tasis (G. *ektasis*, extension). Distension; dilatation.

ectat·ic (G. *ektasis*, extension). Distended; dilated.

ecthȳ·ma (G. *ekthuma*, a pustule). A form of impetigo characterized by the eruption of large superficial pustules, developing into superficial ulcers covered with dark crusts, occurring chiefly on the lower limbs. **E. terebrans:** a fulminating type of e. in young children, superimposed on the lesions of vaccinia or chickenpox.

ec·toblast (G. *ektos*, outside; *blastos*, germ). Ectoderm, *q.v.*

ectocar·dia (G. *ektos*, outside; *kardia*, heart). An abnormal position of the heart.

ec·tochoroi·dea (G. *ektos*, outside; *choris*, membrane; *eidos*, form). The external surface of the choroid coat of the eye.

ectodac·tylism (G. *ektos*, outside; *daktulos*, finger). Lacking one or more digits.

ec·toderm (G. *ektos*, outside; *derma*, skin). The external germinal layer in the gastrula, giving rise to epidermis and its derivatives (hair, nails, epithelium of sebaceous, sweat and mammary glands), epithelium of mouth and its derivatives (enamel, taste buds, epithelium of salivary and other buccal glands, anterior portion of the pituitary gland), epithelium of anus, distal portion of the male urethra, nostrils, cranial sinuses, conjunctiva, lacrimal glands, lens, and of pars nervosa, ciliaris and iridica retinae, of the membranous labyrinth, and lining of external ear, of the central spinal canal and the cerebral vesicles, to all neurons and neuroglia, to pineal gland, posterior portion of the pituitary gland, adrenal medulla, and the paraganglia, and possibly to smooth muscle associated with sweat glands and the iris. Syn. ectoblast, epiblast.

ectoder·mal (G. *ektos*, outside; *derma*, skin). 1. Relating to the ectoderm. 2. Derived from the ectoderm.

ecto-entad (G. *ektos*, out; *entos*, in; L. *ad*, to). From without inward.

ectŏ·genous (G. *ektos*, out; *gennan*, to produce). Capable of growth outside the body; applied especially to certain parasites or micro-organisms.

ectoglute·us (G. *ektos*, outside; L. *gluteus*). The gluteus maximus muscle.

ectŏ·gony (G. *ektos*, outside; *goneus*, parent). The influence of the immature zygote on the mother.

ectokelŏ·stomy (G. *ektos*, outside; *kēlē*, hernia; *stoma*, mouth). An operation in which the sac of an infected inguinal hernia is kept open by drainage.

ec·tomere (G. *ektos*, outside; *mĕros*, part). Any of the cells of the ovum that take part in the formation of the ectoderm.

ectonū·clear (G. *ektos*, outside; L. *nux*, a nut). Any part of the cell outside the nucleus.

ectŏ·pagus (G. *ektos*, outside; *pēgnunai*, to fix). A twin monster, united laterally along the chest.

ectopă·rasite (G. *ektos*, outside; *para*, for; *sitos*, food). A parasite that lives on the surface of its host.

ectopectŏrā·lis (G. *ektos*, outside; L. *pectus*, chest). The pectoralis major muscle.

ectoperitonī·tis (G. *ektos*, outside; *peritonaion*, surrounding membrane). Inflammation of the parietal peritoneum.

ec·tophyte (G. *ektos*, out; *phuton*, plant). A vegetable ectoparasite.

ectŏ·pia (G. *ektopos*, displaced). Abnormal position of an organ. **E. pupillae:** see corectopia.

ectop·ic (G. *ektopos*, displaced). In an abnormal position. **E. pregnancy:** extra-uterine pregnancy, *q.v.*

ec·toplasm (G. *ektos*, out; *plassein*, to form). 1. The peripheral, concentrated, viscid, relatively homogeneous or hyaline protoplasmic layer of the cytosome. 2. More especially in protozoa, the peripheral layer of the cytoplasm, forming the various organs of motion, contraction and prehension.

ectopŏ·tomy (G. *ektopos*, out of place; *tomē*, section). Operation for the removal of an extra-uterine pregnancy.

ectoptĕ·rygoid (G. *ektos*, outside; *pteruga*, wing; *eidos*, form). The outer pterygoid muscle.

ectorĕ·tina (G. *ektos*, outside; L. *retina*). The external layer of the retina.

ectorhī·nal (G. *ektos*, outside; *rhis*, nose). Situated at the outside of the nose.

ec·tosarc (G. *ektos*, outside; *sarx*, flesh). The ectoplasm, *q.v.*

ectŏ·scopy (G. *ektos*, outside; *skopein*, to view). Outlining the lungs by the method of inspection.

ec·tosome (G. *ektos*, outside; *sōma*, body). Any of the specific cytoplasmic granules, as in primordial germ cells.

ectosphĕ·noid (G. *ektos*, outside; *sphainos*, wedge; *eidos*, form). The outer cuneiform bone.

ectostŏ·sis (G. *ektos*, outside; *osteon*, bone). The growth of bone from the outside or perichondrium.

ec·tothrix (G. *ektos*, outside; *thrix*, hair). A group of trichophytes, *q.v.*, growing mainly on the surface of hairs of the host, comprising *Trichophyton asteroides*, *T. lacticolor*, etc.

Ec·totrichŏ·phyton (G. *ektos*, outside; *thrix*, hair; *phuton*, a plant). A species of fungi which invades the outer part of human hair.

ectrim·ma (G. *ektrimma*, an excoriation). A bedsore.

ectrŏ·geny (G. *ektrōma*, abortion; *gennan*, to produce). Congenital absence of a part or organ.

ectromē·lia (G. *ektrōma*, an abortion; *mĕlos*, a limb). Congenital absence of limbs.

ectrŏ·melus (G. *ektrōma*, abortion; *mĕlos*, limb). A monster with no limbs, or with rudimentary or defective limbs.

ectrop·ic (G. *ek*, out; *trepein*, to turn). Everted.

ectrŏ·pion, ectrŏ·pium (G. *ek*, out; *trepein*, to turn). Eversion of a part, especially of an eyelid, or of the uterine cervix.

ec·zema (G. *ek*, out; *zein*, to boil). An acute or chronic inflammatory disease of the skin, characterized by multiformity of lesions, which may include any combination of papules, vesicles and pustules on a more or less erythematous base, resulting in weeping, crusted or scaly, itching or burning lesions; due partly to a constitutional diathesis, partly to exogenous stimuli, such as ingested food. **E., erythematous:** first stage of an e. in which the skin is reddened and swollen. **E. fissum:** e. characterized by linear cracks in the epidermal surface. **E., herpetoid:** a form of e. characterized by round or oval patches of groups of itching vesicles or papules, especially on the dorsal surfaces of hands or other parts of the extremities. **E. madidans**: weeping e. **E. marginatum**: a form of epidermophytosis, affecting especially the groins, characterized by rounded, red areas surrounded by a well-marked raised eczematous margin. **E., nummular**: e. herpetoid. **E. sclerosum**: e. characterized by marked thickening of the skin due to papillary hypertrophy resulting in rough horny verrucose patches, especially on palmar and plantar surfaces and about the ankles. **E. seborrhoicum**: chronic e., originating from seborrhoea, affecting especially the head, chest, interscapular region and articular folds.

eczĕ·matoid (G. *ek*, out; *zein*, to boil; *eidos*, form). Resembling an eczema.

eczĕ·matous. Pertaining to or affected with eczema.

Edebohl's posture (Edebohl, G. M., American surgeon, 1853–1908). Simon's posture, *q.v.*

eden·tate, eden·tulous (L. *e*, out of; *dens*, tooth). Without teeth.

edes·tin. The protein of the seeds of the sunflower, hemp and castor-oil bean.

Edinger's nucleus (Edinger, L., German neurologist, 1855–1918). The nucleus of the posterior longitudinal bundle, an aggregation of ganglion-cells in the grey matter of the third ventricle; the dorsal acoustic nucleus.

Edinger-Westphal's nucleus (Edinger, L.; Westphal, A. K. O., German neurologist, born 1862). An accessory bulbar nucleus of the third cranial nerve in the region of the anterior corpora quadrigemina.

effect. Result or consequence.

effec·tor (L. *efficere*, to make). Applied to the endings of nerve fibrils in muscles, glands, etc., which effect the functional activity of the organ.

effĕ·minate (L. *femina*, female). Unmanly.

ef·ferent (L. *efferre*, to bear away). Carrying away, as e. blood-vessels, conveying blood away from the tissues; e. nerves, centrifugal nerves.

effervesce (L. *effervescere*, from *fervēre*, to be hot). To foam with the escape of gas.

efferves·cent. Effervescing; capable of becoming effervescent when dissolved.

effleurage (Fr. *effleurer*, to touch lightly). In massage, the stroking movement.

efflores·cence. 1. An eruption; a rash. 2. Conversion of a crystalline substance into powder by a loss of its water of crystallization on exposure to air.

efflu·vium (L.). An evil-smelling exhalation.

efflux·ion (L. *effluere*, to flow out). 1. An outflow. 2. That which flows out.

effort syndrome. A condition characterized by attacks of fatigue, dyspnoea, palpitations and precordial pains after bodily or emotional exertion, occurring especially in young adults. Syn. neurocirculatory asthenia; Da Costa's syndrome; disordered action of the heart; soldier's heart.

effū·sion (L. *effusio*, a pouring out). 1. A pouring out, especially of a transudate or an exudate, into serous cavities. 2. The effused fluid.

efuni·culate (L. *e*, neg.; *funiculus*, a little cord). Having no navel cord.

ēgagrop·ilus (G. *aigagros*, a wild goat; L. *pĭla*, a ball). Hair ball formed in the stomach or intestine.

eger·sis (G., a waking). Wakefulness.

eges·ta (L. *e*, out; *gerere*, to bear). Excretions.

egg. See ovum. **E. albumin**: albumin in white of egg.

ēgil·ops (G. *aix*, goat; *ops*, eye). Inflammation of the inner canthus of the eye due to lacrimal fistula.

ego (L. *ego*, I). In psychoanalysis, that part of the mental apparatus which results from the influence of the external world on the more primal structure Id.

While never entirely differentiated from the Id, it serves to hold the Id in check.

egocen·tric (L. *ego*, I; *centrum*, centre). Self-centred.

Ehrenritter's ganglion (Ehrenritter, J., Austrian anatomist, died 1790). The jugular ganglion.

Ehret's disease (Ehret, H., German physician, born 1870). Paralysis of the peronei muscles with spasmodic contracture of their antagonists.

Ehrlich's anaemia (Ehrlich, P., German physician, 1854–1915). Aplastic anaemia; a rapidly progressing anaemia accompanied by hyperplasia of the bone-marrow and haemorrhages into the mucous membrane. **E.'s biochemical theory**: that a specific chemical affinity exists between specific living cells and specific chemical substances. **E.'s diazo reagent**: a solution of sulphanilic acid and sodium nitrite used in the van den Bergh liver function test to measure bilirubin. **E.'s reagent**: a solution of *p*-dimethylaminobenzaldehyde in acetic acid/hydrochloric acid mixture. Syn. Rosindol reaction; Böhme's Indol test. **E.'s side-chain theory**: a hypothesis which is based on the phenomena of immunity. **E.'s solution**: a solution of a basic aniline dye in aniline oil and water.

Ehrlich-Hata preparation. '606' Salvarsan.

Eichhorst's corpuscles (Eichhorst, H., Swiss physician, 1849–1921). Small globular blood corpuscles found in pernicious anaemia. **E.'s neuritis**: n. fascians, in which the morbid process involves both the nerve-sheath and the interstitial tissues of muscles. **E.'s type of progressive muscular atrophy**: the femorotibial type, with contracture of the toes.

Eichstedt's disease (Eichstedt, K. F., German physician, 1816–92). Pityriasis versicolor.

eidet·ic (G. *eidētikos*, scientific, from *eidenai*, lit. to have seen, hence, to know). Having in a high degree the power to retain sensory, especially visual, perceptions.

eighth nerve. Auditory nerve.

Eijkman's test (Eijkman, C., Dutch physiologist, 1858–1930). A test for phenol. A red colouration is produced if a few drops of an alcoholic solution of nitrous acid, ethyl ether, and sulphuric acid are added to the phenol solution.

Eimeria. A genus of coccidians.

Eimer's organ, body (Eimer, G. H. T., Swiss anatomist, 1843–98). The sensory end organ first observed in the skin of the snout of the common mole (*Talpa europea*).

Einthoven's string galvanometer (Einthoven, W., Dutch physiologist, 1860–1927). An instrument for measuring electric currents by their magnetic effects.

Eitelberg's test (Eitelberg, A. Austrian physician, born 1847). A tuning fork test in cases of deafness.

e.j. Abbreviation for elbow jerk.

ejă·culate (L. *ex*, out; *jaculare*, from *jaculum*, a dart). To throw out suddenly.

ejaculā·tion (L. *ex*, out; *jaculare*, to throw). Ejecting suddenly, especially ejection of seminal fluid.

ejaculā·tory (L. *ex*, out; *jaculare*, to throw). Throwing out suddenly.

ejec·ta (L. past part. of *ejicere*, to cast out). Matter thrown out; excretions.

ejec·tion (L. *ejicere*). 1. The casting out of excretions. 2. Ejecta.

elastic (G. *elaunein*, to beat out, lit. to drive). Having the quality of elasticity, *q.v.* **E. fibres**: fibres with e. properties within the intercellular substance of connective tissue.

elasti·city (G. *elaunein*, to beat out). The property of a body to resist a deforming force in returning to its original shape after the removal of that force.

elas·tin (G. *elaunein*, to beat out). The characteristic constituent of yellow elastic connective tissue, a protein mainly composed of glycine, leucine, alanine, phenylalanine, proline and valine, differing from collagen especially by containing leucine in a much larger proportion.

elastō·sis. Any deterioration of elastic tissues.

elatē·rium (L.). The extract from the juice of the squirting cucumber. A powerful cathartic.

Elaut's triangle (Elaut, L. Belgian anatomist). Between the common iliac arteries and the promontory of the sacrum.

elbow. The joint at the bend of the arm.

elder flowers. The dried corollas and stamens of the *Sambucus nigra*, growing in Europe. The flowers produce a volatile oil and are used for dressings.

elec. Abbreviation for electricity.

elec·tosomes (L. *eligere*, to choose; G. *sōma*, body). Mitochondria as structures of specific chemical action.

elec·trencĕ·phalogram. See electro-encephalogram, electro-encephalography.

electric (G. *ēlektron*, amber). Producing, charged with, produced or operated by electricity. **E. bath:** application of galvanic or slow sinusoidal current to the body or the limbs (four-cell bath) while immersed in water. **E. chorea:** see chorea, e. **E. conduction:** flow of an e. charge between two points of different e. potential. **E. current:** 1. any motion of an e. charge. 2. Abbreviated for intensity or strength of e. current; the amount of e. charge passing through an area in a unit of time. **E. density:** intensity of e. charge per unit of area. **E. field:** any field in which e. forces may be shown to exist, such as the portion of space around an electrically charged body. **E. intensity:** the mechanical force at a point that a unit charge would experience if placed at that point. **E. potential:** a characteristic point in an e. field, *q.v.*, measured by the energy necessary to move a positive unit of e. charge from outside the field to the point in question without altering the field itself. See also difference of potential.

elec·trical (G. *ēlektron*, amber). Pertaining to electricity.

electri·city (G. *ēlektron*, amber). 1. A general term covering any electric phenomenon. 2. More specifically, electric charge.

electrizā·tion (G. *ēlektron*, amber). The application of an electric charge, as to the body.

electrobiŏ·logy (G. *ēlektron*, amber; *bios*, life; *logos*, a treatise). The branch of biology dealing with electric phenomena of organisms.

elec·trocar·diogram (G. *ēlektron*, amber; *kardia*, heart; *gramma*, from *graphein*, to mark). The record made by an electrocardiograph.

elec·trocar·diograph (G. *ēlektron*, amber; *kardia*, heart; *graphein*, to mark). An instrument for recording the changes of electric potential, caused by contraction of the heart muscles, by means of either a string galvanometer or a cathode ray oscillograph which is connected with two different parts of the body (cf. lead) and the vibrations of which are photographed.

elec·trocardiŏ·graphy (G. *ēlektron*, amber; *kardia*, heart; *graphein*, to mark). The method of recording an electrocardiogram.

elec·trocau·tery (G. *ēlektron*, amber; *kauterion*, from *kaiein*, to burn). Cautery by means of heat developed by a galvanic current.

elec·trochĕ·mistry. The study of chemical changes produced by electricity.

elec·trocoă·gulation (G. *ēlektron*, amber; L. *coagulare*, from *cogere*, to collect). Coagulation of tissues by electric current.

elec·trode (G. *ēlektron*, amber; *hodos*, road). Any terminal by which an electric current passes in and out of a body, such as an electrolyte, vacuum tube or animal body.

elec·trodiagnō·sis. The diagnosis of disease by means of electricity.

elec·trodī·aphane (G. *ēlektron*, amber; *diaphanēs*, translucent). An instrument for illuminating the stomach.

elec·trodynă·mics (G. *ēlektron*, amber; *dunamis*, power). The science pertaining to electric currents, electrically or magnetically charged moving bodies, electrons and varying electric or magnetic fields.

elec·trodynamŏ·meter (G. *ēlektron*, amber; *dunamis*, power; *metron*, measure). An instrument for measuring electric currents by the force produced between two coils passed by currents.

electro-encephalogram (G. *ēlektron*, amber; *egkephalos*, brain; *gramma*, from *graphein*, to mark). A record of cerebral action currents.

electro-encephalŏ·graphy (G. *ēlektron*, amber; *egkephalos*, brain; *graphein*, to mark). Method of recording cerebral action currents.

electrŏ·lysis (G. *ēlektron*, amber; *luein*, to loosen). 1. The decomposing effect of an electric current on a conducting medium (the electrolyte); the dissociation of ions, *q.v.*, of an electrolyte and their migration to the electrodes. 2. Destruction of tissue, such as hair roots or warts, by an electric current.

elec·trolyte (G. *ēlektron*, amber; *luein*, to loosen). Any acid, base, salt or other substance which when dissolved in water or certain other fluids or when melted dissociates into ions, rendering the liquid thereby electrically conductive.

elec·trolyze. To subject to electrolysis.

elec·tromag·net (G. *ēlektron*, amber; *Magnēsia*, in Lydia). A core of soft iron, surrounded by insulated wire, which is magnetic as long as an electric current is passing through the wire.

elec·tromag·netism. Magnetism produced by an electric current or an electric field.

electromas·sage (G. *ēlektron*, amber; Fr. *masser*, to massage). The transmission of an electric current through a kneading instrument; a combination of electro-therapy with massage.

electrŏ·meter (G. *ēlektron*, amber; *metron*, measure). An instrument for measuring the differences of electric potential used for indication of electric charges.

electromō·tive (G. *ēlektron*, amber; L. *movēre*, to move). Producing an electric current; causing electric effects. **E. force:** the voltage between externally unconnected terminals of an electric source. Abbreviation e.m.f.

elec·tromȳ·ogram (G. *ēlektron*, amber; *mus*, muscle; *gramma*, from *graphein*, to mark). A record of the action currents of muscles.

elec·tron (G. *ēlektron*, amber). A particle of negative electric charge, being the smallest known amount both of electric charge and mass; a constituent of the atom of any chemical element, the valency of the latter depending on the number of extranuclear electrons in its atoms; any increase above, or decrease below, the normal number of electrons of a body or part of a body represents a negative or positive charge, respectively, while moving electrons constitute an electric current.

elec·tronarcō·sis. Narcosis produced by means of electric currents.

elec·tronĕ·gative (G. *ēlektron*, amber; L. *negare*, to deny). Pertaining to or charged with negative electricity; tending to pass to the anode in electrolysis.

electron·ic. Relating to electrons.

electro-osmō·sis (G. *ēlektron*, amber; *ōsmos*, a thrust). The movement of a conducting solvent through a membrane.

electropathŏ·logy (G. *ēlektron*, amber; *pathos*, disease; *logos*, a discourse). The study of morbid conditions by means of electric irritation.

elec·trophorē·sis (G. *ēlektron*, amber; *pherein*, to carry). Movement of electrically charged suspended particles.

elec·tropnēu·mograph (G. *ēlektron*, amber; *pneuma*, breath; *graphein*, to write). An instrument for recording breathing.

electropŏ·sitive (G. *ēlektron*, amber; L. *positivus*, from *ponere*, to place). Pertaining to or charged with positive electricity; tending to pass to the cathode in electrolysis.

elec·tropuncture (G *ēlektron*, amber; L. *pungere*, to penetrate). The application of galvanic current to a part through a needle serving as electrode.

elec·tropyrĕx·ia (G. *ēlektron*, amber; *puressein*, to be feverish). The artificial raising of the temperature by means of electric currents.

electrorĕ·tinogram (G. *ēlektron*, amber; Mediaeval L. *retina*, perh. from L. *rete*, a net; G. *gramma*, mark). A record of the retinal action currents.

elec·troscope (G. *ēlektron*, amber; *skopein*, to view). An instrument for detecting the presence of small electric charges.

elec·trosol. A colloidal metal.

elec·trosome (G. *ēlektron*, amber; *sōma*, body). Part of the cytoplasm which is capable of chemical action.

electrostat·ic (G. *ēlektron*, amber; *statikos*, from *histanai*, to cause to stand). Pertaining to static or stationary electricity.

electrostat·ics (G. *ēlektron*, amber; *statikos*, from *histanai*, to cause to stand). The science of static or stationary electricity.

electrosur·gery. The use of electric currents in surgery.

elec·trosyn·thesis (G. *ēlektron*, amber; *suntiathenei*, to put together). Synthesis of a chemical compound by the use of electricity.

electrothĕ·rapy (G. *ēlektron*, amber; *therapeia*, treatment). The application of electricity for therapeutic purposes.

elec·trotherm (G. *ēlektron*, amber; *thermē*, heat). A heat-producing apparatus used to relieve pain by the application of an electric current to the skin.

elec·trotome (G. *ēlektron*, amber; *tomē*, section). An electric surgical knife.

electrŏ·tonus (G. *ēlektron*, amber; *tonos*, tone). The change of condition in a nerve during the passage of a constant galvanic current. See also anelectrotonus; catelectrotonus.

elec·trotrĕ·phine. A trephine operated by an electric current.

elec·trovā·gogram (G. *ēlektron*, amber; *L. vagus*; G. *gramma*, a writing). The electrical changes occurring in the vagus nerve as recorded by a string galvanometer.

elec·tuary (Late L. *electuarium*, an electuary; from G. *ekleikhein*, to lick up). A medicinal preparation containing as base honey or syrup to form a paste-like mass.

elĕ·idin (G. *elaia*, olive-tree). A protein (or protein-like substance) of oily consistency occurring in and between the cells of the stratum lucidum of the epidermis.

element (L. *elementum*). 1. Any one of the ultimate parts of which anything is supposed to be composed. 2. In chemistry, a substance that cannot be decomposed into simpler substances by ordinary chemical means (i.e., excluding radio-activity or bombardment of atoms) and that consists of atoms of one type only. The recognized elements number 92. Their arrangement according to their atomic numbers constitutes the series of the periodic law of Mendeleev (Dmitri Ivanovich) and Mendel (Lothar). 3. A component.

elemen·tary (L. *elementum*). 1. Ultimate. 2. Pertaining to elements. **E. bodies:** small intracellular bodies, $0.1\,\mu$ to $0.25\,\mu$ in size, found in many diseases caused by viruses, and probably consist of aggregations of virus particles. Syn. Paschen bodies.

elĕŏ·meter (G. *elaion*, oil; *metron*, measure). An apparatus for the determination of the specific gravity of oil.

el·eosac·charum (G. *elaion*, oil; *sakkhar*, sugar). An oil-sugar.

elephanti·asis (G. *elephas*, elephant). A chronic condition characterised by diffuse fibromatosis of the cutaneous and sub-cutaneous tissues and gross enlargement of the affected parts (i.e., mainly the lower limbs and external genitals); mostly due to obstruction of lymph-flow, as caused by filariasis, *q.v.* **E. nervosum:** neurofibromatosis, *q.v.*, involving a limited region in a diffuse manner so that the affected part is grossly enlarged or deformed.

elevā·tor (L. *elevare*, to lift up). An instrument used as a lever for raising a part.

eliminā·tion (L. *eliminare*, from *e*, out, and *limen*, threshold). Casting out, removing, especially waste products.

elix·ir (Arab. *al*, *iksir*). A sweetened, aromatic preparation containing alcohol or glycerin used as a vehicle for bitter or nauseous drugs.

Elliot's operation (Elliot, R. H., Colonel, Indian Medical Service, 1864–1936). Corneo-scleral trephining for chronic glaucoma.

Elliot-Smith, area paraterminalis of (Elliot-Smith, Sir L. G., Australian anatomist, 1871–1937). A space on the mesial aspect of the embryonic cerebral hemisphere. **Fasciculus praecommissuralis of E.-S.:** the peduncle of the corpus callosum in the embryo.

ellip·soid. A geometrical surface all plane sections of which are ellipses or circles.

Ellis's ligament (Ellis, C., American physician, 1826–83). The rectovesical fascia at its attachment to the rectum. **E.'s line:** the upper limit of a pleural effusion. **E.'s sign:** a curved line of dullness found on percussion of the chest, during the absorption of a pleural exudate.

Ellis's muscle (Ellis, G. V., English anatomist, 1812–1900). The subcutaneous external sphincter or corrugator cutis ani, an annular muscle about $\frac{1}{4}$ inch in diameter situated beneath the skin at the anal margin.

Ellis-Damoiseau's curve. Ellis's line and sign, *q.v.*

elm. A tree of the *Ulmus* family. **E., slippery:** the dried inner bark of the *U. fulva*. The resulting powder is used as a demulcent in catarrhal affections, diarrhoea, etc.

Elsberg's solution (Elsberg, C. L., American surgeon, born 1871). A 20 per cent solution of iodine in alcohol and ether.

Elsner's asthma (Elsner, C. F., German physician, 1749–1820). Angina pectoris.

Elsner's medium (Elsner, M., German bacteriologist, 1861–1935). A special culture medium composed of Holz's acid potato-gelatin with 1 per cent of potassium iodide.

elute (L. *eluere*, to wash off). To wash out.

elu·tion (L. *eluere*, to wash off). Separation of substances by washing.

elutriā·tion (L. *elutriare*, to wash out). 1. Separation of substances by repeated washing and decanting. 2. In pharmacy, the method of repeated washing and decanting for obtaining a fluid containing an insoluble powder of a certain fineness.

elytri·tis (G. *elutron*, a sheath). Inflammation of the vagina.

ĕ·lytrocele (G. *elutron*, a sheath; *kēlē*, hernia). Vaginal hernia.

elytroclā·sia (G. *elutron*, a sheath; *klasis*, a fracture). Vaginal rupture.

elytroclei·sis (G. *elutron*, a sheath; *kleisis*, closure). Closure of the vagina.

ĕ·lytroplasty (G. *elutron*, a sheath; *plassein*, to form). Plastic surgery of the vagina.

ĕ·lytroptō·sis (G. *elutron*, a sheath; *piptein*, to fall). Vaginal prolapse.

elytror·rhaphy (G. *elutron*, a sheath; *rhaphē*, suture). Suture of the vagina.

elytrŏ·tomy (G. *elutron*, a sheath; *tomē*, section). Incision into the vagina.

Em. Symbol for Emanation (2). It is the decomposition product of radium. Syn. radon.

emaciā·tion (L. *emaciare*, to make lean). Wasting.

emaculā·tion (L. *e*, out; *macula*, spot). The removal of spots or freckles from the face.

email·loid (Fr. *émail*, enamel). A tumour growing from tooth enamel.

emanā·tion (L. *emanare*, to flow out). 1. Emission. 2. A gaseous element produced by disintegration of radio-active substances. Symbol. Em.

emasculā·tion (L. *emasculare*, to castrate). Removal or absence of the male genitals.

Embadomonas intestinalis. A protozoan flagellate.

embalm (Fr. *embaumer*, from L. *balsamum*, balsam). To treat a cadaver with antiseptic and preservative substances to prevent putrefaction.

embedding. The fixation of a specimen in a medium such as paraffin for its support during the cutting of thin sections.

embolec·tomy (G. *en*, in; *ballein*, to throw; *ektomē*, excision). Removal of an embolus.

embol·ic (G. *en*, in; *ballein*, to throw). Relating to or caused by an embolus or embolism.

em·bolism (G. *en*, in; *ballein*, to throw). The obstruction or occlusion of a blood-vessel, especially an artery, by a transported clot. E., paradoxical: e. in which the embolus has arisen in a vein or in one of the right chambers of the heart, but becomes impacted in a systemic artery owing to passage of the embolus either through a defect of the cardiac septa, especially a patent foramen ovale, or through the pulmonary capillaries. In venous thrombophlebitis, emboli may, however, also originate from a secondary pulmonary infarction or a secondary endocarditis on the left side of the heart.

em·bololā·lia (G. *emballein*, to throw in; *lalia*, a talking). The inclusion of meaningless words into the speech.

em·bolus (G. *en*, in; *ballein*, to throw). Any foreign particle, such as a detached part of a thrombus, a collection of fat globules, air bubbles or tumour cells, circulating in the blood and forming an obstruction to the bloodflow at the place of its lodgment. E., infective: an e. containing pathogenic micro-organisms which cause the development of an abscess at the site of its lodgment.

em·boly (G. *embolē*, a throwing in). The process of invagination of the wall of the blastula, giving rise to the gastrula.

embrocā·tion (G. *embrokhē*, a fomentation). 1. The application, especially by rubbing, of a lotion to a part of the body. 2. The liquid so applied.

em·bryo (G. *embruon*). 1. A developing organism prior to its emergence from the egg membranes, or (in plants) from the seed. 2. In viviparous animals, an organism during its early stages of intra-uterine development; in man, up to the end of the second month.

embryocar·dia (G. *embruon*; *kardia*, heart). A condition in which the heart-sounds resemble those of the foetus, the first and second sounds being almost alike and the long pause shortened.

em·bryogen·esis, embryŏ·geny (G. *embruon*; *gennan*, to produce). Origin and development of the embryo.

embryŏ·logy (G. *embruon*; *logos*, a treatise). The science of the development of the embryo.

embryŏ·ma (G. *embruon*). 1. A rudimentary parasitic foetus in a double monster. 2. A teratoid tumour of eventually malignant character in a sex gland, arising probably from primitive germinal cells, composed of structures derived from any of the three germinal layers. 3. Wilm's tumour, *q.v.*

embryŏ·matous (G. *embruon*). Pertaining to an embryoma. E. cyst: a cyst of the ovary or the testicle containing rudimentary parts of a parasitic twin embryo. See also embryoma (2).

embrȳ·onal, embryŏn·ic (G. *embruon*). Pertaining to an embryo.

embryotŏ·cia (G. *embruon*; *tokein*, to give birth). An abortion.

em·bryotome (G. *embruon*; *tomē*, section). Instrument for performing embryotomy.

embryŏ·tomy (G. *embruon*; *tomē*, section). Instrumental dismemberment of a foetus in the uterus for reducing its size when its removal is otherwise impossible.

em·bryotox·on (G. *embruon*; *toxon*, a bow). Impaired transparency of the corneal margin in the newborn.

embryot·rophy (G. *embruon*; *trophē*, from *trephein*, nourish). The nutrition of the foetus.

embryul·cia (G. *embruon*; *helkein*, to drag). Surgical instrument for the withdrawal of the foetus from the uterus.

emedul·late (L. *ē*, out; *medulla*, marrow). To extract marrow.

emergency (L. *emergere*, to come forth). An urgent and sudden need.

em·esis (G. *emeein*, to vomit). Vomiting.

em·etatrō·phia (G. *emeein*, to vomit; *atrophia*, atrophy). The wasting that accompanies continuous vomiting.

emet·ic (G. *emeein*, to vomit). Promoting emesis.

emetine. An alkaloid derived from ipecacuanha. Principally used in medicine in the treatment of amoebic dysentery.

E.M.F. Abbreviation for electromotive force.

emic·tory (L. *e*, out; *mingere*, to urinate). A diuretic.

emigrā·tion (L. *emigrare*, to depart). See diapedesis.

eminence (L. *eminentia*, prominence). A projecting part of an organ, especially of a bone.

emissā·rium (L. *emittere*, to send out). An outlet.

em·issary (L. *emittere*, to send out). Applied to the veins which pierce the cranial bones, forming an anastomosis between the veins of the cranial surface and the dural sinuses.

emission (L. *emittere*, to send out). 1. An ejaculation, *q.v.* 2. Radiation of light- or heat-rays.

emmen·agogue (G. *emmēna*, menses; *agōgos*, leading). 1. Promoting menstrual flow. 2. An agent promoting menstrual flow.

emmē·nia (G. *emmēna*, menses). The menses.

emmen·ic. Pertaining to the menses.

emmeniŏ·pathy (G. *emmēna*, menses; *pathos*, disease). Any menstrual disorder.

Emmerich's bacillus (Emmerich, R., German bacteriologist, 1852–1914). *Bacillus coli communis*.

Emmet's operation (Emmet, T. A., American gynaecologist, 1828–1919). Trachelorrhaphy.

em·metrope (G. *en*, in; *metron*, measure; *ops*, eye). A person whose eyes are emmetropic.

emmetrō·pia (G. *en*, in; *metron*, measure; *ops*, eye). The normal condition of refraction in which, with suspended accommodation, parallel rays of light are accurately focused on the retina.

K

emmetrop·ic. Relating to emmetropia.

emol. A powder of talc, silica, aluminium and a trace of lime.

emol·lient (L. *emollire*, from *mollis*, soft). 1. Softening; soothing. 2. A softening or soothing preparation.

emō·tion (L.L. *emotio*, from *emovēre*, to agitate). The totality of both mental and bodily responses to a situation involving an excitation of, or marked change of feeling in association with a change in neuro-endocrine activity (of sometimes mainly sympathetico-mimetic, sometimes mixed character) and sometimes with increased motor activity.

emō·tional (L.L. *emotio*, from *emovēre*, to agitate). Pertaining to or manifesting emotion.

emphysē·ma (G. *emphusan*, to inflate). Any abnormal distension of a tissue by air or some other gas. E., **compensatory**: e. of an area of the lung developing while another portion has become consolidated. E., **interstitial**: distension of the interstitial tissue of the lung by air which has escaped from ruptured pulmonary alveoli; the air usually collecting in the lymph spaces may pass to the mediastinum and from there to the tissues of the neck and chest wall. E., **pulmonary**: abnormal distension of the pulmonary alveoli by air with consequent destruction of their walls and narrowing or obliteration of the blood-vessels in the remaining septa, causing serious impairment of the elasticity of the lung tissue and of the pulmonary circulation and thereby respiratory embarrassment, dilatation and hypertrophy of the right heart and systemic venous congestion, leading to systemic circulatory insufficiency; also giving rise to barrel-shaped deformity of the chest, the antero-posterior diameter of which approximates to the transverse diameter, to enlargement of the intercostal spaces, to a low position of the inferior pulmonary borders, and to increased resonance on percussion and indistinctness of the breathing sounds. E., **surgical**: distension of subcutaneous tissue by air penetrating from wounds of air-containing organs, or from without.

emphysē·matous (G. *emphusan*, to inflate). Pertaining to, or affected with, emphysema.

empi·ric, empi·rical (G. *empeirikos*, experienced). Pertaining to or based on actual experience only.

empi·ricism (G. *empeirikos*, experienced). Dependence upon experience only.

Empir's 'granulie'. Acute miliary tuberculosis of the lungs.

emplā·stic (G. *emplastron*, a plaster). Adhesive.

emplā·strum (G. *emplastron*, a plaster). A plaster; a hard adhesive preparation softening under the heat of the body surface.

emprosthŏ·tonos, emprŏs·thotŏ·nus (G. *emprosthen*, before; *tōnos*, tone). Tonic muscular spasm, affecting especially the flexor muscles, so that the body is bent forward.

emp·tysis (G. *emptusis*, a spitting). Spitting, especially spitting of blood.

empyē·ma (G. *en*, in; *puon*, pus). Purulent pleurisy.

em·pyocele. A septic scrotal tumour.

emulsificā·tion (L. *emulgere*, to milk; *facere*, to make). The process of making or becoming an emulsion.

emul·sify. To change into an emulsion.

emul·sin. An enzyme splitting amygdalin and other beta glycosides. Syn. synaptase.

emul·sion (L. *emulgere*, to milk). 1. A suspension of a liquid dispersed in form of droplets or fine particles in another liquid, the former acting as dispersed, the latter as continuous phase. See also colloid. 2. In pharmacy, a suspension of an oil or resin in water, e.g. by means of gum arabic, effecting a very fine division of the oleaginous or resinous particules.

emul·soid (L. *emulgere*, to milk; G. *eidos*, form). Term applied to colloids forming semi-solid or solid gels, e.g., protein colloids, starch, gum arabic. Syn. hydrophilic or graphilic colloid.

emul·sum (L. *emulgere*, to milk). An emulsion.

enă·mel. The vitreous calcareous substance covering the crown of the teeth, formed from the enamel organ. **E. organ**: the structure composed of adamantoblasts and formed from an ingrowth of the oral epithelium (dental lamina of the labiodental stratum).

enan·thema (G. *en*, in; *anthēma*, an offering). An eruption on a mucous membrane.

enan·thrope (G. *en*, in; *anthrōpos*, man). The source of disease commencing internally.

enan·tiobiō·sis (G. *enantios*, opposite; *bios*, life). Symbiosis, *q.v.*

enan·tiomor·phous (G. *enantios*, opposite; *morphē*, form). Similar but contrasted or reversed in form, as either of the two hands or of two opposite optically active substances.

Enan·tiotham·nus. A genus of fungi.

enar·kyochrome (G. *en*, in; *arkūs*, a net; *khrōma*, colour). A term used by Nissl for a nerve cell taking the stain best in the cell body.

enarthrō·dial (G. *en*, in; *arthron*, joint). Relating to an enarthrosis.

enarthrō·sis (G. *en*, in; *arthron*, joint). A ball-and-socket joint, admitting of movement in any direction, e.g. that of the hip.

en bissac (Fr.). A diverticulum in a hernial sac.

en bloc (Fr.). As a whole.

encan·this (G. *en*, in; *kanthos*, the angle of the eye). A new growth occurring in the inner canthus of the eye.

encapsulā·tion (L. *in*; *capsula*, dim. of *capsa*, a box). The surrounding of a part by a capsule.

encap·suled (L. *in*; *capsula*, little box). Enclosed.

enceinte (Fr.). Pregnant.

encephal·ic (G. *egkephalos*, brain). Pertaining to the brain.

encephalit·ic (G. *egkephalos*, brain). Relating to or affected with encephalitis.

encephalī·tis (G. *egkephalos*, brain). Inflammation of the brain. E., **epidemic**: a virus disease, of sometimes epidemic character, characterized by vascular congestion, perivascular round-cell infiltration, degeneration of the nerve-cells and glial proliferation mainly of the midbrain and the basal ganglia and clinically by an acute stage of widely varying severity and symptoms (such as fever, lethargy or inversion of sleep, oculomotor paresis usually with diplopia, pareses of other cranial or peripheral nerves, extrapyramidal rigidity or hyperkinesis) often followed after varying intervals by a chronic stage in which parkinsonism, *q.v.*, and also oculogyric spasms, mental deterioration and change of personality are the most frequent symptoms. Syn. E. lethargica; von Economo's e. E., **haemorrhagic**: see polio-encephalitis, haemorrhagic. E., **Japanese**: a virus disease of which two types are recognized: a Type A largely resembling epidemic e. of von Economo (see above), and a Type B of more acute nature and a higher mortality, involving higher age groups and affecting the entire brain, but in the survivors rarely leaving serious sequelae. **E. periaxialis diffusa**: See Schilder's disease. E. **post-vaccinalis**: an acute disseminated encephalomyelitis, *q.v.*, appearing within the second week after vaccination against smallpox; extremely rarely in infants vaccinated during the first six months of life. E., **St. Louis**: a virus disease differing from epidemic e. of von Economo mainly by the frequent occurrence of meningeal irritation, its shorter course and a low incidence of sequelae.

encě·phalocele (G. *egkephalos*, brain; *kēlē*, hernia). A protrusion of a portion of the brain through a cranial fissure.

encĕ·phalodiăl·ysis (G. *egkephalos*, brain; *dia*, through; *lusis*, loosening). Softening of the brain.

encephalŏ·graphy (G. *egkephalos*, brain; *graphein*, to write). X-ray investigation of the brain after replacement by air of some cerebrospinal fluid by (usually) ventricular, suboccipital or lumbar puncture, whereby the ventricular spaces become opaque to X-rays.

encĕ·phaloid (G. *egkephalos*, brain; *eidos*, form). 1. Resembling brain tissue. 2. Medullary carcinoma, *q.v.*

encephalŏ·logy (G. *egkephalos*, brain; *logos*, a treatise). The science pertaining to a study of the brain.

encephalŏ·ma (G. *egkephalos*, brain). A brain tumour.

encĕ·phalomalā·cia (G. *egkephalos*, brain; *malakia*, softness). Softening of brain substance due to cerebral thrombosis or embolism, with resulting ischaemia and degeneration of the involved area.

encĕ·phalomeningī·tis (G. *egkephalos*, brain; *mēnigx*, membrane). Inflammation of both brain and meninges.

encĕ·phalomenin·gocele (G. *egkephalos*, brain; *mēnigx*, membrane; *kēlē*, hernia). Protrusion of both brain and meninges through a cranial fissure.

encĕ·phalomere (G. *egkephalos*, brain; *meros*, part). A segment in the cranial portion of the neural tube.

encĕ·phalomyelī·tis (G. *egkephalos*, brain; *muelos*, marrow). Inflammation of both brain and spinal cord. E., acute disseminated: a condition characterized by scattered patches of perivascular demyelinization in both grey and white matter of brain and spinal cord, and infiltration of perivascular spaces with lymphocytes and plasma cells, especially marked in pons, medulla and lumbar region of the cord; and clinically by fever, headache, vomiting, cerebral and/or spinal pareses, meningeal symptoms or convulsions; occurring as primary disease or following vaccination or measles, mumps, smallpox, typhus fever, pertussis or other infectious diseases; possibly due to the virus causing the primary disease or to its stimulating effect on another virus latent in the central nervous tissue. E., equine: a virus disease transmitted by several species of mosquitoes, affecting mainly horses, rarely man, in whom it resembles a severe form of epidemic encephalitis, *q.v.*, Syn. Borna disease.

encĕ·phalomyelŏ·pathy (G. *egkephalos*, brain; *muelos*, marrow; *pathos*, disease). Any disease affecting both the brain and the spinal cord.

encĕ·phalon (G. *egkephalos*, brain). The brain.

encephalopath·ic (G. *egkephalos*, brain; *pathos*, disease). Relating to a brain disease.

encephalŏ·pathy (G. *egkephalos*, brain; *pathos*, disease). Any disease of the brain. See also Wernicke's e. E., hypertensive: the cerebral syndrome due to acute or chronic arterial hypertension (as in essential hypertension, malignant hypertension, eclampsia, chronic glomerulo-nephritis), characterized by headache and/or vomiting, convulsions, coma, or other signs of focal or diffuse cerebral disturbance, including cerebral vascular lesions. E., lead: a condition characterized by epileptic fits, and/or acute mania, delirium, coma and optic neuritis, due to chronic lead poisoning.

encephalopă·thia satur·nia (G. *egkephalos*, brain; *pathos*, disease; L. *Saturnus*, Saturn, astrological symbol of lead). Encephalopathy, lead, *q.v.*

encephalorrhā·gia (G. *egkephalos*, brain; *rhēgnunai*, to burst out). Cerebral haemorrhage.

encĕ·phalosclerŏ·sis (G. *egkephalos*, brain; *sklerōsis*, hardening). Hardening of the brain.

encĕ·phalothlip·sis (G. *egkephalos*, brain; *thlibein*, to press). Pressure on the brain.

encephalŏ·tomy (G. *egkephalos*, brain; *tomē*, section). 1. Surgical incision of the brain. 2. Craniotomy, *q.v.*

encheirē·sis (G. *en*, in; *kheir*, hand). Any manipulative action.

enchon·dral (G. *en*, in; *khondros*, cartilage). 1. Lying within cartilage. 2. Originating from cartilage.

enchondrŏ·ma (G. *en*, in; *khondros*, cartilage). A chondroma growing in tissue not ordinarily containing cartilage, as in the interior of a bone.

enchondrŏ·sis (G. *en*, in; *khondros*, cartilage). Any cartilaginous outgrowth of tumour.

enchylē·ma (k) (G. *en*, in; *khulos*, juice). The cell-sap, or fluid granular substance filling the interstices of the cell-body and the nucleus.

encys·ted (G. *en*, in; *kustis*, the bladder). Enclosed in a cyst or capsule.

Endamoeba. See entamoeba.

endangiī·tis. Inflammation of the endangium.

endan·gium (G. *endon*, within; *aggeion*, a vessel). The inner lining of a blood vessel.

en·daortī·tis (G. *endon*, within; *aortē*, aorta). Inflammation of the innermost coat of the aorta.

end·arteri·tis (G. *endon*, within; *artēria*, artery). Inflammation of the innermost layer of the arterial wall. E. obliterans: a group of conditions characterized by the thickening of the arterial intima with narrowing or obliteration of the lumen, occurring in granulomatous tissues (as those affected by tuberculosis, syphilis or lepra) and in organs undergoing involution.

end-artery (G. *artēria*, artery). An a. that has no adequate anastomoses with another a., so that in cases of occlusion a collateral circulation cannot develop.

end-bulb of Krause. Encapsulated terminal arborization of freely anastomosing varicose and knobbed nerve fibrils in the corium, conjunctiva and certain other mucous membranes, and in connective tissues of glans penis, clitoris, tendons and striated muscle.

endem·ic (G. *en*, in; *dēmos*, people). Applied to any disease that is constantly prevalent in a particular area, sometimes in varying degrees.

endemiŏ·logy (G. *en*, in; *dēmos*, people; *logos*, discourse). The science of endemic diseases.

endermatic, ender·mic (G. *en*, in; *derma*, skin). Situated on or applied to the true skin; within the skin.

en·deron (G. *en*, in; *derma*, skin). The deeper part of the skin, beneath the epidermis. Hence enderonic, relating to enderon.

end-fibril (L. *fibrilla*, dim. of *fibra*, fibre). 1. A type of intra-epithelial nerve-ending, a naked terminal fibre forming a delicate plexus between the epithelial cells. 2. The terminal fibril of a neuron ending within the cytoplasm of another nerve-cell.

end-gut. The distal part of the large intestine and the rectum; the hind-gut.

end-lobe. The occipital lobe.

Endo's medium (Endo, S., Japanese physician, 1869–1937). Culture medium consisting of lactose agar with sodium hydroxide, phenolphthalein, fuchsin and sodium sulphate.

end-abdŏ·minal (G. *endon*, within; L. *abdomen*). Relating to the inner abdomen.

en·do-aneurysmŏr·rhaphy (G. *endon*, within; *aneurusma*, aneurysm; *rhaphē*, suture). Any one of the three following surgical methods: (1) Obliterative: incision of the aneurysmal sac, emptying of its contents, suturing from within of the openings of the parent artery and all other communicating vessels, obliteration of the sac by layers of invaginating sutures. (2) Restorative: used for saccular aneurysms with one opening into the parent artery; incision and evacuation of the sac, suturing from within of the opening into the artery without narrowing the restored artery, obliteration of the sac. (3) Reconstructive: used especially for fusiform aneurysms in which the two openings of the parent artery are closed together: incision and evacuation of the sac, insertion of a rubber tube into the two openings of the parent artery, suturing the adjacent parts of the sac over the tube, removal of the tube just before completion of the sutures.

endobiŏt·ic (G. *endon*, within; *bios*, life). Living in the tissues of the host.

en·doblast (G. *endon*, within; *blastos*, germ). Entoderm, *q.v.*

endocar·dial (G. *endon*, within; *kardia*, heart). Pertaining to the endocardium.

en·docardī·tis (G. *endon*, within; *kardia*, heart). A condition characterized by inflammatory changes of the endocardium, particularly, or limited to that, of the valves; usually due to rheumatic fever or to a bacterial infection. **E., bacterial:** e. due to a bacterial infection. **E., infective:** e., ulcerative, *q.v.* **E., malignant:** e., ulcerative, *q.v.* **E., rheumatic:** e. associated with rheumatic fever, usually accompanied by some inflammatory changes of the myocardium and less frequently also of the pericardium by the presence of Aschoff bodies, *q.v.*, in the myocardium and other vascular tissues; affecting particularly children and young adults; characterized by fever, tachycardia, heart murmurs and other cardiac disturbances such as palpitations, precordial pain, cardiac dilatation, and by moderate leucocytosis; frequently resulting in the establishment of a progressive valvular heart failure. **E., subacute bacterial:** a form of e. usually (i.e., in about 90 per cent of cases) due to *Streptococcus viridans* infection, characterized by remittent fever, constant or transitory presence of the causative micro-organism in the blood, progressive wasting and exhaustion, hypochromic anaemia with leucocytosis, petechiae, splenic enlargement, infarctions of spleen and/or lungs and kidneys, sometimes by eruptions of Osler's nodes, *q.v.*, and nearly always fatal outcome. Syn. E. lenta. **E., ulcerative:** bacterial e. characterized by ulceration of the inflammatory foci, giving rise to spread of infective emboli. Syn. infective e., malignant e. **E., verrucous:** rheumatic e. characterized by the development of wart-like vegetations from the inflammatory foci along the rims of the valves (mainly aortic and mitral).

endocar·dium (G. *endon*, within; *kardia*, heart). The serous membrane lining the interior of the heart.

endocel·lular (G. *endon*, within; L. *cellula*). Within a cell.

endocervī·cal (G. *endon*, within; L. *cervix*, neck). Relating to the inner parts of the cervix uteri.

endocervici·tis (G. *endon*, within; L. *cervix*, neck). Inflammation of the mucous membrane of the uterine cervix.

endochon·dral (G. *endon*, within; *khondros*, cartilage). Situated within a cartilage; arising from the interior of a cartilage.

endochŏ·rion (G. *endon*, within; *khorion*, membrane). The vascular layer of the allantois on the inner surface of the chorion.

en·docoli·tis (G. *endon*, within; *kolon*, colon). Inflammation of the internal coat of the colon.

en·docolpī·tis (G. *endon*, within; *kolpos*, a hollow). Inflammation of the innermost coat of the vagina.

en·docorpus·cular (G. *endon*, within; L. *corpusculum*, dim. of *corpus*, body). Contained in a corpuscle.

endocrā·nial (G. *endon*, within; *kranion*, skull). Contained inside the cranium.

en·docrani·tis (G. *endon*, within; *kranion*, skull). Inflammation of the endocranium.

endocrā·nium (G. *endon*, within; *kranion*, skull). 1. The dura mater, *q.v.* 2. The inner surface of the skull.

en·docrine (G. *endon*, within; *krinein*, to separate). 1. Secreting internally. 2. Pertaining to a product of internal secretion. **E. gland:** any gland forming one or several hormones which are passed to the body not by any excretory duct but by way of the blood-stream ('internal secretion'). Syn. ductless gland.

end·ocrinŏ·logy (G. *endon*, within; *krinein*, to separate; *logos*, a discourse). The science of the endocrine glands.

end·ocrinŏ·pathy (G. *endon*, within; *krinein*, to separate; *pathos*, disease). Any disease caused by disorder of the endocrine glands.

endocrinŏ·sis (G. *endon*, within; *krinein*, to separate). Disorder due to malfunctioning of the endocrine glands.

endocrinothĕ·rapy (G. *endon*, within; *krinein*, to separate; *therapeia*, treatment). The giving of endocrine gland preparations in the treatment of disease.

endŏ·crinous (G. *endon*, within; *krinein*, to separate). Relating to the endocrine glands or to internal secretions.

en·docystī·tis (G. *endon*, within; *kustis*, bladder). Inflammation of the innermost lining of the bladder.

en·docyte (G. *endon*, within; *kutos*, cell). Any foreign substance which may be found inside a cell.

Endoderm. Entoderm, *q.v.*

Endodermŏ·phyton (G. *endon*, within; *derma*, skin; *phuton*, a plant). A genus of fungus which invades and damages the skin.

endodia·scopy (G. *endon*, within; *dia*, through; *skopein*, to view). Examination of any of the body cavities by means of a tube illuminated at its distal end.

endodontī·tis (G. *endon*, within; *odous*, tooth). Inflammation of the pulp of a tooth.

endo-ectothrix (G. *endon*, within; *ektos*, outside; *thrix*, hair). Trichophyton fungi developing within the hair as well as (usually at a later stage) on the surface of the hair follicle of the host; comprising *T. cerebriforme* and *T. plicatile*, producing ringworm of the scalp, beard and glabrous skin. Syn. neo-endothrix.

endo·enteri·tis (G. *endon*, within; *enteron*, intestine). Inflammation of the innermost lining of the intestine.

endo-en·zyme (G. *endon*, within; *en*, in; *zumē*, leaven). An intracellular enzyme; an enzyme obtained from the phagocytic cells.

endŏ·gamy (G. *endon*, within; *gamos*, marriage). 1. Conjugation between gametes descended from the same ancestor. 2. The custom of marriage within a particular group (family, clan, etc.).

endogas·tric (G. *endon*, within; *gastēr*, stomach). Relating to the interior of the stomach.

endogastri·tis (G. *endon*, within; *gastēr*, stomach). Inflammation of the innermost lining of the stomach.

endŏ·genous (G. *endon*, within; *gennan*, to produce). Produced within, e.g. within the body.

endoglob·ular (G. *endon*, within; L. *globus*, a sphere). Within the blood corpuscles.

endognā·thion (G. *endon*, within; *gnathos*, jaw). The middle quadrant of the upper jaw.

endo·intoxication (G. *endon*, within; *toxikon*, poison). The absorption of an endogenous toxin causing poisoning.

en·dolabyrinthī·tis (G. *endon*, within; *laburinthos*, maze). Inflammation of the lining membranes of the labyrinth.

en·dolaryn·geal (G. *endon*, within; *larugx*, larynx). Within the larynx.

Endolimax nana (G. *endon*, within; L. *limax*, a snail; *nanus*, a dwarf). A non-tissue-invading protozoon, found as a parasite in the intestines in man.

en·dolymph (G. *endon*, within; L. *lympha*, water). The fluid of the membranous labyrinth of the ear.

endoly̆·sin (G. *endon*, within; *luein*, to loosen). Relatively thermostable non-specific bactericidal intracellular antibody, especially in leucocytes.

en·dometrec·tomy (G. *endon*, within; *metra*, womb; *ektome*, excision). Excision of the uterine mucosa.

endome·trial (G. *endon*, within; *metra*, womb). Pertaining to the endometrium.

endometriŏ·ma (G. *endon*, within; *metra*, womb). A tumour thought to arise from endometrial tissue implanted on the serous surface of pelvic viscera or into an abdominal organ or from other epithelial tissue of the female genital organs which has undergone metaplastic change, or perhaps from atretic ovarian follicles occurring most commonly in the ovary but also in the Fallopian tubes, the rectovaginal septum, pelvic ligaments, umbilicus, groin, 'or intestinal wall, forming cysts with haemorrhagic contents ('chocolate-coloured cysts') which are renewed at each menstrual period, rupture of the cysts being followed by development of particularly dense adhesions.

endometriŏ·sis (G. *endon*, within; *metra*, womb). The condition characterized by the presence of endometriomata.

en·dometri·tis (G. *endon*, within; *metra*, womb). Inflammation of the endometrium.

endome·trium (G. *endon*, within; *metra*, womb). The mucous membrane of the uterus.

endomix·is (G. *endon*, within; *mixis*, mixture). A process of reproduction in protozoa analogous to parthenogenesis in multicellular organisms in which the macro-nucleus is replaced by material derived from micro-nucleus or micro-nuclei which undergo(es) two maturation divisions; occurring sometimes periodically, alternating with amphimixis in which reproduction is effected by syngamy (conjugation).

Endomy̆·ces (G. *endon*, within; *mukes*, mushroom). Yeast-like fungi characterized by presence of asci, budding forms and well-developed mycelium.

endomycŏ·sis. Infection with Endomyces.

endomy̆·sium (G. *endon*, within; *mus*, muscle). The connective tissue septa originating from the perimysium separating small bundles of muscle cells.

endona·sal (G. *endon*, within; L. *nasus*, nose). The interior of the nose.

endoneū·ral (G. *endon*, within; *neuron*, sinew). Pertaining to the interior of a nerve.

endoneurī·tis (G. *endon*, within; *neuron*, sinew). Inflammation of the endoneurium.

endoneū·rium (G. *endon*, within; *neuron*, sinew). The connective tissue septa originating from the perineurium, forming a framework for the support of individual nerve fibres.

endopă·rasite (G. *endon*, within; *parasitos*, parasite). A parasite living within its host.

endopel·vic (G. *endon*, within; L. *pelvis*). Situated within the pelvis.

en·dopericar·dial (G. *endon*, within; *peri*, around; *kardia*, heart). Relating to both the endocardium and the pericardium.

en·dopericardi·tis (G. *endon*, within; *peri*, around; *kardia*, heart). Inflammation of endo- and pericardium.

en·dophlebi·tis (G. *endon*, within; *phleps*, vein). Inflammation of the inner coat of a vein. E. obliterans hepatica: thrombophlebitis causing obstruction of the hepatic veins. Syn. Chiari's disease.

en·doplasm (G. *endon*, within; *plassein*, to form). The main central portion of the cytoplasm, consisting of hyaloplasm with the spongioplasm.

en·doplast (G. *endon*, within; *plassein*, to form). A cell nucleus.

end-organ (O. E. *endian*, end; G. *organon*, organ). Ensheathed terminal arborization of a nerve fibre at the junction of the corium and the subcutaneous tissue and in the connective tissue septa of the latter. E. of Golgi; neurotendineus E.: fusiform nerve-ending in muscle tendons near the junction of tendon-bundles with muscle fibres. E., neuromuscular: sensory nerve-endings in muscle tissue. Syn. muscle spindle.

endorhă·chis (G. *endon*, within; *rhakhis*, spine). The dura mater of the spine.

en·dosarc (G. *endon*, within; *sarx*, flesh). The central portion of the protoplasm in some protozoa.

en·doscope (G. *endon*, within; *skopein*, to view). An instrument for examining visually the interior of a hollow organ, such as the bladder, respiratory, or intestinal tract.

endoscop·ic. Relating to endoscopy.

endŏ·scopy (G. *endon*, within; *skopein*, to view). Examination with an endoscope.

endosecrē·tory (G. *endon*, within; L. *secreta*, from *secernere*, to separate). Relating to the internal secretions.

endosep·sis. Septicaemia arising within the body.

endoskel·eton (G. *endon*, within; *skeletos*, skeleton). An internal supporting structure of an animal, consisting usually of cartilage and/or bone, but sometimes of spicules of carbonate of lime or of a siliceous material.

endosmŏ·meter (G. *endon*, within; *osmos*, a thrust; *metron*, measure). An instrument for measuring endosmosis.

endosmŏ·sis (G. *endon*, within; *osmos*, a thrust). Osmosis, *q.v.*, from without inward.

endosmot·ic. Pertaining to endosmosis.

endosŏ·ma (G. *endon*, within; *soma*, body). The contents of an erythrocyte.

en·dospore (G. *endon*, within; *spora*, seed). 1. An asexual spore formed within the parent cell. 2. The inner coat of the sporocyst in sporozoa.

endŏ·steal (G. *endon*, within; *osteon*, bone). Pertaining to the endosteum.

endostĕi·tis (G. *endon*, within; *osteon*, bone). Inflammation of the endosteum.

endostĕŏ·ma (G. *endon*, within; *osteon*, bone). A tumour within a bone cavity.

endŏ·steum (G. *endon*, within; *osteon*, bone). The fibro-vascular membrane lining the medullary cavity of bones.

endostī·tis. Endosteitis, *q.v.*

endothē·lial (G. *endon*, within; *thele*, nipple). Pertaining to the endothelium.

endothēlii·tis. Inflammation of the endothelium.

en·dothēlio·ma (G. *endon*, within; *thele*, nipple). A tumour derived from endothelial cells; the group of endotheliomata is rather ill-defined and authors differ considerably as to what particular tumours they include in this group.

endothē·lium (G. *endon*, within; *thele*, nipple). The single-celled layer forming the inner lining of heart, blood and lymph vessels, and the walls of capillaries, lymph spaces and serous cavities. See also mesothelium.

endother·mic (G. *endon*, within; *therme*, heat). 1. Relating to a process in which heat is being absorbed from the surrounding medium. 2. Relating to endothermy.

en·dothermy (G. *endon*, within; *therme*, heat). Surgical diathermy; use of diathermy, *q.v.*, through a knife or needle for surgical purposes.

En·dothrix (G. *endon*, within; *thrix*, hair). A group of Trichophyton fungi developing exclusively within the hair of the host, comprising *T. tonsurans*, *T. sabouraudi* and *T. violaceum*, which cause tinea capitis, tinea circinata and onychomycosis.

endotoxicŏ·sis (G. *endon*, within; *toxikon*, poison). Poisoning resulting from an endotoxin.

endotox·in (G. *endon*, within; *toxikon*, poison). A toxin obtained by extraction or disintegration of certain bacteria, possibly a cleavage product of bacterial protoplasm developed in the infected host, not freely excreted by the micro-organism; stimulating the production of various anti-bacterial antibodies.

end-plate. Intramuscular ending of a motor axon.

enelectrŏ·lysis (G. *en*, in; *ēlektron*, amber; *luein*, to loosen). A method of removing superfluous hair by pulling it out and applying an electric needle to the cavity.

en·ema (G. *en*, in; *hienai*, to send). Liquid introduced into the rectum for therapeutic or nutritive purposes. **E. syringe:** instrument for introducing a liquid into the rectum.

energet·ics (G. *energētikos*, active, ult. from *ergon*, work). Branch of physics dealing with the transformation of energy from one form to another.

energŏ·meter (G. *energeia*, energy; *metron*, measure). Apparatus for measuring output of energy, especially for studying, through the pulse, the work of the heart.

energy (G. *energeia*). The capacity for doing work. **E., conservation of:** the conception that while e. may be transformed from one form to another, it cannot be destroyed or created. **E., free:** e. which can be utilized for work. **E., kinetic:** e. of a body resulting from its motion. **E., potential:** e. of a body resulting from its position, composition or condition.

enervā·tion (L. *ē*, from; *nervus*, power). Lack of energy.

engage·ment. Act of engaging. One bone articulating with another in a joint.

engas·trius (G. *en*, in; *gaster*, stomach). A double monster, in which one foetus is enclosed in the abdomen of the other.

Engelmann's intermediate disc (Engelmann, T. W., German histologist, 1843–1909). A narrow zone of transparent homogeneous substance lying on each side of Krause's membrane.

Englisch's sinus (Englisch, J. Austrian physician, 1835–1915). The petro-occipital venous sinus.

englobing (L. *in*, in; *globus*, globe). The taking in of an object, e.g. by a phagocyte.

Engman's disease (Engman, M. F., American dermatologist, born 1868). Infectious eczematoid dermatitis.

engorge·ment (Fr. *engorger*). 1. Stasis of blood-flow. 2. Enlargement and induration of an organ due to (1). Syn. congestion.

en·gram (G. *eggraphein*, to inscribe). The impression left by mental experience. See mneme.

enophthal·mos (G. *en*, in; *ophthalmos*, eye). Recession of the eyeball into the orbital cavity.

enostō·sis (G. *en*, in; *osteon*, bone). A circumscribed mass of hyperplastic bone tissue lying within compact or cancellous bone.

en·siform (L. *ensis*, sword; *forma*, shape). Shaped like a sword.

ensister·num (L. *ensis*, sword; G. *sternon*, breast). The xiphoid process of the sternum.

ensom·phalus (G. *en*, in; *sōma*, body; *omphalos*, navel). A double monster the partners of which are only more or less superficially united.

en·strophe (G. *en*, in; *strephein*, to turn). Inversion.

E.N.T. Abbreviation for ear, nose and throat.

en·tad (G. *entos*, within; L. *ad*, towards). From without inward; towards a centre.

Entamōe·ba (G. *entos*, within; *amoibē*, change). A genus of protozoa of the order Amoebida. **E. coli:** a species of e., a non-pathogenic intestinal parasite in man; trophozoites, spherical precystic forms and the spherical or ovoid cysts (1-8 nuclei) are found in the lumen of the large intestine. **E. histolytica:** species of

e., causing amoebic dysentery in man. The trophozoites (indistinct nucleus, active mobility) invade the submucous layers of the large intestine, ingest red blood corpuscles, multiply by division, cause formation of intestinal ulcers (localized lesions surrounded by healthy tissue), and may penetrate the smaller radicles of the portal system, through which they are carried to the liver (especially upper part of right lobe) causing hepatitis, which may progress to abscess formation (characterized by debris of liver cells); a liver abscess may rupture into the lung, or organisms may be carried to the brain through the systemic circulation. Spread of disease occurs probably entirely by the cystic forms which are present in the stools in the chronic or carrier stages of the disease.

entā·sia (G. *entasis*, a stretching). Muscle spasm.

entĕ·lechy (G. *entelekheia*, actuality). Completion.

entepicon·dyle (G. *enton*, within; *epi*, upon; *kondulos*, knuckle). Internal condyle of the humerus.

enteradenī·tis (G. *enteron*, intestine; *adēn*, gland). Inflammation of the glands of the intestine.

en·teral (G. *enteron*, intestine). Intestinal.

enteral·gia (G. *enteron*, intestine; *algos*, pain). Pain in the intestine.

enterangiĕmphrax·is (G. *enteron*, intestine; *aggeion*, vessel; *emphraxis*, stoppage). Obstruction to the intestinal blood-vessels.

enteraux·ē (G. *enteron*, intestine; *auxē*, increase). Hypertrophy of the unstriped muscles of the intestinal wall.

enterec·tasis (G. *enteron*, intestine; *ektasis*, extension). Dilation of the intestines.

enterec·tomy (G. *enteron*, intestine; *ektomē*, excision). Excision of a part of the intestine.

entĕ·ric (G. *enteron*, intestine). Pertaining to the intestine. **E. fever:** paratyphoid fever (see fever, typhoid, paratyphoid).

enterī·tis (G. *enteron*, intestine). Inflammation of the intestine, especially of the small intestine.

entero-anastomō·sis (G. *enteron*, intestine; *ana*, upon; *stoma*, mouth). Intestinal anastomosis.

En·terobacteriā·ceæ. A genus of Eubacteriales, some of which inhabit the intestinal tract in man and other vertebrates.

en·terocele (G. *enteron*, intestine; *kēlē*, hernia). A hernia of a portion of the intestine.

entero-cholecystŏ·stomy (G. *enteron*, intestine; *khole*, gall; *kustis*, bladder; *stoma*, mouth). Cholecystenterostomy, *q.v.*

enterochrŏ·maffin cell (G. *enteron*, intestine; *khroma*, colour). Argentaffin cells in the small intestine.

en·terococ·cus (G. *enteron*, intestine; *kokkos*, berry). A streptococcus found in the intestinal tract, which is thought sometimes to cause appendicitis or cholecystitis. Syn. Streptococcus faecalis.

en·terocōele (G. *enteron*, intestine; *koilos*, hollow). The abdominal cavity.

en·terocoli·tis (G. *enteron*, intestine; *kolon*, colon). Inflammation of both small intestine and colon.

en·terocolŏ·stomy (G. *enteron*, intestine; *kolon*, colon; *stoma*, mouth). Artificial anastomosis between the small and the large intestine.

en·terocyst (G. *enteron*, intestine; *kustis*, bladder). An intestinal cyst.

en·terocyst·ocele (G. *enteron*, intestine; *kustis*, bladder; *kēlē*, hernia). Hernia involving both the urinary bladder and an intestinal loop.

en·terocystō·ma (G. *enteron*, intestine; *kustis*, bladder). A teratoid cyst lined by ciliated epithelium occurring along the gastro-intestinal canal and in organs such as brain, lung or genital organs, where an enteric or entodermal origin is improbable.

enterody̆·nia (G. *enteron*, intestine; *odune*, pain). Pain in the intestines.

entero-enterŏ·stomy (G. *enteron*, intestine; *stoma*, mouth). Artificial anastomosis between two intestinal loops.

entero-epip·locele (G. *enteron*, intestine; *epiploon*, omentum; *kēlē*, hernia). Hernia involving both omentum and a portion of the intestine.

en·terogastri·tis (G. *enteron*, intestine; *gastēr*, stomach). Gastro-enteritis, *q.v.*

en·terogă·strocele (G. *enteron*, intestine; *gastēr*, stomach; *kēlē*, hernia). A hernia containing parts of both stomach and intestine.

enterogă·sterone. A hormone found in the walls of the foregut.

enterŏ·genous (G. *enteron*, intestine; *gennan*, to produce). Originating in the intestine.

en·terograph (G. *enteron*, intestine; *graphein*, to write). An apparatus used to record intestinal movements.

en·terohepati·tis (G. *enteron*, intestine; *hēpar*, liver). Inflammation of both the intestine and the liver.

en·terohȳ·drocele (G. *enteron*, intestine; *hudōr*, water; *kēlē*, hernia). Hydrocele complicated with intestinal hernia.

en·terokī·nase (G. *enteron*, intestine; *kinein*, to move). An enzyme, present in duodenal mucous membrane, increasing, when mixed with pancreatic juice, the proteolytic action of the latter.

en·terolith (G. *enteron*, intestine; *lithos*, stone). A concretion formed within the intestine.

en·terolithī·asis (G. *enteron*, intestine; *lithos*, stone). The formation of intestinal concretions.

enterŏ·logist (G. *enteron*, intestine; *logos*, a discourse). A specialist in intestinal diseases.

enterŏ·logy (G. *enteron*, intestine; *logos*, a discourse). Branch of medicine pertaining to the intestines.

enterŏ·lysis (G. *enteron*, intestine; *lusis*, release). The surgical removal of adhesions from the intestines.

en·teromeg·aly (G. *enteron*, intestine; *megas*, large). Enlargement of the intestines.

en·teromere (G. *enteron*, intestine; *meros*, part). One of the primitive transverse divisions of the alimentary tract of the embryo.

en·teromē·rocele (G. *enteron*, intestine; *mēros*, thigh; *kēlē*, hernia). Femoral hernia.

en·teromycŏ·sis (G. *enteron*, intestine; *mukēs*, mushroom). Intestinal mycosis.

en·teromyī·asis (G. *enteron*, intestine; *muia*, fly). Disease of the intestine due to the presence of the larvae of flies.

en·teron (G., intestine). 1. The intestinal or alimentary canal, excluding parts of ectodermal origin. 2. The intestine.

en·teroneuri·tis (G. *enteron*, intestine; *neuron*, nerve). Inflammation of the intestinal nerves.

enterŏ·pathy (G. *enteron*, intestine; *pathos*, disease). Any disease of the intestine.

en·teropexy (G. *enteron*, intestine; *pēxis*, fixation). Artificial fixation of a part of the intestine to the abdominal wall.

en·teroplasty (G. *enteron*, intestine; *plassein*, to form). A plastic operation on the intestine.

en·teroplē·gia (G. *enteron*, intestine; *plēgē*, stroke). Intestinal paralysis.

en·teroplex (G. *enteron*, intestine; *plekein*, to weave). An instrument consisting of two aluminium rings fitting into each other, for rejoining divided ends of intestine.

en·teroplexy (G. *enteron*, intestine; *plekein*, to weave). A method of joining divided ends of intestine by which continuity of the intestinal canal is again obtained.

enteroptŏ·sis (G. *enteron*, intestine; *ptōsis*, fall). The condition in which the intestinal loops, especially the transverse colon, are in a rather low position.

enterorrhā·gia (G. *enteron*, intestine; *rhēgnunai*, to burst out). Intestinal haemorrhage.

enteror·rhaphy (G. *enteron*, intestine; *rhaphē*, suture). Suture of the intestine.

enterorrhex·is (G. *enteron*, intestine; *rhēxis*, a breaking). Intestinal rupture.

en·teroscope (G. *enteron*, intestine; *skopein*, to view). Instrument for examining the interior of the intestine.

en·terosep·sis (G. *enteron*, intestine; *sēpsis*, putrefaction). Sepsis of the intestine.

en·terospasm (G. *enteron*, intestine; *spasmos*, spasm). Intestinal spasm.

en·terostā·sis (G. *enteron*, intestine; *stasis*, a standing still). Intestinal stasis.

en·terostax·is (G. *enteron*, intestine; *staxis*, a dripping). Loss of blood from the intestinal mucous membrane.

en·terostenŏ·sis (G. *enteron*, intestine; *stenos*, narrow). Stricture of the intestinal canal.

enterŏ·stomy (G. *enteron*, intestine; *stoma*, mouth). Formation of an artificial opening into the intestine through the abdominal wall.

en·terotome (G. *enteron*, intestine; *tomē*, section). A surgical knife used in opening up the intestine.

enterŏ·tomy (G. *enteron*, intestine; *tomē*, section). Incision of the intestine.

en·terozŏ·on (G. *enteron*, intestine; *zōon*, animal). Any animal parasite of the intestine.

en·thelminth (G. *entos*, within; *helmins*, an intestinal worm). Any parasitic intestinal worm.

en·theomā·nia (G. *entheos*, inspired; *mania*, madness). Religious mania.

en·toderm (G. *entos*, within; *derma*, skin). The inner germinal layer in the gastrula, giving rise to epithelium of digestive tract (excluding mouth and anus) and associated glands (pharyngeal, oesophogeae, gastric, intestinal; pancreas and liver with gallbladder), middle ear and pharyngotympanic tube, respiratory tract (except nostrils), thyroid, parathyroid, thymus, female urethra, proximal part of male urethra, urinary bladder, prostatic and Cowper's glands, Bartholin's glands, nuclei pulposi of intervertebral discs, remains of embryonic notochord.

entoder·mal (G. *entos*, within; *derma*, skin). Relating to or derived from entoderm.

ento·ectad (G. *entos*, within; *ektos*, without; L. *ad*, to). From within outwards.

en·tomere (G. *entos*, within; *meros*, part). One of the central blastomeres.

entŏ·mion (G. *entomē*, notch). The point where the parietal notch of the temporal bone is crossed by the anterior extension of the mastoid angle of the parietal bone.

entomŏ·logy (G. *entoma*, insects; *logos*, discourse). The part of zoology dealing with insects.

en·tophyte (G. *entos*, within; *phuton*, plant). Any vegetable organism living within the body of an animal or plant.

entop·ic (G. *en*, in; *topos*, place). Situated in the usual place.

en·toplasm (G. *entos*, within; *plassein*, to form). Endoplasm, *q.v.*

entop·tic (G. *entos*, within; *optikos*, of sight). Pertaining to the interior of the eye. E. phenomena: visual sensations arising from objects situated within the eye itself.

entoptŏ·scopy (G. *entos*, within; *ops*, eye; *skopein*, to view). Examination of the interior of the eye.

entoret·ina (G. *entos*, within; L. *rete*, a net). The inner portion of the retina.

Entorula. A genus of fungi, of which certain kinds have been found in human lesions.

en·tosarc (G. *entos*, within; *sarx*, flesh). The inner protoplasm of a protozoan.

entŏs·thoblast (G. *entos*, within; *blastos*, germ). The inner portion of a nucleolus.

entot·ic (G. *entos*, within; *ōtĭkos*, of the ear). Pertaining to the internal ear. **E. sounds:** sounds originating within the ear itself.

entotympan·ic (G. *entos*, within; *tumpanon*, drum). Inside the tympanum of the ear.

entozō·on (G. *entos*, within; *zōon*, animal). Any animal parasite living within another animal.

entrip·sis (G. *en*, in; *tripsis*, rubbing). Rubbing in of oil.

entrō·pion (G. *en*, in; *trepein*, to turn). Inversion of the border of the eyelid towards the globe.

en·tropy (G. *en*, in; *trepein*, to turn.) That fraction of the energy produced by a system (e.g. a cell) which, being retained within the cell, is not available for external work.

enucleā·tion (L. *ex*, from; *nucula*, dim. of *nux*, nucleus). 1. Deprivation of a nucleus. 2. Shelling out, e.g., of a tumour or organ from its capsule. 3. Excision of the eyeball.

enurē·sis (G. *enourein*, urinate). Involuntary emptying of the bladder.

envī·ronment (Fr. *environ*). The sum total of external influences acting on the organism.

enzymat·ic (G. *en*, in; *zumē*, leaven). Enzymic, *q.v.*

en·zyme (G. *en*, in; *zumē*, leaven). Any of a class of catalytic substances occurring in vegetable and animal tissues which are produced by cells and accelerate specific conversions of more or less complex organic material.

enzym·ic (G. *en*, in; *zumē*, leaven). Pertaining to an enzyme.

enzymŏ·logy (G. *en*, in; *zumē*, leaven; *logos*, discourse). The science of enzymes and enzymic action.

enzymō·sis (G. *en*, in; *zumē*, leaven). Ferment produced by an enzyme.

enzymū·ria (G. *en*, in; *zumē*, leaven; *ouron*, urine). The presence of enzymes in urine.

ē·onism (Chev. d'Eon de Beaumont, 1728–1810). Assumption of the dress of the opposite sex.

ē·osin (G. *eos*, dawn). Tetrabromofluorescein, used as a (acid) dye as an indicator in histology.

eosinopē·nia (G. *eōs*, dawn; *penia*, poverty). A decrease of the normal number of eosinophile cells in the peripheral blood.

eosi·nophil, eosĭ·nophile (G. *eōs*, dawn; *philein*, to love). Staining readily with eosin or with acid dyes generally. **E. cells:** (1) polymorphonuclear leucocytes possessing numerous coarse acidophile granules. (2) Acidophile cells of the anterior pituitary gland producing the growth hormone.

ēosinophĭ·lia (G. *eōs*, dawn; *philein*, to love). 1. An abnormal increase in the number of eosinophile cells in the circulating blood. 2. The property of microbes or tissue elements to be readily stained by eosin or acid dyes generally.

epac·tal (G. *epaktos*, brought in). Intercalated; supernumerary.

Epanutin. A proprietary preparation of sodium diphenylhydantoinate, used in the treatment of epilepsy.

epen·dyma (G. *ependuma*, an upper garment). The epithelial membrane lining the cerebral ventricles and cisternae and the central canal of the spinal cord.

epen·dymal (G. *ependuma*, an upper garment). Pertaining to the ependyma.

ependymi·tis (G. *ependuma*, an upper garment). Inflammation of the ependyma.

epen·dymoblastō·ma (G. *ependuma*, an upper garment; *blastos*, germ). A tumour derived from primitive ependymal spongio-blasts, resembling otherwise ependymoma, *q.v.*

ependymō·ma (G. *ependuma*, an upper garment). A benign tumour derived from ependymal cells, developing usually in children, especially in the floor or roof of the fourth ventricle and in the filum terminale of the cord, and tending to calcify.

ephē·bic (G. *ephēbos*, a youth). Relating to puberty.

eph·edrine. An alkaloid, $C_{10}H_{15}NO$, obtained from various species of ephedra and also prepared synthetically. Its action is similar to adrenaline.

ephē·lis (G. *epi*, upon; *hēlios*, sun). A freckle.

ephem·eral (G. *epi*, upon; *hēmera*, day). Of short duration; lasting not more than a day.

ephiāl·tes (G. *epi*, upon; *hiallein*, to send). Nightmare.

ephidrō·sis (G. *ephidrōsis*, superficial perspiration). Profuse sweating.

ephip·pium (G. *epi*, upon; *hippos*, horse). The sella turcica.

ĕ·piblast (G. *epi*, upon; *blastos*, germ). Ectoderm, *q.v.*

epiblast·ic (G. *epi*, upon; *blastos*, germ). Ectodermal, *q.v.*

epiblĕ·pharon (G. *epi*, upon; *blepharon*, eyelid). See epicanthus.

epi·bole, epi·boly (G. *epi*, upon; *ballein*, to throw). A process of gastrula formation in certain metazoa, characterized by expansion of the ectoderm around the endoderm and mesoderm.

epican·thus (G. *epi*, upon; *kanthos*, corner of the eye). Congenital, half-moon-shaped skin-fold covering the inner angle, or both angles, of the eye.

epicar·dia (G. *epi*, upon; *kardia*, heart). The portion of the oesophagus between the diaphragm and the stomach.

epicar·dial. 1. Relating to the epicardium. 2. Relating to the epicardia.

ep·icardiĕc·tomy (G. *epi*, upon; *kardia*, heart; *ektomē*, excision). Excision of the pericardium.

epicar·dium (G. *epi*, upon; *kardia*, heart). The visceral layer of the pericardium.

epicen·tral (G. *epi*, upon; *kentron*, centre). Adjoined to a vertebral centrum.

ep·icoēle, epicoē·lia (G. *epi*, upon; *koilia*, a ventricle). The anterior part of the fourth ventricle of the brain.

epicome (G. *epi*, upon; *komē*, hair). A monster having united to its head that of a rudimentary twin.

epicon·dyle, epicon·dylus (G. *epi*, upon; *kondulos*, a knuckle). 1. Bony eminence upon either of the femoral condyles. 2. Either of the (lateral and medial) condylar projections at the lower end of the humerus.

epicŏ·racoid (G. *epi*, upon; *korax*, crow; *eidos*, form). Having a position above the coracoid process.

epicos·tal (G. *epi*, upon; *costa*, rib). Placed upon a rib.

epicrā·nium (G. *epi*, above; *kranion*, skull). The structures covering the cranium.

epicrī·sis (G. *epi*, upon; *krisis*, crisis (of a disease)). A second crisis.

epicrit·ic (G. *epi*, upon; *krinein*, to separate). Pertaining to the perception of slight changes of pressure, temperature or pain.

epicrū·sis (G. *epi*, upon; *krousis*, a striking). Massage by strokes or blows.

epicysti·tis (G. *epi*, above; *kustis*, bladder). Inflammation of the structures in the abdomen around the bladder.

epicystŏ·tomy (G. *epi*, above; *kustis*, bladder; *tomē*, section). Suprapubic incision of the bladder.

epidem·ic (G. *epi*, on; *dēmos*, people). Term applied to an infectious disease affecting large numbers at the same time or spreading within a short time over a wide area. **E. encephalitis:** see encephalitis, e. **E. erythema:** see erythema infectiosum. **E. myalgia:** an acute infectious disease perhaps of virus origin, characterized by abrupt onset of fever, headache and severe paroxysmal pain in the regions of the attachment of the diaphragm lasting a few days but frequently recurring one to three times at intervals of one to two days. Syn. Bornholm disease; E. pleurodynia. **E. parotitis**: mumps. **E. pleurodynia**: E. myalgia.

epidemĭŏ·logy (G. *epi*, upon; *dēmos*, people; *logos*, a discourse). The science pertaining to epidemics.

epider·mal (G. *epi*, upon; *derma*, skin). Relating to or composed of epidermis.

epider·malizā·tion (G. *epi*, upon; *derma*, skin). The conversion of columnar into stratified epithelium.

epidermă·toplasty (G. *epi*, upon; *derma*, skin; *plassein*, to form). Skin-grafting by transplantation of strips or patches of epidermis with the underlying layer of the corium.

epider·mic (G. *epi*, upon; *derma*, skin). Relating to or composed of epidermis.

epider·mis (G. *epi*, upon; *derma*, skin). The outer nonvascular layer of the skin, consisting of stratum corneum or horny layer, stratum lucidum, stratum granulosum, prickle-cell layer or stratum spinosum, and cylindrical cell layer or stratum cylindricum.

epidermizā·tion (G. *epi*, upon; *derma*, skin). The formation, especially new formation, of epidermis.

epider·moid (G. *epi*, upon; *derma*, skin; *eidos*, form). 1. Resembling epidermis. 2. A teratoma derived from epidermal cells, differing from a dermoid by absence of true dermal structures. **E. carcinoma**: see carcinoma, squamous-celled.

ep·idermŏ·lysis (G. *epi*, upon; *derma*, skin; *luein*, to loosen). Separation of the epidermis with formation of bullae. **E. bullosa hereditaria**: dominantly or recessively transmitted disease, characterized by the development of vesicles and bullae on slightest pressure; usually subsiding at puberty. **E. bullosa dystrophica**: a type of E. b. hereditaria in which the vesicles are often haemorrhagic and heal under scarring resulting in atrophic or other changes of the skin.

epidermŏ·ma (G. *epi*, upon; *derma*, skin). A wart.

epider·momycŏ·sis (G. *epi*, upon; *derma*, skin; *mukēs*, mushroom). Dermatomycosis, *q.v.*

Epider·mophyte, Epidermophy̆·ton (G. *epi*, upon; *derma*, skin; *phuton*, plant). Any fungus parasitic upon the epidermis. **E. cruris**: a member of the group of fungi producing epidermophytosis, favouring intertriginous positions (tinea cruris, tinea axillaris, dhobie itch, athlete's foot.) **E. inguinale, e. cruris.** *q.v.*

epidermophytŏ·sis (G. *epi*, upon; *derma*, skin; *phuton*, plant). Any skin disease caused by an epidermophyte.

epidi·ascope (G. *epi*, upon; *dia*, through; *skopein*, to view). An optical projector which can be used both for ordinary (transparent) slides and for opaque objects.

epidi·dymal. Relating to the epididymis.

epididymec·tomy (G. *epi*, upon; *didumoi*, testicles, lit. twins; *ektomē*, excision). Excision of the epididymis.

epidi·dymis (G. *epi*, upon; *didumoi*, testicles, lit. twins). The small structure lying at the back of and above the testis, mainly composed of the convoluted tubes arising from the testis; divided into the head or globus major and the tail or globus minor.

epididymī·tis (G. *epi*, upon; *didumoi*, testicles, lit. twins). Inflammation of the epididymis.

epididymo-orchitis (G. *epi*, upon; *didumoi*, testicles, lit. twins; *orkhis*, testicle). Inflammation of the epididymis and testis.

epidū·ral (G. *epi*, upon; L. *durus*, hard). Situated upon or over the dura. **E. injection**: an injection, e.g. of an anaesthetic, through the sacrococcygeal ligament into the e. space. **E. space**: the space between the two layers of the dura mater, of limited extension in the cranium, but relatively large in the spinal canal.

epĭ·gamous (G. *epi*, upon; *gamos*, marriage). Pertaining to anything occurring after fertilization.

epigă·ster (G. *epi*, upon; *gastēr*, belly). The large intestine or hind gut.

epigastral·gia (G. *epi*, upon; *gastēr*, belly; *algos*, pain). Epigastric pain.

epigă·stric (G. *epi*, upon; *gastēr*, belly). Referring to the epigastrium.

epigă·strium (G. *epi*, upon; *gastēr*, belly). The upper middle part of the abdomen.

epigă·strius (G. *epi*, upon; *gastēr*, belly). A double monster in which an undeveloped foetus is united to the epigastric region of the autosite.

epigă·strocele (G. *epi*, upon; *gastēr*, belly; *kēlē*, hernia). Epigastric hernia.

epigĕ·nesis (G. *epi*, upon; *gennan*, to produce). The theory that the development of the embryo and of each of its parts takes place by progressive differentiation of an originally simple structure, the embryonic parts not being preformed as such in either of the parental germ-cells.

epiglot·tic (G. *epi*, upon; *glōttis*). Relating to the epiglottis.

epi·glottidi·tis (G. *epi*, upon; *glōttis*). Inflammation of the epiglottis.

epiglot·tis (G. *epi*, upon; *glōttis*). A fibrocartilaginous structure, behind the tongue in front of the glottis, towards which the arytaenoid cartilages are drawn during swallowing, thus closing the larynx towards the pharynx.

epi·glotto-hyoi·dean (G. *epi*, upon; *glōttis*; *huoeidēs*, shaped like the letter Y.) Pertaining to both epiglottis and hyoid bone.

epĭ·gnathous (G. *epi*, upon; *gnathos*, jaw). Having the maxilla protruding over the mandible.

epĭ·gnathus (G. *epi*, on; *gnathos*, jaw). A monster in which a parasitic foetus is united to the base of the skull or to the maxillary bone of the autosite, protruding from its pharynx.

epiguă·nin (Sp. *guano*, dung). A xanthin base.

epihy̆·al bone (G. *epi*, upon; *huoeidēs*, like the letter Y). The stylohyoid ligament when it is ossified.

epihy̆·oid (G. *epi*, upon; *huoeidēs*, like the letter Y). Located on the hyoid bone.

epilamel·lar (G. *epi*, upon; *lamella*, dim. of *lamina*, a plate). Upon a basement membrane.

ĕ·pilate (L. *e*, from; *pilus*, hair). To remove hair by the destruction of its roots.

epilā·tion (L. *e*, from; *pilus*, hair). Removal of hair by destruction of its roots.

epi·latory (L. *e*, from; *pilus*, hair). Removing hair permanently.

epilem·ma (G. *epi*, upon; *lemma*, husk). The neurilemma of the branches of nerve-filaments.

epilem·mal. Relating to the epilemma.

ĕ·pilepsy (G. *epilēpsia*, seizure). A condition characterized by recurring attacks consisting in typical forms of sudden loss of consciousness accompanied by generalized convulsions which are at first (for some seconds) of a tonic type (with arms commonly flexed and lower limbs rigidly extended) and for the following 1 to 3 minutes of clonic form, followed by some degree of stupor, the whole attack being sometimes preceded by an auditory, visual, olfactory, gustatory, cutaneous, visceral or kinaesthetic sensation or hallucination ('aura'); probably conditioned by increased excitability of the cerebral cortex, which may itself be related to a change in the acid-base equilibrium of the blood towards alkalosis, or to retention of tissue fluid, defective oxygenation of the blood, or impairment of intracranial circulation. **E., Jacksonian** (Hughlings Jackson, English neurologist, 1834–1911): condition characterized by epileptic seizures due to a lesion of the cerebral motor cortex, starting in (and sometimes confined to) the region of the body related to the irritated cortical area, usually spreading soon to adjoining regions in an order frequently corresponding to that of their cortical representation. E., minor: see petit mal. E., myoclonic : hereditary disease, characterized by the association of epileptiform fits and myoclonus, *q.v.* E., reflex: a form of e. in which the attacks are excited by some peripheral irritation.

epilep·tic (G. *epilēpsia*, seizure). 1. Relating to epilepsy. 2. One affected with epilepsy. E. **equivalent:** physical or mental disturbance, such as attacks of perspiration, of hemicrania, hallucinations, impulses to violent actions, and dipsomania, which replace the outbreak of a typical e. attack. E. **psychoses:** mental disturbances such as automatism, confusion, depression, mania and dream-state, which occur transiently or periodically, in association with or replacing an e. attack, or which develop as final condition (e. dementia) in epileptics.

epilep·tiform (G. *epilēpsia*, seizure; L. *forma*, form). Resembling an epileptic attack.

epileptogen·ic, epileptŏ·genous (G. *epilēpsia*, seizure; *gennan*, to produce). Producing epilepsy.

epilep·toid (G. *epilēpsia*, seizure; *eidos*, form). Resembling epilepsy.

Epilobium. A genus of plants which includes the common willow-herb and which yields an astringent useful in diarrhoea.

epiloi·a (G. *epilēpsia*, seizure). A term coined by E. B. Sherlock, English physician, who held that it 'has some of the features which characterize a good name: it is short, unmeaning, distinctive and capable of forming an adjective'; (*The Feeble-minded*, 1911, p. 243). A condition characterized by the association of tuberous sclerosis, *q.v.*, epileptic fits, mental deficiency and adenoma sebaceum, *q.v.*, usually beginning in childhood or adolescence, often associated with retinal phacomata, *q.v.*, and mixed tumours of kidney, heart, and other organs.

ĕ·pilose (L. *ex*, from; *pilosus*, from *pilus*, hair). Bald; without hair.

ĕ·pimenorrhă·gia (G. *epi*, upon; *mēn*, month; *rhegnunai*, to burst out). Excessive menstruation.

epimenorrhœ·a (G. *epi*, upon; *mēn*, month; *rheein*, to flow). Over-frequent recurrence of the menstrual period.

ĕ·pimere (G. *epi*, upon; *meros*, part). In chordates, the dorsal region of the mesoderm on each side of the neural tube.

epimỹ·sium (G. *epi*, upon; *mus*, muscle). The fibroelastic tissue ensheathing a muscle.

epinephrec·tomy (G. *epi*, upon; *nephros*, kidney; *ektomē*, excision). Excision of the suprarenal gland.

epinĕ·phrin, epinĕ·phrine (G. *epi*, upon; *nephros*, kidneys). Adrenalin, *q.v.*

epinephrī·tis (G. *epi*, upon; *nephros*, kidneys). Inflammation of the suprarenal capsule.

epineph·ros (G. *epi*, upon; *nephros*, kidney). The suprarenal gland.

epineū·ral (G. *epi*, upon; *neuron*, sinew). Derived from a neural arch.

epineū·rium (G. *epi*, upon; *neuron*, sinew). The connective tissue sheath of a nerve-trunk.

epinŏ·sic (G. *epi*, upon; *nŏsos*, disease). Unhealthy.

epiŏt·ic (G. *epi*, upon; *ous*, ear). 1. Situated above the ear. 2. Pertaining to the upper outer portion of the bony capsule of the inner ear.

epipharyngī·tis (G. *epi*, upon; *pharugx*, throat). Inflammation of the nasopharynx.

epiphă·rynx (G. *epi*, upon; *pharugx*, throat). The nasopharynx.

epi·phora (G. *epi*, upon; *pherein*, to carry). Overflow of tears due to excessive secretion or, especially, to impeded outflow.

epiphrē·nal (G. *epi*, upon; *phrēn*, diaphragm). Above the diaphragm.

epiphylax·is (G. *epi*, upon; *phulaxis*, a guarding). Increase of the defensive agencies of the body.

epiphỹ·seal (G. *epi*, upon; *phusis*, nature). Referring to or of the nature of an epiphysis. E. **line:** a line of unossified cartilage at the proximal end of an epiphysis, present until growth of bone is completed.

epiphysiŏ·lysis (G. *epi*, upon; *phusis*, nature; *luein*, to loosen). Separation of the epiphysis from the metaphysis.

epi·physis (G. *epi*, upon; *phusis*, nature). 1. The distal parts of a long bone which are united to the diaphysis at first by cartilage, later by osseous bone. 2. The pineal body.

epiphysī·tis (G. *epi*, on; *phusis*, nature). Inflammation of an epiphysis. See also Perthes's disease.

ĕ·piphyte (G. *epi*, on; *phuton*, plant). A vegetable ectoparasite, *q.v.*

epiplasm (G. *epi*, on; *plassein*, to form). In ascomycetes, a part of the protoplasm remaining after the formation of the spores.

epipleū·ral. Located on the side of the thorax.

epip·locele (G. *epiploon*, omentum; *kēlē*, hernia). A hernia containing part of the omentum.

ĕ·piplo·ec·tomy (G. *epiploon*, omentum; *ektomē*, excision). Excision of the omentum.

epiplŏ·ic (G. *epiploon*, omentum). Relating or belonging to the omentum.

ĕ·piplo·ï·schiocele (G. *epiploon*, omentum; *iskhion*, hip-joint; *kēlē*, hernia). Hernia through the sciatic notch or foramen containing part of the omentum.

ĕ·piploï·tis (G. *epiploon*, omentum). Inflammation of the omentum.

ĕ·piplomē·rocele (G. *epiploon*, omentum; *mēros*, thigh; *kēlē*, hernia). Femoral hernia containing part of the omentum.

epiplomphă·locele (G. *epiploon*, omentum; *omphalos*, navel; *kēlē*, hernia). Umbilical hernia containing omentum.

epip·lŏŏn (G. *epiploon*, omentum). The omentum.

epip·lopexy (G. *epiploon*, omentum; *pegnunai*, to fix). Morison's operation of suturing the great omentum to the anterior abdominal wall in order to establish a collateral venous circulation in cirrhosis of the liver.

epiplŏr·rhaphy (G. *epiploon*, omentum; *rhaphē*, suture). Epiplopexy, *q.v.*

epiplŏ·scheocele (G. *epiploon*, omentum; *oskhē*, scrotum; *kēlē*, hernia). Hernia of the scrotum, containing omentum.

episclē·ra (G. *epi*, on; *skleros*, hard). The loose connective tissue lying between the conjunctiva and the sclera.

episclē·ral (G. *epi*, on; *skleros*, hard). 1. Pertaining to the episclera. 2. Situated upon the sclera.

ep·isclerī·tis. Inflammation of the conjunctival tissues between the conjunctiva and the sclera.

epi·siocele (G. *episeion*, the region of the pubes; *kēlē*, hernia). Pudendal hernia.

epi·sioclī·sia (G. *episeion*, the region of the pubes; *kleisis*, closure). Surgical closure of the vagina.

epi·sio-elytror·rhaphy (G. *episeion*, the region of the pubes; *elutron*, sheath; *rhaphē*, suture). Operation for the repair of the perineum.

epi·sion-haematŏ·ma (G. *episeion*, the region of the pubes; *haima*, blood). Haematoma of the labia major.

epi·sioplasty (G. *episeion*, the region of the pubes; *plassein*, to form). A plastic operation upon the vulva.

episior·rhagy (G. *episeion*, the region of the pubes; *rhēgnunai*, to burst out). Haemorrhage from the vulva.

episior·rhaphy (G. *episeion*, the region of the pubes; *rhaphē*, suture). Repair of a lacerated vulva.

epi·siostenō·sis (G. *episeion*, the region of the pubes; *stenos*, narrow). Stenosis of the vulva.

episiŏ·tomy (G. *episeion*, the region of the pubes; *tomē*, section). Incision through the vulva in child-birth, to prevent laceration of the perineum.

epispā·dias (G. *epi*, on; *spaein*, to tear). Congenital deformity in which the urethra opens on the dorsal surface of the penis. Hence **epispadiac**: pertaining to epispadias.

epispăs·tic (G. *epi*, on; *spaein*, to tear). 1. Blistering. 2. Any blistering agent.

epispi·nal (G. *epi*, upon; L. *spina*). Located upon the spinal cord.

epispleni·tis (G. *epi*, on; *splēn*, spleen). Inflammation of the capsule of the spleen.

epi·stasis (G. *epi*, on; *stasis*, a standing). The halting of any kind of discharge.

epistat·ic. Superimposed.

epistax·is (G. *epistazein*, to bleed at the nose again, from *epi*, upon; *stazein*, to drip). Nasal haemorrhage.

epister·nal (G. *epi*, on; *sternon*, breast). 1. Above the sternum. 2. Pertaining to the sternum.

epister·num (G. *epi*, upon; *sternon*, chest). The manubrium.

episthŏ·tonos (G. *epi*, on; *tonos*, tone). Emprosthotonos, *q.v.*

epistrŏ·pheus (G. *episthropheus*, pivot). The second cervical vertebra. Syn. axis.

epitendi·neum (G. *epi*, on; L. *tendo*, from *tendere*, to stretch). The dense fibro-elastic tissue ensheathing a tendon. Syn. vagina fibrosa.

epitĕ·non (G. *epi*, on; *tenōn*, tendon). Epitendineum.

epithalam·ic (G. *epi*, upon; *thalamos*, chamber). Situated on the thalamus.

epithă·lamus (G. *epi*, on; *thalamos*, a chamber). The structure forming the roof of the third cerebral ventricle, including the tela choroidea superior and the pineal gland.

epithē·lial (G. *epi*, on; *thēlē*, nipple). Relating to or composed of epithelium. **E. pearls**: cell nests, *q.v.*

epithē·lioblastō·ma (G. *epi*, on; *thēlē*, nipple; *blastos*, germ). An epithelial tumour.

epithē·liogenet·ic, **epithē·liogen·ic** (G. *epi*, on; *thēlē*, nipple; *gennan*, to produce). Originating from epithelial proliferation.

epithē·lioid (G. *epi*, on; *thēlē*, nipple; *eidos*, form). Resembling epithelium. **E. cell**: large polymorphous mononuclear cell with pale acidophile protoplasm and oval or elongated nucleus poor in chromatin; resembling some types of epithelial cells, derived from mesenchymal tissue (endothelium, macrophage, fibroblast) and found around foci of granulation tissue, especially in tuberculosis, sarcoidosis of Boeck and syphilis.

ĕ·pithelioly·sin (G. *epi*, upon; *thēlē*, nipple; *luein*, to loosen). A cytolysin produced by inoculation with epithelial cells.

epitheliŏ·ma (G. *epi*, on; *thēlē*, nipple). 1. Squamous-celled carcinoma, syn. epidermoid carcinoma. 2. Any tumour derived from epithelial cells. **E. adenoides cysticum**: a form of squamous-celled carcinoma of low malignancy, composed of epithelial masses showing both glandular arrangement and cyst formation. Syn. Brooke's tumour; acanthoma adenoides cystica.

epithē·lium (G. *epi*, on; *thēlē*, nipple). A cellular avascular layer covering the surfaces and lining the internal cavities of the body; classified, according to arrangement and shape of cells, into simple and stratified, into squamous, columnar and transitional, and into ciliated, pyramidal, goblet and neuro-epithelium.

epithelizā·tion (G. *epi*, on; *thēlē*, nipple). The growth of epithelium over a raw surface.

epi·thesis (G., an application). Surgical correction of deformities.

epiton·ic (G. *epitonos*, strained). Abnormally tense.

epitri·chium (G. *epi*, on; *trikhion*, dim. of *thrix*, hair). Superficial layer of foetal epidermis.

epitrŏch·lea (G. *epi*, on; *trokhilia*, the sheaf of a pulley). The internal condyle (epicondylus medialis) of the humerus.

epituberculō·sis. A radiological phenomenon, characterised by the presence of a large opacity in the lung, arising in the course of a tuberculous infection and believed to be a form of tuberculous pneumonia.

ep·itympan·ic (G. *epi*, on; *tumpanon*, a kettledrum). Relating to the epitympanum.

epitympani·tis (G. *epi*, on; *tumpanon*, a kettledrum). Inflammation of the epitympanum.

epitym·panum (G. *epi*, on; *tumpanon*, a kettledrum). The space of the middle ear above the tympanic membrane. Syn. the attic; epitympanic recess.

epity·phlon (G. *epi*, on; *tuphlon*, the caecum). The vermiform appendix.

epizō·ic. Relating to an epizoon.

epizō·on (G. *epi*, on; *zōon*, animal). An animal parasite living on the exterior of the host.

epizōŏt·ic (G. *epi*, on; *zōon*, animal). Relating to infectious diseases affecting large numbers of animals at the same time.

epluchage (Fr.). The excision of contaminated wound tissue.

eponў·chium (G. *epi*, on; *onux*, nail). The horny layer covering the nailbed from the 2nd to the 8th month of foetal life.

ĕ·ponym (G. *epōnumos*, named after). Name, e.g. of an organ or disease, which is derived from the name of a person or place as organ of Corti and Bornholm disease.

eponym·ic. Relating to an eponym.

ep·ōŏphorec·tomy (G. *epi*, on; *ōon*, egg; *pherein*, to carry; *ektomē*, excision). Removal of the epoophoron.

epōŏph·oron (G. *epi*, on; *ōon*, egg; *pherein*, to carry). The parovarium, *q.v.*

Epsom salts. Magnesium sulphate.

Epstein's pearls (Epstein, A., Austrian paediatrician, 1849–1918). The small, slightly elevated, yellowish-white masses on each side of the median line of hard palate of the newborn.

Epstein's nephrosis (Epstein, A. A., American physician, born 1880). Chronic nephritis associated with various forms of endocrine disorder especially hyperthyroidism.

epū·lis (G. *epi*, on; *oula*, gums). 1. A term covering any tumour or inflammatory hyperplastic swelling upon the gums. More specifically, either 2. A fibroma, or particularly, 3. A benign giant cell tumour arising from the periodontal membrane of deciduous teeth, especially the canine and bicuspid teeth.

ep·ulofibrō·ma (G. *epi*, upon; *oula*, gums; L. *fibra*, fibre). Fibroma of the gums.

epuloid (G. *epi*, upon; *oula*, gums; *eidos*, form). Resembling an epulis.

equā·tion (L. *aequare*, to equal). 1. An expression of equality. 2. In chemistry, an expression by symbols representing a reaction quantitatively. **E., personal**: a deviation in the result of a scientific observation due to the personal peculiarities of the observer.

equā·tor (L. *aequum*, equal). An imaginary line drawn through the centre of a sphere. **E. of a cell**: the boundary of the plane through which cell-division takes place.

equator·ial. Relating to an equator. **E. division**: mitosis with longitudinal division of the chromosomes. **E. plane of the eye**: plane dividing the anterior and posterior halves of the eye. **E. plate:** the structure at the equator of the spindle formed by the chromosomes during the metaphase.

Equidae (L. *equus*, horse). A genus of mammals, which includes the horse.

equilibra·tion (L. *aequum*, equal; *librare*, to weigh). The maintenance of equilibrium.

equilib·rium. 1. An even balance between opposing forces or actions. 2. Any state in which no spontaneous change can take place.

equimo·lar (L. *aequus*, equal; *moles*, mass). Containing quantities of substances proportional to their molecular weights.

equimole·cular (L.*aequus*, equal; Fr.*molécule*, dim. from L. *moles*, mass). Applied to solutions which contain in equal volumes of the solvent an equal number of molecules of the dissolved substance.

equi·nia (L. *equus*, horse). Glanders, *q.v.*

equi·noca·vus (L. *equus*, horse; *cavus*, hollow). A form of talipes presenting the characteristics of both talipes equinus and cavus, *q.v.*

equi·nova·rus (L. *equus*, horse; *varus*, bent). A form of talipes, *q.v.*, presenting the characteristics of both talipes equinus and varus.

equipoten·tial (L. *aequum*, equal; *potens*, able). 1. Having the same potentiality or the same prospective capability. 2. Having the same electric potential.

Equisetum (L. *equus*, horse). Mare's tail; a class of seedless plants related to the club-mosses and ferns.

equi·valence (L. *aequus*, equal; *valere*, to be worth). 1. Equality of valence. 2. Equivalent (3, 4).

equi·valent (L. *aequus*, equal; *valere*, to be worth). 1. Of equal valency or value; equal with regard to a particular property. 2. A symptom taking the place of another (more usual) one in a given disease. 3. The weight of an element that combines with or displaces 8 parts by weight of oxygen; the atomic weight of an element divided by its valency.'4. The combining weight of a compound or radical; the molecular weight of a compound divided by the valency of its principal atom.

Er. Symbol of erbium.

era·sion (L. *ex*, from; *radere*, to scrape). The act of scraping away or curetting.

Erb's disease (Erb, W. H., German physician, 1840–1921). Severe pseudo-paralytic myasthenia; asthenic bulbar paralysis. **E.'s juvenile form of progressive muscular atrophy:** the scapulo-humeral form. **E.'s paralysis:** paralysis of the muscles of the upper arm, caused by a lesion of the fifth and sixth cervical nerve-roots. **E.'s point:** a p. situated about two finger-breadths above the clavicle and one finger-breadth external to the sternomastoid. Electric stimulation at this point contracts the deltoid biceps, brachialis anticus and supinator longus. **E.'s symptom:** 1. Increase of electric irritability of the motor nerves in tetany. 2. Dullness on percussion over the manubrium sterni in acromegaly. **E.'s waves:** undulations produced in a muscle by passing a fairly strong constant current through it and leaving the electrodes in place, the circuit remaining closed. They are sometimes observed in Thomsen's disease.

Erb-Charcot's disease. Spastic spinal paralysis; spasmodic tabes dorsalis.

Erb-Goldflam's symptom-complex. See Erb's disease.

Erb-Westphal's symptom. See Westphal's sign.

Erben's phenomenon (Erben, S., Austrian neurologist, born 1863). 1. A temporary slowing of the pulse on bending forward or trying to sit down; has been observed in neurasthenia. 2. In sciatica the pain is increased by hyperflexion of the leg on the sound side. 3. The local temperature of the knee in sciatica is reduced on the painful side.

erbium. A rare element, symbol Er. It is found at Ytterby, Sweden, in the mineral gadolinite.

Erdmann's reagent (Erdmann, H., German chemist, 1862–1910). A mixture of nitric acid and sulphuric acid, used in testing alkaloids.

erect (L. *erigere*, to erect). 1. To raise, e.g. through engorgement of erectile tissues. 2. Upright; in the state of erection.

erec·tile (L. *erigere*, to erect). 1. Capable of becoming erect. 2. Inducing erection. **E. tissue:** cavernous tissue, engorgement of which renders the part containing the tissue firm and erect.

erec·tion (L. *erigere*, to erect). Act of erecting; state of being erect, as the erection of the penis or clitoris due to engorgement of its erectile tissue.

erec·tor (L.). 1. A muscle raising a part. 2. A prism attached to the eyepiece of a microscope to annul the inversion of the image.

eremopho·bia (G. *ĕrēmos*, solitary; *phobos*, fear). A morbid dread of being alone.

erep·sin (G. *ereipein*, to throw down). A peptidase, or mixture of peptidases, found in intestinal mucous membrane, but also widely distributed throughout other tissues, hydrolyzing peptides to amino-acids.

erep·tic. Relating to erepsin.

ere·thic (G. *erethizein*, to excite). Pertaining to erethism.

erethism (G. *erethizein*, to excite). 1. Excessive irritability. 2. Excessive irritability with regard to sexual libido. **E. mercurialis:** condition due to chronic mercury poisoning, characterized by ready mental excitability, insomnia, headache, vertigo, shyness, and sometimes by hallucinations.

erethro·phoby, ereuto·phoby. Erythrophobia, *q.v.*

erg (G. *ergon*, work). A unit of work or energy; the work done in moving a body by one centimetre against the force of one dyne.

erga·sia (G. *ergon*, work). The totality of functions and reactions of an individual.

ergasiopho·bia (G. *ergon*, work; *phobos*, fear). A dread of operations.

ergas·tic (G. *ergon*, work). Applied to certain lifeless protoplasmic products such as cellulose or starch.

er·gogram (G. *ergon*, work; *gramma*, a mark). A graphic record of muscular work.

er·gograph (G. *ergon*, work; *graphein*, to write). An instrument for recording muscular work.

ergo·meter (G. *ergon*, work; *metron*, measure). A variety of dynamometer.

ergomet·rine. The alkaloid responsible for the oxytocic activity of aqueous extract of ergot.

ergopho·bia (G. *ergon*, work; *phobos*, fear). A morbid dread of work.

ergos·terol (Old Fr. *argot*, ergot, *q.v.*; G. *stereos*, solid; L. *oleum*, oil). $C_{28}H_{43}OH$; a sterol, *q.v.*, derived from ergot, yeast and other fungi; activated by ultra-violet rays to vitamin D.

ergot (Old Fr. *argot*, spur, or excrescence). The growth produced by the fungus *Claviceps purpurea* on rye, consisting of the fungal sclerotium, yielding various alkaloids and amines.

ergo·tamine. An alkaloid obtained from ergot, used in the treatment of migraine.

er·gotism. Condition due to poisoning with either rye products contaminated with ergot or with any of the toxic constituents of ergot, affecting mainly the posterior columns of the spinal cord, clinically characterized by (*a*) numbness and paraesthesia of the distal parts of the extremities, progressing to gangrene which is at first markedly painful (St. Anthony's fire) but later accompanied by complete anaesthesia, or (*b*) numbness of the mentioned parts followed by spasms of the muscles of the limbs and eventually of the whole body, accompanied by severe giddiness and/or blindness, deafness, delirium and dementia.

ergotox·ine. The alkaloid responsible for ergotism, *q.v.*

Erichsen's disease (Erichsen, J., English surgeon, 1818–96). Railway spine; railway brain. A series of symptoms following accidents, which may assume the form of traumatic hysteria, neurasthenia, hypochondriasis or melancholia. Syn. Page's disease. **E.'s ligature:** one consisting of a double thread, one half of which is white, the other black; used in ligation of naevi. **E.'s sign:** to differentiate coxalgia from sacroiliac disease: compression of the two iliac bones causes pain in the latter disease but not in the former.

erigens (L. *erigere*, to raise). Producing erection.

Erigeron. Fleabane, a plant having various species used as diuretics.

erode (L. *erodere*, to eat away). To wear down.

erŏ·dent (L. *erodere*, to eat away). 1. Caustic; causing erosion. 2. A caustic agent.

erogen·ic, erŏ·genous (G. *erōs*, love; *gennan*, to produce). Arousing or promoting sexual sensations. **E. zones:** parts of the body invested with libidinous properties.

erŏ·sion (L. *erodere*, to eat away). 1. Localized loss of epithelium. 2. Localized decalcification of enamel and dentine, occurring especially on labial and buccal surfaces of teeth, characterized by a smooth-bottomed, more or less shallow cavity.

erŏ·sive. Relating to or producing erosion.

erot·ic (G. *erōs*, love). Relating to sexual feeling.

erŏ·ticism, ĕ·rotism (G. *erōs*, love). 1. Condition characterized by sexual love feelings. 2. Exaggerated display of sexual feelings.

erotogen·ic. Erogenic, *q.v.*

erotomā·nia (G. *erōs*, love; *mania*, madness). Excessive sexual feelings.

erŏ·topath (G. *erōs*, love; *pathos*, disease). An individual with maladjusted sexual impulses.

erotophō·bia (G. *erōs*, love; *phobos*, fear). Neurotic fear of developing sexual feelings.

errat·ic (L. *errare*, to wander). 1. Irregular. 2. Moving about. 3. Deviating from a rational course.

errhine (G. *en*, in; *rhis*, nose). Causing discharge from the nose.

erubes·cence (L. *erubescere*, to redden). Flushing.

eructā·tion (L. *eructare*, to belch). Belching.

erup·tion (L. *erumpere*, to break out). 1. A bursting forth. 2. The breaking out of a skin rash; a skin rash. 3. The emergence of a tooth through the gum.

erup·tive. Pertaining to or attended by an eruption.

Erysimum. A genus of plants, of which some varieties yield a cardiac stimulant.

erysi·pelas (G. *eruthros*, red; *pella*, skin). An acute inflammation of the skin and subcutaneous tissues, due to local infection with haemolytic streptococci (group A), characterized by fever, malaise, uniform redness, swelling and tenderness of the affected parts, spread of the sharply limited inflammatory changes by continuity through the lymph spaces, the involution of the changes beginning in the first involved areas. **E. perstans faciei:** a form of lupus erythematosus disseminatus, *q.v.*

erysipĕ·latous (G. *eruthros*, red; *pella*, skin). Affected with or resembling erysipelas.

erysi·peloid (G. *eruthros*, red; *pella*, skin; *eidos*, form). An infectious disease resembling erysipelas but slower in onset and without systemic symptoms; occurring especially in butchers, fishmongers and cooks, and caused by the *Bacillus erysipelatus suis* (*Erysipelothrix rhusiopathiae*), the organism causing erysipelas in swine. Syn. erythema migrans.

Erysi·pelothrix (G. *eruthros*, red; *pella*, skin; *thrix*, hair). A genus of higher bacteria forming rod-shaped organisms with only an occasional long filament which may show slight branches. **E. rhusiopathiae:** the organism causing swine erysipelas and human erysipeloid.

erythē·ma (G. *eruthainein*, to dye red). Diffuse or patchy redness of the skin, blanching on pressure, due to congestion of cutaneous capillaries. **E. ab igne:** e. due to exposure to artificial heat. **E. annulare:** annular form of e. exudivatum multiforme. **E. caloricum:** e. due to heat. **E. exudivatum multiforme:** acute skin disease characterized by usually bilateral and symmetrical erythematous eruptions of maculopapular or vesico-bullous type, occurring particularly on face, neck and back of hands, forming sometimes annular or gyrate lesions with more or less marked exudation of serum in the corium. **E. fugax:** transitory blushing. **E. induratum:** tuberculide characterized by painless bluish red firm nodules in cutis and subcutaneous tissues of the lower extremities, with usually necrotic changes. Syn. Bazin's disease. **E. infectiosum:** an acute infectious disease, usually occurring in epidemics and affecting children, characterized by dusky flushing of the cheeks and a rose-red, more or less well defined maculo-papular eruption, especially on the face, buttocks and limbs, of a circular or crescentic and later annular arrangement, slight fever and mild leukopenia. Syn. epidemic e.; fifth disease. **E. iris:** a form of e. multiforme, the lesions forming reddish concentric circles with a bluish centre. **E. marginatum:** a condition characterized by flat-topped disc-shaped papular lesions enlarging at the periphery while regressing centrally, forming large circinate patches. **E. migrans:** erysipeloid, *q.v.* **E. nodosum:** an illness usually associated with a change in allergic condition especially in tuberculosis, or sometimes, especially in adults, with some rheumatic conditions, characterized by initial fever and the eruption, particularly over the tibial surface of the lower legs, of rounded or oval slightly elevated, bluish-red, painful nodules within the cutis and the subcutaneous tissue. **E. of the ninth day:** generalized e., occurring occasionally 8 to 10 days after administration of neoarsphenamine. **E. pernio:** chilblain, *q.v.* **E. serpens:** erysipeloid, *q.v.* **E. solare:** e. due to exposure to sunrays. **E. venenata:** e. due to any mineral or vegetable poison.

erythē·matous (G. *eruthainein*, to dye red). Pertaining to or marked by erythema.

erythraē·mia (G. *eruthros*, red; *haima*, blood). Abnormal increase in the number of red blood corpuscles. See also polycythaemia.

erythras·ma (G. *eruthros*, red). A mycotic affection of the epidermis caused by *Microsporon minutissimum*, characterized by well-defined reddish or brownish, slightly scaly patches occurring especially at the upper inner part of the thigh, axillae, submammary folds or other moist regions.

erythraē·moid (G. *eruthros*, red; *eidos*, form). Bearing a resemblance to erythraemia.

ĕ·rythrism (G. *eruthros*, red). Condition of having red hair or red plumage.

erỹ·thritol tetrani·trate. A substance used in the treatment of angina pectoris. It lowers blood pressure by dilating the peripheral arterioles.

erỹ·throblast (G. *eruthros*, red; *blastos*, germ). Any nucleated red blood corpuscle. See also megaloblast, normoblast. **E., primary:** the nucleated red blood corpuscles preceding in development the basophile normoblast; pro-erythroblast.

erythroblastaē·mia (G. *eruthros*, red; *blastos*, germ; *haima*, blood). A condition in which an abnormal number of erythroblasts is found in the blood.

erythroblas·tic. Relating to an erythroblast.

erythroblastō·ma (G. *eruthros*, red; *blastos*, germ). A type of myeloma derived from red-blood-cell-forming tissues.

erythroblastō·sis (G. *eruthros*, red; *blastos*, germ). The presence of nucleated erythrocytes in the circulating blood. **E. foetalis:** see haemolytic disease of the newborn.

ery̆·throchlorŏ·pia (G. *eruthros*, red; *khloros*, green; *ōps*, eye). Colour-blindness in respect of blue and yellow, so that green and red are the only colours distinguished.

erythrŏ·clasis (G. *eruthros*, red; *klaein*, to break). Erythronoclasis, *q.v.*

erythroclăs·tic (G. *eruthros*, red; *klaein*, to break). Erythronoclastic, *q.v.*

ery̆·throconte. Erythrokont, *q.v.*

ĕ·rythrocy̆anō·sis (G. *eruthros*, red; *kuanos*, blue). Any condition characterized by areas of bluish-red discoloration of the skin. **E. crurum (puellarum):** a condition occurring especially in girls and young women, characterized by purplish, more or less uniform or mottled, discoloration of the skin or parts inadequately protected against cold, i.e. especially of feet and legs, usually more marked over the calves and the insertion of the tendo Achilles, accompanied by a burning or itching sensation and swelling of the affected areas.

ery̆·throcyte (G. *eruthros*, red; *kutos*, cell). A red blood-corpuscle; the fully mature, anuclear, non-motile cell which has lost nucleus, Golgi net, mitochondria and centrioles during maturation (in mammals), averaging in man 7.74μ in surface area, probably of biconcave disc-form, carrying the pigment haemoglobin which combines with oxygen in the lungs and carries CO_2 from the tissues to the lungs.

erythrocy̆tŏ·lysis (G. *eruthros*, red; *kutos*, cell; *luein*, to loosen). Disintegration of the red blood corpuscles.

erythrocy̆tŏ·meter (G. *eruthros*, red; *kutos*, cell; *metron*, measure). A graduated glass capillary tube for counting erythrocytes.

erythrocy̆tō·sis (G. *eruthros*, red; *kutos*, cell). Abnormal increase in the number of erythrocytes in the circulating blood.

erythroder·ma (G. *eruthros*, red; *derma*, skin). Reddening of the skin with more or less infiltration. **E. desquamativa:** an inflammatory condition of the skin occurring in young seborrhoeic infants (1st to 3rd month), usually starting at the scalp and tending to involve gradually the whole body; characterized by marked epidermal desquamation and always associated with nutritional disturbance. Syn. Leiner's disease. **E. ichthyosiformis congenita:** a congenital affection of the skin characterized by generalized erythema, especially marked over the front of the neck and the flexor surfaces of the large joints, and associated with hyperkeratosis of the soles of the feet, seborrhoea of scalp and face, deformities of the nails and sometimes with a pemphigus-like eruption.

erythroedē·ma (G. *eruthros*, red; *oidein*, to swell). A disease in infants marked by photophobia, muscular weakness, swollen red hands and feet and disordered digestion. Syn. pink disease.

erythrogen·ic (G. *eruthros*, red; *gennan*, to produce). Producing red blood cells.

erythroid (G. *eruthros*, red; *eidos*, form). Having a red colour.

eryth·rokont (G. *eruthros*, red; *kontos*, a pole). A small rod-shaped body in red blood corpuscles, found especially in untreated pernicious anaemia.

erythroleukae·mia (G. *eruthros*, red; *leukos*, white; *haima*, blood). An anaemia with an excess of immature red cells and leucocytes in the blood.

erythromā·nia (G. *eruthros*, red; *mania*, madness). Distressing and uncontrollable blushing.

ĕ·rythromelal·gia (G. *eruthros*, red; *melos*, limb; *algos*, pain). A chronic condition characterized by paroxysmal attacks of flushing with throbbing and burning pain and intense hyperaesthesia, affecting mainly regions on one or both lower extremities, aggravated by heat, exertion or dependent posture; probably due to a local obliterative disease of the arteries and arterioles.

ĕ·rythron (G. *eruthros*, red). Red blood corpuscles and their precursors conceived as a single functional unit.

ery̆·throneocy̆tō·sis (G. *eruthros*, red; *neos*, new; *kutos*, cell). Presence of regenerative forms of red blood cells in the circulating blood.

erythronoclā·sis (G. *eruthros*, red; *klaein*, to break). Disintegration of red blood corpuscles.

erythronoclas·tic (G. *eruthros*, red; *klaein*, to break). Characterized by or causing disintegration of red blood corpuscles.

erythronopoiē·sis (G. *eruthros*, red; *poiein*, to make). Formation of red blood corpuscles.

erythronopoiĕt·ic (G. *eruthros*, red; *poiein*, to make). Pertaining to erythronopoiesis.

ĕ·rythropar·asite. A parasite of red blood cells.

erythrŏ·pathy (G. *eruthros*, red; *pathos*, disease). Any disease of the red blood corpuscles.

ĕ·rythropē·nia (G. *eruthros*, red; *penia*, poverty). Diminished amount of red blood corpuscles.

ĕ·rythrophă·gia (G. *eruthros*, red; *phagein*, to eat). Phagocytic destruction of red blood corpuscles.

ĕ·rythrophile (G. *eruthros*, red; *philein*, to love). Staining readily with red dyes.

ĕ·rythrophō·bia (G. *eruthros*, red; *phobos*, fear). Neurotic fear of blushing.

ĕrythrŏ·pia. Erythropsia, *q.v.*

ĕ·rythropla·kia (G. *eruthros*, red; *plax*, anything flat). Early stages of squamous carcinoma on a mucous membrane.

erythropoiē·sis (G. *eruthros*, red; *poiein*, to make). Erythronopoiesis, *q.v.*

erythrop·sia (G. *eruthros*, red; *ops*, the eye). Perverted visual perception in which all objects appear red.

erythrop·sin (G. *eruthros*, red; *ops*, the eye). Visual purple, *q.v.*

erythrosedimentā·tion (G. *eruthros*, red; L. *sedimentum*, from *sedēre*, to sit). The sedimentation of red blood cells.

Esbach's reagent (Esbach, G. H., French physician, 1843–90). Solution consisting of picric acid 1, citric acid 2, water to 100. It is used as a test for albumin in the urine.

Esch. Abbreviation for Escherichia.

es·char (G. *eskhara*, scab). A dry slough.

escharot·ic (G. *eskhara*, scab). Caustic; producing a slough.

Escherich's bacillus (Escherich, T., German physician, 1857–1911). The *Escherichia coli*.

Escherĭ·chia. A group of bacteria comprising mainly the colon and lactic acid bacilli.

Eschscholtzia. A genus of plants. It includes the Californian poppy from which a hypnotic extract is obtained.

es·culent (L. from *esca*, food). Edible.

esep·tate (L. *e*, from; *septum*, from *sepire*, to enclose). Without a septum.

eser·idine. An alkaloid $C_{15}H_{23}N_3O_3$ from the Calabar bean.

ĕ·serine (W. African native *éséré*). An alkaloid obtained from the Calabar bean, identical with physostigmine, *q.v.*

Esmarch's bandage (Esmarch, J. F. A. von, German surgeon, 1823–1908). An elastic rubber bandage, wound tightly about a limb from the periphery towards the centre in order to present a bloodless field for operation.

esŏd·ic (G. *ēsō*, inward; *hodos*, road). Afferent.

eso-ethmoidī·tis. Inflammation of the ethmoid sinuses.

esogastri·tis. Inflammation of the innermost lining of the stomach.

esophor·ia (G. *ĕsō*, inward; *pherein*, to bear). Tendency to squint inwards.

esophor·ic. Characterized by or relating to esophoria.

esoter·ic (G. *esoterikos*, inner). Intended only for the initiate.

esotrŏ·pia (G. *ĕsō*, inward; *trepein*, to turn). Convergent squint.

espŭn·dia (Sp.). A leishmaniasis, *q.v.*, affecting skin and secondarily buccal and nasal mucous membranes, endemic in South America.

essence (L. *essentia*, from *esse*, to be). A solution of an essential oil in alcohol.

essential. 1. Relating to the essence of a substance. 2. Not due to another disease. E. oil: a volatile oil from an aromatic plant; syn. volatile oil. E. hypertension: see hypertension, e.

ester (Term coined by the German chemist Gmelin from G. *aithēr*, ether, and Germ. *Säure*, acid). A compound formed from an alcohol and an acid with elimination of water.

esterase. Any enzyme hydrolyzing (saponifying) esters.

esterificā·tion. Conversion into an ester.

esthiŏ·mene (G. *esthiomenos*, eating). 1. Any ulcerative condition of the vulva. 2. Lupus vulgaris of the vulva. 3. Pudendal elephantiasis, usually due to lymphogranulomatosis inguinalis.

Estlander's operation (Estlander, J. A., Finnish surgeon, 1831–81). Excision of portions of one or more ribs in the treatment of empyema.

estrangement. In psychiatry, loss of sense of the environment.

Et. Symbol for ethyl.

état (Fr., from L. *stare*, to stand). E. criblé: status cribrosus, *q.v.* E. mamelonné: a condition of the stomach due to chronic gastritis, characterized by wart-like hypertrophy of the mucous membrane. E. marbré: status marmoratus, *q.v.* E. vermoulu: worm-eaten appearance of the cerebral cortex, due to arteriosclerotic lesions causing focal disintegration of cortical substance.

ethanol. Ethyl alcohol.

Eternod's sinus (Eternod, A. F. C., Swiss histologist, 1854–1932). A loop of vessels connecting the vessels of the chorion to those in the yolk sac.

ethane. A saturated hydrocarbon having the formula C_2H_6.

etheogĕ·nesis (G. *ētheas*, young man; *genesis*, development). Non-sexual development by male gametes of protozoa.

ether (G. *aither*, upper air). Two members of this general class of compounds are in use as anaesthetics: diethyl ether $(C_2H_5)_2O$ and divinyl ether, $CH_2=CH.O.CH=CH_2$.

ethereal (G. *aithēr*, upper air). Relating to or containing ether.

ē·therize (G. *aithēr*, upper air). 1. To convert into ether. 2. To anaesthetize with ether.

ē·theromā·nia (G. *aithēr*, upper air; *mania*, madness). Ether-addiction.

etherŏ·meter (G. *aithēr*, upper air; *metron*, measure). An apparatus used in the administration of ether anaesthetic by means of which the amount used can be measured.

ethics (G. *ēthikos*, moral). The science of morals.

ethi·sterone. A synthetic compound derived from testosterone showing progesterone-like activity. Syn. Pregneninolone; ethynyl testosterone.

eth·mocardī·tis (G. *ēthmos*, sieve; *kardia*, heart). Inflammation of the connective tissue of the heart.

ethmocĕ·phalus (G. *ēthmos*, sieve; *kephalē*, head). A monster with a rudimentary nose like a proboscis.

ethmofron·tal (G. *ēthmos*, sieve; L. *frons*, forehead). Relating to the ethmoid and frontal bones.

ethmoid (G. *ēthmos*, sieve; *eidos*, form). 1. The bone at the base of the skull forming part of the walls and septum of the nasal cavity, composed in man of the perforated cribriform plate, a median plate and the superior and middle conchae. 2. Relating to the e. bone.

ethmoi·dal (G. *ēthmos*, sieve; *eidos*, form). Relating to the ethmoid bone. E. cells; E. sinuses: air-containing cavities in the ethmoid bone communicating with the nasal fossae. E. notch: the space between the orbital plates of the frontal bone, occupied by the cribriform plate.

ethmoidec·tomy (G. *ēthmos*, sieve; *eidos*, form; *ektomē*, excision). Excision of the ethmoid cells.

ethmoidī·tis (G. *ēthmos*, sieve; *eidos*, form). Inflammation of the ethmoid bone or of the ethmoid sinuses.

ethmoidŏ·tomy (G. *ēthmos*, sieve; *eidos*, form; *tomē*, section). Incision into an ethmoid sinus.

eth·nic (G. *ethnos*, a nation). Pertaining to racial characters.

ethnŏ·graphy (G. *ethnos*, a nation; *graphein*, to write). Description of the races or peoples of the world.

ethnŏ·logy (G. *ethnos*, a nation; *logos*, a discourse). The science dealing with the human races.

ethocaine hydrochloride. A local anaesthetic. Syn. procaine hydrochloride, *q.v.*

ethyl (G. *aithēr*, upper air; *hulē*, matter). Monovalent radical, C_2H_5. E. alcohol: ordinary alcohol, C_2H_5OH, a product of vinous fermentation.

ethylă·mine. A ptomaine found in putrefying yeast.

ethylate (G. *aithēr*, upper air; *hulē*, matter). 1. A compound derived from ethyl alcohol by substitution of the hydroxyl hydrogen by a metal. 2. To introduce one or more ethyl groups.

ethylene. Olefiant gas, colourless and inflammable.

ethyl·ic. Relating to ethyl.

ē·tiolā·tion (Fr. *étiole*, from L. *stipula*, straw). Pallor caused by the exclusion of light.

etiŏ·logy. See aetiology.

etrŏ·tomy (G. *ētron*, hypogastrium; *tomē*, section). General term for lower abdominal and pelvic operations.

euaesthē·sia (G. *eu*, well; *aisthēsis*, feeling). The sense of wellbeing; vigour and normal condition of the senses.

Eubacteriales. An order of relatively simple microorganisms of the class of Schizomycetes.

Eucalyptus (G. *eu*, well; *kaluptos*, covered). A genus of myrtaceous trees, chiefly found in Australia. Oil of e.: a volatile oil obtained from various species of e. trees, but principally from the E. globulus. The oil has antiseptic and stimulant properties.

Eucatropine hydrochloride. A synthetic mydriatic.

euchromatop·sia (G. *eu*, well; *khrōma*, colour; *opsis*, vision). Normal colour vision.

euchromosome (G. *eu*, well; *khrōma*, colour; *sōma*, body). Autosome, *q.v.*

eudiŏ·meter (G. *eudia*, fair weather; *metron*, measure). An instrument used for measuring and analysing gases.

eu·flavine. An acridine antiseptic for topical application.

eugen·ics (G. *eu*, well; *gennan*, to produce). The science dealing with influences that improve the inborn characters of a race, especially in man.

Eugĕnol. 2-methoxy-4ⁿ-allylphenol. An oily liquid obtainable from oil of cloves and having similar properties.

euglŏ·bulin (G. *eu*, well; L. *globus*, globe). A small fraction of serum globulin which can be separated by dialysis of the serum.

eukinē·sia (G. *eu*, well; *kinein*, to move). Normal power of movement.

Eulenburg's disease (Eulenburg, A., German neurologist, 1840–1917). Congenital paramyotonia.

Eumycē·tes (G. *eu*, well; *mukēs*, mushroom). A class of Thallophytes, *q.v.*, comprising the higher fungi, characterized by the presence of a thallus in the form of hyphae, and by branching and reproduction by various forms of spores, sometimes sexual.

eunoi·a (G. *eu*, well; *nous*, mind). Normal condition of mind and will.

eu·nuch (G. *eunoukhos*, from *eunē*, bed; *ekhein*, to have charge of). A castrated male.

eu·nuchoidism (G. *eunoukhos*, eunuch; *eidos*, form). A condition characterized by hypoplasia of the testes and penis, deficiency in secondary sex characters, delay in fusion of the epiphyses of the long bones, a tendency to excessive growth in length of the extremities, and sometimes by obesity of the female type.

eupareū·nia (G. *eu*, well; *pareunos*, bedfellow). Sexual compatibility.

eupep·sia (G. *eu*, well; *peptein*, to digest). Normal digestion.

eupep·tic (G. *eu*, well; *peptein*, to digest). 1. Characterized by a good digestion. 2. Promoting digestion.

euphor·ia (G. *eu*, well; *pherein*, to bear). Sense of feeling well.

euphor·ic. Relating to euphoria.

euplas·tic (G. *eu*, well; *plassein*, to form). Capable of being transformed into organized tissue.

eupnōē·a (G. *eu*, well; *pnein*, to breathe). Normal or quiet respiration.

euprax·ia (G. *eu*, well; *prassein*, to do). Normal performance of co-ordinated movements.

eupȳ·rene (G. *eu*, well; *purēn*, fruit-stone). The normal type of sperm.

eu·ryon (G. *eurus*, wide). Either of the points at the end of the greatest transverse diameter of the skull.

euryprosō·pic (G. *eurus*, wide; *prosōpon*, face). Having a facial index, *q.v.*, between 80 and 85.

euryther·mic (G. *eurus*, broad; *thermē*, heat). Capable of surviving and growing in considerable ranges of temperature.

eusol. Dakin's solution, *q.v.*

Eustachian artery (Eustachi, B., Italian anatomist, 1513–74). 1. A branch of the Vidian artery. 2. A branch of the pterygopalatine artery. **E. catheter:** an instrument for distending or making applications to the E. tube. **E. muscle:** the laxator tympani. **E. tube:** the canal, partly bony and partly cartilaginous, connecting the pharynx with the tympanic cavity. **E. valve:** the fold of the lining membrane of the right auricle of the heart, between the opening of the inferior vena cava and the auriculo-ventricular orifice.

eustā·chium. The pharyngotympanic tube. Syn. Eustachian tube, *q.v.*

eusys·tole. A normal condition of the heart's systole.

eutec·tic (G. *eu*, well; *tēkein*, to melt). Melting easily.

euthanā·sia (G. *eu*, well; *thanatos*, death). 1. An easy or calm death. 2. The practice of painlessly killing people suffering from incurable disease.

eutō·cia (G. *eu*, well; *tokos*, childbirth). Normal childbirth.

eutrichō·sis (G. *eu*, well; *thrix*, hair). A normal condition of the hair.

eutroph·ic (G. *eu*, well; *trephein*, to nourish). 1. Relating to eutrophy. 2. Promoting nutrition.

eu·trophy, eutrō·phia (G. *eu*, well; *trephein*, to nourish). A state of healthy nutrition.

evă·cuant (L. *evacuare*, to empty). 1. Emptying. 2. An agent that causes the emptying of an organ.

evacuā·tion (L. *evacuare*, to empty). 1. The act of emptying, as of the bowels. 2 The evacuated matter.

evaginā·tion (L. *e*, out; *vagina*, sheath). Protrusion from a sheath or other structure.

evanes·cent (L. *evanescere*, to vanish). To disappear quickly.

evaporā·tion (L. *e*, out; *vaporare*, to steam). The conversion of a substance from a liquid or solid state into vapour.

Eve's method (Eve, F. C., contemporary English physician). A method of artificial respiration in which the patient is rocked upwards and downwards, the diaphragm being forced up and down by these movements.

eventratio diaphragmatica (L. *e*, from; *venter*, bowels; G. *dia*, through; *phragma*, a fence). Protrusion of a relaxed diaphragm (and therefore of abdominal viscera) into the thoracic cavity.

eventrā·tion (L. *e*, from; *venter*, belly). 1. Protrusion of the abdominal viscera through the abdominal wall. 2. Extensive hernia of abdominal organs.

ever·sion (L. *e*, from; *vertere*, to turn). A turning outward, or a state of being turned outward, e.g., e. of the eyelid.

evidement (Fr.). The operation of scraping away a diseased part of any organ or cavity.

evideur (Fr.). A surgical instrument used in the performance of évidement.

evirā·tion (L. *e*, from; *vir*, man). Castration.

eviscerā·tion (L. *e*, from; *viscus*, inner part). To remove viscera, or the contents of an organ.

evocā·tion (L. *e*, from; *vocare*, to call). That part of the morphogenetic effect of an organism which is related to the action of the evocator.

evocā·tor (L. *e*, from; *vocare*, to call). The chemical substance emitted by the organism, acting as the morphogenetic stimulus.

evolution (L. *evolvere*, to roll out). The process of development, especially of a race of species.

evulsio nervi optici (L.). Evulsion of the optic nerve.

evul·sion (L. *evulsio*, a plucking out). A forcible extraction or tearing away of a part.

Ewald's test meal (Ewald, C. A., German physician, 1846–1915). A method not now used in ascertaining the condition of the gastric juice.

Ewart's sign (Ewart, W., English physician, 1848–1929). In marked pericardial effusion the left clavicle is so elevated that the upper border of the first rib can be felt with the finger as far as the sternum.

Ewing's tumour (Ewing, J., American pathologist, 1866–1943). A rare type of bone tumour.

exacerbā·tion (L. *exacerbare*, to exasperate). An increase in the severity of a disease.

exā·crinous (G. *exō*, outside; *krinein*, to separate). Relating to external secretions.

exaē·mia (G. *ex*, from; *haima*, blood). A term denoting oligaemia and reduction of venous return due to loss or prolonged deprivation of fluid.

exal·gin. Acetylmethylanilide; an antipyretic.

exaltā·tion (L. *ex*, from; *altus*, high). An abnormal condition of mental and spiritual ecstasy.

exanimā·tion (L. *ex*, from; *anima*, air). Coma.

exan·thema, exan·them (G. *exanthēma*, eruption). 1. An eruption of the skin. 2. Any disease, especially an infectious fever, characterized by a skin rash. **E. subitum:** an acute infectious disease, affecting children only up to 2 to 3 years of age, characterized by sudden onset of fever with signs of malaise, lasting for 3 to 4 days, falling then abruptly, being immediately followed by a morbilliform, erythematous or rubella-like rash which usually spreads from back and shoulders to abdomen and lastly to face and limbs, fading after about 2 days without desquamation or pigmentation. Syn. sixth disease; three day fever.

exanthemat·ic, exanthē·matous. Pertaining to or characterized by exanthema.

ex·anthrope (G. *ex*, out; *anthrōpos*, man). Any source of disease originating externally.

exarterī·tis (G. *ex*, out; *arteria*, artery). Inflammation of the outer coat of an artery.

exarticulā·tion (L. *ex*, from; *articulus*, joint). Amputation at a joint.

excavā·tion (L. *excavare*, to hollow out). A hollow or cavity, such as the cupping of the optic disc.

ex·cavator (L. *excavare*, to hollow out). 1. An instrument for scraping away tissue. 2. A dental instrument for opening or making cavities to remove decayed matter from them.

excen·tric (G. *ex*, away; *kentron*, centre). Out of the centre or median line.

excerebrā·tion (L. *ex*, from; *cerebrum*, brain). Removal of the brain, especially of the foetal brain to facilitate delivery of the foetus from the uterus.

exci·pient (L. *excipere*, to take out). An inert substance combined with a drug to render the latter suitable for administration.

excise (L. *excidere*, to cut out). To cut out or off; to remove.

exci·sion (L. *excisio*). The cutting out or off of a part.

excītabi·lity (L. *excitare*, to stimulate). 1. Property of reacting to a stimulus. 2. Property of becoming unduly excited readily.

exci·table (L. *excitare*, to stimulate). 1. Capable of reacting to a stimulus. 2. Readily excited.

exci·tant (L. *excitare*, to stimulate). 1. Stimulating. 2. An agent which stimulates the activity of an organ.

excitā·tion (L. *excitare*, to stimulate). 1. Act of stimulating or exciting. 2. Condition due to stimulation.

exci·tatory (L. *excitare*, to stimulate). Characterized by excitation; tending to excite. **E. wave**: wavelike involvement of successive muscle fibres by the e. process.

excite (L. *excitare*, to stimulate). To call forth or to cause increase in activity; to stimulate.

excite·ment (L. *excitare*, to stimulate). Any aroused or increased activity in an organ or of an organism.

exci·ting (L. *excitare*, to stimulate). Calling forth directly; causing or increasing activity.

exci·toglan·dular (L. *excitare*, to stimulate; *glans*, an acorn). Stimulating the functions of glands.

exci·tometabol·ic (L. *excitare*, to stimulate; G. *metabolē*, change). Stimulating metabolic activity.

exci·tomō·tor (L. *excitare*, to stimulate; *motor*, from *movere*, to move). Exciting motor function.

exci·tor (L. *excitare*, to stimulate). Any nerve, which when stimulated, causes activity in the part of the body which it supplies.

ex·clave (L. *ex*, out; *clavus*, an excrescence). A detached portion of any organ; an accessory organ.

exclū·sion (L. *exclusio*, a shutting out). Rejection.

excochlēā·tion (L. *ex*, out; *cochlear*, spoon). To curette or scrape out material from a cavity.

excoriā·tion (L. *excoriare*, to flay). Abrasion of a portion of the skin.

excorticā·tion (L. *ex*, out; *cortex*, rind). Decortication, *q.v.*

ex·crement (L. *excrementum*, from *excernere*, to separate out). Excreted waste matter; the faecal matter.

excremen·tal, excrementī·tious. Relating to excrement.

excres·cence (L. *excrescere*, to grow out). 1. An outgrowth. 2. An abnormal outgrowth.

excrē·ta (L. *excernere*, to separate out). Excreted waste matter, such as urine; excretions.

excrete (L. *excernere*, to separate out). To expel waste matter from the body.

excrē·tion (L. *excernere*, to separate out). 1. Process of excreting. 2. Excreted waste matter.

ex·cretory. Relating to or serving for excretion.

excur·sion (L. *excursio*, from *ex*, out; *currere*, to run). A departure, or a wandering off. This term may be applied to the eyes as from a midposition.

excurvā·tion (L. *ex*, out; *curvare*, to curve). Outward curvature.

exencē·phalus (G. *ex*, out; *egkephalos*, brain). A monster with a cranial defect exposing the cerebral surface.

exen·terate (G. *ex*, out; *enteron*, bowel). Eviscerate; enucleate.

exenterā·tion (G. *ex*, out; *enteron*, bowel). Evisceration; enucleation.

exenterī·tis (G. *ex*, out; *enteron*, bowel). Inflammation of the peritoneal or outer covering of the bowel.

exer·esis (G. *ex*, out; *haireein*, to take). Removal, especially by evulsion.

exfoetā·tion (L. *ex*, out; *foetus*). Ectopic foetation.

exflagellā·tion (L. *ex*, out; *flagellum*, a whip). 1. The casting off of flagella or cilia. 2. The breaking away of 6-8 whip-shaped microgametes from the residual mass of a male malarial gametocyte.

exfoliā·tion (L. *ex*, out; *folium*, leaf). 1. Lamellar desquamation of the upper layers of the skin. 2. Lamellar separation of a surface from the underlying tissue.

exfō·liative. Characterized by or causing exfoliation.

exhā·lent (L. *exhalare*, to breath out). Exhaling; serving for exhalation.

exhalā·tion (L. *exhalare*, to breath out). 1. Giving off in the form of vapour; expiration. 2. The substance thus given off, as the breath.

exhaustion (L. *exhaurire*, to drain out). 1. Loss of strength, as from fatigue. 2. To extract completely the active constituents of a crude drug by percolation, maceration or successive treatment with differently acting solvents. 3. Process of exhausting a vessel of air.

exhibit (L. *exhibēre*). To administer a medicine.

exhibi·tionism (L. *exhibēre*, to show). The gratification of sexual impulses by displaying the erotogenic zones.

exhibi·tionist (L. *exhibēre*, to show). A person addicted to exhibitionism.

exhi·larant (L. *exhilarare*, to gladden). Animating.

exhumā·tion (L. *ex*, out; *humus*, earth). The removal of a corpse from the place of burial; disinterment.

ex·itus (L. *exire*, to go out). Death.

Exner's plexus (Exner, S. Austrian physiologist, 1846–1926). A plexus formed by horizontal fibres (axis-cylinder terminals) in the superficial layer of the cerebral cortex. **E.'s nerve**: the nervus laryngeus medius.

exocar·dia (G. *exō*, outside; *kardia*, heart). Displacement of the heart.

exocar·dial (G. *exō*, outside; *kardia*, heart). Outside the heart. **E. murmurs**: murmurs synchronous with the cardiac action but originating outside the cardiac cavities, such as pericardial or cardiopulmonary murmurs.

exodon·tia (G. *ex*, out; *odous*, tooth). Branch of dentistry pertaining to extraction of teeth.

exō·gamy (G. *exō*, outside; *gamos*, marriage). 1. Conjugation between gametes descending from different ancestors. 2. The custom of marriage outside a certain group (family, clan, etc.).

exogas·tric (G. *exō*, outside; *gastēr*, belly). Relating to the outside coats of the stomach.

exogastrī·tis (G. *exō*, outside; *gastēr*, belly). Inflammation of the outermost coat of the stomach.

exogenet·ic, exō·genous (G. *exō*, outside; *gennan*, to produce). 1. Not arising within the organism; due to an external cause. 2. Growing on the exterior.

exometrī·tis (G. *exō*, outside; *mētra*, womb). Inflammation of the external coat of the uterus.

exŏ·pathy (G. *exō*, outside; *pathos*, disease). Any disease due to a cause outside the body.

exom·phalos (G. *exō*, outside; *omphalos*, navel). Congenital umbilical hernia.

L

exophor·ia (G. *exō*, outside; *phoros*, bearing). Tendency to squint outward.

exophthal·mic (G. *exō*, outside; *ophthalmos*, eye). Relating to exophthalmos. **E. goitre:** see goitre, e. **E. ophthalmoplegia:** ophthalmoplegia associated with exophthalmos and usually with disordered thyroid function (hyperthyroidism, status after thyroidectomy), affecting usually one eye more than the other (if not one eye exclusively), occurring more frequently in individuals of over 40 and resulting commonly in diplopia.

exophthal·mos, exophthal·mus (G. *exō*, outside; *ophthalmos*, eye). Abnormal prominence or protrusion of the eyeball.

exoplasm. Ectoplasm, *q.v.*

exor·bitism. Exophthalmos, *q.v.*

exor·mia (G. *ex*, out; *horman*, to rush). Any papular skin disease.

exosep·sis (G. *exō*, outside; *sēpsis*, decay). Any septic condition due to causes outside the body.

exoserō·sis (G. *exō*, outside; L. *serum*). A discharging of serum.

exoskě·leton (G. *exō*, outside; *skeleton*). System of hard, bony or horny structures on or near the outside of an animal body.

ex·osmose, exosmō·sis (G. *exō*, outside; *ōsmos*, impulsion). Outward osmosis.

exosplē·nopexy (G. *exō*, outside; *splēn*, spleen; *pēxis*, fixation). An operation whereby the spleen is attached to the anterior abdominal wall by its capsule.

exostosec·tomy (G. *exō*, outside; *osteon*, bone; *ektomē*, excision). Surgical removal of an exostosis.

exostō·sis (G. *exō*, outside; *osteon*, bone). A circumscribed mass of hyperplastic or neoplastic bone tissue projecting above the surface of a bone.

exotě·ric (G. *exōtěrikos*, outer). Developed outside the body.

exother·mal, exother·mic (G. *exō*, outside; *thermē*, heat). Characterized by release of heat.

ex·othyropex·ia (G. *exō*, outside; *thura*, door; *pēxis*, fixation). The exposure of an enlarged thyroid gland and fixing it outside the neck.

exot·ic (G. *exōtikos*). Foreign.

exotox·in (G. *exō*, outside; *toxikon*, poison). A toxin freely excreted by a micro-organism, e.g., by *Bacillus diphtheriae*, *B. tetani*, *B. botulini* and some other anaerobic bacteria and by the haemolytic streptococcus, having usually a selective action on certain tissues.

exotrō·pia (G. *exō*, outward; *trepein*, to turn). Divergent squint.

expan·sion (L. *expandere*, to spread). Increase in size.

expec·tancy, expectā·tion. The state of watching for or awaiting an event. **E. of life:** the number of years that a person may be presumed to live, according to statistical probability.

expec·tant (L. *expectare*, to await). Awaiting. **E. mother:** pregnant woman. **E. treatment:** a watching of the progress of a disease without gross or specific interference.

expec·torant (L. *expectorare*, from *ex*, out; *pectus*, breast). Promoting expectoration.

expec·torate. To eject from the lungs or trachea.

expectorā·tion. 1. Ejection from the lungs or trachea. 2. The matter so ejected.

expě·riment (L. *experimentum*). A trial or special observation made to confirm or disprove something doubtful.

expirā·tion (L. *ex*. out; *spirare*, breathe). The act of expelling air from the lungs through nose or mouth.

expira·tory. Relating to expiration.

expire. 1. To breathe out. 2. To die.

explantā·tion (L. *ex*, out; *planta*, a sprout). Growth of cells outside the organism from which they were derived, and in isolation from other tissue. See tissue culture.

exploration (L. *explorare*, to search out). Investigation.

explor·atory. Relating to exploration. **E. puncture:** a puncture made for diagnostic purposes.

expression (L. *expressio*). The act of pressing out.

expul·sion (L. *expellere*). 1. The act of driving out. 2. The state of being driven out.

expul·sive (L. *expellere*). 1. Relating to expulsion. 2. Capable of expelling.

exsan·guinate (L. *ex*, out; *sanguis*, blood). 1. To render bloodless. 2. Bloodless.

exsanguinā·tion (L. *ex*, out; *sanguis*, blood). The act of making bloodless.

exsan·guine, exsangui·neous (L. *ex*, out; *sanguis*, blood). Bloodless.

exsic·cant (L. *exsiccare*, to dry out). A drying agent.

ex·siccate (L. *exsiccare*, to dry out). To evaporate moisture from a substance.

exsiccā·tion (L. *exsiccare*, to dry out). Act of drying.

exsic·cative (L. *exsiccare*, to dry out). Drying; tending to make dry.

exstrophy (G. *ex*, out; *strephein*, to turn). The turning inside out of a part. **E. of bladder:** a congenital condition in which the base of the bladder opens on the anterior abdominal wall.

extend (L. *extendere*, to stretch out). To stretch; to straighten out.

exten·sion (L. *extendere*, to stretch out). 1. A stretching out, particularly the muscular movement by which a flexed limb is straightened. 2. Traction upon a fractured or dislocated limb to restore it to its normal position.

exten·sor (L. *extendere*, to stretch out). That which serves to extend, e. g. e. muscles. **E. plantar response:** dorsiflexion (plantar extension) of the great toe on stimulation of the lateral border of the sole of the foot. Syn. positive Babinski reflex.

exterior (L.). Outside.

exter·nal (L. *externus*, outward). 1. On the exterior. 2. Away from the mesial plane or centre of the body. 3. Acting from without.

ex·terocep·tive (L. *exterus*, on the outside; *capere*, to take). 1. Pertaining to an exteroceptor. 2. Pertaining to stimuli acting upon an exteroceptor.

ex·terocep·tor (L. *exterus*, on the outside; *capere*, to take). A sense organ responding to stimuli arising outside the body, such as acoustic, visual, thermal, tactile stimuli. The term is sometimes confined to sense organs situated in the supporting tissues of ectodermal tissue.

ex·tima (L. *extimus*, outermost). The external coat of an artery.

extinguish (L. *extinguere*, to quench). To put out.

extinc·tion (L. *extinguere*, to quench). 1. Act of destroying. 2. State of being destroyed.

ex·tirpate (L. *extirpare*, to root out). To remove entirely; to eradicate.

extirpā·tion (L. *extirpare*, to root out). Entire removal of a part.

extor·sion (L. *ex*, out; *torsio*, a griping). External rotation of a part.

extra (L). Beyond.

extra-arti·cular (L. *extra*, beyond; *articulus*, joint). Outside the proper structure of a joint.

extrabron·chial (L. *extra*, outside; G. *brogkhos*, trachea). Outside the bronchial tubes.

extrabuc·cal (L. *extra*, outside; *bucca*, cheek). Outside the mouth.

extracap·sular (L. *extra*, outside; *capsula*, little box). Outside a capsule; outside the capsular ligament of a joint.

extracar·dial (L. *extra*, outside; G. *kardia*, heart). Exocardial, *q.v.*

extracel·lular (L. *extra*, outside; *cellula*). Outside a cell, or cells.

extracorpor·eal (L. *extra*, outside; *corpus*, body). Outside the body.

extracrā·nial (L. *extra*, outside; *kranion*, head). Outside the cranium.

extract (L. *extrahere*, to draw out). In pharmacy, a solid preparation made by evaporating the alcoholic, aqueous or ethereal solution of a drug.

extrac·tion (L. *extrahere*, to draw out). 1. The act of drawing out, or of removing. 2. The process of making an extract.

extrac·tor (L. *extrahere*, to draw out). An instrument for extracting sequestra, foreign bodies, etc.

extradū·ral (L. *extra*, beyond; *durus*, hard). Outside the dura mater.

extra·epiphy·seal (L. *extra*, outside; G. *epi*, on; *phusis*, from *phuein*, to grow). Outside the epiphysis.

extrage·nital (L. *extra*, outside; *genitus*, begotten). Outside the genital organs.

extrahepat·ic (L. *extra*, outside; G. *hepar*, liver). Outside the liver.

extramalleō·lus (L. *extra*, outside; *malleolus*, hammer). The lateral or outer malleolus of the tibia.

extramar·ginal (L. *extra*, outside; *margo*, edge). Outside consciousness.

extrame·dullary (L. *extra*, outside; *medulla*, marrow). Outside the medulla.

extramū·ral (L. *extra*, beyond; *murus*, wall). Situated outside a wall.

extrā·neous (L. *extraneus*, external). Existing or belonging outside the organism.

extranū·clear (L. *extra*, outside; *nucula*, dim. of *nux*, nut). Outside the nucleus of a cell.

extra-ŏ·cular (L. *extra*, outside; *oculus*, eye). Outside the eyeball.

extraparen·chymal (L. *extra*, outside; *paregkuma*, poured in beside). Outside the parenchyma.

extrapericar·dial (L. *extra*, outside; *peri*, about; *kardia*, heart). Outside the pericardium.

extraplacen·tal (L. *extra*, outside; *placenta*). Outside the placenta.

extrapleū·ral (L. *extra*, outside; *pleura*, rib). Outside the parietal layer of the pleura.

extrapō·lar (L. *extra*, outside; *polus*, pole). Not lying between the poles, as of an electric battery.

extrapul·monary (L. *extra*, outside; *pulmo*, lung). Outside the lungs.

extrapyrǎ·midal (L. *extra*, outside; G. *puramis*, pyramid). Outside the pyramidal system. **E. system:** the central nervous pathways related to muscular tonus, originating perhaps in the premotor area and possibly other parts of the cerebral cortex and partly in various subcortical masses of grey matter (striatum, amygdaloid nucleus, red nucleus, substantia nigra, corpus Luysii, thalamic nuclei).

extrarē·nal (L. *extra*, outside; *rēn*, kidney). Outside, or independent of, the kidneys.

extrasomat·ic (L. *extra*, outside; *soma*, body). Outside the body.

extrasȳs·tole (L. *extra*, outside; G. *sustolē*, contraction). A premature contraction of the heart, replacing the normal systole, due to a stimulus from some abnormal focus arising before the normal impulse.

extratrǎ·chĕal (L. *extra*, outside; *trachea*). Outside the trachea.

extratympan·ic (L. *extra*, outside; G. *tumpanon*, drum). Outside the tympanum of the ear.

extra-ū·terine (L. *extra*, outside; *uterus*). Outside the uterus. **E.-u. pregnancy:** pregnancy in which the foetus is situated outside the uterus, e.g. in the Fallopian tube or in the ovary.

extravagī·nal (L. *extra*, outside; *vagina*, sheath). Outside the vagina.

extrǎ·vasate (L. *extra*, outside; *vas*, vessel). 1. Of a fluid, to pass out of a normal channel, especially into the surrounding tissues. 2. The extravasated fluid.

extrǎvasā·tion (L. *extra*, outside; *vas*, vessel). 1. The passing of fluid outside its normal channel. 2. The extravasated fluid.

extravas·cular (L. *extra*, outside; *vascularis*, from *vas*, vessel). Outside a vessel.

extraventrī·cular (L. *extra*, outside; *ventriculus*, dim. of *venter*, belly). Outside a ventricle.

extrĕ·mity (L. *extremus*, outermost). A limb; the distal or terminal part of any organ.

extrin·sic (L. *extrinsecus*, from without). External; originating or lying outside a part but acting on it, e.g. e. ocular muscles, the four recti and the two oblique muscles of the eyeball. **E. factor:** term applied to the not yet clearly defined substance present, e.g. in beef-muscle and autolyzed yeast, which when acted upon by the intrinsic factor, *q.v.*, produces the haemopoietic substance (anti-pernicious-anaemia factor) which is stored in the liver.

extrō·phia. Deformity of any internal organ.

extrover·sion (L. *extra*, outside; *vertere*, to turn). 1. State of being turned inside out. 2. A mental attitude in which the person's interests are mainly directed to objects other than himself.

ex·trovert (L. *extra*, outside; *vertere*, to turn). A person who is mainly interested in objects other than himself.

extrude. Thrust out.

extrū·sion. A thrusting out or expulsion.

extuba·tion (L. *ex*, out; *tubus*, tube). The removal of a (e.g. laryngeal) tube.

exu·berant (L. *exuberare*, to abound). Prolific; copious.

ex·udate (L. *exudare*, to sweat out). The matter which has passed out by exudation.

exudā·tion (L. *exudare*, to sweat out). 1. The passing out of serous fluid and cells (mainly leucocytes) through unruptured walls of capillaries and venules. 2. Increased secretion of mucous matter.

ex·udative (L. *exudare*, to sweat out). Characterized by exudation. **E. diathesis:** constitutional anomaly in children characterized by abnormal function of skin and mucous membranes, resulting in infantile eczema, and/or urticarial strophulus, prurigo, catarrhs of the mucous membranes and exuberant growth of lymphatic tissue.

exumbilicā·tion (L. *ex*, out; *umbilicus*). Marked protrusion of the umbilicus.

exu·viāe. The sloughing off of the epidermis.

eye. The organ of vision. **E., artificial:** a thin shell of glass or plastic material coloured like the natural eye, which is placed in the conjunctival sac after removal of the eye. **E., black:** a haematoma of the periorbital tissues following trauma.

eyeball. The globe of the eye.

eyebrow. The supercilium.

eyelash. The hair growing from the eyelid.

eyelid. One of the two (upper and lower) covers protecting the eye.

Eysson's bone (Eysson, H., Dutch anatomist, 1620–1690). The ossa mentalia at the symphysis menti.

eye-strain. Fatigue of the eye caused by over-use or uncorrected ocular defect.

eye tooth. A canine tooth.

F

F. Symbol for an atom of fluorine.

F_1. The ' first filial generation'. The offspring of a given mating.

F_2. The 'second filial generation' produced by mating two members of the F_1 generation, so producing an inbred grandchild.

F.A. Abbreviation for fatty acid.

fabel·la (L. *faba*, bean). A sesamoid fibro-cartilage sometimes present in the gastrocnemius muscle.

Faber's anaemia (Faber, K., Danish physician, born 1862). Achylanaemia, a simple anaemia marked by achylia gastrica, *q.v.*

fabricā·tion. The retailing of imaginary happenings as if they were facts.

Fabricius's ship (Fabricius, H., ab Aquapendente, Italian anatomist, ca. 1533–1619). The fanciful resemblance of the contours of the occipital, sphenoid and frontal bones to the outline of a ship.

face (L. *facies*). The front of the head from forehead to chin. F., mask-like: expressionless, immobile facies often seen in alcoholic multiple neuritis.

fa·cet (Fr. *facette*, from L. *facies*, face). A small plane surface.

fā·cial (L. *facies*, face). Pertaining to (1) the face or (2) the seventh cranial (facial) nerve. F. index: see index, f.

fā·ciēs (L.). 1. The face. 2. The appearance of the face. 3. A surface. F. Hippocratica: see Hippocratic face.

facilitā·tion (L. *facilis*, easy). The act of making easy, or promoting.

fā·ciocervi·cal (L. *facies*, face; *cervix*, neck). Relating to the face and the neck.

fā·ciolin·gual (L. *facies*, face; *lingua*, tongue). Relating to the face and the tongue.

facioplas·ty (L. *facies*, face; G. *plassein*, to shape). Plastic surgery of the face.

fā·cioplē·gia (L. *facies*, face; G. *plēgē*, a stroke). Paralysis of the face.

facti·tious (L. *facere*, to make). Artificial.

factor (L., a maker). Unit of inheritance transmitted in the germ cells (see gene). F., filtrate: component of vitamin B_2 promotes growth in rats. F., extrinsic: in food which functions with intrinsic factor producing haematopoiesis. See Castle's factors.

făc·ultative (L. *facultas*, capability). 1. Optional. 2. Being able to thrive under different conditions.

faē·cal (L. *faex*, dregs). Relating to faeces.

faeces (L. *faex*, dregs). Excrement; the discharge of the bowels.

faē·colith (L. *faex*, dregs; G. *lithos*, stone). A stone-like concretion of faeces.

faē·culent (L. *faex*, dregs). Containing faecal matter.

Faget's sign (Faget, J. C., French physician, 1818–84). A fall in the pulse rate with a rise in temperature seen in cases of yellow fever.

fā·gin (L. *fagus*, beech). A narcotic obtained from beechnuts.

Fahraeus's sedimentation test (Fahraeus, R., contemporary Swedish pathologist). A quick settling of the erythrocytes in citrated blood indicates pregnancy.

Fahrenheit (Fahrenheit, G. D., German physicist, 1686–1736). Pertaining to the thermometric scale introduced by F., in which the zero point represents the temperature produced by mixing equal quantities (weight) of snow and salt. Abbrev. F. F.'s thermometer: a thermometer with freezing point at 32° and boiling point at 212°.

faint. To lose consciousness.

fal·cial (L. *falx*, sickle). Relating to a falx.

fal·ciform (L. *falx*, sickle, *forma*, shape). Sickle-shaped.

fal·cula (L. *falx*, sickle). The falx cerebelli.

fallec·tomy. Excision of any portion of the Fallopian tube.

Fallopian aqueduct or canal (Falloppio, G., Italian anatomist, 1523–63). A canal in the petrosa, from the internal auditory meatus to the stylomastoid foramen, transmitting the facial nerve. F. gestation: tubal gestation. F. hiatus: an opening in the anterior surface of the petrosa, transmitting the petrosal branch of the vidian nerve. F. ligament: 1. See Poupart's ligament, inguinal ligament. F. muscle: the pyramidalis. F. tube: the oviduct. F. valve: see Bauhin's valve.

Fallot's tetralogy (Fallot, L. A., French physician, 1850–1911). Four commonly associated congenital heart defects. 1. Dextro-position of the aorta. 2. Right ventricle hypertrophy. 3. Intraventricular septal defect. 4. Stenosis of the pulmonary artery.

Falret's type of mania of persecution (Falret, J. P., French psychiatrist, 1794–1870). A form of paranoia occurring in degenerates.

false (L. *falsus*, from *fallere*, to deceive). Not true; not real; imitating. F. image: the image of the deviating eye in diplopia. F. joint: see ankylosis, false. F. membrane: a fibrinous exudate, devoid of any tissue-structure. Syn. pseudomembrane. F. pains: labour-like pains not followed by labour movements. F. passage: a passage formed by instrumental laceration of a natural passage. F. ribs: the five lower ribs. Syn. costae spuriae.

falx (L. *falx*, sickle). Any sickle-shaped organ. F. cerebelli: the dural fold between the two lobes of the cerebellum, separated from the f. cerebri by the tentorium cerebelli. F. cerebri: the dural fold between the two cerebral hemispheres, containing in its upper margin the superior sagittal and in its lower margin the inferior sagittal sinus.

fā·mēs (L). Hunger.

fami·lial (L. *familia*, from *famulus*, servant). Pertaining to, or occurring in several members of, a family.

family. 1. In biology, a category intermediate between order (higher category) and genus (lower category). 2. In chemistry, a sub-group in the periodic table of elements.

fang. The root of a tooth.

Fannia. A genus of flies. F. canicularis: the lesser house fly.

far point. The most distant point which is focused with completely relaxed accommodation.

Farabeuf's triangle (Farabeuf, L. H., French surgeon, 1841–1910). The upper part of the neck. The sides of the triangle are formed by the internal jugular vein and the facial vein, and its base by the hypoglossal nerve.

farad (Faraday, M.). The unit of electric capacity: the capacity, charged with one coulomb, giving a difference of potential of one volt.

Faraday's laws of electrolysis (Faraday, M., English physicist, 1791–1867). 1. The mass of a substance decomposed by passing an electric current through a solution is directly proportional to the quantity of electricity passing. 2. When an electric current is passed through a series of several different substances the mass of each substance decomposed is proportional to its chemical equivalent.

farad·ic. Pertaining to induced electric currents.

faradi·meter. An instrument used in measuring faradic currents.

faradism. The application of induced currents.

faradizā·tion. Faradism; stimulation with faradic currents.

fă·radother·apy. Treatment by means of faradic currents.

farcy (L. *farcire*, to stuff). Glanders, *q.v.*, especially the more chronic form. **F. bud:** cutaneous swelling in glanders. **F. pipe:** hard swelling of subcutaneous lymphatics in glanders.

farī·na (L). Flour.

farinā·ceous (L. *farina*, flour). Consisting of or yielding flour.

Farre's tubercles (Farre, J. R., English physician, 1775–1862). Cancerous nodules on the surface of the liver.

Farre's white line (Farre, F. J., English gynaecologist, 1804–86). The boundary line at the hilum of the ovary between the germ epithelium and the squamous epithelium of the broad ligament. It marks the insertion of the mesovarium.

Farre-Waldeyer's line. See Farre's white line.

farsightedness. Hyperopia.

fă·scia (L. *fascia*, band). The fibro-elastic tissue ensheathing muscles. **Abernethy's:** extraperitoneal fatty tissue which covers the external iliac artery. **Anal:** a thin sheet of fascia that is an offshoot from the parietal pelvic fascia just below the origin of the levator ani muscle. **Axillary:** stretches from the anterior to the posterior fold of the axilla and forms the floor of the space. It is continuous anteriorly with the deep pectoral fascia and posteriorly it blends with the deep fascia covering the latissimus dorsi muscle. **Buccopharyngeal:** is an offshoot of the prevertebral layer of the deep cervical fascia along the medial aspect of the carotid sheath. **Bulbi** (Tenon's capsule): consists of a condensation of the connective tissue round the eyeball for which it forms a complete bursal envelope. **Camper's:** the subcutaneous fatty layer of the lower part of the anterior abdominal wall. **Clavipectoral:** is that part of the deep pectoral fascia that occupies a triangular interval bounded above by the subclavius muscle, below by the superior edge of the pectoralis minor and at the apex of which is the coracoid process. **Colles's:** the deep layer of the superficial fascia in the perineum. **Cooper's:** the subperitoneal areolar tissue found in the scrotum. **Cremasteric:** is composed of two layers of striated muscle, forming the cremaster. **Cribriform:** superficial fascia in the upper part of the thigh, attached to the margins of the saphenous ring ; it is interrupted by numerous holes or passages for the transmission of vessels, hence its name. **Deep cervical:** deep fascia of the neck and it is divided into: (1) a superficial investing layer, which completely invests the neck in the form of a collar; and (2) deep processes or laminae, which invest the muscles, viscera, and chief blood vessels and nerves. **Dentate:** a band of grey matter extending from the upper surface of the gyrus hippocampi and the fimbria hippocampi. **Endothoracic:** a thin layer of connective tissue that lies between the deep stratum of muscles and the pleura and corresponds to the transversalis fascia of the abdomen. **External spermatic:** connective tissue derived from the intercrural fibres that extend between the columns of the superficial inguinal rings. **Forearm, f. of:** deep fascia of considerable strength, its fibres being mainly transverse; some, however, are disposed longitudinally and obliquely. **Gerota's** or **Renal fascia:** which surrounds the perirenal fat. It consists of two layers, a posterior layer or fascia of Zuckerkandl, and an anterior layer, or fascia of Toldt. **Iliac:** covers the iliacus and psoas major muscles. Above the level of the iliac crest it is related only to the psoas major and the part covering the muscle is spoken of as the psoas fascia. **Infundibuliform:** part of the internal spermatic fascia in the region of deep inguinal ring. **Internal spermatic:** part of the fascia transversalis. **Interosseous:** deep fascia of the hand which crosses the dorsal aspect of the metacarpal bones. **Lata:** the deep fascia of the thigh, it is a dense fibrous membrane ensheathing the muscles of the thigh like a stocking. **Lumbar** (aponeurosis): is situated between the last rib and the iliac crest and is often regarded as the posterior aponeurosis of the transversus abdominis muscle. **Lunate:** part of the fascia which covers the obturator internus muscle and forms the roof of the ischiorectal fossa. **Masseteric:** is an upward prolongation of the deep cervical fascia. It is attached superiorly to the zygoma, and laterally and posteriorly is continuous with the parotid fascia. **Obturator:** the lateral portion of the parietal pelvic fascia which covers the obturator internus muscle. **Orbital:** covers the bony walls of the orbit and forms a sheath for the contents of the cavity. **Parotid:** a process of deep cervical fascia which is given off a little inferior to the angle of the mandible, and it passes superiorly on the deep surface of the parotid gland to the skull. **Pectoral:** is a layer situated on the deep aspect of pectoralis major muscle, taking part in the formation of the deep layer of its sheath. **Pelvic:** clothes the inner wall of the pelvis, and gives medial expansions, which have an intricate connection with, and serve to support, the contained viscera. It is divisible into two portions—parietal and visceral. **Pharyngobasilar** (pharyngeal aponeurosis): is situated between the muscular layer of the pharynx and the mucous membrane. **Pretracheal:** part of the cervical fascia, which is at first intimately connected with the anterior wall of the carotid sheath, passes medially deep to the infrahyoid muscles and splits to ensheathe the thyroid gland, trachea and oesophagus, and then it passes to the median plane, where it is continuous with the fascia of the opposite side. **Prevertebral:** part of the deep cervical fascia which is connected with the posterior wall of the carotid sheath, passes medially deep to the pharynx and oesophagus and superficial to the prevertebral muscles. **Propria:** see Cooper. **Psoas:** part of the iliac fascia which covers the psoas major muscle. **Renal:** see Gerota's fascia. **Scarpa's:** deep layer of the superficial layer of fascia in the upper part of the thigh. **Sibson's** (suprapleural membrane): covers the cupola of the pleura, and extends from the medial border of the first rib to the front of the transverse process of the seventh cervical vertebra. **Tegmental:** part of the lunate fascia which is reflected across the ischiorectal fossa. **Temporal:** a strong aponeurosis which covers the temporal muscle. **Toldt's:** anterior layer of the renal fascia. **Transversalis:** thick fascia which is situated deep to the transversus abdominis muscle. It is of greatest strength over the lower part of the abdominal wall. **Triangular:** the reflected part of the inguinal ligament and is also known as the ligament of Colles. It is situated behind the spermatic cord and superior crus of the superficial inguinal ring. **Zuckerkandl's:** the posterior layer of the renal fascia.

fă·scial. Pertaining to a fascia.

făs·cicle (L. *fasciculus*, from *fascis*, bundle). A bundle of fibres.

fasci·cular. Bundle-shaped; pertaining to a fasciculus.

fasci·culus (L.). A fascicle. **F. cuneatus:** (tract of Burdach) of the spinal cord is situated on the lateral side of the tract of Goll and is separated from the posterior horn by the tract of association fibres known as the posterior fasciculus proprius. **F. gracilis:** (tract of Goll) of the spinal cord occupies the medial part of the posterior white column in the cervical and upper thoracic parts of the cord. It is formed by the long ascending branches of the medial divisions of the posterior roots of the coccygeal, sacral, lumbar and lower thoracic nerves. **F. interfascicularis** (comma tract or semilunar tract): of the spinal cord is located in the middle of the posterior white column between the fasciculus gracilis and fasciculus cuneatus and is well defined in the thoracic region of the cord. **F. posterolateral** (Lissauer's tract) of the spinal cord lies along the apex of the posterior horn between the posterolateral sulcus and the substantia gelatinosa Rolandi. **F. retroflexus:** a small tract of fibres in the brain passing from the habenular nucleus to the interpeduncular nucleus.

fasciec·tomy (L. *fascia*, band; G. *ektomē*, excision). Excision of a fascia.

fascio·desis (L. *fascia*, band; G. *deein*, to bind). An operation in which a tendon is sutured to a fascia.

Fasci·ola. A genus of flukes. **F. hepatica:** liver fluke, a member of the family Fasciolidae; a trematode parasitic in sheep, cattle and occasionally in man; usually found in extra- and intra-hepatic bile ducts. May also occur as wandering parasite in lungs and elsewhere; intermediary host, water snails.

fasci·ola (L. dim. of *fascia*, band). A tract of grey matter, the dorsal continuation of the fascia dentata of the cerebrum.

fasci·olar. Relating to the fasciola.

fascioli·asis (L. *fascia*, band). Infestation with flukes of the family Fasciolidae.

Fasciolidae. Family of digenetic trematodes of the sub-order of Distomata, *q.v.*

Fasciolopsis burki. A trematode of the sub-order of Distomata; the largest trematode parasitic in man; found in small intestine and stomach (pig, man); intermediary host, snails.

fascio·tomy (L. *fascia*, band; G. *tomē*, section). The division of a fascia.

fasci·tis (L. *fascia*, band). Inflammation of a fascia.

fast. Resisting destruction or staining; term applied to bacteria: e.g. acid-fast, resistant to the action of acids.

fastiga·tum (L. *fastigare*, to sharpen). The nucleus fastigii.

fasti·gium (L. *fastigium*, top). 1. The acme; the summit. 2. The angle between the anterior and posterior medullary vela in the roof of the fourth ventricle.

fat. 1. Obese. 2. A solid or liquid neutral compound of glyceryl esters of the higher fatty acids, as stearic, palmitic and oleic acid, soluble in ether but not in water. **F. embolism:** obstruction of an arterial vessel by fatty globules, e.g. in a case of fracture, the fat globules reaching the blood-stream from the bone-marrow. **F. necrosis:** necrosis of fatty tissue, occurring mainly in the abdomen in acute pancreatitis owing to liberation of pancreatic lipolytic enzymes into the pancreatic tissue and surrounding parts. **F. phanerosis:** unmasking of normally invisible fat, as in fatty degeneration. **F.-soluble vitamins:** Vitamins A, D and E. **F., neutral:** a compound of one of the fatty acids and glycerin. **F., split:** fat hydrolyzed by a fat-splitting enzyme, such as lipase. **F., unsplit:** unhydrolysed fat.

fatal (L. *fatalis*, fated). Causing death.

fatigue (L. *fatigare*, to fatigue). Weariness.

fatty. Containing or derived from fat. **F. acids:** (1) Any one of the series of the formula $C_nH_{2n}O_2$,

so-called because some of them, e.g., palmitic, stearic or oleic acid, combine with glycerol to form fats. (2) Any organic acid occurring in neutral fats or fatty substances. **F. degeneration:** See degeneration, f. **F. heart:** (1) Fatty degeneration of the heart muscle, as occurring in pernicious anaemia, phosphorus poisoning, cachexia; (2) F. infiltration of the heart muscle, due to obesity. **F. infiltration:** excessive deposition of fat in the connective tissue of an organ or, in the case of the liver, within the parenchymatous cells. **F. liver:** (1) F. degeneration or (2) F. infiltration of the liver cells, or a combination of both, as occurring in obesity, chronic alcoholism, delayed chloroform poisoning, phosphorus poisoning, etc. **F. series:** see aliphatic series.

fau·ces (L. *fauces*, the throat). The throat, from the mouth to the pharynx.

Fauchard's disease (Fauchard, P., French dentist, 1678–1761). Alveolar periostitis; pyorrhoea alveolaris: progressive necrosis of the dental alveoli; Riggs's disease.

fau·cial (L. *fauces*, throat). Pertaining to the fauces.

fauci·tis (L. *fauces*, throat). Faucial inflammation.

fauna (L.). The animal life of a locality, country, continent, etc.

Fauvel's granules (Fauvel, S. A., French physician, 1813–84). Small peribronchial abscesses.

fa·vus (L. *favus*, honeycomb). A contagious disease of the skin, affecting most commonly the scalp, characterized by yellowish cup-shaped friable crusts (scutulae) which tend to coalesce, forming mortar-like masses; caused by fungi of the genus Achorion, usually by *Achorion schoenleinii*.

Fe. Symbol of ferrum (iron).

febricide (L. *febris*, fever; *caedere*, to destroy). Destroying fever.

febri·city (L. *febris*, fever). Feverishness.

febrifa·cient (L. *febris*, fever; *facere*, to make). Producing fever.

febri·ferous (L. *febris*, fever). Febrifacient, *q.v.*

febri·fugal (L. *febris*, fever; *fugare*, to put to flight). Abolishing or reducing fever.

feb·rifuge (L. *febric*, fever). 1. Abolishing or reducing fever. 2. An agent that abolishes or reduces fever.

feb·rile (L. *febris*, fever). Pertaining to or characterized by fever.

fe·bris (L.). Fever.

Fechner's law (Fechner, G. T., German naturalist, 1801–87). The intensity of a sensation is proportional to the logarithm of the stimulus.

FeCl₂. Ferrous chloride.

FeCl₃. Ferric chloride.

FeCO₃. Ferrous carbonate.

fe·cundate (L. *fecundare*, to impregnate). To fertilize; to impregnate.

fecunda·tion (L. *fecundare*, to impregnate). Fertilization; impregnation.

fecun·dity (L. *fecundus*, fertile). The power of producing offspring.

Fede's disease (Fede, F., Italian physician, 1832–1913). A papillomatous ulceration of the frenum of the tongue.

Federici's sign (Federici, C., Italian physician, 1832–92). Perception of the heart sounds over the abdominal wall following the perforation of a hollow viscus.

feeble-mindedness. Congenital mental deficiency not amounting to imbecility.

feeding. Giving or taking of food. **F., artificial:** the artificial introduction of food, e.g. by means of a stomach tube or an enema. 2. The feeding of an infant by food other than mother's milk.

feeling tone. A pleasant or unpleasant attribute of a sensation.

Fehleisen's streptococcus (Fehleisen, F., German physician, 1854–1924). Streptococcus erysipelatis.

Fehling's solution (Fehling, H. von, German chemist, 1812–85). A solution of cupric sulphate mixed with alkali and Rochelle salt. Largely used as an oxidising agent, and as a test for reducing sugar.

fel (L. *fel*, gall). Bile.

fellā·tio (L. *fellare*, to suck). The introduction of the penis into the mouth of the sexual partner.

felo de se (L.). 1. One who intentionally kills himself. 2. An act of suicide.

felon. A whitlow. See paronychia.

female (L. *femella*, dim. of *femina*, woman). 1. Relating to the sex that conceives and bears young. 2. Denoting the hollow portion of a double-limbed instrument which receives the complementary or male part.

fem·inism (L. *femina*, woman). Mental and/or physical approximation in the male to female characters.

feminizā·tion (L. *femina*, woman). Development by male subjects of female characters.

fem·oral (L. *femur*, thigh). Pertaining to the femur.

femorā·lis muscle (L. *femur*, thigh). The cruraeus.

fem·orocele (L. *femur*, thigh; G. *kēlē*, hernia). A femoral hernia.

femoro-iliac (L. *femur*, thigh; *ilium*). Relating to both the femur and the ilium.

fem·orotib·ial (L. *femur*, thigh; *tibia*). Relating to both the femur and the tibia.

fē·mur (L. *femur*, thigh). The thigh-bone; the proximal bone of the hind limb of animals.

fenes·tra (L. *fenestra*, window). 1. A window or opening. 2. An opening in a dressing or plaster. 3. A window-like opening in an instrument, as in the blade of a forceps. **F. ovalis**: the small oval opening, covered by a membrane, between the tympanum and vestibule. **F. rotunda**: the small round opening, covered by a membrane, between the tympanum and the scala tympani of the cochlea.

fen·estrated (L. *fenestra*, window). Having openings or windows.

fenestrā·tion (L. *fenestra*, window). An operation on the internal ear for deafness.

fennel. An umbelliferous herb, *Foeniculum vulgare*, from the fruit of which a stimulant and carminative substance is extracted.

Fenwick's disease (Fenwick, S., English physician, 1821–1902). Primary atrophy of the stomach.

Fe₂O₃. Ferric oxide.

Fe(OH)₃. Ferric hydroxide.

Féréol's nodosities (Féréol, L. H. F., French physician, 1825–91). Ephemeral subcutaneous nodosities observed in acute articular rheumatism.

Fereol-Graux's type of ocular palsy. Associated paralysis, of nuclear origin, of the internal rectus muscle of one side and the external rectus of the other.

Fergusson's operation (Fergusson, Sir W., English surgeon, 1808–77). Excision of the upper jaw. **F.'s speculum**: A tubular vaginal speculum.

fer·ment (L. *fermentum*, leaven). 1. To undergo fermentation. 2. Substance which causes fermentation. Syn. enzyme.

fermentā·tion (L. *fermentum*, leaven). Decomposition, especially of carbohydrate, by enzymes.

fermen·tative (L. *fermentum*, leaven). 1. Caused by a ferment. 2. Causing fermentation.

ferrated (L. *ferrum*, iron). Charged with iron.

Ferrein's cords (Ferrein, A., French physician, 1693–1769). True vocal cords. **F.'s pyramids**: the medullary rays in the kidney which take the form of pyramidal bundles of uriniferous tubules, which are separated from each other by portions of the labyrinth.

ferric (L. *ferrum*, iron). 1. Pertaining to or containing iron. 2. Applied to compounds containing iron with a valence of more than two.

ferrŏ·meter (L. *ferrum*, iron; G. *metron*, measure). An instrument for measuring the iron content of blood.

fer·ropexy (L. *ferrum*, iron; G. *pēxis*, fixation). The fixation of iron.

ferrothĕ·rapy (L. *ferrum*, iron; G. *therapeia*, treatment). The use of iron in the treatment of disease.

ferrous (L. *ferrum*, iron). Applied to compounds containing bivalent iron.

ferrū·ginous (L. *ferrugo*, rust, from *ferrum*, iron). 1. Containing iron. 2. Resembling iron-rust.

ferrum (L.). Iron. Symbol Fe.

fer·tile (L. *fertilis*, fruitful). 1. Fertilized. 2. Capable of conceiving and bearing young.

fertilizā·tion (L. *fertilis*, fruitful). 1. Impregnation; fecundation. 2. Union of a male and a female germ cell.

Ferula. A genus of umbelliferous plants, which includes several varieties yielding asafoetida.

ferves·cence (L. *fervescere*, to become hot). Rise in temperature.

fervor (L.). Fever heat.

fester (Old Fr. *festrir*, from L. *fistula*, an ulcer). 1. To suppurate. 2. A small ulcer; a pustule.

festinā·tion (L. *festinare*, to hasten). Acceleration of gait to prevent a falling forward, as in paralysis agitans. Syn. propulsive gait.

fetish (Port. *feitico*, from L. *facticius*, from *facere*, to make). A non-living object to which supernatural powers are attributed.

fetishism. 1. The veneration of a fetish. 2. Fixation of a sexual libido to, and therefore stimulation of it by, a certain part of the body or article of clothing.

fetishist. A person addicted to fetishism.

fever (L. *febris*, fever). 1. Abnormal increase in body temperature. 2. A systemic disease, associated with increased body temperatures. 3. An infectious disease, especially one of those characterized by an eruption on skin or mucous membranes. **African tick f.**: a disease closely allied to relapsing f., *q.v.*, caused by *Spirochaeta Duttoni* and transmitted by ticks. **Blackwater f.**: malaria, nearly always of subtertian type, complicated by acute intravascular haemolysis of the red blood corpuscles with haemoglobinuria and haemolytic jaundice, accompanied by marked prostration, rigors, restlessness, vomiting, oliguria; due to repeated attacks of or continuous infection with subtertian malaria and apparently sometimes precipitated by taking quinine. **Catheter f.**: infection of the lower urinary tract due to the use of catheters or bougies in non-aseptic circumstances. **Cerebrospinal f.**: meningococcal meningitis. **Childbed f.**: puerperal f. **Continued f.**: a fever without remissions or intermissions. **Enteric f.**: typhoid or paratyphoid f. **Glandular f.**: infective mononucleosis, *q.v.* **Haverhill f.**: (Haverhill, town in Massachusetts) an infectious disease, characterized by f., maculopapular, sometimes haemorrhagic, rash and arthritis; caused by *Haverhillia multiformis*, possibly conveyed by milk. **Hay f.**: See hay f. **Intermittent f.**: any f. with intermediate afebrile periods. **Malta f.**: See undulant f. **Mediterranean f.**: See undulant f. **Neurogenic f.**: f. apparently due to an idiopathic disturbance of certain cerebral centres, i.e. not caused by any infection of micro-organisms or other toxic products. **Oroya f.**: an acute infectious disease prevalent in the Peruvian Andes, characterized by f. with rapidly developing anaemia, splenomegaly and enlargement of lymph nodes and the presence of rod-shaped bodies (*Bartonella bacilliformis* or Barton's bodies) in the red blood corpuscles, probably transmitted by one of the phlebotomus species. **Para-**

typhoid f.: acute febrile disease with symptoms and signs of acute gastroenteritis, or with those of typhoid f.; due to oral infection with one of the bacteria paratyphosa. **Phlebotomus f.**: an acute, practically never fatal disease, characterized by sudden fever of 3–4 days' duration, headache, general malaise; caused by a virus and transmitted by the sandfly, *Phlebotomus papatasii*. Syn. Papataci f.; sandfly f. **Puerperal f.**: see puerperal f. **Rat-bite f.**: an infectious disease, characterized by relapsing f., lymphangitis and a reddish or purple eruption; caused by *Spirillum minus* and transmitted by rats. **Relapsing f.**: an acute febrile disease, characterized by alternate periods of f. and apyrexia of 5–10 days' duration; caused by the *Spirochaeta Obermeieri* and transmitted by lice or ticks of the genus *Ornithodorus*. **Remittent f.**: any f. with daily differences in temperature of more than 1°F. **Rheumatic f.**: an acute disease, characterized by f., sweating, swelling and tenderness of joints, and especially in children and adolescents often associated with endocarditis and/or pericarditis, or pancarditis, and/or chorea, the involvement of the joints not being a constant feature. **Rocky mountain f.**: an acute infectious disease, characterized by sudden onset, f. of 2–3 weeks' duration, generalized pains, nervous prostration, maculopapular or petechial eruption; probably caused by *Rickettsia rickettsi* transmitted by a tick. In the western part of the United States it is usually transmitted by the wood tick, *Dermacentor Andersoni*; in the eastern part by the common dog tick, *Dermacentor variabilis*. **Sandfly f.**: see F., phlebotomus above. **Scarlet f.**: an acute infectious febrile disease, due to haemolytic streptococcus; characterized by pharyngitis and a punctiform scarlet red eruption on the skin, followed by desquamation. Syn. scarlatina. **Spotted f.**: (1) Cerebrospinal f. (2) Typhus f. **Three day f.**: see phlebotomus fever. **Trench f.**: an infective disease, characterized by relapsing f. and tenderness of the shins; caused by a virus and transmitted by lice. **Typhoid f.**: an acute disease of very variable symptomatology, but often characterized by f., relative bradycardia, rose-coloured eruption, enlargement of the spleen, diarrhoea or constipation, persistent headache, anorexia and abdominal tenderness; pathologically mainly by hyperplasia leading to necrosis and ulceration of intestinal lymphoid tissue, especially in the distal part of the ileum; caused by infection (contaminated food, water; contagion) with the typhoid bacillus. **Typhus f.**: an acute infectious disease characterized by sudden onset, macular (sometimes morbilliform) later often petechial eruption (appearing on 4th to 7th day), continuous f., enlargement of the spleen, marked restlessness, and later prostration, terminated by crisis or rapid lysis usually about the 16th to 17th day; caused by *Rickettsia prowazeki* and transmitted by lice and sporadically by rat fleas. Syn. jail f. **Hospital f.**: exanthematic typhus. **Undulant f.**: group of diseases comprising Mediterranean f. and abortus f. Both are characterized by more or less wave-like bouts of pyrexia without corresponding increase in the pulse-rate, malaise, enlargement of the spleen, muscle- and joint-pains, sweats; caused by *Brucella melitensis* and *Brucella abortus*, respectively, and conveyed by milk of infected goats or cows. **Yellow f.**: an infectious disease, characterized by f., bradycardia, jaundice, tendency to haemorrhages, haematemesis, albuminuria, severe prostration; caused by a virus and transmitted by mosquitoes of the genus Aedes.

fiat, fiant (Pres. subj., 3rd pers. sing. and pl., of *fieri*, to be made). Latin terms used in recipes=let it, them, be made.

fibrae‧mia (L. *fibra*, fibre; G. *haima*, blood). A condition in which fibrin is found in the blood.

fibre (L. *fibra*, fibre). A thread-like structure such as a muscle cell or the axis cylinder process of a nerve cell.

fi‧bril (L. *fibrilla*, dim. of *fibra*, fibre). 1. A small fibre. 2. A neuro-fibril. 3. A fibre-like uni-directional chain of molecules.

fibril‧lar (L. *fibrilla*, dim. of *fibra*, fibre). Pertaining to fibrils.

fibrillā‧tion (L. *fibrilla*, dim. of *fibra*, fibre). 1. The formation of fibrils. 2. Localized irregular twitchings of muscle fibres, occurring, e.g., in progressive muscular atrophy, amyostatic lateral sclerosis, syringomyelia, uraemia. **F., auricular**: see auricular f.

fibrillŏ‧lysis (L. *fibrilla*, little fibre; G. *luein*, to loosen). The destruction of fibrils.

fi‧brin (L. *fibra*, fibre). A protein-containing double-refracting substance formed during coagulation of blood and related substances.

fibrinā‧tion (L. *fibra*, fibre). The production of abnormal quantities of fibrin.

fibri‧nogen (L. *fibra*, fibre; G. *gennan*, to produce). One of the blood proteins (0·1 per cent to 0·2 per cent in mammalian blood), formed in the liver; becoming converted into fibrin by the action of thrombin in the presence of calcium and thromboplastin (from platelets).

fibrinoly‧sis (L. *fibra*, fibre; G. *luein*, to loosen). Hydrolysis of fibrin; the spontaneous resolution of fibrin in shed blood.

fibrinō‧sis (L. *fibra*, fibre). A condition in which abnormally large amounts of fibrin are present in the blood.

fi‧brinous (L. *fibra*, fibre). 1. Containing fibrin. 2. Characterized by fibrosis. **F. bronchitis**: bronchitis characterized by the expectoration of fibrous casts of the bronchioles.

fibrinū‧ria (L. *fibra*, fibre; G. *ouron*, urine). The presence of fibrin in the urine.

fibro-adē‧nia (L. *fibra*, fibre; G. *adēn*, gland). Fibrous degeneration of a gland.

fibro-adenō‧ma (L. *fibra*, fibre; G. *adēn*, gland). A benign neoplasm composed of adenomatous and connective tissue. **F. of breast**: a f. occurring chiefly in young women, commonest in nulliparae, predominantly of either intracanalicular (more common) or pericanalicular (much rarer) growth.

fibroblast (L. *fibra*, fibre; G. *blastos*, germ). A mesenchymal cell giving rise to connective tissue.

fibroblastō‧ma (L. *fibra*, fibre; G. *blastos*, germ). A tumour composed of fibroplastic or connective tissue cells.

fibrocarcinō‧ma (L. *fibra*, fire; G. *karkinos*, crab). Any carcinoma containing a proportion of fibrous tissue.

fibro-car‧tilage (L. *fibra*, fibre; *cartilago*, cartilage). Cartilage containing collagenous fibres.

fibrochondrī‧tis (L. *fibra*, fibre; G. *khondros*, rib). Inflammation of fibrocartilage.

fi‧brochondrō‧ma (L. *fibra*, fibre; G. *khondros*, cartilage). A tumour composed of fibrous tissue and cartilage.

fibrocȳs‧tic (L. *fibra*, fibre; G. *kutis*, bladder). Fibrous degeneration with true or apparent cystic degeneration. **F. disease of pancreas**: disease of infants and young children characterized by fibrosis and cyst-formation in the pancreas, steatorrhea and chronic pulmonary sepsis. **F. disease of bone**: see osteitis fibrosa cystica generalisata.

fibro-enchondrō‧ma (L. *fibra*, fibre; G. *en*, in; *khondros*, cartilage). An enchondroma containing some fibrous elements.

fibrō‧glia (L. *fibra*, fibre; G. *glia*, glue). The basement substance of connective tissue.

fi‧brogliō‧ma (L. *fibra*, fibre; G. *glia*, glue). A glioma in which there are some fibrous elements.

fi·broid (L. *fibra*, fibre; G. *eidos*, form). 1. Composed of fibrous tissue. 2. A fibroma. 3. A uterine benign tumour, occurring mainly during the reproductive phase of life, related in growth to disturbances of ovarian hormone secretion; usually retrogressing after the menopause; composed of plain muscle and fibrous tissue and occurring chiefly in the body of the uterus, either interstitial, submucous, subperitoneal or subserous.

fibroidec·tomy (L. *fibra*, fibre; G. *ektomē*, excision). Surgical removal of a fibroid.

fi·brolipō·ma (L. *fibra*, fibre; G. *lipos*, fat). A benign neoplasm composed of fibrous and fatty tissue.

fibrō·ma (L. *fibra*, fibre). A benign neoplasm composed of fibrous tissue. **F. molluscum:** see neurofibromatosis. **F. perineural:** benign tumour of nerves, forming round or fusiform white masses on the course of larger peripheral nerves, originating usually from Schwann's sheath (Schwannoma).

fibromatō·sis (L. *fibra*, fibre). 1. Diffuse hypertrophy of fibrous tissue. 2. Neurofibromatosis, *q.v.*

fibromec·tomy (L. *fibra*, fibre; G. *ektomē*, excision). The surgical removal of a fibroma.

fibromyōsitis (L. *fibra*, fibre; G. *mus*, muscle). Inflammation of a muscle fibre.

fibromyō·ma (L. *fibra*, fibre; G. *mus*, muscle). A benign tumour of the uterus containing myomatous and fibrous tissue. Syn. uterine fibroid.

fi·bromyōmec·tomy (L. *fibra*, fibre; G. *mus*, muscle; *ektomē*, excision). Excision of a fibromyoma.

fibromyxō·ma (L. *fibra*, fibre; G. *muxa*, mucus). A tumour composed of fibrous tissue and myxomatous tissue.

fibroplas·tic (L. *fibra*, fibre; G. *plassein*, to form). Fibre-forming.

fibroplate (L. *fibra*, fibre; G. *platus*, flat). A disc of interarticular fibro-cartilage.

fibropŏ·lypus (L. *fibra*, fibre; G. *polus*, many; *pous*, foot). A fibroid polypus.

fibropū·rulent (L. *fibra*, fibre; *purulentus*, foul). Composed of pus and fibrin.

fibrosarcō·ma (L. *fibra*, fibre; G. *sarx*, flesh). A sarcoma composed of either large or small spindle cells (more malignant in the latter case).

fibrō·sis (L. *fibra*, fibre). Abnormal increase of fibrous tissue in an organ; fibrous degeneration.

fibrosī·tis (L. *fibra*, fibre). Inflammatory proliferation of fibrous tissue, e.g. in ligaments, tendons, muscle sheaths, fasciae; muscular rheumatism.

fibrot·ic (L. *fibra*, fibre). Pertaining to fibrosis.

fibrous (L. *fibra*, fibre). Consisting of or pertaining to fibres. **F. tissue:** connective tissue.

fi·bula (L. *fibula*, buckle). The slender outer bone of the lower leg, articulating above with the tibia and below with the talus.

fi·bular. Pertaining to the fibula.

Fick's bacillus (Fick, R. A., German physician, 1866–1939). The bacillus *proteus vulgaris*.

Ficker's diagnosticum (Ficker, P. H., German bacteriologist, born 1868). An emulsion of dead typhoid bacillus culture.

Ficus (L. *ficus*, fig). A genus of trees, which includes the fig.

fidicinā·lēs (L. *fidicen*, lute-player). The lumbricales muscles of the hand.

Fiedler's disease (Fiedler, C. L. A., German physician, 1835–1921). Acute infectious jaundice.

field. A space within which a phenomenon takes place. **F., electrical:** the space surrounding a charged body in which its action is perceptible. **F. of vision:** the totality of the visual stimuli acting on the fixed eye at a given moment.

Fielding's membrane (Fielding, G. H., English anatomist, 1801–71). The tapetum of the retina.

fifth disease. A mild infectious disease in childhood, characterized by a macular or maculopapular eruption, commencing over cheeks and forehead, soon becoming confluent, forming rose-red patches with raised edges, fading in the centre. Syn. erythema infectiosum. **F. cranial nerve:** the trigeminal nerve. **F. ventricle:** see ventricle, fifth.

filament (L. *filum*, a thread). A thread-like structure.

Fila·ria. A genus of thread worms. See under Filarioidea.

filarial. Pertaining to or caused by Filariae.

filari·asis. Any disease due to infestation with Filariae, producing blocking and inflammation of the lymph vessels and thus elephantiasis and chyluria.

Filarī·idae. Family of Filarioidea; usually with filiform bodies, in adult stage a parasite of vertebrates in connective tissue, blood-vessels and serous cavities.

Filari·ina. Sub-family of Filariidae; in larval stage (microfilariae) parasitic in circulating blood; containing the species *Wuchereria bancrofti* and *W. loa loa.*

Filarioi·dea. Order of nematode parasites, requiring an intermediate host for development and transmission (usually mosquitoes).

Filatov's disease (Filatov, N. F., Russian physician, 1847–1902). Acute febrile cervical adenitis of children.

filiform (L. *filum*, thread; *forma*, shape). Thread-like.

Filipowicz's sign (Filipowicz, C., contemporary Polish physician). Palmoplantar phenomenon; a yellowish discoloration of the prominent portions of the palmar and plantar surfaces, seen in typhoid fever, articular rheumatism and tuberculosis.

fi·lipuncture (L. *filum*, thread; *punctura*, a pricking). A method of treating an aneurysm by inserting a steel wire in order to promote coagulation.

filix mas. Male fern.

fillet. 1. A band of fibres. 2. A band of afferent fibres arising in the cuneate and gracilis nuclei, ascending in the medulla just behind the pyramidal tracts, crossing the sensory decussation. Cf. lemniscus.

filopō·dium (L. *filum*, thread; G. *pous*, foot). A thread-like pseudopodium.

fi·lopressure (L. *filum*, thread; *pressura*, from *pressere*, to press). The manual compression of a blood vessel.

filter. 1. A porous structure used for separating solid particles from a liquid. 2. To pass something through a filter (1.). 3. In X-ray therapy, metal screen that holds back rays of certain wavelengths whilst allowing others to pass. **F., Berkefeld:** a tubular filter composed of diatomaceous earth. **F., Chamberland:** a filter composed of porous clay. **F., Pasteur:** a filter of unglazed porcelain. **F., Seitz:** bacterial filter comprising an asbestos disc in a suitable holder. **F., Wood's:** light filter, transmitting ultra-violet rays, but holding back visible light rays.

filter-passing. Filtrable, *q.v.*

fil·trable. Capable of passing through a filter. **F. virus:** any virus of a size smaller than the minute pores of an unglazed porcelain or diatomaceous earth filter; such filters cannot be passed by organisms or particles large enough to be seen through an ordinary microscope.

filtrate. The liquid that has passed through a filter.

filtrā·tion. The separation of solid particles from a liquid by means of a filter.

filtrum ventriculi (L.). Small channels on the back of the larynx.

filum (L. *filum*, thread). A thread-like structure. **F. terminale:** the tapering distal end of the conus medullare.

fim·bria (L.). A fringe. **F. hippocampi:** a narrow band of white matter near the medial border of the hippocampus.

fim·briāted (L. *fimbria*, fringe). Fringed.

fimbri·ātum (L. *fimbria*, fringe). The corpus fimbriatum.

fimbriocele (L. *fimbria*, fringe; G. *kele*, hernia). Hernia enclosing some of the fimbriae of the Fallopian tube.

finger. Any of the five digits of the hand.

finger-agnō·sia. Inability to recognise the individual fingers; usually associated with agraphia, acalculia and failure to discriminate between right and left; due to lesion of the angular gyrus of the left cerebral hemisphere.

Finkler-Prior spirillum (Finkler, D., German bacteriologist, 1852–1912). A spirillum found in the faeces in cholera patients.

Finney's operation (Finney, J. M. T., American surgeon, 1863–1942). A form of gastro-duodenostomy in which a large opening is formed, ensuring free drainage from the stomach.

Finsen light treatment (Finsen, N. R., Danish physician, 1860–1904). 1. A method of treatment of skin diseases by exposure of the diseased part to the violet and ultra-violet rays of the sun or of the electric arc-light. 2. Prevention of pitting in smallpox by keeping the patient in a red-lighted room from which the chemical rays at the other end of the spectrum are excluded.

fireman's cramp. Tetany in stokers due to loss of sodium chloride by excessive sweating.

first aid. Emergency treatment or assistance in accidents, injuries, etc.

first cranial nerve. The olfactory nerve.

first intention. Healing of a wound by immediate union without suppuration.

Fischer's brain murmur (Fischer, L., American paediatrician, born 1864). A systolic murmur heard over the anterior fontanelle or in the temporal region in rachitic infants. **F.'s sign:** a pre-systolic murmur heard in cases of adherent pericardium without valvular disease.

Fischer's tufts. Also called 'bouquet de Fischer'. The terminal expansions of nerve fibres between tactile end organs.

Fiske-Bryson's symptom. See Bryson's sign.

fission (L. *fissio*, from *findere*, to cleave). Reproduction by division into two or more equal parts; the common mode of reproduction in bacteria and protozoa. **F., atomic:** the energetic splitting of uranium or plutonium nuclei produced by the action of neutrons.

fissi·parous (L. *fissus*, from *findere*, to cleave; *parere*, to produce). Propagating by fission.

fissū·ra (L.). A fissure.

fissure (L. *fissura*). 1. A groove or cleft, e.g., f. of Silvius (fissura Sylvii), the cleft separating the temporal from frontal and parietal lobes of the brain. 2. A cleft-like lesion, e.g. anal f., a painful cleft-like lesion at the mucocutaneous junction of the anus. **F., palpebral:** the space between the upper and lower eyelids.

fī·stula (L. *fistula*, pipe). Abnormal channel between two hollow organs or between one hollow organ and the surface.

fistulŏ·tomy (L. *fistula*, pipe; G. *tomē*, section). The surgical opening up of a fistula.

fistulec·tomy (L. *fistula*, pipe; G. *ektomē*, excision). The surgical removal of a fistula.

fistulo-enterŏ·stomy (L. *fistula*, pipe; G. *enteron*, intestine; *stoma*, mouth). An operation in which a permanent fistula between the bile ducts and the small intestine is made.

fī·stulous. Pertaining to or affected with a fistula.

fit. A convulsion; a sudden paroxysm.

Fitz's syndrome (Fitz, R. H., American physician, 1843–1913). In cases of acute pancreatitis, intense pain in the epigastrium and vomiting.

fix (L. *fixus*, from *figere*, to fasten). 1. To hold firm. 2. To harden tissues or to kill organisms for microscopic or other study.

fixā·tion (L. *fixus*, from *figere*, to fasten). 1. A making firm. 2. The operation of rendering fixed, by means of sutures, a displaced organ. 3. Central vision, i.e., the looking at an object so that its image falls upon the macular area of the retina. 4. In microscopy, the preparation of tissues in their original form. 5. The prevention of haemolysis by a complement. 6. Arrest of sexual libido at an immature stage of its development (e.g. mother f.) preventing the direction of libido to another object.

fix·ative (L. *fixus*, from *figere*, to fasten). A substance for making an object permanent, or for preventing damage to it by certain treatment, such as staining.

fixed (L. *fixus*, from *figere*, to fasten). Held fast. **F. idea:** a morbid belief or conception which permanently dominates the entire mind.

flabel·lum (L. *flabellum*, fan). 1. A fan-like structure. 2. A group of divergent fibres in the corpus striatum.

flac·cid (L. *flaccidus*, from *flaccus*, flabby). Flabby; relaxed; characterized by diminution of muscle tone.

Flack's node (Flack, M., English physiologist, born 1882). The sino-atrial node in the heart—the Keith and Flack node.

flagel·lar (L. *flagellum*, a whip). Pertaining to a flagellum.

Flagella·ta. A group of the class of Mastigophora, *q.v.*, including the Trypanosoma, *Trichomonas vaginalis* and *Giardia lamblia*; micro-organisms characterized by the presence of one or more flagella.

flagel·late. Furnished with flagella; applied to certain micro-organisms.

flagellā·tion (L. *flagellum*, a whip). 1. Formation of flagella. 2. Flogging. 3. Sexual perversion where libido is stimulated by flogging.

flagel·lum (L.). A whip-like appendage; a long mobile cilium; the organ of locomotion of certain micro-organisms.

flail joint. An abnormally mobile joint.

Flajani's disease (Flajani, G., Italian surgeon, 1739–1808). Exophthalmic goitre.

flap. A partly detached portion of skin or other soft tissue.

flari·meter (L. *flare*, to blow; G. *metron*, measure). A device for measuring shortness of breath.

flat foot. A foot with depressed plantar arch; pes planus.

flash point. The temperature at which a combustible liquid gives off a vapour producing an inflammable mixture with air when the mixture is momentarily exposed to a flame.

flask. A narrow-necked glass or metal bottle.

Flatau's law (Flatau, E., Polish neurologist, 1868–1932). The greater the length of the fibres in the spinal cord, the nearer to the periphery are they situated.

flā·tulence (L. *flatus*, a snorting). The presence of abnormal amounts of gas in the bowels.

flā·tulent. Characterized by flatulence.

flā·tus (L.). 1. Gas, especially in the alimentary canal. 2. Expulsion of gas from stomach or bowel.

flatworm. See Platyhelminthes.

flā·veoprotein (L. *flavus*, yellow; G. *prōtos*, first). A yellow pigment, an enzyme acting as reducing agent in the presence of suitable dehydrogenases, occurring widely in living tissues.

flavĕ·scent (L. *flavescere*, to grow yellow). Yellowish.

fla·vine (L. *flavus*, yellow). See flaveoprotein.

Flavobacte·rium. A genus of Bacteriaceae which become orange yellow in cultures.

flā·vone. $C_{15}H_{10}O_2$. Parent substance of certain yellow dyes found in plants, many as glycosides.

flavour. Taste.

fla·vus (L.). Yellow.

fl. dr. Abbreviation for fluid drachm.

flea. Any insect belonging to the order *Siphonaptera*.

Flechsig's areas (Flechsig, P. A., Bohemian neurologist, 1847–1929). The subdivisions of the substance of the medulla cerebri, caused by the passage of the root bundles of the hypoglossal and vagus nerves. F.'s tract: the tractus spinocerebellaris dorsalis. F.'s association centres: centres of the cortex cerebri.

Fleischl's haemometer (Fleischl, E. von, von Marxow, Austrian pathologist, 1846–91). A special haemoglobinometer.

Fleischmann's bursa (Fleischmann, G., German anatomist, 1777–1853). The spaces on each side of the septum of the tongue at the anterior extremities of the genioglossus muscles.

Fleming's tincture of aconite (Fleming, A., English physician, 1824–75). A tincture about five times as strong as ordinary tincture, and never used internally.

Flemming's solution (Flemming, W., German anatomist, 1843–1905). A solution consisting of 15 parts of 1 per cent solution of chromium trioxide, 4 parts of a 2 per cent solution of osmic acid, 1 part of glacial acetic acid; used as a tissue fixative.

flesh. The soft parts of the animal body.

flex (L. *flexus*, from *flectere*, to bend). To bend.

flexibilitas cerea (L.). Wax-like flexibility of the limbs in catalepsy.

flexibility (L. *flectere*, to bend). The quality of being able to bend or yield.

flexion (L. *flectere*, to bend). The process of bending.

Flexner's bacillus (Flexner, S., American pathologist, born 1863). *Shigella paradysenteriae*. A bacillus causing dysentery. F.'s serum: antimeningococcus serum, used in the treatment of epidemic cerebrospinal meningitis.

flexor (L., from *flectere*, to bend), A muscle that bends a limb or a part.

flexū·ra (L.). A bending or curve in an organ.

flex·ure. A bending, e.g., hepatic f. of the colon.

Flindt's spots (Flindt, N., Danish physician, 1843–1913). See Koplik's spots.

Flint's arcade (Flint, A., American physician, 1812–86). The vascular arches at the bases of the pyramids of the kidney, situated between the rounded base of the pyramid and the cortical substance. F.'s murmur. A presystolic apical murmur heard occasionally in cases of aortic regurgitation.

floating. 1. Free to move about. 2. Abnormally mobile. F. rib: the most caudal two or three ribs which are neither attached to the sternum nor to another rib.

floccilā·tion (L. *floccus*, a lock of wool). Picking of bedclothes.

floc·cular (L. *floccus*, lock of wool). Relating to the flocculus.

flocculā·tion (L. *floccus*, lock of wool). Precipitation of a solution (especially of a sol) in flakes. F. test: see Kahn's test.

floc·culence (L. *floccus*, lock of wool). Flakiness.

floc·culent (L. *floccus*, lock of wool). Containing small lumps; flaky; woolly.

floc·culus (L.). 1. A small tuft or flake. 2. A lobe on the inferior cerebellar surface.

Flood's ligament (Flood, V., Irish surgeon, 1800–47). The superior glenohumeral ligament of the shoulder joint.

flooding. Severe haemorrhage from the uterus.

floor of the pelvis. The tissue forming the inferior boundary of the pelvis.

Flor. Abbreviation for *flores*, L. for flowers.

flora (L.). 1. The entire vegetation of a given area. 2. A reference book for systematic identification of flowering plants.

Florence's reaction (Florence, A., French physician, 1851–1927). On treating semen with a strong solution of iodine and potassium iodide brown crystals are formed in the shape of needles or plates.

flores (L. pl. of *flos*, flower). 1. Flowers. 2. Applied to some substances obtained in flake-like form by sublimation, e.g., flores sulphuris.

florid (L. *floridus*, blooming). Of a bright pink or red colour.

Flourens's doctrine (Flourens, M. J. P., French physiologist, 1794–1867). A theory that the whole cerebrum is concerned in every psychic process.

Flower's angle (Flower, Sir W. H., English anatomist, 1831–99). The nasomalar angle. F.'s bone: the epipteric bone; wormian bone at pterion of mammals.

fl. oz. Abbreviation for fluid ounce.

fluctuā·tion (L. *fluctuare*, from *fluctus*, from *fluere*, to flow). A wave-like to and fro motion, or the variation of any property with time, e.g. fluctuation of a patient's temperature.

Fluhrer's probe (Fluhrer, W. F., American physician, 1870–1932). A probe made of aluminium which was used in investigating gunshot wounds of the brain.

fluid (L. *fluidus*, from *fluere*, to flow). 1. A substance whose particles change freely their relative position without a separation of the mass. 2. Form of matter that cannot permanently resist any force tending to alter its shape. 3. Liquid or gaseous. Cerebrospinal f.: the f. contained in the subarachnoidal space, in the cerebral ventricles and in the central canal of the spinal cord.

fluid drachm. A measure for liquids; $\frac{1}{8}$ of a fl. ounce, or 3·55 cc.

fluid extract. Liquid preparation containing the active principles of a crude drug freed from vegetable tissues and prepared by extraction with suitable solvents.

fluid ounce. Eight fluid drachms, or 28·41 cc.

fluke. Any trematode worm.

fluor (L. from *fluere*, to flow). 1. A liquid condition. 2. The menstrual flow. F. albus: leucorrhoea.

fluorene. A coal tar hydrocarbon $C_6H_4CH_2.C_6H_4$.

fluoresce. To exhibit fluorescence.

fluorĕ·scein. Fluorescent organic compound prepared from phthalic anhydride and resorcinol. The sodium salt is used in ophthalmic practice for detecting lesions and foreign bodies. Formula $C_{20}H_{10}O_5$.

fluorĕ·scence (L. *fluere*, to flow). 1. The property of certain bodies (first discovered in calcium fluoride) to emit light rays so long as they are absorbing radiation from some other source, the emitted light being usually of a longer wave length, and therefore of a different colour, than the absorbed rays. 2. The radiation due to fluorescence (1).

fluorĕ·scent (L. *fluere*, to flow). Having a different colour by transmitted and by reflected light. F. screen: a glass plate coated on one side with a f. substance emitting light under the action of X-rays.

fluoride (L. *fluere*, to flow). A compound of fluorine with another element.

fluorine (L. *fluere*, to flow). An element of the halogen family. Symbol F.

fluŏr·oscope (L. *fluere*, to flow; G. *skopein*, to view). An apparatus used for examining internal organs and structures by means of X-rays.

fluorŏ·scopy (L. *fluere*, to flow; G. *skopein*, to view). Examination of an object through a fluorescent screen, *q.v.*

flush. Redness of the face.

flutter, auricular. A form of cardiac irregularity in which the auricle contracts rhythmically at a rate of from 200 to 350 per minute and the ventricles respond to a certain proportion of the auricular stimuli.

flux (L. *fluere*, to flow). Any excessive discharge.

fluxion (L. *fluere*, to flow). Congestion; hyperaemia.

fly. A two-winged insect, especially of the genus *Musca*.

foamy liver. A liver full of gas bubbles produced by anaerobic micro-organisms.

focal (L. *focus*, fire-place). Pertaining to a focus. **F. depth:** the power of a lens to give clear images of objects at different distances from it. **F. infection:** a localized infection acting as focus for the dissemination of infected matter to other parts of the body. **F. length:** distance of the focus from the surface of the lens. **F. lesion:** a lesion limited to a small focus. **F. nephritis:** see nephritis, focal. **F. plane:** a plane passing through the focus and parallel to the surface of a lens. **F. reaction:** a reaction in a diseased part due to the administration of a test substance.

Fochier's abscess (Fochier, A., French gynaecologist, 1845–1903). Fixation abscess.

foci·meter (L. *focus*, hearth; G. *metron*, measure). A device used to discern the focus of a lens.

focus (L. *focus*, fire-place). 1. The principal seat of a disease. 2. The meeting point of rays made convergent by a convex lens or a concave mirror. **F., principal:** point on which parallel rays converge after passing through a lens. **F., real:** meeting point of convergent rays.

foe·tal (L. *foetus*, offspring). Pertaining to a foetus.

foetā·tion. 1. The formation of a foetus. 2. Gestation; pregnancy.

foe·ticide (L. *foetus*, offspring; *caedere*, to destroy). The intentional killing of the foetus *in utero*.

foe·tid (L. *foetidus*, stinking). Having an offensive odour.

foe·tor (L. *foetor*, a stench). Offensive odour.

foe·tus (L. *foetus*, offspring). An embryo, especially in vertebrates, in the later stages of development, e.g. in man from the fourth month of pregnancy.

fold. The infolding of two surfaces or membranes such as the gluteal folds, the axillary fold and the amniotic fold.

foliā·ceous (L. *folium*, leaf). Leaf-like; laminated.

fō·lic acid. Pteryol glutamic acid. It exists in two forms, free and conjugated, depending on the number of glutamic acid radicals in the molecule. Obtained from liver and yeast. It is a vitamin essential for the growth of chicks and monkeys and necessary for the growth of some strains of lactobacilli. In humans it is therapeutically effective in most megaloblastic anaemias but is without effect on their neurological complications.

folie (Fr. *folie*, madness). Insanity. **F. à deux:** insanity in two closely associated persons, e.g. man and wife. **F. brightique:** mental disorder in Bright's disease.

Folin's tests (Folin, O., American chemist, 1867–1934). Tests for 1. urea; 2. uric acid; 3. sugar; 4. amino acids.

folium (L. *folium*, leaf). A leaf; a thin plate.

Folli's process (Folli, C., Italian anatomist, 1615–60). The processus anterior mallei (auditory ossicle).

follicle (L. *folliculus*, dim. of *follis*, a bag). 1. A small secretory cavity. 2. A simple tubular gland, especially of the skin. 3. A circumscribed mass of lymphoid cells. **F., graafian:** an ovarian f. containing liquor folliculi, and when mature the following layers (from without inwards): theca folliculi, membrana granulosa, liquor folliculi occupying the antrum folliculi, discus proligerus, corona radiata, zona pellucida, perivitelline space, vitelline membrane, egg cytoplasm (vitellus), the germinal vesicle (nucleus) and the germinal spot (nucleolus). **F., nabothian:** a tubule of a gland of the uterine cervix enlarged owing to occlusion of its outlet.

folliclis. Acne scrofulosorum, *q.v.*

folli·cular. Pertaining to a follicle or characterized by follicles; follicle-like. **F. tonsillitis:** inflammation of the tonsil(s) confined to the lymph follicles surrounding the tonsillar crypts.

folliculi·tis (L. *folliculus*, little bag). Inflammation of a follicle, especially of a hair follicle.

folliculō·ma (L. *folliculus*, little bag). A tumour originating in a follicle.

folliculō·sis (L. *folliculus*, little bag). A condition in which there is an excessive development of follicles.

folli·culus (L.). A follicle.

Follin's grains (Follin, F. A. E., French surgeon, 1823–67). The small bodies consisting of isolated portions of the Wolffian tubules in the parovarium.

Foltz's valvules (Foltz, J. C. E., French anatomist, 1822–76). The valvules or constrictions just within the mouths of the lacrimal ducts.

fomentā·tion (L. *fomentum*, from *fovēre*, to warm). The application of moist heat to a part of the body to relieve pain by hyperaemia. 2. The substance thus applied.

fō·mēs (L. *fomes*, tinder). Any substance, such as bedding or clothing, capable of acting as a medium for transmitting infectious organisms.

fō·mites. Plural of fomes, *q.v.*

Fontana's spaces (Fontana, A. F., Italian philosopher, 1720–1805). Small spaces in the angle of the iris and communicating with the aqueous chamber and the canal of Schlemm.

fontanel, fontanelle (Fr. *fontanelle*, dim. of *fontaine*, little fountain). The space covered by a membranous structure between cranial bones in an infant which are not yet completely ossified.

fonti·culus (L. *fonticulus*, dim. of *fons*, fountain). The depression in the neck, just above the sternum.

food. Any substance which, when introduced into the body, is capable of being utilized to build up tissues or to supply heat. **F. poisoning:** an acute disease caused by food contaminated with pathogenic bacilli or containing bacillary toxins.

foot. The terminal portion of the leg below the ankle; the organ which supports the body in walking.

foot and mouth disease. An infectious virus disease of cattle and rarely of man, characterized in man mainly by stomatitis.

foot drop. Extension of the foot due to paresis of the extensor muscles of the leg.

foot, Madura. See Madura foot.

forage. Fodder. **F. poisoning:** epizootic cerebrospinal meningitis of horses.

forā·men (L. *foramen*, a hole). A small opening; a hole. **Anterior condylar:** a small opening situated in front of the condylar portion of the occipital bone. It transmits the hypoglossal nerve and a meningeal branch of the ascending pharyngeal artery. **Caecum:** a small depression in the mid-line of the posterior third of the tongue. It is situated behind the vallate papillae. **Caroticoclinoid:** a foramen which transmits the internal carotid artery in the cavernous sinus. An inconstant opening. It is only present when the caroticoclinoid ligament is ossified. **Centrale:** a small foramen in the cochlear area of the lamina cribrosa in the inner ear. It transmits nerve filaments. **Entepicondylar:** only present in man when a supracondylar process is present and a fibrous band passes from this process to the internal epicondyle of the humerus. The foramen is present in many vertebrates. **Ethmoidal** (internal orbital): two in number. Anterior, in the inner wall of the orbit and transmits the anterior ethmoidal vessels and nerve. Posterior, in the inner wall of the orbit behind the anterior and transmits the posterior ethmoidal vessels and nerve. **Hypoglossal:** see anterior condylar. **Incisive:** 4 in number. *Lateral* in the hard palate one on each side, they transmit a branch of the greater palatine vessels. *Median* situated in the midline of the hard palate, one anterior, and one posterior, the anterior transmits the left long spheno-palatine nerve, the posterior the right nerve. **Infra-orbital:** a foramen in the maxilla which transmits the infra-orbital nerve and vessels. **Internal orbital:** see anterior and posterior ethmoidal. **Interventricular** (foramina of Monro): lead from the third ventricle of the brain into the lateral ventricles. Each foramen is bounded posteriorly by the anterior tubercle of the thalamus, anteriorly by the anterior pillar of the fornix and above by the apex of the tela choroidea where the choroid plexuses of the two lateral ventricles are continuous with each other and with the choroid plexuses of the third ventricle. **Jugular:** is situated between the petrous portion of the temporal bone and the jugular process of the occipital bone. It lodges the commencement of the internal jugular vein and transmits the glossopharyngeal, vagus, and spinal accessory nerves; the inferior petrosal sinus; and meningeal branches of the ascending pharyngeal and occipital arteries. **Lacerum:** an opening in the base of the skull situated between the basilar process of the occipital, the apex of the petrous portion of the temporal, and the greater wing of the sphenoid near the root of the pterygoid process. **Magnum:** situated in the occipital bone in the mid-line it transmits the central nervous axis and its membranes, the accessory nerves, the vertebral arteries, the anterior spinal and posterior meningeal arteries, parts of the cerebellar amygdalae, and the membrana tectoria. **Mandibular:** an opening on the inner side of the lower jaw leading to the mandibular canal which lodges the inferior dental nerve and vessels. **Mastoid:** a large opening on the outer surface of the mastoid process of the temporal bone through which passes a large emissary vein. **Mental:** an opening on the outer surface of the mandible for the exit of the mental nerve and vessels. **Obturator** (thyroid foramen): lies below, and medial to, the acetabulum of the hip bone, its boundaries being formed by the ischium and pubis. It is covered by the obturator membrane which closed the opening, except opposite the obturator groove superiorly, where it converts that groove into the obturator canal. **Of Hüschke:** a small deficiency at the centre of the tympanic plate which is present until about five years of age. It may in rare cases persist throughout life. **Of Luschka** (lateral apertures of the fourth ventricle): are two small openings one in the extremity of each lateral recess situated immediately behind the posterior margins of the valves of Tarin. **Of Magendie** (median aperture of the fourth ventricle): is a small longitudinal slit in the inferior angle of the roof of the fourth ventricle of the brain. **Of Munro** (interventricular foramina): lead from the third ventricle of the brain into the two lateral ventricles. **Of Winslow** (opening into the lesser sac of peritoneum): is situated behind the right or free border of the lesser omentum, on a level with the body of the twelfth thoracic vertebra. **Optic:** a circular aperture between the upper and lower roots of the small wing of the sphenoid bone which leads forwards and outwards into the orbit, and transmits the optic nerve and ophthalmic artery. **Ovale** (skull): a large opening in the greater wing of the sphenoid for the passage of the mandibular division and the motor root of the fifth cranial nerve, the accessory meningeal artery, the middle meningeal vein, and sometimes the lesser superficial petrosal nerve. (Heart) an opening in the inferior part of the atrial septum in the foetal heart. It may persist throughout life. (Shoulder joint) (the foramen ovale of Weitbrecht) a triangular interval between the superior and middle glenohumeral ligaments. **Parietal:** a small opening near the superior border of the parietal bone for the transmission of an emissary vein which passes between the intracranial superior sagittal sinus and one of the tributaries of the extracranial occipital vein. **Posterior condylar:** an inconstant opening behind the occipital condyle which when present transmits an emissary vein passing between the intracranial transverse sinus and the extracranial suboccipital venous plexus. **Pterygospinous:** an inconstant opening in the lateral pterygoid plate of the sphenoid, it transmits muscular branches of the mandibular nerve. **Rotundum:** a circular opening at the base of the greater wing of the sphenoid bone which transmits the maxillary division of the fifth cranial nerve. **Sciatic** (greater): is formed by the greater sciatic notch, the spine of the ischium, the sacrotuberous ligament, and the sacro-spinous ligament. **Sciatic** (lesser): is formed by the lesser sciatic notch, the spine of the ischium, the sacro-tuberous ligament, and the sacrospinous ligament. **Singulare:** a small opening at the bottom of the internal auditory meatus which transmits the nerves and arteries to the ampulla of the posterior semicircular canal. **Sphenopalatine:** a small opening on the medial wall of the pterygo-palatine fossa for the sphenopalatine branches of the spheno-palatine ganglion and the sphenopalatine artery. **Spinosum:** a small opening in the spine of the sphenoid bone; it transmits the middle meningeal artery. **Sternal:** an inconstant opening in the body of the sternum, the result of imperfect ossification. **Stylomastoid:** an opening on the inferior surface of the temporal bone, it is the outlet of the facial canal, and by it the facial nerve makes its exit, and the stylomastoid branch of the posterior auricular artery passes in. **Supra-orbital:** an inconstant opening in the supra-orbital margin of the frontal bone for the passage of the supra-orbital nerve and artery. **Supratrochlear:** an inconstant opening in the lower end of the humerus, when the thin sheet of bone dividing the olecranon and coronoid fossae is absent. **Thyroid:** see obturator foramen. **Transversarium:** an opening in the transverse process of the cervical vertebrae, it transmits the vertebral artery, part of the vertebral plexus of veins and the vertebral sympathetic plexus of nerves. **Tympanohyal:** an opening at the base of the foetal temporal bone which closes as the base of the styloid process becomes ossified. **Vesalii** (emissary sphenoidal foramen): an inconstant opening at the base of the great wing of the sphenoid bone and transmits an emissary vein from the cavernous sinus. **Zygomaticofacial:** a small opening on the anterior surface of the skull situated above the zygomatic tuberosity and transmits the zygomaticofacial branch of the zygomatic nerve.

forä·mina. Plural of foramen. **Ethmoidal** (anterior and posterior): these open upon the inner wall of the orbit, the anterior transmits the anterior ethmoidal vessels and nerve, whilst the posterior gives passage to the posterior ethmoidal vessels and nerve. **Incisive:** see Scarpa's and Stenson's foramina. **Intervertebral:** are formed by the apposition of the superior and inferior vertebral notches of contiguous pedicles of the vertebrae, each transmits a spinal nerve. **Nutrient:** small or large openings in the bones for the passage of nutrient vessels. **Palatine:** two small openings in the tubercle of the palate bone, the greater and lesser palatine foramina. These canals transmit the greater and lesser palatine nerves and arteries. **Scarpa's** (median incisive foramina): two small openings in the incisive fossa of the maxilla, they transmit the long sphenopalatine nerves, the left nerve passing through the anterior and the right through the posterior opening. **Stenson's** (lateral incisive foramina): two lateral openings in the incisive fossa of the maxilla. Each transmits a branch of the greater palatine artery from the incisive fossa to the nasal fossa. **Thebesius** (foramina venarum minima): are several minute openings on the wall of the atrium of the heart. Some of these are simply blind recesses while others are the orifices of minute veins called the venae cordis minimae which return the blood from the wall of the atrium.

force (L. *fortis*, strong). Any interaction between two bodies altering their rest or motion, or form, or size; $\frac{mass \times velocity.}{time}$

forced (L. *fortis*, strong). Accomplished by an exertion of force. **F. feeding:** 1. Forcible feeding against the individual's will. 2. Systematic over-feeding as a therapeutic measure.

for·ceps (L. *forceps*). Pincers; a two-bladed instrument for grasping, extracting or compressing. **Artery f.:** used to grasp and compress an artery. **Aural f.:** curved forceps used in ear surgery. **Axis-traction f.:** used in obstetrics for pulling in the direction of the pelvic axis. **Dental f.:** used to extract teeth. **Dissecting f.:** forceps with blades but no handles. **Dressing f.:** forceps with handles like scissors. **Lane-Fagge's bone-holding f.:** used in orthopaedic surgery. **Lion f.:** forceps used in operations on bones and joints. **Obstetrical f.:** forceps applied to the head of the foetus to complete a delivery in a difficult labour. **Rat-tooth f.:** forceps with two or more teeth at their tips. **Sequestrum f.:** forceps with strong serrated jaws to remove portions of bone. **Strabismus f.:** forceps used in the operation for squint. **Sinus f.:** forceps with long, slender blades for entering into a sinus. **Tenaculum f.:** forceps with a hook at the end of each blade. **Tongue f.:** used to grasp the tongue. **Uterine f.:** forceps used in gynaecological operations. **Vulsellum f.:** forceps with hooks at the end of each blade. **Willett's f.:** used to grasp and pull on the foetal scalp to stop haemorrhage in certain cases of placenta praevia.

Forchheimer's sign (Forchheimer, F., American physician, 1853–1913). A rose red eruption of the soft palate and uvula seen in cases of rubella.

for·cipressure (L. *forceps*, pincers; *pressura*, from *premere*, to press). The arrest of a haemorrhage by a spring forceps.

Fordyce's disease (Fordyce, J. A., American dermatologist, 1858–1925). A disease of the mucous membrane of the lips in which patches of milium-like bodies are seen.

forearm. The arm between the elbow and the wrist.

forebrain. See prosencephalon.

forefinger. The first finger.

foregut. The cephalic end of the embryonic tube that develops into the digestive tract.

forehead. The face above the eyes.

Forel's decussation (Forel, A., Swiss psychiatrist, 1848–1931). The ventral tegmental decussation (between the red nuclei).

foren·sic (L. *forensis*, from *forum*, a public place). Pertaining to a court of law. **F. medicine:** medicine applied to legal questions.

foreskin. The prepuce.

Forlanini's treatment (Forlanini, C., Italian physician, 1847–1918). Artificial pneumothorax in cases of pulmonary tuberculosis.

Formad's kidney (Formad, H. F., American physician, 1847–92). Enlarged kidneys of chronic alcoholism.

formal·dehyde. A gas, H.CHO, used as a disinfectant for rooms and for large objects where heat is unsuitable. Soluble in water: a 40% solution is known as formalin, *q.v.*

formalin. A 40% solution of formaldehyde gas in water. Used occasionally as an antiseptic and for checking perspiration; more commonly as a 10% solution (4% formaldehyde) in saline or alcohol as a fixative and a preservative in anatomy and histology.

formate. Any salt of formic acid.

formā·tio (L. *formatio*, from *forma*, shape). A formation. **F. reticularis:** a term applied to certain areas of the central nervous system characterized by a lattice-like arrangement of nerve fibres, e.g., the network of grey matter in the cervical cord extending from the base of the dorsal grey column to the white substance.

for·mative (L. *forma*, shape). Influencing or giving form; capable of development.

forme fruste (Fr. from L. *forma*, shape; *frustra*, in vain). An incomplete form of a disease; term especially used in relation to endocrine diseases.

for·mic, formi·cic (L. *formica*, an ant). Pertaining to formic acid, H.COOH.

For·mica (L.). A genus of ants.

formicā·tion (L. *formica*, ant). A sensation as of ants creeping over the skin; 'pins and needles'—paraesthesia.

formol. Shortened form of formalin. **F.-gel test:** see Napier's aldehyde test. **F. saline, F.-sublimate:** histological fixatives, solutions of formol, in saline and mercuric chloride respectively. **F.-toxoid:** a solution of bacterial toxins rendered harmless for injection purposes by incubation with formaldehyde.

formolise. To render harmless, e.g. a bacterial culture, by treatment with formol.

for·mula (L. *formula*, dim. of *forma*, shape). 1. Prescribed form for making up a medicine. 2. A symbolic representation of the chemical composition of a compound showing the numbers of the various atoms which constitute a molecule of the compound. **F., electronic:** a structural f. in which the electrons which constitute the various types of bonds are represented symbolically—usually by dots. **F., empirical:** a f. showing the smallest numbers of the various atoms which could constitute a molecule of the compound. **F., molecular:** a f. showing the true composition of a molecule of a compound in terms of the numbers of the various constituent atoms. These are equal to or simple multiples of the numbers used in the empirical f. **F., stereochemical:** a structural f. in which the spatial directions of the various bonds are shown. Used mainly for representation of optically active compounds. **F., structural:** a f. in which the linking of the atoms is shown by symbolic representation of the valency bonds—usually by lines.

for·mulary. A collection of formulae for making medical preparations.

Fornet's reaction (Fornet, W., German physician, born 1877). A precipitation test used in cases of typhoid and syphilis.

for·nicolumn (L. *fornix*, arch; *columna*, pillar). The anterior pillar of the fornix.

fornicom·missure (L. *fornix*, arch; *committere*, to bring together). The commissure uniting the two hemifornices of the brain.

for·nix (L. *fornix*, arch). 1. An arched structure, a vault; e.g., the vault of the vagina around the uterine cervix. 2. A triangular structure of white matter connecting the cornu Ammonis and gyrus fornicatus with the basal ganglia of interbrain, midbrain and subthalamic region.

Förster's operation (Förster, O., German neurologist, 1873–1941). Division of the posterior nerve roots in cases of spastic paralysis.

fortification figures. See teichopsia.

fortū·itous (L. *fors*, chance). Relating to chance.

fossa (L. *fossa*, from *fodere*, to dig). A depression. **Canine:** a small depression on the outer surface of the maxilla just lateral to the canine ridge, the depression gives origin to the levator anguli oris muscle. **Cerebellar, of the skull:** two in number, they lodge the hemispheres of the cerebellum. **Coronoid:** a depression in the anterior surface of the lower end of the humerus, it receives the coronoid process of the ulna in flexion of the elbow joint. **Cubital:** a triangular hollow on the anterior aspect of the elbow. In the roof of the space are the skin, the median basilic and median cephalic veins, the medial cutaneous nerve, the musculocutaneous nerve and deep fascia. The floor is formed by the brachialis and a part of the supinator muscles. **Digastric:** an oval depression on the inner side of the mandible just lateral to the symphysis, it gives origin to the anterior belly of the digastric muscle. **Digital, of the femur:** a deep depression on the medial surface of the great trochanter for the attachment of the obturator externus tendon. **Digital, of the peritoneum:** a depression in the parietal peritoneum just posterior to the deep inguinal ring. **Floccular:** a trivial depression occurring in the foetal chondrocranium in the region of the auditory capsule. **F. for Gall-bladder:** a large depression on the inferior surface of the liver which lodges the gall-bladder. **Hypophyseal** (sella turcica): situated in the body of the sphenoid bone, it lodges the hypophysis cerebri or pituitary body. **Hypotrochanterica:** an uncommon condition in which the lower part of the gluteal tuberosity of the femur may assume the form of a depression. **Iliac:** large concave inner surface of the hip bone which lodges the iliacus muscle. **Incisive:** a small depression on the outer surface of the maxilla which gives origin to the depressor septi muscle. **Incudis:** a depression on the posterior wall of the middle ear, it receives the short process of the incus. **Infraclavicular:** a depression below the centre of the clavicle corresponding to a variable interval between the deltoid and pectoralis major muscle. **Infraspinous:** the lower division on the posterior surface of the scapula; it lodges the infraspinatus muscle. **Interpeduncular, of the brain:** is a diamond-shaped depression situated above and in front of the pons. It forms the floor of the third ventricle. **Intrabulbar:** the dilated part of the spongy portion of the urethra. It is about 1¼ inches in length. **Ischiorectal:** a triangular space between the rectum and the tuberosity of the ischium. It contains fat and the inferior rectal vessels. **Jugular:** forms part of the jugular foramen in the posterior fossa of the skull. **Lacrimal:** a depression within the zygomatic process of the frontal bone; it lodges the lacrimal gland. **Malleolar:** a depression in the posterior part of the external malleolus of the fibula. It gives attachment to the posterior fasciculus of the lateral ligament of the ankle joint. **Mandibular:** a deep depression behind the anterior root of the zygoma of the temporal bone. It articulates with the condyle of the mandible. **Nasal:** two in number, right and left, and they lie on each side of the median plane. They extend horizontally from before backwards, opening on the face by means of the anterior bony aperture of nose, and communicating posteriorly with the nasopharynx by the posterior bony aperture of nose. **Navicularis:** a small depression that lies between the hymen and the frenulum labiorum. **Of Rosenmuller:** a recess in the pharyngeal wall in the region of the Eustachian tube. **Olecranon:** a large depression on the posterior surface of the lower end of the humerus, it receives the olecranon process of the ulna in extension of the elbow joint. **Ovalis:** is situated upon the inferior part of the atrial septum a little superior and to the left of the orifice of the in-ferior vena cava. It indicates the position of the foramen ovale of the foetal heart. **Ovarian:** a peritoneal depression on the lateral wall of the pelvis for the ovary. **Parafloccular:** depression on the inferior part of the temporal bone in foetal life, it is represented by the subarcuate fossa in adult life. **Patellaris** (hyaloid fossa): the posterior part of the hyaloid membrane which receives the crystalline lens of the eye. **Popliteal:** a diamond-shaped depression situated posterior to the knee joint. It is bounded on the outer side by the biceps above and the lateral head of the gastrocnemius below; on the inner side above by the semitendinosus and semimembranosus and below by the inner head of the gastrocnemius. **Posterior condylar:** a small depression behind each condyle of the occipital bone, it may be pierced by a posterior condylar canal, on one or both sides, for an emissary vein passing between the sigmoid sinus and the suboccipital venous plexus. **Pterygoid:** a depression at the posterior part of the pterygoid processes of the sphenoid, it contains the medial pterygoid and tensor palati muscles. **Pterygopalatine:** a space situated at the base of the pterygomaxillary fissure. It contains the third part of the maxillary artery, the maxillary nerve and the sphenopalatine ganglion. **Pyriform:** a depression situated on either side of the inlet of the larynx. **Radial:** a small depression on the anterior surface of the lower end of the humerus which receives the anterior margin of the head of the radius in complete flexion of the elbow joint. **Retromolar:** a concavity on the inner surface of the mandible opposite the third molar socket; some fibres of the temporal muscle are attached to this fossa. **Rotunda:** a funnel-shaped depression situated on the inner wall of the middle ear just behind and below the promontory. **Scaphoid:** a depression at the base of the medial pterygoid plate which gives origin to the tensor palati muscle. **Subarcuate:** a depression on the internal surface of the temporal bone just above the internal auditory meatus. It represents the parafloccular fossa of early life. **Sublingual:** a fossa on the inner surface of the mandible above the mylohyoid muscle for the sublingual gland. **Submandibular:** a large depression on the inner surface of the mandible below the mylohyoid line, for the submandibular (submaxillary) gland. **Supraspinous:** the upper smaller depression on the posterior surface of the scapula. It gives origin over its inner two thirds to the supraspinatus muscle. **Suprasternal:** a deep depression above the upper border of the manubrium sterni, lying between the sternal heads of attachment of the sternomastoid muscles. **Supratonsillar** (intratonsillar cleft): a small recess above the tonsil, it is the remains of the medial portion of the second visceral depression. **Temporal:** of the skull is bounded above by the superior temporal lines of the frontal and parietal bones and below by the upper border of the zygomatic arch laterally, and the infratemporal crest of the greater wing of the sphenoid medially. **Terminal** (fossa navicularis): a dilatation about ½ inch long in the anterior part of the spongy part of the urethra in the male. **Trochanteric:** see digital fossa of femur. **Trochlear:** is a depression on the orbital plate of the frontal bone close to the medial angular process. The fibrocartilaginous pulley or trochlea is attached by fibrous tissue to this fossa. **Vermian:** a depression in the posterior fossa of the skull near the foramen magnum it receives part of the vermiform process of the cerebellum.

fosset, fossette (Fr. *fossette*, from L. *fossa*, ditch). 1. A dimple; a small depression. 2. A small deep ulcer of the cornea.

fos·sula, fos·sulet (L. dim. of *fossa*, ditch). A small fossa.

Fothergill's disease (Fothergill, J., English physician, 1712–80). Scarlatina anginosa.

Fothergill's neuralgia (Fothergill, S., English physician. Treatise published 1804). Trigeminal neuralgia.

Fouchet's test (Fouchet, A., contemporary French physician). A test to determine the presence of excess of bilirubin in the blood.

foudroyant (Fr. *foudre*, lightning). Fulminant, fulminating; overwhelming.

foundling. An abandoned infant.

fourchet, fourchette (Fr. *fourchette*, dim. of *fourche*, from L. *furca*, fork). A fold of mucous membrane in the posterior commissure of the vulva.

Fournier's disease (Fournier, J. A., French dermatologist, 1832–1914). Idiopathic gangrene of the scrotum.

fourth. Next after the third. **F. cranial nerve:** the trochlear nerve. **F. disease:** Duke-Filatow's disease. **F. ventricle:** one of the internal spaces of the brain; enclosed by the medulla oblongata, connected with the third ventricle, *q.v.*, by the aquaeductus Sylvii and distally continuous with the central canal of the spinal cord.

fō·vea (L. *fovea*, pit). A small fossa or dimple; term applied particularly to the f. centralis retinae, a small area in the macula lutea, the site of most distinct vision.

fō·veal (L. *fovea*, pit). Pertaining to a fovea.

fō·veate (L. *fovea*, pit). Having foveae.

fovē·ola (L. *fovea*, pit). A small fovea.

Foville's fasciculus (Foville, L., French neurologist, 1799–1878). The taenia semicircularis between the ventricular surfaces of the nucleus caudatus and the thalamus.

Fowler's position (Fowler, G. R., American surgeon, 1848–1906). Sitting position in bed with a pillow beneath the knees to maintain the position.

Fowler's solution (Fowler, T., English physician, 1736–1801). Liquor arsenicalis, containing 1 per cent of arsenic trioxide in neutral solution. Used orally in some tonics and for some forms of dermatitis, and locally in conjunction with tincture of ipecacuanha in the treatment of Vincent's angina.

Fox's impetigo (Fox, W. T., English dermatologist, 1836–79). Impetigo contagiosa.

foxglove. A flowering plant of the genus Digitalis. The leaves of the purple-flowered *D. purpurea* contain glycosides having an action on the heart. Their effect is to decrease the rate but increase the force of the beat.

f.p. Abbreviation for freezing point.

f.r. Abbreviation for flocculation reaction.

fract. dos. Abbreviation for L. *fracta*, broken; G. *dosis*, dose; in divided doses.

frac·tional (L. *fractio*, from *frangere*, to break). Pertaining to a fraction. **F. cultivation:** the cultivation of one micro-organism from a growth of several. **F. distillation:** a method of separating volatile substances of different boiling points by collecting separately the distillates evaporating at certain temperatures. **F. sterilization:** intermittent sterilization used for killing spores of micro-organisms, heating (streaming steam or water bath) to 100° C. on three or more successive days for a certain period.

frac·tionate (L. *frangere*, to break). To separate into different fractions.

fractū·ra (L. *fractura*, from *frangere*, to break). A fracture, *q.v.*

fracture (L. *fractura*, from *frangere*, to break). A breaking, especially of a bone. **Chauffeur's f.:** f. of the outer part of the lower end of the radius and styloid process caused by backfiring of a motor engine while the chauffeur is starting it with a handle. **Colles's f.:** see Colles's f. **Complicated f.:** f. with injury of important adjacent structures. **Compound f.:** a f. complicated by wound of the parts overlying the fractured part of the bone. **Depressed f.:** a f. in which the fractured part has become depressed beneath the normal level. **Greenstick·f.:** a f. in which the bone is broken on one side only and bent on the other side; occurring mainly in children. **Impacted f.:** a f. where one part is driven into the other. **Pott's f.:** see Pott's f. **Simple f.:** a f. without laceration of the overlying soft issues.

frae·num (L. *fraenum*, bridle). A fold of skin or mucous membrane, limiting movements of or supporting an organ.

fragi·litas (L. *fragilis*, brittle). Fragility; brittleness. **F. ossium:** see osteogenesis imperfecta.

fragmentā·tion (L. *fragmentum*, fragment). A separation or decomposition into fragments.

framboe·sia (Fr. *framboise*, raspberry). Yaws, *q.v.*

Frank's operation (Frank, F., German gynaecologist, 1856–1923). An opening into the stomach. Gastrostomy by means of a cone of stomach brought through the abdominal wall.

Fränkel's treatment (Fränkel, A., German physician, 1864–1938). The use of strophanthin in cases of cardiac failure.

Frankenhäuser's ganglion (Frankenhäuser, F., German gynaecologist, died 1894). The cervical sympathetic ganglion of the uterus.

frankincense. An oleo gum resin from various species of Borwelli, which burns with a pleasant odour.

Franklin's glasses. Bifocal spectacles named after Benjamin Franklin, American scientist, 1706–90.

Frasera. A genus of plants of the gentian family.

Frauenhofer's lines (Frauenhofer, J. von, German optician, 1787–1826). Black lines in the solar spectrum.

F.F.R. Fellow of the Faculty of Radiologists.

F.R.C.O.G. Fellow of the Royal College of Obstetricians and Gynaecologists.

F.R.C.P. Fellow of the Royal College of Physicians. **F.R.C.P.E.,** Fellow of the Royal College of Physicians of Edinburgh. **F.R.C.P.I.,** Fellow of the Royal College of Physicians of Ireland.

F.R.C.S. Fellow of the Royal College of Surgeons. **F.R.C.S.E.,** Fellow of the Royal College of Surgeons of Edinburgh. **F.R.C.S.I.,** Fellow of the Royal College of Surgeons of Ireland.

F.R.C.V.S. Fellow of the Royal College of Veterinary Surgeons.

F.R.F.P.S. Fellow of the Royal Faculty of Physicians and Surgeons of Glasgow.

freckle. See lentigo.

free. In chemistry, uncombined. **F. association:** a psycho-analytic method in which the spontaneous flow of words associated with a test word, and brought forward without conscious restraint, is used for investigating the origin and development of ideas.

freemartin. An hermaphrodite female twin born with a perfect male. Term usually applied to cattle.

freeze. To produce an effect by the action of intense cold.

freezing mixture. A mixture for producing intense cold, as by a mixture of salt and snow.

freezing point. The temperature at which a liquid is converted into a solid state.

Frei's bubo (Frei, W. S., German dermatologist, 1885–1943). Inguinal lymphogranulomatosis.

frĕ·mitus (L. *fremitus*, from *fremere*, to growl). A palpable vibration, e.g. of the chest walls. **F., friction:** a rubbing sensation sometimes felt by the palpating hand in dry pleurisy or dry pericarditis over the affected part. **F., vocal:** vibration felt over the lung when the hand is placed flat upon the chest wall and the patient says 'ninety-nine' or some other resonant syllables.

Frenkel's sign (Frenkel, H. S., Berlin neurologist, 1860–1931). Hypotonia of the lower extremities in tabes dorsalis.

frenzy. Violent excitement.

fre·quency (L. *frequentia*, from *frequens*, frequent). 1. The number of occurrences of a phenomenon (such as oscillations or cycles of electric current) in a unit of time. 2. In statistics, the ratio of the number of events, values or individuals in a single class to the total number of events, values or individuals observed or classified. **F. distribution:** distribution of values or individuals among the various classes.

Freudian. Relating to or one who follows the doctrines of Sigmund Freud (Austrian neurologist 1856–1939), especially that many psychological disorders result from unconscious sexual impressions in childhood and can be cured by bringing these to conscious notice by psycho-analysis; and that dreams are the symbolic fulfilment of suppressed, often sexual desires.

Freund's anomaly (Freund, H. W., German gynaecologist, 1859–1925). A small thoracic inlet is a predisposing cause of pulmonary tuberculosis. **F.'s reaction:** the serum from a non-cancerous patient will cause lysis of cancer cells.

Freund's operation (Freund, A., German gynaecologist, 1833–1917). Section of the first rib and costal cartilage.

Frey's gastric follicles (Frey, H., German histologist, 1822–1900). The crypts at the bottom of which the gastric glands open.

Freyer's operation (Freyer, Sir P. J., English surgeon, 1852–1921). Suprapubic prostatectomy.

fri·able (L. *friabilis*, from *friare*, to crumble). Easily crumbled.

friar's balsam. Tinctura benzoini composita; a compound tincture of benzoin 10 per cent, with storax, aloe and balsam of tolu in alcohol 90 per cent. Used as an inhalant in bronchitis and laryngitis; can be used internally in the treatment of chronic bronchitis.

Fricke's bandage (Fricke, J. K. G., German surgeon, 1790–1841). Scrotal bandage by means of strips in cases of orchitis.

fric·tion (L. *frictio*, from *fricare*, to rub). 1. Resistance to motion between two bodies in contact. 2. Rubbing; inunction by rubbing. 3. A method of massage in which circular and centripetal strokings are used. **F. fremitus:** see fremitus, f. **F. sound:** the sound heard in auscultation caused by the rubbing together of two inflamed and loosely adherent serous membranes.

Friedländer's bacillus (Friedländer, C., German pathologist, 1847–87). *Klebsiella pneumoniae.* **F.'s decidual cells:** the large connective tissue cells of the uterine mucosa that form the compact layer of the uterine decidua.

Friedman's test (Friedman, M. H., contemporary American physician). Modified Aschheim-Zondek test using rabbits.

Friedmann's disease (Friedmann, M., German physician, 1858–1925). Relapsing infantile spastic paralysis.

Friedreich's disease (Friedreich, N., German physician, 1825–82). Hereditary ataxia. **F.'s sign:** collapse of the internal jugular veins in cases of adherent pericardium.

fright neurosis. A neurosis conditioned by an experience of fright.

frigi·dity (L. *frigidus*, from *frigus*, cold). Coldness; absence of sexual libido.

frigori·fic (L. *frigus*, cold; *facere*, to make). Producing cold.

Friteau's triangle (Friteau, E., born 1867). The area on the cheek devoid of branches of the facial nerve.

Fröhlich's syndrome (Fröhlich, A., Austrian neurologist, born 1871). Dystrophia adiposogenitalis.

Froin's syndrome (Froin, G., French physician, born 1874). Found in cases where communication between ventricles and spinal fluid is obstructed; the lumbar cerebrospinal fluid is yellow, coagulates quickly and contains much globulin.

Frommann's striae (Frommann, C., German anatomist, 1831–92). The striations in the axis cylinders of nerves stained by silver nitrate.

frons (L.). The forehead.

fron·tad (L. *frons*, forehead; *ad*, to). Toward the frontal aspect.

fron·tal (L. *frons*, forehead). 1. Pertaining to the anterior part or aspect of an organ or of the body. 2. Relating to the forehead. 3. Relating to the f. bone or f. lobe. **F. eminence:** the prominence of the f. bone above each superciliary ridge. **F. lobe:** portion of the brain in front of the Rolandian fissure and above the horizontal limb of the Sylvian fissure.

frontā·lis muscle (L. *frons*, forehead). The anterior or frontal part of the occipito-frontalis muscle.

fron·tocerebel·lar (L. *frons*, forehead; *cerebellum*, dim. of *cerebrum*, brain). Relating to the frontal lobe and the cerebellum.

frontomā·lar (L. *frons*, forehead; *mala*, cheek). Relating to the frontal and the malar bones.

frontomax·illary (L. *frons*, forehead; *maxilla*, jaw). Relating to the frontal and the upper jaw-bones.

fronto-occip·ital (L. *frons*, forehead; *occiput*). Relating to the forehead and the occiput.

frontoparī·etal (L. *frons*, forehead; *paries*, a wall). Relating to the frontal and parietal bones.

frontopon·tine (L. *frons*, forehead; *pons*, a bridge). Relating to the frontal lobe and the pons.

frontotem·poral (L. *frons*, forehead; *tempora*, pl. of *tempus*, the temples). Relating to the frontal and temporal bones.

Froriep's ganglion (Froriep, A., German physiologist, 1849–1917). The rudimentary, transient and inconstant dorsal root ganglion on the posterior aspect of the hypoglossal nerve.

frostbite. An injury to the skin or a part from extreme cold especially when combined with rapid loss of heat by wind; characterized by redness, swelling and pain (capillary damage) which may go on to the necrosis of superficial and deeper tissues.

fruc·tose (L. *fructus*, fruit). Fruit-sugar; laevulose. $C_6H_{12}O_6$, a carbohydrate present in all sweet fruits and in honey.

fructosū·ria (L. *fructus*, fruit; G. *ouron*, urine). Urinary excretion of fructose. **F., essential:** a recessively hereditary anomaly of metabolism characterized by urinary excretion of about 13 per cent of ingested fructose (including the fructose resulting from the breakdown of cane sugar), probably due to failure of normal hydrolysis of fructose to lactic acid.

fruc·tus (L. fruit). Fruit; the ripened ovary of a plant together with parts of the flower which take part in its development.

fruit. See fructus.

frustrā·tion (L. *frustra*, in vain). State induced by preventing the achievement of some desired object.

Fuchs's colobō·ma (Fuchs, E., Austrian oculist, 1851–1930). A small defect of the choroid at the lower border of the optic disc. **F.'s stomata:** the depressions on the anterior surface of the iris near to the pupillary border.

fuch·sin, fuch·sine. A red dye consisting of hydrochlorides or acetates of rosaniline or pararosaniline, a staining agent.

fuchsi·nophil, fuchsi·nophile. Stainable with fuchsin.

fuchsinŏ·philous. Easily stained with fuchsin.

Fucus. A genus of seaweeds, including *F. vesiculosus*, used in the treatment of goitre.

M

fū·gitive (L. *fugitivus*, from *fugere*, to take to flight). Fleeting; wandering; transient.

fugue (L. *fuga*, a taking to flight). An abnormal mental condition characterized by apparently rational behaviour during a period of impulsive activity (such as wandering about) for which the individual has afterwards complete amnesia.

Fukala's operation (Fukala, V., Austrian ophthalmologist, 1847–1911). Extraction of the crystalline lens in cases of myopia of high degree.

ful·gurant (L. *fulgur*, lightning). Like lightning.

fulgurā·tion (L. *fulgur*, lightning). 1. Lightning stroke. 2. Surgical diathermy; electrosurgery.

Fullers earth. A natural, porous, colloidal aluminium silicate. Used for clarifying and decolourising oils and fats.

ful·minant, ful·minating (L. *fulmen*, a thunderbolt). Sudden and severe.

fumă·ric acid. A dibasic unsaturated organic acid $(CH.COOH)_2$. Occurs naturally in some plants and fungi.

fū·migant. Material used in fumigation.

fumigā·tion (L. *fumigare*, from *fumus*, smoke). Exposure to fumes, especially disinfection by exposure to the fumes of a disinfectant.

fuming (L. *fumus*, smoke). Smoking, as of certain acids.

function (L. *functio*, a performing). 1. The normal or special action of an organ or part. 2. The characteristic properties of a chemical compound, due to the presence of a particular atom or group or arrangement of atoms.

functional (L. *functio*, a performing). Relating to the special action of an organ. **F. albuminuria:** albuminuria, orthostatic. **F. disease:** a disease caused by disturbance of the function of one or more parts which has not led to and is not caused by any detectable structural alteration. **F. group:** term used in chemistry to denote a group of atoms which give to a compound certain characteristic properties, e.g. the aldehyde amine group.

fun·dal (L. *fundus*, bottom). Pertaining to the fundus.

fundamen·tal. 1. Relating to the base. 2. The essential basic principles or rules as in "the fundamentals of chemistry".

fundec·tomy (L. *fundus*, bottom; G. *ektomē*, excision). Surgical removal of the fundus of an organ.

fun·dus (L., bottom). 1. The enlarged or arched portion of certain hollow organs. 2. The base of an organ. 3. The part of the eye opposite the pupil (retina, choroidea).

fun·gal. Relating to a fungus.

fun·gate (L. *fungus*). Of granulation or malignant tissue, to grow rapidly, like a fungus, or to assume the form of a fungus (mushroom).

fungi. Pl. of fungus.

fun·gicide (L. *fungus*; *caedere*, to kill). A fungus-destroying agent.

fun·giform (L. *fungus*; *forma*, shape). Of mushroom-like shape.

fun·gistat·ic (L. *fungus*; *stare*, to stand). Inhibiting the growth of fungi.

fun·goid (L. *fungus*; G. *eidos*, form). Mushroom-like.

fungō·sity. A soft excrescence.

fungous (L. *fungus*). Of spongiose or mushroom-like appearance.

fungus (L.). 1. Non-chlorophyll-producing thallophytes, *q.v.*, including the phycomycetes, ascomycetes, basidiomycetes and myxomycetes. 2. A spongy, morbid growth of granulation or malignant tissue. **F. cerebri:** see hernia cerebri.

fū·nicle (L. *funiculus*, dim. of *funis*, a cord). A slender cord, a fascicle.

funǐ·cular (L. *funis*, a cord). Pertaining to the umbilical or spermatic cord.

funiculī·tis (L. *funis*, a cord). Inflammation of the spermatic cord.

funǐ·culus (L. *funiculus*, dim. of *funis*, a cord). 1. A cord-like structure, such as the umbilical cord. 2. A bundle of nerve fibres in a sheath of perineurium. 3. Any of the three main columns of white matter of each lateral half of the spinal cord.

fū·niform (L. *funis*, cord; *forma*, shape). Like a cord.

fu·nis (L.). A cord; the umbilical cord.

funnel (L. *infundibulum*, from *in*, into; *fundere*, to pour). A cone-shaped vessel with an apical tube. **F. chest:** a depression of the central part of the anterior wall of the chest.

fur. A morbid coating of the tongue.

fur·ca (L., fork). Any forked process.

furcal, furcate (L. *furca*, fork). Forked.

fur·cula, fur·culum (L. *furcula*, dim. of *furca*, fork). 1. A forked elevation in the floor of the embryonic pharynx, giving rise to the epiglottis. 2. The wishbone.

furfur (L., bran). Dandruff; scurf.

furfurā·ceous (L. *furfur*, bran). Resembling the scales of bran.

fū·ror (L.). Fury; rage.

furred. Having a morbid coating, as of the tongue.

furrow. A groove.

Fürstner's disease (Fürstner, C., German psychiatrist, 1848–1906). Pseudo-spastic paralysis with tremor.

furun·cle (L. *furunculus*, a boil; dim. of *fur*, a thief). A boil. See furunculus.

furun·cular. Pertaining to a furuncle.

furunculō·sis (L. *furunculus*, a boil). The condition characterized by the presence of boils.

furun·culus (L. *furunculus*, a boil; dim. of *fur*, a thief). A furuncle; a local inflammatory condition of the integument, ordinarily involving a skin-gland or hair-follicle and ending in suppuration. **F. orientalis:** see Oriental sore.

Fusarium. A genus of moulds of the Ascomycetes class.

fū·sein (L. *fucus*, red cosmetic). Melanin pigment of the retinal cells.

fuse (L. *fusus*, from *fundere*, to melt). 1. A thin metal wire inserted as a safety precaution in an electric circuit. 2. To melt.

fū·sible (L. *fusus*, from *fundere*, to melt). That which can be easily fused or melted.

fū·siform (L. *fusus*, spindle; *forma*, form). Spindle-shaped.

Fusiformis. See fusobacterium, fuso-spirillary. Caused by fusiform organisms and spirillae, as in Vincent's angina.

fū·sion (L. *fundere*, to melt). 1. The process of liquefying or melting. 2. The process of uniting; in psychoanalysis specifically union of (life and death) instincts. 3. Perception resulting from combination of stimuli, e.g. binaural or binocular fusion.

Fusobacterium. A genus of bacteria.

fuso-spirillary. Caused by fusiform bacilli and spirillae as in Vincent's angina.

G

G. An abbreviation for gramme.

γ. Greek symbol. See gamma.

Ga. The symbol for gallium.

Gabbett's method (Gabbett, H. S., British physician). A method of staining tubercle bacilli. **G.'s stain**: for tubercle bacilli, consisting of fuchsin 1 part, alcohol 1 part, phenol 5 parts, distilled water 100 parts.

gabǐ·anol. A compound of an oily character obtained from shale and used in the treatment of lung diseases.

Gabler's hemiplegia (Gabler, A., French physician, 1821–79). A hemiplegia associated with crossed paralysis of the cranial nerves.

Gaboon ulcer (Gaboon, the French Congo). Tropical ulcer, very similar to syphilitic ulcer.

gă·duin. A fatty principle, $C_{36}H_{46}O_9$, obtained from cod-liver oil.

Gadus. A genus of fish, including *G. morrhua*, the codfish.

Gaffky scale (Gaffky, G. T. A., German bacteriologist, 1850–1918). Used in the prognosis of phthisis, based on the number of tubercle bacilli in the sputum.

Gaff·kўa. A genus of Micrococcaceae, including the micrococcus tetragenus.

gag. 1. Apparatus for holding open the mouth. 2. To retch or try to vomit.

gait. The manner of walking.

galactacrā·sia (G. *gala*, milk; *crasis*, mixture). Abnormality in the composition of milk.

galactae·mia (G. *gala*, milk; *haima*, blood). A condition in which milk is present in the blood.

galac·tagogue (G. *gala*, milk; *ăgōgŏs*, leading). Promoting the secretion of milk; an agent that does this.

galac·tase (G. *gala*, milk). A proteolytic enzyme of milk; a rather unfortunate term suggesting as it does a hydrolytic effect on the carbohydrate galactose.

galac·tic (G. *gala*, milk). Relating to milk.

galactidrō·sis (G. *gala*, milk; *hidrōs*, sweat). The sweating of a fluid resembling milk.

galac·tin (G. *gala*, milk). The lactogenic hormone, for which the name prolactin is usually used. It has been used successfully to promote lactation in cases of failure or deficient secretion.

galac·toblast (G. *gala*, milk; *blastos*, germ). A colostrum corpuscle.

galac·tocele (G. *gala*, milk; *kēlē*, tumour). 1. Milk-containing retention cyst or dilatation of the main milk ducts of the lactating female breast. 2. Hydrocele with milky contents.

galactŏ·meter (G. *gala*, milk; *metron*, measure). Apparatus used to measure the specific gravity of milk.

galac·topexy (G. *gala*, milk; *pexis*, fixation). A plastic operation on the breast.

galactŏ·phagous (G. *gala*, milk; *phagein*, to eat). Feeding on milk.

galac·tophore (G. *gala*, milk; *pherein*, to carry). A duct conveying milk.

galac·tophori·tis (G. *gala*, milk; *pherein*, to carry). Inflammation of the milk glands.

galactŏ·phorous (G. *gala*, milk; *pherein*, to bear). Conveying milk.

galactŏ·phygous (G. *gala*, milk; *phuge*, flight). Arresting milk secretion.

galac·topoiē·sis (G. *gala*, milk; *poiein*, to make). Formation of milk.

galactorrhoē·a (G. *gala*, milk; *rhoia*, flow). Excessive secretion of milk.

galac·tose (G. *gala*, milk). A hexose, $C_6H_{12}O_6$, derived by hydrolysis from lactose.

galac·toside (G. *gala*, milk). Cerebroside, *q.v.*

galactō·sis (G. *gala*, milk). Secretion of milk.

galactostā·sis (G. *gala*, milk; *stasis*, stationariness). Stasis of milk in the breast.

galactosū·ria (G. *gala*, milk; *ouron*, urine). The excretion of galactose in the urine.

galactotrŏ·phic (G. *gala*, milk; *trephein*, to rear). 1. Promoting the flow of milk. 2. Applied to a hormone of the anterior pituitary gland stimulating mammary secretion. Syn. lactotropic.

galactū·ria (G. *gala*, milk; *ouron*, urine). The secretion of milk-like urine. See chyluria.

gă·lalith (G. *gala*, milk; *lithos*, stone). A product of casein and formol which is absorbent, and is used in vascular surgery.

gal·banum. Gum resin from *Ferula galbaniflua* and other species. It is expectorant and stimulant.

Galbiati's operation (Galbiati, G., Italian surgeon, 1776–1844). Symphysiotomy.

gă·lea (L., helmet). The aponeurotic structure of the scalp, connecting the frontal and occipital muscles.

Galeati's glands (Galeati, Italian physician, 1686–1775). Lieberkuhn's crypts, *q.v.*

galĕā·tus (L. *galea*, helmet). Born with a caul.

Galen's nerve (Galen, C., Greek anatomist and physiologist, A.D. 131–200. He settled in Rome in 164). A branch of the superior laryngeal nerve, ramus anastomoticus cum nervo laryngo inferiore. **G.'s great vein**: the vena cerebri magna. **G.'s veins**: venae choroideae.

galē·na. Naturally occurring lead sulphide.

Galen·ic, Galen·ical. Of, or according to, Galen. **G. medicines**: 1. Those of vegetable as distinguished from chemical or spagyric origin. 2. Those designed for the use of human patients, i.e. not veterinary. 3. Those prepared according to an official formula.

galeophĭ·lia (G. *gălē*, cat; *philein*, to love). Love of cats.

galeophō·bia (G. *gălē*, cat; *phobos*, fear). Fear of cats.

galerŏ·pia, galerop·sia (G. *gălĕrŏs*, cheerful; *opsis*, vision). Supernormal clarity of vision.

gall. Bile. **G.-stone**: concretion in the gall-bladder or bile ducts.

Gall's craniology (Gall, F. J., Austrian anatomist, 1758–1828). Phrenology.

gallate. Any salt of gallic acid.

gall-bladder. The pear-shaped vessel containing bile and situated on the under side of the liver. **Hydrops of G.**: condition characterized by the presence of a colourless mucoid fluid in the gall-bladder, due to absorption of bile and its replacement by the secretion of gall-bladder epithelium in cases of complete obstruction of the cystic duct.

gallic acid. $C_7H_6O_5$. Acid found in nutgalls and tea. Obtained from tannic acid by boiling it with dilute acids.

gal·lipot (Old Dutch *gleypot*). A small pot, especially as used for holding medical preparations.

gal·lium. A rare metal occurring in iron ores. Symb. Ga.

gallon, imperial. A measure of capacity, equal to 4 quarts, or 4·546 litres.

gallop rhythm. Term applied to the auscultatory finding of 3 (instead of 2) well heard heart sounds, resembling the sound of a galloping horse; when the third sound is heard during diastole (especially when protodiastolic) over the heart apex it denotes right ventricular strain in the presence of left ventricular failure; a systolic third sound is of no significance, and a presystolic third sound is usually due to slight delay in auriculo-ventricular conduction or occasionally to very forceful auricular contraction. A third heart sound is to be distinguished from a reduplicated second sound which is always best heard over the base of the heart, and which is due to asynchronous closure of the aortic and pulmonary valves.

gall-stone. See gall.

Galton's whistle (Galton, F., English scientist, 1822–1911). An instrument used for detecting the perception of high tones by the ear.

galvan·ic (Galvani, L., Italian anatomist, 1737–98). Pertaining to galvanism. **G. battery:** a series of cells generating electricity by chemical reaction and so disposed as to secure the combined effect of the various units. **G. electricity:** Galvanism, *q.v.*

gal·vanism. Electricity generated by chemical action.

gal·vaniză·tion. Subjection to the action of a galvanic current; application of an electric current to the body for therapeutic or diagnostic purposes.

gal·vanocau·tery. Division or destruction of tissues by means of a platinum-loop heated by a galvanic current.

gal·vanocontracti·lity. Contractility under stimulation by the galvanic current.

gal·vanofaradiză·tion (Galvani, L.; Faraday, M.). The simultaneous excitation of a nerve or muscle by both galvanic and faradic current.

galvanŏ·meter (Galvani, L.; G. *metron*, measure). An instrument for detecting (presence or direction) or for measuring the magnitude of electric currents.

gal·vanopuncture. The introduction of needles that complete an electric circuit.

galvă·noscope (Galvani, L.; G. *skopein*, to view). An instrument for detecting the presence and direction of an electric current, e.g. by its effect on a magnetic needle.

gal·vanosurgery. The use of galvanic currents for surgical purposes.

gal·vanotax·is (Galvani, L.; G. *tassein*, to arrange). Taxis induced and directed by galvanic current.

gal·vanothĕ·rapy (Galvani, L.; G. *therapeia*, treatment). Treatment by means of a galvanic current.

gal·vanothermy (Galvani, L.; G. *thermē*, heat). The production of heat by means of a galvanic current.

gal·vanotŏ·nus (Galvani, L.; *tonos*, tone). 1. Electrotonus, *q.v.* 2. The continued tetanus of a muscle between the make and break contraction.

galvanotrŏ·pism (Galvani, L.; G. *trephein*, to turn). Tropism caused and directed by a galvanic current.

gam·bir. Syn. for catechu.

gă·mete (G. *gamein*, to marry). 1. A sex-cell; a mature germ cell. 2. Either of the two germ cells undergoing conjugation, *q.v.*

gamēt·ic. Referring to a gamete.

gamē·toblast (G. *gamein*, to marry; *blastos*, germ). A sporozoite.

gamē·tocide (G. *gamein*, to marry; L. *caedere*, to kill). Destroying gametes or gametocytes; an agent that does this.

gamē·tocyte (G. *gamein*, to marry, *kutos*, a container). 1. Mother cell of a gamete, *q.v.* 2. Sexual form of a merozoite.

gamē·togĕ·nesis, gametŏ·geny (G. *gamein*, to marry; *gennan*, to produce). 1. Production of gametes. 2. The development of gametocytes into macro- or micro-gametes.

gamē·togenic (G. *gamein*, to marry; *gennan*, to produce). Conducive to the production of gametes and gametocytes.

gamē·tophyte (G. *gamein*, to marry; *phuton*, plant). The sexual form of such plants as exhibit alternate generation.

Gamgee tissue. Gauze and cotton tissue.

gamma. 1. The third letter of the Greek alphabet, γ. 2. A unit of weight, equal to one millionth part of a gramme. **G. rays:** rays emitted by radio-active substances of shorter wavelength than X-rays. **G. streptococci:** non-haemolytic streptococci.

gam·macism (G. *gamma*, g., *akkizesthai*, to affect indifference). Difficulty in articulating the letters g and k.

Gamna disease. A form of splenomegaly.

gamogĕ·nesis (G. *gamos*, marriage; *genesis*, production). Sexual reproduction.

gă·mogenet·ic (G. *gamos*, marriage; *genesis*, production). Relating to gamogenesis.

gamomă·nia (G. *gamos*, marriage; *mania*, madness). Insane desire for marriage.

Gandy-Gamna nodule. Yellow nodules seen sometimes in cases of splenomegaly.

gang·lial, gang·liar (G. *gagglion*, a tumour). Relating to a ganglion or ganglia.

gang·liăte, gang·liăted (G. *gagglion*, a tumour). Furnished with ganglia.

gangliĕc·tomy (G. *gagglion*, a tumour; *ektomē*, excision). Excision of a ganglion.

gang·liform (G. *gagglion*, a tumour; L. *forma*, shape). Having the shape of a ganglion.

gangliī·tis (G. *gagglion*, a tumour). Inflammation of a ganglion.

gang·lioblast (G. *gagglion*, a tumour; *blastos*, germ). An embryonic ganglion cell.

gang·liocyte (G. *gagglion*, a tumour; *kutos*, a container). A ganglion cell; a nerve cell.

gangliŏ·ma (G. *gagglion*, a tumour). A tumour originating from ganglion cells; a ganglionic neuroma.

gang·lion (G. *gagglion*, a tumour). 1. The normal tumescence of certain nerves consisting of nerve cells, nerve fibres and a supporting framework of dense fibro-elastic connective tissue, and forming a subsidiary nerve centre. 2. A mass of grey matter, *q.v.*, forming a structural and functional unit. 3. A localized swelling due to a chronic effusion within a tendon sheath occurring mainly on the wrist or back of the foot. **Cardiac** (ganglion of Wrisberg): a small g. situated in the thorax just anterior to the arch of the aorta. It contains fibres from the sympathetic and vagus nerves. **Ciliary** (lenticular g.): is a small quadrilateral body about the size of a large pin-head and is situated in the posterior part of the orbit. It is a g. of the parasympathetic division of the autonomic nervous system. **Compound palmar:** tuberculous tenosynovitis. **Diaphragmaticum:** a small g. situated on the deep aspect of the diaphragm just below the opening for the vena cava. It is the communication between the right phrenic nerve and the right phrenic sympathetic plexus. **Facial** (geniculate g.): an enlargement of the facial nerve and lies in the aqueduct of Falloppius in the temporal bone. **Gasserian** (trigeminal g.): a g. associated with the sensory root of the fifth cranial nerve; it lies on the superior surface of the apex of the petrous part of the temporal bone. **Geniculate:** see facial g. **Impar:** the small g. which constitutes the fusion of the chain of vertebral ganglia in front of the coccyx. **Inferior cervical:** is situated between the transverse process of the seventh cervical vertebra and the neck of the first rib. It forms part of the sympathetic chain in the neck. **Inferior, of vagus** (g. of the trunk): is the larger of the two ganglia of the vagus and is situated just below the jugular foramen. **Jugular:** superior g. on the glossopharyngeal nerve, situated in the superior part of the jugular foramen in the skull. **Lenticular:** see ciliary g. **Middle cervical:** is situated opposite the sixth cervical vertebra and is the smallest of the cervical ganglia. **Of Bochdalek:** a small g. on the middle superior dental branch of the maxillary nerve. **Of Corti** (spiral g.): situated in the spiral canal of the modiolus of the bony cochlea in the temporal bone of the skull. **Of Froriep:** a minute swelling on the hypoglossal nerve. **Of Meckel** (sphenopalatine): a small triangular body situated in the upper part of the pterygopalatine fossa close to the sphenopalatine foramen. **Of Scarpa** (vestibular): an enlargement of the vestibular part of the auditory nerve; it is situated in the internal auditory meatus. **Of Valentin:** a small swelling on the middle superior dental branch of the maxillary nerve where a communication takes place with the posterior superior dental branch of the maxillary. **Otic:** is a small oval body situated close to the foramen ovale on the deep surface of the mandibular nerve at the place of origin of the nerve to the pterygoid muscle. **Petrous:** a swelling on the glossopharyngeal nerve, it lies in the inferior part of the jugular foramen where it occupies a groove on the petrous portion of the temporal bone. **Phrenic:** a small enlargement on the termination of the phrenic nerve, it is situated on the diaphragm. **Sphenopalatine:** see g. of Meckel. **Spinal:** a swelling on the posterior root of the spinal nerves. The ganglion is situated in the intervertebral foramen. **Spiral:** see g. of Corti. **Splanchnic:** a small swelling on the right greater splanchnic nerve just before the nerve leaves the thorax. **Stellate:** the g. on the first thoracic sympathetic chain. **Submandibular** (submaxillary): is a small swelling connected with the lingual nerve in the submandibular region. **Superior cervical:** is part of the cervical portion of the sympathetic trunk. It is fusiform and more than an inch long. It is situated anterior to the transverse process of the second and third cervical vertebrae. **Superior mesenteric:** two ganglia situated in the superior mesenteric plexus of the sympathetic. **Superior, of vagus** (g. of the root): a small enlargement of the vagus nerve which is situated in the jugular foramen. **Trigeminal:** see Gasserian. **Vestibular:** see g. of Scarpa. **Wrisberg's:** see cardiac g.

gang·lionec·tomy (G. *gagglion*, a tumour; *ektomē*, excision). Excision of a ganglion.

gang·lioneuro·ma (G. *gagglion*, a tumour; *neuron*, nerve). A tumour composed of differentiated (mature) nerve cells occurring mainly in the sympathetic ganglionic chain or the adrenal medulla, rarely also in the central nervous system (especially the brain-stem).

ganglioneū·ron (G. *gagglion*, a tumour; *neuron*, nerve). A neuron the cell-body (nerve-cell) of which lies within the spinal or cerebral ganglia.

ganglion·ic (G. *gagglion*, a tumour). Ganglial, *q.v.*

ganglioni·tis (G. *gagglion*, a tumour). Inflammation of a ganglion (1).

Gangolphe's sign (Gangolphe, L., contemporary French surgeon). In intestinal obstruction, a serosanguineous effusion in the abdomen arising soon after strangulation has occurred.

gangō·sa (Sp. *gangoso*, speaking through the nose). A distinctive type of rhino-pharyngitis, probably always due to yaws.

gangrene (G. *gaggraina*, a gangrene). Necrosis of a part of the body, due to failure of arterial blood supply. **Diabetic g.:** gangrene occurring in arteriosclerotic diabetics. **Dry g.:** g. with exsiccation of the involved tissues. **Gas g.:** see under gas. **Moist g.**

g. in which liquefaction of tissues with or without gas-production is caused by the rapid growth of putrefacient micro-organisms; usually also characterized by destruction of venous as well as arterial blood flow, the venous stasis causing oedema of the affected part. **Senile g.:** g. due to arteriosclerosis of the involved parts.

gangrenes·cent. Tending to become gangrenous.

gang·renous (G. *gaggraina*, a gangrene). Relating to or characterized by gangrene.

Gant's line (Gant, F. J., English surgeon, 1825–1905). An imaginary line below the great trochanter, serving as a guide in section of the femur.

Gantzer's accessory bundle (Gantzer, C. F. L., German anatomist, qualified 1813). The muscle fibres joining the flexor pollicis longus, arising variably from the humerus or ulna. **G.'s muscle:** The musculus accessorius ad flexorem digitorum profundum—complete isolation of the normal junctional fibres between the superficial and deep flexors of the digits of the manus.

Gardiner-Brown's test (Gardiner-Brown, A., English otologist). In diseases of the labyrinth the bone conduction is not so good as normal.

Garel's sign (Garel, J., French physician, 1852–1931). Luminous perception by the eye on the sound side only when an electric light is placed within the mouth; seen in empyema or tumour of the antrum of Highmore.

gar·garism, gargaris·ma (G. *gargarizein*, to gargle). A gargle.

gar·gle. 1. To rinse the mouth and throat. 2. A solution for rinsing the mouth and throat.

gar·goylism. A congenital abnormality of the metabolism of one of the phospholipoids, characterized by a chondro-osteodystrophy with kyphosis, corneal opacities, hepatomegaly, and mental deficiency; so-called because of the resemblance of the facial features to those of a gargoyle. Syn. Hurler's disease.

Garland's S-curve (Garland, G. M., U.S. physician, 1848–1926). See Ellis's sign.

Garrod's test (1) (Garrod, Sir A. B., English physician. 1819–1907). For uric acid in the blood: take 30 cc. of serum and add 0·5 cc. of acetic acid, and immerse a fine thread. The thread becomes incrusted with uric acid crystals. This test is positive in gout.

Garrod's test (2) (Garrod, Sir A. E., English physician. 1857–1937). For haematoporphyrin in the urine: take 100 cc. of urine and add 20 cc. of a 10 per cent solution of caustic soda, and filter. Wash the filtrate, add absolute alcohol and enough hydrochloric acid to dissolve the precipitate. Examine with spectroscope for the two bands of haematoporphyrin.

gar·rot (Fr. *garrotter*, to pinion). A tourniquet, *q.v.*

garrot·ting. Killing by strangulation.

Gärtner's cyst (Gärtner, H. T., Danish anatomist, 1785–1827). A cystic tumour developed from G.'s duct. **G.'s duct:** a tubule extending from the broad ligament to the walls of the uterus and vagina during intra-uterine life, being a vestige of the main portion of the Wolffian duct.

gas (word invented by F. Van Helmont, Flemish chemist, 1577–1644, from G. *khaos*, chaos, the void). 1. An air-like fluid; especially applied to those substances which are normally uniform; those which can be readily condensed to liquids or normally in a liquid or solid state are called vapours. 2. Any gas used for producing general anaesthesia, particularly nitrous oxide. **G. bacilli:** *Clostridium Welchii, Cl. oedematiens, Cl. sporogenes, Cl. oedematis maligni.* **G. gangrene:** gangrene caused by infection of necrotic muscle with one of the gas bacilli, *q.v.*, characterized by rapid spread of subcutaneous emphysema and gangrene.

gā·seous. Of the nature of gas.

Gaskell's bridge (Gaskell, W. H., English physician, 1847–1914). The atrioventricular bundle. **G.'s nerves:** the accelerator nerves of the heart.

gassed. Injured or overcome by poisonous gas.

gasserec·tomy. Excision of the Gasserian ganglion, the ganglion of the sensory root of the fifth cranial nerve.

Gasserian ganglion (Gasser, J. L., Professor of Anatomy in Vienna, fl. 1757–65). The ganglion (ganglion semilunare of nervus trigeminus) was named *after* him and not *by* him. (The ganglion is sometimes said to have been named after A. P. Gasser, also a professor of Vienna, but was not named until 200 years after his time, 1505–77.)

gaster (G., belly). The stomach.

gastră·denītis (G. *gastēr*, stomach, *adēn*, gland). Inflammation of the stomach glands.

gas·tral (G. *gastēr*, stomach). Gastric.

gastral·gia (G. *gastēr*, stomach; *algos*, pain). Pain in the stomach.

gastratrō·phia (G. *gastēr*, stomach; *atrophia*, starvation). Atrophy of the stomach.

gastrectā·sia, gastrec·tasis (G. *gastēr*, stomach; *ektasis*, extension). Dilatation of the stomach.

gastrec·tomy (G. *gastēr*, stomach; *ektomē*, excision). Excision of the whole (total g.) or part (partial or sub-total g.) of the stomach.

gastric (G. *gastēr*, stomach). Relating to the stomach. **G. crisis:** paroxysmal epigastric pain with vomiting in tabes dorsalis. **G. influenza:** an imprecise term used to cover feverish conditions characterized by malaise with abdominal pain and/or vomiting and diarrhoea. **G. juice:** the secretion of the glands of the stomach, normally containing free hydrochloric acid, pepsin and Castle's intrinsic haemopoietic factor. **G. tetany:** tetany due to alkalosis, produced by continued loss of hydrochloric acid through vomiting or repeated gastric lavage, especially in pyloric stenosis. **G. ulcer:** acute or chronic disease, characterized by the formation of one or (less commonly) several ulcers of the mucous membrane (but when progressive involving the more external coats) of the stomach, situated commonly at the lesser curvature or near the pylorus.

gastrin (G. *gastēr*, stomach). Hormone in the pyloric glands of the stomach which excite secretion of the cells in the fundus.

gastrī·tis (G. *gastēr*, stomach). Inflammation of the gastric mucous membrane. **G., acute:** acute inflammation of the gastric mucous membrane, often associated with acute enteritis. **G., chronic:** chronic inflammation of the gastric mucous membrane, leading to either hypertrophy or atrophy of the mucous coat; in the latter case usually to decrease or loss of secretion of hydrochloric acid and sometimes of gastric enzymes. **G., phlegmonous:** a severe disease characterized by acute bacterial inflammation, starting in the submucous layer of the stomach.

gastro·anastomō·sis (G. *gastēr*, stomach; *anastomosis*, an opening). In hourglass contraction of the stomach, the formation of a communication between the pyloric and cardiac portions of the stomach.

gas·trocele (G. *gastēr*, stomach; *kēlē*, hernia). Hernia of the stomach.

gastrocnē·mius (G. *gastēr*, stomach; *knēme*, leg). A muscle in the calf of the leg.

gastrocŏl·ic (G. *gastēr*, stomach; *kŏlon*, colon). Relating to both stomach and colon.

gas·trocoloptō·sis (G. *gastēr*, stomach; *kŏlon*, colon; *ptosis*, a falling). Visceroptosis of stomach and colon.

gas·trocolŏ·stomy (G. *gastēr*, stomach; *kŏlon*, colon; *stoma*, mouth). The artificial formation of a communication between the stomach and the colon.

gas·trocolpŏ·tomy (G. *gastēr*, stomach; *kolpos*, womb; *tomē*, section). Caesarean section, incising through the linea alba into the upper part of the vagina.

gastrodĭ·dymus (G. *gastēr*, stomach; *didumos*, twin). A double monster, with one abdominal cavity.

gas·troduodē·nal (G. *gastēr*, stomach; L. *duodeni*, twelve each). Relating to both stomach and duodenum.

gas·troduodenī·tis (G. *gastēr*, stomach; L. *duodeni*, twelve each). Inflammation of mucous membranes of the stomach and duodenum.

gas·troduodenŏ·stomy (G. *gastēr*, stomach; L. *duodeni*, twelve each; G. *stoma*, mouth). The artificial formation of a communication between the stomach and duodenum.

gastrodў·nia (G. *gastēr*, stomach; *odunē*, pain). Stomach pain.

gastro-entĕ·ric (G. *gastēr*, stomach; *enteron*, intestine). Relating to both the stomach and intestine, especially the small intestine.

gastro·enterī·tis (G. *gastēr*, stomach; *enteron*, intestine). Acute, usually febrile, disease characterized by inflammation of the mucous membranes of stomach and small intestine, causing abdominal pain, nausea, diarrhoea; caused by food contaminated with pathogenic micro-organisms.

gastro·enterŏ·logy (G. *gastēr*, stomach; *enteron*, intestine; *logos*, treatise). That branch of medicine relating to diseases of the stomach and intestines.

gastro·enteroptō·sis (G. *gastēr*, stomach; *enteron*, intestine; *ptosis*, a falling). Downward displacement of the stomach and intestines.

gastro-enterŏ·stomy (G. *gastēr*, stomach; *enteron*, intestine; *stoma*, mouth). The artificial formation of a communication between the stomach and small intestine.

gastro-epiplō·ic (G. *gastēr*, stomach; *epiploon*, caul). Relating to both stomach and omentum.

gastrogastrŏ·stomy (G. *gastēr*, stomach; *stoma*, mouth). Gastro-anastomosis, *q.v.*

gastrŏ·genous (G. *gastēr*, stomach; *gennan*, to produce). Due to gastric function or dysfunction.

gas·trohelcō·sis (G. *gastēr*, stomach; *helkos*, ulcer). Ulceration of the stomach.

gas·trohepat·ic (G. *gastēr*, stomach; *hēpar*, liver). Relating to both stomach and liver.

gas·trohysterec·tomy (G. *gastēr*, stomach; *hustera*, womb; *ektomē*, excision). Abdominal hysterectomy; removal of the uterus through the abdominal wall.

gas·trohysterŏ·tomy (G. *gastēr*, stomach; *hustera*, womb; *tomē*, section). The Caesarean section; surgical delivery of the foetus by means of abdominal incision.

gastro-intĕ·stinal (G. *gastēr*, stomach; L. *intestinum*, an intestine). Relating to both stomach and intestines.

gastro·jĕ·junal (G. *gastēr*, stomach; L. *jejunus*, hunger). Relating to both the stomach and the jejunum.

gas·trojejunŏ·stomy (G. *gastēr*, stomach; L. *jejunus*, hunger; G. *stome*, mouth). The artificial formation of a direct communication between stomach and jejunum.

gas·trokinē·sograph (G. *gastēr*, stomach; *kinēsis*, motion; *graphein*, to write). A gastrograph. An apparatus for recording peristaltic movements of the stomach.

gas·trolith (G. *gastēr*, stomach; *lithos*, stone). A calcareous formation in the stomach.

gas·trolithī·asis (G. *gastēr*, stomach; *lithos*, stone). Morbid condition associated with the formation of gastroliths.

gastro·logy (G. *gastēr*, stomach; *logos*, treatise). That section of medicine relating to the stomach and its diseases.

gastro·lysis (G. *gastēr*, stomach; *luein*, to loosen). Division of adhesions between the stomach and adjacent viscera.

gastromalā·cia (G. *gastēr*, stomach; *malakia*, softness). Softening of the walls of the stomach.

gastromĕ·galy (G. *gastēr*, stomach; *mĕgas*, large). Enlarged stomach.

gastromĕ·lus (G. *gastēr*, stomach; *melos*, limb). A monster with one or two accessory limbs attached to the abdomen.

gas·tronephrī·tis (G. *gastēr*, stomach; *nephros*, kidney). Inflammation of both stomach and kidneys.

gastro-oesophagē·al (G. *gastēr*, stomach; *oisophagos*, gullet). Relating to both the stomach and oesophagus.

gas·tropară·lysis (G. *gastēr*, stomach; *paraluein*, to loosen). Paralysis of the stomach.

gastro·pathy (G. *gastēr*, stomach; *pathos*, disease). Any disease or disorder of the stomach.

gas·tropexis, gas·tropexy (G. *gastēr*, stomach; *pexis*, fixation). The surgical fixation of a displaced stomach to the abdominal wall.

gas·trophore (G. *gastēr*, stomach; *phoros*, bearing). An instrument for fixing the stomach during gastric operations.

gastrophrĕ·nic (G. *gastēr*, stomach; *phrēn*, diaphragm). Relating to both the stomach and diaphragm.

gas·troplasty (G. *gastēr*, stomach; *plassein*, to form). Plastic surgery of the stomach.

gastroplē·gia (G. *gastēr*, stomach; *plēgē*, stroke). Paralysis of the stomach.

gastroptō·sis (G. *gastēr*, stomach; *ptosis*, a falling). A downward displacement of the stomach.

gastrorrhā·gia (G. *gastēr*, stomach; *rhēgnunai*, a bursting forth). Gastric haemorrhage.

gastror·rhaphy (G. *gastēr*, stomach; *rhaphē*, suture). Suture of the stomach.

gastrorrhex·is (G. *gastēr*, stomach; *rhēxis*, rupture). Rupture of the stomach.

gastrorrhœ·a (G. *gastēr*, stomach; *rhoia*, flow). Hypersecretion of gastric juice.

gastro·schisis (G. *gastēr*, stomach; *skhisis*, a cleavage). Congenital deformity in which the abdominal cavity is open, due to defect in abdominal wall.

gas·troscope (G. *gastēr*, stomach; *skopein*, to view). An instrument for visual examination of the interior of the stomach, into which it is introduced via mouth and oesophagus.

gastro·scopy (G. *gastēr*, stomach; *skopein*, to view). Examination of the stomach by means of the gastroscope.

gastrosplĕ·nic (G. *gastēr*, stomach; *splēn*, spleen). Relating to both stomach and spleen.

gas·trostenō·sis (G. *gastēr*, stomach; *stenos*, narrow). Stricture of the stomach.

gastro·stomy (G. *gastēr*, stomach; *stoma*, mouth). The establishment of a fistulous opening into the stomach.

gas·trosuccorrhœ·a (G. *gastēr*, stomach; L. *succus*, juice; G. *rhoia*, flow). Hypersecretion of gastric juice.

gastro·tomy (G. *gastēr*, stomach; *tomē*, section). Incision of the stomach.

gas·trotrachelŏ·tomy (G. *gastēr*, abdomen; *trakhēlos*, neck; *tomē*, section). Opening the uterus and removing the foetus through a transverse incision of the cervix.

gas·trotympanī·tēs (G. *gastēr*, stomach; *tumpanon*, a drum). Gaseous distension of the stomach.

gas·trula (G. *gastēr*, stomach). The embryonic stage of development following the blastula when the embryo is composed of two cellular layers (epiblast and hypoblast).

gastrulā·tion (G. *gastēr*, stomach). The process of the formation of the gastrula.

gathering. A collection of pus beneath a surface.

Gaucher's disease (Gaucher, P. C. E., French physician, 1854–1918). An affection described by G. as 'primary epithelioma of the spleen', now regarded as a metabolic disorder in which a lipoid (kerasin) is deposited in large cells in the spleen.

gaulthē·ria oil. Oil of wintergreen obtained from the tree *Gaultheria procumbens.*

gauntlet. A bandage covering the hand and fingers like a glove.

gauze. A thin open-meshed cloth used for surgical purposes. **Antiseptic g.:** g. impregnated with an antiseptic substance.

gă·vage (Fr.). Feeding through a stomach tube.

Gavard's muscle (Gavard, H., French anatomist, 1753–1802). Oblique fibres in the muscular coat of the stomach.

Gay's glands (Gay, A. H., Austrian anatomist, 1842–1907). The circumanal glands.

Gay-Lussac's law (Gay-Lussac, J. L., French naturalist, 1778–1850). Same as Charles's law in physics.

Gee's disease (Gee, S. J., English physician, 1839–1911). Coeliac disease, *q.v.*

Gegenbaur's cells (Gegenbaur, C., German anatomist, 1826–1903). Osteoblasts.

Geigel's reflex (Geigel, R., German physician, 1859–1930). The inguinal reflex in the female, corresponding to the cremasteric reflex in the male.

Geiger-Müller counter. Instrument for detecting and counting charged particles emitted from a radioactive source.

gel. See under colloid.

gĕ·latin, gĕ·latine (L. *gelare*, to congeal). A protein substance obtained by boiling connective tissues in water, forming a jelly on cooling and becoming hard and flexible when dry.

gelā·tinous. Having the nature of or resembling gelatine.

gelā·tion (1). Formation of a gel.

gelā·tion (2). (L. *gelatio*, frost). 1. Freezing. 2. Frostbite.

Gellé's test (Gellé, M. E., French ear specialist, 1834–1923). Tuning-fork test for diseases of the auditory ossicles.

Gély's suture (Gély, J. A., French surgeon, 1806–61). An intestinal suture of thread.

gĕ·mellary (L. *gemellus*, twin). Relating to twins; paired.

gemel·lus. (L.) See under muscles.

gĕ·minate, gĕ·minous (L. *gemini*, twins). In pairs; relating to twin formation.

gemmā·tion (L. *gemmare*, to bud). Budding; a form of reproduction in certain micro-organisms.

gĕ·na (L., cheek). The cheek.

gene (G. *gennan*, to produce). A chromosomal factor reproduced at each cell division and carrying a hereditarily transmissible character. **Genes, multiplex:** applied to genes which, although present in different chromosomes, produce similar effects.

general. Common to a class; diffuse. **G. anatomy:** anatomy of the tissues in general, distinguished from that dealing with special organs. **G. paralysis of the insane:** see paralysis, g., of the insane. **G. pathology:** pathology of the tissues in general, as distinguished from that dealing with special organs.

generalize. To make general; to spread.

gĕ·nerate (L. *generare*, to beget). To produce offspring; to originate.

generā·tion. 1. The act of producing offspring. 2. A period extending from the birth of an individual to the birth of his offspring, usually reckoned at 30 years. 3. Formation.

gĕ·nerative (L. *generare*, to beget). Relating to generation.

genĕ·ric (L. *genus*, race, stock). 1. Relating to the same genus. 2. General.

gĕ·nesis (G.). Origin; formation.

genet·ic (G. *genesis*, production). 1. Pertaining to development. 2. Pertaining to genes or genetics.

genet·ics (G. *genesis*, production). That section of biology relating to the process and characters of inheritance.

genī·al (G. *geneion*, chin). Relating to the chin.

geni·culate (L. *geniculatus*, bent, from *genu*, knee). Bent abruptly, as the bent knee. **G. bodies:** four protuberances on the posterior end of the thalamus, the medial g. bodies receiving fibres from the inferior corpora quadrigemina and from the lateral lemniscus, and sending axons to the cortex of the temporal lobes; the lateral g. bodies receiving the optic tract fibres from the superior corpora quadrigemina. Syn. the metathalamus.

genioglos·sal (G. *geneion*, chin; *glōssa*, tongue). Relating to both the chin and the tongue.

genioglos·sus. See under muscles.

geniohӯ·oid. See under muscles.

geni·on (G. *geneion*, chin). 1. The chin. 2. In craniometry, the apex of the lower genial tubercle.

gĕ·nioplasty (G. *geneion*, chin; *plassein*, to form). Plastic operation on chin.

gĕ·nital (L. *genitalis*, generative). Relating to the genitalia or to generation.

genitā·lia, gĕ·nitals (L. *genitalis*, generative). The organs of generation.

gĕ·nitofĕ·moral (L. *genitalis*, generative; *femur*, thigh). Relating to both the genitalia and the thigh.

gĕ·nito·ū·rinary (L. *genitalis*, generative; *urina*, urine). Relating to the genitalia and to the urinary organs.

gĕ·nius (L.). An inborn dominant and distinctive power.

Gennari's band, line or layer (Gennari, F., Italian anatomist of the 18th century). The outer band of Baillarger, *q.v.*

gĕ·noblast (G. *gennan*, to produce; *blastos*, germ). The nucleus of the fertilized ovum, supposedly bisexual.

gĕ·notype (G. *genos*, race, stock; *tupos*, model). A type determined, i.e. transmitted, by a gene or genes.

gen·tian. The common name for plants of the genus Gentiana, yielding an excellent bitter tonic and stomachic.

gĕ·nu (L.). 1. The knee. 2. Any structure bent like the knee. **G. recurvatum:** backward curvature of the leg at the knee joint, caused by paresis of the flexor muscles, or slackness of the posterior wall of the articular capsule. **G. valgum:** knock-knee, knee curved inwards. **G. varum:** bowed leg, knee curved outwards.

gĕ·nuclast (L. *genu*, knee; G. *klaein*, to break). A surgical instrument used in the removal of knee joint adhesions.

gĕ·nuflex (L. *genu*, knee; *flexus*, a bending). Bent at the knee, or bent like the knee.

genupec·toral (L. *genu*, knee; *pectus*, breast). Relating to the posture in which the patient rests upon the knees and the chest.

genus (L., race, stock; pl. *genera*). A group of living organisms with common morphological or phylogenetic characteristics; usually comprising several species.

gĕ·nyantri·tis (G. *genus*, jaw; *antron*, cave). Inflammation of the antrum of Highmore.

Geocyclus. A genus of schizomycetes.

gĕŏ·phagism (G. *gē*, earth; *phagein*, to eat). The eating of earth. Hence, **geophagist,** a habitual earth eater.

Georget's stupidity. A state of simple mental confusion unaccompanied by hallucination.

gĕrat·ic (G. *gēras*, old age). Relating to old age.

geratŏ·logy, gerĕŏ·logy (G. *gēras*, old age; *logos*, a discourse). That branch of medicine which relates to old age.

Gerdy's fibres (Gerdy, P. N., French pathologist and surgeon, 1797–1856). The sparse inconstant superficial transverse ligaments of the fingers. **G.'s ligament:** the lower part of the clavipectoral fascia which joins the axillary fascia.

Gerhardt's sign (Gerhardt, C., German physician, 1883–1903). A systolic murmur heard between the mastoid process and the vertebral column in aneurysm of the vertebral artery.

Gerhardt's test (Gerhardt, C. F., French chemist, 1816–56). For urobilin. Take some urine and shake with chloroform to extract urobilin. Take extract and add some iodine solution and a solution of caustic potash. If urobilin is present a green fluorescence will appear.

geria·trics (G. *gēras*, old age; *iatrikē*, medicine). That branch of medicine that relates to the diseases of old age.

Gerlach's valve (Gerlach, J. von, Professor of Anatomy and Physiology in Erlangen, 1820–96). An occasional fold of mucous membrane which guards the opening of the apendix into the caecum.

Gerlier's disease (Gerlier, F., Swiss physician, 1840–1914). Paralysing vertigo, an endemic disease characterized by vertigo, ptosis, paresis of the extremities, pains in the head and neck and severe depression.

germ (L. *germen*, a sprout). 1. A spore or seed; an embryo in its early stage. 2. A microbe.

German measles. See under rubella.

Germanin. See suramin.

germicī·dal (L. *germen*, a sprout; *caedere*, to destroy). Destroying germs.

ger·micide (L. *germen*, a sprout; *caedere*, to destroy). An agent capable of destroying germs.

ger·miculture (L. *germen*, a sprout; *cultura*, from *colere*, to tend). The artificial growing of germs.

ger·mifuge (L. *germen*, a sprout; *fugare*, to dispel). An agent capable of expelling germs.

ger·minal (L. *germen*, a sprout). Relating to a germ or to the development of an embryo, an organ or tissue.

germinā·tion (L. *germinatio*, a budding). 1. The development or budding of a seed or spore. 2. The development of an embryo from an impregnated ovum.

ger·minative (L. *germinatio*, a budding). Relating to germination.

geroder·ma (G. *gerōn*, old man; *derma*, skin). Atrophy of the skin, as in old age.

geromor·phism (G. *gēras*, old age; *morphē*, form). Condition of premature old age.

geron·tic (G. *gerōn*, old man). Relating to old age.

gerontŏ·logy (G. *gerōn*, old man; *logos*, a discourse). The branch of medical science relating to old age.

gerontox·on (G. *gerōn*, old man; *toxon*, bow). The arcus senilis.

Gerota's capsule (Gerota, D., Roumanian surgeon, 1867–1939). The fascia renis.

Gersuny's symptom (Gersuny, R., Austrian surgeon, 1844–1924). A sensation of adhesion of the mucosa of the bowel to the faecal mass when pressure is applied with the tips of the fingers. It is noted in cases of constipation.

gestalt (Ger.). Form; figure; shape; pattern. In psychology structures or phenomena conceived as whole (organized or functional) units, i.e. the effect or behaviour the qualities of which are not determined by that/those of their individual elements. **G. theory:** psychological theory according to which all mental experience is derived from, or presents itself in the form of, wholes (organized or functional units), i.e. not from the separation of isolated elements—such wholes when relatively incomplete tending to be 'automatically' completed.

gestā·tion (L. *gestare*, to carry). Pregnancy.

geūmaphō·bia (G. *geuma*, taste; *phobos*, fear). Neurotic fear of tastes.

ghatti gum. A gum derived from the Indian tree, *Anogeissus latifolia*, and used for the same purpose as acacia.

Ghon-Sachs bacillus. *Clostridium septicum.*

Giacomini's band (Giacomini, C., Italian anatomist, 1840–98). The terminal part of the dentate gyrus of the brain.

giant. A person of exceptionally large size. **G. cell:** a multinuclear cell formed by fusion of two or more macrophages or by nuclear division of the cell body, a characteristic element of granulomatous tissue, also found around foreign bodies or sites of haemorrhage (in these cases they are characterized by peripherally arranged nuclei. Syn. Langhan's g.c.); in rheumatic nodules (Aschoff's cells); in tissues affected by Hodgkin's disease (Sternberg-Dorothy Reed cells); finally the typical cell in osteoclastoma (g.c. tumour of bone). **G. cell sarcoma, G. cell tumour:** Osteoclastoma, *q.v.*

giantism. Gigantism, *q.v.*

Giannuzzi's cells (Giannuzzi, Italian anatomist of the 19th century). Small flattened granular cells with a spherical nucleus, found in the submaxillary and parotid glands of the dog and rabbit; demilune cells.

Giardia Lamblia (Giard, A., French biologist, 1896–1908; Lambl, W. D., Austrian physician, 1824–1895). A species of flagellata, parasitic in the small intestine of man, infection taking place by ingestion of food contaminated by the parasite in its cyst stage; sometimes causing a form of dysentery or steatorrhoea. Syn. *G. intestinalis.*

giardi·asis. Infestation with *Giardia Lamblia.*

Gibbon's hernia (Gibbon, E., English historian, 1737–94, who suffered from this complaint). A large inguinal hernia associated with a hydrocele.

gibbŏ·sity (L. *gibber*, hump). The state of being hump-backed.

gib·bous (L. *gibbus*, hump-backed). Humpbacked.

gibbus (L., hump-backed). 1. A hump. 2. An angular kyphosis.

Gibert's disease (Gibert, C. M., French physician, 1797–1866). Pityriasis rosea.

Gibson's bandage (Gibson, W., U.S., surgeon, 1788–1865). A bandage used in cases of fracture of the lower jaw.

Gibson's rule (Gibson, A., British physician, 1854–1913). In cases of lobar pneumonia if the systolic blood pressure (in mm. of Hg.) falls below the pulse rate per minute, the prognosis is bad.

gid·diness. Sensation of whirling or unsteadiness of the body. See also under vertigo.

Giemsa's stain (Giemsa, G., German bacteriologist, born 1867). A compound of Azur II eosin, anhydrous glycerin and absolute methyl alcohol. Used in haematology and as a stain for inclusion bodies, *q.v.*

Gierke's corpuscles (Gierke, H. P., German anatomist, 1847–86). Roundish colloid bodies, sometimes found in the central nervous system. They appear to be identical with Hassall's corpuscles. **G.'s respiratory bundles:** tractus solitarius.

Gierke's disease (Gierke, E. von, German pathologist, born 1877). See glycogen disease.

Gifford's reflex (Gifford, H., American oculist, 1858–1929). The contraction of the pupil which occurs when an endeavour is made to close the lids, the patient attempting to keep them open. **G.'s sign:** in early cases of Graves' disease the patient cannot evert the upper eyelid.

gigant·ism (G. *gigas*, giant). Abnormal overgrowth of the whole or part of the body.

gigan·toblast (G. *gigas*, giant; *blastos*, germ). A large nucleated red blood corpuscle.

gigan·tocyte (G. *gigas*, giant; *kutos*, container). A large non-nucleated red blood corpuscle.

gigantosō·ma (G. *gigas*, giant; *sōma*, body). Gigantism.

Gigli's operation (Gigli, L., Italian gynaecologist, 1863–1908). Pubiotomy. **G.'s saw:** a chain saw used in G.'s operation.

Gilbert's sign (Gilbert, N. A., French physician, 1858–1927). In hepatic cirrhosis the urine is excreted more quickly during a fast than after a meal.

gilbert (Gilbert, W., English physicist, 1544–1603). The unit of magnetomotive force; its symbol is F.

Gilchristia dermatitidis (Gilchrist, T. C., American dermatologist, 1862–1927). A species of tissue-invading blastomycotic fungi, the organism causing American blastomycosis.

gill. One of the respiratory organs of animals breathing in water.

gill or **gille** (Old Fr. *gille*). One-fourth of a pint.

Gilles de la Tourette's disease (Gilles de la Tourette, G., French physician, 1857–1904). A form of tic with motor incoordination, echolalia and coprolalia. **G.'s sign:** inversion of the ratio existing normally between the earth phosphates and alkaline phosphates in urine; found in paroxysms of hysteria.

Gillette's suspensory ligament (Gillette, E. P., French surgeon, 1836–86). The longitudinal fibres of the oesophagus passing to the posterior aspect of the larynx—suspensory ligament of the oesophagus.

Gimbernat's ligament (Gimbernat, A. de, Spanish surgeon, 1742–90). Pectineal part of the inguinal ligament. Syn. lacunar ligament.

gin. Common grain spirit distilled with juniper berries.

ginger. The dried rhizome (scraped) of *Zingiber officinale*. Ginger is carminative in its action and the tincture is useful in relieving acute flatulent distension or colic.

gin·gĭva (L., gum). The vascular tissue surrounding the necks of the teeth and covering the alveoli.

gin·gival (L. *gingiva*, gum). Relating to the gum. **G. line:** a line along the teeth-bearing gums seen in chronic metallic poisoning, as the blue line in lead poisoning.

gingivī·tis (L. *gingiva*, gum). Inflammation of the gums.

gin·givoglossī·tis (L. *gingiva*, gum; G. *glossa*, tongue). Inflammation of both the gums and the tongue.

ging·lymoid (G. *gigglumos*, hinge-joint; *eidos*, form). Resembling a hinge joint.

ginglymus (G. *gigglumos*, a hinge-joint). A hinge joint. Syn. diarthrosis.

Giovannini's disease (Giovannini, S., Italian dermatologist, 1851–1920). A rare nodular disease of the hair caused by a fungus; a fungus form of monilethrix.

Giraldès's bonnet à poil (Giraldès, J. A., Portuguese surgeon, 1808–75). Widening of the frontal part of the cranium; seen in chronic hydrocephalus. **G.'s organ:** the paradidymis, a small tube-like organ situated at the junction of the spermatic cord and epididymis. It corresponds to the female parovarium.

girdle. A band to go around the body. **G. anaesthesia:** an anaesthetic ring around the body. **G. pain:** or **G. sensation:** the sensation of constriction around the abdomen, or some other part, as in tabes dorsalis and other spinal cord diseases.

Girdner's probe (Girdner, J. H., American physician, 1856–1933). Used in war surgery. A metal probe is attached to one end of a telephone wire, the other end of the wire is fixed to a metal disc. The disc is placed on the skin. If the probe comes into contact with a bullet in the body, the surgeon hears a click in the receiver.

Giuffrida-Ruggieri stigma of degeneration (Giuffrida-Ruggieri, V., Italian anthropologist, 1872–1922). Absence or incompleteness of the glenoid fossa.

glabel·la, glabel·lum (L. *glaber*, bald). A point midway between the two supra-orbital ridges; the convex part of the forehead immediately above the nasal root.

glabrificā·tion (L. *glaber*, smooth; *facere*, to make). The process of becoming smooth and hairless.

glā·brous (L. *glaber*, smooth). Smooth; hairless.

glā·cial (L. *glacies*, ice). Icy; ice-like. **G. acetic acid:** concentrated acetic acid, so-called because it forms ice-like crystals at room temperature.

glā·diate (L. *gladius*, sword). Shaped like a sword.

glā·diōlus. The second or middle part of the sternum.

glair (Old Fr. *glaire*, white of egg). The white of egg, or matter resembling this in viscosity and appearance.

glairy (Old Fr. *glaire*, white of egg). Viscous; mucoid.

gland (L. *glans*, acorn). A secreting organ formed in the embryo by invagination of the epithelial surfaces of the mucous membranes, classified according to form of invagination into tubular, alveolar (or saccular), and tubulo-alveolar (or racemose) types, and into simple, convoluted, branched and compound sub-types. **Adrenal g.** (suprarenal): are two in number and are situated, one on each side, in the epigastric region. They are compressed from before backwards, broad from side to side, and set upon the superior extremity of the corresponding kidney, to which they are bound by connective tissue. **Bartholin's g.:** racemose or acino-tubular gland. Two in number and are variable in size. They lie on each side of the external orifice of the vagina. They lie in the same anatomical plane as the corresponding glands (Cowper's glands) in the male. **G. of Blandin:** anterior lingual glands situated beneath the apex of the tongue. (See glands of Nuhn.) **Bowman's g.:** nasal glands. Found in the olfactory mucous membrane. **Brunner's g.** (duodenal glands): are confined to the duodenum, and are serially continuous with the pyloric glands of the stomach. **Buccal g.:** mucous glands situated between the mucous membrane of the cheek and the deep surface of the buccinator muscle. **Bulbo-urethral g.** (Cowper's): are two in number, right and left. They are situated above the perineal membrane and the bulb, lying slightly posterior to the urethra. **Ceruminous g.:** situated in the skin of the external auditory meatus. They are convoluted tubular glands, similar in structure to sweat glands and they secrete the earwax. **Ciliary g.** (Glands of Moll): modified sweat glands situated in the eyelids at the attachment of the eyelashes. **Cloquet's g.:** lymphatic gland lying in the femoral ring and draining the external urinary meatus. **Cowper's g.:** see bulbo-urethral glands. **Duodenal g.:** see Brunner's glands. **Ebner's g.:** acinous glands found in the tongue in the region of the vallate papillae. **Endocrine g. or g., ductless:** a g. containing secreting epithelium in a more or less distinct tubular arrangement, having no excretory duct, the specific product (hormone) being directly secreted into the blood. **Excretory g.:** a g. having a duct conveying the secretion to the free surface of the mucous membrane. **Gastric g.:** mucous glands of the stomach. They are of two kinds, cardiac and pyloric. **Greater vestibular g.:** Bartholin's glands. **Haemal g.:** small glands scattered among the tissue covering the thymus. **Haversian g.:** the so-called Haversian gland which occupies the acetabular fossa. It is simply a mass of fat invested by the ligament of the head of the femur and the synovial membrane. **Intestinal g.:** crypts of Lieberkühn. Simple tubular glands found in large numbers over the whole of the mucous membrane of the small intestine, as well as that of the large bowel. **Labial g.:** mucous glands situated on the deep surface of the mucous membrane of the lips, where they lie in the mucous membrane and the orbicularis oris muscle. **Lacrimal g.:** small disc-shaped gland situated in the anterior and lateral part of the orbit. It secretes the tears. **Littre's g.:** urethral glands; compound mucous glands situated in the mucous membrane of the urethra. **Mammary g.:** a compound racemose gland, composed of 15 to 20 lobes, each representing a number of lobules. It is situated on the front of the chest. **Meibomian g.:** tarsal glands. Modified sebaceous glands situated on the deep surface of each tarsus and lying between the plate and the conjunctiva. Their secretion lubricates the margins of the eyelids, and prevents them from adhering. **Molar g.:** molar mucous glands lie both superficial and deep to the buccinator muscle in the vicinity of the terminal part of the parotid duct. **G. of Moll:** ciliary glands. Modified sweat glands in the eyelids. **Nasal g.:** see Bowman's glands. **G. of Nuhn:** anterior lingual glands; see glands of Blandin. **Parathyroid g.:** four in number and arranged in pairs. The upper pair are related to the dorsal borders of the lobes of the thyroid gland, and the lower pair are placed posterior to the inferior ends of the lobes. **Parotid g.:** salivary gland situated in the space between the ramus of the mandible anteriorly, the sternomastoid muscle posteriorly, the styloid process medially, and the articular eminence and the root of the zygoma superiorly. **Prostate g.:** gland surrounding the neck of the urinary bladder and related to the first inch of the urethra. **Sublingual g.:** smallest of the salivary glands, and resembles an almond in shape. It is situated beneath the mucous membrane of the floor of the mouth. **Submandibular g.:** submaxillary gland. Salivary gland situated in the anterior part of the digastric triangle of the neck. **Submaxillary g.:** see submandibular gland. **Suprarenal g.:** see adrenal gland. **Tarsal g.:** see meibomian gland. **Thymus g.:** ductless gland situated in the anterior mediastinum. Attains its full size at about two years, after which it gradually shrinks away. **Thyroid g.:** ductless gland situated in the neck. Its size is subject to much variation. It weighs about an ounce. **Urethral g.:** glands of Littre. Compound mucous glands in the mucous membrane of the urethra. **G. of uterus:** utricular glands. Mucous glands in the mucous membrane of the cavity of the body of the uterus. **Weber's g.:** mucous glands in the tongue.

glanders. An acute or chronic contagious disease of the horse, ass, guinea-pig, cat and dog, communicable to man, in whom it is characterized by inflammatory purulent lesions, especially of the nasal mucous membranes and subcutaneous tissues. It is caused by the *Malleomyces mallei*. See also farcy.

glandilem·ma (L. *glans*, acorn; G. *lemma*, husk). The capsule of a gland.

glandiform (L. *glans*, acorn; *forma*, shape). 1. Acorn-shaped. 2. Adenoid.

glan·dula, glan·dule (L. *glandulae* (pl.), dim. of *glans*). A small gland.

glan·dular (L. *glandulae*, small glands). Relating to a gland or of the nature of a gland. **G. fever:** see under mononucleosis, infectious.

glans (L.). The bulbous extremity of the penis or of the clitoris.

Glaser's artery (Glaser, J. H., Swiss anatomist and botanist, 1629–75). The tympanic artery. **G.'s fissure:** the glenoid fissure, which divides the glenoid fossa of the temporal bone.

glass. A brittle, transparent substance consisting of fused sand and soda or potash (or both) and other materials.

glassy. Resembling glass; vitreous; hyaline.

Glauber's salt (Glauber, J. R., German physician and chemist, 1604–68). Sodium sulphate decahydrate, $Na_2SO_4 + 10H_2O$.

glaucō·ma (G. *glaukos*, grey-green). A disease of the eye characterized by increased intra-ocular pressure, resulting in hardness of the globe, excavation ('cupping') of the optic disc, restriction of the field of vision, corneal anaesthesia, coloured halo about lights, and a lessening of the visual power that may result in blindness; due either to increased production of aqueous humour with normal or decreased outflow (at the angle of the anterior chamber) or to decrease in outflow with normal or increased inflow of aqueous humour.

gleet. Chronic urethritis, marked by a slight mucopurulent discharge.

gleety. Resembling or relating to gleet.

Glénard's disease (Glénard, F., French physician, 1848–1920). Enteroptosis.

glenohū·meral (G. *glēnē*, socket; L. *humerus*, shoulder). Relating to the glenoid cavity of the scapula and the humerus.

glē·noid (G. *glēnē*, socket; *eidos*, form). Having, or resembling a shallow cavity or socket; e.g., **G. cavity:** the depression in the scapula articulating with the head of the humerus.

Gley's glands (Gley, M. E. E., French physiologist, 1857–1930). The parathyroid glands.

glī·a (G., glue). The interstitial tissues of the central nervous system. Syn. neuroglia.

glī·al. Relating to glia.

glī·obactē·ria (G. *glia*, glue; *bakterion*, little stick). Bacteria embedded in a gelatinous substance, zooglea.

glī·oblastō·ma multiforme (G. *glia*, glue; *blastos*, germ; L. *multiformis*, many-shaped). Spongioblastoma multiforme, *q.v.*

gliocytō·ma (G. *glia*, glue; *kutos*, cell). A cerebral tumour composed of relatively mature glial elements, i.e. astrocytes, oligodendrocytes.

gliō·ma (G. *glia*, glue). A tumour of the central nervous system, originating from neuroglial cells (astrocytes or ependymal cells) or their precursors, classified as astrocytoma, medulloblastoma, ependymoblastoma, oligodendroglioma, medullo-epithelioma, and mixed glioma.

gliomatō·sis (G. *glia*, glue). Proliferation of neuroglia, replacing the nerve-cell tissue.

gliō·matous (G. *glia*, glue). Relating to 1. glioma, and 2. gliomatosis.

glī·omyō·ma (G. *glia*, glue; *mus*, muscle). Combined glioma and myoma.

glī·omyxō·ma (G. *glia*, glue; *muxa*, mucus). A glioma accompanied by mucoid degeneration.

glī·oneurō·ma (G. *glia*, glue; *neuron*, nerve). Neuroglioma, *q.v.*

gliō·sa (G. *glia*, glue). The grey matter of the spinal cord situated around the head of the dorsal horn and the central canal.

glī·osarcō·ma (G. *glia*, glue; *sarx*, flesh). A tumour consisting of the neuroglia cells of glioma and the fusiform cells of sarcoma.

gliō·sis (G. *glia*, glue). Gliomatosis, *q.v.*

glī·osome (G. *glia*, glue; *sōmă*, body). An astrocytal granule.

glis·chrin. A nitrogenous type of mucus produced in the urine by the presence of *Bact. gliscrogenum.*

glischrū·ria. Glischrin in the urine.

Glisson's capsule (Glisson, F., English physician and anatomist, 1597–1677). The connective tissue of the liver which enfolds the portal vein, hepatic artery and hepatic duct. **G.'s sphincter:** the sphincter of Oddi of the bile duct.

glissoni·tis. Inflammation of Glisson's capsule.

globate (L. *globus*, sphere). Of a globe; shaped like a globe.

globe (L. *globus*, sphere). The globe of the eye; the eyeball.

globin. A constituent of haemoglobin; a histone.

globinŏ·meter (L. *globus*, globe; G. *metron*, measure). An instrument for determining the percentage of oxyhaemoglobin present in a given quantity of blood.

glŏ·bular (L. *globulus*, a globule). Of a globe-like form.

glŏ·bule (L. *globulus*). 1. A small more or less spherical structure, such as a blood corpuscle. 2. A small pill.

glŏ·bulin (L. *globulus*, a globule). A protein coagulated by heat, insoluble in water, soluble in diluted solutions of salts of strong bases and acids. Globulins have approximately spherical molecules.

glŏ·bulinū·ria (L. *globulus*, a globule; G. *ouron*, urine). The presence of globulins in the urine.

glŏ·bulism. Homeopathy.

glŏ·bus (L., globe). A ball or globe. **G. hystericus:** the neurotic sensation of having a lump in the throat. **G. pallidus:** the medial portion of the lenticular nucleus of the corpus striatum; so-called because of its paler tint as compared with the lateral portion.

glomangiō·ma. See glomus tumour.

glŏ·merate (L. *glomerare*, to form into a ball). Rolled together like a coil of thread.

glomĕ·rular (L. *glomus*, a ball of thread, etc.). Relating to a glomerule.

glomĕ·rule, glomĕ·rulus (L. *glomus*, a ball of thread, etc.). 1. A small rounded mass. 2. A spherical coil of capillary vessels in the renal cortex, invaginated into the end of a uriniferous tubule (Bowman's capsule). About 800,000 to 1,000,000 glomerules are contained in a normal kidney in man; this glomerular apparatus serves to produce a protein-free filtrate of the blood which is converted chiefly into urine by subsequent re-absorption of water and certain solutes by the epithelium of the renal tubules. Other names for Bowman's capsule are: renal capsule; Malpighian body.

glomerulī·tis (L. *glomus*, a ball of thread, etc.). Inflammation of the glomerules of the kidney.

glomĕ·rulonephrī·tis (L. *glomus*, a ball of thread, etc.). G. *nĕphros*, kidney). See nephritis.

glŏ·mus (L., a ball of thread, etc.). 1. A coil. 2. A small conglomeration of minute arterioles and venules. 3. The glomerule of the primitive embryonic kidney (pronephron). 4. The part of the choroid plexus covering the optic thalamus. **G., caroticum:** a structure situated at the bifurcation of the common carotid artery, containing chromaffine cells, non-medullated nerve fibres and blood vessels belonging to the chromaffine system, *q.v.* **G. cell:** cell surrounding the arterio-venous channels in the skin of extremities, especially of the fingers and toes. **Coccygeal g.:** a structure situated at the tip of the coccyx, belonging to the chromaffine system. **G. tumour:** a small, benign, exquisitely tender, purplish tumour composed of minute blood vessels surrounded by plain muscle and epithelial cells, non-medullated nerve fibres arising from peripheral anastomoses between arterioles and venules, occurring mostly under a finger or toenail or, more rarely, on the skin of a limb.

glos·sa (G., tongue). The tongue.

glos·sal (G. *glōssa*, tongue). Relating to the tongue.

glossal·gia (G. *glōssa*, tongue; *algos*, pain). Any pain in the tongue.

glossec·tomy (G. *glōssa*, tongue; *ektomē*, excision). Amputation or excision of the tongue.

Glossī·na (G. *glōssa*, tongue). A genus of blood-sucking flies, of the family Muscidae (tsetse flies). **G. morsitans**: species of G., the usual vector of *Trypanosoma brucei*, the organism causing nagana. **G. rhodesiensis**: species of G., vector of *Trypanosoma rhodesiense*, the organism causing sleeping sickness in Rhodesia.

glossi·tis (G. *glōssa*, tongue). Inflammation of the tongue.

glos·socele (G. *glōssa*, tongue; *kele*, tumour). Swelling of the tongue due to oedema.

glosso-epiglottidě·an (G. *glōssa*, tongue; *epi*, on; *glottis*). Pertaining to both tongue and epiglottis.

glos·sograph (G. *glōssa*, tongue; *graphein*, to write). An instrument for recording the movements of the tongue.

glossohȳ·al, glossohȳ·oid (G. *glōssa*, tongue; *huoeidēs*, shaped like the letter Y). Relating to both tongue and hyoid bone.

glos·soid (G. *glōssa*, tongue; *eidos*, form). Resembling a tongue.

glossŏ·logy (G. *glōssa*, tongue; *logos*, a discourse). A book concerning nomenclature.

glossŏ·lysis (G. *glōssa*, tongue; *luein*, to loosen). Paralysis of the tongue.

glosson·cus (G. *glōssa*, tongue; *ogkos*, tumour). Swelling of the tongue.

glossopǎ·latine (G. *glōssa*, tongue; *pǎlātum*, palate). Relating to both the tongue and the palate.

glos·sopalati·nus (G. *glōssa*, tongue; L. *pǎlātum*, palate). See palatoglossus muscle.

glossŏ·pathy (G. *glōssa*, tongue; *pathos*, disease). Any disease of the tongue.

glos·sopharyngē·al (G. *glōssa*, tongue; *pharugx*, pharynx). 1. Relating to the tongue and the pharynx. 2. Relating to the glossopharyngeal or ninth cranial nerve.

glos·soplasty (G. *glōssa*, tongue; *plassein*, to form). Plastic surgery applied to the tongue.

glossoplē·gia (G. *glōssa*, tongue; *plēgē*, stroke). Paralysis of the tongue.

glossoptō·sis (G. *glōssa*, tongue; *ptōsis*, a fall). Displacement downwards of the tongue.

glossor·rhaphy (G. *glōssa*, tongue; *rhaphē*, suture). Suturing of the tongue.

glos·sospasm (G. *glōssa*, tongue; *spasmos*, spasm). Spasm of the tongue.

glossŏ·tomy (G. *glōssa*, tongue; *tomē*, section). Surgical incision into the tongue.

glossotri·chia (G. *glōssa*, tongue; *thrix*, hair). Hairy tongue.

glossy skin. A painful condition of the skin, usually of the digits, characterized by atrophy and shiny appearance of the skin.

glot·tic (G. *glōttis*). Relating to the glottis.

glot·tis (G.). 1. The vocal apparatus of the larynx. 2. The rima glottidis, the space between the right and left arytenoid cartilages and the vocal cords. 3. The structures around this space.

glover's stitch or suture. A form of continuous wound suture.

glucae·mia, glycae·mia (G. *glukus*, sweet; *haima*, blood). Condition in which sugar is present in the blood.

glū·cide (G. *glukus*, sweet). A term comprising the carbohydrates and glucosides; an organic substance consisting wholly or partly of sugars.

glucohae·mia (G. *glukus*, sweet; *haima*, blood). Condition in which sugar is present in the blood.

glucŏ·lysis (G. *glukus*, sweet; *luein*, to loosen). Enzymatic decomposition of glucose and other sugars.

glū·conē·ogě·nesis (G. *glukus*, sweet; *neos*, new; *genesis*, production). Formation of glucose from non-carbohydrate substances.

glucŏ·nic acid (G. *glukus*, sweet). $C_6H_{12}O_7$. Formed by the oxidation of glucose.

glū·coprŏ·tein (G. *glukus*, sweet; *prōtos*, first). Group of proteins containing a carbohydrate radical and a simple protein (conjugated proteins); e.g., mucin.

glucosǎ·mine (G. *glukus*, sweet). A glucoprotein; component of mucin and mucoids; constituent of cell walls of fungi and of hard shell of crustaceae.

glū·cose (G. *glukus*, sweet). A naturally occurring sugar. Syn. dextrose; grape sugar; $C_6H_{12}O_6$. It is found in fruits, in blood and in the urine of diabetics.

glūcosū·ria (G. *glukus*, sweet; *ouron*, urine). Excretion of glucose in the urine. **G., renal**: permanent excretion of glucose in the urine, not associated with hyper-glycaemia or other signs of diabetes mellitus.

glucotrop·ic (G. *glukus*, sweet; *trephein*, to turn). Promoting the formation of glucose.

glū·cyl (G. *glukus*, sweet). The univalent radical of glucin.

glue. Hard brittle gelatin substance derived from the boiling of animal substances, such as hoofs and hides, in water. When warmed, the preparation acts as a cement.

Gluge's corpuscles (Gluge, G., German pathologist, 1812–98). Migratory connective tissue cells containing a nucleus, fat and granular detritus.

glū·side. Saccharin.

glutǎ·mic acid (L. *gluten*, glue). An amino-acid, alpha-amino-glutaric acid, $C_5H_9NO_4$.

glutǎ·mine (L. *gluten*, glue). A mono-amide from glutamic acid; widely distributed in plants.

glutathī·one (L. *gluten*, glue; G. *theion*, sulphur). A tripeptide of cystine, glutamic acid and glycine widely distributed (animal tissues, germinating plants) oxidizing tissue enzymes, acting by virtue of the (-S-S-) group as a hydrogen acceptor.

glū·teal (G. *gloutos*, buttock). Relating to the buttocks.

glū·teī (G. *gloutos*, buttock). The muscles of the buttocks.

glū·ten (L., glue). The viscid substance in dough, especially from wheat flour; originating from the saturation of some of the cereal proteins with water.

glū·teofě·moral (G. *gloutos*, buttock; L. *femur*, thigh). Relating to the buttocks and the thigh.

glū·teo-in·guinal (G. *gloutos*, buttock; L. *inguen*, groin). Relating to the buttocks and the groin.

glū·teus (G. *gloutos*, buttock). One of the large muscles of the buttock.

glū·tinous (L. *gluten*, glue). Glue-like.

glū·toid (L. *gluten*, glue). A gelatin and formaldehyde preparation used for coating capsules intended to pass through the stomach and dissolve in the intestine.

glȳcae·mia. Glucaemia, *q.v.*

glȳ·case (G. *glukus*, sweet). An enzyme acting on maltose converting it into dextrose. Usually called maltase.

glȳ·cerate (G. *glukus*, sweet). Any salt of glyceric acid.

glȳ·ceride (G. *glukus*, sweet). An ester of glycerol.

glȳ·cerin, glycerine (G. *glukus*, sweet). A syrupy liquid, $CH_2OH.CHOH.CH_2OH$, produced by decomposing fats with alkali or super-heated steam. Miscible with water and alcohol, but not with ether or chloroform. Used internally as a demulcent and laxative, as a sweetening agent, and as an ingredient in linctuses. Has little effect externally on whole skin, but is hygroscopic when used on broken skin, and has value in the treatment of chapped hands and chilblains.

glȳ·cerol (G. *glukus*, sweet). A trihydric alcohol, $CH_2OH.CHOH.CH_2OH$. The same as glycerin, *q.v.*

glȳ·cerose (G. *glukus*, sweet). $C_3H_6O_3$. A derivative of glycerol.

glў·ceryl (G. *glukus*, sweet). The trivalent radical ·CH₂·C·H·CH₂ of glycerol, combining with the fatty acids to form neutral fats. **G. trinitrate:** nitric ester of glycerin $C_3H_5(NO_3)_3$; used in the treatment of angina pectoris.

glў·cin, glў·cine (G. *glukus*, sweet). Amino-acetic acid $CH_2(NH_2)COOH$.

glў·cogen (G. *glukus*, sweet; *gennan*, to produce). A carbohydrate (polyhexose) normally present in nearly all animal tissues, but especially in liver and muscles. It is synthesized from carbohydrates, proteins, glycerol and probably also from fatty acids and catabolised into glucose as required to create energy. **G. disease:** an inborn disease in children, characterized by abnormal accumulation of glycogen in, and therefore enlargement of, the liver and/or kidney (epithelium of convoluted tubules), heart muscle and other organs, resulting in infantilism with hypoglycaemia and tendency to ketosis. Syn. von Gierke's disease.

glў·cogĕ·nase (G. *glukus*, sweet; *gennan*, to produce). Enzyme hydrolyzing glycogen.

glў·cogĕ·nesis (G. *glukus*, sweet; *gennan*, to produce). Formation of the polymerized form of glycogen from glucose.

glў·cogenŏ·lysis (G. *glukus*, sweet; *gennan*, to produce; *luein*, to loosen). The breaking down of glycogen into glucose.

glў·cogenŏ·sis. Glycogen disease, *q.v.*

glycogeū·sia (G. *glukus*, sweet; *geusis*, taste). A condition characterized by the presence of a sweet taste in the mouth.

glycohaē·mia (G. *glukus*, sweet; *haima*, blood). A condition in which sugar is present in the blood.

glў·col (G. *glukus*, sweet). A dihydric alcohol.

glў·colate. Any salt of glycolic acid.

glycŏ·lic acid. $C_2H_4O_3$; oxyacetic acid.

glycoli·pid (G. *glukus*, sweet; *lipos*, fat). Any lipid liberating on acid hydrolysis a carbohydrate, an alcohol (sphingosinol), and a fatty acid, e.g. phrenosin, kerasin.

glycŏ·lysis. Glucolysis, *q.v.*

glў·cone·ogĕ·nesis. Gluconeogenesis, *q.v.*

glycopĕ·nia (G. *glukus*, sweet; *pĕnia*, poverty). Hypoglycaemia; low sugar content of the blood.

glycopex·is (G. *glukus*, sweet; *pexis*, fixation). Storage of glucose or glycogen.

glycophĕ·nol (G. *glukus*, sweet; *phoinix*, purple). Saccharin.

glў·coside (G. *glukus*, sweet). A glucide yielding on hydrolysis sugar and a non-sugar substance called the 'aglucone' or 'genin', a compound of some alcohol and the aldehyde group of a carbohydrate; widespread in animal and vegetable tissues.

glycosŏ·meter (G. *glukus*, sweet; *metron*, measure). An instrument for quantitative estimation of sugar in urine.

glycosū·ria (G. *glukus*, sweet; *ouron*, urine). Excretion of glucose in the urine.

glycurŏ·nic acid. (G. *glukus*, sweet; *ouron*, urine). An oxyaldehyde acid, an intermediary product of metabolism, occurring normally in the urine in small amounts in paired or conjugated form.

glycuronū·ria (G. *glukus*, sweet; *ouron*, urine). Excretion of glycuronic acid in the urine.

Glycyrrhi·za (G. *glukus*, sweet; *rhiza*, a root). A genus of leguminous plants including the **G. glabra:** the root of which yields liquorice.

glўŏx·al. $C_2H_2O_2$; an amorphous substance formed by oxidizing acetaldehyde with HNO_3.

glўŏx·alase. An enzyme occurring in all animal tissues except pancreas and lymph nodes, hydrolyzing a simple or substituted glyoxaldehyde into the corresponding glycolic acid, e.g., methyl glyoxal to lactic acid.

G.M.C. General Medical Council (of Great Britain).

Gmelin's test (Gmelin, L., German physiologist, 1788–1853). A test for bile pigments in the urine. Strong nitric acid is added to urine. A coloured layer is formed.

gnat. A small dipterous insect, resembling the common mosquito, with which it is often confused. The gnat has no sting.

gnā·thic (G. *gnathos*, jaw). Relating to the jaw. **G. index:** see under index, g.

gnā·thion (G. *gnathos*, jaw). The lowest point in the median line of the inferior maxilla.

gnathocĕ·phalus (G. *gnathos*, jaw; *kephalē*, head). A monster lacking all parts of the head except the jaws.

gnathŏ·schisis (G. *gnathos*, jaw; *skhĭsis*, cleavage). Congenital cleft jaw.

Gnathŏ·stoma (G. *gnathos*, jaw; *stoma*, mouth). A genus of nematodes, parasitic in some animals and occasionally in man.

G.N.C. General Nursing Council (of Great Britain).

Godélier's law (Godélier, C. P., French physician, 1813–77). Tuberculous disease of the peritoneum is always associated with tuberculous disease of the pleura.

godemiche (L. *gaudium mihi*, my delight). An artificial penis, used in sapphism.

Godman's fascia (Godman, J. D., U.S. anatomist, 1794–1830). A continuation of the pretracheal fascia to the thorax and pericardium.

Goethe's bone (Goethe, J. W. von, German poet and philosopher, 1749–1832). The large wormian bone at the lambda, not necessarily representing the true os interparietale.

goggles. Spectacles with coloured lenses and cloth sides to protect the eyes from glare or dust.

goi·tre (F. *goitre*, from L. *guttur*, throat). Any enlargement of the thyroid gland. **Colloid g.:** g. characterized by distended acini filled with 'colloid' of high iodine content. **Exophthalmic g.:** toxic g., *q.v.* **Intrathoracic g.:** a g. partly situated in the thoracic cavity, tending to press upon the trachea. **Simple g.:** a chronic diffuse or nodular enlargement of the thyroid gland without functional disturbance. Endemic in certain parts of Europe (Tyrol, Switzerland) and U.S.A. (g.-belt), due to lack of iodine in water or food, **Substernal g.:** a g. partly situated behind the upper part of the sternum. See also intrathoracic g. **Toxic g.:** a condition characterized by diffuse enlargement of the thyroid gland and epithelial hypertrophy and hyperplasia, and disappearance of 'colloid', and by increased metabolic rate leading to loss of body weight, by tachycardia with or without the signs of circulatory insufficiency, exophthalmos, increased perspiration, peristalsis and emotional instability. Syn. exophthalmic g.; Graves' disease; hyperthyroidism. **Toxic g., secondary:** toxic g. which has developed many years after the establishment of a symptomless goitre, occurring usually about the 40th or 50th year of life, and clinically mainly characterized by loss of weight (due to increased metabolic rate) and cardiac signs (especially auricular fibrillation), the ocular signs often remaining in abeyance.

goitrogĕ·nic (L. *guttur*, throat; G. *gennan*, to produce). Producing goitre.

goi·trous. Pertaining to or affected with goitre.

gold. A precious, yellow-coloured, malleable and non-rusting metal, having a high specific gravity. Gold and a large number of gold compounds are used in medicine.

Goldflam's disease (Goldflam, S. V., Polish neurologist, 1852–1932). See Erb's disease.

Golgi's apparatus (Golgi, C., Italian histologist, 1844–1926). An anastomosing network of delicate fibrils of varying thickness found in nearly all cells. In nerve cells the apparatus is usually perinuclear. The chemical nature of the structure is probably lipo-protein. Syn. internal reticular apparatus. **G.'s cells:** large nerve cells with greatly branching processes found in the cortex of the brain. **G.'s funnels:** fibrillary coils supposed by G. to enclose myelinated nerve fibres.

Golgi-Mazzoni's corpuscles. See Mazzoni.

Golgi-Rezzonico's funnels. Golgi's funnels, *q.v.*

Goll's column (Goll, F., Swiss anatomist, 1829–1904). A tract which occupies the medial part of the posterior white column in the cervical and upper thoracic parts of the spinal cord. Syn. fasciculus gracilis. **G.'s nucleus:** a small nucleus in the medulla oblongata in which the fasciculus gracilis ends. Syn. gracilis tubercle.

Goltz's experiment (Goltz, F. L., German physician, 1834–1902). Stoppage of the heart's action of a frog, produced by repeated tapping of the abdomen.

Gombault's triangle (Gombault, A. F., French physician, 1844–1904). The septo-marginal tract in the sacral region of the cord where it forms a triangular area at the dorso-medial angle of the posterior funiculus.

gomphi·asis (G. *gomphios*, molar teeth). The condition of having loose teeth.

gŏ·nad (G. *gŏnē*, semen). A sexual gland: a testicle, an ovary.

gŏ·nadal (G. *gŏnē*, semen). Relating to a gonad.

gonadec·tomy (G. *gŏnē*, semen; *ektomē*, excision). Excision of a testicle or of an ovary.

gonadŏ·pathy (G. *gŏnē*, semen; *pathos*, disease). Any gonadal disease.

gonadotrō·phins (G. *gŏnē*, semen; *trephein*, to increase). Gonad stimulating substances obtained from pregnancy urine or serum. See hormone.

gonadotrŏ·pic (G. *gŏnē*, semen; *trepein*, to direct). Stimulating gonadal function.

gonag·ra (G. *gonu*, knee; *algos*, pain). Gouty arthritis of the knee joint.

gŏ·nangiĕc·tomy (G. *gŏnē*, semen; *aggeion*, vessel; *ektomē*, excision). Excision of a part of the vas deferens.

gonarthri·tis (G. *gonu*, knee; *arthron*, joint). Inflammation of the knee joint.

gonarthrŏ·tomy (G. *gonu*, knee; *arthron*, joint; *tomē*, section). Incision into the knee joint.

Gongylonē·ma. A genus of nematodes. **G. pulchrum:** a parasite of the upper alimentary tract of various ruminants, horses, pigs, and very occasionally man.

gŏ·nid, goni·dium (G. *gŏnē*, semen). 1. An asexually reproductive cell or spore. 2. A unicellular alga in the thallus of a lichen.

gŏ·niocraniŏ·metry (G. *gōnia*, angle; *kranion*, head; *metron*, measure). Measurement of the angles of the skull.

gōniŏ·meter (G. *gōnia*, angle; *metron*, measure). An instrument used in the measuring of angles.

gŏ·nion (G. *gōnia*, angle). A point at the outer side of the angle of the mandible.

gŏ·nioscope (G. *gōnia*, angle; *skopein*, to view). An instrument used in recording the varying angles made by the optical axis with the lines of muscle action.

gŏ·nite (G. *gŏnē*, semen). The reproductive elements of bacteria.

goni·tis (G. *gonu*, knee). An inflammation of the knee.

gŏ·noblennorrhoe·a (G. *gŏnē*, semen; *blennos*, mucus; *rhoia*, a flowing). Gonorrhoea.

gŏ·nocele (G. *gonu*, knee; *kēlē*, hernia). Swelling of the knee.

gŏ·nicide (G. *gŏnē*, semen; L. *caedere*, to kill). Anything which is destructive to the gonococcus.

gonococcae·mia (Gonococcus; G. *haima*, blood). A condition when gonococci are found in the blood.

gonococ·cal. Relating to gonococcus.

gonococ·cus (G. *gŏnē*, semen; *kokkos*, berry). The diplococcus causing gonorrhoea and ophthalmia neonatorum, the *Neisseria gonorrhoeae*.

gŏ·nocyte (G. *gŏnē*, semen; *kutos*, cell). The name given by Van Beneden for an ovum which contains only the female pronucleus.

gonohae·mia (G. *gŏnē*, semen; *haima*, blood). Generalized gonorrhoea.

gonorrhoe·a (G. *gŏnē*, semen; *rhoia*, a flow). An infectious disease characterized by inflammation of the mucous membrane of the urethra and, unless cured at an early stage, of other parts of the urogenital system (especially the epididymis, seminal vesicles, prostate). It occasionally leads to septicaemia or endocarditis and much more rarely to gonococcal arthritis. It is caused by the gonococcus, *Neisseria gonorrhoeae*.

gonorrhoe·al (G. *gŏnē*, semen; *rhoia*, flow). Relating to gonorrhoea.

gonotoxae·mia (G. *gŏnē*, semen; *toxikon*, poison; *haima*, blood). Toxaemia due to gonococcal infection.

gonotox·in (G. *gŏnē*, semen; *toxikon*, poison). A gonococcal toxin.

Goodell's sign (Goodell, W., U.S. gynaecologist, 1829–94). A soft cervix means a probable pregnancy.

goose-flesh. The erection on the skin of small rough papillae—usually caused by cold and sometimes also by fright. Syn. cutis anserina.

Gordon's reflex (Gordon, A., U.S. neurologist, born 1874). Extension of great toe or sometimes of all the toes when the deep flexor muscles of the leg are compressed; found in disease of the pyramidal tract.

Gordon's sign (Gordon, W., English physician, 1863–1929). The area of cardiac dullness is diminished in cases of carcinoma if the patient is in a recumbent position.

gor·get (Fr. *gorge*, throat). A grooved instrument employed in lithotomy.

Gosselin's fracture (Gosselin, L. A., French surgeon, 1815–87). A conical or V-shaped fracture of the lower end of the tibia.

Gossÿ·pium. A genus of malvaceous plants. The root bark of some species is useful in dysmenorrhoea and amenorrhoea. The common name for this is cotton root bark.

Gottschalk's operation (Gottschalk, S., German surgeon, 1860–1914). An operation performed through the vagina in which the uterosacral ligaments are shortened.

Gottstein's process (Gottstein, J., German otologist, 1832–95). The slender process of an outer hair-cell, joining it to the basal membrane of Corti's organ.

gouge (Fr.). A chisel-like instrument for cutting or removing bone or other hard structure.

Goulard's cerate (Goulard, T., French surgeon, 1724–84). A mixture of lead subacetate 20 and cerate of camphor 80.

Gould's bowed-head sign (Gould, G. M., U.S. ophthalmologist, 1848–1922). In diseases affecting the peripheral part of the retina the patient often bends his head low to enable the functioning part of the retina to focus to the ground.

goundou. An affection occurring in Central Africa and South America, probably associated with yaws and characterized by bilateral hyperostosis either of the ascending or nasal process of the maxilla, or affecting other cranial bones as well. Syn anákhré.

Gouraud's disease (Gouraud, V. O., French surgeon, 1772–1848). Inguinal hernia.

gout. A disease, mainly confined to males, characterized by a paroxysmal and painful inflammation of joints, especially the great toe, accompanied by an excess of uric acid in the blood.

gouty. Relating to or of the nature of gout.

Gower's column (Gowers, Sir W. R., British neurologist, 1845-1915). The anterior spinocerebellar tract of the spinal cord. It lies for the most part in the anterior section of the lateral white column. **G.'s intermediate process:** the lateral horn in the dorsal region of the spinal cord. **G.'s. paraplegia:** a paraplegia due to caries of the spine. **G.'s tract:** see G.'s column.

Goyrand's hernia (Goyrand, J. G., French surgeon, 1803-66). Inguino-interstitial hernia; incomplete inguinal hernia, not descending into the scrotum.

G.P.I. Abbreviation for general paralysis of the insane.

Gr., gr. Abbreviation for grain.

Graafian follicles (Graaf, R. de, Dutch physician, 1641-73). Small spherical vesicular bodies found in the cortical layer of the ovary, each containing an ovule. **G. oviduct:** see Fallopian tube.

grăˑcile (L. *gracilis*). Slender.

gracilis (L.). See under muscles.

gradăˑtim (L.) Gradually

grăˑduate (L. *gradus*, a step). 1. To take a degree from a university. 2. A person upon whom a degree has been conferred. 3. To mark with degrees; a vessel marked on its sides with lines or figures indicating the volume of its contents at the respective levels.

Graefe's disease (Graefe, A. von, German ophthalmologist, 1828-70). Progressive ophthalmoplegia. **G.'s sign:** inability of the upper eyelid to follow the downward movement of the eyeball; most frequently seen in exophthalmic goitre. **G.'s spots:** spots close to the supra-orbital foramen or over the vertebrae which, when pressed, cause relaxation of the spasm of the eyelids in blepharofacial spasm.

Grafenberg's ring (Grafenberg, E., German gynaecologist, in U.S.A.). A flexible silver wire ring, inserted within the uterus well above the cervical canal, and left there indefinitely as a contraceptive.

graft. 1. A portion of skin and/or muscle, bone, periosteum, nerve, etc., taken from a living organism and employed to replace a defect in a corresponding structure. 2. To implant living tissue.

Graham's law (Graham, T., English chemist, 1805-69). The rate of diffusion of gases through porous membranes is in inverse ratio to the square root of their density.

grain (L. *granum*, a grain). 1. Seed, as that of cereals. 2. Any small hard body resembling a seed; a granule. 3. The unit of weight of the troy (5,760 gr. = 1 pound troy) and avoirdupois (7,000 gr. = 1 pound avoirdupois) systems.

Gram's method (Gram, H. C. J., Danish physician, 1853-1938). A method of staining bacteria. The film of organisms is first treated with methyl violet, which is replaced, without washing, by Gram's solution, a dilute solution of iodine in potassium iodide. This combination produces a dark-purple colour which is retained by Gram-positive organisms after washing with alcohol, but disappears from Gram-negative organisms. The latter are demonstrated by counterstain (usually neutral red).

Gram-negative, Gram-positive. Incapable, capable of being stained by Gram's method.

gramme (G. *gramma*, written mark). The gravimetric unit of the metric system of weights and measures, equivalent to the quantity of a cubic centimetre of distilled water at 4° C. equal to 15.432356 grains.

Grancher's disease (Grancher, J. J., French physician, 1843-1907). Massive or spleno-pneumonia; a form of p. with splenization of the lung, the exudate filling the alveoli and the large bronchi. **G.'s sign:** a raised pitch of inspiratory murmur, indicating pulmonary consolidation. **G.'s system:** Control of juvenile tuberculosis by removal of susceptible children from tuberculous households. **G's triad:** the three symptoms pointing to incipient pulmonary tuberculosis: decreased strength of vesicular murmur, augmented vocal fremitus and Skodaic resonance.

grand mal (Fr., great sickness). Fully developed epilepsy. See also petit mal.

grandeur (Fr.). Greatness.

Grandry's corpuscles (Grandry, M., French 19th century physician of Liège). The sensory end-organs in the skin of the bills of ducks and geese.

grăˑnula (L. *granulum*, a small grain). A granule.

grăˑnular (L. *granulum*, a small grain). 1. Marked by granulations. 2. Having a structure or surface as if consisting of granules. 3. Containing granules. **G. kidney:** applied to the appearance of the kidney in the end stages of chronic nephritis in which the organ has a granular (2) surface owing to diffuse destruction, with fibrous replacement of parenchymatous tissue.

grăˑnulate. To undergo granulation.

granulăˑtion (L. *granulum*, a small grain). 1. Any of the small, soft, reddish nodules, mainly consisting of capillaries, histiocytes and lymphocytes, forming in the repair of a wound or ulcer, or an area of chronic inflammation of an internal organ, as the early stage of cicatricial tissue. 2. The formation of tissue characterized by granulation (1).

grăˑnule (L. *granulum*, a small grain). 1. A small grain or particle. 2. A small pill.

grăˑnulocytopēˑnia (L. *granulum*, a small grain; G. *kutos*, cell; *penia*, poverty). Abnormally low number of white blood cells of the myeloid series in the peripheral blood. Syn. neutropenia.

grăˑnulocȳˑtopoiēˑsis (L. *granulum*, a small grain; G. *kutos*, cell; *poiein*, to make). Producing granulocytes.

granulōˑma (L. *granulum*, a small grain). Tumour-like tissue, composed of granulation tissue. **G. annulare:** a chronic skin disease, characterized by the formation of firm, keloid-like, reddish nodules, especially at the back of hand or fingers, forming circles by confluence, and histologically by granulomatous tissue differing from tuberculous tissue by the eventual development of fibrous and not caseous degeneration. **G. infectiosum:** blastomycosis, American, *q.v.* **Paracoccidioidal g.:** a mild type of granuloma due to fungus infection, and occurring in South America. Also called Almeida's disease. **G. pyogenicum:** a small pedunculated, highly vascular, tender granuloma developing at the site of an injury, probably resulting from infection with *Staph. pyogenes*. Syn. botryomycosis hominis: granuloma telangiectaticum.

granulōˑmatous. Characterized by granulation tissue.

granˑulopēˑnia. Granulocytopenia, *q.v.*

granˑulopoiēˑsis (L. *granulum*, a small grain; *poiein*, to make). The formation of white blood corpuscles of the myeloid series.

grăˑnulose (L. *granulum*, a small grain). The inner and soluble portion of starch-granules.

granulōˑsis (L. *granulum*, a small grain). The development of multiple granules. **G. rubra nasi:** a condition characterized by intense redness of the distal part of the nose with small non-confluent dark-red nodules and constant hyperhidrosis, gradually disappearing during puberty, and perhaps due to some disturbance of cerebral vasomotor centres.

grăˑnum (L.). A grain.

Granville's hammer (Granville, J. M., English physician, 1833-1900). An instrument used in the treatment of neuralgia.

Granville's lotion (Granville, A. B., English physician, 1783-1872). Compound ammonia liniment.

graph (G. *graphein*, to write). A diagrammatic recording of data.

grǎ·phic (G. *graphein*, to write). Relating to writing; the record of the results of quantitative observations in a system of co-ordinates.

graphomā·nia (G. *graphein*, to write; *mania*, madness). An insane desire to write.

grǎ·phospasm (G. *graphein*, to write; *spasmos*, spasm). Writer's cramp.

Grashey's aphasia (Grashey, H. von, German psychologist, 1839–1911). A curious form of aphasia caused by a diminution in the duration of sensory impressions, causing disturbance of perception and association. It occurs as a sequel to cerebral trauma.

Grasset's sign (Grasset, J., French physician, 1849–1918). A condition seen in incomplete hemiplegia; the patient lying on his back cannot raise both legs at the same time, though he can raise each one separately.

Gratiolet's optic radiation (Gratiolet, L. P., French anatomist, 1815–65). The radiatio occipitothalamica, a bundle of fibres passing from the lateral geniculate body and the pulvinar through the internal capsule to the visual centre in the occipital lobe.

grating (1) (Mediaeval L. *grata*, from L. *crates*, a hurdle). 1. A glass ruled with equidistant parallel lines to produce diffraction of rays passing through it. 2. A frame or screen composed of parallel or crossed bars.

grating (2) (Fr. *gratter*, to scratch). A sound produced by the friction of rough surfaces against each other.

grattage (Fr. *gratter*, to scratch). A method of removing morbid growths by friction with a harsh sponge or brush.

grave (L. *gravis*, heavy). Serious or dangerous.

gravel (Fr. *gravelle*). Sand-like concretions found (abnormally) in the urinary tract.

Graves' disease (Graves, R. J., Irish physician, 1797–1853). Exophthalmic goitre; Basedow's disease. **G.'s sign:** increase of the systolic impulse, often observed in the beginning of pericarditis.

grǎ·vid (L. *gravidus*). Pregnant.

grǎ·vida (L. *gravidus*, pregnant). A pregnant woman.

gravǐ·ditas (L.). Pregnancy.

gravi·dity (L. *graviditas*). The state of being pregnant.

grǎ·vidocar·diac (L. *gravidus*, pregnant; G. *kardia*, heart). Relating to cardiac conditions in pregnancy.

gravǐ·meter (L. *gravis*, heavy; G. *metron*, measure). An instrument used in ascertaining specific gravities.

gravimě·tric (L. *gravis*, heavy; G. *metron*, measure). Relating to measurement by weight.

gravitā·tion (L. *gravitas*, weight). The force by which bodies are drawn towards the earth or towards each other.

grǎ·vity (L. *gravitas*, weight). Weight. **Specific g.:** the proportion of the weight of a substance to that of an equal volume of another (e.g., water) taken as a standard.

Grawitz's granules (Grawitz, P., German pathologist, 1850–1932). Basic granules which can be seen in the red blood corpuscles in certain pathological conditions. **G.'s tumour:** hypernephroma; carcinoma of the renal tubules.

green. The colour of grass.

Greenhow's disease (Greenhow, E. H., English physician, 1814–88). Vagabonds' disease. Chronic irritation due to pediculi.

gref·fotome (Fr. *greffe*, graft; G. *tomē*, section). A knife used in cutting skin grafts.

Grě·garina (L. *grex*, flock). Simple sporozoa, common parasites in the digestive tracts and body cavities of insects.

Gregory's powder (Gregory, J., Scottish physician, 1753–1821). Pulvis rhei compositus (rhubarb 25% with heavy and light magnesium carbonates, and ginger).

grenz rays (Ger. *grenze*, boundary). X-rays with a length of about 2 Angströms, used mainly in the treatment of superficial (skin) lesions.

grey. The colour obtained by mixing black and white. **G. matter:** the brownish-grey substance forming the cortex of the brain and cerebellum, the cerebral basal ganglia, and the inner part of the spinal cord. It consists of nerve cells and fibres. **G. powder:** finely divided mercury with chalk. Used as a purgative.

Griesinger's sign (Griesinger, W., German neurologist, 1817–68). A retromastoid oedematous swelling seen in cases of thrombosis of the lateral or transverse sinus.

Griffith's mixture (Griffith, R. E., U.S. physician, 1798–1850). Mistura ferri composita (iron sulphate, 6; myrrh, 18; sugar, 18; potassium carbonate, 8; lavender, 50; rosewater, 900).

grinder. A molar tooth.

grip, grippe (Fr. *grippe*). Influenza, *q.v.*

gripe. Severe pain or spasm in the bowel.

gristle. Cartilage, *q.v.*

Gritti's amputation (Gritti, R., Italian surgeon, 1857–1920). An amputation above the knee, the patella is preserved and secured on to the cut surface of the divided femur.

groan. 1. To utter a moaning sound when in distress or pain. 2. The sound thus uttered.

groin. The depression between the abdomen and thigh.

groove. A furrow or channel. **Auricular g.:** a small depression in front of the sacroiliac joint in the female. **Basilar g.:** a depression on the inner surface of the basilar portion of the occipital bone. **Bicipital g.:** a deep depression between the tuberosities of the humerus in which the tendon of the biceps lies. **Carotid g.:** on the body of the sphenoid; it contains the cavernous sinus and the internal carotid artery. **Clement Lucas g.:** situated on the inner surface of the spine of the sphenoid bone in which the chorda tympani nerve is found. **Dental g.:** small groove found in the developing maxilla. **Infra-orbital g.:** found on the superior or orbital surface of the maxilla. **Lacrimal g.:** found on the nasal surface of the maxilla, transmitting the nasolacrimal duct. **Meningeal g.:** on the inner side of the parietal bone caused by the meningeal vessels. **Mylohyoid g.:** caused by the inferior dental nerve on the inner surface of the mandible. **Nasal g.:** on the inner surface of the ethmoid bone caused by the anterior ethmoidal nerve. **Nuchal g.:** the median furrow in the mid-line of the neck posteriorly. **Obturator g.:** a depression on the inner surface of the pelvis which lodges the tendon of the obturator externus muscle. **Occipital g.:** a shallow depression on the inner surface of the mastoid process which lodges the occipital artery. **Olfactory g.:** on the superior surface of the lesser wing of the sphenoid bone for the olfactory tract. **Optic g.:** transverse furrow on the superior surface of the body of the sphenoid bone. **Peroneal g.:** shallow groove on the posterior surface of the lower end of the fibula for the tendons of the peronei muscles. **Popliteal g.:** deep depression on the outer surface of the lateral condyle of the femur, it lodges the tendon of the popliteus muscle. **Sigmoid g.:** deep groove on the inner surface of the mastoid portion of the temporal bone, lodges the sigmoid venous sinus. **Spiral g.:** winding groove on the posterior surface of the middle third of the shaft of the humerus, lodges the radial nerve and the profunda brachii vessels. **Subclavian g.:** depression on the inferior surface of the clavicle for the insertion of the subclavius muscle. **Ulnar g.:** shallow depression on the posterior surface of the medial epicondyle of the humerus in which the ulnar nerve passes.

gross (Fr. *gros*, large). Coarse; large. **G. lesion:** a lesion perceptible to the naked eye.

Gross's disease (Gross, S. D., U.S. surgeon, 1805–84). See Physick's encysted rectum.

Grossich's method (Grossich, A., Italian surgeon, 1849–1926). The use of tincture of iodine as an antiseptic.

ground itch. An itching lesion of the skin of the feet, due to infestation with larvae of hookworms. See ankylostomiasis.

group. A collection of organisms or objects possessing common characteristics. **G. practice:** practice of medicine by a group of associated specialists each dealing with his own field of experience.

Grove's cell (Grove, Sir W. R., English physicist, 1811–96). A two-fluid battery cell, the fluids being dilute solutions of sulphuric and nitric acids, and the metals immersed in them being zinc and platinum.

growth. 1. The increase in size of an organism or one of its parts in the process of development. 2. New-growth, see neoplasm. **G. hormone:** the hormone formed by the eosinophilic cells of the pituitary gland, promoting body growth.

Gruber's bursa (Gruber, J., Austrian aurist, 1827–1900). The synovial cavity of the tarsal sinus.

Gruber's fossa (Gruber, W. L., Russian anatomist, 1814–90). A small recess at the inner end of the clavicle, in the suprasternal space.

Gruber's reaction (Gruber, M. von, German bacteriologist, 1853–1927). See Widal's reaction.

Gruby's disease (Gruby, D., Hungarian physician, 1810–98). Alopecia areata.

gruel. A thin porridge made of oatmeal or other cereal and water.

grumous (L. *grumus*, hillock). Clotted.

Grunbaum-Widal test. See Widal's reaction.

Grynfelt's triangle (Grynfelt, J. C., French surgeon, 1840–1913). A small triangular muscular space below the 12th rib, bounded behind by the quadratus lumborum and anteriorly by the internal oblique. Lumbar abscess or hernia may occur in this space.

grȳ·ochrom (G. *grū*, morsel; *khrōma*, colour). Term applied to structures having no specific arrangement, as the spinal ganglia.

grypō·sis (G. *grupōsis*, a hooking). Abnormal curvature of the nails.

Gt., gt. Abbreviation for L. *gutta*, drop.

guai·acol. Catechol monomethyl ether $C_6H_4(OCH_3)$ OH, occurring in wood tar creosote. Can be produced synthetically by methylation of catechol. Is used as its carbonic ester orally in treatment of phthisis and bronchiectasis.

guard. An appliance on a surgical knife or on a trocar to prevent too deep an incision or puncture.

Gubaroff's fold or valve (Gubaroff, A. P. von, Russian gynaecologist, born 1855). The site of the cardiac sphincter of the stomach.

gubernă·culum (L. *gubernaculum*, a rudder). A guiding structure, e.g., **G. testis:** a cord attached to the scrotum, serving to direct the descent of the testis from the abdominal cavity to the scrotum.

Gudden's commissure (Gudden, B. A. von, Professor of Psychiatry in Zurich and later in Munich, 1824–86). Fibres of the medial root of the optic tract passing from the internal geniculate body of one side to that of the other side via the chiasma.

Guéneau de Mussy's point (Guéneau de Mussy, N. F. O., French physician, 1813–85). A painful area in cases of diaphragmatic pleurisy which is found along the inner border of the sternum.

Guérin's glands (Guérin, A. F. M., Professor of Surgery at Hôtel Dieu, Paris, 1816–95). See Skene's glands. **G.'s valve:** the mucous membrane which surrounds the lacuna magna of the male urethra.

Guidi's canal. See Vidian canal. (The Italian Guidi is latinized Vidius).

guil·lotine (Fr.). A surgical instrument for removal of tonsils, growth in the larynx, etc.

Guinard's method (Guinard, A., French surgeon, 1856–1911). Treatment of growths by the application of calcium carbide.

guinea-pig. A small rodent from South America, now extensively bred in Europe. It is much used in laboratories in experimental work.

guinea worm. The *Dracunculus medinensis*. **G. W. disease:** Dracontiasis, *q.v.*

Guinon's disease (Guinon, G. French physician, 1859–1929). Tic de Guinon. See Gilles de la Tourette's disease.

gula (L., gullet). The pharynx and oesphagus.

Gull's disease (Gull, Sir W. W., English physician, 1816–90). Myxoedema. **G.'s renal epistaxis:** haematuria of renal origin.

Gull-Sutton's disease (Gull, Sir W. W., English physician, 1816–90, and Sutton, H. G., English physician 1837–91). Arteriocapillary fibrosis; diffuse arteriosclerosis.

gullet. The oesophagus, *q.v.*

Gullstrand's slit lamp (Gullstrand, A., Swedish ophthalmologist, 1863–1930). A lamp for examination of the eye.

gum (G. *kommi*, gum). Amorphous translucent solids consisting of calcium, potassium and magnesium salts of aldobionic acids. They are produced from the old walls of various plants as results of injuries.

gumma (G. *kommi*, gum). A localized syphilitic (tertiary syphilis) lesion, of a consistency resembling that of india-rubber, characterized by granulomatous tissue with endarteritis and periarteritis, by necrobiosis with formation of a fibrous capsule or by tendency to necrosis and caseation.

gum·matous. Of the nature of or affected with gumma.

gums. Gingiva, *q.v.*

Gunn's dots (Gunn, R. M., English ophthalmologist, 1850–1909). Bright white dots observed on oblique illumination around the macula lutea; they do not appear to be pathological.

Günz's ligament (Günz, J. G., German anatomist, 1714–89). The ligamentous fibres of the obturator membrane forming the inner wall of the canal transmitting the obturator vessels and nerves.

gurgling (L. *gurgulio*, gullet). The sound produced by the passage of gas through a fluid, e.g. by palpation of the abdomen when a bowel containing fluid matter is distended with gas.

gustā·tion (L. *gustare*, to taste). The sense of taste or the act of tasting.

gus·tatory (L. *gustare*, to taste). Relating to the sense of taste.

gut. The intestine.

Guthrie's muscle (Guthrie, G. J., English surgeon, 1785–1856). The deep transverse perineal muscle.

gutta (L.). A drop.

guttis quibusdam (L.). With a few drops.

guttatim (L.). Drop by drop.

guttur (L.). The throat.

gut·tural (L. *guttur*, throat). Relating to the throat.

Guyon's isthmus (Guyon, F. J. C., French surgeon, 1831–1920). A prolongation and narrowing of the internal os uteri.

gymnas·tics (G. *gumnos*, naked). Physical exercise, for the restoration or maintenance of bodily health.

gym·nobactē·ria (G. *gumnos*, naked; *bakterion*, stick). Nonflagellate bacteria.

gym·nocyte (G. *gumnos*, naked; *kutos*, cell). Unicellular organism.

gymnophō·bia (G. *gumnos*, naked; *phobos*, fear). A neurotic dislike of seeing a naked person or a naked part of the body.

N

gymnŏ·sophy (G. *gumnos*, naked; *sophos*, wise). The nudist cult.

gȳnaecolŏ·gic, gȳnaecolŏ·gical (G. *gunē*, woman; *logos*, a discourse). Relating to gynaecology.

gȳnaecŏ·logist (G. *gunē*, woman; *logos*, a discourse). A specialist in gynaecology.

gȳnaecŏ·logy (G. *gunē*, woman; *logos*, a discourse). That part of medicine relating to diseases peculiar to woman, especially those affecting the organs of generation.

gȳnaephō·bia (G. *gunē*, woman; *phobos*, fear). Neurotic aversion from the society of women.

gȳnan·der (G. *gunē*, woman; *anēr*, man). A male pseudohermaphrodite, an individual with male gonads and female secondary sex characters.

gynan·dria, gynan·drism (G. *gunē*, woman; *anēr*, man). Male pseudohermaphroditism.

gȳnatrē·sia (G. *gunē*, woman; *atrētos*, not perforated). Vaginal imperforation.

gȳnopǎ·thic (G. *gunē*, woman; *pathos*, disease). Relating to women's diseases.

gȳnŏ·pathy (G. *gunē*, woman; *pathos*, disease). Any kind of woman's disease.

gȳnoplǎ·stics (G. *gunē*, woman; *plassein*, to form). Plastic surgery performed on the female generative organs.

gȳp·sum (G. *gupsos*, chalk). Native calcium sulphate.

gyrate (L. *gyrare*, to turn round). To spin round.

gyrā·tion (L. *gyrare*, to turn round). A turning in a circle.

gyre (G. *guros*, round). See gyrus.

gȳrencephal·ic (G. *guros*, round; *egkephalos*, brain). Relating to a brain with a convoluted cortex.

gyrō·ma (G. *guros*, round). Myoma of the ovary.

gyrŏ·meter (G. *guros*, round; *metron*, measure). An instrument for measuring the gyri of the brain.

gyrō·sa. Gastric vertigo.

gȳ·rospasm (G. *guros*, round; *spasmos*, spasm). Spasmodic rotary movement of the head.

gȳ·rus (G. *guros*, round). The term applied to the convolutions of the brain.

H

H. The symbol for an atom of Hydrogen.

H. The symbol for oersted.

H^+. The symbol for hydrogen ion.

$[H^+]$. The symbol for hydrogen ion concentration.

h. Abbreviation for Planck's constant.

H-agglutinin (Abbrev. from Ger. *Hauch*). A floccular agglutinin, stimulated by the flagella of organisms, reacting specifically on the corresponding antigen. H-antigen: a variant in antigenic constitution of different single-cell cultures from the same strain or species, heat-labile; characteristic of motile organisms and many other species of enteric bacteria. H. substance: a substance resembling in its effects, if not identical with, histamine, thought to be liberated in the skin on mechanical stimulation of the skin.

Haab's pupil reflex (Haab, O., Swiss ophthalmologist, 1850–1931). If a bright object already present in the visual field be looked at, the pupils contract without there being any appreciable change during convergence or accommodation. This indicates a cortical lesion.

habe·na (L., rein). A fraenum.

habe·nula (L. dim. of *habena*, rein). 1. A fraenum. 2. A strip; a ribbon-like structure; a term used for any of the fibres of the basilar membrane of the internal ear. 3. One of the peduncles of the pineal gland.

habit (L. *habitus*, from *habere*, to hold). A constant or often repeated action or condition. H. spasm: a neurotic tic: often recurring co-ordinated movements, usually limited to one muscle group, capable of suppression by will and ceasing during sleep.

hab·itat (L. "it inhabits"). The natural home of an animal or plant.

habromā·nia (G. *habros*, graceful; *mania*, madness). Mental disturbance characterized by a disposition to cheerful gaiety.

Haeckermann's area. The area known as the Laimer-Haeckermann area at the junction of the pharynx and the oesophagus.

haem (G. *haima*, blood). A complex pyrrol derivative containing iron; one of the constituents of haemoglobin.

hae·machrome. Haematin, *q.v.*

haemachrō·sis (G. *haima*, blood; *khrōsis*, a colouring). A condition characterized by abnormal redness of the blood.

haemacytozō·ŏn (G. *haima*, blood; *kutos*, cell; *zōon*, animal). A protozoon present in red blood corpuscles.

hae·mad (G. *haima*, blood; L. *ad*, to). 1. Toward the haemal or ventral side; opposed to the neurad. 2. A blood cell.

haemagglutinā·tion (G. *haima*, blood; L. *agglutinare* from *gluten*, glue). Agglutination of red blood corpuscles.

haemagglū·tinin (G. *haima*, blood; L. *agglutinare* from *gluten*, glue). An agglutinin acting on red blood corpuscles.

hae·magogue (G. *haima*, blood; *agōgos*, leading). 1. Promoting menstrual or haemorrhoidal flow of blood. 2. Any agent promoting the discharge of blood.

hae·mal (G. *haima*, blood). Relating to the blood or vascular system. H. node: see haemolymph node.

haemagō·nium. Haemohistioblast, *q.v.*

haemamoe·ba (G. *haima*, blood; *amoibē*, change). An amoeboid parasite of blood-cells.

haeman·gioblastō·ma (G. *haima*, blood; *aggeion*, vessel; *blastos*, germ). An angioblastoma; malignant tumour of the endothelium of blood vessels.

haeman·gio-endotheliō·ma (G. *haima*, blood; *aggeion*, vessel; *endon*, within; *thēlē*, nipple). A tumour derived from vascular endothelial cells.

haem·angiō·ma (G. *haima*, blood; *aggeion*, vessel). A neoplasm originating from blood vessels. Syn. angioma.

haem·angiomatō·sis (G. *haima*, blood; *aggeion*, vessel). The condition characterized by the presence of multiple haemangiomata.

haeman·giosarcō·ma. See angiosarcoma.

haemaphō·bia (G. *haima*, blood; *pgobos*, fear). Morbid fear of seeing blood.

haemarthrō·sis (G. *haima*, blood; *arthron*, joint). Haemorrhage into a joint.

haematĕ·mesis (G. *haima*, blood; *ĕmeein*, to vomit). The vomiting of blood.

haematencĕ·phalon (G. *haima*, blood; *egkephalos*, brain). Haemorrhage into the brain.

haemathĕ·rapy (G. *haima*, blood; *thĕrapeia*, treatment). The treatment of disease by the use of blood or plasma.

haemather·mous (G. *haima*, blood; *thermos*, hot). Warm-blooded.

haemat·ic (G. *haima*, blood). Relating to blood.

hae·matin (G. *haima*, blood). An iron-containing pyrrole derivative of oxy-haemoglobin. It is bluish-black in colour, amorphous, and soluble in dilute alkalis and acids. It is not soluble in water, alcohol and ether. Syn. methaeme.

haematinae·mia (G. *haima*, blood). Condition in which haematin is present in the blood.

hae·matoblast (G. *haima*, blood; *blastos*, germ). An undeveloped red blood corpuscle.

hae·matocele (G. *haima*, blood; *kēlē*, tumour). 1. A haematoma in the tunica vaginalis testis or in the spermatic cord. 2. A haematoma in the pelvic cavity.

haematocoē·lia (G. *haima*, blood; *koilia*, cavity). Haemorrhage into the peritoneal cavity.

hae·matochē·zia (G. *haima*, blood; *khēzein*, to ease the bowels). The passing of bloodstained stools.

hae·matochylū·ria (G. *haima*, blood; *khulos*, juice; *ouron*, urine). The presence of blood and chylous material in the urine, as e.g. in filariasis.

hae·matocol·pos (G. *haima*, blood; *kolpos*, womb). A collection of blood within the vagina.

hae·matocrit (G. *haima*, blood; *krinein*, to separate). An instrument for the estimation of the relative proportions of red cells and plasma in blood by centrifugal separation.

haematō·cryal (G. *haima*, blood; *kruos*, cold). Cold-blooded.

hae·matocyst (G. *haima*, blood; *kustis*, bladder). A cyst containing blood.

hae·matocyte (G. *haima*, blood; *kutos*, cell). A blood corpuscle.

hae·matocytŏ·lysis (G. *haima*, blood; *kutos*, cell; *luein*, to loosen). Haemolysis.

hae·matocytŏ·meter. The same as haemocytometer, *q.v.*

hae·matodes (G. *haimatōdēs*, blood-red). Bloody; filled with blood.

haemato-encephă·lic barrier (G. *haima*, blood; *egkephalos*, brain). Term applied to the areas in which penicillin, for example, is unable to pass from the blood stream to the cerebro-spinal fluid.

hǎe·matogĕ·nesis (G. *haima*, blood; *gennan*, to produce). The development of blood.

hǎe·matogĕ·nic (G. *haima*, blood; *gennan*, to produce). Relating to the formation of blood or blood corpuscles.

hǎe·matŏ·genous (G. *haima*, blood; *gennan*, to produce). Derived from blood; or blood-forming.

hǎe·matoglŏbin. Haemoglobin, *q.v.*

hǎematoi·din (G. *haima*, blood; *eidos*, form). An iron-free derivative of haemoglobin, crystallising in rhomboidal prisms or amorphous granules occurring, mainly extracellularly, in areas of old haemorrhage; possibly identical with biliverdin.

hǎe·matokrit. Haematocrit, *q.v.*

hǎematŏ·logy (G. *haima*, blood; *logos*, a discourse). That section of medicine dealing with the blood and its diseases. Thus **Haematologist**, one versed in haematology.

hǎe·matolymph·angĭo·ma (G. *haima*, blood; L. *lympha*, water; G. *aggeion*, vessel). A neoplasm originating from both blood- and lymph-vessels.

hǎemato·ma (G. *haima*, blood). A collection of extravasated blood in the body.

hǎe·matomēdiasti·num (G. *haima*, blood; L. *in medio stare*, to stand in the middle). An effusion of blood into the mediastinal spaces.

hǎe·matomē·tra (G. *haima*, blood; *mētra*, uterus). An accumulation of blood within the cavity of the uterus.

hǎe·matomphǎ·locele (G. *haima*, blood; *omphalos*, navel; *kēlē*, tumour). A haemorrhage into an umbilical hernia.

hǎe·matomȳe·lia (G. *haima*, blood; *muelos*, marrow). Haemorrhage into the spinal cord.

hǎe·matomȳeli·tis (G. *haima*, blood; *muelos*, marrow). Acute haemorrhagic myelitis of the spinal cord.

hǎe·matomȳ·elopore (G. *haima*, blood; *muelos*, marrow; *pŏros*, a passage). A cavity in the spinal cord the result of haemorrhage.

hǎe·matonephrŏ·sis (G. *haima*, blood; *nephros*, kidney). Blood in the pelvis of the kidney.

hǎe·matophathŏ·logy (G. *haima*, blood; *pathos*, disease; *logos*, a discourse). That branch of medical science dealing with disease of the blood.

hǎe·matopericar·dium (G. *haima*, blood; *peri*, around; *kardia*, heart). Haemorrhage into the pericardium.

hǎe·matoperitonē·um (G. *haima*, blood; *pĕri*, around; *teinein*, to stretch). Haemorrhage into the peritoneum.

hǎe·matopex·is (G. *haima*, blood; *pēxis*, coagulation). Coagulation of the blood.

hǎe·matophage (G. *haima*, blood; *phagein*, to eat). A phagocytic cell which is destructive to red blood corpuscles.

hǎematŏ·phagous (G. *haima*, blood; *phagein*, to eat). Feeding on blood; blood sucking.

hǎe·matoplas·tic (G. *haima*, blood; *plassein*, to form). Blood-forming.

hǎe·matopoiē·sis (G. *haima*, blood; *poiēsis*, formation). The formation of blood corpuscles; usually applied only to the formation of red blood corpuscles.

hǎe·matopoiĕt·ic (G. *haima*, blood; *poiētikos*, formative). Relating to the formation of blood, especially to that of red blood cells.

hǎe·matoporphȳr·in (G. *haima*, blood; *porphura*, purple). A red pigment not occurring naturally, prepared from blood by the action of concentrated sulphuric acid.

haemator·rhachis (G. *haima*, blood; *rhakhis*, spine). Haemorrhage into the vertebral canal.

hǎe·matorrhoē·a (G. *haima*, blood; *rhoia*, flow). A copious flow or discharge of blood.

hǎe·matosal·pinx (G. *haima*, blood; *salpigx*, tube). A collection of blood in the Fallopian tube.

hǎe·matosper·mia (G. *haima*, blood; *sperma*, seed). The discharge of blood-stained semen.

hǎe·matothor·ax. Haemothorax, *q.v.*

hǎe·matotox·ic (G. *haima*, blood; *toxikon*, poison). Relating to a poisoned state of the blood.

hǎe·matotȳm·panum (G. *haima*, blood; *tumpanon*, a drum). Haemorrhage into the tympanic cavity.

hǎe·matox·ylin (G. *haima*, blood; *xulon*, wood). The colouring matter of logwood; a crystalline substance, used as a nuclear stain in histology.

hǎe·matozē·mia (G. *haima*, blood; *zēmia*, loss). A slow loss of blood.

hǎe·matozō·on (G. *haima*, blood; *zōon*, animal). Any animal parasite in the blood. Hence **Haematozoic**, living in the blood.

hǎe·matū·ria (G. *haima*, blood; *ouron*, urine). The discharge of blood-containing urine. See also haemoglobinuria.

hǎe·mic (G. *haima*, blood). Relating to or caused by the blood.

hǎemo-agglū·tinin. An agglutinin specific for red blood corpuscles.

hǎe·moblast (G. *haima*, blood; *blastos*, germ). Erythroblast. Primitive form of erythrocyte or immature red blood corpuscle.

hǎe·moblastŏ·sis (G. *haima*, blood; *blastos*, germ). State in which excess of haemoblasts exist in blood stream.

hǎemochrō·mogen (G. *haima*, blood; *khrōma*, colour; *gennan*, to produce). Compound of a ferrous protoporphyrin with denatured globulin.

hǎemŏ·clasis (G. *haima*, blood; *klasis*, fracture). Haemolysis; destruction of the erythrocytes.

hǎemoclas·tic (G. *haima*, blood; *klasis*, fracture). Haemolytic, *q.v.*

hǎe·mocō·nia (G. *haima*, blood; *konia*, dust). Haemokonia, *q.v.*

hǎemo-concentration. Condition in which, due to loss of plasma, as in burns, the ratio $\dfrac{\text{volume of blood cells}}{\text{volume of plasma}}$ in the blood stream, is increased.

hǎe·mochromatŏ·sis (G. *haima*, blood; *khroma*, colour). An inborn error of metabolism, characterized by excessive deposition of haemosiderin and haemofuscin in some organs. Bronze diabetes, *q.v.*

hǎe·mocyte (G. *haima*, blood; *kutos*, cell). A blood corpuscle.

hǎemocy·toblast (G. *haima*, blood; *kutos*, cell; *blastos*, germ). A primitive basophile, agranular, mononuclear cell regarded by Ferrata and those adhering to the monophyletic theory of blood-cell origin as the stem-cell of all blood cells, developing by different processes of differentiation into a myeloid h. (supposed to give rise to both red and myeloid cells); a lymphoid h. (believed to give rise to the cells of the lymphocytic series); or into a monoblast, being itself derived from the haemohistioblast, *q.v.*

hǎe·mocytŏ·lysis (G. *haima*, blood; *kutos*, cell; *luein*, to loosen). Dissolution of red blood corpuscles.

hǎe·mocyto·meter (G. *haima*, blood; *kutos*, cell; *metron*, measure). An instrument used for counting blood corpuscles.

hǎemodynam·ics (G. *haima*, blood; *dunamis*, power). The physical laws governing the circulation of blood.

Hǎe·moflagella·ta (G. *haima*, blood; L. *flagella*, whip). Various genera of flagellated protozoa, including trypanosoma and leishmania, members of which spend at least part of their life cycle in the blood of vertebrates.

hǎemofus·cin (G. *haima*, blood; L. *fuscus*, tawny). A yellowish-brown iron-free pigment, derived from haemoglobin, found in increased amounts in certain organs in haemochromatosis.

hāēmogen·esis (G. *haima*, blood; *gennan*, to produce). Haematogenesis, *q.v.*

hāēmoglō·bic (G. *haima*, blood; L. *globus*, globe). Producing haemoglobin.

hāēmoglō·bin (G. *haima*, blood; L. *globus*, globe). A compound of a pigment of the pyrrol group (a protoporphyrin) with iron and globin; the respiratory pigment of the red corpuscles; combining readily with oxygen to form oxyhaemoglobin, the loose chemical combination by which oxygen is carried from the lungs to the tissues and which gives the brighter red colour to the arterial as compared with the venous blood. Abbrev. Hb.

hāē·moglobināē·mia (G. *haima*, blood; L. *globus*, globe; G. *haima*, blood). The condition characterized by the presence in the blood of free haemoglobin (i.e., dissolved out of the red corpuscles).

hāē·moglobinŏ·meter (G. *haima*, blood; L. *globus*, globe; G. *metron*, measure). An instrument for the quantitative measurement of haemoglobin in the blood.

hāē·moglobinū·ria (G. *haima*, blood; L. *globus*, globe; G. *ouron*, urine). The presence of dissolved haemoglobin in the urine. H., cold: h. conditioned by exposure of the body (whole or part) to cold. H., paroxysmal, nocturnal: recurrent nocturnal paroxysms of h., probably at least partly conditioned by decrease in CO_2 combining power of the blood at night, no abnormal haemolysis having so far been found in the blood. Syn. Marchiafava-Micheli's disease.

haēmohĭ·stioblast (G. *haima*, blood; *histion*, a web; *blastos*, germ). A primitive undifferentiated mesenchymal cell, regarded by Ferrata and those adhering to the monophyletic theory of blood-cell origin as giving rise to the myeloid and lymphoid haemocytoblast, *q.v.*, and to the monoblast.

hāē·moid (G. *haima*, blood; *eidos*, form). Having the appearance of blood; like blood.

haēmokō·nia (G. *haima*, blood; *konia*, dust). 1. Fragments of disintegrated red blood cells. 2. In a wider sense also including other granular particles in the blood, especially certain spheroidal lipoid granules.

hāē·mokonio·sis (G. *haima*, blood; *konia*, dust). A condition in which abnormally large quantities of haemokoniae are present in the blood.

hāē·molymph (G. *haima*, blood; L. *lympha*, water). Referring to both blood and lymphatic tissue or fluid. H. node: millet-seed- to pea-sized nodes, occurring in prevertebral connective tissue, in subcutaneous tissue, etc., having essentially lymph-node structure and representing probably a regressing lymph-node.

hāēmŏly·sin (G. *haima*, blood; *lusis*, dissolution). A substance producing haemolysis.

haēmŏ·lysis (G. *haima*, blood; *lusis*, dissolution). Liberation of haemoglobin from red blood corpuscles.

haēmoly·tic (G. *haima*, blood; *luein*, to dissolve). Relating to, or causing, haemolysis. H. anaemia: See anaemia, h. H. disease of the newborn: a haemolytic anaemia of late foetal life or of newborn resulting from agglutination by abnormal antibody in maternal serum, commonly Rh. incompatibility.

hāē·momediasti·num (G. *haima*, blood; L. *in medio stare*, to stand in the middle). Haemorrhage into the mediastinum.

haēmomē·tra (G. *haima*, blood; *metra*, womb). See haematometra.

haēmŏ·metry (G. *haima*, blood; *metron*, measure). Estimation of the quantity of haemoglobin or of the number of corpuscles in the blood.

hāē·mopathŏ·logy (G. *haima*, blood; *pathos*, disease; *logos*, a discourse). The pathology of the blood.

haēmŏ·pathy (G. *haima*, blood; *pathos*, disease). Any blood disease.

hāē·mopericar·dium (G. *haima*, blood; *pĕri*, around; *kardia*, heart). Haemorrhage into the pericardial cavity.

hāē·moperitonē·um (G. *haima*, blood; *peri*, around; *teinein*, to stretch). Haemorrhage into the peritoneal cavity.

haēmopex·ia (G. *haima*, blood; *pēxis*, coagulation). A general term used for disorders and diseases in which there is a tendency for the blood to coagulate.

haēmopex·in (G. *haima*, blood; *pēxis*, coagulation). A blood-coagulating ferment.

haēmophi·lia (G. *haima*, blood; *philein*, to love). A recessively transmitted condition characterized by excessive haemorrhage from very trivial injuries and by prolonged coagulation (and normal bleeding) time; occurring practically only in males, although transmitted by the female.

haēmophil·ic (G. *haima*, blood; *philein*, to love). Relating to haemophilia.

Haēmŏ·philus (G. *haima*, blood; *philein*, to love). Generic term for bacilli not growing in pure culture without the presence of haemoglobin or a related substance; including *H. Ducreyi*, the organism causing soft chancre; *H. influenzae*, an organism associated with respiratory lesions in influenza; *H. of Koch-Weeks*, an organism causing conjunctivitis; *H. pertussis*, the organism causing whooping cough.

haēmophō·bia (G. *haima*, blood; *phobos*, fear). Morbid fear of the sight of blood.

haēmophthal·mos (G. *haima*, blood; *ophthalmos*, eye). Haemorrhage into the vitreous chamber.

haē·mopneumothor·ax (G. *haima*, blood; *pneuma*, breath; *thōrax*, thorax). A collection of blood and air within the pleural cavity.

hae·mopoiē·sis. Haematopoiesis, *q.v.*

haēmopoiē·tin (G. *haima*, blood; *poiēsis*, formation). See intrinsic factor.

haēmoptý·sic (G. *haima*, blood; *ptuein*, to spit). Relating to haemoptysis.

haēmŏ·ptȳsis (G. *haima*, blood; *ptuein*, to spit). Haemorrhage from the larynx, trachea, bronchi or lungs.

haē·morrhage (G. *haima*, blood; *rhegnunai*, to break). An escape of blood from the vessels, either by diapedesis through the intact walls or by rhexis through the ruptured walls. Unavoidable h.: uterine h. due to detachment of a placenta praevia.

haēmorrhā·gic (G. *haima*, blood; *rhēgnunai*, to break). Relating to or characterized by haemorrhage.

haē·morrhoid (G. *haimorrhoides*, plural of *haimorrhois*). A pile; a varicose condition of the veins of the lower portion of the rectum. External h.: situated outside the anus; Internal h.: situated within the anal canal.

haēmorrhoi·dal. 1. Relating to or affected with haemorrhoids. 2. Applied to blood vessels, nerves, etc., about the anus.

haēmorrhoidec·tomy (G. *haimorrhoides*, haemorrhoids; *ektomē*, excision). Surgical removal of haemorrhoids.

haē·mosal·pinx. Blood in the uterine (Fallopian) tube.

haēmosĭd·erin (G. *haima*, blood; *sidēros*, iron). A product of the decomposition of haemoglobin, found mainly intercellularly in areas of old haemorrhage and in parenchymatous tissues in conditions of excessive haemolysis.

haēmosiderō·sis (G. *haima*, blood; *sidēros*, iron). The condition characterized by abnormal deposits of haemosiderin in parenchymatous tissues.

haēmospā·sia (G. *haima*, blood; *spaein*, to draw). The drawing of blood to a part, as e.g., by dry cupping.

haēmospas·tic. Relating to haemospasia.

haēmosper·matism. Haematospermia, *q.v.*

Haēmospori·dia (G. *haima*, blood; *sporidion*, dim of *sporos*, seed). A sub-order of sporozoa living in the blood, penetrating the blood cells of vertebrates where they pass through schizogony; they pass another part of their life-cycle in invertebrate hosts where they undergo sporogony; comprising families of plasmodiadae, haemoproteidae and babesidae.

haemŏ·stasis, haemostā·sia (G. *haima*, blood; *stasis*, a halt). The stagnation or arrest of a flow of blood.

hae·mostat (G. *haima*, blood; *stasis*, a halt). Haemostatic forceps.

haemostat·ic (G. *haima*, blood; *stasis*, a halt). Arresting haemorrhage.

hae·motachŏ·meter (G. *haima*, blood; *takhus*, swift; *metron*, measure). An instrument for measuring the rate of the flow of blood.

haemother·apy (G. *haima*, blood; *therapeia*, treatment). Treatment by the intramuscular injection of blood.

haemothor·ax (G. *haima*, blood; *thōrax*, thorax). An accumulation of blood in the pleural cavity.

haemotym·panum (G. *haima*, blood; *tumpanon*, a drum). Accumulation of blood in the tympanic cavity.

Haffkine's vaccine or serum (Haffkine, W. M. W., Russian bacteriologist, 1860–1930). A preparation of plague bacilli used by inoculation as a preventive of plague.

haf·nium (L. *Hafnia*, Copenhagen). A rare element, occuring in zirconium ores. Symbol Hf.

Hagedorn's needle (Hagedorn, W., German surgeon, 1831–94). A triangular surgical needle for suture purposes.

Haglund's disease (Haglund, S. E. P., Swedish orthopaedist, born 1870). Bursitis in connection with the tendo Achillis.

Hahnemannism (Hahnemann, C. F. S., German physician and founder of homoeopathy, 1755–1843). Homoeopathy.

hair. A delicate filament, appendage of the skin.

hairy tongue. See black tongue.

hä·lazone. *p*-sulphondichloroamidobenzoic acid, $C_7H_5O_4NCl_2S$. Synthetic organic compound used for sterilization of drinking water.

Halban's sign (Halban, J., Austrian gynaecologist, 1870–1937). Growth of fine hair on face and body during pregnancy.

Haldane's chamber (Haldane, J. S., English physiologist, 1860–1936). Chamber used in study of physiology of respiration and cardiovascular system under conditions of decreased atmospheric pressure.

Hales's piezometer (Hales, S., English physiologist, 1677–1761). Apparatus used by Hales to measure blood pressure in carotid artery of the horse.

halibut liver oil. Oil extracted from fresh or suitably preserved liver of the halibut, *Hippoglossus hippoglossus*. There are many commercial preparations of the oil, which is particularly rich in vitamins A and D.

hä·listerē·sis (G. *hals*, salt; *sterēsis*, privation). The loss of calcium salts from bone.

halitō·sis (L. *halitus*, exhalation). Foul breath.

hä·litus (L.). A vapour.

Hall's disease. See Marshall Hall.

Haller's ansa (Haller, A. von, Swiss anatomist, 1708–77). A loop formed anterior to the internal jugular vein by a small nerve diverging from the facial immediately below the stylomastoid foramen, and uniting with the glossopharyngeal slightly below Andersch's ganglion. It is not constant. **H.'s circle:** see Zinn's circle. **H.'s colic omentum:** a process of the upper boundary of the greater omentum which may become attached to the testis during foetal life and be comprised in the sac of an inguinal hernia. **H.'s cones:** the coni vasculosi of the epididymis. **H.'s congenital hernia:** See Malgaigne's hernia. **H.'s**

fretum: see H.'s isthmus. **H.'s habenula:** the slender cord formed when the canal connecting the cavities of the peritoneum and tunica vaginalis in early life is effaced. **H.'s isthmus:** fretum Halleri, the constriction which separates the ventricle from the aortic bulb during early foetal life. **H.'s network:** the rete vasculosum of the testis. **H.'s plexus:** the interlacement (H.'s laryngeal plexus) formed by branches of the external laryngeal and sympathetic nerves on the exterior surface of the inferior constrictor pharyngis. **H.'s splendid line:** the linea splendens, the longitudinal fibrous band of the pia answering to the site of the anterior median fissure of the spinal cord. **H.'s tripod:** tripus Halleri, the coeliac axis. **H.'s tunica vasculosa:** the lamina vasculosa of the choroid. **H.'s vas aberrans:** a small convoluted duct united with the tail of the epididymis or the commencement of the vas deferens. **H.'s venous circle:** a broken circle of superficial veins often visible through the integument of the mammae, especially during lactation.

hallucinā·tion (L. *halucinatio*). A delusional perception of an object or phenomenon which has no external existence.

hallucinō·sis. A psychosis in which hallucinations form the main symptom.

hal·lux (L. *allex*, pl. *allices*). The great toe. **H. flexus:** the deformity of fixed extension of first metatarsophalangeal joint and flexion of the interphalangea joint: a hammer toe applied to the hallux. **H. valgus:** deviation of the great toe towards the others, i.e. lateral deviation. **H. varus:** deviation of the great toe away from the others, i.e. medially towards the midline of the body.

halo (G. *halōs*, a circle). A circle; the pigmented areola of the nipple. **H. glaucomatosus:** a yellowish white circle round the optic disc in glaucoma.

hă·logen (G. *hals*, salt; *gennan*, to produce). The collective term for the four elements, chlorine, fluorine, bromine and iodine, which form salts by direct union with metals.

halŏ·genous, halogen·ic (G. *hals*, salt; *gennan*, to produce). Producing saline compounds.

hă·loid (G. *hals*, salt; *eidos*, form). Resembling common salt.

ham. 1. The back portion of the knee; the popliteal space. 2. The buttock, hip and thigh.

Hamamē·lis (G. *hama*, together; *mēlon*, apple). A genus of shrubs. The leaves and bark of the *H. virginiana* (the witch hazel) are used as a haemostatic and astringent.

hamartō·ma (G. *hamartein*, to err). Developmental defect in tissue combination, with limited tendency for tumour-like growth.

hamate bone. Unciform, a small carpal bone.

hamā·tum (L.). The unciform bone.

Hamberger's schema (Hamberger, G. E., German physician, 1697–1755). Postulates that the external intercostal muscles are inspiratory, and the internal intercostal muscles are expiratory in function.

Hamilton-Irving's box. Apparatus used for suprapubic drainage of the bladder. It consists of an oval box with a brim which fits over the wound. Urine collects into the box from which it is drained by two holes into tubing which passes into a urinal. The box is kept in position by a rubber belt which the patient wears round his trunk.

hammer. In anatomy, the malleus. **H.-nose:** rhinophyma. **H.-toe:** a permanent hyper-extension of the first phalanx and flexion of the distal phalanges. Syn. mallet toe.

Hammond's disease (Hammond, W. A., American neurologist, 1828–1900). Athetosis.

hamstring. The tendons bounding the ham above on the outer and inner side.

hă·mular (L. *hamus*). Shaped like a hook.

hă·mulus (L. dim. of *hamus*, hook). A hook-like process, as of a bone.

hand. The distal part of the arm in man, composed of the carpus, metacarpus and phalanges.

hangnail. A loose fragment of epidermis at the root of the nail accompanied by inflammation.

Hannover's canal (Hannover, A., Danish anatomist, 1814–94). The space between the zonule of Zinn and the vitreous.

Hanot's cirrhosis or disease (Hanot, V. C., French physician, 1844–95). Hypertrophic cirrhosis of the liver with jaundice.

hă·palonў·chia (G. *hapalos*, soft; *onux*, finger-nail). Soft finger-nails.

haphalgē·sia (G. *haphē*, touch; *algos*, pain). Pain on merely touching objects.

haploid (G. *haploos*, simple). Having half the number of chromosomes of the normal somatic cell, as most gametes; applied to the number of chromosomes after reduction-division.

haplŏ·pathy (G. *haploos*, simple; *pathos*, disease). A disease without complications.

hap·loscope (G. *haploos*, simple; *skopein*, to view). A stereoscopic instrument used for determining the visual axes.

hapten (G. *haptein*, to touch). 1. A receptor in cells combining with microbial products; cf. haptophore. 2. Substance capable of forming conjugates with proteins of antigenic character, but not capable of stimulating antibodies.

haptic (G. *haptein*, to touch). Relating to touch.

haptine (G. *haptein*, to touch). A receptor which has been set free in Ehrlich's side-chain hypothesis.

hap·tophil, hap·tophile (G. *haptein*, to touch; *philein*, to love). A receptor with an affinity for a haptophore.

hap·tophore (G. *haptein*, to touch; *pherein*, to carry). That portion of a toxin molecule that tends to become attached to the cell receptor (hapten).

haptophor·ic, haptŏ·phorous (G. *haptein*, to touch; *pherein*, to bring). 1. Pertaining to haptophores. 2. Having combining powers.

Harder's gland (Harder, J. J., Swiss anatomist, 1656–1711). The accessory lacrimal gland of the orbit; the Harderian gland; glandula palpebrae tertiae profunda.

hare lip. A congenital fissure of the upper lip, due to arrested facial development. Syn. cheiloschisis.

harlequin foetus. A foetus affected with universal ichthyosis.

Harley's disease (Harley, G., English physician, 1829–96). Paroxysmal haemoglobinuria; Dressler's disease.

Harris's lines (Harris, H. A., contemporary Professor of Anatomy at Cambridge, born 1886). The transverse lines in long bones near the epiphysis.

Harrison's groove (Harrison, E., English physician, 1766–1838). A curve extending from the level of the ensiform cartilage towards the axilla and answering to the insertion of the diaphragm. It is seen in adenoids and in rickets.

Hartmann's critical point (Hartmann, H., French surgeon, born 1860). The site on the large intestine where the lowest sigmoid artery meets the superior rectal arterial branch.

Hartmann's pouch (Hartmann, R., German anatomist, 1831–93). A dilatation of the neck of the gallbladder.

Hartmann's solution (Hartmann, A. F., contemporary American physician). A form of Ringer's solution with added sodium lactate. Used in treatment of gastro-enteritis in infants and diabetic coma. Usually given by intravenous infusion.

hartshorn. 1. Cornu cervi, the horn of the stag, from which formerly ammonia, or spirit of hartshorn, was obtained. 2. Popular name for ammonia water.

harvest mite. Minute red mite attacking man and animals; the six-legged larval stage of the mites of the genus *Trombicula*.

Hashimoto's disease (Hashimoto, H., contemporary Japanese surgeon). Chronic thyroiditis. A diffuse lymphoid hyperplasia produces symmetrical enlargement and hardness of the thyroid gland. May be associated with myxoedema. Some authorities consider that the condition is related to Riedel's thyroiditis.

hashish. The top leaves and tender parts of hemp (*Cannabis indica*). Used as an intoxicant. Term also applied to the product of digesting the plant with butter.

Hasner's fold (Hasner, J. Ritter von, Austrian ophthalmologist, 1819–92). A fold of mucous membrane at the lower end of the nasolacrimal duct. Syn. plica lacrimalis.

Hassall's corpuscles (Hassall, A. H., English physician, 1817–94). Concentrically striated corpuscles, apparently of a degenerative character, found in the medulla of the follicles of the thymus gland.

haunch bone. The ilium.

haustration. The sacculations of the colon as seen in X-ray films.

haustrum (L., a machine for drawing water). The pouch of the wall of the colon between the semilunar plicae.

haustus (L., a draught of liquid). A draught (of medicine).

haut mal. (Fr.). Severe epilepsy.

Havers's canals (Havers, C., English anatomist, 1650–1702). Spaces in the compact tissue of bone; they contain blood- and lymph-vessels. H.'s glands: retrosynovial pads or fringes of synovial membrane consisting of intra-articular fat. H.'s lamellae: bony septa surrounding the canals. H.'s system: the concentric arrangement of the bony lamellae around a Haversian canal.

hawking. Clearing phlegm from the throat.

Hay diet (Hay, W. H., American dietician, born 1866). A selective diet intended to promote health and weight control.

hay fever. A condition characterized by hyper-secretion of nasal and conjunctival mucous membranes caused by hypersensitiveness to the pollen of grasses and other plants.

Hay's test (Hay, M., Scottish physician, 1855–1932). Test for bile salts in urine. Flowers of sulphur sprinkled on the top of a tube of urine sink if bile salts are present, owing to the lowering of the surface tension.

Hayem's corpuscles (Hayem, G., French physician, 1841–1933). See Bizzozero's blood-platelets. H.'s disease: apoplectiform myelitis.

Haygarth's nodes (Haygarth, J., English physician, 1740–1827). Exostoses of the joints of the fingers in arthritis deformans.

Hb. Symbol of Haemoglobin.

H_3BO_3. Boric Acid.

HCHO. Formaldehyde.

HCl. Hydrochloric acid.

HCO_3. The bicarbonate radical.

HCO_3^-. Bicarbonate ion.

h.d. Abbreviation of *hora decubitus*, (L.), 'at bedtime'.

He. Symbol of Helium.

head. That portion of the body containing the brain.

Head's areas (Head, Sir H., English neurologist, 1861–1940). The cutaneous areas of sensory nerve root (segmental) distribution.

headache. Any pain in the head.

healing. The curing of wounds; any curing procedure. H. by first intention: healing of a wound when the parts unite spontaneously without granulation of tissue.

health. Condition of being well, with all organs functioning properly.

hearing. The sense of sound.

heart. The strongly muscular organ at the centre of the circulatory system in the middle mediastinum. **H. failure cell:** a histiocyte from the alveolar wall filled with haemosiderin derived from red blood cells in pulmonary alveoli, found in the sputum in cases of passive pulmonary congestion. **H. murmur:** See murmur, cardiac.

heart-block. A disturbance of cardiac rhythm, due to impairment of conduction of stimuli from the auricle to the ventricle in which the ventricle contracts less frequently than the auricle. **H.-B., complete:** h.-b. in which ventricle and auricle beat with independent rhythm, no auricular stimuli reaching the ventricle, the latter contracting at its 'autonomous' rate (i.e. above 30 times per minute). **H.-B., partial:** h.-b. in which only every second, third or fourth etc., auricular contraction is followed by a ventricular contraction.

heartburn. A burning sensation felt in the epigastric or lower oesophageal region, usually due to hyperchlorhydria.

heat. 1. Warmth. 2. Period of sexual excitement of female mammals. **H. apoplexy,** or **H. stroke:** a condition characterized by severe prostration, high temperature, which may progress to coma, convulsions and death, due to exposure to extreme heat, with insufficient loss of heat. **H., specific:** the amount of heat necessary to raise one gramme of substance through 1°C. **H. unit:** see calorie.

Heath's operation (Heath, C., English surgeon, 1835–1905). Division of the mandible in front of the masseter muscle in cases of ankylosis of the mandibular joint.

heavy hydrogen. Deuterium (an isotope of hydrogen).

heavy water. Deuterium oxide. Water in which the hydrogen in combination is replaced by deuterium.

hebephrē·nia (G. hēbē, puberty; phrēn, mind). A form of schizophrenia usually occurring in young adults, characterized by rapid mental deterioration.

Heberden's disease (Heberden, W., English physician, 1710–1801). 1. Angina pectoris. 2. Arthritis deformans. **H.'s nodes:** deformity of the fingers in arthritis deformans.

Heberden-Rosenbach's nodes. Heberden's nodes, q.v.

hebet·ic (G. hēbē, puberty). Relating to puberty.

hebetude (L. hebetudo, dullness). Blunting of the intellect in some acute fevers.

hē·bin (G. hēbē, puberty). A hormone from the anterior lobe of the pituitary body which stimulates the gonads.

Hebra's erythema (Hebra, F. von, Austrian dermatologist, 1816–80). Polymorphous erythema. **H.'s pityriasis:** pityriasis rubra. **H.'s prurigo:** true prurigo.

hectic (G. hektikos, habitual). 1. Habitual. 2. Characterized by progressive loss of power and weight; hence, morbidly flushed; mainly applied to the fever or countenance of a person affected with phthisis.

hectine. The sodium salt of the benzene sulphonyl derivative of para-amino-phenyl-arsonic acid.

hectogramme (G. hekaton, hundred; gramma, a small weight). One hundred grammes, or 1543·2340 grains.

hectolitre (G. hekaton, hundred; litra, a weight of one pound). One hundred litres, or 22·009 imperial gallons.

hectometre (G. hekaton, hundred; metron, measure). One hundred metres, or 328 feet 1 inch.

hedō·nia (G. hēdŏnē, pleasure). Exaggerated cheerfulness.

hē·donism (G. hēdŏnē, pleasure). The cult of pleasure.

hedrocele (G. hedra, anus; kēlē, hernia). Anal prolapse.

heel. The back part of the foot.

Hegar's sign (Hegar, A., German gynaecologist, 1830–1914). Softening and compressibility of the lower segment of the uterus and the upper half of the cervix, encountered on bimanual examination during the first two or three months of pregnancy.

Heidenhain's demilunes (Heidenhain, R., German physiologist, 1834–97). See Giannuzzi's cells. **H.'s rods** or **striae:** columnar cells of the uriniferous tubules.

Heim's pill (Heim, E. L., German physician, 1747–1834). A pill consisting of ½ gr. powdered digitalis, ¼ gr. ipecacuanha, ¼ gr. powdered opium and ½ gr. extract of helenium used in allaying the fever of phthisis.

Heim-Kreysig's sign (Heim, E. L., German physician, 1747–1834; Kreysig, F. L., German physician, 1770–1839). See Kreysig's sign.

Heine-Medin disease (Heine, J. von, German physician, 1800–79; Medin, O., Swedish physician, 1847–1928). A group of paralyses including infantile spinal, Landry's, bulbar, pontine, cerebral, ataxic, neuritic and meningitic forms, presumed to be various localizations of action by the same infective agent. See also poliomyelitis.

Heineke-Mikulicz operation (Heineke, W. H., German surgeon, 1834–1901; Mikulicz-Radecki, J. von, Polish surgeon, 1850–1905). Plastic operation on the pylorus.

Heinz's bodies (Heinz, R., German pathologist, 1865–1924). The small bodies occasionally seen in red blood corpuscles after staining with Azure I.

Heister's diverticulum (Heister, L., German anatomist, 1683–1758). The sinus of the jugular vein. **H.'s valves:** the transverse valvular folds of the mucous membrane of the cystic bile-duct.

hel·coid (G. helkos, ulcer; eidos, form). Like an ulcer.

helcō·ma (G. helkos, ulcer). An ulcer.

helcō·sis (G. helkōsis, ulceration). The formation and growth of an ulcer.

Held's decussation (Held, H., German anatomist, born 1886). The decussation of certain fibres of the acoustic nerve to reach the lateral fillet. **H.'s ground net:** a hypothetical terminal reticulum of the nervous system.

hĕ·licoid (G. hĕlix, coil; eidos, form). Coiled like a helix; spiral.

helicotrē·ma (G. hĕlix, coil; trēma, hole). The opening between the two scales of the cochlea.

Helie's bundle of fibres (Helie, L. T., French anatomist, 1804–67). The fasciculus ansiforme; vertical and ansiform bundle of the superficial musculature of the anterior uterus.

hē·liencephalī·tis (G. hēlios, sun; egkephalos, brain). Encephalitis due to exposure to the sun.

hē·liopă·thia (G. hēlios, sun; pathos, disease). Any disorder caused by exposure to the sun's rays.

hē·liophĭ·lia (G. hēlios, sun; philein, to love). Exaggerated affinity for sunlight, resulting sometimes in ecstasies and muscular contractions.

hē·liophō·bia (G. hēlios, sun; phŏbos, fear). A morbid fear of sunlight.

heliotax·is (G. hēlios, sun; tăxis, arrangement). Taxis, q.v., in which sunlight is the orienting stimulus.

hē·liothĕ·rapy (G. hēlios, sun; therapeia, treatment). The treatment of disease by exposure to sunlight.

heliŏ·tropism (G. hēlios, sun; trepein, to turn). Tropism, q.v., in which sunlight is the orienting stimulus.

helium (G. hēlios, sun). A light, inert gaseous element. Symbol He. Atomic weight 4·003.

helix (G. helix, coil). The rounded convex margin of the external ear.

Heller's plexus (Heller, A. L. G., German pathologist, born 1840). The arterial plexus in the intestinal wall.

Heller's test (Heller, J. F., Austrian pathologist, 1813–71). Test for albumin in the urine. To some nitric acid in a test-tube urine is added by pouring it down the side of the tube; the development of an opaque white ring indicates that albumin is present.

Helmholtz's ligament (Helmholtz, H. L. F. von, German anatomist, 1821–94). The axial ligament of the malleus; the anterior and posterior ligaments considered as a single ligament elongated in the line of rotation of the malleus.

hel·minth (G. *helmins*, worm). A general term covering certain low forms of parasitic worms of the Platyhelminthes (flat-worms) and Nemathelminthes (thread-worms).

helminthi·asis (G. *helmins*, worm). The condition of harbouring worms in the body, and its sequelae.

helmin·thic (G. *helmins*, worm). Same as anthelmintic, *q.v.*

helmintho·logy (G. *helmins*, worm; *logos*, a discourse). That section of zoology relating to helminths.

helminthopho·bia (G. *helmins*, worm; *phŏbos*, fear). A morbid fear of being worm-infested.

Helmont's mirror or speculum (Helmont, J. B. van, Belgian surgeon and scientist, 1577–1644). The centrum tendinosum of the diaphragm.

helŏ·ma (G. *hēlos*, a nail). A corn.

helŏ·tomy (G. *hēlos*, a nail; *tomē*, section). The surgical removal of corns.

Helvetius's ligaments (Helvetius, J. C. A., French physician and anatomist, 1685–1755). The lateral bands of muscular fibres and connective tissue of the stomach wall producing sacculation of the antrum; pyloric ligaments.

Helweg's bundle or triangular tract (Helweg, H. K. S., Danish psychiatrist, 1847–1901). The tractus olivospinalis, a continuation of the tractus thalamoolivaris or central tegmental tract.

heme. See haem.

hē·meralŏ·pia (G. *hēmera*, day; *alaos*, blind; *ōps*, eye). Night-blindness; the condition of having normal vision in daylight, diminished vision in twilight and insufficient illumination. Due to vitamin A deficiency. (The term originally meant day-blindness).

hĕ·miachromatop·sia (G. *hēmi*, half; *a*, neg; *khroma*, colour; *opsis*, vision). Colour-blindness in one half of the field of vision.

hĕ·miageu·sia (G. *hēmi*, half; *a*, neg.; *geusis*, taste). Loss of taste in one lateral half of the tongue.

hemial·gia (G. *hēmi*, half; *algos*, pain). One-sided neuralgia.

hemianacū·sis (G. *hēmi*, half; *an*, neg.; *akouein*, to hear). Loss of hearing in one ear.

hemianaesthē·sia (G. *hēmi*, half; *an*, neg.; *aisthēsis*, feeling). Anaesthesia of one lateral half of the body.

hemianalgē·sia (G. *hēmi*, half; *an*, neg.; *algos*, pain). Insensibility to pain throughout one lateral half of the body and limbs.

hemianō·pia, hemianop·sia (G. *hēmi*, half; *an*, neg.; *opsis*, vision). Blindness in one-half of the visual field. **H. unilateral:** h. affecting one eye only.

hemiatax·ia (G. *hēmi*, half; *a*, neg.; *taxis*, arrangement). Unilateral ataxia.

hemiăthetŏ·sis (G. *hēmi*, half; *athetos*, displaced). Unilateral athetosis.

hemiă·trophy (G. *hēmi*, half; *atrophia*, atrophy). Atrophy of one side of the body, or of one part of the body.

hemibăl·lism (G. *hēmi*, half; *ballismos*, dancing). Unilateral chorea.

hemicĕ·phalus (G. *hēmi*, half; *kephalē*, head). A monster in which the cerebral hemispheres and skull are partially lacking.

hemichorē·a (G. *hēmi*, half; *khoreia*, a dance). Chorea of one side of the body.

hemicrā·nia (G. *hēmi*, half; *kranion*, skull). Paroxysmal headache confined to one side of the head, often accompanied by nausea, scotomata and oliguria. Syn. migraine.

hemihȳ·peraesthē·sia (G. *hēmi*, half; *huper*, above; *aisthēsis*, feeling). Hyperaesthesia confined to one lateral half of the body.

hemihȳper·trophy (G. *hēmi*, half; *huper*, above; *trophē*, nutrition). Hypertrophy of one lateral half of the body.

hemĭ·melus (G. *hēmi*, half; *melos*, limb). A monster with imperfectly developed extremities.

hemĭō·pia (G. *hēmi*, half; *ōps*, eye). See hemianopia.

hemĭō·pic (G. *hēmi*, half; *ōps*, eye). Relating to hemianopia.

hemĭ·pagus (G. *hēmi*, half; *pēgnunai*, to fix). A double monster united at the thorax and with a common mouth.

hemiparaesthē·sia (G. *hēmi*, half; *para*, beyond; *aisthēsis*, feeling). Paraesthesia affecting part of one lateral half of the body only.

hemipărē·sis (G. *hēmi*, half; *parēsis*, paralysis). Paresis of one side of the body.

hemiplē·gia (G. *hēmi*, half; *plēgē*, a blow). Paralysis of one side of the body. **Alternate h.:** paralysis of a part on one side of the body and of another part on the other side. Also called **Crossed h.** and Gubler's paralysis.

Hemip·tera (G. *hēmi*, half; *pteron*, wing). True bugs; order of arthropods, members of which are mostly adapted to feed upon juices of plants or animals.

hemisphere (G. *hēmi*, half; *sphaira*, sphere). Half a sphere; e.g. **Cerebral h.:** one lateral half of the cerebrum.

hemlock. Conium.

Henke's space (Henke, P. J. W., German anatomist, 1834–96). The interval between the vertebral column and the pharynx; retropharyngeal space. **H.'s triangle:** that between the descending part of the inguinal fold, the lateral part of the fold and the lateral border of the rectus abdominis.

Henle's ampulla (Henle, F. G. J., German anatomist, 1809–85). The ampulla of the uterine tube. **H.'s layer:** the outer layer of cells in the root sheath of a hair. **H.'s loop:** the looped portion of the uriniferous tubules of the kidney. **H.'s membrane:** see Bruch's layer. **H.'s spine:** the suprameatal spine, processus auditorius of the temporal bone. It serves as a point of reference in trephining the mastoid process.

henna. The powdered, dried leaves of *Lawsonia alba*, used as a dye for hair.

Henoch's purpura (Henoch, E. H., German paediatrist, 1820–1910). Purpura associated with symptoms of gastro-intestinal upset.

henogĕ·nesis (G. *hĕn*, one; *genesis*, origin). Ontogenesis.

henō·sis (G. *henōsis*, union). Healing.

henŏ·tic (G. *henōtikos*, unifying). Attempting to heal.

Henry's law (Henry, W., English chemist, 1775–1837). See Dalton's law.

Hensen's canal (Hensen, V., German physiologist, 1835–1924). Canalis reuniens which joins the cochlear canal to the saccule. **H.'s knot or node:** a thickening at the site of the first formation of the primitive streak; protochordal knot of Hubrecht.

Hensing's ligament (Hensing, F. W., German anatomist, 1719–45). Left superior colic ligament; phrenicocolic ligament or sustentaculum coli linealis.

hepar (G. *hēpar*, liver). 1. The liver. 2. A substance with the colour of liver, such as **H. sulphuris.**

hĕ·parin (G. *hēpar*, liver). A substance secreted by basophile cells in the walls of arteries, liver capsule and other parts; acting as anticoagulant by inhibiting the conversion of prothrombin into thrombin.

hĕ·parinate (G. *hēpar*, liver). Any heparin salt.

hĕ·parinize (G. *hēpar*, liver). The use of heparin to prevent coagulation of the blood.

hepatal·gia (G. *hēpar*, liver; *algos*, pain). Pain in the liver.

hepatar·gia (G. *hēpar*, liver; *argia*, idleness). Insufficiency of liver function.

hepatec·tomy (G. *hēpar*, liver; *ektomē*, excision). Total or partial excision of the liver.

hepat·ic (G. *hēpar*, liver). Relating to or belonging to the liver.

hĕ·paticogastrŏ·stomy (G. *hēpar*, liver; *gaster*, stomach; *stoma*, mouth). An anastomosis between the bile duct and the stomach.

hepä·ticolĭ·thotripsy (G. *hēpar*, liver; *lithos*, stone; *tribein*, to crush). Crushing of a stone in the hepatic duct.

hepä·ticŏ·stomy (G. *hēpar*, liver; *stoma*, mouth). The formation of a fistula in the hepatic duct.

hepati·tis (G. *hēpar*, liver). Inflammation of the parenchymatous tissue of the liver.

hepatizā·tion (G. *hēpar*, liver). The change of lung tissue into a condition in which it resembles the liver in consistency, as in lobar pneumonia.

hepä·tocele (G. *hēpar*, liver; *kēlē*, hernia). Hernia of the liver.

hĕ·patocirrhŏ·sis (G. *hēpar*, liver; *kirrhos*, tawny). Cirrhosis of the liver.

hepatogĕ·nic, hepatŏ·genous (G. *hēpar*, liver; *gennan*, to produce). Produced by or in the liver.

hepatŏ·graphy (G. *hēpar*, liver; *graphein*, to write). A description of the liver.

hepato-lenti·cular (G. *hēpar*, liver; L. *lenticularis*, lentil-like). Pertaining to both liver and the lenticular nucleus of the brain.

hepato-lenticular-degeneration (G. *hēpar*, liver; L.L. *lenticularis*, lentil-like; *degenerare*, to degenerate). A familial disease of progressive character, usually starting during adolescence, characterized by the association of a multilobular cirrhosis of the liver with degenerative changes in the lenticular and caudate nuclei and in cortical nerve cells, resulting in nerve lesions of the extrapyramidal type with defects of articulation and deglutition and mental debility, and by the formation of the pigmented ring of Kayser-Fleischer, *q.v.* Syn. Wilson's disease; progressive lenticular degeneration.

hĕ·patolith (G. *hēpar*, liver; *lithos*, stone). Biliary calculus.

hĕ·patolithĭ·asis (G. *hēpar*, liver; *lithos*, stone). A condition characterized by the formation of gallstones in the intrahepatic bile ducts.

hĕ·patomĕ·galy (G. *hēpar*, liver; *mĕgas*, great). Enlargement of the liver.

hepatŏ·ma (G. *hēpar*, liver). A tumour of the liver.

hĕ·patopexy (G. *hēpar*, liver; *pēxis*, fixation). Surgical fixation of the liver.

hĕ·patoptŏ·sis (G. *hēpar*, liver; *ptōsis*, a falling). Abnormally low position of the liver.

hĕ·patorē·nal (G. *hēpar*, liver; L. *rēn*, kidney). Pertaining both to the liver and the kidney. **H. syndrome:** severe disorder of kidney function due to degeneration of renal tubules, occurring in acute stages of liver disease or following operation on biliary passages.

hepatŏr·rhaphy (G. *hēpar*, liver; *rhaphē*, suture). Suture of the liver.

hepatorrhex·is (G. *hēpar*, liver; *rhēxis*, rupture). Rupture of the liver.

herb (L. *herba*). A plant of which the stem contains no wood and which dies down to the ground at the end of its season.

herbal (L. *herba*, herb). 1. An old term for a book on herbs, especially one describing their pharmacological properties. 2. Pertaining to herbs.

herbalist. A professional healer, using mainly herbs.

herbi·vorous (L. *herba*, herb; *vorare*, to eat). Living on vegetable food.

Herbst's bodies, corpuscles (Herbst, E. F., German physician, 1803–93). The sensory terminals in the skin of the beaks of birds.

herĕ·ditary (L. *hereditarius*). Transmitted from parent to offspring.

herĕ·dity (L. *hereditas*). The transmission of bodily or mental characters from ancestor to offspring.

hĕ·redosў·philis (L. *heres*, heir; *syphilis*). Congenital syphilis.

Hering's theory of colour sensation (Hering, E., German physiologist, 1834–1918). Three primary substances in the retina which are constantly undergoing a reciprocal process of breaking down and reformation. These substances are respectively broken down by red, yellow and white light and built up by green, blue and black. There are therefore 6 primary sensations arranged in antagonistic pairs. When light falls on the retina they are broken down and built up in varying quantities. When no light falls on the retina they neutralize each other.

hĕ·ritable (L. *heres*, heir). Any quality or character capable of being inherited.

Hermann's fluid (Hermann, F., German anatomist, 1859–1920). A hardening fluid for body tissues, consisting of glacial acetic acid 4 parts, 2 per cent solution of osmic acid 8 parts, 1 per cent solution of platinum chloride 60 parts.

hermaph·rodism, hermaph·roditism (G. *Hermēs*, Mercury; *Aphroditē*, Venus). The co-existence in an individual of gonads of either sex, resulting in a mixture of male and female characteristics varying according to the relative preponderance of male or female sex-hormone production. See also pseudohermaphroditism.

hermaph·rodite. An individual affected with hermaphroditism.

hermet·ic (G. *Hermes*, a divine name used as alchemical symbol). Airtight.

hernia (L). The protrusion of a viscus or portion of a viscus through the walls of a cavity it normally occupies into a sac. **H. cerebri:** protrusion of the brain substance through the skull.

her·nial. Relating to hernia. **H. sac:** the membrane which the organ pushes before it or into which it descends.

her·niate. To form a hernia.

herŏ·ic (G. *hērōs*, hero). Bold or daring; severe; usually applied to medical treatments or surgical measures involving a risk.

heroin, heroine (G. *hērōs*, hero). The diacetic-acid ester of morphine, used as an anodyne or sedative. The action of h. is similar to that of morphine but the effect on the respiratory centre is more powerful.

hĕ·roinism. Addiction to the use of heroin.

Herophilus, torcular of (Herophilus, Greek physician of Alexandria, 335–280 B.C.). The dilatation at the junction of the superior longitudinal, straight, two lateral and occipital sinuses; the confluens sinuum.

herpes (G. *herpein*, to creep). An acute inflammatory disease of the skin or mucous membrane, characterized by the development of vesicles in a cluster-like arrangement. **H. zoster:** see zoster.

herpet·ic. Relating to herpes.

herpĕ·tiform (G. *herpein*, to creep; L. *forma*, shape). Resembling herpes.

her·sage (Fr. from *herse*, a harrow). Splitting up a nerve into its segmental fibres.

Hertwig's epithelial sheath (Hertwig, R., German zoologist, 1850–1937). The cells of the enamel organ of the tooth germ persisting around the roots of teeth.

Herxheimer's spirals (Herxheimer, K., German dermatologist, born 1861). Minute spiral fibres found in the rete mucosum of the epidermis.

Heryng's benign ulcer (Heryng, T., Polish laryngologist, 1847–1925). A solitary ulcer of unknown origin on the anterior fauces.

Heschl's convolutions (Heschl, R., Austrian pathologist, 1824–81). The gyri temporales transversi.

Hesselbach's fascia (Hesselbach, F. K., German surgeon, 1759–1816). The fascia cribriformis. **H.'s hernia**: a plurilobular hernia passing through the cribriform fascia. **H.'s ligament**: the ligamentum interfoveolare. **H.'s triangle**: triangular area bounded by the inferior epigastric artery, the margin of rectus abdominis and the inguinal ligament, externally.

hĕ·teradel·phus (G. *heteros*, other; *adelphos*, brother). A double monster the acephalic parasite of which is joined to the autosite at the ventral aspect.

heteradē·nia (G. *heteros*, other; *adēn*, gland). Abnormal glandular tissue.

hĕ·teraden·ic (G. *heteros*, other; *adēn*, gland). Pertaining to abnormal glandular tissue.

hĕ·teradenō·ma (G. *heteros*, other; *adēn*, gland). Any tumour composed of heteradenic tissue.

hĕ·terauxē·sis (G. *heteros*, other; *auxēsis*, growth). The relation of the growth rate of a part of a developing organism (whether morphological or chemical) to the growth rate of the whole or of another part; a comparison between organisms of the same group but of different ages and hence sizes.

hĕ·terocĕ·phalus (G. *heteros*, other; *kephalē*, head). A monster with two heads of unequal size.

hĕ·terochrō·mia (G. *heteros*, other; *khrōma*, colour). Difference of colour, applied to structures normally of the same colour, especially the irides of the two eyes or two different parts of the same iris. Syn. anisochromia.

hĕ·terochrō·mosome (G. *heteros*, other; *khrōma*, colour). Allosome, *q.v.*

hĕ·terochrō·mous (G. *heteros*, other; *khrōma*, colour). Having different colours.

hĕ·terochrō·nia, **hĕterŏ·chronism**, **heterŏ·chrony** (G. *heteros*, other; *khronos*, time). Development or occurrence of a phenomenon at an abnormal time.

hĕ·terochron·ic, **heterŏ·chronous** (G. *heteros*, other; *khronos*, time). 1. Irregular in occurrence; occurring at an abnormal sequence. 2. Difference in chronaxie, *q.v.*, amongst related neurons.

heterocȳ·clic (G. *heteros*, other; *kuklos*, circle). Applied to cyclic compounds in which the ring is formed of atoms of different kinds.

heterŏ·dymus (G. *heteros*, other; *didumos*, twin). A double monster the parasitic part of which has only a head, neck, and rudimentary thorax.

heteroe·cious (G. *heteros*, other; *oikos*, house). Applied to parasites which live upon different hosts at different stages of growth.

hetero-ĕ·rotism (G. *heteros*, other; *erōs*, love). Sexual feeling directed towards another individual.

heterogă·metous, **heterŏ·gamous** (G. *heteros*, other; *gamos*, marriage). Having, or producing, unlike gametes.

heterŏ·gamy (G. *heteros*, other; *gamos*, marriage). A type of conjugation in which fusing gametes differ from each other in structure and function.

hĕ·terogē·neous (G. *heteros*, other; *genos*, kind). Differing in kind or nature; dissimilar; composed of different substances; not homogeneous.

hĕ·terogĕ·nesis (G. *heteros*, other; *genesis*, generation). A mode of reproduction in which the offspring do not emulate the development of the ancestors, as in mutation or in alteration (sexual and asexual) in the mode of reproduction.

hetero-inoculation (G. *heteros*, other; L. *in*, in; *oculus*, eye). Inoculation of one person with virus taken from another.

heterŏ·logous (G. *heteros*, other; *logos*, a discourse). 1. Characterized by heterology. 2. Derived from an individual of another species.

heterŏ·logy (G. *heteros*, other; *logos*, a discourse). 1. Lack of correspondence between parts. 2. Atypical or abnormal.

heterŏ·lysin (G. *heteros*, other; *lusis*, dissolution). A lysin acting on cells in individuals of another species.

heterŏ·lysis (G. *heteros*, other; *lusis*, dissolution). Destruction by a lysis derived from another organismal species.

heterolyt·ic (G. *heteros*, other; *lusis*, dissolution). Relating to or produced by heterolysis or a heterolysin.

hĕ·teromĕ·ric (G. *heteros*, other; *mĕros*, part). Applied to axones crossing to the opposite side of the spinal cord.

hĕ·terometrŏ·pia (G. *heteros*, other; *metron*, measure; *ōps*, eye). Dissimilarity in refraction of the two eyes.

hĕ·teromor·phism (G. *heteros*, other; *morphē*, form). 1. The property of crystallizing in different forms. 2. A deviation from type or norm; property of exhibiting different forms at different stages in the life-history.

hĕ·teromorphō·sis (G. *heteros*, other; *morphōsis*, a forming). 1. Malformation. 2. Malplacement; especially with regard to the new formation of an organ which has been lost.

hĕ·teromor·phous (G. *heteros*, other; *morphē*, form). 1. Atypical in form. 2. Relating to heteromorphism.

heterŏ·nomous (G. *heteros*, other; *nomos*, law). Growing according to a different type.

heterŏ·nomy (G. *heteros*, other; *nomos*, law). 1. Subordination to a law of adaptive modification. 2. Condition of being heteronomous.

heterŏ·nymous (G. *heteros*, other; *onuma*, name). Crossed double visual images.

heterŏ·pagus (G. *heteros*, other; *pagos*, fixture). A double monster in which the rudimentary parasite is attached to the anterior abdominal wall of the autosite.

hĕ·terophor·ia (G. *heteros*, other; *phoros*, bearing). Latent squint; tendency to squint.

heterophthal·mia (G. *heteros*, other; *ophthalmos*, eye). Difference in colour of the two eyes. Also called heterochromia.

hĕ·teroplā·sia (G. *heteros*, other; *plassein*, to form). 1. Abnormal tissue formation. 2. Malplaced tissue.

hĕ·teroplasm (G. *heteros*, other; *plassein*, to form). Malplaced tissue.

hĕ·teroplas·tic (G. *heteros*, other; *plassein*, to form). 1. Relating to heteroplasia. 2. Differing in structure.

hĕ·teroplasty (G. *heteros*, other; *plassein*, to form). 1. Heteroplasia. 2. The transplantation of grafts taken from another individual.

hĕ·terosex·ual (G. *heteros*, other; L. *sexus*, sex). Relating to the opposite sex.

heterŏ·sporous (G. *heteros*, other; *sporos*, seed). Having two types of spore.

hetero-suggestion (G. *heteros*, other; L. *suggerere*, to suggest). Suggestion by another person.

hĕ·terotax·is (G. *heteros*, other; *taxis*, arrangement). Abnormal position or transposition of organs.

hĕ·terotŏ·pia (G. *heteros*, other; *tŏpos*, place). 1. Displacement 2. Congenital displacement of tissue.

hĕ·terotox·in (G. *heteros*, other; *toxikon*, poison). Any toxin formed outside the body.

hĕt·erotrichŏ·sis (G. *heteros*, other; *trikhōsis*, hairgrowth). Hair of different colours on the body.

hĕ·terotrō·phic (G. *heteros*, other; *trophein*, to nourish). Applied to bacteria which are (1) capable of existence and growth only in media containing one or more organic substances; or (2) existing as parasites.

hĕ·terotrō·pia (G. *heteros*, other; *trŏpos*, turn). Incapacity for bifocal fixation owing to the deviation of one eye.

hĕ·terotryp·sin (G. *heteros*, other; *tripsis*, from *tribein*, to rub). A pancreatic juice enzyme.

hĕ·terotyp·ical (G. *heteros*, other; *tupos*, type). 1. Differing from type. 2. Heterologous.

hĕ·terozȳ·gote (G. *heteros*, other; *zugon*, yoke). A heterozygous individual.

he·terozȳ·gous (G. *heteros*, other; *zugon*, yoke). Term used in genetics to describe the offspring of crossbreeding two pure but different strains.

Heuber-Herter's disease. See coeliac disease.

Heubner's disease (Heubner, J. O. L., German paediatrician, 1843–1926). Endarteritis of the brain due to syphilis.

Hewlett's stain (Hewlett, R. T., English pathologist, 1865–1940). Hewlett's method of staining bacterial capsules. Carbol fuchsin with a weak solution of gentian violet as counter-stain.

hexachrō·mic (G. *hex*, six; *khrōma*, colour). Capable of recognizing only six of the seven colours of the spectrum; being therefore unable to distinguish violet from indigo.

hexadac·tylism (G. *hex*, six; *daktulos*, finger). Having six fingers or toes on a hand or foot.

hexamethonium. Hexamethonium and pentamethonium are salts of bromine and iodine which diminish synaptic conduction throughout the autonomic nervous system. They cause a marked lowering of blood pressure and on this account are used in the treatment of hyperpiesis and by anaesthetists in certain operations to reduce the liability to haemorrhage. They also diminish gastric secretion and mobility and are used in the treatment of peptic ulcer. Clinically, hexamethonium salts are preferred to those of pentamethonium.

hexamine. A crystalline substance used as a urinary antiseptic. Formula $(CH_2)_6N_4$.

hex·ane. A paraffin hydrocarbon used as a solvent.

hexă·valent (G. *hex*, six; L. *valere*, to be strong). Having a valency of six.

hexes·trol, hexōe·strol (G. *hex*, six; *oistros*, orgasm). A synthetic oestrogen obtained by the hydrogenation of stilboestrol in presence of palladium.

hexobar·bitone. A barbiturate drug. See barbiturate.

hexoki·nase (G. *hex*, six; *kinēsis*, movement). A yeast derivative which helps to convert glucose into lactic acid.

hĕx·osamine. A sugar with the amine group replacing a hydroxyl group.

hexose (G. *hex*, six). Any monosaccharide which contains six carbon atoms in the molecule; typically of the formula $C_6H_{12}O_6$.

hexosephos·phate. An ester of a hexose with phosphoric acid.

hex·ylresor·cinol. A crystalline substance used as a urinary disinfectant; also used externally and as an anthelmintic. Formula $C_{12}H_{18}O_2$.

Hey's infantile hernia (Hey, W., English surgeon, 1736–1819). Cooper's hernia, *q.v.* H.'s ligament: the femoral ligament, a falciform expansion of the fascia lata.

Hg. The symbol for mercury.

Hgb. Abbreviation for haemoglobin.

$HgCl_2$. Mercuric chloride or corrosive sublimate.

H.+Hm. Compound hypermetropic astigmatism.

hiā·tal. Relating to a hiatus.

hiā·tus (L.). An empty space or opening. H. hernia: a protrusion of part of the fundus of the stomach through the oesophageal hiatus of the diaphragm into the thorax.

hibernā·tion (L. *hibernus*, wintry). The condition of passing the winter, especially that of passing it in a sleeping state.

hiccup, hiccough. A spasmodic contraction of the diaphragm, producing inspiration associated with a sudden closure of the glottis. H., epidemic: a disease characterized by h., possibly related to epidemic encephalitis.

Hick's sign. See under Braxton Hicks.

hī·drocystō·ma (G. *hidrōs*, sweat; *kustis*, bladder). An affection of the skin of the face characterized by deep-seated pseudo-vesicles believed to be due to cystic dilatation of sweat-ducts or sweat-glands.

hī·dropoiē·sis (G. *hidrōs*, sweat; *poiēsis*, formation). The formation of sweat.

hī·dropoiet·ic (G. *hidrōs*, sweat; *poiēsis*, formation). Relating to hidropoiesis.

hidrorrhoē·a (G. *hidrōs*, sweat; *rhoia*, a flow). Profuse sweating.

hidrō·schĕsis (G. *hidrōs*, sweat; *skhesis*, retention). Retention of sweat.

hidrose (G. *hidrōs*, sweat). Relating to sweat.

hidrō·sis (G. *hidros*, sweat). 1. The excretion of sweat. 2. Extreme sweating.

hieral·gia (G. *hieros*, holy; *algos*, pain). Any pain in the sacrum.

Higginson's syringe (Higginson, A., English 19th-century surgeon). A rubber enema syringe.

high frequency treatment. Short wave diathermy.

higher bacteria. Bacteria showing increased complexity of structure and function, i.e. forming irregularly segmented filaments which may branch, or developing certain portions of their substance into productive bodies; comprising actinobacteria, leptotrichia, actinomyces, and erysipelothrix.

Highmore, antrum of (Highmore, N., English anatomist, 1613–85). The sinus maxillaris, a cavity in the superior maxillary bone communicating with the middle meatus of the nose. H.'s corpus: the mediastinum testis.

highmori·tis. Inflammation of the antrum of Highmore.

hī·lar. Relating to the hilus; e.g. H. glands: lymph nodes at the pulmonary hilum.

Hildebrand's disease (Hildebrand, J. V., Austrian physician, 1763–1818). Typhus fever.

Hilton's muscle (Hilton, J., English surgeon, 1804–78). The inferior aryteno-epiglottideus muscle. H.'s sac: the sacculus laryngis. H.'s white line: marks the junction of the mucous lining of the bowel and the cutaneous tissue.

hilum, hilus (L. *hilum*, a trifle). 1. A recess at the surface of an organ at which vessels, nerves and ducts enter or leave. 2. Scar on seed coat where the seed has broken away from its stalk.

hind. Relating to a part behind, e.g. Hindbrain: the cerebellum and medulla oblongata. H.-gut: that part of the primitive gut which is supplied by the inferior mesenteric artery, i.e. the left side of the transverse colon, the descending colon, the pelvic colon, and rectum.

hip. 1. The part of the body formed by and covering the lateral portion of the pelvis and the cranial end of the femur. H.-joint: the joint between the innominate bone and the femur. H.-j. disease: tuberculosis of the hip joint.

hippocam·pal (G. *hippos*, horse; *kampos*, a seamonster). Relating to the hippocampus.

hippocam·pus (G. *hippos*, horse; *kampos*, a seamonster). A name given to two elevations, h. major and h. minor, situated in the middle and posterior horns respectively of the lateral ventricles of the brain.

Hippocas·tanum (G.). The horse-chestnut.

Hippocrates. The great Greek physician born in 460 B.C., and called the 'Father of Medicine'.

Hippocrat·ic (Hippocrates, Greek physician, 5th century, B.C.). Relating to, or described by Hippocrates. **H. chorda** or **funis:** the tendo Achillis. **H. facies:** an anxious, pinched expression seen especially in those dying of cholera and acute general peritonitis. **H. corpus:** the collection of Greek medical texts, which includes the genuine writings of Hippocrates. **H. finger:** hypertrophy of the ungual phalanx and nail in phthisis and other wasting diseases. **H. morbus sacer:** epilepsy. **H. Oath:** has been since his time the accepted embodiment of medical ethics. **H. succussion:** succussion employed to obtain a splashing sound in seropneumothorax and pyopneumothorax.

hippurate (G. *hippos*, horse; *ouron*, urine). Any salt of hippuric acid.

hippū·ria (G. *hippos*, horse; *ouron*, urine). Excessive amounts of hippuric acid in the urine.

hippuric acid. $C_9H_9NO_3$ sometimes found in human urine; it occurs normally in urine of herbivorous animals, especially in horses.

hippus (G. *hippos*, horse). Alternate dilatation and constriction of the pupil due to iridal spasm.

hircis·mus (L. *hircus*, goat). A goatlike odour from the human axilla.

hircus (L., goat). An axillary hair.

Hirschfeld's disease (Hirschfeld, F., German physician, born 1863). A form of diabetes of rapid progress, usually ending in death in three months.

Hirschfeld's ganglion (Hirschfeld, L. M., Austrian anatomist, 1816–76). The posterior renal sympathetic ganglion. **H.'s nerve:** the lingual branch of the facial nerve; the branch that goes to form the ansa of Haller.

Hirschsprung's disease (Hirschsprung, H., Danish physician, 1830–1916). Congenital hypertrophic dilatation of the lower part of the colon in young children.

hir·sute (L. *hirsutus*, shaggy). Hairy.

hir·suties (L.), **hir·sutism.** 1. Excessive growth of hair. 2. Abnormal growth of hair as in female virilism.

hirū·din (L. *hirudo*, leech). The extract of the buccal glands of the pond-leech.

Hirudi·nea (L. *hirudo*, leech). Leeches; a family of Annelida.

hirū·do (L. pl. *hirudines*). The leech.

His's canal (His, W., German anatomist, 1831–1904) The thyroglossal duct of the foetus. **H.'s cells:** parablast cells; specialized cells formative of blood vessels and held to be distinct from ordinary mesoderm cells. **H.'s perivascular spaces:** lymph spaces surrounding the blood-vessels of the brain and spinal cord. **H.'s stroma:** the supporting framework of the mammary gland.

His's muscle bundle (His, W., junior, German physician, 1863–1934). This arises from the atrioventricular node and conveys the stimuli to both ventricles.

hi·stamine (G. *histos*, web). An amine formed from histidine. Formula $C_5H_9N_3$. Can be made synthetically and is a powerful vasodilator. **H. test:** estimation of hydrochloric acid in gastric secretion following subcutaneous injection of histamine, which has the effect of powerfully promoting gastric secretion. Anti-histaminics are substances which antagonise histamine and are used in allergic conditions, e.g. Antistin, Benadryl, Histantin.

histă·minase. An enzyme acting on histamine.

histidine (G. *histos*, web). An amino acid; $C_6H_9N_3O_2$.

hi·stiocyte (G. *histos*, web; *kutos*, cell). A connective tissue cell.

hi·stioïd (G. *histos*, web; *eidos*, form). Histoid, *q.v.*

histochemistry (G. *histos*, web; *khumeia*, alchemy). Chemistry pertaining to composition of and changes in the tissues of an organism.

hi·stoclā·sis (G. *histos*, web; *klasis*, a breaking). The breaking down of tissue.

histocyte. Histiocyte, *q.v.*

hi·stodiă·lysis (G. *histos*, web; *dialusis*, dissolution). The dissolution of tissues.

hi·stogĕ·nesis (G. *histos*, web; *gennan*, to produce). The formation of tissue.

hi·stogenet·ic (G. *histos*, web; *gennan*, to produce). Relating to histogenesis.

histoid (G. *histos*, web; *eidos*, form). 1. Resembling tissue. 2. Proceeding from one tissue only. **H. tumour:** a t. composed of only one type of tissue.

histŏ·logist (G. *histos*, web; *logos*, a discourse). An expert in histology.

histŏ·logy (G. *histos*, web; *logos*, a discourse). The science of tissue structure; microscopic anatomy of tissues.

histŏ·lysis (G. *histos*, web; *lusis*, solution). Disintegration and dissolution of organic tissues.

histō·ma (G. *histos*, web). Any tissue tumour.

hi·stone (G. *histos*, web). Any of the group of simple proteins which are not coagulable by heat; which are soluble in water and dilute acid; strongly basic; and insoluble in ammonia.

Hi·stoplasma capsulā·tum (G. *histos*, web; *plasma*, a formation; L. *capsula*, a small box). A protozoan parasite in man in Central and South America.

histoplasmō·sis. Diseased condition brought about by infestation with *Histoplasma capsulatum*.

history (G. *historia*, a learning by enquiry). **Family h.:** details as to illnesses or abnormalities of the patient's relatives. **Medical h.:** an account of a patient's symptoms and signs and previous illnesses.

hi·stotome (G. *histos*, web; *tomē*, section). An apparatus for cutting tissue for the study of its minute structure; a microtome.

histŏ·tomy (G. *histos*, web; *tomē*, section). The dissection of tissues.

histriŏ·nic (L. *histrio*, actor). Dramatic.

hives. 1. Urticaria. 2. Term also given to laryngitis, croup and skin eruptions.

HNO₂. Nitrous acid.

HNO₃. Nitric acid.

H₂O. Water.

H₂O₂. Hydrogen dioxide or peroxide.

hobnail liver. Alcoholic cirrhosis of the liver.

Hoboken's valves (Hoboken, N., von, Dutch anatomist, 1632–78). The twistings of the umbilical vessels in the cord, causing depressions externally and valve-like projections internally.

Hocevar's 'sterile' glands (Hocevar, M., Austrian ophthalmologist; research published 1900). The Krause's glands that lack secretory ducts.

Hoche's tract (Hoche, A., German psychiatrist, 1865–1943). The septo-marginal tract in the dorsal region of the spinal cord. In the lumbar region it is known as the 'centrum ovale' of Flechsig and in the sacral region as the tract of Gombault and Philippe.

Hochsinger's phenomenon (Hochsinger, K., Austrian paedriatician, born 1860). Pressure on the inner side of the biceps muscle causes closure of the fist in tetany.

Hodara's disease (Hodara, M., Turkish physician, died 1926). A form of trichorrhexis nodosa seen by H. in Turkish women.

Hodgkin's disease (Hodgkin, T., English physician, 1798–1866). A disease of the reticulo-endothelial system, causing progressive hyperplasia of the lymphatic glands associated with anaemia. Syn. lymphadenoma.

Hodgson's disease (Hodgson, J., English physician, 1788–1869). Dilatation of the arch of the aorta, with consequent lesion of the aortic valves.

Hofer's nerve (Hofer, G., Austrian laryngologist, born 1887). The depressor nerve, represented in man by a branch of the superior laryngeal nerve to the cardiac plexus.

Hoffa's operation (Hoffa, A., German orthopaedist, 1859–1907). Hollowing out the acetabulum and reduction of the head of the femur, after severing the muscles inserted into the upper portion of the bone, in congenital dislocation of the hip.

Hoffmann's anodyne (Hoffmann, F., German physician, 1660–1742). A compound of ether, 30; alcohol, 67; ethereal oil, 3. **H.'s symptom**: increase of mechanical irritability of the sensory nerves in tetany.

Hoffmann's duct (Hoffmann, M., German anatomist, 1622–98). The ductus pancreaticus.

Hoffmann's type of progressive muscular atrophy (Hoffmann, J., German physician, 1857–1919). See under Charcot-Marie.

Hoffmann's violet (Hoffmann, W. W., German chemist, 1818–92). The stain also known as Dahlia.

hog cholera. An infectious epizootic virus disease of swine, resembling cholera, q.v., in its symptoms.

Högyes's treatment (Högyes, E., Hungarian physician, 1847–1906). Treatment of hydrophobia by immunization after exposure, using virus fixé in decreasing dilutions.

Hohl's method (Hohl, A. F., German physician, 1789–1862). A method of preserving the perineum in labour.

Holden's line (Holden, L., English surgeon, 1815–1905). An indistinct furrow below Poupart's ligament, passing over the capsule of the hip-joint; it serves as a guide in amputation.

Holl's ligament (Holl, M., Austrian surgeon, 1852–1920). The intercrural ligament joining the two corpora cavernosa clitoridis in front of the urinary meatus in the female.

hollow. 1. Empty. 2. A depression. **H.-back:** Lordosis, q.v. **H.-foot:** talipes cavus, q.v.

Holmes's operation (Holmes, T., English surgeon, 1825–1907). Excision of the os calcis.

Holmgren's canals (Holmgren, E. A., Swedish histologist, 1866–1922). The canaliculi within the cell protoplasm.

hŏ·loblast (G. holos, whole; blastos, germ). An ovum which undergoes complete segmentation.

holoblast·ic (G. holos, whole; blastos, germ). Applied to ova undergoing complete segmentation, practically the whole amount of yolk being included in the process of cleavage.

holocain. A compound formed by condensation of paraphenetidin with acetphenetidin. **H. hydrochloride** is used as an anaesthetic in the practice of ophthalmology, in 1 per cent solution.

hŏ·locrine (G. holos, whole; krinein, to separate). Applied to a gland the secretory product of which consists mainly of disintegrated cells of the gland itself, as the sebaceous glands.

holodiă·stolic (G. holos, entire; diastŏle, a drawing apart). Throughout diastole—usually applied to particular heart sounds.

holŏ·gamy (G. holos, entire; gămos, a marriage). Macrogamy, q.v.

ho·lorhachi·schisis (G. holos, whole; rhakhis, spinal column; skhizein, to cleave). Congenital fissure of the entire spinal cord.

Holŏ·tricha (G. holos, whole; thrix, hair). An order of protozoa showing a nearly complete covering of the surface with cilia.

Holthouse's hernia (Holthouse, C., English surgeon, 1810–90). An inguinal hernia which has taken a course outwards along the groin.

hoarse. Rough-voiced.

hŏ·malcě·phalus (G. hŏmălos, level; kephalē, head). A flat-headed person.

homă·tropine (G. homoios, like; atropos, inflexible). An alkaloid derived from atropine. It is used to produce dilatation of the pupil and paralysis of accommodation. Its effects pass off more quickly than those of atropine, which is used in the same way. Formula $C_{16}H_{21}O_3N$.

Home's lobe (Home, Sir E., English surgeon, 1756–1832). The median (third) lobe of the prostate.

home-sickness. Nostalgia; urgent desire to return home.

homici·dal (L. homo, man; caedere, to destroy). Relating to homicide. **H. mania:** insanity characterized by murderous impulses.

hŏ·micide (L. homo, man; caedere, to destroy). 1. The killing of a human being without malice or intent, as distinguished from murder or manslaughter. 2. A general term for the killing of a human being by another.

hŏ·miculture (L. homo, man; cultura, cultivation). The improvement of the human species by following the laws of breeding; stirpiculture.

hŏ·minal (L. homo, man). Relating to human beings.

homocen·tric (G. homos, same; kentron, centre). Having the same centre. **H. rays:** light rays having a common centre.

homoclad·ic (G. homos, the same; klădos, branch). Relating to the anastomosis between the branches of the same artery.

homoeŏ·chronous (G. homoios, like; khronos, time). Similar in time or periodicity.

homoeomor·phous (G. homoios, like; morphē, shape). Having a similar appearance.

hō·moeopath (G. homoios, like; pathos, disease). A practitioner of homoeopathy.

homoeopă·thic (G. homoios, like; pathos, disease). Relating to homoeopathy.

homoeŏ·pathy (G. homoios, like; pathos, disease). A system of treatment by the administration of very small amounts of drugs or agents which, if given in large doses to healthy subjects, would produce in these the symptoms from which the patient is suffering.

homoeoplă·sia (G. homoios, like; plassein, to form). 1. The growth of tissue resembling normal tissue, or matrix, in its properties and form. 2. The tissue thus formed.

homoeoplas·tic (G. homoios, like; plassein, to form). Relating to a neoplasm resembling in structure that of the tissue from which it originates.

hō·moeotransplanta·tion (G. homoios, like; L. trans, across; plantare, to plant). The transplantation of tissue taken from one individual to another of the same species.

homogenē·ity (G. homos, same; genos, kind). The character of being homogeneous.

homogē·neous (G. homos, same; genos, kind). Having the same nature or qualities; of uniform character or structure.

homogē·nesis (G. homos, same; genesis, generation). Reproduction in which the offspring passes through the same cycle as the parent.

homŏ·genizā·tion (G. homos, same; gennan, to produce). The act or process of rendering or becoming homogeneous; e.g., pertaining to a process by which fat is distributed equally to all parts of milk.

homogentisic acetic acid. A product of oxidation of tyrosine and perhaps of phenylalanine, present in the urine in alkaptonuria, q.v.

hŏ·mogentisū·ria. Alkaptonuria, q.v.

homoglan·dular (G. homos, same; L. glans). Relating to the same gland.

hō·mohaemothĕ·ra·py (G. *homos*, same; *haima*, blood; *therapeia*, treatment). Treatment of disease by the injection of blood from a donor.

homoiother·mal (G. *homoios*, like; *thermē*, heat). 1. Warm-blooded. 2. Maintaining a uniform temperature.

homolǎ·teral (G. *homos*, the same; L. *latus*, side). Relating to the same side.

homŏ·logous (G. *homos*, the same; *logos*, treatise). Corresponding or identical in structure or belonging to the same type. In chemistry, pertaining to organic series the members of which differ by a multiple or an arithmetical ratio in certain constituents.

hō·mologue (G. *homos*, the same; *logos*, treatise). An organ which corresponds to another in structure, function, position and development.

homŏ·logy (G. *homos*, the same; *logos*, treatise). The quality of being homologous.

homŏ·nymous (G. *homos*, the same; *onuma*, name). Having the same name. H. hemianopia: that affecting the nasal half of the visual field on one side and the temporal half on the other.

homoplā·sia (G. *homos*, the same; *plǎsis*, a moulding). Normal development.

Homop·tera (G. *homos*, same; *pteron*, wing). An order of arthropods closely related to the order of Hemiptera.

homosexuǎ·lity (G. *homos*, the same; L. *sexualis*, sexual). Sexual perversion in which desire is directed towards an individual of the same sex.

homother·mal (G. *homos*, the same; *thermē*, heat). Warm-blooded.

homoton·ic (G. *homos*, the same; *tonos*, tone). Relating to or following a uniform course.

hō·motransplantā·tion (G. *homos*, same; L. *trans*, across; *plantare*, to plant). The transfer of tissues from one animal to another of the same species; usually applied to a nerve, tendon or bone graft.

homŏ·tropism (G. *homos*, the same; *tropos*, a turning). An instinctive turning of like towards like.

hō·motype (G. *homos*, the same; *tupos*, type). A part resembling and corresponding to another part; e.g., the humerus and the femur.

homozȳ·gous (G. *homos*, the same; *zugon*, yoke). Having received the same gene from both parental germ cells.

hood. An apparatus with a chimney designed to draw away vapours produced by various chemical and pharmaceutical processes.

hook. A curved instrument.

hookworm. Parasite of the species *Ankylostoma duodenale* or *Uncinaria americana*. H. disease: see ankylostomiasis; uncinariasis.

Hoover's sign (Hoover, C. F., American physician, 1865–1927). 1. If a normal person or a hemiplegic in a supine position raises one leg, the other presses downward in a degree proportional to its strength. This does not occur in hysteria or malingering. 2. A modification in the movements of the costal margin during respiration caused by a flattening of the diaphragm; this suggests empyema or other intrathoracic condition producing a change in the contour of the diaphragm.

Hope's sign (Hope, J., English physician, 1725–86). Double cardiac beat in aneurysm of the aorta.

Hopmann's polyp (Hopmann, C. M., German rhinologist, 1849–1925). Papillary hypertrophy of the nasal mucous membrane, somewhat resembling a papilloma.

Hoppe-Goldflam's symptom complex (Hoppe, J. I., Swiss physiologist, 1811–91; Goldflam, S., Polish physician). Myasthenia gravis; Erb's disease, *q.v.*

hor. decub. L. *hora decubitus*, at bedtime.

hordē·olum (L. *hordeolus*, dim. of *hordeum*, grain of barley). A sty; a boil of the connective tissue of the eyelids, near to a hair-follicle.

hor·monal. Relating to hormones.

hor·mone (G. *horman*, to set in motion). Chemical substance secreted by an endocrine gland into the blood stream in order to bring about specific changes in distant cells and organs: e.g. adrenocorticotrophic hormone of pituitry which influences the activity of the adrenal cortex. For individual hormones see under proper names.

horn. 1. A substance mainly composed of keratin. 2. cornu.

Horne, saccus of van (Horne, J. van, Dutch anatomist and surgeon, 1621–70). The saccus lacteus; receptaculum chyli.

Horner's muscle (Horner, W. E., American anatomist, 1793–1853). The tensor tarsi. H.'s teeth: incisors with horizontal grooves due to a deficiency of enamel.

Horner's ptosis or symptom-complex (Horner, J. F., Swiss ophthalmologist, 1831–86). A slight ptosis, with miosis, retraction of the eyeball and flushing of the face on the affected side; caused by lesions of the cervical sympathetic.

horny. Composed of or resembling horn. H. layer: the stratum corneum of the skin.

horop·ter (G. *horos*, limit; *optēr*, observer). All the points seen singly by the two retinae when the fixation-point remains static.

hor·ripilā·tion (L. *horrēre*, to bristle; *pilus*, hair). Cutis anserina; goose-flesh.

Horrocks's maieutic (Horrocks, P., English obstetrician, 1852–1909). A rubber bag attached to the end of a catheter and used for dilating the cervix.

horse-shoe kidney. A developmental error in which the lower ends of both kidneys are fused across the midline.

Horsley's putty or wax (Horsley, Sir V., English surgeon, 1857–1916). A compound of beeswax, oil and carbolic acid used to stop haemorrhage from bone especially the skull during brain operations. H.'s trephine: a circular trephine.

Hortega cell (Hortega, P. del R., Spanish histologist, 1882–1945). Variety of neuroglial cell described by Hortega. Its action is phagocytic. Syn. microglia. H.'s method: various methods devised to demonstrate specialized cells of the central nervous system by silver impregnation.

hor. un. spatio. L. *horae unius spatio*, after one hour.

hospital (Mediaeval L. *hospitale*, from *hospes*, host or guest). A building used for the care and treatment of the sick.

hos·pitalism (L. *hospes*, host or guest). The morbid conditions accruing from the gathering together of diseased people in a hospital.

hos·pitalize (L. *hospes*, host or guest). To send a patient to hospital.

host (L. *hospes*, host). The organism upon which a parasite is living. H., definitive: organism harbouring the adult stage of a parasite. H., intermediary: organism harbouring the larval stage of parasite.

hot. Possessing or producing the sensation of heat; stimulating.

Houston's folds (Houston, J., Irish surgeon, 1802–45). Three oblique folds of the mucous membrane of the rectum. H.'s muscle: the part of the ischiocavernosus passing to the dorsum of the penis.

Hovius's canal (Hovius, J. Dutch physician of the 17th century). Fontana's spaces, *q.v.*

Howell's bodies (Howell, W. H., American physiologist, 1860–1945). Ovular or globular bodies sometimes found in erythrocytes.

Howship's lacunae or foveolae (Howship, J., English surgeon, 1781–1841). Absorption spaces in bone.

H.-Romberg's sign: see under Romberg.

Hoyer's canals (Hoyer, H., Polish anatomist and histologist, 1834–1907). The communications between small arteries and small veins without the intervention of capillaries.

H₃PO₂. Hypophosphorous acid.

H_3PO_2. Hypophosphorous acid.

H_3PO_3. Phosphorous acid.

$H_4P_2O_6$. Hypophosphoric acid.

$H_4P_2O_7$. Pyrophosphoric acid.

h.s. L. *hora somni*, at bedtime.

H_2S. Hydrogen sulphide.

H_2SO_4. Sulphuric acid.

Ht. Symbol for total hypermetropia.

Hubrecht's protocordal knot (Hubrecht, A. A. W., Dutch anatomist, 1853–1915). The knot or node of Hensen.

Huchard's disease (Huchard, H., French physician, 1844–1910). Arterial hypertension caused by spasm of the vasoconstrictors, which H. believed produced general arteriosclerosis. **H.'s sign:** a change from the standing to the lying posture not followed by a lessening of the pulse rate is a sign that arterial hypertension is present. **H.'s treatment:** the treatment of dilatation of the stomach by almost excluding liquids from the diet.

Hueck's ligament (Hueck, A. F., German anatomist, 1802–42). The pectinate ligament of the iris; ligamentum pectinatum iridis.

Hueppe's disease (Hueppe, F., German bacteriologist, 1852–1938). Haemorrhagic septicaemia.

Hueter's sign (Hueter, K., German surgeon, 1838–82). There is no transmission of osseous vibration in cases of fracture with fibrous interposition between the fragments.

Huguenin's projection systems (Huguenin, G., Swiss psychiatrist, 1841–1920). The upper and lower motor and upper, middle and lower sensory neurones. A system of 'levels' in sensory and motor activities.

Huguier's canal (Huguier, P. C., French surgeon, 1804–73). Iter chordae anterius, a subdivision of the fissure of Glaser. **H.'s disease:** 1. Hypertrophic elongation of the supravaginal portion of the cervix uteri. 2. Lupus of the vulva. **H.'s fossa:** the sinus tympani. **H.'s glands:** see Bartholin's glands.

humanized (L. *humanus*, human). Term applied to viruses that have been passed through the human organism. **H. milk:** cow's milk modified by reduction of fat and increase of lactose content to resemble human milk.

humec·tant (L. *humectare*, to moisten). 1. Moistening. 2. A diluent; a substance used for moistening.

humectā·tion (L. *humectare*, to moisten). The process of moistening.

hū·meral (L. *humerus*, shoulder). Relating to the humerus.

hū·merus (L.). The bone of the upper arm.

humid (L. *humidus*). Moist.

humi·dity (L. *humidus*, moist). The state of being moist; moisture. **Absolute h.:** the actual amount of water present in the air at a particular moment. **Relative h.:** the percentage of water in the air compared with that which would be present under the condition of saturation with water.

hū·mour (L. *humor*, fluid). 1. Old term denoting any body fluid. 2. Temperament, disposition, as the four humours of Galen, the choleric, melancholic, phlegmatic and sanguine. **Aqueous h.:** the transparent structureless fluid of the anterior and posterior chambers of the eye. **Crystalline h.:** Lens, crystalline, *q.v.* **Vitreous h.:** the transparent, jelly-like substance filling the eye cavity behind the lens and the ora serrata. Syn. vitreous body; corpus vitreum.

hū·moral (L. *humor*, fluid). Relating to the natural fluids of the body. **H. pathology:** a system of pathology which maintains that disease is primarily due to an abnormal condition of the body humours.

Humphry's ligament (Humphry, Sir G. M., English anatomist, 1820–96). Associated with the posterior cruciate ligament in the knee joint.

hunger. Longing for food. **Air h.:** breathlessness. **H. pain:** in cases of duodenal ulcer comes on in the early hours of the morning and is relieved by taking food.

Hunter's canal (Hunter, John, Scottish surgeon and anatomist, 1728–93. Founder of the Hunterian Museum at the Royal College of Surgeons, London). A triangular muscular canal in the middle of the thigh. It is bounded anteriorly and laterally by the vastus medialis, posteriorly by the adductor longus and superficially by the sartorius. It transmits the femoral vessels and the internal saphenous nerve. **H.'s gubernaculum:** gubernaculum testis. **H.'s chancre:** primary syphilitic ulcer. **H.'s method:** a method of treating aneurysm by proximal ligation of the artery.

Hunter's membrane (Hunter, W., English anatomist, 1718–83). The uterine decidua to which he gave the name.

Huntington's chorea (Huntington, G., American physician, 1850–1916). Chronic progressive hereditary chorea.

Hurler's disease (Hurler, Gertrud, contemporary German paediatrician). Lipochondrodystrophy. See gargoylism.

Hürthle's cell (Hürthle, K., German histologist, born 1860). A large eosinophilic cell rich in cytoplasm found by Hürthle on the outer surfaces of follicles of the thyroid gland.

Huschke's canal or foramen (Huschke, E., German anatomist, 1797–1858). A foramen formed by the fusion of the tubercles of the annulus tympanicus. It is generally obliterated at puberty, but may persist through life. **H.'s cartilage:** see Jacobson's cartilage. **H.'s valve:** prominent lower margin of the opening of the lacrimal ducts into the lacrimal sac (opposite the valve of Rosenmüller).

Hutchinson's disease (Hutchinson, Sir J., English surgeon, 1828–1913). 1. See Tay's choroiditis. 2. Solar dermatitis of a recurrent nature. **H.'s facies:** the distinctive facial expression caused by drooping eyelids and immobility of the eyeballs seen in ophthalmoplegia externa. **H.'s patch:** a salmon-coloured patch on the cornea in syphilitic keratitis. **H.'s prurigo:** the prurigo of dentition. **H.'s pupil:** one dilated on the side of the lesion in traumatic meningeal haemorrhage, with contraction of the other pupil. **H.'s teeth:** peg-shaped incisor teeth notched at the cutting edge, seen in hereditary syphilis. **H.'s triad:** diagnostic of hereditary syphilis: 1. Diffuse interstitial keratitis. 2. Disease of the labyrinth. 3. H.'s teeth.

Hutinel's disease (Hutinel, V. H., French paediatrician, 1849–1933). Cirrhosis of the liver in childhood with ascites, and oedema of lower extremities.

Huxham's tincture (Huxham, J., English physician, 1692–1768). Compound tincture of cinchona bark.

Huxley's layer or membrane (Huxley, T. H., English biologist, 1825–95). A layer of nucleated, elongated polygonal cells forming the inner portion of the inner root-sheath of the hair follicle.

Hy. Abbreviation for hypermetropia.

hȳ·alin (G. *hualos*, glass). An albuminoid substance.

hȳ·aline (G. *hualos*, glass). 1. Translucent; glass-like. 2. Hyaline change—a degenerative process during which collagenous connective tissue and fibrous tissue loses structure and becomes homogeneous. It then stains well with acid dyes. Tissue cells may also undergo a similar change after death.

hȳalĭ·nogen (G. *hualos*, glass; *gennan*, to produce). 1. Insoluble substances found in the walls of hydatid cysts, etc.; the parent substance of hyalin. 2. An albuminoid in cartilage.

hȳalinū·ria (G. *hualos*, glass; *ouron*, urine). The presence of hyalin in the urine.

hȳ·aloid (G. *hualos*, glass; *eidos*, form). Transparent; glass-like.

hȳ·alonyx·is (G. *hualos*, glass; *nuxis*, puncture). Puncture of the vitreous body of the eye.

hȳ·alophā·gia (G. *hualos*, glass; *phagein*, to eat). Glass-eating.

hȳ·aloplasm (G. *hualos*, glass; *plasma*, anything moulded). The fluid, finely granulated ground substance of the endoplasm. Syn. enchylema; cytolymph.

hȳ·aluro·nidase. An enzyme used to facilitate diffusion of injected drugs. The enzyme is found in mammalian seminal fluid and is produced in small amounts by certain micro-organisms. It is also found in leeches, in snake and viper venoms and in various tissues.

hybrid (L. *hybrida*, mongrel). The offspring of parents who differ in one or several distinctive characters.

hȳ·bridism, hybrĭ·dity (L. *hybrida*, mongrel). Crossbreeding; being hybrid.

hydan·tōin. Glycolyl urea, a substance derived from allantoin. Formula $C_3H_4O_2$. Derivative, sodium diphenyl hydantoin, used in the treatment of epilepsy.

hydantō·inate. Any salt of hydantoin.

hȳdăt·id (G. *hudation*, a drop of water). 1. The cyst formed by the larva of Taenia echinococcus. 2. Remnants of embryonic structures. **H. cyst**: caused by the Taenia echinococcus, the sites of election being the liver, lungs and muscles. **H. disease**: the condition of being infected by the larvae of Taenia echinococcus. **H. mole**: see under mole. **H. of Morgagni**: see under Morgagni.

hydă·tidiform (G. *hudation*, a drop of water; L. *forma*, shape). Resembling a hydatid.

Hydatĭ·gena. A genus of tapeworm resembling *Taenia*. Has large head but no neck. Found in intestines of Carnivores.

hydă·toid (G. *hudōr*, water; *eidos*, form). 1. Hydatidiform. 2. Aqueous humour.

hydnocar·pate. Any salt of hydnocarpic acid.

hydnocar·pic acid. An unsaturated fatty acid obtained from chaulmoogra and hydnocarpus oils. The ethyl ester is used in the treatment of leprosy. Formula $H_{16}H_{28}O_2$.

Hydnocar·pus wightiana (G. *hudnos*, truffle; *karpos*, fruit). A tree found in tropical regions. The seeds yield an oil that has been used in the treatment of leprosy.

hydradeni·tis (G. *hudōr*, water; *aden*, gland). Inflammation of the sweat glands of the axilla.

hydrae·mia (G. *hudōr*, water; *haima*, blood). Increase in the water-content of the blood.

hydrāe·roperitonē·um (G. *hudōr*, water; *aēr*, air; *peri*, around; *teinein*, to stretch). A collection of fluid and gas in the peritoneal cavity.

hȳ·dragogue (G. *hudōr*, water; *agōgos*, leading). Applied to drugs which effect an increase in the secretion of water from the kidneys.

hydram·nion, hydram·nios (G. *hudōr*, water; *amnion*, the membrane round the foetus). The presence of an abnormal amount of amniotic fluid.

hydrar·gyrate (G. *hudrarguros*, mercury). Relating to or containing mercury.

hydrargȳ·ria, hydrargyrĭ·asis, hydrar·gyrism (G. *hudrarguros*, mercury). Chronic mercurial poisoning. Syn. mercurialism.

hydrar·gyrum (G. *hudrarguros*). Mercury.

hydrarthro·sis (G. *hudōr*, water; *arthron*, joint). An accumulation of fluid in a joint.

o

hydras·tine. An alkaloid obtained from the root of *Hydrastis canadensis* (Golden Seal). Formula $C_{21}H_{21}O_6N$.

hydras·tinine. An artificial alkaloid derived from hydrastine and used as a haemostatic and a cardiac stimulant. Formula $C_{11}H_{11}O_2N$.

Hydră·stis. The plant Golden Seal, of the order *Ranunculaceae*. The rhizome of *H. canadensis* yields the alkaloids hydrastine and berberine, which have tonic and diuretic properties.

hȳ·drate (G. *hudōr*, water). A compound containing water in chemical combination.

hȳ·drated (G. *hudōr*, water). Chemically combined with water.

hydrā·tion (G. *hudōr*, water). The action of combining chemically with water.

hydrau·lics (G. *hudōr*, water; *aulos*, pipe). That part of physics which deals with the statics and dynamics of fluids.

hȳ·drazine (G. *hudōr*, water; G. *azein*, to dry up). A colourless, poisonous liquid, strongly alkaline and a powerful reducing agent. Phenyl hydrazine is hydrazine with one hydrogen atom replaced by a phenyl radicle.

hȳ·drencephalĭ·tis (G. *hudōr*, water; *egkephalos*, brain). Inflammatory hydrocephalus.

hȳ·drencĕ·phalocele (G. *hudōr*, water; *egkephalos*, brain; *kēlē*, hernia). Hernia of the brain containing part of a cerebral ventricle.

hydrencĕ·phalus (G. *hudōr*, water; *egkephalos*, brain). Hydrocephalus, q.v.

hydren·terocele (G. *hudōr*, water; *enteron*, gut; *kēlē*, hernia). Hernia of the intestine in which the sac contains extravasated fluid.

hydriă·tic, hydriă·tric (G. *hudōr*, water; *iatros*, healer). Relating to the treatment of disease with water.

hydriă·trics (G. *hudōr*, water; *iatros*, healer). Hydrotherapy, q.v.

hȳ·dric (G. *hudōr*, water). Relating to water.

hȳ·dride (G. *hudōr*, water). A chemical compound containing hydrogen united to an element or radical.

hydrĭŏ·dic acid. An inorganic acid containing hydrogen and iodine. Formula HI.

hȳ·driodide. A salt of any amine or alkaloid with hydriodic acid.

hydrō·a (G. *hudōr*, water; *ōon*, egg). A general term applied to skin disease characterized by vesicle formation. **H. aestivale** or **H. vacciniforme**: a recurrent skin disease appearing in periods of intense sunlight-radiation, characterized by papules, papulo-vesicles or bullae, by superficial ulceration and scarring on parts exposed to sunlight, sometimes associated with porphyrinuria, and always present in the congenital type of the latter disease.

hydrobrō·mic acid (G. *hudōr*, water; *brōmos*, a foetid odour). HBr. A solvent for quinine and given for headaches and neuralgia.

hydrobrō·mide. Any salt of an amine or alkaloid with hydrobromic acid.

hydrocar·bon (G. *hudōr*, water; L. *carbo*, coal). Any compound composed only of hydrogen and carbon.

hydrocar·bonism (G. *hudōr*, water; L. *carbo*, coal). Poisoning from hydrocarbons, chiefly found in miners and petroleum refinery workers.

hȳ·drocele (G. *hudōr*, water; *kēlē*, tumour). A collection of serous fluid between the two membranes of the tunica vaginalis of the testicle or spermatic cord. The term is also sometimes applied to serous swellings in other parts of the body.

hydrocenō·sis (G. *hudōr*, water; *kenōsis*, an emptying). The removal of fluid either by means of hydragogue cathartics or by the operation of 'tapping' the cavity containing the fluid accumulations.

hȳ·drocephal·ic (G. *hudōr*, water; *kephalē*, head). Relating to or affected by hydrocephalus.

hȳ·drocĕ·phalocele (G. *hudōr*, water; *kephalē*, head; *kēlē*, hernia). Hydrencephalocele, *q.v.*

hydrocĕ·phaloid (G. *hudōr*, water; *kephalē*, head; *eidos*, form). 1. Relating to or resembling hydrocephalus. 2. A disease of infants resembling hydrocephalus.

hydrocĕ·phalus (G. *hudōr*, water; *kephalē*, head). An abnormal accumulation of fluid in the cerebral ventricles (internal hydrocephalus) or in the subarachnoid space of the brain (external hydrocephalus). The symptoms include progressive enlargement of the head, bulging of the fontanelles, thinning of the skull, atrophy of the brain, distension of the superficial veins, mental impairment and convulsions.

hydrochlor·ic acid (G. *hudōr*, water; *khlōros*, greenish-yellow). A gaseous compound of hydrogen and chlorine. Strong hydrochloric acid contains 35-38% w/w of HCl. Syn. muriatic acid.

hyrochlor·ide. Any salt of an amine or alkaloid with hydrochloric acid.

hȳ·drocholecys·tic (G. *hudōr*, water; *khŏlē*, bile; *kustis*, bladder). Dropsy of the gall-bladder.

hydrocir·socele (G. *hudōr*, water; *kirsos*, enlargement of a vein; *kēlē*, hernia). Hydrocele associated with varicose veins of the spermatic cord.

hȳ·drocoelia (G. *hudōr*, water; *koilia*, belly). Dropsy of the belly.

hydrocol·pocele (G. *hudōr*, water; *kolpos*, womb; *kēlē*, tumour). A serous tumour of the vagina.

hydro-elec·tric (G. *hudōr*, water; *elektron*, amber). Relating to electricity generated by water power.

hydrogen (G. *hudōr*, water; *gennan*, to produce). Symbol H. The lightest element, with an atomic weight of 1·008; valency 1. H. is a gaseous element, occurring in nature, e.g. combined with oxygen in the form of water, H_2O. It is to be found in practically all organic compounds and is a constant constituent of acids. **H.-esis:** 1. The collecting or forming of a watery fluid. 2. Any disease marked by a predominance of mucous secretion, fat or bile. **H. peroxide:** H_2O_2; peroxide of hydrogen. (The normal oxide is water, H_2O.) Used as an antiseptic and bleaching agent.

hydroglos·sa (G. *hudōr*, water; *glōssa*, tongue). Ranula.

hȳ·drogymnas·tics. Gymnastics performed in water.

hydrohae·mia (G. *hudōr*, water; *haima*, blood). Hydraemia, *q.v.*

hȳ·drohymenī·tis (G. *hudōr*, water: *humēn*, membrane). Inflammation of a serous membrane or surface.

hydrohys·tera. See under hydrometra.

hydrokinet·ics (G. *hudōr*, water, *kinein*, to move). The study of fluids in motion.

hydrolactŏ·meter (G. *hudōr*, water; L. *lac*, milk; G. *metron*, measure). An instrument used in estimating the percentage of water in milk.

hȳ·drolymph (G. *hudōr*, water; L. *lympha*, water). A term given to the blood of certain lower animals, which is chiefly composed of the salt or fresh water in which they live and contains only a small quantity of corpuscular elements.

hydrŏ·lysis (G. *hudōr*, water; *lusis*, a loosening). The process by which a chemical compound unites with water and then divides into smaller molecules.

hydrolyt·ic. Relating to hydrolysis.

hydrŏ·ma (G. *hudōr*, water). 1. A tumour containing water. 2. A cyst or swelling containing water or serous fluid. 3. The cystlike dilatation of a lymph vessel of the neck.

hȳ·dromel (G. *hudōr*, water; *mĕli*, honey). A mixture of honey and water, sometimes with a medicinal substance added.

hȳ·dromenin·gocele (G. *hudōr*, water; *mēnigx*, membrane; *kēlē*, hernia). A meningocele protruding through the skull.

hydrŏ·meter (G. *hudōr*, water; *metron*, measure). An apparatus for estimating the specific gravities of liquids.

hydromē·tra (G. *hudōr*, water; *mētra*, uterus). An abnormal accumulation of mucus or watery fluid in the uterus.

hȳ·dromē·trocol·pos (G. *hudōr*, water; *mētra*, uterus; *kolpos*, vagina). Distension of vagina and uterus with accumulated fluid.

hydrŏ·metry (G. *hudōr*, water; *metron*, measure). Measurement of specific gravity of fluids.

hȳ·dromicrocĕ·phaly (G. *hudōr*, water; *mikros*, small; *kephalē*, head). Microcephaly with internal hydrocephalus.

hydrom·phalus (G. *hudōr*, water; *omphalos*, navel). A tumour-like protrusion of the umbilicus.

hȳ·dromyē·lia (G. *hudōr*, water; *muelos*, marrow). Dilatation of the central canal of the spinal cord.

hȳ·dromyĕ·locele (G. *hudōr*, water; *muelos*, marrow; *kēlē*, hernia). A variety of spina bifida in which the hernial sac contains cerebrospinal fluid as well as spinal cord.

hydron·cus (G. *hudōr*, water; *ogkos*, mass). A swelling caused by an accumulation of water.

hȳ·dronephrectā·sia (G. *hudōr*, water; *nephros*, kidney; *ektasis*, extension). Dropsical distension of the kidney.

hydroneph·ros (G. *hudōr*, water; *nephros*, kidney). A dropsical kidney.

hȳ·dronephrō·sis (G. *hudōr*, water; *nephros*, kidney). A distension of the kidney by urine as a result of obstruction to the outflow.

hȳ·dronephrot·ic. Relating to hydronephrosis.

hydrō·nium ion. Hydrogen ion associated with water molecule.

hydro-ŏ·ligocythae̅·mia (G. *hudōr*, water; *oligos*, few; *kutos*, cell; *haima*, blood). A type of anaemia characterized by an increase in the proportion of serum to blood cells.

hȳ·dropancreatō·sis (G. *hudōr*, water; *pancreas*). A condition in which serous fluid is present in the pancreas.

hȳ·droparasal·pinx (G. *hudōr*, water; *para*, beside; *salpigx*, tube). The presence of water in the accessory tubes of the oviduct.

hydropath·ic (G. *hudōr*, water; *pathos*, disease). Relating to hydropathy; hydrotherapeutic.

hydrŏ·pathy (G. *hudōr*, water; *pathos*, disease). Hydrotherapy, *q.v.*

hȳ·dropericardī·tis (G. *hudōr*, water; *peri*, around; *kardia*, heart). Pericarditis with serous effusion into the pericardial cavity.

hȳ·dropericar·dium (G. *hudōr*, water; *peri*, around; *kardia*, heart). A collection of serous fluid within the pericardial cavity.

hydropĕ·rion (G. *hudōr*, water; *peri*, around; *ōon*, egg). Fluid between decidua vera and decidua reflexa.

hȳ·droperitonē·um (G. *hudōr*, water; *peri*, around; *teinein*, to stretch). Ascites.

hydropex·ia (G. *hudōr*, water; *pexis*, fixation). The holding of water.

hydrŏ·philous (G. *hudōr*, water; *philein*, to love). Absorbing water.

hydrophŏ·bia (G. *hudōr*, water; *phobos*, fear). 1. Fear of water, a symptom of rabies. 2. Rabies, *q.v.*, in man.

hydrophŏ·bic. Relating to hydrophobia.

hȳ·drophobopho·bia (G. *hudōr*, water; *phobos*, fear). Intense fear of becoming affected with hydrophobia. The condition sometimes results in a state which simulates true hydrophobia.

hȳ·drophone (G. *hudōr*, water; *phōnē*, voice). An instrument used in auscultatory percussion.

hydrophthal·mia (G. *hudōr*, water; *ophthalmos*, eye). Abnormal distension of the ocular bulbs by serous fluid or by increased intraocular pressure. Syn. infantile glaucoma.

hȳ·drophysomē·tra (G. *hudōr*, water; *phusa*, bellows; *mētra*, uterus). The presence of water and gas *in utero*.

hydrop·ic (G. *hudrōps*, dropsy). Relating to dropsy; dropsical.

hy·droplasm (G. *hudōr*, water; *plasma*, something formed). The fluid consituent of protoplasm.

hydroplas·mia (G. *hudōr*, water; *plassein*, to form). A condition in which the blood plasma is thinned by the presence of water.

hydropleuri·tis (G. *hudōr*, water; *pleura*, rib). Pleurisy accompanied by effusion.

hȳ·dropneumatō·sis (G. *hudōr*, water; *pneuma*, breath). A collection of gas or air and fluid in the tissues.

hydropneumō·nia (G. *hudōr*, water; *pneumōn*, the lungs). Pulmonary oedema.

hȳ·dropneū·moperitonē·um (G. *hudōr*, water; *pneuma*, air; *peri*, around; *teinein*, to stretch). The presence of both serous fluid and air or gas within the peritoneum.

hȳ·dropneumothor·ax (G. *hudōr*, water; *pneuma*, air; *thōrax*, chest). The presence of both serous fluid and air or gas in the pleural cavity.

hȳ·drops (G. *hudrōps*, dropsy). Dropsy; an abnormal accumulation of serous fluid in any tissue or cavity of the body.

hȳ·dropȳ·onephrō·sis (G. *hudōr*, water; *puŏn*, pus; *nephros*, kidney). Dilatation of the renal pelvis with pus and urine.

hydroquinone. A dihydric phenol, formula $C_6H_6O_2$ used in photography in conjunction with metol. Can be made from arbutin by hydrolysis. It is a patent bacteriostatic.

hydror·rachis (G. *hudōr*, water; *rhakhis*, spine). An abnormal accumulation of cerebrospinal fluid within the central canal or in the subarachnoid space of the spinal cord.

hydrorrhoē·a (G. *hudōr*, water; *rhoia*, a flowing). A discharge of watery fluid.

hydrosal·pinx (G. *hudōr*, water; *salpigx*, trumpet). Distension of the uterine tube with fluid.

hȳ·drosar·cocele (G. *hudōr*, water; *sarx*, flesh; *kēlē*, hernia). A sarcocele accompanied by hydrocele.

hydrŏ·scheocele (G. *hudōr*, water; *oskhe*, scrotum; *kēlē*, hernia). Dropsical hernia of the scrotum.

hȳ·drosol. Any colloid sol in aqueous solution.

hydrostat·ic (G. *hudōr*, water; *statikos*, standing). Relating to hydrostatics.

hydrostat·ics (G. *hudōr*, water; *statikos*, standing). The science dealing with the properties of liquids in a state of equilibrium.

hydrothē·rapy (G. *hudōr*, water; *therapeia*, treatment). The treatment of disease by baths and external application of water.

hydrothor·ax (G. *hudōr*, water; *thōrax*, chest). An accumulation of a serous fluid in the pleural cavity, occurring especially in cardiac and renal diseases.

hydrō·tis (G. *hudōr*, water; *ous*, ear). Dropsy of or effusion of serous fluid into the ear.

hydrotym·panum (G. *hudōr*, water; *tumpanon*, a drum). The presence of a watery effusion in the tympanic cavity.

hydro-ūrĕ·ter (G. *hudōr*, water; *ourēter*, ureter). Condition in which the ureter is dilated due to obstruction lower down the urinary tract.

hydrox·ide (G. *hudōr*, water; *oxus*, acid). A compound containing the radical – OH in ionic combination.

hydrox·yl (G. *hudōr*, water; *oxus*, acid). The univalent radical OH.

hydrox·ybutȳ·ric acid (*G. hudōr*, water; *oxus*, acid; *bouturon*, butter). Intermediate product of metabolism present in cases of disturbed metabolism, in urine and blood, e.g., diabetes.

hydroxylă·mine (G. *hudōr*, water; *oxus*, acid; *ammoniakon*, sal ammoniac). Colourless solid, formula NH_2OH. A basic substance and a strong reducing agent.

hydrū·ria (G. *hudōr*, water; *ouron*, urine). The discharge of large quantities of urine having low specific gravity.

hydrū·ric. Relating to or characterized by hydruria.

hȳĕtŏ·metry (G. *huĕtos*, rain; *metron*, measure). Rainfall measurement.

Hygēī·a (G.). Goddess of health, a daughter of Aesculapius.

hygeniŏ·latry (G. *hugiēs*, healthy; *latreuein*, to worship). Preoccupation with one's own health.

hȳ·giene (G. *hugieinos*, healthy). The science dealing with the conditions necessary for maintaining the health of individuals and populations. Syn. public health.

hygien·ic (G. *hugieinos*, healthy). Relating to hygiene.

hȳ·gienist (G. *hugieinos*, healthy). A person skilled in hygiene.

hygrŏ·ma (G. *hugros*, moist). A swelling caused by chronic bursitis. H., cystic: congenital lymphangioma.

hygrŏ·meter (G. *hugros*, moist; *metron*, measure). An instrument for the estimation of the amount of moisture in the air.

hygromet·ric (G. *hugros*, moist; *metron*, measure). 1. Relating to hygrometry. 2. Hygroscopic.

hygrŏ·metry (G. *hugros*, moist; *metron*, measure). The measurement of moisture in the air.

hygrophō·bia (G. *hugros*, moist; *phobos*, fear). Insane dread of liquids.

hȳ·groscope (G. *hugros*, moist; *skopein*, to view). An instrument that indicates variations in the moisture of the air.

hygroscop·ic (G. *hugros*, moist; *skopein*, to view). Capable of absorbing moisture from the air.

hygrostō·mia (G. *hugros*, moist; *stoma*, mouth). Chronic excessive salivation.

hyla. See paraqueduct.

hyle (G. *hulē*, matter). The primitive undifferentiated matter in nature.

hȳ·lic (G. *hulē*, matter). Relating to primitive matter.

hylō·ma (G. *hulē*, matter). A tumour growing in a primal pulp-tissue.

hylŏ·pathism (G. *hulē*, matter; *pathos*, disease). A disease caused by defect or disorder of the body-substance.

hylozō·ism (G. *hulē*, matter; *zōē*, life). The theory that all matter is living.

hȳ·men (G. *humēn*, membrane). The fold of mucous membrane which more or less occludes the vaginal entrance.

hȳ·menal (G. *humēn*, membrane). Relating to the hymen.

hymenec·tomy (G. *humēn*, membrane; *ektomē*, excision). Excision of the hymen.

hymenī·tis (G. *humēn*, membrane). Inflammation of the hymen.

Hymenŏ·lepis (G. *humēn*, membrane; *lĕpis*, rind). A genus of Cestoda or tapeworms.

hymenŏ·logy (G. *humēn*, membrane; *logos*, treatise). The science relating to the structure, functions and diseases of membranes.

hymenŏr·rhaphy (G. *humēn*, membrane; *rhaphē*, suture). More or less complete closure of the vagina by suture at the hymen.

hymen·otome (G. *humēn*, membrane; *tomē*, section). A surgical instrument used for cutting membranes.

hymenŏ·tomy (G. *humēn*, membrane; *temnein*, to cut). Surgical incision of the hymen.

hȳ·obasi·oglos·sus. The basal portion of the hyoglossus muscle.

hyoglos·sal (G. *huoeides*, shaped like the letter Y; *glōssa*, tongue). Relating to the hyoglossus.

hyoglos·sus (G. *huoeides*, shaped like the letter Y; *glōssa*, tongue). The muscle extending from the hyoid bone to the tongue.

hy·oid (G. *huoeides*, shaped like the letter Y). **H. bone:** a bone between [the root of the tongue and the larynx.

hyomandĭ·bular (G. *huoeides*, shaped like the letter Y; L. *mandere*, to chew). Relating to the hyoid bone and the inferior maxilla.

hyopharўn·geus (G. *huoeides*, shaped like the letter Y; *pharugx*, throat). The middle pharyngeal constrictor.

hyoscine (G. *huoscuamos*, henbane). Formula $C_{17}H_{21}O_4N$. A liquid alkaloid, syn. scopolamine, derived from hyoscyamus and usually employed as hyoscine hydrobromide. It is an effective depressant of the cerebrum and motor centres of the spinal cord and used to allay insomnia, mania and sexual excitement. Obtained from various solanaceous plants particularly species of Datura, Scopola and Duboisia.

hyoscŷ·amine (G.). Symbol $C_{17}H_{23}NO_3$. An alkaloid found in hyoscyamus. It is isomeric with atropine; used as a narcotic and sedative.

Hyoscŷ·amus (G.). A plant of the family Solanaceae; henbane. The leaves and flowering tops of *H. niger* produce the alkaloids hyoscine and hyoscyamine. These are sedative to the nervous system and are used in the treatment of a variety of complaints, such as hysteria and cough. They are also used to allay pain in rheumatism and malignant tumours.

hyothŷ·roid (G. *huoeides*, shaped like the letter Y; *thureos*, a shield; *eidos*, form). Relating to the hyoid bone and the thyroid cartilage.

hypacĭ·dity (G. *hupo*, under; L. *acidus*, sour). Subacidity; deficiency in acids.

hypacou·sis, hypacū·sis (G. *hupo*, under; *akousis*, a hearing). Impairment of hearing due to diminished sensibility of the auditory nerves.

hypaē·mia. Hyphaemia, *q.v.*

hȳp·aesthesia (G. *hupo*, under; *aisthēsis*, feeling). Impairment of sensation; diminished tactile sensibility.

hȳp·albuminō·sis (G. *hupo*, under; L. *albus*, white). Diminution of the proportion of albumin in the blood.

hȳpalgē·sia (G. *hupo*, under; *algēsis*, sense of pain). Diminished sensitiveness to pain.

hȳpal·gia (G. *hupo*, under; *algos*, pain). Diminished sensitiveness to pain.

hypam·nios (G. *hupo*, under; *amnion*, the membrane round the foetus). Insufficient quantity of amniotic fluid.

hypasthē·nia (G. *hupo*, under; *astheneia*, weakness). Loss of strength in a small degree.

hypax·ial (G. *hupo*, under; L. *axis*, axis). Situated below the body-axis.

hyperă·cid (G. *huper*, over; L. *acidus*, acid). Excessively acid.

hyperacĭ·dity (G. *huper*, over; L. *acidus*, acid). Excessive acidity.

hyperacoū·sis, hyperacū·sia, hyperacū·sis (G. *huper*, over; *akousis*, a hearing). Abnormal acuteness of the sense of hearing; auditory hyperaesthesia.

hyperactĭ·vity (G. *huper*, over; L. *activus*, active). Excessive or abnormal activity.

hyperacū·ity (G. *huper*, over; L. *acuere*, to sharpen). Abnormal perception of sound.

hyperadenō·sis (G. *huper*, over; *adēn*, gland). An enlarged lymph-gland.

hyperadipō·sis (G. *huper*, over; L. *adeps*, fat). Extreme fatness.

hyperadrē·nia (G. *huper*, over; L. *ad*, to; *ren*, kidney). The symptoms appearing in cases of over-activity of the adrenal gland.

hyperaē·mia (G. *huper*, over; *haima*, blood). Localized congestion with blood. **Active h.:** h. due to increased arterial flow. **Passive h.:** h. due to obstruction to venous flow.

hyperaesthē·sia (G. *huper*, over; *aisthesis*, feeling). Increased sensitivity.

hȳ·peralbuminō·sis (G. *huper*, over; L. *albus*, white). An abnormal increase in the amount of albumin in the blood.

hyperalgē·sia, hyperal·gia (G. *huper*, over; *algos*, pain). Increased sensibility to pain.

hyperamnesia. Hypermnesia, *q.v.*

hyperă·phia (G. *huper*, over; *haphē*, touch). Abnormal sensitiveness to touch.

hȳ·peraphrodĭ·siac (G. *huper*, over; *Aphroditē*, Venus). An exaggerated venereal appetite.

hȳ·perbilirubinaē·mia (G. *huper*, over; L. *bilis*, bile; *ruber*, red; G. *haima*, blood). Increased amount of bilirubin in the blood.

hȳ·perbrachycephal·ic (G. *huper*, over; *brakhus*, short; *kephalē*, head). Excessively brachycephalic.

hypercap·nia (G. *huper*, over; *kapnos*, smoke). An abnormal increase of carbon dioxide in the blood, producing over-activity in the respiratory centre.

hypercar·dia (G. *huper*, over; *kardia*, heart). Cardiac hypertrophy.

hypercathar·sis (G. *huper*, over; *katharsis*, purge). Excessive purging.

hȳ·perchlorhŷ·dria (G. *huper*, over; *khlōros*, green; *hudōr*, water). The presence of an abnormal amount of hydrochloric acid in the gastric secretion.

hȳ·perchromăt·ic (G. *huper*, over; *khrōmă*, colour). Applied to nuclei of cells which stain more deeply than normal, particularly in neoplastic tissue.

hȳ·percinē·sis Hyperkinesis, *q.v.*

hypercrĭ·nia (G. *huper*, over; *krinein*, to separate). Abnormal or excessive secretion, especially of the endocrine glands.

hȳ·percryalgē·sia (G. *huper*, over; *kruos*, cold; *algēsis*, sense of pain). Abnormal sensitiveness to cold.

hypercyē·sis (G. *huper*, over; *kuēsis*, conception). 1. Superfoetation. 2. The state of mind in which conceptions follow quickly one upon another.

hȳ·perdicrot·ic (G. *huper*, over; *dikrotos*, double-beating). Affected with marked or delayed dicrotism; a condition in which the aortic notch is below the base-line.

hyperdĭ·crotism (G. *huper*, over; *dikrotos*, double-beating). Excessive dicrotism.

hyperdisten·sion (G. *huper*, over; L. *distendere*, to distend). Abnormal distension.

hyperdiurē·sis (G. *huper*, over; *dioureein*, to urinate). Excessive secretion of urine.

hyperdynă·mia (G. *huper*, over; *dunamis*, force). Excessive strength.

hȳ·perē·mesis (G. *huper*, over; *emesis*, a vomiting). Excessive vomiting. **H. gravidarum:** h. in pregnancy. See also morning sickness.

hyperencē·phalus (G. *huper*, over; *egkephalos*, brain). A monster foetus lacking the whole upper part of the skull, so that the brain is exposed.

hȳ·perephidrō·sis (G. *huper*, over; *ephidrōsis*, sweating). Excessive sweating.

hȳ·perergă·sia (G. *huper*, over; *ergon*, work). Increased functional activity.

hȳ·peresophor·ia (G. *huper*, over; *esō*, inward; *phoros*, bearing). Heterophoria, *q.v.*

hȳ·perexophor·ia (G. *huper*, over; *exo*, outward; *phoros*, bearing). A tendency to turn the eyes outward and upward.

hȳ·perexten·sion (G. *huper*, over; L. *extendere*, to extend). Over-extension, e.g. of a joint.

hyperflex·ion (G. *huper*, over; L. *flectere*, to bend). Over-flexion.

hypergĕ·nesis (G. *huper*, over; *genesis*, generation). Excessive development of the organs or parts of the body.

hȳ·pergeusaesthē·sia (G. *huper*, over; *geusis*, taste; *aisthēsis*, feeling). Abnormal acuteness of the sense of taste.

hyperglobū·lia (G. *huper*, over; L. *globus*, globe). Abnormal increase in the number of red blood corpuscles.

hȳ·perglobulinae·mia (G. *huper*, over; L. *globus*, globe; G. *haima*, blood). Increase in level of globulin in the blood.

hȳ·perglucō·sic (G. *huper*, over; *glukus*, sweet). A term applied to any diabetic diet which includes an amount of carbohydrates greater than the patient's tolerance.

hyperglycae·mia (G. *huper*, over; *glukus*, sweet; *haima*, blood). The presence of an increased amount of sugar in the blood.

hyperglycĭ·stia (G. *huper*, over; *glukus*, sweet; *histos*, web). Excess of sugar in the tissues.

hypergō·nadism (G. *huper*, over; *gonē*, seed). Excessive internal secretion of the sexual glands.

hyperhĕdo·nia (G. *huper*, over; *hēdonē*, pleasure). Excessive pleasure in gratifying desires.

hyperhē·donism (G. *huper*, over; *hēdonē*, pleasure). 1. Excessive sensation of libido. 2. Sexual erethism.

hyperhidrō·sis, hyperidrō·sis (G. *huper*, over; *hidrōs*, sweat). Excessive sweating.

hyperhor·monal (G. *huper*, over; *hormone*). Hormone excess.

hyperhydrae·mia (G. *huper*, over; *hudōr*, water; *haima*, blood). Abnormal increase of water in the blood.

hyperhypnō·sis (G. *huper*, over; *hupnos*, sleep). Excessive sleepiness.

hyperin·sulinism. Hypoglycaemia, spontaneous, *q.v.*

hy·perinvolū·tion (G. *huper*, over; L. *involvere*, to wrap up). Excessive involution of an organ, especially after enlargement, e.g. of the uterus after pregnancy.

hȳ·perkeratō·sis (G. *huper*, over; *keras*, horn). 1. Hypertrophy of the horny layer of the skin. 2. Hypertrophy of the cornea.

hȳ·perkinē·sis (G. *huper*, over; *kinēsis*, motion). A condition characterized by excessive movement.

hyperkinet·ic (G. *huper*, over; *kinēsis*, motion). Relative to hyperkinesis.

hyperlactā·tion (G. *huper*, over; L. *lactare*, to have milk). Abnormal prolongation of lactation.

hȳ·perleū·cocytō·sis (G. *huper*, over; *leukos*, white; *kutos*, cell). Increase in the number of leucocytes.

hyperlipae·mia (G. *huper*, over; *lipos*, fat; *haima*, blood). Excess of fat in the blood; lipaemia.

hypermă·stia (G. *huper*, over; *mastos*, breast). 1. Hypertrophy of mammary gland. 2. Presence of supernumerary mammary glands.

hȳ·permature (G. *huper*, over; *maturus*, ripe). Over-ripe.

hypermetrō·pia (G. *huper*, over; *metron*, measure; *ōps*, eye). Anomaly of ocular refraction in which parallel rays of light are, with suspended accommodation, focussed below the retina. This is due to an abnormally short longitudinal diameter of the eye or, rarely, to a diminished refraction power of its media. Syn. longsightedness.

hypermnē·sia, hypermnē·sis (G. *huper*, over; *mnēsis*, memory). Abnormal exaltation of the faculty of memory.

hypermoti·lity (G. *huper*, over; L. *motio*, movement). Excessive increase in motor activity.

hypermyŏ·trophy, hypermyotrō·phia (G. *huper*, over; *mus*, muscle; *trophē*, nourishment). A state of increased development or size of muscles.

hypermyotō·nia (G. *huper*, over; *mus*, muscle; *tonos*, tone). State of increased muscle tone.

hypernephrī·tis (G. *huper*, over; *nephros*, kidney). Inflammation of adrenal body.

hypernephroma (G. *huper*, over; *nephros*, kidney). Name given to malignant tumour of kidney on account of resemblance of some of its cells to adrenal cortex. Now thought to be carcinoma of kidney tubule cells. Syn. Grawitz's tumour.

Hyperol. Proprietary compound of urea and hydrogen peroxide yielding hydrogen peroxide on hydrolysis.

hȳ·peronȳ·chia (G. *huper*, over; *onux*, nail). Hypertrophy of the nails.

hȳ·perope (G. *huper*, over; *ōps*, eye). One who is affected with hyperopia.

hyperō·pia (G. *huper*, over; *ōps*, eye). Longsightedness. See hypermetropia.

hyperos·mia (G. *huper*, over; *osmē*, smell). An abnormally acute sense of smell.

hȳ·perostĕŏ·geny (G. *huper*, over; *osteon*, bone; *gennan*, to produce). Hypertrophy of bones.

hȳ·perostō·sis (G. *huper*, over; *osteon*, bone). Diffuse thickening of a bone.

hȳ·perparathȳ·roidism (G. *huper*, over; *para*, beside; *thureos*, shield; *eidos*, form). Abnormally increased function of the parathyroid gland, usually due to an adenoma of the gland. The condition causes generalized osteitis fibrosa, spontaneous fractures, pain and weakness of bones and muscles and there is a tendency for the formation of renal calculi.

hyperpă·thia (G. *huper*, above; *pathos*, disease). Unpleasant sensation derived from tactile impulses.

hyperpep·sia (G. *huper*, over; *pepsis*, digestion). Dyspepsia characterized by excessive amounts of chlorides in the gastric juice.

hȳ·perperistal·sis (G. *huper*, over; *peri*, around; *stalsis*, compression). Abnormally increased peristalsis.

hyperphă·gia (G. *huper*, over; *phagein*, to eat). Excess in eating.

hyperphō·nia (G. *huper*, over; *phonē*, voice). Stammering caused by over-irritability of voice production muscles.

hyperphor·ia (G. *huper*, over; *phoros*, bearing). Tendency of the visual axis of one eye to be above or below that of the other.

hyperpiē·sia, hyperpiē·sis (G. *huper*, over; *piĕsis*, compression). Hypertension; high blood pressure.

hyperpigmentā·tion (G. *huper*, over; L. *pigmentum*, paint). Marked pigmentation.

hyperpi·nealism (G. *huper*, over; L. *pineus*, pine cone). Over secretion of the pineal gland.

hȳ·perpitū·itarism (G. *huper*, over; L. *pītūīta*, slime). Abnormal over-function of the pituitary gland, sometimes due to an adenoma of the cells of the anterior lobe, resulting in gigantism or acromegaly.

hȳ·perplā·sia (G. *huper*, over; *plasis*, formation). An increase in the size of a tissue or an organ, due to increase in the number of cells.

hyperplas·tic. Relating to hyperplasia.

hyperpnoē·a (G. *huper*, over; *pnoē*, breath). Over-breathing; over-ventilation of the lungs.

hyperporō·sis (G. *huper*, over; *pōrōsis*, callus formation). Excessive callus formation in the union of fractured bones.

hyperprā·xia (G. *huper*, over; *praxis*, exercise). The restless movements seen in certain types of mania.

hyperprotĕŏ·sis (G. *huper*, over; *prōtos*, first). A condition brought about by excessive proteins in the diet.

hyperpselaphē·sia (G. *huper*, over; *psēlaphēsis*, touching). Extreme sensitiveness to touch.

hyperpyret·ic (G. *huper*, over; *purĕtos*, fever). Relating to hyperpyrexia.

hyperpȳrĕx·ia (G. *huper*, over; *purĕtos*, fever). Exceedingly high body temperature.

hyperrĕ·sonance (G. *huper*, over; L. *resonare*, to resound). An increased resonance on percussion.

hypersecrē·tion (G. *huper*, over; L. *secernere*, to set apart). Abnormally increased secretion.

hypersen·sitiveness (G. *huper*, over; L. *sentire*, to feel). Abnormally increased sensibility, e.g., to the ingestion of some foodstuffs.

hypersom·nia (G. *huper*, over; L. *somnus*, sleep). An excessive amount of sleep.

hypersthē·nia (G. *huper*, over; *sthěnos*, strength). A state of exalted body strength.

hypertară·chia (G. *huper*, over; *tărăkhē*, confusion). Excessive nervous irritability.

hyperten·sion (G. *huper*, over; L. *tendere*, to stretch). Increased tension, especially of the arterial system; high blood pressure. Essential h.: h. of unknown origin.

hyperten·sive (G. *huper*, over; L. *tendere*, to stretch). Characterized by high blood pressure.

hyperthē·lia (G. *huper*, over; *thēlē*, nipple). A condition in which supernumerary nipples are present.

hyperthermalgē·sis (G. *huper*, over; *thermē*, heat; *algos*, pain). Abnormal sensitiveness to heat.

hyperther·mia (G. *huper*, over; *thermē*, heat). Rise of body temperature not due to bacterial invasion.

hyperthỹ·mia (G. *huper*, over; *thumos*, mind). A condition characterized by a tendency to perform impulsive actions.

hyperthỹ·rea (G. *huper*, over; *thureos*, shield). The condition caused by over-activity of the thyroid gland.

hyperthỹ·roid (G. *huper*, over; *thureos*, shield; *eidos*, form). Characterized by hyperthyroidism.

hyperthỹ·roidism (G. *huper*, over; *thureos*, shield; *eidos*, form). The condition due to abnormally increased function of the thyroid gland, including both exophthalmic and toxic goitre. Syn. thyrotoxicosis.

hypertō·nia (G. *huper*, over; *tonos*, tone). Abnormal increase of muscular tonicity.

hyperton·ic (G. *huper*, over; *tonos*, tone). Characterized by hypertonia.

hypertox·ic (G. *huper*, over; *toxikon*, poison). Excessively poisonous.

hypertrichi·asis, hypertrichō·sis (G. *huper*, over; *thrix*, hair). Abnormal growth of hair on a part or on the whole of the body.

hypertrŏ·phic (G. *huper*, over; *trophē*, nutrition). Characterized by hypertrophy.

hyper·trophy (G. *huper*, over; *trophē*, nutrition). Increase in the size of tissue, due to enlargement of its individual cells or fibres. H., compensatory: an increase in size of an organ due to physiological stimulus, i.e., enlargement of one kidney when the other has been removed. H., simple: an increase in size of the individual cells. H., true: an increase in size of all the component tissues of a muscle or any organ often due to excessive use.

hypertrŏ·pia (G. *huper*, over; *trěpein*, to turn). The deviation of one visual line above the other.

hỹ·pha (G. *huphē*, a web). Multinucleate filament with or without septa found in fungi.

hyphae·mia (G. *hupo*, under; *haima*, blood). 1. Insufficiency of blood. 2. Haemorrhage into the anterior chamber of the eye.

hy·phal (G. *hupo*, under). Applied to species of fungi. See Hyphomycetes.

hyphedō·nia (G. *hupo*, under; *hēdonē*, pleasure). Morbid state, characterized by greatly decreased pleasure in the fulfilment of desires.

hyphidrō·sis (G. *hupo*, under; *hidrōs*, sweat). Deficiency of perspiration.

Hyphomycē·tes (G. *huphē*, web; *mukēs*, mushroom). A group of Fungi Imperfecti in which the asexual spores are not produced in specialized structures.

hypnaesthē·sia (G. *hupnos*, sleep; *aisthēsis*, feeling). Drowsiness.

hypnagŏ·gic (G. *hupnos*, sleep; *ăgōgŏs*, bringing). 1. Inducing sleep. 2. Induced by sleep.

hyp·nagogue (G. *hupnos*, sleep; *ăgōgŏs*, bringing). Hypnotic.

hypnal·gia (G. *hupnos*, sleep; *algos*, pain). Neuralgia occurring during sleep.

hyp·napagŏ·gic (G. *hupnos*, sleep; *apo*, away; *ăgōgŏs*, bringing). Inhibiting sleep.

hypnic (G. *hupnikos*, of or for sleep). Relating to or causing sleep.

hypnogen·ic, hypnŏ·genous (G. *hupnos*, sleep; *gennan*, to produce). 1. Producing sleep. 2. Inducing a state of hypnotism.

hypnoi·dal (G. *hupnos*, sleep; *eidos*, form). Resembling or simulating sleep.

hypnolep·sy (G. *hupnos*, sleep; *lēpsis*, seizure). Narcolepsy; abnormal sleepiness.

hypnŏ·logy (G. *hupnos*, sleep; *logos*, treatise). The science pertaining to sleep and hypnotism.

hypnŏ·pathy (G. *hupnos*, sleep; *pathos*, disease). Sleep caused by a diseased state of the mind or body.

hypnopom·pic (G. *hupnos*, sleep; *pompē*, procession). Relating to condition in which a person on awakening from sleep sees dream figures persisting.

hypnŏ·sia (G. *hupnos*, sleep). A condition of overpowering sleepiness.

hypnŏ·sis (G. *hupnos*, sleep). A sleep-like condition induced by suggestion, and characterized by abnormally increased suggestibility in the patient.

hypnot·ic (G. *hupnos*, sleep). 1. Inducing sleep. 2. Relating to hypnotism. 3. A drug or other remedy promoting sleep.

hyp·notism (G. *hupnos*, sleep). 1. The science of hypnosis. 2. Hypnosis, *q.v.*

hyp·notist (G. *hupnos*, sleep). One skilled in carrying out hypnotism.

hyp·notize (G. *hupnos*, sleep). To induce a state of hypnosis.

hypo (G. *hupo*, under). An abbreviation for sodium thiosulphate.

hypo-aci·dity (G. *hupo*, under; L. *acidus*, acid). Deficiency of normal acid in the system.

hypo-actĭ·vity (G. *hupo*, under; L. *activus*, active). Abnormal decrease in activity.

hypo-adē·nia (G. *hupo*, under; *adēn*, gland). Abnormally decreased glandular functioning.

hypo-adrē·nia (G. *hupo*, under; L. *ad*, to; *rēnes*, kidneys). Abnormal diminishing of adrenal activity.

hypo-albuminae·mia (G. *hupo*, under; L. *albumen*; G. *haima*, blood). A condition characterized by abnormally diminished amounts of albumin in the blood.

hypo-alimentā·tion (G. *hupo*, under; L. *alimentum*, nourishment). The condition resulting from undernourishment.

hypo·alonae·mia (G. *hupo*, under; *hals*, salt; *haima*, blood). A condition in which there is a deficiency of salts in the blood.

hypo-azotū·ria (G. *hupo*, under; *a*, neg.; *zoē*, life; *ouron*, urine). The condition resulting from diminished amounts of urea in the urine.

hypobarŏ·pathy (G. *hupo*, under; *barus*, heavy; *pathos*, disease). Mountain or air sickness.

hỹ·poblast (G. *hupo*, under; *blastos*, germ). Entoderm, *q.v.*

hypobla·stic (G. *hupo*, under; *blastos*, germ). Relating to the hypoblast.

hypobrō·mite (G. *hupo*, under; *bromos*, a foetid odour). Any salt of hypobromous acid. Sodium hypobromite is used in the estimation of urea in the urine.

hypobromous acid. HBrO. An unstable acid that has not yet been isolated. It forms hypobromites.

hypocap·nia (G. *hupo*, under; *kapnos*, smoke). A condition in which there is a moderate diminution of carbon dioxide in the blood.

hypocathar·sis (G. *hupo*, under; *kathairein*, purge). A mild purgation.

hypochlorae·mia (G. *hupo*, under; *khlōros*, green; *haima*, blood). Deficiency of chlorides in the blood.

hypochlorae·mic. Relating to or characterized by hypochloraemia.

hypochlorhȳ·dria (G. *hupo*, under; *khlōros*, green; *hudōr*, water). Deficiency of hydrochloric acid in the gastric juice.

hypochlorhȳ·dric. Characterized by hypochlorhydria.

hypochlor·ite. A salt of hypochlorous acid.

hypochloriza·tion. Treatment by reduction of intake of sodium chloride.

hypochlorous acid. HClO, an unstable compound used for bleaching and as a disinfectant.

hypocholesterae·mia (G. *hupo*, under; *cholesterin*; G. *haima*, blood). A deficiency of cholesterin in the blood.

hȳpochon·driac (G. *hupo*, under; *khondros*, cartilage). 1. Relating to the hypochondrium. 2. A person affected with hypochondriasis.

hȳpochondrī·acal (G. *hupo*, under; *khondros*, cartilage). Pertaining to or affected with hypochondriasis.

hȳpochondrī·asis (G. *hupo*, under; *khondros*, cartilage). A condition of mental depression caused by the patient's belief that he is suffering from a grave organic disease.

hypochon·drium (G. *hupo*, under; *khondros*, cartilage). The upper lateral region of the abdomen beneath the costal cartilages.

hypochor·dal (G. *hupo*, under; *khordē*, cord). Ventral, applied to the vertebral column.

hypochrō·mia (G. *hupo*, under; *khrōma*, colour). Abnormally decreased pigmentation or unusual transparency of the skin.

hypochrō·mic. Characterized by hypochromia.

hypochrō·sis (G. *hupo*, under; *khrōsis*, a colouring). Pallor of the skin.

hypochȳ·lia (G. *hupo*, under; *khulos*, juice). A condition in which there is a deficiency of chyle.

hypocoe·lom (G. *hupo*, under; *koilos*, hollow). The ventral portion of the coelom.

hypocystō·tomy (G. *hupo*, under; *kustis*, bladder; *tomē*, a cutting). Opening the urinary bladder through the perineum.

hypocytō·sis (G. *hupo*, under; *kutos*, cell). Decline in the number of blood corpuscles.

Hypoderma (G. *hupo*, under; *derma*, skin). A genus of warble flies of the Oestridae family.

hȳ·podermă·tomy (G. *hupo*, under; *derma*, skin; *tomē*, section). Subcutaneous surgical section.

hypoder·mic (G. *hupo*, under; *derma*, skin). 1. Beneath the skin. 2. Applied beneath the skin.

hypoder·mis (G. *hupo*, under; *derma*, skin). The subcutaneous tissue.

hȳ·podermŏ·clȳsis (G. *hupo*, under; *derma*, skin; *klusis*, injection). The subcutaneous injection of considerable amounts of fluid, especially of normal saline solution.

hypodȳ·nia (G. *hupo*, under; *odunē*, pain). Slight pain.

hypo-exophor·ia (G. *hupo*, under; *exo*, outside; *phoros*, bearing). A tendency for the visual axis of one eye to deviate downward and outward.

hypofunc·tion (G. *hupo*, under; L. *fungi*, to perform). Abnormally diminished function.

hy·pogalac·tia (G. *hupo*, under; *gala*, milk). Diminished milk secretion.

hypogas·tric (G. *hupo*, under; *gastēr*, stomach). Relating to the hypogastrium.

hypogas·trium (G. *hupo*, under; *gastēr*, stomach). That part of the central abdomen below a line joining the intertubercular plane.

hypogas·trocele (G. *hupo*, under; *gastēr*, stomach; *kēlē*, hernia). A hernia in the hypogastric area.

hypogě·nitalism (G. *hupo*, under; L. *genitalis*, generative). Deficient development of the sexual organs.

hypogeu·sia (G. *hupo*, under; *geusis*, taste). Diminution of the sense of taste.

hypoglan·dular (G. *hupo*, under; L. *glans*, acorn). Abnormally diminished glandular activity.

hypoglobū·lia (G. *hupo*, under; L. *globus*, globe). Decreased number of red blood corpuscles.

hypoglos·sal (G. *hupo*, under; *glōssa*, tongue). Situated under the tongue.

hypoglos·sus (G. *hupo*, under; *glōssa*, tongue). The twelfth cranial nerve.

hypoglot·tis (G. *hupo*, under; *glōttis*, mouth of the windpipe). The under part of the tongue.

hypoglycae·mia (G. *hupo*, under; *glukus*, sweet; *haima*, blood). Deficiency of sugar in the blood. **H., spontaneous:** the condition due to over-function of the internal secretion of the pancreatic glands, caused either by a pancreatic neoplasm or by a functional disturbance of the endocrine equilibrium. H. is characterized by the following symptoms: a feeling of hunger, perspiration, tremors, mental confusion, convulsions, and coma.

hypognā·thus (G. *hupo*, under; *gnathos*, jaw). A double monstrosity in which the parasite is attached to the lower jaw of the autosite.

hypogŏ·nadism (G. *hupo*, under; *gŏnē*, seed). Diminished internal secretion of the sexual glands.

hypohidrō·sis (G. *hupo*, under; *hidrōs*, sweat). Abnormally diminished perspiration.

hypokinē·sia, hypokinē·sis (G. *hupo*, under; *kinēsis*, movement). Deficiency of motor reactions.

hypokolā·sia (G. *hupo*, under; *kŏlazein*, to correct). A condition of defective inhibition.

hȳ·poleū·cocytō·sis (G. *hupo*, under; *leukos*, white; *kutos*, cell). An abnormal diminution of white blood cells.

hypoleukae·mia (G. *hupo*, under; *leukos*, white; *haima*, blood). Syn. hypoleucocytosis.

hypolipae·mia (G. *hupo*, under; *lipos*, fat; *haima*, blood). Deficiency of fat in the blood.

hypolymphae·mia (G. *hupo*, under; L. *lympha*, water; G. *haima*, blood). An abnormal diminution in the number of lymphocytes in the blood.

hypomā·nia (G. *hupo*, under; *mania*, madness). A moderate degree of mania.

hypomă·stia (G. *hupo*, under; *mastos*, breast). Abnormal smallness of the mammary gland.

hypomelanchŏ·lia (G. *hupo*, under; *melas*, black; *kholē*, gall). A moderate degree of melancholia.

hypomenorrhoe·a (G. *hupo*, under; *mēn*, month; *rhoia*, a flow). Deficiency of menstrual discharge.

hypometă·bolism (G. *hupo*, under; *mĕtăbolē*, change). Diminished metabolism.

hypomnē·sis (G. *hupo*, under; *mnesis*, memory). Deficiency in the powers of memory.

hypomȳ·xia (G. *hupo*, under; *muxa*, mucus). Deficiency in the secretion of mucus.

hȳ·ponanosō·ma (G. *hupo*, under; *nanos*, dwarf; *sōma*, body). Very small dwarf.

hyponeū·ria (G. *hupo*, under; *neuron*, nerve). Diminished nerve power.

hypō·nomous (G. *hupo*, under; *nŏmas*, wandering). Spreading beneath the surface.

hyponȳ·chial (G. *hupo*, under; *onux*, finger-nail). Underneath a nail.

hyponȳ·chium (G. *hupo*, under; *onux*, finger-nail). The thickened part of the horny layer of the epidermis at the tip of the finger, adjacent to the free border of the nail.

hȳ·poparathȳ·roid. Characterized by hypoparathyroidism.

hȳ·poparathȳ·roidism (G. *hupo*, under; *para*, beside; *thureos*, shield; *eidos*, form). Diminished function of the parathyroid glands, usually occurring only as a sequel to surgical interference, characterized by hypocalcaemia, tetany, and sometimes by cataract.

hypopep·sia (G. *hupo*, under; *pepsis*, digestion). Impaired powers of digestion.

hypoperistal·sis (G. *hupo*, under; *peri*, around; *stalsis*, contraction). Abnormally diminished powers of peristalsis.

hypophă·rynx (G. *hupo*, under; *pharugx*, throat). The inferior part of the pharynx which is situated behind the larynx.

hypophŏ·nia (G. *hupo*, under; *phonē*, voice). Partial loss of voice owing to lack of coordination of the voice-production muscles.

hypophor·ia (G. *hupo*, under; *phoros*, bearing). A tendency of the visual axis of one eye to deviate below that of the other.

hypophosphoric acid. H_2PO_3, a crystalline, hygroscopic acid of phosphorus which forms hypophosphates.

hypophosphorous acid. H_3PO_2. A monobasic acid of phosphorus which forms hypophosphites. A powerful reducing agent.

hypophos·phate. Any salt of hypophosphoric acid.

hypophos·phite. Any salt of hypophosphorous acid.

hypophy·sĕăl (G. *hupo*, under; *phuein*, to produce). Pertaining to the pituitary gland.

hypophysec·tomy (G. *hupo*, under; *phuein*, to produce; *ektomē*, excision). The operation for removal of the pituitary gland.

hypŏ·physis (G. *hupo*, under; *phuein*, to produce). An outgrowth. **H. cerebri:** the pituitary gland.

hȳ·popitū·itarism (G. *hupo*, under; L. *pītūīta*, slime). The condition due to deficiency in one or more of the functions of the anterior lobe of the pituitary gland.

hypoplā·sia (G. *hupo*, under; *plassein*, to form). Defective development of a tissue or organ.

hypŏ·pyon (G. *hupo*, under; *puon*, pus). The presence of pus in the anterior chamber of the eye.

hyposalaē·mia (G. *hupo*, under; L. *sal*, salt; G. *haima*, blood). Abnormal deficiency of blood salts.

hyposecrē·tion (G. *hupo*, under; L. *secernere*, to separate). Deficiency of secretion.

hyposexuă·lity (G. *hupo*, under; L. *sexus*, sex). Deficient sexual development.

hypos·mia (G. *hupo*, under; *osmē*, smell). Impairment of the sense of smell.

hyposō·mia (G. *hupo*, under; *soma*, body). Deficiency in bodily development.

hypospā·dia, hypospā·dias (G. *hupo*, under; *spaein*, to draw out). A congenital deformity in which the external orifice of the urethra is situated at the under surface of the penis.

hypŏ·stasis (G. *hupo*, under; *stasis*, halt). 1. A sediment or deposit. 2. Stasis of the blood in dependant parts of an organ or of the body.

hypostat·ic (G. *hupo*, under; *stasis*, halt). Characterized by or due to hypostasis.

hyposthē·nia (G. *hupo*, under; *sthenos*, strength). Subnormal strength; weakness.

hyposthē·nic. Characterized by hyposthenia.

hyposthenū·ria (G. *hupo*, under; *sthenos*, strength; *ouron*, urine). Inability of functionally deranged kidney to elaborate a concentrated urine.

hypostyp·tic (G. *hupo*, under; *stuptikos*, astringent). Mildly styptic.

hyposul·phite. A salt of hyposulphurous acid. Also known as hydrosulphite. Sodium hyposulphite is used as a reducing agent in the dyeing industry.

hyposulphurous acid. Dithionous acid. Formula $H_2S_2O_4$.

hypoten·sion (G. *hupo*, under; *teinein*, to stretch). Subnormal pressure; low blood pressure.

hypoten·sive. Characterized by hypotension.

hypothă·lamus (G. *hupo*, under; *thalamos*, an inner chamber). Area of the midbrain beneath the thalamus, comprising optic chiasma, infundibular process and stalk, corpora mammillaria, tuber cinereum and the postinfundibular eminence.

hypothē·nar (G. *hupo*, under; *thenar*, palm of the hand). The eminence of soft tissue on the palm of the hand over the metacarpal bone of the little finger.

hypother·mal (G. *hupo*, under; *thermē*, heat). Tepid.

hypother·mia, hypother·my (G. *hupo*, under; *thermē*, heat). Subnormal temperature.

hypŏ·thesis (G. *hupo*, under; *thĕsis*, position). A theory not absolutely proved by facts set forth for the explanation of a phenomenon.

hȳ·pothyrĕŏ·sis, hypothy·roidism (G. *hupo*, under; *thureos*, shield; *eidos*, form). Deficient functional activity of the thyroid gland and the condition caused by it. See also myxoedema, cretinism.

hypotō·nia, hypŏ·tonus (G. *hupo*, under; *tonos*, tone). Diminished tonicity or tension.

hypotŏ·nic (G. *hupo*, under; *tonos*, tone). 1. Below the normal tonicity or tension. 2. Applied to solutions having a lesser osmotic pressure than isotonic solutions.

hȳ·potoxi·city (G. *hupo*, under; *toxikon*, poison). Reduced toxicity.

hypotri·chous (G. *hupo*, under; *thrix*, hair). Partial or total absence of hair due to developmental abnormality.

hypŏ·trophy (G. *hupo*, under; *trophein*, to nourish). 1. Defective nutrition. 2. Defective development.

hypotrō·pia (G. *hupo*, under; *tropē*, a turning). A squint causing the eye to look downwards.

hypovā·ria (G. *hupo*, under; L. *ovum*, egg). Deficient ovarian secretion causing delayed puberty in girls.

hȳ·povitaminō·sis (G. *hupo*, under; L. *vita*, life). A clinical condition due to lack of vitamins in the food.

hypoxan·thine (G. *hupo*, under; *xanthos*, yellow). $C_5H_4N_4O$. A non-toxic leucomaine, found in most animal tissues well supplied with nucleated cells.

hypsicĕ·phaly (G. *hupsi*, aloft; *kephalē*, head). A condition in which the skull has a cephalic height index of over 75.

hypur·gia (G. *hupourgia*, medical attendance). Medical assistance.

hypur·gic (G. *hupourgikos*). Helping; administering.

hȳ·stera (G. *hustera*, womb). The uterus or womb.

hysteral·gia (G. *hustera*, womb; *algos*, pain). Pain in the uterus.

hysteratrē·sia (G. *hustera*, womb; *atrētros*, not perforated). An imperforate condition of the external orifice of the uterus.

hysterec·tomy (G. *hustera*, womb; *ektomē*, excision). Excision of the uterus. **Abdominal h.:** h. by laparotomy. **h., vaginal :** h. performed through the vagina.

hystereuryn·ter (G. *hustera*, womb; *eurunein*, to extend). An instrument for dilating the os uteri.

hysterĕū·rysis (G. *hustera*, womb; *eurunein*, to extend). Dilatation of the cervix of the uterus.

hystĕ·ria (G. *hustera*, womb). A form of neurosis characterized by the presence of various disturbances of psychic, motor, sensory, visual, etc., functions, predominantly occurring in young women.

hystĕ·ric, hystĕ·rical (G. *hustera*, womb). Relating to or affected with hysteria.

hystĕ·riconeural·gic (G. *hustera*, womb; *neuron*, nerve; *algos*, pain). Like neuralgia, but having its origin in hysteria.

hystĕ·rics. An attack of hysteria.

hysterī·tis (G. *hustera*, womb). Inflammation of the uterus.

hysterobubon·ocele (G. *hustera*, womb; *boubōn*, groin; *kēlē*, hernia). An inguinal hernia, the sac of which contains the uterus.

hysterocarcinŏ·ma (G. *hustera*, womb; *karkinos*, crab). Carcinoma of the uterus.

hy·sterocă·talepsy (G. *hustera*, womb; *katalambanein*, to seize). A type of hysteria in which catalepsy is a marked feature.

hy·sterocele (G. *hustera*, womb; *kēlē*, hernia). A hernia containing the uterus.

hy·steroklei·sis (G. *hustera*, womb; *kleisis*, a closure). The closing of the uterus by suturing the os.

hysterocỹē·sis (G. *hustera*, womb; *kuēsis*, conception). Uterine pregnancy.

hy·sterodỹ·nia (G. *hustera*, womb; *odunē*, pain). Pain in the uterus.

hystero-epilepsy (G. *hustera*, womb; *epilēpsis*, a seizure). A form of hysteria characterized by convulsions resembling those of epilepsy.

hy·sterogastror·rhaphy (G. *hustera*, womb; *gastēr*, stomach; *rhaphē*, suture). Hysteropexy, *q.v.*

hysterogen·ic (G. *hustera*, womb; *gennan*, to produce). Causing or inducing a hysterical attack.

hysteroid (G. *hustera*, womb; *eidos*, form). 1. Resembling hysteria. 2. Relating to hystero-epilepsy.

hy·sterokataphrax·is (G. *hustera*, womb; *kataphraxis*, a stopping up). An operation for supporting the uterus.

hy·sterolaparŏ·tomy (G. *hustera*, womb; *lapara*, flank; *tome*, section). Abdominal hysterotomy.

hy·sterolith (G. *hustera*, womb; *lithos*, stone). Calculus in the uterus.

hysterŏ·logy (G. *hustera*, womb; *logos*, treatise). The total of what is known of the anatomy, physiology and pathology of the uterus.

hy·sterolox·ia (G. *hustera*, womb; *loxos*, oblique). Displacement of the uterus laterally.

hysterŏ·lysis (G. *hustera*, womb; *lusis*, solution). An operation in which the uterus is freed and fixed in an anteflexed position.

hy·steromalā·cia (G. *hustera*, womb; *malakia*, softness). Softening of the uterus.

hy·steromā·nia (G. *hustera*, womb; *mania*, madness). Nymphomania.

hysterŏ·meter (G. *hustera*, womb; *metron*, measure). An instrument for the measurement of the uterus.

hy·steromyŏ·ma (G. *hustera*, womb; *mus*, muscle). Uterine myoma.

hy·steromyomec·tomy (G. *hustera*, womb; *mus*, muscle; *ektomē*, excision). Surgical removal of a uterine fibroid or myoma.

hy·steromyŏ·tomy (G. *hustera*, womb; *mus*, muscle; *tome*, section). Operation in which the body of the uterus is incised for the removal of fibroids.

hy·steroneurasthē·nia (G. *hustera*, womb; *neuron*, nerve; *a*, neg.; *sthenos*, strength). 1. Neurasthenia caused by uterine disease. 2. The stage at which neurasthenia ends and hysteria begins.

hy·steroneurŏ·sis (G. *hustera*, womb; *neuron*, nerve). A reflex neurosis due to irritation of the uterus.

hystero·ŏŏphorec·tomy (G. *hustera*, womb; *ōon*, egg; *pherein*, to carry; *ektomē*, excision). Removal of uterus and ovaries.

hystero-ovariŏ·tomy. Hystero-oophorectomy, *q.v.*

hy·steropară·lysis (G. *hustera*, womb; *para*, beside; *luein*, to loosen). Paralysis of the uterine walls.

hysterŏ·pathy (G. *hustera*, womb; *pathos*, disease). A disease or disorder of the uterus.

hy·steropexy (G. *hustera*, womb; *pēxis*, fixation). Surgical fixation of the uterus to correct displacement.

hysterŏ·pia (G. *hustera*, womb; *ōps*, eye). A disorder of vision caused by hysteria.

hy·steropsychŏ·sis (G. *hustera*, womb; *psukhē*, mind). Mental disorder associated with uterine disease.

hysterŏ·ptosis (G. *hustera*, womb; *ptōsis*, a fall). A falling or prolapse of the uterus.

hysteror·rhaphy (G. *hustera*, womb; *rhaphē*, suture). 1. The suture of a uterine wound. 2. Hysteropexy.

hy·sterorrhex·is (G. *hustera*, womb; *rhēxis*, a rent). Rupture of the uterus.

hy·steroscope (G. *hustera*, womb; *skopein*, to view). A uterine speculum.

hy·sterospasm (G. *hustera*, womb; *spasmos*, contraction). Spasm of the uterus.

hysterŏ·tomy (G. *hustera*, womb; *tome*, section). Incision of the uterus.

hy·sterotrachelor·rhaphy (G. *hustera*, womb; *trakhēlos*, neck; *rhaphē*, suture). A plastic operation for the restoration of a lacerated cervix uteri.

hy·sterotrachelo·tomy (G. *hustera*, womb; *trakhēlos*, neck; *tome*, section). Surgical incision of the uterine cervix.

hy·sterotrau·matism (G. *hustera*, womb; *trauma*, injury). Hysterical symptoms due to or following traumatism.

hy·sterotris·mus (G. *hustera*, womb; *trismos*, a rasping). Spasm of the uterus.

hystricī·asis (G. *hustrix*, hedgehog). 1. A disease of the hairs, causing them to stand erect. 2. Ichthyosis hystrix.

I

I. The symbol for an atom of iodine.

ĭăn·thinop·sia (G. *ianthos*, the violet; *ōps*, eye). A visual condition in which objects appear to be violet coloured.

ĭătē·ria (G. *iatērion*, a cure). Healing.

ĭătralip·tic (G. *iatros*, physician; *aleiphein*, to anoint). Treatment by the use of ointments and frictions.

ĭăt·ric (G. *iatros*, physician). Relating to the physician or to medical science.

ĭăt·rochĕ·mical (G. *iatros*, physician; *khumeia*, alchemy). A theory of the 17th century according to which vital processes in general, and therefore also the action of drugs, depend upon chemical processes.

ĭ·ătrol. Oxy-iodo-methyl-anilide. An antiseptic agent.

iatrŏ·logy (G. *iatros*, physician; *logos*, treatise). Medical science.

ĭ·atrophy·sics (G. *iatros*, physician; *phusikos*, natural). A theory of the 17th century according to which vital processes can be explained by the laws of physics.

ibid. Abbreviation for L. *ibidem*, in the same place.

ĭ·bite. Syn. bismuth oxy-iodotannate, an antiseptic.

ibō·găin. An alkaloid, $C_{52}H_{66}O_2N_6$, obtained from the plant *Tabernanthe Iboga* (of the Acanthaceae family) growing in West Africa. It is supposed to have aphrodisiac and sustaining properties. Ibogaine hydrochloride has been used for angina pectoris and other cardiac conditions.

ice. Water in the solid state, i.e. at or below a temperature of 0° C. or 32° F.

ĭ·chor (G. *ikhōr*, serous matter). The watery fluid escaping from a wound.

ĭ·choroid (G. *ikhōr*, serous matter; *eidos*, form). Like pus.

ichorrhoē·a (G. *ikhōr*, serous matter; *rhoia*, flow). A discharge of ichor.

ichtham·mol (G. *ikhthus*, fish; L. *oleum*, oil). A viscous, almost black, substance consisting mainly of the ammonium salts of the sulphonic acids of an oil prepared from a bituminous schist. It is used externally for eczema, psoriasis, etc., and in a 10 per cent solution for pruritus and ulcers. Syn. ichthyol.

ĭch·thyocol·la (G. *ikhthus*, fish; *kolla*, glue). Isinglass. The dried, prepared swimming bladder of the sturgeon.

ĭch·thyoid (G. *ikhthus*, fish; *eidos*, form). Resembling a fish.

ĭch·thyol. Syn. ichthammol.

ichthyŏ·phagy (G. *ikhthus*, fish; *phagein*, to eat). The habit of living on fish flesh.

ĭch·thyophō·bia (G. *ikhthus*, fish; *phobos*, fear). An abnormal dislike of fish.

ichthyō·sis (G. *ikhthus*, fish). A congenital disease of the skin, characterized by dryness and scaliness. **I. hystrix:** linear warty naevus, its distribution often corresponding apparently to that of a cutaneous nerve.

ĭch·thyosul·phonate. A salt of ichthyosulphonic acid.

ichthyŏt·ic (G. *ikhthus*, fish). Affected with ichthyosis.

ĭch·thyotox·icum (G. *ikhthus*, fish; *toxikon*, poison). Ptomaine poisoning from eating fish.

ĭch·thyotox·ism (G. *ikhthus*, fish; *toxikon*, poison). Fish poisoning.

icŏ·nolagny (G. *eikōn*, image; *lagnos*, lewd). Sexual desires produced by looking at works of art.

ictĕ·ric (G. *ikteros*, jaundice). Pertaining to jaundice. **I. index:** a measure of the intensity of the yellow colour of serum which is in most cases mainly due to bilirubin. Estimated by comparing the serum with a standard solution of 1:10000 potassium dichromate, the colour intensity of which is taken as unity.

ictero·anāe·mia (G. *ikteros*, jaundice; *a*, neg.; *haima*, blood). Jaundice associated with anaemia.

ic·terogen·ic (G. *ikteros*, jaundice; *gennan*, to produce). Producing jaundice.

ic·terohaem·oglobinū·ria (G. *ikteros*, jaundice; *haima*, blood; L. *globus*, globe; G. *ouron*, urine). Jaundice and haemoglobinuria.

ic·terohepati·tis (G. *ikteros*, jaundice; *hēpar*, liver). Jaundice accompanying inflammation of the liver.

ic·teroid (G. *ikteros*, jaundice; *eidos*, form). Like jaundice.

ic·terus (G. *ikteros*, jaundice). Jaundice, *q.v.* **I. gravis:** due to acute hepatitis or a toxic necrosis as in acute yellow atrophy. **I. gravis neonatorum:** a severe sometimes familial condition of jaundice beginning a few days after birth, characterized by a persistence of erythroblasts in the peripheral blood, resulting from serological (Rh) incompatibility between maternal and foetal blood. **I. neonatorum:** the physiological jaundice appearing in a high percentage of infants 3–7 days after birth, lasting about a fortnight and not accompanied by any other symptoms. It is due to haemolysis.

ic·tus (L., a blow). Sudden attack. **I. laryngis:** laryngeal vertigo; a violent attack of coughing followed by glottis spasm and momentary loss of consciousness.

Id. Abbreviation for L. *idem*, the same.

id (G. *idios*, private; or L. *id*, it). 1. A psychoanalytic term denoting the 'deep' obscure part of a person's mind. 2. A granule of a chromosome.

idea (G., form). A mental conception.

ideā·tion (G. *idea*, form). The mental process of forming an idea or conception.

ideā·tional (G. *idea*, form). Pertaining to ideation or to ideas.

identificā·tion (L. *idem*, same; *facere*, to make). A method whereby certain physical peculiarities of the body may be used to identify a person.

iden·tical (L. *idem*, the same). The same; precisely corresponding. **I. points:** any pair of retinal points in the two eyes which receive stimuli from the same point of an object at infinite distance, *q.v.*

ĭ·deomō·tor (G. *idea*, form; L. *movere*, to move). Psychomotor, *q.v.*

ĭ·deomus·cular (G. *idea*, form; *mus*, muscle). Relating to the influence exerted upon the muscular system by a mental concept.

ĭ·deophrē·nia (G. *idea*, form; *phrēn*, mind). A form of insanity in which there is marked perversion of ideas.

ĭ·deophrē·nic. Characterized by ideophrenia.

ĭ·deoplā·sia (G. *idea*, form; *plassein*, to form). Giving shape to the ideas in the hypnotic state.

ĭ·deovă·scular (G. *idea*, form; L. *vasculum*, dim. of *vas*, vessel). Relating to vascular changes resulting from a dominant idea.

ĭ·dio-agglutinā·tion (G. *idios*, own; L. *ad*, to; *glutinare*, to glue). Self-agglutination.

ĭ·dioblast (G. *idios*, own; *blastos*, germ). A cell having a character different from that of the surrounding cells, due to a difference either in its form or its contents.

ĭ·diocy (G. *idiōtēs*, an unskilled person). A congenital condition of an extreme degree of mental deficiency. **I., amaurotic:** a congenital, developmental, recessively inherited disease characterized by the association of severe progressive mental deterioration, disturbances of motor and visual function with retinal changes, probably due to a disorder of lipoid metabolism; becoming manifest either shortly after birth (syn. Tay-Sachs's disease) during later childhood (juvenile type, Spielmayer-Vogt-Batten-Mayou type) or later in life (Kufs type). **I., Mongolian:** a form of i. associated with a mongolian appearance of the face, i.e. obliquely placed eyes with prominence of the epicanthi, with a thick, protruding tongue, short, broad fingers, umbilical hernia, etc.

ĭ·dĭogĕ·nesis (G. *idios*, own; *genesis*, generation). The origin of diseases of an idiopathic nature.

id·iogĕ·nic (G. *idios*, own; *gennan*, generation). Relating to idiogenesis.

ĭ·dioglos·sia (G. *idios*, own; *glōssa*, tongue). Disorder of speech, characterized by substitutions and transpositions of sounds.

idiohyp·notism (G. *idios*, own; *hupnos*, sleep). Self-induced hypnotism.

idĭolў·sin (G. *idios*, own; *luein*, to dissolve). A lysin normally present in the blood.

ĭ·diometrī·tis (G. *idios*, own; *mētra*, womb). Inflammation of the substance of the uterus.

ĭ·diomus·cular (G. *idios*, own; *mus*, muscle). Pertaining to muscle tissue only and not involving any nerve stimulus. **I. contraction:** the contraction of part of a tired or degenerated muscle on mechanical stimulation.

ĭ·diopă·thic (G. *idios*, own; *pathos*, disease). Of spontaneous origin; primary; applied to diseases which are not the sequel to any other disease, e.g., i. epilepsy; i. hypertrophy of the heart.

idĭŏ·pathy (G. *idios*, own; *pathos*, disease). Any pathological condition of spontaneous origin.

idiophrĕ·nic (G. *idios*, own; *phrēn*, mind). A form of insanity due to disease of the brain.

ĭ·dioplasm (G. *idios*, own; *plasma*, anything formed). The substance contained in the chromosomes which mediates the transmission of hereditary characters. Syn. germ-plasm.

idiorĕ·tinal (G. *idios*, own; L. *retina*, from *rete*, net). Peculiar to the retina.

ĭ·diosome (G. *idios*, own; *sōma*, body). The attraction sphere of a spermatoblast.

ĭ·diosyn·crasy (G. *idios*, own; *sun*, with; *krasis*, combination). 1. A mental or physical trait or characteristic peculiar to the individual. 2. Peculiar sensitivity in an individual to the ingestion or application of some particular food, drug or medicament.

ĭ·diosyncrat·ic. Relating to or characterized by idiosyncrasy.

idiot (G. *idiōtēs*, an unskilled person). A person suffering from idiocy, *q.v.* **I., Aztec type:** an i. characterized by having an abnormally small head. **Kulmuk i.:** an i. with Mongolian type of idiocy. **Profound i.:** an i. with practically no mental powers at all, and usually with physical abnormalities. **Superficial i.:** an i. with some few limited powers (of speech, etc.) and possessed of some ability to coordinate movements.

ĭ·diotism. Idiocy, *q.v.*

ĭ·dioventri·cular (G. *idios*, own; L. *ventriculus*, dim. of *venter*, stomach). Peculiar to and originating in a ventricle of the heart, esp. of abnormal rhythm.

ignā·tia. The seed of *Strychnos ignatii*.

igni-operā·tion (L. *ignis*, fire; *opus*, work). Operation performed by the cautery.

ig·nipedi·tēs (L. *ignis*, fire; *pes*, foot). Burning sensation in the feet symptomatic of beri-beri.

ig·nipuncture (L. *ignis*, fire; *punctura*, puncture). Cauterization by puncture with needles brought to a white heat.

ignis Sancti Ignatii (L. St. Ignatius's fire). Erysipelas.

ignī·tion (L. *ignis*, fire). The act of making fire.

il·eac (L. *ilia*, entrails). Relating to the ileum.

ilĕĕc·tomy (L. *ilia*, entrails; G. *ektomē*, excision). Excision of the ileum.

ilĕi·tis (L. *ilia*, entrails). Inflammation of the ileum. **I., regional:** a chronic disease affecting usually the terminal part of the ileum, characterized by the development of granulomatous tissue within the intestinal walls, often leading to intestinal obstruction and fistula formation. Syn. Crohn's disease; Terminal i.

ĭ·leocae·cal (L. *ilia*, entrails; *caecus*, blind). Relating to the ileum and the caecum jointly.

ĭ·leocaecŏ·stomy (L. *ilia*, entrails; *caecus*, blind; G. *stoma*, mouth). An operation in which the ileum is joined to the caecum after excision of a portion of the terminal ileum.

ĭl·eocŏ·lic (L. *ilia*, entrails; G. *kŏlon*, colon). Relating both to the ileum and the colon.

ĭ·leocoli·tis (L. *ilia*, entrails; G. *kŏlon*, colon). Inflammation of both the ileum and the colon.

ĭ·leocolŏ·stomy (L. *ilia*, entrails; G. *kŏlon*, colon; *stoma*, mouth). The surgical formation of a fistula between the ileum and colon.

ĭ·leŏ·ilĕŏ·stomy (L. *ilia*, entrails; G. *stoma*, mouth). The surgical formation of a fistula between two parts of the ileum.

ĭ·leoproctŏ·stomy (L. *ilia*, entrails; G. *proktos*, rectum; *stoma*, mouth). An operation in which the ileum is joined to the rectum.

ĭ·leosigmoidŏ·stomy (L. *ilia*, entrails; G. *sigma*, the letter S; *eidos*, form; *stoma*, mouth). An operation in which the ileum is joined to the sigmoid colon.

ĭlĕŏ·stomy (L. *ilia*, entrails; G. *stoma*, mouth). The surgical formation of a passage through the abdominal wall into the ileum.

ilĕŏ·tomy (L. *ilia*, entrails; G. *tomē*, section). An opening into the ileum through the abdominal wall.

ĭ·lĕŭm (L. *ilia*, entrails). The lower half of the small intestine, between jejunum and caecum.

ĭ·lĕŭs (G. *eileos*, colic). Intestinal obstruction.

Ilex. A genus of shrubs, including the holly, of which the leaves yield a tonic.

ĭ·lĭăc (L. *ilium*, the groin). Relating to the ilium.

ilī·acus. A muscle arising from the iliac fossa and inserted into the upper end of the femur.

ĭ·liadel·phus (L. *ilium*, flank; G. *adelphos*, brother). A monster which is double in the upper part and single below.

ĭ·liocapsula·ris (L. *ilium*, flank; *capsula*, little box). Part of the iliacus muscle.

ĭ·liocolŏ·tomy (L. *ilium*, flank; G. *kolon*, colon; *tomē*, a cutting). An incision into the colon in the iliac region.

ĭ·liocos·tal (L. *ilium*, flank; *costa*, rib). Relating to the ilium and the ribs.

ĭ·liocostā·lis (L. *ilium*, flank; *costa*, rib). A muscle situated on the back of the spine.

ĭ·liofĕ·moral (L. *ilium*, flank; *femur*, thigh). Relating to the ilium and the femur.

ĭ·liohypogas·tric (L. *ilium*, flank; G. *hupo*, under; *gaster*, stomach). Relating to the ilium and hypogastrium.

ĭ·lio-in·guinal (L. *ilium*, flank; *ingue*, groin). Relating to the ilium and the groin.

iliolum·bar (L. *ilium*, flank; *lumbus*, loin). Pertaining to the iliac and lumbar regions.

ĭ·liopectin·eal (L. *ilium*, flank; *pecten*, comb). Relating to the ilium and pectineus muscle.

iliopel·vic (L. *ilium*, flank; *pelvis*, basin). Relating to the iliac muscle and the pelvis.

iliopso·as (L. *ilium*, flank; G. *psoa*, muscles of the loins). The psoas and iliacus muscles considered together.

iliosa·cral (L. *ilium*, flank; *sacrum*, holy). Relating to the ilium and the sacrum.

ilioti·bial (L. *ilium*, flank; *tibia*, shin-bone). Relating to the ilium and the tibia.

i·liotrochantĕ·ric (L. *ilium*, flank; G. *trochanter*, runner). Relating to the ilium and a trochanter.

iliospi·nal. Relating to the ilium and the spine.

i·lĭum (L.). 1. The flank. 2. The upper broad portion of the innominate bone.

ill. 1. Sick, in bad health. 2. A disorder.

illegi·timacy (L. *in*, un-; *legitimus*, lawful). The state of being unlawful, of having been born out of wedlock.

illegi·timate. Not in accordance with statutory law. **l. child:** a child born out of wedlock.

illumina·tion (L. *illuminare*, from *lumen*, light). 1. The lighting up of an object. 2. The amount of light thrown upon an object. **I., dark ground:** a method of making visible microscopic objects which are not visible on ordinary illumination: they are lit up from the side by the peripheral rays of the source of light and are seen brightly on a dark ground.

illu·sion (L. *illusio*, mockery). A false interpretation of a sensual perception.

illŭ·sional (L. *illusio*, mockery). Pertaining to or characterized by illusions.

illuta·tion (L. *in*, in; *lutum*, mud). Mud-bath treatment of disease.

i·ma (L. *imus*, lowest). Lowest; last; deepest; e.g. thyroidea ima, the lowest thyroid artery.

im·age (L. *imago*). The picture of an object caused by rays of light emanating or reflected from it.

imă·ginary (L. *imago*). Present only in the imagination of a person.

ima·go (L.). 1. The insect after the completion of its metamorphosis. 2. An uncorrected memory of a beloved person formed in childhood.

imbă·lance (L. *in*, un-; *bilanx*, having two scales). Lack of balance.

im·becile (L. *imbecillis*, weak). Affected by imbecility.

imbeci·lity (L. *imbecillis*, weak). A degree of mental deficiency not amounting to idiocy.

imbed. In histology, to fix an object in some hard substance such as paraffin, to facilitate the cutting of sections of it.

imbibi·tion (L. *in*, in; *bibere*, drink). The penetration of a fluid into solid substance; absorption of a liquid.

im·bricated (L. *imbrex*, tile). Overlapping; arranged like tiles on a roof.

i·mide, i·mid. Any compound of the radical NH united to a bivalent acid radical.

imino. The bivalent NH group which may be attached to one or two carbon atoms.

Imlach's fat pad (Imlach, F., Scottish surgeon, who qualified in 1872). The fat surrounding the round ligament. **I.'s ring:** a subdivision of the crural canal in which the round ligament lies surrounded by fat.

immă·culate (L. *in*, un-; *macula*, a spot). Spotless.

im·mature (L. *in*, un-; *maturus*, ripe). Unripe.

immē·diate (L. *in*, un-; *mediatus*, halved). Direct; not mediated.

immer·sion (L. *in*, in; *mergere*, to dip). 1. The plunging of a body into a liquid; e.g., i. bath, a plunge bath. 2. The method of dipping the lens of a microscope into a drop of a liquid placed on the slide; used to bring light rays from the object under examination into the microscope which would otherwise be reflected by the layer of air between object and lens.

im·minent (L. *imminere*, to overhang). Impending.

immis·cible (L. *in*, un-; *miscere*, to mix). Not capable of being mixed.

immis·sio (L. *in*, in; *mittere*, to send). Insertion.

immobĭ·lity (L. *immobilis*, immovable). The state of being fixed.

immobiliza·tion (L. *immobilis*, immovable). Fixing; rendering immobile, as of a joint.

immune (L. *immunis*, exempt). Protected, especially against infectious disease. **I. body:** Antibody, *q.v.*

immu·nity (L. *immunitas*, immunity). The state of increased resistance to the effects of absorption of foreign toxic substances (micro-organisms, viruses, and some vegetable poisons). **I., active:** i. obtained either from recovery from an infectious disease or by inoculation with the specific infective organism or the toxic substance produced by this organism. **I., passive:** i. obtained from the introduction of an antitoxic serum.

immuniza·tion (L. *immunis*, exempt). The act of rendering or method of rendering immune.

immunŏ·logy (L. *immunis*, exempt; G. *logos*, treatise). The science concerned with the study of immunity.

immunotox·in (L. *immunis*, exempt; G. *toxikon*, poison). See antitoxin.

immunotransfū·sion (L. *immunis*, exempt; *trans*, across; *fundere*, to pour). Transfusion with blood from a donor previously immunized against the infection from which the recipient is suffering.

impac·ted (L. *impactus*, from *impingere*, to push in). Wedged in tightly.

impac·tion (L. *impactus*, from *impingere*, to push in). 1. The state of being wedged or fixed, e.g., i. of faeces in the rectum; i. of a calculus in the ureter; i. of an unerupted tooth within the jaw. 2. Concussion.

impal·pable (L. *in*, un-; *palpare*, to stroke). Not felt by touch.

impă·ludism (L. *in*, in; *palus*, a marsh). Chronic malaria.

im·par (L. *impar*, uneven). Odd; unequal; without a fellow.

impĕ·rative (L. *imperare*, to order). Compulsory; absolute.

impercep·tion (L. *in*, un-; *percipere*, to perceive). Defective perception.

imper·forate (L. *in*, in; *perforare*, to perforate). Characterized by imperforation, e.g., i. anus; i. hymen.

imperfora·tion (L. *in*, in; *perforare*, to perforate). Congenital absence of a natural opening. Syn. atresia.

imperial drink. A refreshing alkaline drink made with a teaspoonful of cream of tartar, 3–4 oz. of sugar and the juice of 1 lemon to 1 pint of boiling water.

imper·meable (L. *in*, un-; *per*, through; *meare*, to pass). Impenetrable.

imper·vious (L. *in*, un-; *pervius*, passable). Impenetrable.

impeti·ginous (L. *impetere*, to assail). Pertaining to impetigo.

impeti·go (L. *impetere*, to assail). Inflammatory and pustular disease of the skin. **I. bullosa:** bullous type of i. contagiosa, *q.v.* **I. contagiosa:** an infectious skin disease involving the superficial layer of the epidermis, characterized by the development of vesicles and pustules from small erythematous spots, which after rupturing form brownish scabs; caused by *Streptococcus pyogenes*. **I. follicularis:** superficial pustular folliculitis, *q.v.*, which may occur on any hairy area. Syn. Bockhart's impetigo. **I. herpetiformis:** a skin disease characterized by the development of small greenish pustules arranged in groups on an inflamed base, often accompanied by general symptoms.

implacen·tal (L. *in*, un-; *placenta*, a flat cake). Having no placenta.

implantă·tion (L. *in*, in; *plantare*, to plant). The act of setting in or of grafting a tissue. **I. cone:** see axon hillock. **I. cyst:** see dermoid (3).

im·potence (L. *in*, un-; *potens*, powerful). Lack of power; especially lack of sexual power.

im·potency. Impotence.

impoten·tia coeun·di (L. *in*, un-; *potens*, powerful, *coire*, to copulate). Inability to perform coitus. **I. erigendi** (L. *erigere*, to raise): incapability of induction of penile erection.

impreg·nate (L. *impraegnare*, to make pregnant). 1. To make pregnant. 2. To saturate with.

impregnă·tion (L. *impraegnare*, to make pregnant). 1. Fertilization. 2. The process of saturating.

impres·sio (L.). An impression, e.g., i. gastrica, an impression made on the liver by the stomach.

impres·sion (L. *impressio*). 1. A hollow or depression. 2. The effect upon the mind by a perception or an idea. **Is, digital:** small pits on the inner surface of the skull.

impulse (L. *impellere*, to push against). 1. A force acting during a short interval. 2. A sudden mental feeling which urges one on to an action. **I., cardiac:** the palpable impulse of the apex, or any other part of the heart, on the anterior wall of the chest. **I., morbid:** a sudden and, as it were, uncontrollable desire not amounting to an obsession to commit an unlawful act.

impul·sion (L. *impellere*, to push against). Action under an impulse.

impū·rity (L. *impurus*, unclean). 1. The state of being not pure or clean. 2. The substance that causes such a state.

in. Abbreviation for inch.

inaci·dity (L. *in*, un-; *acidus*, acid). The condition of being free from acidity.

inactivā·tion (L. *in*, un-; *activus*, active). The process of destroying a specific property of a body fluid, e.g. inactivated serum, of which the thermolabile complement has been destroyed by heat.

ină·dequacy (L. *in*, not; *adaequare*, to equalize). Insufficiency.

ină·nimate (L. *in*, not; *animus*, soul). Without life.

inanĭ·tion (L. *inanis*, empty). 1. Lack of food. 2. Exhaustion, especially from starvation.

inartĭ·culate (L. *in*, not; *articulus*, joint). Not jointed or articulated—especially applied to speech.

in articulo mortis (L.). At the point of death.

inassi·milable (L. *in*, not; *assimilis*, similar). Applied to substances which cannot be assimilated.

inax·on (G. *inĕs*, pl. of *is*, muscle fibres; *axon*, axis). A neuron with a long axon.

inborn. Congenital.

incandes·cent (L. *incandescere*, to glow). Glowing; heated to a degree of emitting light.

incar·cerated (L. *in*, in; *carcer*, a prison). Imprisoned; wedged; locked, e.g., i. hernia, a hernia which cannot be pushed back without surgical interference.

incarcerā·tion (L. *in*, in; *carcer*, a prison). The state of being wedged or locked.

incă·rial bone. The interparietal bone, generally part of the occipital bone; so called because found as a distinct bone in ancient Incas.

incarna·tio (L. *in*, in; *caro*, flesh). Conversion into flesh. **I., unguis:** see unguis incurvatus.

incarnā·tus (L. *in*, in; *caro*, flesh). Converted into flesh; growing into flesh.

incen·diarism (L. *incendere*, to kindle). Criminal fireraising.

ia·cest (L. *incestus*, sinful). Sexual intercourse between nearest relatives, such as between a brother and sister.

in·cidence (L. *incidere*, to fall upon). 1. A falling upon; the direction in which one body strikes another, e.g.

angle of i., the angle at which a ray of light strikes a surface. 2. The range of occurrence, such as age i.

incinerā·tion (L. *in*, into; *cineres*, ashes). Cremation; reduction to ashes.

inci·pient (L. *incipere*, to begin). Beginning to develop.

incised (L. *incidere*, to cut into). 1. Cut. 2. Notched.

incĭ·sion (L. *incisio*, cut). 1. The act of cutting into. 2. A knife wound or one made with another cutting instrument. **I., crucial:** two incisions crossing each other at right angles.

incĭ·sive (L. *incidere*, to cut). 1. Cutting. 2. Relating to the incisor teeth.

incĭ·sor teeth. *Dentes incisivi*, the four anterior teeth in each jaw.

incisū·ra (L. *incidere*, to cut). 1. An incision. 2. A notch. 3. A fissure. 4. A sulcus.

incĭ·sure (L. *incidere*, to cut). A notch or fissure.

inclu·sion (L. *includere*, to enclose). 1. The state of being enclosed or included. 2. The act of enclosing. 3. That which is enclosed. **I. body:** certain intracellular structures found, e.g., in virus diseases, such as smallpox, herpes, etc., in the affected tissues. Some of these bodies represent probably the virus itself. **I., foetal:** a monster in which one foetus is enclosed within another.

incohē·rence (L. *in*, not; *cohaerere*, to hold together). Lack of systematic connection, e.g., of ideas or of language.

incohē·rent (L. *in*, *cohaerere*, to hold together). Not connected or coherent.

incombus·tible (L. *in*, not; *comburere*, to burn up). Incapable of burning.

incompă·tibility (L. *in*, not; *cum*, together; *pati*, to suffer). The property of being incompatible.

incompă·tible (L. *in*, not; *cum*, together; *pati*, to suffer). Applied to substances which when mixed lose their original properties or usefulness and may become toxic, and which must not therefore be administered together.

incom·petence, incom·petency (L. *in*, not; *competens*, competent). Incapability. **I., mitral:** incapability of closure of the mitral valves.

incompress·ible (L. *in*, not; *comprimere*, to squeeze). Not compressible.

incon·gruence (L. *incongruens*, inconsistent). Lack of congruence or correspondence.

incon·tinence (L. *in*, not; *continere*, to contain). Lack of voluntary power to control the excretion of faeces from rectum or urine from bladder. **I., paradoxical:** i. of urine due to over-distension of the bladder with urine. Syn. false i.

inco·ordinā·tion (L. *in*, not; *cum*, together; *ordinare*, to arrange). Lack of co-ordination, especially in regard to muscular movements. See also ataxia.

incorporā·tion (L. *in*, into; *corpus*, body). The thorough union of one substance with another.

in·crement (L. *incrementum*). Increase.

incrē·tion (L. *in*, into; *cernere*, to separate). Internal secretion.

incretŏ·logy (L. *in*, into; *cernere*, to separate; G. *logos*, discourse). Endocrinology.

in·cretory (L. *in*, into; *cernere*, to separate). Pertaining to incretion.

incrustā·tion (L. *in*, on; *crusta*, crust). The formation of a crust; deposition of mineral salts at a surface.

incubā·tion (L. *in*, into; *cubare*, to lie down). 1. The period between the invasion of pathogenic microorganisms into the body and the clinical manifestation of the disease caused thereby. 2. The culture of micro-organisms in an incubator.

in·cubator (L. *in*, into; *cubare*, to lie down). 1. An apparatus for the cultivation of micro-organisms under a temperature favourable to their growth. 2. An apparatus for rearing prematurely born infants under a favourable temperature.

in·cubus (L. *incubare*, to lie down). Nightmare.

in·cudal (L. *incus*, anvil). Pertaining to the incus.

incudec·tomy (L. *incus*, anvil; G. *ektomē*, excision). The operation of removing the incus.

incū·dius (L. *incus*, anvil). The laxator tympani muscle.

incū·rable (L. *in*, not; *curare*, to cure). Not curable.

incur·vate (L. *incurvatus*). Curved inward.

incus (L., anvil). The central of the three bones of the middle ear.

indagā·tion (L. *indagare*). Investigation or examination.

indentā·tion (L. *in*, into; *dens*, tooth). 1. A notch; a sulcus. 2. The state of being notched.

index (L.). 1. That which indicates a condition or a process. 2. The ratio of measurement of a part compared with an arbitrarily fixed standard. 3. A list. **I., cardiac:** the volume of blood per minute per square metre of body surface. **I., cephalic:** the ratio between the breadth of the cranium multiplied by 100 and its length. **I., cephalic height:** the ratio between the basi-bregmatic height multiplied by 100 and the greatest length. **I., colour:** the ratio between the percentage of haemoglobin and the first two figures of the number of erythrocytes per cmm. **I., dental:** the ratio between the combined length of premolar and molar teeth multiplied by 100 and the basi-nasionic length (the distance from basion to nasion) **I., facial:** the ratio between the nasoprosthionic length (distance from nasion to prosthion) multiplied by 100 and the greatest width between the two zygomatic zones. **I. finger:** the forefinger. **I., gnathic:** the ratio between the basi-prosthionic length (distance from basion to prosthion) multiplied by 100 and the basi-nasionic length. **I., icteric:** see icteric index. **I., nasal:** the ratio between the width of the pyriform aperture multiplied by 100 and its height. **I., orbital:** the ratio between the height of the orbit multiplied by 100 and its width.

indexŏ·meter (L. *index*; G. *metron*, measure). An instrument for the estimation of the index of refraction of fluids.

Indian hemp. Cannabis.

in·dican (G. *indikon*, indigo). A glucoside occurring in indigo plants.

indicanae·mia (G. *indikon*, indigo; *haima*, blood). A condition in which indican is found in the blood.

indicanu·ria (G. *indikon*, indigo; *ouron*, urine). Urinary excretion of an abnormal amount of indican (1).

indicā·tion (L. *indicare*, to indicate). 1. A sign. 2. The circumstances by which the particular form of treatment may be determined.

in·dicator (L.). 1. That which indicates something. 2. A substance indicating change in chemical reaction by a change of colour. 3. A substance showing the beginning or end of a chemical reaction.

indif·ferent (L. *in*, not; *differre*, to differ). 1. Harmless, without effect, neutral, not readily influenced. 2. Not differentiated, as of tissues.

indi·genous (L. *indigena*, native). Native to a country or place.

indigĕ·stible (L. *in*, not; *digerere*, to dissolve). Not able to be digested.

indigĕ·stion (L. *in*, not; *digerere*, to dissolve). A disturbance of digestion.

indigitā·tion (L. *in*, into; *digitus*, finger). Invagination.

in·digo. 1. A dark blue dye obtained from various plants and also produced synthetically. 2. The sixth colour in the spectrum. **I. carmine:** the sodium salt of indigotin disulphonic acid. Used in kidney efficiency tests.

indirect (L. *in*, not; *directus*, straight). Not straight.

indiscrim·inate. Promiscuous; affecting more than one part of the body.

in·disposi·tion (L. *indispositus*, disordered). Any slight ailment.

individual psychology. See psychology, individual.

indole (G. *indikon*, indigo). A substance derived from pyrrol, originating in intestinal fermentation of proteins. Formula C_8H_7N.

in·dolent (L. *indolentia*, freedom from pain). Painless; sluggish; indifferent.

indolyl acetic acid. An organic acid occurring in traces in normal urine. It is an auxin, i.e., it stimulates plant growth.

indophenol-oxidase. An oxidation-reduction enzyme occurring in living tissues. It is so called because it is investigated by its ability to oxidise *p*-phenylenediamine in the presence of *a*-naphthol to give a blue indophenol derivative.

indox·yl (G. *indikon*, indigo; *oxus*, sharp). Prepared from indole by various methods as an intermediate in indigo synthesis. Indoxyl is readily oxidised to indigo.

indoxylae·mia (G. *indikon*, indigo; *oxus*, sharp; *haima*, blood). A condition in which indoxyl is present in the blood.

indoxylu·ria (G. *indikon*, indigo; *oxus*, sharp; *ouron*, urine). A condition in which indoxyl is present in the urine.

induced (L. *inducere*, to lead on). 1. Produced or brought on from without. 2. Produced artificially, as i. labour.

induc·tion (L. *inducere*, to lead on). 1. The drawing of general conclusions from empirical facts. 2. The production of an electric current in a body which is in proximity to, but not in direct contact with, an electrical body. 3. The act of inducing or causing.

in·dulin. A coal-tar dye.

induli·nophil (*Indulin*; G. *philein*, to love). Staining with indulin.

in·durated (L. *in*, in; *durare*, to harden). Hardened, e.g., i. chancre, the primary syphilitic ulcer.

indurā·tion (L. *in*, in; *durare*, to harden). The state of being, or the process of becoming, hard; a hardened area of tissue.

in·durative (L. *in*, in; *durus*, hard). Pertaining to induration.

indusium griseum (L.). Marginal portion of the corpus callosum in the brain.

inĕ·briant (L. *inebriare*, to make drunken). Intoxicant; causing inebriation.

inebriā·tion (L. *inebriare*, to make drunken). The condition of being intoxicated.

inēbri·ety (L. *inebrietas*). Habitual alcoholism.

inelas·tic (L. *in*, not; G. *elaunein*, to drive). Not elastic.

inert (L. *iners*, idle). Inactive.

iner·tia (L.). The property of a body to remain in the same condition, such as rest or uniform motion. **I., uterine:** absence or insufficiency of uterine contractions during labour.

in extre·mis (L.). At the end; dying.

in·fancy (L. *infans*, unable to speak). Early childhood, especially the first year of life.

in·fant (L. *infans*, unable to speak). 1. A baby; a child during his first year of life. 2. Under English law, a person under the age of 21.

infan·ticide (L. *infans*, unable to speak; *caedere*, to kill). 1. Murder of an infant. 2. The murderer of an infant.

in·fantile. Pertaining to infancy. **I. paralysis:** poliomyelitis, acute anterior, *q.v.*

in·fantilism (L. *infans*, unable to speak). The persistence of the characteristics of childhood into adult life. **I., hepatic:** i. associated with disturbance of liver function. **I., renal:** i. associated with chronic nephritis. **I., Levi-Lorain type:** ateleiosis, *q.v.* **I., intestinal:** coeliac disease, *q.v.*

in·farct (L. *infarcire*, to stuff into). A usually wedge-shaped area of necrotic tissue due to obstruction of a terminal artery. **I., uric acid:** the accumulation of uric acid crystals in the renal tubules of the newborn.

infarc·tion (L. *infarcire*, to stuff into). 1. An infarct. 2. The development of an infarct.

infect (L. *inficere*, to infect). To induce infection by communicating the specific pathogenic micro-organism.

infec·tion (L. *inficere*, to infect). 1. The communicating of a disease by micro-organisms. 2. An infectious disease. **I., mixed:** infection by more than one species of micro-organism.

infec·tious (L. *inficere*, to infect). 1. Caused by an infection. 2. Communicating pathogenic micro-organisms.

infec·tive (L. *inficere*, to infect). Infectious. **I. endocarditis:** malignant or ulcerative endocarditis, *q.v.* **I. mononucleosis:** an acute i. disease characterized by fever, glandular enlargement and an increase of somewhat atypical lymphocytes in the blood. Syn. glandular fever.

infecun·dity (L. *infecundus*, unfruitful). Sterility; barrenness.

infē·rior. (L.). Lower.

inferiority complex. The sum total of more or less subconscious and mentally insufficiently compensated feelings about an actual or supposed bodily or mental inferiority.

in·ferolǎ·teral (L. *inferus*, below; *lateralis*, at the side). Situated below and to the outer side.

in·feromē·dian (L. *inferus*, below; *medius*, middle). Situated below and in the middle line.

in·feropostē·rior (L. *inferus*, below; *posterior*, behind). Situated below and behind.

infestā·tion (L. *infestare*, to molest). 1. The communication of a disease caused by metazoan parasites. 2. The state of being infested.

infē·sted (L. *infestare*, to molest). Harbouring metazoan parasites, such as insects or nematodes.

infibulā·tion (L. *in*, into; *fibula*, a brooch). An operation in which the prepuce is stitched over the glans penis.

in·filtrate (L. *in*, into; L.L. *filtrare*, to strain). 1. To produce infiltration. 2. The substance deposited in the tissues during infiltration (1).

infiltrā·tion (L. *in*, into; L.L. *filtrare*, to strain). 1. The entering into cells or intercellular spaces of some abnormal substance or an abnormal amount of substance usually there present. 2. The state thus produced.

in·finite (L. *infinitus*, boundless). Not limited; greater than any given amount. **I. distance:** in optics, a distance of 20 feet or more, so called because rays entering the eye from an object at that distance are practically parallel and parallel rays are defined as rays coming from a point at an infinite distance.

infirm (L. *in*, not; *firmus*, strong). Weak; feeble.

infir·mary (L. *infirmus*, weak). A hospital.

infir·mity (L. *infirmus*, weak). Any weakening disease.

inflame (L. *inflammare*, to set on fire). To suffer inflammation.

inflammā·tion (L. *inflammare*, to set on fire). The totality of reactions of a living tissue upon injury, comprising mainly hyperaemia, exudation of plasma and migration of leucocytes from blood vessels, and proliferation of certain cells.

inflam·matory (L. *inflammare*, to set on fire). Relating to inflammation.

inflā·tion (L. *inflatio*, swelling). Distension with air.

inflec·tion, inflex·ion (L. *inflectere*, to bend in). 1. A bending inward. 2. Modification of the voice when speaking.

influēn·za (Ital. *influenza*, influence). An acute infectious and often epidemic disease, characterized by inflammation of the mucous membrane of the respiratory tract, fever, prostration and other variable symptoms.

influēn·zal. Relating to influenza.

influx (L. *influere*, to flow in). An inflow.

infra-axil·lary (L. *infra*, below; *axilla*, armpit). Below the axilla.

in·fraclavi·cular (L. *infra*, below; *clavicula*, a small key). Below the collar-bone.

infracom·missure (L. *infra*, below; *commissura*). The inferior commissure of the brain.

infraconstric·tor (L. *infra*, below; *constringere*, to bind). The inferior constrictor muscle of the pharynx.

infracor·tical (L. *infra*, below; *cortex*, rind). Below the cortex of the brain or kidney.

infracos·tal (L. *infra*, below; *costa*, rib). Below the ribs.

infracŏ·tyloid (L. *infra*, below; G. *kotule*, cup; *eidos*, form). Below the acetabulum of the hip bone.

infrac·tion (L. *infringere*, to break). Incomplete fracture of a bone.

in·fradiaphragmat·ic (L. *infra*, below; G. *diaphragma*, barrier). Below the diaphragm.

infraglě·noid (L. *infra*, below; G. *glene*, cavity; *eidos*, form). Below the glenoid cavity of the scapula.

infraglot·tic (L. *infra*, below; G. *glottis*). Below the glottis.

infrahȳ·oid (L. *infra*, below; G. *huoeidēs*, shaped like the letter Y). Below the hyoid bone.

inframam·mary (L. *infra*, below; *mamma*, breast). Below the mamma.

inframandi·bular (L. *infra*, below; *mandere*, to chew). Below the lower jaw.

inframaxil·lary (L. *infra*, below; *maxilla*, jaw). Below or under the jaw.

infra-or·bital (L. *infra*, below; *orbita*, a track). Below the floor of the orbit.

infrapatel·lar (L. *infra*, under; *patella*, kneecap). Below the patella.

infrapū·bic (L. *infra*, below; *pubes*, adult). Below the os pubis.

infra-red. Electro-magnetic radiations of the same character as X-rays, light waves and wireless waves, but with a wave-length longer than those of visible light and shorter than those of wireless waves. This radiation is concerned with the propagation of heat.

infrascǎ·pular (L. *infra*, below; *scapulae*, shoulder-blades). Below the shoulder-blade.

infraspinā·tus muscle (L. *infra*, below; *spina*, spine). A muscle on the back of the scapula.

infraspī·nous (L. *infra*, under; *spina*, spine). Below a spine, as of the scapula or a vertebra.

infraster·nal (L. *infra*, under; G. *sternon*, chest). Below the sternum.

infratem·poral (L. *infra*, below; *tempora*, the temples). Situate below the temporal bone.

infraton·sillar (L. *infra*, below; *tonsilla*). Below the tonsil.

infratroch·lear (L. *infra*, under; G. *trokhilia*, hoisting tackle). Subtrochlear, *q.v.*

infratur·binal (L. *infra*, below; *turbo*, a whirl). The inferior turbinal bone in the nose.

infra-umbili·cal (L. *infra*, below; *umbilicus*, navel). Below the navel or umbilicus.

infravagi·nal (L. *infra*, below; *vagina*, a sheath). Situated below the vaginal vault.

infundi·bular (L. *infundibulum*, a funnel). 1. Relating to the infundibulum. 2. Funnel-shaped.

infundi·buliform (L. *infundibulum*, funnel; *forma*, shape). Funnel-shaped.

infundi·bulin (L. *infundibulum*, funnel). Extract of the posterior lobe of the pituitary body.

infundi·bulum (L.). 1. A funnel-shaped passage or part, e.g., ethmoidal i., the tube passing from the ethmoidal cells to the middle of the nose. 2. The stalk of the pituitary gland.

infused (L. *infundere*, to pour into). 1. Extracted by infusion (1). 2. Injected.

infū·sion (L. *infusio*, a pouring in). 1. The process of extracting the active principles of a vegetable substance by water that has been heated to boiling point. 2. The product resulting from this process; syn. infusum, *q.v.* 3. The slow injection of a liquid into a vein or into subcutaneous tissue.

Infusor·ia (L.). A class of Protozoa, so called because first observed in organic infusions.

infū·sum (L. *infundere*, to pour into). An aqueous extract of the active principles of a vegetable substance obtained by the process of infusion (1).

ingě·sta (L. *ingerere*, to carry into). Food substances introduced into the body.

ingě·stion (L. *ingerere*, to carry into). The act of taking food or other substances, in solid or liquid form, into the body.

Ingrassia, process of (Ingrassia, G. F., Italian anatomist, 1510–80). The orbitosphenoid element of the sphenoid bone.

ingravě·scent (L. *ingravescere*, to grow heavy). Growing more severe; increasing in weight.

ingrē·dient (L. *ingredi*, to enter). Any substance forming part of a compound.

in·guen (L.). The groin.

in·guinal (L. *inguen*, groin). Relating to the groin, e.g., i. hernia.

inhā·lant, inhā·lent (L. *inhalare*, to breathe upon). See inhalation (2).

inhalā·tion (L. *inhalare*, to breathe upon). 1. The breathing of air or other vapour into the lungs. 2. A medicinal substance to be employed by inhalation (1).

inhale. To breathe in.

inhā·ler. Instrument for administering inhalation.

inhě·rent (L. *inhaerere*, to stick). Native; innate.

inhě·ritance (L. *in*, into; *heres*, heir). 1. The act of inheriting. 2. What is inherited. I., dominant: a mode of transmission in which the hereditary character is transmitted directly from the affected person to some or all of his children, the affected children in turn transmitting it to the next generation. I., holandric: a mode of transmission in which a dominant gene is transmitted by the Y-chromosomes, *q.v.*, to all sons of the affected father. I., hologynic: a mode of transmission in which all females are affected and transmit the affection to all daughters but to none of their sons. I., recessive: a mode of i. in which the hereditary characters fail to become manifest in the presence of the factor for the corresponding dominant character. I., sex-linked: a mode of transmission in which the gene for the respective character is carried in the X-chromosomes, *q.v.*

inhě·rited. Derived from an ancestor.

inhi·bit (L. *inhibere*, to restrain). To restrain or suppress.

inhibi·tion (L. *inhibere*, to restrain). The act of restraining or suppressing; a restraint.

inhi·bitor (L. *inhibere*, to restrain). 1. An agent which suppresses or restrains action. 2. A nerve the function of which is to restrain.

inhi·bitory (L. *inhibere*, to restrain). 1. Restraining, suppressing. 2. Being capable of restraining.

i·niac. Relating to the inion.

i·niad (G. *inion*; L. *ad*, to). Towards the iniac aspect.

inience·phalus (G. *inion*; *egkephalos*, brain). Foetal monstrosity

iniody·mus (G. *inion*; *didumos*, twin). A foetal monstrosity with two heads joined at the occiput.

i·nion (G., occiput). The external protruberance of the occipital bone.

i·niops (G. *inion*, occiput; *ōps*, eye). A foetal monstrosity with parts below the umbilicus double, one thorax, one head with two faces, but the posterior face incomplete.

ini·tial (L. *initium*, a beginning). Beginning; early; primary.

inject (L. *injicere*, to throw into). To pour or force in, as to i. a fluid into a tissue, cavity or vessel.

injec·ted. 1. Filled by injection. 2. Congested.

injec·tion (L. *injicere*, to throw into). 1. The forcing of a liquid into a tissue, cavity or vessel of the body, e.g. hypodermic, intraperitoneal or intravenous injections. 2. The liquid injected.

in·jury (L. *injuria*, wrong). Damage or harm to the body.

inlet. 1. The inlet of the pelvis, the upper limit of the pelvic cavity. 2. The place at which air is admitted into a room for ventilation.

Inman's disease (Inman, T., English physician, 1820–76). Myalgia.

innate (L. *innatus*, inborn). Congenital.

innervā·tion (L. *in*, into; *nervus*, nerve). 1. The nerve-supply of a part. 2. Conduction of nervous energy.

innidā·tion (L. *in*, into; *nidus*, nest). Development of cells in a part to which they have been carried, e.g. by metastasis.

innocent (L. *innocens*, harmless). Not harmful.

innŏ·cuous (L. *innocuus*). Not hurtful.

innŏ·minate (L. *innominatus*, nameless). Without a name. I. artery: the largest branch of the aortic arch. I. bone: that which forms the anterior wall and the sides of the pelvic cavity. I. vein: one of the two veins which form at their junction the superior vena cava.

innŏ·xious (L. *innoxius*, harmless). Harmless; not dangerous to health.

inoblast (G. *iněs*, fibres; *blastos*, germ). Cell from which connective tissue is developed.

inoccipi·tia (L. *in*, not; *occiput*, from *caput*, head). Deficiency of the occipital lobe of the cerebrum.

inochondrō·ma (G. *iněs*, fibres; *khondros*, cartilage). Fibrochondroma.

inŏ·culable (L. *in*, into; *oculus*, eye). Capable of being inoculated.

inŏ·culate. The act of performing inoculation.

inoculā·tion (L. *in*, into; *oculus*, eye). 1. The introduction of micro-organisms, or of a vaccine or serum into living organisms. 2. The introduction of micro-organisms, etc., into a healthy individual to produce a very mild form of disease followed by immunity from this particular disease.

inŏ·perable (L. *in*, not; *opus*, work). That which cannot, or should not, be operated upon.

inopex·ia (G. *iněs*, fibres; *pēxis*, fixation). A tendency to spontaneous coagulation in the blood.

inorgan·ic (L. *in*, not; G. *organon*, instrument). 1. Not of organic origin. 2. Pertaining to chemical substances which do not contain carbon (carbonates and cyanides excepted).

inosclērō·sis (G. *iněs*, fibres; *sklēros*, hard). Sclerosis of fibrous tissue.

inos·culate (L. *in*, in; *osculum*, dim. of *os*, mouth). To anastomose.

inosculā·tion (L. *in*, in; *osculum*, dim. of *os*, mouth). The joining of blood vessels together.

i·nosine. Inosite.

i·nosinate. Any salt of inosinic acid.

inosin·ic acid. $C_{10}H_{13}O_8N_4$ found in muscle tissue. A constituent of nucleic acid.

ĭ·nosite, ĭ·nosit (G. *ĭnĕs*, fibres). Syn. inositol.

inosī·tis (G. *ĭnĕs*, fibres). Inflammation of muscle fibres.

inŏ·sitol (G. *ĭnĕs*, fibres). A cyclic hexahydric alcohol widely distributed in muscle and other animal tissues and in plants, esp. certain seeds. A member of the vitamin B complex and used in bacteriology as a fermentable carbohydrate. It cures mouse alopecia and may inhibit the growth of tumours.

inostĕātō·ma (G. *ĭnĕs*, fibres; *stear*, fat). A fibrous fatty tumour.

inosū·ria (G. *ĭnĕs*, fibres; *ouron*, urine). The excretion of inosite in the urine.

inotrop·ic (G. *ĭnĕs*, fibres; *trepein*, to turn). Pertaining to influences which modify the contractility of the heart muscle.

in·quest (L. *inquirere*, to seek). A judicial enquiry to establish the cause of death of one who has died by violence or in some unknown way.

inquisī·tion (L. *inquirere*, to seek). A systematic legal investigation, more especially one into the mental sanity or insanity of a person.

inructā·tion (L. *in*, into; *ructare*, to belch). The abnormal swallowing of air.

insalivā·tion (L. *in*, into; *saliva*, spittle). The mixture of food with saliva during mastication.

insalū·brious (L. *in*, not; *saluber*, healthful). Unhealthy.

insane (L. *insanus*, mad). Not of sound mind.

insă·nitary (L. *in*, not; *sanitas*, health). Not sanitary; not in a satisfactory condition for the maintenance of health.

insanitā·tion (L. *in*, not; *sanitas*, health). Absence of sanitary conditions.

insă·nity (L. *insania*, madness). Derangement of the mental faculties without loss of consciousness.

inscriptio tendinea (L.). Transverse fibrous septum in the rectus abdominis muscle.

insă·tiable (L. *insatiabilis*). Not capable of being satisfied.

insect (L. *insectum*). Any member of the class Insecta.
I. powder: any insecticidal powder.

Insecta (L.). A class of Arthropoda including the orders Hemiptera, Diptera and Siphonaptera. They are characterized by a division of the body into three parts: head, thorax and abdomen.

insec·ticide (L. *insectum*, an insect; *caedere*, to kill). A preparation for the destruction of insects.

inseminā·tion (L. *inseminare*, to implant). 1. The introduction of semen into the vagina. 2. Impregnation.

insenĕ·scence (L. *insenescere*, to grow old). The process of growing old.

insen·sible (L. *insensibilis*, unfeeling, unfelt). 1. Without the sense of feeling. 2. Not noticeable by sensual perception.

inser·tion (L. *inserere*, to implant). 1. The act of setting in or placing in. 2. That which is set or placed in. 3. The point of attachment, as of a muscle.

insi·dious (L. *insidiae*, ambush). Not manifest; hidden or stealthy.

in situ (L.). In a given or natural position.

insolā·tion (L. *in*, in; *sol*, sun). 1. Exposure to sunrays. 2. Sunstroke or heatstroke, *q.v.*

insŏ·luble (L. *in*, not; *solubilis*, soluble). Incapable of being dissolved.

insom·nia (L. *in*, not; *somnus*, sleep). Inability to fall asleep; want of sleep.

inspec·tion (L. *inspicere*, to look at). Visual examination of the body or of a part.

insper·sion (L. *inspergere*, to sprinkle on). The act of dusting with fine powder.

inspirā·tion (L. *inspirare*, to breathe into). The inhaling of air into the lungs; the drawing in of the breath.

inspirā·tor (L. *inspirare*, to breathe in). An inhaler.

inspi·ratory (L. *inspirare*, to breathe in or into). Pertaining to inspiration.

inspis·sated (L. *in*, into; *spissare*, to thicken). Thickened or rendered dry by inspissation.

inspissā·tion (L. *in*, into; *spissare*, to thicken). The process of rendering dry or thick by evaporation of easily vaporizable parts.

inspis·sator (L.). An instrumen t used for the thickening or drying of liquids by means of evaporation.

instep. The arch on the dorsal surface of the foot.

instillā·tion (L. *instillare*, to pour in by drops). The pouring in of a fluid, drop by drop.

in·stinct (L. *instinguere*, to incite). An alleged faculty of living organisms by which they are enabled to adapt themselves, independently of their experience, to a given stimulus.

instinc·tive. Prompted by instinct.

in·strument (L. *instrumentum*). A tool or implement used in the performance of mechanical or manipulative actions.

instrumen·tal (L. *instrumentum*). Relating to an instrument or performed by instruments.

insuffĭ·ciency (L. *in*, not; *sufficere*, to suffice). Failure of normal action or function, e.g. of circulation.

insufflā·tion (L. *in*, into; *sufflare*, to blow). The blowing of powder, air or a liquid into a cavity or tube.

in·sufflator (L. *in*, into; *sufflare*, to blow). An instrument used for insufflation.

in·sula (L.). 1. An island. 2. The island of Reil, a cerebral area situated in the depth of the Sylvian fissure. 3. Any one of the islands of Langerhans in the pancreas.

in·sular (L. *insula*, island). 1. Isolated. 2. Relating to the island of Reil. 3. Relating to the islands of Langerhans in the pancreas.

in·sulate (L. *insula*, island). 1. To isolate; to separate from surroundings. 2. To surround a substance conducting electricity or heat with a non-conducting substance.

insulā·tion (L. *insula*, island). 1. The state of being insulated. 2. The act of insulating.

in·sulātor (L. *insula*, island). A substance not conducting, or not easily conducting, electricity or heat.

insulin (L. *insula*, island). An extract of the islands of Langerhans of the pancreas using 60% acid alcohol, containing a hormone, a protein, which is essential for the normal control of carbohydrate metabolism; a deficiency of insulin causes diabetes mellitus. **Protamine zinc i.:** a preparation of i. with protamine and zinc which retards its absorption after injection, and enables it to be actively absorbed over a period of 24 hours or more. **Globin i.:** a preparation of i. combined with beef globin which prolongs its action up to 24 hours or more by being slowly absorbed. **I. reaction or shock:** a state of hyperinsulinism which may occur spontaneously or more commonly as a result of overdosage, causing a sudden reduction in the blood sugar with circulatory insufficiency. Intentionally produced hyperinsulinism is sometimes used in the treatment of schizophrenia.

insulinae·mia (*insulin*; G. *haima*, blood). The condition caused by the presence of insulin in the blood.

in·sulinoid (*insulin*; G. *eidos*, form). Resembling insulin.

insulinō·ma (L. *insula*, island). Adenoma of the islets of Langerhans.

insult (L. *insultare*, to spring upon). Trauma.

insusceptibĭ·lity (L. *in*, neg.; *suscipere*, to receive). Lack of susceptibility; e.g., immunity.

integrā·tion (L. *integratio*, a unifying). 1. The process of systematically arranging data into sets of higher order. 2. Co-ordination of neural function.

P

intĕ·grity (L. *integer*, unimpaired). Wholeness or soundness.

intĕ·gument (L. *integumentum*). A covering, especially the skin.

integument·ary (L. *integumentum*, a covering). Relating to the skin.

integumen·tum commu·ne (L.). The skin.

in·tellect (L. *intellectus*, understanding). The mind or the faculty of thinking.

intel·ligence (L. *intelligere*, to understand). The ability to respond successfully to a new situation. **I. quotient:** the ratio of the i. of an individual as determined by i. tests to the normal i. of his age. **I. test:** the estimation of the i. of an individual by his response to a series of problems.

intem·perance (L. *in*, not; *temperare*, to regulate). Lack of moderation, e.g., with regard to alcohol, or to eating or drinking in general.

intensi·meter (L. *intensus*, tight; G. *metron*, measure). An instrument used to measure the intensity of X-rays.

inten·sity (L. *intensus*, tight). 1. The quantitative degree attributed to a phenomenon. 2. The quantity of energy per unit of space.

inten·sive (L. *intensus*, tight). Increasing in force or intensity.

inten·tion (L. *intensus*, tight). Purpose. See also under healing. **I. tremor:** a tremor induced by attempts at voluntary motion.

interacces·sory (L. *inter*, between; *accessio*, addition). Situated between the accessory processes of the lumbar vertebrae.

interaci·nar, interaci·nous (L. *inter*, between; *acinus*, berry). Situated between acini.

interal·veolar (L. *inter*, between; *alveolus*, stomach). Between alveoli.

in·terartí·cular (L. *inter*, between; *articulus*, joint). Situated between joints.

in·terarȳtēn·oid (L. *inter*, between; G. *arutaina*, a ladle; *eidos*, form). Between the two arytenoid cartilages.

in·teraurí·cular (L. *inter*, between; *auricula*, ear-lobe). Between the auricles.

in·terbrain. The thalamencephalon. The posterior part of the anterior vesicle of the brain.

intercã·dence (L. *inter*, between; *cadere*, to fall). An irregular pulse, in which an extra beat is interposed between two pulsations.

inter·calary (L. *intercalare*, to insert). Placed between.

intercanali·cular (L. *inter*, between; *canaliculus*, a small channel). Between canaliculi.

intercapil·lary (L. *inter*, between; *capillus*, hair). Between capillaries.

intercar·pal (L. *inter*, between; *carpus*). Between the carpal bones.

intercel·lular (L. *inter*, between; *cellula*, a small storeroom). Situated between cells.

intercen·tral (L. *inter*, between; *centrum*). Between nerve centres.

intercĕ·rebral (L. *inter*, between; *cerebrum*). Between the two cerebral hemispheres.

interchon·dral (L. *inter*, between; G. *khondros*, cartilage). Between cartilages.

interclavi·cular (L. *inter*, between; *clavicula*, collarbone). Between the clavicles.

interclin·oid (L. *inter*, between; G. *klinē*, bed; *eidos*, form). Between the clinoid processes of the sphenoid bone.

in·tercolum·nar (L. *inter*, between; *columna*). Between columns or pillars. **I. fascia:** the cremasteric fascia.

in·tercon·dylar, in·tercon·dyloid (L. *inter*, between; G. *kondulos*, knuckle). Between the condyles.

intercos·tal (L. *inter*, between; *costa*, rib). Between the ribs.

intercos·tohū·meral (L. *inter*, between; *costa*, rib; *humerus*, shoulder). Between the arm and the ribs.

in·tercourse (L. *intercursus*). Communication. **I., sexual:** coitus.

intercrā·nial (L. *inter*, between; G. *kranion*, skull). Pertaining to the inner portion of the skull.

intercri·cothyrŏ·tomy (L. *inter*, between; G. *krikos*, a ring; *thureos*, a shield; *tome*, section). Laryngotomy by transverse section of the cricothyroid membrane.

intercrū·ral (L. *inter*, between; *crus*, leg). Between the legs.

intercur·rent (L. *inter*, between; *currere*, to run). Occurring between. **I. disease:** a disease occurring in a person already suffering from another disease.

interden·tal (L. *inter*, between; *dens*, tooth). Between the teeth or between two adjacent teeth.

interdic·tion (L. *interdictio*, a prohibiting). A legal process depriving an insane person, or one suspected of insanity, of the control of his own affairs or those of others.

interdí·gital (L. *inter*, between; *digitus*, finger). Between the fingers.

in·terdigitā·tion (L. *inter*, between; *digitus*, finger). The interlocking of two similar parts, e.g. of the fingers of the two hands.

in·terface (L. *inter*, between; *faciēs*, face). Boundary, usually between two liquids which will not mix.

interfā·cial (L. *inter*, between; *faciēs*, face). Relating to an interface.

interfascí·cular (L. *inter*, between; *fasciculus*, bundle). Situated between fasciculi.

interfĕ·moral (L. *inter*, between; *femur*, thigh). Situated between the thighs.

interfe·rence (L. *inter*, between; *ferire*, to strike). 1. Prevention. 2. In optics and acoustics, the phenomenon that two waves which meet while being in different phases annul each other.

interfíbril·lar (L. *inter*, between; *fibra*, a fibre). Situated between the fibrils of tissues.

interfron·tal (L. *inter*, between; *frons*, forehead). Between the two halves of the frontal bone. **I. suture:** the metopic suture.

in·terganglĭŏ·nic (L. *inter*, between; G. *gagglion*, a tumour under the skin). Between ganglia; connecting ganglia.

interglū·teal (L. *inter*, between; G. *gloutos*, buttock). Situated between the buttocks.

intergō·nial (L. *inter*, between; G. *gonia*, angle). Between the angles of the lower jaw.

interkinē·sis (L. *inter*, between; G. *kinein*, to move). 1. The resting stage of a cell-nucleus. 2. The stage between the first and second mitotic division.

interlŏ·bar (L. *inter*, between; G. *lobos*, lobe). Situated between the lobes. **I. pleurisy:** inflammation of the pleura between two adjacent pulmonary lobes.

interlŏ·bular (L. *inter*, between; L.L. *lobulus*, lobe). Between lobules.

interlocking of twins. Twins which become interlocked during delivery.

intermam·mary (L. *inter*, between; *mamma*, breast). Between the breasts.

intermar·ginal (L. *inter*, between; *margo*, edge). Lying between two margins.

intermarriage. 1. Marriage between persons of different races. 2. Marriage between persons related by consanguinity.

intermaxil·la (L. *inter*, between; *maxilla*). The intermaxillary bone.

intermaxil·lary (L. *inter*, between; *maxilla*, jaw). Between the maxillary bones.

intermĕ·diate (L. *inter*, between; *medius*, middle). Situated between; intervening.

intermen·strual (L. *inter*, between; *mensis*, month). Occurring between two menstrual periods.

intermen·strūŭm (L. *inter*, between; *mensis*, mouth). The period between two menstrual periods.

inter·ment (L. *in*, into; *terra*, earth). Burial of a corpse.

intermis·sion (L. *intermittere*, to let pass). An interval, e.g. between the paroxysms of a fever or the beats of a pulse.

intermit·tent (L. *intermittere*, to let pass). Characterized by intervals, e.g., i. fever.

intermus·cular (L. *inter*, between; *musculus*, muscle). Between muscles.

internal capsule. A band of white nerve fibres between the optic thalamus and the caudate and lenticular nuclei.

inter·nus (L.). 1. Internal. 2. The rectus internus muscle of the eye.

in·terocep·tor (L. *inter*, between; *capere*, to take). A receptor which is stimulated by mechanical impulses from entodermal organs, especially from viscera.

interor·bital (L. *inter*, between; *orbita*). Situated between the orbits.

interos·seous (L. *inter*, between; *os*, bone). Situated between two bones.

interosseus muscles. Small muscles situated in the foot and hand.

in·terpari·etal (L. *inter*, between; *paries*, wall). Between the parietal bones, e.g., i. suture; i. fissure.

interpedun·cular (L. *inter*, between; *pedunculus*, a little foot). Situated between the cerebral or cerebellar peduncles of the brain **I. space:** the posterior perforated space in the floor of the third ventricle of the brain.

interpō·lar (L. *inter*, between; G. *pŏlos*, axis). Between two poles.

interpolā·tion (L. *interpolare*, to interrupt). The surgical removal of tissue to a new situation.

in·terprotomĕ·tamere (L. *inter*, between; G. *prōtŏs*, first; *mĕta*, among; *mĕros*, part). In an embryo, that part situated between the primary segments.

interpū·bic (L. *inter*, between; *pubes*, adult). Situated between the pubic bones.

interrē·nal (L. *inter*, between; *rēn*, kidney). Between the kidneys.

interrup·ted (L. *interrumpere*, to break up). Broken; irregular; not continuous.

interrup·ter (L. *interrumpere*, to break up). That which interrupts; applied to an apparatus for interrupting an electric current.

interscă·pular (L. *inter*, between; *scapulae*, shoulder-blades). Between the shoulder-blades.

in·terspace (L. *inter*, between; *spatium*, space). A space between two parts, e.g. the space between two adjacent ribs.

interspi·nal (L. *inter*, between; *spina*, spine). Between the vertebral spines.

inter·stices (L. *interstitium*, a space between). Small intervals or spaces in a structure.

interstĭ·tial (L. *interstitium*, a space between). 1. Situated in the interspaces of a part. 2. Relating to i. tissue, *q.v.* **I. hernia:** a congenital oblique hernia in which the sac has an extra diverticulum. **I. keratitis:** keratitis of the middle and posterior layers of the cornea, usually occurring in both eyes and mostly caused by congenital syphilis. **I. pregnancy:** tubo-uterine pregnancy, a form of extra-uterine pregnancy. **I. tissue:** the connective tissue situated in the interspaces of the parenchymatous tissue of an organ.

intersys·tolĕ (L. *inter*, between; G. *sustolē*, contraction). The interval between the end of the auricular and the beginning of the ventricular systole.

intertră·gicus muscle (L. *inter*, between; *tragikos*, goat like). A small muscle of the external ear.

intertransversā·lis muscle (L. *inter*, between; *transversus*, turned across). A small muscle between the transverse processes of the vertebrae.

in·tertransverse (L. *inter*, between ; *transversus*, turned across). Connecting the transverse processes of adjacent vertebrae.

intertri·ginous (L. *inter*, between; *terere*, to rub). Relating to intertrigo.

intertri·go (L. *inter*, between; *terere*, to rub). An erythematous state of the skin produced by friction of opposed surfaces.

in·tertrochanter·ic (L. *inter*, between; G. *trokhantēr*, a runner). Between the trochanters.

in·terval (L. *intervallum*, interval). A space either of distance or of time; a gap.

interventri·cular (L. *inter*, between; *ventriculum*, dim. of *venter*, belly or ventricle). Situated between the ventricles.

interver·tebral (L. *inter*, between; *vertebra*, vertebra). Situated between the vertebrae. **I. discus:** the cartilaginous discs between adjacent vertebrae.

intestī·nal (L. *intestinum*, intestine). Relating to the intestine.

intes·tine (L. *intestinum*, intestine). The part of the digestive tract extending from the duodenum to the anus. **I., large:** that part of the i. consisting of caecum, colon, sigmoid and rectum. It is about five feet long. **I., small:** that part of the i. consisting of duodenum, jejunum and ileum, and is approximately twenty feet in length.

intesti·num (L.). The intestine. **I. crassum:** the large intestine. **I. tenue:** the small intestine.

in·tima (L. *intimus*, innermost). The innermost of the three coats of a blood-vessel.

in·timal. Relating to the intima.

intimī·tis. Inflammation of an intima.

intŏ·lerance (L. *in*, not; *tolerare*, to bear). Inability to tolerate, e.g. a particular drug.

intox·icant (L. *in*, into; G. *toxikon*, poison). Capable of producing intoxication.

intoxicā·tion. Poisoning; inebriation.

intra-abdŏ·minal (L. *intra*, within; *abdomen*, abdomen). Within the abdominal cavity.

intra-artē·rial (L. *intra*, within; G. *arteria*). Within an artery.

intra-arti·cular (L. *intra*, within; *articulus*, joint). Within a joint.

intracap·sular (L. *intra*, within; *capsula*, small box). Within the capsular ligament of a joint, e.g., i. fracture.

intracar·diac (L. *intra*, within; G. *kardia*, heart). Within the heart.

in·tracartilă·ginous (L. *intra*, within; *cartilago*, cartilage). Endochondral, *q.v.*

intracel·lular (L. *intra*, within; *cellula*, small storeroom). Within a cell.

intracrā·nial (L. *intra*, within; G. *kranion*, skull). Within the skull.

in·trad (Early L.). Within.

intrader·mal (L. *intra*, within; G. *derma*, skin). Within the skin.

intraduodē·nal (L. *intra*, within; *duodenum*). Within the duodenum.

intradū·ral (L. *intra*, within; *dura*, hard). Inside the dura mater.

intrafoetā·tion (L. *intra*, within; *foetus*). The formation of a foetus within another foetus.

intragas·tric (L. *intra*, within; G. *gastēr*, belly). Within the stomach.

intragland·ular (L. *intra*, within; *glandula*, dim. of *glans*). Within a gland.

intraglŏ·bular (L. *intra*, within; *globus*). Within a blood corpuscle.

intrahepat·ic (L. *intra*, within; G. *hepar*, liver). Within the liver.

intra-intesti·nal (L. *intra*, within; *intestinum*, intestine). Within the gut.

intralamel·lar (L. *intra*, within; *lamella*, a thin plate). Within the lamellae.

intralaryn·ge͞al (L. *intra*, within; G. *larugx*, larynx). Within the larynx.

in·traligamen·tous (L. *intra*, within; *ligamentum*, bandage). Situated within, or in the folds of, a ligament.

intralŏ·bular (L. *intra*, within; L.L. *lobulus*, small lobe). Within a lobule.

intramam·mary (L. *intra*, within; *mamma*, breast). Within the breast.

intramar·ginal (L. *intra*, within; *margo*, edge). Within margins.

intramedul·lary (L. *intra*, within; *medulla*, marrow). Within the medulla.

intramem·branous (L. *intra*, within; *membrana*, membrane). Within a membrane.

intramu͞·ral (L. *intra*, within; *murus*, wall). Within the substance of the walls of an organ; e.g., i. fibroid of the uterus.

intramus·cular (L. *intra*, within; *musculus*, muscle). Within the substance of a muscle.

intrana͞·sal (L. *intra*, within; *nasus*, nose). Within the nasal cavity.

intrane͞u·ral (L. *intra*, within; G. *neuron*, nerve). Within a nerve.

intranu͞·clear (L. *intra*, within; *nucleus*, kernel). Within a nucleus.

intra-ŏ·cular (L. *intra*, within; *oculus*, eye). Within the globe of the eye.

intra-oral (L. *intra*, within; *ōs*, mouth). Situated within the mouth.

intra-or·bital (L. *intra*, within; *orbita*). Within the orbit.

intra͞-ŏs·tĕăl (L. *intra*, within; *os*, bone). Within bone.

in·traparenchy̆·matous (L. *intra*, within; G. *para*, beside; *egkheein*, to pour in). Situated within the parenchyma, between the elements of a tissue.

intraparī·etal (L. *intra*, within; *paries*, wall). Intramural, *q.v.*

intrapel·vic (L. *intra*, within; *pelvis*, basin). Within the pelvis.

in·traperi·cardial (L. *intra*, within; G. *peri*, around; *kardia*, heart). Within the pericardium.

in·traperitone͞·al (L. *intra*, within; G. *peri*, around; *teinein*, to stretch). Within the peritoneal cavity.

intraple͞u·ral (L. *intra*, within; G. *pleura*, rib). Within the pleural cavity.

in·trathŏra͞·cic (L. *intra*, within; G. *thōrax*, chest). Within the thoracic cavity.

intratra͞·cheal (L. *intra*, within; G. *trakhus*, rough). 1. Within the trachea. 2. Through the trachea. **I. insufflation:** insufflation through a tube introduced into the trachea.

intratympăn·ic (L. *intra*, within; G. *tumpanon*, a drum). Within the tympanic cavity.

intra-ure͞·thral (L. *intra*, within; G. *ourethra*, the urethra). Situated within the urethra.

intra-u͞·terine (L. *intra*, within; *uterus*, womb). Within the uterus.

intravagī·nal (L. *intra*, within; *vagina*, sheath). Within the vagina.

intravasā·tion (L. *intra*, within; *vas*, vessel). The entry of pus or other foreign matter into a blood-vessel.

intravas·cular (L. *intra*, within; *vasculum*, a small vessel). Within a blood-vessel.

intrave͞·nous (L. *intra*, within; *vena*, vein). Within or into a vein. **I. injection:** the injection of a fluid into a vein.

intraventrī·cular (L. *intra*, within; *ventriculus*, ventricle). Within a ventricle.

intravĕsī·cal (L. *intra*, within; *vēsīca*, bladder). Within the bladder.

intra vi·tam (L. *intra*, within; *vita*, life). Occurring during life.

intravit·reous (L. *intra*, within; *vitrum*, glass). Within the vitreous humour.

intrin·sic (L. *intrinsecus*, inward). 1. Situated within. 2. Characterizing the value of an object irrespective of its relations to other objects. **I. factor:** (Castle), a substance of probably enzymic character contained in normal gastric juice; absent in pernicious anaemia.

introdū·cer (L. *introducere*, to lead in). An instrument used for inserting anything into a cavity.

introgas·tric (L. *intro*, within; G. *gastēr*, stomach). Put into the stomach.

intrō·itus (L., entry). An entrance; an inlet.

intromis·sion (L. *intromittere*, to send in). The introduction of one part into another; e.g. of the penis into the vagina.

introspec·tion (L. *introspicere*, to look into). Contemplation of an experience or an idea.

introver·sion (L. *intro*, within; *vertere*, to turn). 1. A turning within; invagination. 2. A mental attitude in which the attention of the individual is directed to himself rather than to the external world.

in·trovert (L. *intro*, within; *vertere*, to turn). An introspective person.

intubā·tion (L. *in*, into; *tubus*, tube). 1. The insertion of a tube into a part as, e.g., into the larynx to make possible the entry of air into the lungs.

intumes·cence (L. *intumescere*, to swell). A swelling or an increase in the volume of an organ.

intumescen·tia (L.). A swelling. **I. cervicalis:** the normal enlargement of the cervical part of the spinal cord.

in·tussuscep·tion (L. *intus*, within; *suscipere*, to receive). Invagination or prolapse of one part of the intestine into an immediately adjoining part of it, causing intestinal obstruction and clinically characterized by sudden onset of abdominal pain or tenesmus, vomiting, passage of frequent bloody and mucous stools, abdominal tenderness and the presence of a sausage-shaped, curved abdominal tumour.

in·tussuscep·tum (L. *intus*, within; *suscipere*, to receive). The invaginated portion of the intestine in intussusception.

in·tussuscip·iens (L. *intus*, within; *suscipere*, to receive). The invaginating part of the intestine in intussusception.

inunc·tion (L. *inunguere*, to anoint). The rubbing of an ointment into the skin.

in utero (L.). Within the uterus.

invă·ginated (L. *in*, into; *vagina*, sheath). Ensheathed.

invaginā·tion (L. *in*, into; *vagina*, sheath). 1. The act of becoming ensheathed. 2. The condition of being ensheathed.

in·valid (L. *invalidus*, weak). 1. Not well. 2. One who is not well or is infirm.

in·validism. The condition of being an invalid.

invā·sion (L. *invadere*, to enter into). The onset, particularly of disease.

inver·sion (L. *invertere*, to turn upside down). 1. The act of turning inward, or upside down, or in any direction contrary to the existing one. 2. The turning of a dextro-rotatory into a laevo-rotatory compound, or *vice versa*. 3. The turning of an optically active disaccharide into two optically inactive monosaccharides. **Sexual i.:** sexual interest and attraction towards one of the same sex; homosexuality.

in·vert (L. *invertere*, to turn upside down). A person addicted to homosexuality. **I. sugar:** a mixture of equal parts of glucose and laevulose.

inver·tase. A ferment present in yeast and pancreatic juice, converting cane sugar into invert sugar. Also called invertin.

Invertebra·ta (L. *in*, not; *vertebra*, vertebra). Animals without a spinal column.

inver·tebrate (L. *in*, not; *vertebra*, from *vertere*, to turn). 1. Without a spinal column. 2. Any animal not possessing vertebrae.

inver·tin. Invertase, *q.v.*

invest·ing (L. *investire*, to surround). Ensheathing; surrounding.

invĕ·terate (L. *inveterare*, to render old). Long-established; chronic; obstinate.

in vitro (L. in glass). Applied to phenomena observed in test-tubes, in contradistinction to those observed *in vivo, q.v.*

in vivo (L.). Within the living body, as distinguished from phenomena observed *in vitro, q.v.*

involū·crum (L. *involucrum*, a wrapping). A sheath; the layer of bone enveloping a sequestrum, *q.v.*

invŏ·luntary (L. *in*, not; *voluntarius*, from *volo*, I wish). Not voluntary; independent of the will. **I. muscles**: those which are not governed by the will, i.e. are innervated by the autonomous nervous system.

involū·tion (L. *involvere*, to roll up). 1. A turning inward. 2. The retrogressive change of the organism in old age, or of an organ, e.g. of the uterus during puerperium or after the menopause. **I. melancholia**: melancholia beginning in advanced age.

ī·odal. The iodine analogue of chloral.

ī·odate (G. *iōdēs*, rust-coloured). Any salt of iodic acid.

iŏ·dic acid. HIO_3. A colourless, crystalline, hygroscopic acid—a strong oxidising agent.

ī·odide (G. *iōdēs*, rust-coloured). A compound of iodine with another element or radical.

ī·odine (G. *iōdēs*, rust-coloured). A non-metallic element belonging to the halogen group. It volatilizes at a low temperature, giving off a purple vapour. Symbol I.

ïodi·nophil (G. *iōdēs*, rust-coloured; *philein*, to love). Any body staining readily with iodine.

ī·odism (G. *iōdēs*, rust-coloured). Chronic iodine poisoning, characterized by headache, coryza and skin eruptions, especially acne. Enlargement of the salivary glands with increased salivation is also seen.

ī·odized. Containing iodine.

ī·ododer·ma (G. *iōdēs*, rust-coloured; *derma*, skin). Any skin disease or disorder due to iodism.

io·doform. CHI_3. Yellow crystalline substance having a strong penetrating smell. It contains about 96·7 per cent of iodine by weight and is used as an antiseptic.

iodogal·licin. Bismuth oxyiodo-methyl gallol. C_6H_2(OH)$_3$COOBi·OH·I, dark grey powder containing iodine and bismuth. It is used as an antiseptic.

iodoglŏ·bulin. One of the active principles of the thyroid gland.

ī·odophil (G. *iōdēs*, rust-coloured; *philein*, to love). Staining readily with iodine.

ī·odophil·ia (G. *iōdēs*, rust-coloured; *philein*, to love). Readiness to stain with iodine.

iodophthā·lein. Sodium salt of tetraiodophenolphthalein. Used in radiography of the biliary tract. $C_2H_8O_4I_4Na_23H_2O$.

iodosobenzoic acid. $C_6H_4(IO)COOH$. A compound resembling iodoform.

iodothȳ·rin. The iodine compound normally found in the body. Syn. thyrein.

iodox·yl. Synthetic iodine containing compound $C_8H_3O_5NI_2Na_2$. Used in radiography of the biliary tract.

iō·dum (L.). Iodine.

ī·on (G., going). An electricity charged atom, radical or molecule.

iŏn·ic. Relating to ions.

ionizā·tion (G. *iōn*, going). Production of ions; electrolytic dissociation.

ionogen·ic (G. *iōn*, going; *gennan*, to produce). Ion-forming.

ionŏ·meter (G. *iōn*, going; *metron*, measure). An instrument used in estimating the amount of X-rays.

ī·onone (G. *ion*, violet). A hydro-aromatic ketone smelling of violets.

i·onothĕ·rapy (G. *iōn*, going; *therapeio*, treatment). The treatment of disease by means of violet rays.

iophŏ·bia (G. *iŏs*, poison; *phobos*, fear). An abnormal fear of poisons.

iō·tacism (G. *iōta*, the letter I). Inability to pronounce distinctly the 'l' sound.

ipecacuā·nha. The dried root and rhizome of *Cephaēlis Ipecacuanha* (Rubiaceae) from Brazil containing at least 2 per cent total alkaloids. It is employed in small doses as an expectorant in bronchitis, but large doses produce vomiting and diarrhoea.

ipsā·tion (L. *ipse*, he himself). Masturbation.

ipsilā·teral (L. *ipse*, himself; *latus*, side). Situated on the same side; applied, e.g. to paralytic signs present on the same side of the body as the cerebral lesion by which they are caused.

I.Q. Intelligence quotient, *q.v.*

irascibi·lity (L. *irascibilis*, quick tempered). Abnormal irritability of temperament.

i·ridadenō·sis (G. *iris*; *adēn*, gland). Glandular affection of the iris.

ī·ridal. Relating to the iris.

i·ridauxē·sis (G. *iris*; *auxēsis*, increase). Tumefaction of the iris.

iridec·tome (G. *iris*; *tomē*, a cutting). A surgical instrument employed in the operation of iridectomy.

iridec·tomy (G. *iris*; *ektomē*, excision). The excision of a part of the iris.

iridectrŏ·pium (G. *iris*; *ektrŏpē*, a turning off). Eversion of part of the iris.

iridaē·mia (G. *iris*; *haima*, blood). Iridal haemorrhage.

i·ridenclei·sis (G. *iris*; *egkleinin*, to shut in). Incarceration of the iris in a wound.

i·riderē·mia (G. *iris*; *eremia*, absence). Total or partial absence of the iris.

iri·dēsis. Iridodesis, *q.v.*

iri·dic (G. *iris*). Relating to the iris.

iri·dium. A hard white metal of the platinum group. Symbol Ir.

i·rido-avul·sion (G. *iris*; L. *a*, from; *vellere*, to tear). Avulsion of the iris.

i·ridocapsuli·tis (G. *iris*; L. *capsula*, little box). Inflammation of the iris and the capsule of the lens of the eye.

i·ridocele (G. *iris*; *kēlē*, hernia). Protrusion of part of the iris through a corneal wound.

iridochoroidi·tis (G. *iris*; *khorion*, intestinal membrane or afterbirth; *eidos*, form). Inflammation of both the iris and choroid of the eye.

iridocycli·tis (G. *iris*; *kuklos*, circle). Inflammation of the iris and the ciliary body.

iridŏ·dēsis (G. *iris*; *dēsis*, a binding). The operation of drawing a portion of the iris through an incision in the cornea and fastening the iris in this position.

iridodiă·lysis (G. *iris*; *dialusis*, dissolution). The separation of the ciliary border of the iris from its attachments.

iridodonē·sis (G. *iris*; *doneein*, to shake). Tremulousness of the iris on rapid ocular movements; present when the ciliary border of the iris is not properly supported by the lens.

iridoplē·gia (G. *iris*; *plēgē*, stroke). Paralysis of the constrictor or dilator muscle of the iris.

iridorhex·is (G. *iris*; *rhēxis*, rupture). Rupture of the iris.

iridosclerŏ·tomy (G. *iris*; *skleros*, hard; *tomē*, section). Puncture of the sclera with division of the iris.

iri·doscope (G. *iris*; *skopein*, to view). An instrument for examining the interior of the eye.

iridosterḗ·sis (G. *iris*; *stĕrēsis*, deprivation). Absence of the iris either partial or complete.

iridŏ·tasis (G. *iris*; *tăsis*, a stretching). Stretching the iris in cases of glaucoma.

iridŏ·tomy (G. *iris*; *tomē*, section). Section of the iris without excision of any portion.

ī·ris (G., rainbow). The coloured circular membrane situated between the cornea and the lens, the central perforation of which represents the pupil. **I.frill**: see collarette.

Irish moss. The dried seaweed *Chondrus crispus* (Gigantinaceae) used in the form of a decoction as an emulsifying agent.

irit·ic. Relating to the iris.

irī·tis (G. *iris*). Inflammation of the iris.

iron. Ferrum. Symbol Fe. An element essential to life.

irrā·diating (L. *in*, into; *radiare*, spread in a circle). Radiating; e.g., pain extending from a localized area to its periphery.

irradiā·tion (L. *in*, into; *radius*, ray). 1. The apparent enlargement of an object owing to differences in illumination of the field of vision. 2. Subjection to the action of rays. 3. Diffusion of a nerve impulse.

irredu·cible (L. *in*, not; *reducere*, to bring back). Not reducible; not capable of being replaced in a normal position.

irrĕ·gular (L. *in*. not; *regula*, rule). Not regular; not rhythmic; not occurring at proper intervals.

irrĕ·spirable (L. *in*, not; *respirare*, to breathe). Not suitable for respiration.

irrigā·tion (L. *irrigare*, to convey water into). The act of washing out by a stream of water; e.g., i. of the bladder.

irritabi·lity (L. *irritare*, to excite). 1. The faculty of responding to stimuli. 2. The functional disturbance of an organ characterized by its reacting to a stimulus in an excessive degree.

ir·ritable (L. *irritare*, to excite). 1. Responding to stimuli. 2. Excitable without an adequate stimulus. **I. bladder:** a condition characterized by frequent micturition in the absence of any organic disease.

ir·ritant (L. *irritare*, to excite). 1. Causing irritation. 2. An agent causing irritation.

irritā·tion (L. *irritare*, to excite). 1. The normal response of a nerve or muscle to a stimulus. 2. The act of stimulation. 3. A condition of undue excitation.

ir·ritative (L. *irritare*, to excite). 1. Having the faculty of irritability. 2. Irritant.

Isambert's disease (Isambert, E., French physician, 1828–76). Tuberculous disease of the oral cavity.

ī·satin. Yellowish-red crystals derived from oxidising indigo with chromic or nitric acid. Formula $C_8H_5NO_2$.

ischae·mia (G. *iskhein*, to hold back; *haima*, blood). Local anaemia.

ischae·mic. Relating to ischaemia.

ischē·sis (G. *iskhein*, to hold back). Retention of a secretion or discharge.

is·chial (G. *iskhion*, hip). Relating to the ischium.

ischidrō·sis (G. *iskhein*, to hold back; *hidrōs*, sweat). Anhidrosis, *q.v.*

is·chiocap·sular (G. *iskhion*, hip; L. *capsula*, little box). Part of the capsular ligament of the hip joint.

is·chiocavernō·sus (G. *iskhein*, to hold back; L. *caverna*, cave). The erector penis muscle or the erector clitoridis muscle.

is·chiocele (G. *iskhion*, hip; *kēlē*, hernia). Sciatic hernia.

is·chiococcȳ·geal (G. *iskhion*, hip; *kokkux*, cuckoo). Pertaining to the ischium and the coccyx.

is·chiococcȳ·geus (G. *iskhion*, hip; *kokkux*, cuckoo). The coccygeus muscle.

is·chiodi·dymus (G. *iskhion*, hip; *didumos*, twin). A double monster joined at the hips.

is·chiofĕ·moral (G. *iskhion*, hip; L. *femur*, thigh). 1. Relating conjointly to the ischium and the femur. 2. The adductor magnus muscle.

ischiŏ·pagus (G. *iskhion*, hip; *pagos*, fixation). A monomphalic monster united by the coccyges and sacra.

is·chiopu·bic (G. *iskhion*, hip; L. *pubes*, adult). Relating conjointly to the ischium and the pubes.

is·chiopubiŏ·tomy (G. *iskhion*, hip; L. *pubes*, adult; *tomē*, section). Division of the ischial and pubic rami in obstructed labour.

is·chiorec·tal (G. *iskhion*, hip; L. *rectus*, straight). Pertaining conjointly to the ischium and rectum; pertaining to the space between the levator ani and obturator internus muscles.

is·chium (G. *iskhion*, hip). The inferior part of the innominate bone; the bone upon which the body rests in sitting.

ischuret·ic (G. *iskhein*, to hold back; *ouron*, urine). Relating to ischuria.

ischū·ria (G. *iskhein*, to hold back; *ouron*, urine). Retention of urine. **I. paradoxa:** see incontinence, paradoxical.

island. Any detached part of an organ. **I. of Langerhans:** in the pancreas. **I. of Reil:** the insula, small convolutions situated at the bottom of the fissure of Sylvius in the brain.

Isle of Man incision. A three-legged incision.

Isle of Wight disease. Found in honey bees and caused by a mite, acarapis woodi, which enters the trachea and causes paralysis of the muscles of flight.

islet. See island etc.

ī·so-agglutinā·tion (G. *isos*, equal; L. *ad*, to; *glutinare*, to glue). The agglutinating action of the blood serum of an animal upon the red corpuscles of any other individual of the same species.

ī·so-agglū·tinin (G. *isos*, equal; L. *ad*, to; *glutinare*, to glue). An agglutinin in the blood serum of an animal acting on the red corpuscles of any other individual of the same species.

ī·sochromat·ic (G. *isos*, equal; *khrōma*, colour). Having the same colour throughout.

ī·sochron (G. *isos*, equal; *khronos*, time). Having equal chronaxie, *q.v.*

isŏ·chronism (G. *isos*, equal; *khronos*, time). 1. The quality of occurring simultaneously. 2. The quality of lasting for equal periods of time.

isŏ·chronous (G. *isos*, equal; *khronos*, time). 1. Simultaneous. 2. Having the same duration.

isocor·ia (G. *isos*, equal; *korē*, pupil of the eye). Equality in the size of the two pupils.

ī·socor·tex (G. *isos*, equal; L. *cortex*, rind). Type of cerebral cortex showing in its early foetal stages arrangement in six layers. See also allocortex.

isodynam·ic (G. *isos*, equal; *dunamis*, power). Having or generating equal amounts of force or energy.

iso-electric point (G. *isos*, equal; *ēlektron*, amber). The *p*H value at which a substance in solution has no resultant electric charge. Used to characterise proteins and amino-acids. The solubility of a protein is negligible at the iso-electric point.

iso·electrical (G. *isos*, equal; *ēlektron*, amber). Being in the same electrical condition.

isŏ·gamy (G. *isos*, equal; *gamos*, marriage). 1. The production of gametes of uniform size which cannot be distinguished as macrogametes and microgametes. 2. Conjugation of similar gametes.

ī·solate (L. *insula*, island). To separate; to place apart.

isolā·tion (L. *insula*, island). 1. The act or process of isolating. 2. The state of being isolated. 3. The separation of individuals with infectious diseases or during the incubation stage of such diseases from others of the community.

isolȳ·sin (G. *isos*, equal; *lusis*, a loosening). A cytolysin acting upon the red corpuscles of any other individual of the same animal species, except those of the animal producing it.

isol͞y·sis (G. *isos*, equal; *lusis*, a loosening). The haemolytic action of the blood-serum of an animal upon the red corpuscles of any other individual of the same species.

isolyt·ic. Relating to isolysis or to an isolysin.

i·somer (G. *isos*, equal; *meros*, part). A compound having the same percentage composition as another compound from which it differs in atomic arrangement. A pair of such compounds have different physical and chemical properties.

isome·ric. Pertaining to or having the qualities of an isomer.

isŏ·merism (G. *isos*, equal; *meros*, part). The quality of being isomeric.

isomet·ric (G. *isos*, equal; *metron*, measure). Of equal measure.

isometrō·pia (G. *isos*, equal; *metron*, measure; *ōps*, eye). Equality of kind or degree in the refraction of the two eyes.

isomor·phic (G. *isos*, equal; *morphē*, shape). 1. Having the same form. 2. Crystallizing in the same form while being of different composition.

isomor·phism (G. *isos*, equal; *morphē*, shape). 1. Equality in form. 2. The quality of being isomorphic (2).

isomor·phous. Isomorphic, *q.v.*

iso-nicotinic acid hydrazide. Chemotherapeutic substance specifically active against infections with mycobacterium tuberculosis. (Syn. isoniazid).

iso-nicotinyl hydrazine. Chemotherapeutic substance resembling iso-nicotinic acid hydrazide in composition and therapeutic activity.

isŏ·pathy (G. *isos*, equal; *pathos*, disease). The treatment of a disease by the administration of the causative agent or its products.

isophor·ia (G. *isos*, equal; *phoros*, bearing). The condition in which the eyes lie in the same horizontal plane.

isŏ·pia (G. *isos*, equal; *ōps*, eye). Equality of visual acuity in the two eyes.

i·soprene. A hemiterpene obtained by destructive distillation of rubber. C_5H_8.

isoprō·pyl alcohol. A secondary alcohol $(CH_3)_2$ CH.OH. Used as a solvent and preservative.

isop·ters (G. *isos*, equal; *optēr*, observer). The curves in the visual field drawn through points of equal visual acuity.

isosē·rum treatment (G. *isos*, equal; L. *serum*). The treatment of a case by the serum of another case having the same disease.

isosmot·ic (G. *isos*, equal; *ōsmŏs*, an impulse). Of equal osmotic pressure.

Isospor·a. A genus of coccidia, of which the non-pathogenic *I. hominis* is sometimes found in the intestinal tract in man.

i·sosthenū·ria (G. *isos*, equal; *sthěnos*, strength; *ouron*, urine). Excretion of urine of a molecular concentration approaching that of blood (spec. grav. 1008–1012). See also hyposthenuria.

isother·mal (G. *isos*, equal; *thermē*, heat). Of equal temperature. **I. lines:** lines drawn on a map through places having the same average temperatures for a given period of time.

isothīocȳ·anate. Any salt of isothiocyanic acid.

isothī·ocyă·nic acid. HNCS. An acid producing isothiocyanates.

isotō·nia (G. *isos*, equal; *tonos*, tone). 1. State of equal tonus. 2. Condition of a solution having an osmotic pressure equal to that of some other fluid with which it is compared.

isoton·ic (G. *isos*, equal; *tonos*, tone). 1. Of equal tonus. 2. Applied to a solution having an osmotic pressure equal to that of some other fluid with which it is compared.

isotonĭ·city (G. *isos*, equal; *tonos*, tone). 1. Isotonia, *q.v.* 2. Equality of osmotic pressure in different solutions.

i·sotope (G. *isos*, equal; *topos*, place). Any one of a number of elements differing in atomic weight but having the same atomic numbers. **Radioactive i.:** an isotope having radioactive properties. Syn. tracer element.

isotox·in (G. *isos*, equal; *toxikon*, poison). A toxin elaborated in the blood of an animal and toxic for animals of the same species.

isotrop·ic, isŏ·tropous (G. *isos*, equal; *tropē*, turn). 1. Having the same refracting power. 2. Having the same properties in every direction.

isŏ·tropy (G. *isos*, equal; *tropē*, turn). 1. The state of having equal or uniform properties throughout. 2. In embryology, having no predetermined axes, especially as applied to the ovum.

issue (Fr. *issue*, from L. *exire*, to go out). 1. Offspring. 2. A serous or purulent discharge.

i·sthmian. Relating to an isthmus.

i·sthmus (G. *isthmos*). The constricted part of an organ.

Itard's catheter (Itard, J. M. G., French otologist, 1774–1838). Eustachian catheter.

Itard-Cholewa sign (Itard, J. M. G., French otologist, 1774–1838; Cholewa, E. R., German physician, born 1845). In cases of otosclerosis the membrana tympani is anaesthetic.

itch. 1. An irritating sensation in the skin. 2. A name for various skin diseases characterized by itching, e.g., barber's itch.

itching. An irritable tickling of the skin; pruritus.

i·ter (L., a way). 1. A passage. 2. The Sylvian aqueduct.

i·teral. Relating to an iter.

i-itis. Abstract suffix indicating a temporarily acute or accentuated condition.

i·vory (L. *ebur*, ivory). 1. The hard bone-like substance, main component of the tusks of elephants and some other animals. 2. Resembling ivory in hardness, e.g., i. exostosis, a compact osteoma. **Dental i.:** dentine, *q.v.*

Ixŏ·des (G. *ixos*, mistletoe; *eidos*, form). A genus of the order Acarina, including the majority of the parasitic ticks.

ixodī·asis (G. *ixos*, mistletoe; *eidos*, form). Any disease caused by infestation with ticks.

J

jaboran·di. The dried leaflets of *Pilocarpus microphyllus*, used as a diaphoretic, sudorific and sialogogue.

Jaccoud's dissociated fever (Jaccoud, S., French physician, 1830–1913). Fever characterized by a slow, irregular pulse occurring in tuberculous meningitis of adult patients.

jacket A fixed bandage, usually made of plaster of paris, applied to a part of the body, especially round the trunk, for keeping it immobilized.

Jackson's epilepsy (Jackson, J. H., English neurologist, 1834–1911). A form of epilepsy which may follow trauma or be produced by a cerebral tumour. It may be focal, or cortical. A group of muscles may be affected, but once the spasm commences there is a tendency to general convulsions. **J.'s syndrome:** a rare form of paralysis including the soft palate and larynx and one half of the tongue, associated with this there is paralysis of the trapezius and sternomastoid muscles.

Jackson's membrane (Jackson, J. N., American surgeon, 1868–1935). A peritoneal fold or adhesion between the caecum or ascending colon and the right abdominal wall.

Jackson's sign (Jackson, Chevalier, American laryngologist, born 1864). 1. An asthmatoid wheeze-sound heard on breathing in cases where a vegetable foreign body is in the trachea. 2. Froth in pyriform fossa.

Jacob's membrane (Jacob, A., Irish ophthalmologist, 1790–1874). The layer of rods and cones of the retina. **J.'s ulcer:** Rodent ulcer of the face, usually near the inner canthus. **J.'s wound:** chancroidal ulcer.

Jacobson's anastomosis or plexus (Jacobson, L. L., Danish anatomist, 1783–1843). The tympanic plexus. **J.'s canal:** a small canal on the ridge between the carotid canal and jugular fossa which transmits the tympanic branch of the glossopharyngeal nerve. **J.'s cartilage:** vomeronasal cartilage. **J.'s nerve:** tympanic branch of glossopharyngeal nerve. **J.'s organ:** a small bilateral depression in the lower part of the nasal septum. **J.'s sulcus:** small vertical groove on the promontory of the tympanum, it contains the tympanic nerve.

Jacobson's retinitis (Jacobson, J., German ophthalmologist, 1828–89). Syphilitic retinitis.

Jacquemet's recess (Jacquemet, M., French surgeon, 1872–1908). The hepatico-cystic recess, a peritoneal pouch between the liver and the gall-bladder.

Jacquemier's sign (Jacquemier, J. M., French obstetrician, 1806–79). Dark blue or purplish coloration of the vaginal mucosa appearing about the 12th week of pregnancy.

Jacques's plexus. The intramuscular nerve plexus in the uterine tube.

Jacquet's erythema. See napkin erythema.

jactitā·tion (L. *jacere*, to throw). Great restlessness in a severely ill patient.

Jadelot's lines (Jadelot, J. F. N., French physician, 1791–1830). Facial furrows believed by J. to indicate the parts of the body in which certain diseases are localized in children.

Jaffé's sign (Jaffé, M., German physician, 1841–1911). There is a heavier flow of pus from a subdiaphragmatic abscess during inspiration than during expiration. The reverse is the case of the collection in a thoracic one.

Jager's diplococcus (Jager, H., German bacteriologist, 1856–1930). *Neisseria meningitidis.*

Jaksch's disease (Jaksch, R. von, Austrian physician, born 1855). Infantile pseudo-leukaemia; anaemia in infants chacterized by some lymphatic enlargement and splenic changes.

jä·lap. The dried tubercles of the *Ipomaea purga* (Convolvulaceae), a powerful purgative.

James's powder (James, R., English physician, 1705–76). Antimonious oxide 33 and calcium phosphate 67; a prompt diaphoretic.

Janet's disease (Janet, P. M., French physician, 1859–1947). Psychasthenia. **J.'s method:** urethral irrigation with potassium permanganate in cases of gonorrhoea.

jä·niceps (L. *Janus*, a god with two faces; *caput*, head). A monster with two faces.

Jarisch's ointment (Jarisch, A., Austrian dermatologist, 1850–1902). An ointment composed of 60 grains of pyrogallol in one ounce of lard. Sometimes applied in chronic eczema, stains the skin and hair black, and has been known to produce severe toxic effects.

Jarjavay's ligament (Jarjavay, J. F., French physician, 1815–68). The posterior ligaments of the broad ligament ; utero-sacral or utero-recto-sacral ligaments. **J.'s muscle:** the musculus ischiobulbosus of the urethra.

Jarmer's suture (Jarmer, K., contemporary dentist of Greifswald). The intra-alveolar suture of the palate.

jaundice (Fr. *jaunisse*, from L. *galbus*, yellow). A yellowish discoloration of the skin and mucous membranes, due to hyperbilirubinaemia. **J., acholuric:** a chronic condition characterized by more or less mild, persistent or intermittent j. with hypochromic spherocytic anaemia, splenomegaly, increased fragility of the red corpuscles and absence of abnormal amounts of bile pigments from the urine. It may be congenital and familial, and is then often associated with turrecephaly, or it may be an acquired anomaly. Syn. haemolytic j. **J., catarrhal:** an acute disease characterized by j. appearing either simultaneously with, or a few days after, a period of gastro-intestinal symptoms, such as anorexia and diarrhoea, and fever, by bilirubinuria, and absence of bile pigments from the stools. It is probably caused by a virus and occurs sometimes in epidemics. Syn. simple j.; acute hepatitis. **J., haemolytic:** (1) Any j. due to excessive intravascular destruction of the red corpuscles. (2) Acholuric j. **J., obstructive:** j. due to obstruction of the common bile duct or of the hepatic ducts by gallstones, tumour, stenosis or atresia of the ducts. **J., physiological:** icterus neonatorum. **J., toxic:** any j. caused by the action of micro-organisms or of a toxic substance on the liver. See also icterus.

Javelle water (Javel, a French town). Liquor potassae chlorinatae.

jaw. Either the maxilla (upper jaw) or mandible (lower jaw).

Jaworski's corpuscles (Jaworski, V., Polish physician, 1849–1925). Spiral, mucous bodies appearing in gastric secretions of patients with severe hyperchlorhydria.

jē·cur (L.). The liver.

jejū·nal (L. *jejunus*, dry). Relating to the jejunum.

jejunec·tomy (L. *jejunus*, dry; G. *ektomē*, excision). Excision of the jejunum or a part of it.

jejunī·tis. Inflammation of the jejunum.

jĕ·junocolŏ·stomy (L. *jejunus*, dry; G. *kŏlon*, colon; *stoma*, mouth). The surgical formation of a fistula between the jejunum and the colon.

jejuno-ilĕi·tis (L. *jejunus*, dry; *ileum*, the groin). Inflammation of both the jejunum and the ileum.

jĕ·juno-ilĕŏ·stomy (L. *jejunus*, jejunum; *ileum*, the groin; G. *stoma*, mouth). The surgical formation of a fistula between the jejunum and the ileum.

jĕ·junojejunŏ·stomy (L. *jejunus*, dry; G. *stoma*, mouth). The formation of a fistula between one loop of jejunum and another.

jejunŏ·stomy (L. *jejunus*, dry; G. *stoma*, mouth). Surgical formation of a fistula through the abdominal wall into the jejunum.

jejunŏ·tomy (L. *jejunus*, dry; G. *tomē*, a cutting). The incision of the jejunum and closing it again. Used in removing a foreign body from this part of the gut.

jejū·num (L. *jejunus*, dry). The part of the small intestine between the duodenum and the ileum, about 8 ft. long.

jelly (L. *gelare*, to freeze). A semi-solid substance containing usually gelatine in colloidal solution.

Jendrassik's manoeuvre (Jendrassik, E., Hungarian physician, 1858–1922). The patient locks the fingers and then attempts to separate the hands, to produce a knee-jerk through withdrawal of attention from the leg muscles.

Jenner's stain (Jenner, L., English physician, 1866–1904). An eosin methylene blue stain widely used in haematology.

Jennerian vaccination (Jenner, E., English physician, 1749–1823). Vaccination against smallpox, which Jenner introduced in 1796.

Jensen's sulcus (Jensen, J., German psychiatrist, 1841–91). The sulcus intermedius primus of the cerebral cortex.

jerk. A sudden muscular contraction. See ankle jerk, knee jerk.

Jobert's fossa (Jobert de Lamballe, A. J., French surgeon, 1799–1867). The fossa in the popliteal area between the adductor magnus above and the gracilis and sartorius below. It is best seen when the knee is bent and the thigh rotated outward.

Joffroy's reflex (Joffroy, A., French physician, 1844–1908). Hip-phenomenon; twitching of the glutei on pressure upon the nates in spastic paralysis and sciatica. **J.'s sign:** 1. Immobility of the facial muscles when the eyeballs are rolled upwards in exophthalmic goitre. 2. Disorder of the arithmetical faculty in the early stages of general paralysis, the patient being unable to do simple sums in addition or multiplication.

Johne's bacillus (Johne, H. A., German pathologist, 1839–1910). Syn. mycobacterium paratuberculosis, pathogenic to cattle and sheep.

Johnson's test (Johnson, Sir G., English physician, 1818–96). A test for albumin in urine. To some urine in a test tube some concentrated picric acid is added. If albumin is present a white ring forms at the junction of the two fluids.

joint (L. *jungere*, to join). An articulation. There are three main classes: (1) Fibrous joint (synarthrosis), the sutures in the skull and the teeth in the jaws. (2) Cartilaginous joint (synchondrosis), spheno-occipital. (3) Synovial joint, elbow or hip.

Jolles's test (Jolles, A., Austrian chemist, born 1864). A test for bile pigments in the urine. To 50 cc. of urine add 5 cc. of 10 per cent barium chloride and 5 cc. chloroform. Shake for several minutes. Set aside for 10 minutes. Chloroform and phosphates fall to bottom carrying bile pigments with them. Draw off chloroform and precipitate with pipette, and evaporate chloroform over a basin of hot water. Allow to cool and pour off any remaining fluid. Place yellow nitric acid here and there on the surface of the pre-cipitate. If bile pigments are present a play of colours appears around each drop.

Jolly's bodies (Jolly, J., French histologist, born 1870). See Howell's bodies.

Jolly's reaction (Jolly, F., German neurologist, 1844–1904). After exhaustion of the contractility of a muscle by a faradic current, it can still be made to contract by the influence of the will.

Jones's position (Jones, Sir R., English surgeon, 1858–1933). In treating fractures of the lower end of the humerus the arm is retained in acute flexion and supination and retained in this position until the fracture has united. **J.'s splint:** a metal splint used in the treatment of fractures of the humerus.

Jonnesco's fossa (Jonnesco, T., Roumanian surgeon, 1860–1926). The duodeno-jejunal peritoneal fossa; a term sometimes applied also to the retro-duodenal fossa.

Jonstoni area (Jonston, J., Polish physician, 1603–75). Celsus's area; alopecia areata.

Jorissenne's sign (Jorissenne, G., Belgian physician). During the early months of pregnancy, rising from the horizontal to the erect does not increase the pulse-rate.

Josseraud's sign. A peculiar metallic sound heard over the pulmonary area in cases of acute pericarditis.

joule (Joule, J. P., English physicist, 1818–89). A unit expressing the amount of work done in one second by an electric current of one ampere against a resistance of one ohm. **J.'s equivalent:** the mechanical equivalent of heat or the amount of work which, converted into heat, will raise 1 gramme of water 1°C. This unit of heat is known as the small calorie, gram calorie or standard calorie.

Jourdain's disease (Jourdain, A. L. B., French physician, 1734–1816). Osteomyelitis of the alveolar margins of the jaws.

ju·gal (L. *jugum*, yoke). Relating to the malar bone.

jugoma·xillary (L. *jugum*, yoke; *maxilla*, jaw). Relating both to the malar bone and the maxilla.

jū·gular (L. *jugulum*, throat). Relating to the neck; e.g., j. foramen; j. process; j. veins.

jū·gulum (L.). The neck or throat.

jū·gum (L.). 1. A yoke. 2. A ridge.

juice (L. *jus*, broth). The liquid extract from plant or animal substance.

Julliard's mask (Julliard, G., Belgian surgeon, 1836–1911). A mask for administering ether.

junc·tion (L. *junctio*). A meeting-point. **J., myoneural:** the end-plate of a motor nerve-fibre in the muscle.

junctū·ra (L. *junctio*). A suture (in the skull).

Jung's method (Jung, C. G., Swiss psychiatrist, born 1875). Psychoanalysis.

Jung's muscle (Jung, K. G., Swiss anatomist, 1793–1864). The musculus pyramidalis auriculae; musculus tragohelicinus.

Jungbluth's vessels (Jungbluth, H., contemporary German physician). Small nutrient blood-vessels found beneath the amnion in the early human embryo.

Juniperus. A genus of coniferous trees, of which the berry of *J. communis* yields a diuretic substance.

junket (L. *junctio*, union). Curds and whey, produced by rennet added to sweet milk warmed to blood heat.

Junod's boot (Junot, V. T., French physician, 1809–81). A case used to enclose the leg, so as to produce passive congestion.

jury (L. *jurare*, to swear). A body of men legally appointed and sworn to render verdict on the guilt or innocence of a prisoner or to determine the facts in judicial inquiries. **J. of matrons:** a body of twelve matrons formerly empanelled to render verdict whether a prisoner pleading pregnancy in stay of execution was or was not pregnant.

jury-mast. An appliance used for extension-treatment of the upper part of the spine.

justo major (L. greater than normal). Generally and equally enlarged pelvis.

justo minor (L. less than normal). Generally and equally contracted pelvis.

juvan·tia (L. *juvare*, to help). Remedies or medicines used to assist the action of others.

jū·venile (L. *juvenis*, young person). Relating to childhood or to young persons.

juxta-arti·cular (L. *juxta*, near; *articulus*, joint). Close to a joint.

jux·taposĭ·tion (L. *juxta*, near; *positio*, situation). An adjacent position.

K

K. The symbol for an atom of Potassium (*Kali*, from Arab. *gali*, glasswork.)

Kaes's feltwork (Kaes, T., German physician, 1852–1913). A plexus of nerve-fibres formed by the intermingling of the projection, commissural and association fibres in the cortex cerebri.

Kaes-Bechterew's layer (Kaes, T., German neurologist, 1852–1913; Bechterew, V. M., Russian neurologist, 1857–1927). A layer of nerve-fibres in the cerebral cortex.

Kahlbaum's disease (Kahlbaum, K. L., German physician, 1828–99). Catatonia.

Kahler's disease (Kahler, O., Austrian physician, 1849–93). Multiple myeloma.

Kahn's test (Kahn, R. L., contemporary American bacteriologist). A test for syphilis. To 3 cc. of serum 0·05 of the diluted antigen is added in a test-tube, which is then shaken for 3 minutes. The tube is incubated overnight at a temperature of 37° C. The presence of flocculation shows that the test is positive.

Kaiserling's solutions (Kaiserling, K., German pathologist, 1869–1942). Three solutions used respectively for fixation, restoration of colour, and mounting of pathological specimens.

kakidrō·sis (G. *kakos*, bad; *hidrōs*, sweat). Ill-smelling perspiration.

kakke. A Japanese term for beri-beri.

kakos·mia (G. *kakos*, bad; *osmē*, smell). Bad odour.

kala-az·ar (Hindustani: 'black disease'). An infectious disease of tropical and sub-tropical countries, characterized by acute pyrexia, splenomegaly, leucopenia, anaemia, diarrhoea and wasting; caused by the *Leishmania Donovani*.

kaliae·mia (Arab. *gali*, glasswork; G. *haima*, blood). A condition in which potash is found in the blood.

Kandahar sore. Furunculus orientalis, *q.v.*

kangaroo ligature. Suture material from the tendons of the kangaroo's tail.

kā·olin. Purified native aluminium silicate. Used as an adsorber of toxins from the alimentary tract in enteritis, dysentery, diarrhoea, etc.

Kaposi's disease (Kaposi, M. K., Austrian dermatologist, 1837–1902). Xeroderma pigmentosum.

karyĕn·chyma (G. *karuon*, nut; *en*, in; *khumos*, juice). Karyolymph, *q.v.*

kă·ryochrome (G. *karuon*, nut; *khrōma*, colour). A nerve-cell the nucleus of which is stainable.

karyŏ·clasis (G. *karuon*, nut; *klasis*, a breaking). The breaking down of the cell nucleus.

kă·ryocyte (G. *karuon*, nut; *kutos*, cell). A nuclear cell.

karyŏ·gamy (G. *karuon*, nut; *gamos*, marriage). A type of cell conjugation in which there is union of their nuclei.

kă·ryogen·esis (G. *karuon*, nut; *genesis*, production). The development of a cell nucleus.

kă·ryogō·nad (G. *karuon*, nut; *gŏnē*, semen). The reproductive nucleus of a cell.

kă·ryokinē·sis (G. *karuon*, nut; *kinēsis*, movement). 1. Indirect nuclear division. 2. Indirect cell-division, the usual method of cell-reproduction. Syn. mitosis.

kă·ryolymph (G. *karuon*, nut; L. *lympha*, water). The fluid constituent of the cell nucleus.

karyŏ·lysis (G. *karuon*, nut; *luein*, to loosen). The breaking down of the cell nucleus.

kă·ryomere (G. *karuon*, nut; *měros*, part). 1. A chromosomal vesicle formed in a certain type of mitosis. 2. The anterior region of the sperm containing the nucleus.

kă·ryomite (G. *karuon*, nut; *mitos*, thread). Chromosome, *q.v.*

karyŏ·mitome (G. *karuon*, nut; *mitos*, thread). The chromatic network of the cell nucleus.

kă·ryon (G. *karuon*, nut). The cell-nucleus.

kă·ryoplasm (G. *karuon*, nut; *plassein*, to form). The protoplasm of a cell nucleus; the substance of a nucleus.

kă·ryoplast (G. *karuon*, nut; *plassein*, to form). 1. The centrosome. 2. The cell-nucleus, as opposed to the protoplast.

kă·ryorrhex·is (G. *karuon*, nut; *rhexis*, a breaking). Rupture or fragmentation of a cell nucleus.

kă·ryosome (G. *karuon*, nut; *soma*, body). 1. A chromatin nucleus or net-work within the cell nucleus. 2. A basophilic cell nucleolus.

kă·ryosphere (G. *karuon*, nut; *sphaira*, sphere). A portion of a cell nucleus, containing the entire group of chromosomes.

kă·ryothē·ca (G. *karuon*, nut; *thēkē*, case). Nuclear membrane.

kata-. See also words beginning with 'cata'.

katathermŏ·meter (G. *kata*, down; *thermē*, heat; *metron*, measure). An apparatus for measuring the cooling power of the atmosphere.

Katayama's test (Katayama, K., Japanese physician, 1856–1931). A test for carbon monoxide in the blood.

kathisophō·bia (G. *kathisis*, a sitting down; *phobos*, fear). Morbid inability to sit still.

katotrō·pia (G. *katō*, below; *trepein*, to turn). The tendency of the visual axes to fall below the object looked at. Syn. cataphoria.

Kayser-Fleischer ring (Kayser, B., German ophthalmologist, born 1869; Fleischer, R., German physician, 1848–1909). A green-coloured ring appearing at the outer edge of the cornea in cases of hepatolenticular degeneration.

Katzenstein's test (Katzenstein, M., German surgeon, 1872–1932). Test for myocardial efficiency. Compression of the femoral arteries causes an increase of systolic blood pressure when the myocardium is efficient.

KBr. The symbol for one molecule of potassium bromide.

KCl. The symbol for one molecule of potassium chloride.

Keating-Hart's treatment (Keating-Hart, W. V. de, French physician, 1870–1922). Fulguration applied to external cancerous growths.

Keen's sign (Keen, W. W., American surgeon, 1837–1932). In cases of Pott's fracture there is an increase in the intermalleolar diameter.

Kehr's operation (Kehr, H., German surgeon, 1862–1916). Cholecystectomy with drainage of the common duct.

Keith's sino-atrial node (Keith, Sir A., English anatomist, born 1866). The node of Keith and Flack, a collection of cells, found in the hearts of all mammals, situated at the junction of the superior vena cava and the terminal band of the right auricle.

kĕ·lectome (G. *kēlē*, tumour; *ektomē*, excision). An instrument used for cutting away a part of a tumour so that its substance may be submitted to examination.

kĕ·loid (G. *kēlis*, stain; *eidos*, form). A fibrous growth occurring at and extending beyond the limits of a skin wound; hyperplastic scar tissue.

Kenny method (Sister E. Kenny, of Brisbane, Australia). A method of treating infantile paralysis. The back and limbs of the patient are wrapped in woollen cloths wrung out in hot water and when pain has ceased passive exercises are begun, the patient being taught to exercise his muscles without help.

kenophō·bia (G. *kenos*, empty; *phŏbos*, fear). Neurotic fear of large empty spaces.

Kent's bundle (Kent, A. F. S., English physiologist, born 1863). The auriculoventricular bundle.

kĕ·phalin. See cephalin.

kĕ·phir, kĕ·phyr (Caucasian, *kephir*). Milk fermented by the *Lactobacillus caucasicus*.

keratal·gia (G. *keras*, horn; *algos*, pain). Pain in the cornea.

keratectā·sia (G. *keras*, horn; *ektasis*, extension). Protrusion of the cornea.

keratec·tomy (G. *keras*, horn; *ektomē*, excision). Excision of part of the cornea.

kerati·asis (G. *keras*, horn). Multiple warts.

kĕ·ratin (G. *keras*, horn). A protein occurring in horny tissues, hair, nails, etc.

kerā·tinous (G. *keras*, horn). Relating to keratin.

kerati·tic (G. *keras*, horn). Pertaining to keratitis. **K. precipitations:** accumulations of leucocytes, pigment or fibrin deposit on the back of the cornea. Abbrev. K.P.

kerati·tis (G. *keras*, horn). Inflammation of the cornea. **K., bullous:** k. characterized by the formation of large vesicles on the cornea, especially on the site of an old scar. **K., dendritic:** a branching form of superficial ulceration of the cornea, usually due to a herpetic infection. **K., interstitial:** infiltration of the deep layers of the cornea, usually due to congenital syphilis. **K., neuroparalytic:** the formation of corneal ulcers following section or injury of the trigeminal nerve. **K., nummulary:** k. characterized by multiple disc-shaped opacities in the superficial layers of the substantia propria of the cornea, occurring usually in one eye only and affecting especially agricultural labourers. **K., phlyctenular:** k. characterized by the formation of yellow phlyctenules, *q.v.*, in the cornea, occurring specially in children, very probably a manifestation of (usually tuberculous) allergy. **K., profunda:** k. characterized by the formation of an opacity in the deeper layers of the cornea about its centre. **K., sclerosing:** non-ulcerative k. due to the spreading of a scleritis; a mild form of scleritis. **K., superficial punctate:** k. characterized by the formation of minute bullae and erosions of the corneal epithelium.

kĕ·ratocele (G. *keras*, horn; *kēlē*, hernia). Prolapse of Descemet's membrane through the cornea.

kĕ·ratocentē·sis (G. *keras*, horn; *kentesis*, a pricking). Puncture of the cornea.

kĕ·ratoconjunctivi·tis (G. *keras*, horn; L. *conjunctivus*, connective). Inflammation of cornea and conjunctiva.

kĕ·ratoconŏ·meter (G. *keras*, horn; *kōnos*, cone; *metron*, measure). An instrument for the estimation of astigmatism by means of the images reflected from the cornea.

kĕ·ratocō·nus (G. *keras*, horn; *kōnos*, cone). A conical protrusion of the cornea.

ke·ratocrī·coid (G. *keras*, horn; *krikos*, ring; *eidos*, form). The cricothyroid muscle.

kĕ·ratoder·ma (G. *keras*, horn; *derma*, skin). 1. A horny skin. 2. The stratum corneum of the skin.

kĕ·ratodermatō·sis (G. *keras*, horn; *derma*, skin). Any skin affection characterized by alteration in the stratum corneum of the skin.

kĕ·ratoder·mia (G. *keras*, horn; *derma*, skin). Hyperkeratosis. **K., gonorrhoeal:** a condition characterized by the development of irregular brownish nodules, especially on the hands or feet, and a parchment-like thickening of the epidermis at the intervening areas; due to gonorrhoea and usually associated with general manifestations of this disease.

kĕ·ratogĕ·nesis (G. *keras*, horn; *genesis*, production). The development of horny growths.

keratŏ·genous (G. *keras*, horn; *genesis*, production). Relating to the formation of horny growths.

kĕ·ratoglō·bus (G. *keras*, horn; L. *globus*, globe). Globular enlargement of the cornea due to congenital glaucoma.

keratohae·mia (G. *keras*, horn; *haima*, blood). The presence of blood in the cornea.

kĕ·ratohȳ·alin (G. *keras*, horn; *hualos*, glass). One of the granular substances present in the cells of the stratum granulosum of the skin.

kĕ·ratoid (G. *keras*, horn; *eidos*, form). Horn-like.

kĕ·rato-īrī·tis (G. *keras*, horn; *iris*, iris). Inflammation of both the cornea and the iris.

ke·ratoleukō·ma (G. *keras*, horn; *leukos*, white). A white opacity in the cornea of the eye.

keratŏ·lysis (G. *keras*, horn; *lusis*, a loosening). Epidermolysis, *q.v.*

keratŏ·ma (G. *keras*, horn). Callosity, *q.v.*

kĕ·ratomalā·cia (G. *keras*, horn; *malakia*, softness). A softening of the cornea, caused by deficiency in intake of vitamin A.

kĕ·ratome (G. *keras*, horn; *tomē*, section). A knife used for incising the cornea in iridectomy.

keratŏ·meter (G. *keras*, horn; *metron*, measure). 1. An instrument for measuring the curves of the cornea. 2. An instrument for measuring the diameter of the cornea.

keratŏ·metry (G. *keras*, horn; *metron*, measure). The measurement of the corneal curves.

kĕ·ratomycō·sis (G. *keras*, horn; *mukēs*, mushroom). Ulcerating or infiltrating keratitis due to infection with certain fungi.

kĕ·ratonyx·is (G. *keras*, horn; *nuxis*, a pricking). The needling of a soft cataract by puncturing the cornea.

kĕ·ratoplasty (G. *keras*, horn; *plassein*, to form). A plastic operation on the cornea.

kĕ·ratoscope (G. *keras*, horn; *skopein*, to view). An instrument for testing the curvature of the cornea.

keratŏ·scopy (G. *keras*, horn; *skopein*, to view). The examination of the cornea with the keratoscope.

keratŏ·sis (G. *keras*, horn). 1. Any skin disease characterized by overgrowth of the horny epithelium; hyperkeratosis. 2. Any condition of a mucous membrane characterized by cornification of its epithelium. **K. follicularis:** a chronic skin disease characterized by single or confluent hard brownish crusts attached to the follicles, projecting above the surface and distributed symmetrically over the body. **K. pharyngis:** a condition of the pharynx characterized by areas where the epithelium has undergone cornification, usually associated with the growth of the leptothrix fungus at these spots. Syn. pharyngomycosis. **K. pilaris:** a skin disease characterized by the formation of horny pointed plugs originating from hair follicles. **K. senilis:** a skin disease occurring in advanced age, characterized by brownish warty growths, especially on the face and the plantar surface of the hands.

kerā·totome. Keratome, *q.v.*

keratŏ·tomy (G. *keras*, horn; *tomē*, section). Incision of the cornea.

keraunophō·bia (G. *keraunos*, thunderbolt; *phŏbos*, fear). Neurotic fear of lightning.

kerec·tomy. Keratectomy, q.v.

kerion Celsi (G. *kērion*, honey-comb; L. Celsus, Roman writer on medicine). A severe form of trichophytosis of the scalp with the formation of abscesses of the hair follicles.

Kerkring's ossicle (Kerkring, T., Dutch anatomist, 1640–93). An occasional centre of ossification in the occipital bone, in the middle of the posterior border of the foramen magnum. K.'s valves: the valvulae conniventes of the small intestine.

kernic·terus (Ger. *kern*, kernel; G. *ikteros*, jaundice). A condition characterized by the selective staining with bile pigment of the basal ganglia of the brain, especially of subthalamic nuclei, lenticular nuclei and the cornu Ammonis, followed by degeneration of these ganglia, occurring during an attack of icterus gravis neonatorum and leading to disturbance of the extra-pyramidal system.

Kernig's sign (Kernig, W., Russian physician, 1840–1917). The inability to extend the leg on the thigh when the thigh is flexed at right angles to the abdomen. The sign is present in meningitis or meningeal irritation.

keto-acid. An organic acid containing the ketone group; e.g., aceto-acetic acid.

ketoge·nesis (L. *acetum*, vinegar; *genesis*, production). The production of ketone or acetone bodies.

kētogen·ic. Pertaining to ketogenesis; producing ketosis.

ketŏ·lysis (L. *acetum*, vinegar; G. *lusis*, loosening). The splitting up of acetone bodies.

ketonāē·mia. Acetonaemia, q.v.

kē·tone (L. *acetum*, vinegar). 1. Organic compounds containing the carbonyl group CO linked to two univalent radicals and derived by oxidation from a secondary alcohol. 2. Acetone. K. bodies: oxybutyric acid, aceto-acetic acid and acetone; the last two substances are formed in the human metabolism only when oxidation of fats is disturbed, e.g. as a sequel to an insufficient catabolism of carbohydrates.

ketonū·ria (L. *acetum*, vinegar; G. *ouron*, urine). The presence of ketone bodies in the urine.

kē·tose. A monosaccharide containing a keto group.

ketō·sis (L. *acetum*, vinegar). The condition characterized by the presence of ketone bodies in the blood, which leads to a decrease in the CO_2 combining power of the blood. See also acidosis.

ketostē·roid. A steroid containing a ketone or ketone groups. Some have marked oestrogenic or androgenic activity.

Key and Retzius's corpuscles (Key, E. A. H., Swedish physician, 1832–1901; Retzius, M. G., Swedish histologist, 1842–1919). Minute corpuscles which are found in the mouths of some aquatic birds. They probably represent transition forms. K. and R.'s foramina: See foramen of Luschka.

kg. Abbreviation for kilogramme.

KHCO₃. Symbol for one molecule of potassium bicarbonate.

khellin. A smooth muscle relaxant obtained from the plant *Ammi visnaga*. Used in the treatment of angina pectoris.

KI. Symbol for one molecule of potassium iodide.

kidney. One of the two glands situated in the upper and posterior part of the abdominal cavity, the function of which is the formation and excretion of urine. K., large white: term applied to the k. as found in subacute glomerulo-nephritis. K., small white: term applied to the k. as found in chronic glomerulo-nephritis. K., red granular: term applied to k. as found in malignant hypertension. K., lardaceous: renal amyloidosis. K., movable: nephroptosis. K., surgical: pyelonephritis. K., horseshoe: congenital fusion of the two kidneys, usually at the inferior pole.

Kiernan's spaces (Kiernan, F., English physician, 1800–74). The interlobular spaces in the liver.

Kiesselbach's area (Kiesselbach, W., German laryngologist, 1839–1902). The area on the nasal septum; site of nasal haemorrhage.

Kilian's line (Kilian, H. F., German obstetrician, 1800–63). Marking the level of the promontory of the sacrum. K.'s pelvis: the osteomalacic pelvis.

Killian's bundle (Killian, G., German laryngo-rhinologist, 1860–1921). 'Fasceau en fronde', the lowest fibres of the inferior constrictor of the pharynx immediately above the true oesophageal musculature. K.'s operation: removal of anterior wall of frontal sinus for inflammatory disease.

kilogramme (G. *khilioi*, thousand; *gramma*, a small weight). One thousand grammes, or 2·2 lb. avoirdupois.

kilolitre (G. *khilioi*, thousand; *litra*, a pound weight). One thousand litres or 35·3171 cubic feet.

kilometre (G. *khilioi*, thousand; *metron*, measure). One thousand metres, or 1093·6 yards.

kilowatt (G. *khilioi*, thousand; watt). One thousand watts of electricity.

kinaesthē·sia (G. *kinein*, to move; *aisthēsis*, feeling). The sense by which movements of any members of the body, weight, position or resistance are perceived, owing to stimulation of specific receptor muscles, tendons and joints.

kinaesthē·tic. Relating to kinaesthesia.

ki·nase (G. *kinein*, to move). Applied to tissue substances which activate pro-enzymes into enzymes.

kinemā·tics (G. *kinein*, to move). The study of motion.

kinemā·tograph (G. *kinein*, to move; *graphein*, to write). An apparatus for making or exhibiting a continuous record of moving objects. Commonly called cinematograph.

kĭ·neplasty (G. *kinein*, to move; *plassein*, to form). An amputation designed to make the stump useful for movement.

kinē·si-aesthesiŏ·meter (G. *kinein*, to move; *aisthēsis*, feeling; *metron*, measure). An instrument for estimating the muscular sense.

kinē·sial·gia (G. *kinein*, to move; *algos*, pain). Pain on muscular movement.

kinesiǎ·trics (G. *kinein*, to move; *iatreia*, medical treatment). Treatment of disease by muscular exercise.

kinesī·meter (G. *kinein*, to move; *metron*, measure). An instrument for measuring threshholds of sensations of movement.

kinesiŏ·logy (G. *kinein*, to move; *logos*, treatise). That part of medical science which pertains to muscular movement and to gymnastics, rhythmical exercises, etc.

kinesŏ·dic (G. *kinein*, to move; *hodos*, way). Relating to motor impulses.

kinĕ·tic (G. *kinein*, to move). Relating to motion. K. energy: the energy possessed by a body due to its motion.

kinĕ·tocyte (G. *kinein*, to move; *kutos*, cell). A roving blood cell.

king's evil. Scrophula; so-called on account of an ancient belief that it could be cured by the touch of a king.

kĭ·noplasm (G. *kinein*, to move; *plasma*, a formation). That constituent of cytoplasm which was believed to give origin to the astral rays, spindle fibres, central bodies, etc.

kĭ·otome (G. *kiōn*, pillar; *tomē*, section). An instrument for amputating the uvula.

kiŏ·tomy (G. *kiōn*, pillar; *tomē*, section). Surgical removal of the uvula.

Kirschner's wire. Special wire used in orthopaedic surgery.

Kitasato's bacillus (Kitasato, S., Japanese bacteriologist, 1852–1931). *Pasteurella pestis*.

Kjeldahl's method (Kjeldahl, J. G. C., Danish chemist, 1849–1900). A method for estimating nitrogen in organic substances, depending on the oxidation of the substance to ammonia with concentrated sulphuric acid in the presence of a catalyst.

Klebs-Loeffler bacillus (Klebs, E., German bacteriologist, 1834–1913; Loeffler, A. J., German physician, 1852–1915). *Corynebacterium diphtheriae.*

Klebsiella (Klebs, E., German bacteriologist, 1834–1913). A genus of Bacteriaceae.

Klein's bacillus (Klein, E. E., Hungarian bacteriologist, 1844–1925). *Bacillus enteritidis sporogenes.* **K.'s muscle**: the musculus compressor labii; marginal bundle of the lips.

Kleinschmidt's glands (Kleinschmidt, A., German ophthalmologist of the 19th century). The conjunctival glands.

kleptolag·nia (G. *kleptein*, to steal; *lagneia*, lust). Sexual gratification obtained by stealing.

kleptomā·nia (G. *kleptein*, to steal; *mania*, madness). Neurotic impulse to steal.

kleptomā·niac. A person affected with kleptomania.

kleptophō·bia (G. *kleptein*, to steal; *phŏbos*, fear). 1. A morbid fear of thieves. 2. A morbid fear of becoming a thief.

Klumpke's paralysis (Klumpke, A. D., French neurologist, 1859–1927). A lower-arm type of paralysis caused by injuries to the eighth cervical and first dorsal nerves, causing paralysis of the flexor muscles to the wrist and fingers.

Km. Abbreviation for kilometre.

knee. The joint between the thigh and foreleg (femur and tibia). **K. -cap**: the patella. **K., housemaid's**: prepatellar bursitis. **K. -jerk**: contraction of the quadriceps femoris upon tapping the patella tendon when the leg is relaxed, a reflex mediated by the 2.–4. lumbar segments of the spinal cord.

knife. A sharp metal instrument for incising the skin or other structures. **Beer's k.**: a small knife with a triangle-shaped blade used for cataract extraction. **Blair k.**: used in plastic surgery. The standard knife for cutting split skin grafts. **Cautery k.**: a knife with its blade connected to an electric battery so that bleeding is prevented by the tissues being seared.

KNO₃. Symbol for one molecule of potassium nitrate.

knock-knee. Genu valgum.

Knoll's glands (Knoll, P., Austrian physiologist, 1841–1900). The special glands in false vocal cords.

knot. 1. An intertwining of the ends of one or more cords so that they cannot easily be separated, e.g. friction k., granny k., reef k., Staffordshire k., among those used in surgery. 2. A circumscribed swelling.

Knox's foramen (Knox, R., Scottish surgeon, 1791–1862). The epitrochlear foramen of the humerus.

knuckle. The dorsal aspect of any of the joints between the phalanges and the metacarpal bones or between the phalanges.

Kobelt's cyst (Kobelt, G. L., German physician, 1804–57). Cystic dilation of a portion of the parovarium. **K.'s muscle**: the 6. compressor venae dorsalis penis. **K.'s network**: the junction of the veins of the bulbs of the vestibule beneath the clitoris. **K.'s tubules**: the tubules of the parovarium.

Kober's test. A chemical test for oestrogens. When these are treated with sulphuric acid and phenolsulphonic acid and then diluted with water, a pink colour is shown.

Kobner's multiple papillary tumours (Kobner, H., German dermatologist, 1838–1904). Alibert's disease, *q.v.*

Koch's bacillus (Koch, R., German bacteriologist, 1843–1910). The *Mycobacterium tuberculosis.* **K.'s**

eruption: a morbilliform eruption following the injection of tuberculin. **K.'s postulates**: certain rules to be applied in considering the claim of a micro-organism to be the cause of a certain disease.

Koch's triangle (Koch, W., German surgeon born 1880). A triangular area of the wall of the right atrium of the heart that marks the situation of the atrio-ventricular node.

Koch-Weeks bacillus (Koch, R., German bacteriologist, 1843–1910; Weeks, J. E., American ophthalmologist, born 1853). A micro-organism of the Haemophilus group which is associated with a certain type of acute conjunctivitis, probably identical with *H. influenzae.*

KOH. Symbol for one molecule of potassium hydroxide.

Kohlrausch's fold (Kohlrausch, O. L. B., German physician, 1811–54). A transverse fold of mucous membrane of the rectum which is situated about 6 cm. above the anal margin.

Kohn's bodies (Kohn, A., Austrian histologist, born 1867). The paraganglia, carotid, coccygeal bodies.

koilonў·chia (G. *koilos*, hollow; *onux*, finger-nail). Concavity of the nail. Syn. spoon-nail.

Kölliker's dental crest (Kölliker, R. A. von, Swiss physiologist and anatomist, 1817–1905). The portion of the maxilla upon which the incisor teeth are developed.

Konstantinovich's artery (Konstantinovich, V. B., Russian surgeon, born 1845). The arteria dorsalis recti; a branch of the superior rectal (haemorrhoidal) artery to the rectum. **K.'s vein**: the marginal vein of the anus.

Koplik's spots (Koplik, H., American physician, 1858–1927). Small whitish spots seen on the mucous membrane of the cheeks and lips during the prodromal stage of measles.

Kopp's asthma (Kopp, J. H., German physician, 1777–1858). Laryngismus stridulus; spasm of the glottis occurring in infants up to two years of age.

Koranyi's auscultation (Koranyi, Baron F. von, Hungarian physician, 1829–1913). A special form of percussion in which the finger is placed perpendicularly during the process.

korō·nion (G. *korŏnē*, a crow). The apex of the coronoid process of the inferior maxilla.

Korsakow's psychosis or syndrome (Korsakow, S., Russian neurologist, 1853–1900). Mental derangement in the form of failure of memory, imaginary reminiscence, sometimes hallucinations with agitation, in polyneuritis; usually of alcoholic origin.

kosher (Heb. *kasher*). Lawful. **K. meat**: the flesh of animals slaughtered in accordance with the Jewish law.

Kovalevsky's canal (Kovalevsky, P., Russian embryologist, 1845–1901). The neurenteric canal.

Koyter's muscle (Koyter, V., Dutch anatomist, 1534–1600). The corrugator supercilii.

K.P. Keratitic precipitates.

kraurō·sis (G. *krauros*, brittle). Shrivelling or atrophy of a part. **K. vulvae**: shrivelling and dryness of the vulva.

Krause's glands (Krause, K. F. T., German anatomist, 1797–1868). The acino-tubular glands of the conjunctiva. **K.'s muscle**: the muscle of the lips.

Krause's membrane (Krause, W. J. F., German anatomist, 1833–1910). A membrane which appears as a dark line on longitudinal section and which limits the sarcomeres of striped muscle. Syn. Dobie's layer or line. **K.'s nerve**: The ulnar collateral branch of the radial nerve. **K.'s ventricle**: the small terminal part of the central canal of the spinal cord.

Kretschmann's space (Kretschmann, F., German otologist, 1858–1934). A small recess in the attic of the middle ear situated below Prussak's space.

Kreysig's sign (Kreysig, F. L., German physician, 1770–1839). In cases of adherent pericardium with each heart beat there is retraction of the epigastric region.

Krishaber's disease (Krishaber, M., French physician, 1836–83). A neurosis of sudden onset, accompanied by cerebral symptoms, neuralgia, syncope and cardiac palpitation.

Kronecker's inhibitory centre (Kronecker, H., Swiss physiologist, 1839–1914). The inhibitory centre of the heart. The dorsal motor nucleus of the vagus.

Krönlein's hernia (Krönlein, R. U., Swiss surgeon, 1847–1910). Properitoneal hernia.

Krukenberg's vein (Krukenberg, A., German anatomist, 1816–77). The central vein of the hepatic lobule.

kryp·ton. Kr. A rare gas occurring in air. (1 part in 2 millions).

K$_2$SO$_4$. Symbol for one molecule of potassium sulphate.

Kuemmell's disease (Kuemmell, H., German surgeon, 1852–1937). Traumatic spondylitis; rarefying spondylitis of the vertebrae.

Kuester's sign (Kuester, O. E., German gynaecologist, 1850–1931). A cystic tumour felt in the median line anterior to the uterus usually indicates ovarian dermoids.

Kulchitsky's cells (Kulchitsky, N., Russian anatomist, 1856–1925). Argentaffin cells in the epithelium of the small intestine.

kumis, kumyss (Tartar, *kumis*). An alcoholic drink made by fermenting milk.

Kulenkampff's anaesthesia (Kulenkampff, D., German surgeon, born 1880). A method of brachial plexus block. It involves blocking the plexus as it lies on the first rib lateral to the subclavian artery.

Kupffer's canals (Kupffer, W., German anatomist, 1829–1902). The embryonic outgrowths from the Wolffian ducts to form ureters. **K.'s cells:** the 'stellate cells' in the lining of blood channels in the liver.

Kussmaul's coma (Kussmaul, A., German physician, 1822–1902). Diabetic coma.

kwashīor·kor (Name used on the Gold Coast, W. Africa). A pellagra-like disease, characterized by anaemia, oedema, skin lesions including loss of pigment, bulky, soft stools and reversal of the albumin/globulin ratio. A cirrhosis of the pancreas and liver is present.

kyllō·sis (G. *kullos*, crooked). Club-foot.

kȳ·mograph, kymogra·phion (G. *kuma*, wave; *graphein*, to write). An instrument for graphical recording of temporal variations of a process.

kymŏ·graphy (G. *kuma*, wave; *graphein*, to write). 1. Recording by kymograph. 2. The recording of the movements of an organ on an X-ray film.

kynophō·bia (G. *kuōn*, dog; *phŏbos*, fear). Neurotic fear of dogs or of becoming affected with rabies.

kyphoscoliō·sis (G. *kuphos*, bent; *skolios*, curved). A condition characterized by both kyphosis and scoliosis.

kyphō·sis (G. *kuphos*, bent). 1. Backward curvature of spine. 2. Humpback or angular curvature.

kyphŏ·tic (G. *kuphos*, bent). Pertaining to or affected with kyphosis.

L

Labarraque's solution (Labarraque, A. G., French chemist; 1777–1850). A solution of sodium carbonate, 10; chloride of lime, 8; water, 100. A disinfectant.

Labbé's triangle (Labbé, L., French surgeon, 1832–1916). A triangular area included between a horizontal line along the lower border of the cartilage of the ninth rib, the line of the false ribs and the line of the liver. It is the area where the stomach lies in contact with the wall of the abdomen. **L.'s vein**: the posterior anastomotic vein of the cortex cerebri.

lă·bial (L. *labium*, lip). 1. Relating to the lips or to a labium. 2. Relating to sounds requiring closure or approximation of the lips.

labia (Pl. of L. *labium*, lip). The lips. **L. majora**: the two cutaneous folds of the female external genital organs. **L. minora**: the nymphae, the two folds of mucous membrane of the female external genital organs.

lă·bialism (L. *labium*, lip). Defective speech characterized by the pronouncing of articulate sounds as labial sounds.

lă·bile (L. *labi*, to slip). Unstable.

labiŏ·logy (L. *labium*, lip; *logos*, a discourse). The study of lip movements.

lă·biomancy (L. *labium*, lip; G. *manteia*, divination). Lip-reading.

lă·bioplasty (L. *labium*, lip; G. *plassein*, to form). Cheiloplasty, *q.v.*

lă·bium (L.). A lip. See labia.

Laborde's method (Laborde, J. B. V., French physician, 1830–1903). Stimulation of respiration by rhythmical traction on the tongue. Used in cases of asphyxia.

labour (L. *labor*, work). Parturition. **L., dry**: l. with more or less complete absence of liquor amnii. **L., induced**: artificially induced l. **L., instrumental**: l. in which instruments are used for the extraction of the foetus. **L., premature**: labour supervening before completion of full term of pregnancy.

lă·brum (L. *labrum*, brim). A lip-like structure. **L. glenoidale**: the fibro-cartilaginous border of a joint cavity.

lă·byrinth (G. *laburhinthos*). The cavities of the internal ear, comprising the vestibule, cochlea and semicircular canals, containing the sensory receptors for hearing and equilibrium.

labyrin·thine (G. *laburhinthos*, maze). Relating to the labyrinth. **L. nystagmus**: nystagmus due to a disorder of the labyrinth.

labyrinthī·tis (G. *laburhinthos*, maze). Inflammation of the labyrinth. See also Menière's syndrome.

labyrinthŏ·tomy (G. *laburhinthos*, maze; *tomē*, section). Opening and drainage of the membranous labyrinth through its outer wall.

lac (L., milk). Milk. **L. sulphuris**: precipitated sulphur.

lă·cerated (L. *lacerare*, to tear). Torn; ruptured.

lacerā·tion (L. *lacerare*, to tear). A tear; a rupture.

lă·chesine. Lachesine chloride. Synthetic substance having mydriatic properties similar to those of atropine.

lachry-. Words having this prefix are spelt 'lacri-' in modern medical writing. Hence 'lacrimal' instead of 'lachrymal'.

lă·crima (L.). A tear.

lă·crimal (L. *lacrima*, tear). Relating to tears. **L. gland**: the gland secreting tears.

lacrimā·tion (L. *lacrima*, tear). 1. Secretion of tears. 2. Excessive secretion of tears; hyperlacrimation.

lactacidae·mia (L. *lac*, milk; *acidus*, bitter; G. *haima*, blood). A condition characterized by the presence of lactic acid in the blood.

lactacidū·ria (L. *lac*, milk; *acidus*, bitter; G. *ouron*, urine). A condition in which lactic acid is excreted in the urine.

lac·tagogue (L. *lac*, milk; G. *agōgos*, leading). Stimulating the secretion of milk.

lactal·bumin (L. *lac*, milk; *albus*, white). A protein contained in milk.

lac·tase (L. *lac*, milk). An enzyme converting lactose into glucose and galactose; present in the intestinal juice of mammals taking milk in their food throughout their lives.

lac·tate (L. *lac*, milk). A salt of lactic acid.

lactā·tion (L. *lactare*, to have or give milk). 1. The secretion of milk. 2. Suckling.

lactā·tional. Relating to lactation.

lac·teal (L. *lacteus*, milky). 1. Relating to milk. 2. Any one of the lymphatic ducts of the small intestine that take up the chyle.

lactĕs·cense (L. *lac*, milk). Milk-like consistency.

lac·tic (L. *lac*, milk). Relating to milk or to derivatives of milk. **L. acid**: $HC_3H_5O_3$, a hydroxy acid occurring in some milk and in muscle tissue; used as a digestive. **L. acid milk**: milk to which l. acid has been added or which has been inoculated with *Streptococcus lacticus*, *Bacillus bulgaricus* or *Bacillus acidophilus*; differing from ordinary cow's milk by its fine, flocculent curds, by its low butter value which approaches that of human milk, and by the fact that growth of contaminating micro-organisms is inhibited if not prevented.

lacti·ferous (L. *lac*, milk; *ferre*, to bear). Secreting or conveying milk.

lac·tifuge (L. *lac*, milk; *fugare*, to put to flight). Diminishing secretion of milk.

lactĭ·genous (L. *lac*, milk; *generare*, to produce). See lactogenic.

lactĭ·gerous (L. *lac*, milk; *gerere*, to convey). Lactiferous, *q.v.*

lac·tin. Lactose, *q.v.*

lactĭ·vorous (L. *lac*, milk; *vorare*, to devour). Feeding on milk.

lac·tocele (L. *lac*, milk; G. *kēlē*, hernia). Galactocele, *q.v.*

lac·toflavin (L. *lac*, milk; *flavus*, yellow). Riboflavin. A member of the vitamin B group.

lactogen·ic (L. *lac*, milk; *generare*, to produce). Promoting the secretion of milk.

lactŏ·meter (L. *lac*, milk; G. *metron*, measure). An instrument for the estimation of the specific gravity of milk.

lactŏ·sazone. A derivative of lactose prepared to demonstrate the presence of lactose in urine.

lac·toscope (L. *lac*, milk; G. *skopein*, to view). An instrument for the estimation of the percentage of fat in milk.

lac·tose (L. *lac*, milk). Milk sugar, the carbohydrate present in the milk of mammals.

lactosū·ria (L. *lac*, milk; G. *ouron*, urine). The presence of lactose in the urine.

lactother·apy (L. *lac*, milk; G. *therapeia*, treatment). The treatment of disease by giving a milk diet.

lac·tovegetar·ian (L. *lac*, milk; *vegēre*, to enliven). Term applied to a diet consisting of milk and vegetable products.

lacu·na (L. *lacus*, lake). A small space, pocket, cavity or depression. L. **magna**: a depression situated on the roof of the fossa navicularis about 1 inch from the urinary meatus. L. **musculosa**: part of the pelvocrural space in the thigh. L. **vasculosa**: small space on the inner side of the thigh.

lacu·nar. Characterized by lacunae.

lacu·nula (L. dim. of *lacuna*). A minute lacuna.

lā·cus (L.). A small space or cavity. L. **lacrimalis**: the space at the inner canthus of the eye, where tears collect.

Laënnec's disease (Laënnec, R. T. H., French physician, 1781-1826). Cirrhosis of the liver due to alcohol. L.'s **pearls**: small gelatinous bodies found in the sputum of asthmatic patients.

laevoduc·tion (L. *laevus*, left; *ducěre*, to lead). The turning of an eye towards the left side.

laevophō·bia (L. *laevus*, left; G. *phobos*, fear). Neurotic fear of objects on the left side of the body.

laevophor·ia (L. *laevus*, left; G. *pherein*, to bear). Tendency of the visual lines to deviate to the left.

laevorotā·tory (L. *laevus*, left; *rotare*, to turn). Turning the rays of polarized light to the left.

lae·vulose (L. *laevus*, left). Fruit sugar, the carbohydrate present in fruits; it turns the rays of polarized light to the left. L. **test**: a test for hepatic function in which the effect of ingestion or intravenous injection of l. is observed by estimation of blood-sugar or by examination of the urine for l.

laevulosae·mia (G. *laevus*, left; *haima*, blood). The presence of laevulose in the blood.

laevulosu·ria (L. *laevus*, left; G. *ouron*, urine). The presence of laevulose in the urine.

lagen·iform (L. *lagēna*, flask; *forma*, shape). Shaped like a flask.

lagnē·sis (G. *lagnes*, salacious). 1. Satyriasis or nymphomania. 2. Coitus.

lagophthal·mos (G. *lagos*, hare; *ophthalmos*, eye). Impossibility of complete closure of the eyelids.

Laimer's area (Laimer, 19th-century Austrian anatomist). The area at the junction of the oesophagus and the pharynx.

lake-coloured (Hind. *lakh*, from Sanskrit *Laksha*). Applied to haemolysed blood.

Lallemand's bodies (Lallemand, C. F., French surgeon, 1790-1853). Concretions in the seminal vesicles.

lalling (G. *lalein*, to babble). An unintelligible stammering; baby-talk.

lalognō·sis (G. *lalos*, loquacious; *gnōsis*, knowledge). Understanding of the spoken word.

lalŏ·pathy (G. *lalos*, loquacious; *pathos*, disease). Any form of speech disorder.

lalophō·bia (G. *lalos*, loquacious; *phobos*, fear). Neurotic dislike of speaking.

laloplē·gia (G. *lalos*, loquacious; *plēgē*, stroke). Paralysis of speech due to a cause other than paralysis of the tongue.

Lalouette's pyramid (Lalouette, P., French physician, 1711–42). The median lobe of the thyroid gland.

lambda (G. Λ, λ, the letter 'l'). The angle of junction of the lambdoid and sagittal sutures.

lamb·dacism (G. *lambda*, letter 'l'). 1. Difficulty in pronouncing the sound of the letter 'l'. 2. Substitution of the letter 'l' for the letter 'r' in speech.

lamb·doid, lambdoi·dal (G. *lambda*, the letter 'l'; *eidos*, form). Resembling the Greek letter Λ. L. **suture**: that between the occipital bone and the two parietal bones.

Lamblia intestinalis (Lambl, W. D., Austrian physician, 1824–95). Giardia Lamblia, *q.v.*

lamblī·asis. Giardiasis, *q.v.*

lamel·la (L. *lamella*, dim. of *lamina*, a plate). 1. A medicated disc, used especially for the application of drugs to the eye. 2. A lamina. 3. A basement membrane.

lamel·lar (L. *lamella*, dim. of *lamina*, a plate). 1. Pertaining to a lamina. 2. Resembling a lamina. 3. Composed of lamellae, as in l. cataract.

lă·mina (L., a plate). A thin plate or layer; a thin membrane. L. **cribrosa**: perforated plate of bone at the bottom of the internal auditory meatus. L. **terminalis**: a thin sheet of nervous tissue passing from the rostrum to the optic chiasma. L. **vasculosa**: the external layer of the choroid of the eye.

Laminaria. A genus of seaweeds.

lă·minated. Composed of laminae.

lă·minal, lă·minae (L. *lamina*, a plate). 1. Resembling a lamina. 2. Composed of laminae.

laminā·tion (L. *lamina*, a plate). Arrangement in layers.

laminec·tomy (L. *lamina*, plate; G. *ektomē*, excision). The surgical removal of the posterior vertebral arches.

lamini·tis. Inflammation of a lamina.

lā·na (L.). Wool.

lance (L. *lancea*). 1. A lancet. 2. To open, with a lancet, scalpel, etc.

Lancereaux's interstitial nephritis (Lancereaux, E., French physician, 1829–1910). Interstitial nephritis resulting from rheumatism.

lan·cet (L. *lancea*, lance). A knife with a two-edged lance-shaped blade.

Lancet coefficient (*The Lancet*, English medical periodical). A measure of the disinfecting power of a substance compared with carbolic acid as the standard.

lan·cinating (L. *lancinare*, to lacerate). Term applied to pains resembling those inflicted by a stab, as the 'shooting' pains in tabes dorsalis.

Lancisi's nerves (Lancisi, G. M., Italian physician, 1654–1720). The striae longitudinales on the upper surface of the corpus callosum.

landmarks. Points, lines, etc., on the surface of an organ, used as guides to deeper-seated parts.

Landolt's clubs (Landolt, E., French oculist, 1846–1926). The 'cellules bipolaires à massue'; retinal nerve cells occurring mainly in amphibia, reptiles and birds.

Landouzy's purpura (Landouzy, L., French physician, 1845–1917). A form of purpura characterized by serious systemic symptoms.

Landouzy-Déjérine's type of progressive muscular atrophy (Landouzy, L., French physician, 1845–1917; Déjérine, J. J., French neurologist, 1849–1917). The facioscapulo humeral type of progressive muscular atrophy.

Landry's paralysis (Landry, J. B. O., French physician, 1826–65). Acute ascending paralysis.

Landzert's canal (Landzert, T., Russian anatomist of the 19th century). The cranio-pharyngeal canal. L.'s **fossa**: a fossa formed by peritoneal folds enclosing the left colic artery and the inferior mesenteric vein respectively, at the side of the duodenum. It is smaller than the fossa duodenalis, which is sometimes found in the same region.

Lane's disease (Lane, Sir W. Arbuthnot, English surgeon, 1856–1943). Chronic stasis of the intestines. L.'s **kinks**: a series of variable flexures in the intestinal canal. L.'s **operation**: ileosigmoidostomy. L.'s **plates**: metal plates used as internal splints in fractures.

Langenbeck's incision (Langenbeck, B. R. K. von, German surgeon, 1810–87). Various incisions used in the treatment of cleft palate. L.'s **operation**: rhinoplasty. L.'s **triangle**: the area over the head of

Q

the femur between the pyriformis and the gluteus medius, employed in arthrotomy of the hip joint.

Langenbeck's nerve (Langenbeck, K. J. M., German surgeon, 1776–1802). The nervus superficialis scapulae—nervi supraclaviculares posteriores.

Langendorff's cells (Langendorff, German physiologist, 1853–1908). The principal cells of the thyroid gland.

Langer's lines (Langer, K. von, Ritter von Edenberg, Austrian anatomist, 1819–87). The cleavage lines of the skin due to the disposition of the subcutaneous fibrous tissue.

Langerhans's bodies or islands (Langerhans, P., German pathologist, 1847–88). Minute isolated masses of spheroidal or polyhedral cells found in the pancreas. **L.'s granular layer:** the stratum granulosum. **L.'s stellate corpuscles:** nerve-fibre ends which have been seen in the rete mucosum of the skin.

Langhans's cells (Langhans, T., German pathologist, 1839–1915). The nucleated epithelial cells, constituting L.'s layer. **L.'s giant cell:** the giant cell seen in tuberculous granuloma. **L.'s layer:** a cellular membrane covering the placental villi beneath the syncytium; it disappears in the later months of pregnancy.

Langley's granulations (Langley, J. N., English physiologist, 1853–1925). The granules seen in secreting gland cells. **L.'s nerves:** the pilomotor nerves.

lan·guor (L.). A sensation characterized by a disinclination to muscular activity, not due to fatigue from any muscular exertion.

Lannelongue's foramina (Lannelongue, O. M., French pathologist, 1840–1911). The venous openings into the right atrium of the heart larger than and distinct from the foramina of Thebesius. **L.'s ligament:** the costo-pericardiac ligament. **L.'s tibia:** deformed tibia due to syphilis.

lă·nolin (L. *lana*, wool). The purified fat from sheep's wool.

Lantermann's incisures (Lantermann, A. J., German anatomist of the 19th century). Oblique partition interrupting the myelin sheath of nerves. **L.'s segments:** each internodal segment of myelin sheath is fragmented into segments of Lantermann.

lanū·go (L., down (substance)). 1. The down-like hair of the human foetus from the 5th to the 9th month. 2. Any down-like hair in children or adults.

Lanz's line (Lanz, O., Dutch surgeon, 1865–1935). A line joining the two anterior superior iliac spines. **L.'s point:** on the line at the junction of the right and middle thirds.

laparŏ·scopy (G. *lapara*, flank; *skopein*, to view). Endoscopic examination of the abdominal cavity through a small incision of the abdominal wall.

laparŏ·tomy (G. *lapara*, flank; *tomē*, section). An incision through the abdominal wall.

la·pis (L.). A stone.

lardā·cĕin (L. *lardum*, lard). A protein substance seen in tissues affected with amyloid degeneration.

lardā·ceous (L. *lardum*, lard). Amyloid or lard-like. **L. degeneration:** a condition characterized by the presence of lardacein deposits in the tissues. Also called amyloid degeneration.

Larrey's amputation (Larrey, J. D., French surgeon, 1766–1842). Method of disarticulation of the humerus at the shoulder joint.

larva (L.). In lower animals undergoing metamorphosis, such as insects, the shape after emergence from the egg. **L. migrans:** creeping disease, *q.v.*

lar·val. 1. Relating to or existing as a larva. 2. Larvate.

lar·vate (L. *larva*, ghost). Concealed; masked; applied to the less obvious forms of a disease.

laryn·geal (G. *larugx*, larynx). Relating to the larynx. **L. crisis:** acute laryngeal spasm due to tabes dorsalis.

laryngec·tomy (G. *larugx*, larynx; *ektomē*, excision). Surgical removal of the larynx.

laryngis·mus. Laryngeal spasm. **L. stridulus:** laryngeal spasm due to infantile tetany, characterized by sudden apnoea followed by crowing inspiration.

laryngī·tis (G. *larugx*, larynx). Inflammation of the larynx.

laryn·gocele (G. *larugx*, larynx; *kēlē*, hernia). A diverticulum of the laryngeal mucosa at the cricothyroid space.

lă·ryngocentē·sis (G. *larugx*, larynx; *kentēsis*, a pricking.) Puncture of the larynx.

laryn·gofis·sure (G. *larugx*, larynx; L. *findere*, to separate). Surgical division of the larynx to remove growths of the vocal cords.

laryn·gograph (G. *larugx*, larynx; *graphein*, to write). An instrument for recording laryngeal movements.

laryngolŏ·gical (G. *larugx*, larynx; *logos*, a discourse). Pertaining to laryngology.

laryngŏ·logist (G. *larugx*, larynx; *logos*, a discourse). A specialist in laryngology.

laryngŏ·logy (G. *larugx*, larynx; *logos*, a discourse). The science of the anatomy and diseases of the larynx.

laryn·gopară·lysis (G. *larugx*, larynx; *paralusis*, paralysis). Paralysis of the muscles of the larynx.

laryngŏ·pathy (G. *larugx*, larynx; *pathos*, disease). Any laryngeal disease.

laryngophan·tom (G. *larugx*, larynx; *phantasma*, phantom). An artificial larynx constructed for didactic purposes.

laryn·gopharyn·geal (G. *larugx*, larynx; *pharugx*, pharynx). Relating to both the larynx and pharynx.

laryn·gopharyngi·tis (G. *larugx*, larynx; *pharugx*, pharynx). Inflammation of the larynx and the pharynx.

laryn·gophă·rynx (G. *larugx*, larynx; *pharugx*, pharynx). The inferior section of the pharynx.

laryngŏ·phony (G. *larugx*, larynx; *phonē*, voice). The sound of the voice as heard on auscultation of the larynx.

laryn·gophthī·sis (G. *larugx*, larynx; *phthisis*, consumption). Tuberculosis of the larynx.

laryn·goplasty (G. *larugx*, larynx; *plassein*, to form). Plastic surgery of the larynx.

lă·ryngoplē·gia (G. *larugx*, larynx; *plēgē*, stroke). Paralysis of the muscles of the larynx.

laryn·gorhinŏ·logy (G. *larugx*, larynx; *rhis*, nose; *logos*, a treatise). Laryngology and rhinology together.

laryngorrhă·gia (G. *larugx*, larynx; *rhegnunai*, to break). Haemorrhage from the larynx.

lă·ryngorrhoe·a (G. *larugx*, larynx; *rhoia*, flow). Excessive secretion of the laryngeal mucosa.

laryn·gosclerŏ·ma (G. *larugx*, larynx; *skleros*, hard). Scleroma of the larynx.

laryn·goscope (G. *larugx*, larynx; *skopein*, to view). A long-handled mirror for examination of the interior of the larynx.

laryn·goscopy (G. *larugx*, larynx; *skopein*, to view). Inspection of the interior of the larynx by a laryngoscope.

laryn·gospasm (G. *larugx*, larynx; *spasmos*, contraction). Spasmodic contraction of the glottis.

laryn·gostenō·sis (G. *larugx*, larynx; *stenos*, narrow). Constriction of the larynx.

laryn·gostrŏ·boscope (G. *larugx*, larynx; *strobos*, a whirling; *skopein*, to view). A laryngoscope combined with an adjustable and intermittent source of illumination, used for observing the vibration of the vocal bands.

laryngŏ·tomy (G. *larugx*, larynx; *tomē*, section). Incision of the larynx.

laryn·gotrachĕi·tis (G. *larugx*, larynx; *trakhus*, rough). Inflammation of both the larynx and trachea.

laryn·gotrachĕŏ·tomy (G. *larugx*, larynx; *trakhus*, rough; *tomē*, section). Laryngotomy with section of the upper tracheal rings.

lă·rynx (G. *larugx*). The voice organ, situated between the trachea and the pharynx.

lasci·via (L.). Excessive libido.

lasci·vious (L. *lascivus*). Excessively libidinous.

Lasègue's sign (Lasègue, E. C., French physician, 1816–83). Test for sciatica. Pain caused by stretching the sciatic nerve. The hip is flexed with the knee held in full extension.

lash. 1. An eyelash. 2. A flagellum.

Lassar's paste (Lassar, O., German dermatologist, 1849–1908). A paste composed of salicylic acid 30 gr., zinc oxide and powdered starch each 6 dr., white soft paraffin 13 dr. It is used in the treatment of erythema intertrigo.

las·situde (L. *lassus*, weary). Weakness not due to over-exertion.

Latarget's nerve (Latarget, A., French anatomist, born 1877). The presacral sympathetic nerve. L.'s vein: the prepyloric vein.

lă·tency (L. *latēre*, to lurk). 1. The state of being latent. 2. The state of apparent inactivity between stimulation of a tissue and its response.

lă·tent (L. *latēre*, to lurk). Not manifest; potential. L. heat: the amount of heat necessary to convert 1 gramme of solid to liquid at the melting point (latent heat of fusion) or 1 gramme of liquid to vapour at the boiling point (latent heat of vaporisation). L. jaundice: hyperbilirubinaemia without visible jaundice of skin or mucous membrane. L. period: (1) the incubation period; (2) the period between stimulation and the corresponding reaction.

lă·tera (L.). Pl. of *latus*, a side.

lă·terad (L. *latus*, side; *ad*, to). Towards the lateral aspect.

lă·teral (L. *latus*, side). At or belonging to the side; away from the median plane. L. column: a column of white matter in each half of the spinal cord situated between dorsal and ventral nerve root fibres. L. pyramidal tract: a tract situated in the distal part of the l. column, *q.v.*, originating from the Betz cells, *q.v.*, of the motor cortex in the Rolandic area, *q.v.*, and ending in the lowest segment of the sacral cord. L. sclerosis, amyotrophic: a chronic disease of the spinal cord characterized by progressive atrophic paresis of the lower limbs, often terminated by bulbar paralysis; due to degeneration of the pyramidal tracts and anterior horn cells. L. sclerosis, primary: an apparently idiopathic chronic disease of the spinal cord, characterized by spastic paraplegia due to degeneration of the l. pyramidal tracts. L. sclerosis, secondary: spastic paraplegia due to some disease affecting the l. pyramidal tracts. L. sinuses: the two veins at the caudal and ventral portions of the cranial cavity between the two layers of the tentorium cerebelli along its attached border. L. ventricle: The space in each cerebral hemisphere filled with cerebrospinal fluid, representing the neural canal.

lă·teris (L.). Genitive of *latus*, side.

lateri·tious, lateri·ceous (L. *later*, brick). Brick-like; of the colour of bricks, e.g. the l. sediment in urine.

lă·teroflex·ion (L. *latus*, side; *flectere*, to bend). A bending to one side.

lă·teropul·sion (L. *latus*, side; *pellere*, to drive). Inability to arrest suddenly the gait on walking sideways, a sign of Parkinson's disease.

lă·terotor·sion (L. *latus*, side; *torquere*, to twist). A twisting to one side.

lă·terover·sion (L. *latus*, side; *vertere*, to turn). A turning to one side.

Latham's circle (Latham, P. M., English physician, 1789–1875). The area on the chest wall corresponding to the area of pericardial dullness.

lă·thyrism (G. *lathuros*, vetchling). Poisoning from the ingestion of certain vetches, e.g. *Lathyrus sativus*, occurring usually through eating adulterated cereals.

latis·simus (L. *latissimus*, superl. of *lātus*, wide). Widest.

latrine (L. *latrina*, or *lavatrina*, water-closet). A water-closet or privy, especially one in the form of a trough which can accommodate several persons at the same time.

lātus¹ (L.). Side.

lātus² (L.). Broad.

lau·danum (Pers. *ladum*, a shrub). Tincture of opium.

laugh. The act of laughter.

laughing gas. Nitrous oxide.

laughter. The sounds involuntarily made to express appreciation of the amusing or of the ridiculous.

Laugier's hernia (Laugier, S., French surgeon, 1799–1872). A form of femoral hernia in which the sac passes through a gap in Gimbernat's ligament.

Laumonier's ganglion (Laumonier, J. B., French surgeon, 1749–1818). The carotid ganglion.

Laura's nucleus (Laura, G. B., Italian anatomist of the 19th century). Deiter's nucleus.

Lauth's canal (Lauth, E. A., Strasbourg physiologist, 1803–37). The canal of Schlemm. L.'s sinus: the sinus venosus sclerae of Schlemm.

Lauth's ligament (Lauth, T., Strasbourg surgeon, 1758–1826). Lauth's name is given, mostly by German writers, to many ligaments including the lateral odontoid ligaments, the cervical portion of the anterior common ligament, the subpubic ligament and the medial ligament of the ankle joint.

lă·vage (L. *lavare*, to wash). Irrigation of an organ. L., colonic: irrigation of the lower bowel.

law. 1. The statement of a fact assumed to occur uniformly. 2. A rule of action prescribed by authority.

lă·xative (L. *laxare*, to slacken). Aperient; a mild purgative.

laxā·tor (L. *laxare*, to slacken). That which loosens. The term is applied to various muscles, e.g. l. tympani, which loosen or relax.

lă·xus (L., slack). Lax; slack; not tense; e.g. cutis laxa.

layer. A mass of nearly uniform thickness. L., cortical: the cerebral cortex.

layette. The clothing outfit of a newly born infant.

lb. Abbreviation for *libra*, Latin for pound.

L.D.S. Licentiate in Dental Surgery.

lead¹. See Plumbum. L. colic: lead-poisoning characterized by severe paroxysmal abdominal pains and obstinate constipation. L. encephalopathy: that form of l. poisoning characterized by morbid symptoms of the central nervous system, such as epileptiform convulsions, acute mania, delirium, coma, etc. L.-poisoning: acute or (usually) chronic poisoning from ingestion or inhalation of lead as contained in dust particles on the hands or in the air.

lead². An electrocardiographic record. L., direct: l. in which one or both contacts are applied directly to the heart muscle. L., indirect: l. in which both contacts are applied to the limbs or to another part at a distance from the heart.

leather-bottle stomach. See linitis plastica.

Leber's corpuscles (Leber, T., German ophthalmologist, 1840–1917). Gierke's corpuscles, *q.v.* L.'s disease: hereditary optic atrophy. L.'s plexus: a plexus of venules between Schlemm's canal and the spaces of Fontana.

Lecat's gulf (Lecat, C. N., French surgeon, 1700–68). The dilatation of the bulbous portion of the urethra.

lĕ·cithin (G. *lekithos*, the inner part of pulse (plant)). A phosphatide occurring in various animal and vegetable tissues.

lĕ·cithinase. An enzyme hydrolyzing lecithin.

lec·tulum (L. *lectus*, a bed). The nail-bed.

Lee's ganglion (Lee, R., English physician, 1793–1877). The sympathetic ganglion of the cervix uteri.

leech. 1. A blood-sucking worm belonging to the class of Hirudinea. 2. An obsolete term for physician.

Leeuwenhoek's canals (Leeuwenhoek, A. van, Dutch microscopist, 1632–1723). The canals in bone now known as the Haversian canals.

leg. The lower extremity, especially from the knee downwards.

Legal's disease (Legal, E., German physician, 1859–1922). Cephalalgia pharyngotympanica; characterized by paroxysmal pains of the scalp in the area of the auriculotemporal nerve.

Le Gendre's nodosities. Bouchard's nodosities, *q.v.*

legi·timacy (L. *legitimus*, lawful). The condition of being legitimate.

legi·timate (L. *legitimus*). 1. Lawful. 2. Born in lawful wedlock.

Legroux's remissions (Legroux, T. de). Lengthy remissions which may occur in the course of phthisis.

legume. The pod (which may be edible) or fruit of leguminous plants, such as beans or peas.

legū·minous. Belonging to the family of Leguminosae, or pulses.

Leiner's disease (Leiner, K., Austrian paediatrician, 1871–1930). See erythroderma desquamativa.

leioder·mia (G. *leiŏs*, smooth; *derma*, skin). Unusual smoothness of the skin.

lei·omȳō·ma (G. *leios*, smooth; *mus*, muscle). A tumour composed of unstriped muscle fibres.

lei·omyosarcō·ma (G. *leios*, smooth; *mus*, muscle; *sarx*, flesh). A tumour composed of unstriped muscle-fibres and sarcomatous cells.

leiŏ·trichy (G. *leios*, smooth; *thrix*, hair). The condition of having straight hair.

Leishman's cells (Leishman, Sir W., Director General R.A.M.C., 1865–1926). Granular basophil leucocytes noted in blackwater fever. **L.'s stain:** a Romanowsky stain widely used for blood.

Leishman-Donovan bodies (Leishman, Sir W., English pathologist 1865–1926; Donovan, C., Irish surgeon, born 1863). Small parasitic bodies found in the liver and spleen of patients with kala-azar.

Leishmā·nia. Genus of Trypanosomidae consisting of *L. Donovani*, the cause of kala-azar *L. tropica*.

Leiter's coil (Leiter, J., Austrian instrument-maker, d. 1892). A flexible metallic tube for bending about any part of the body. Cold water is passed through it to reduce the temperature of the parts encased.

lem·mocyte (G. *lemma*, husk; *kutos*, cell). A cell derived from the neural crest, the precursor of the neurilemma cell. Syn. lemnocyte.

lemnis·cus (G. *lēmniskos*, fillet). 1. A band; a bow. 2. A band of longitudinal sensory fibres extending from the medulla and pons to the thalamus. Syn. fillet.

lem·noblast (G. *lemma*, husk; *blastos*, germ). A primitive lemmocyte.

lemon. The fruit of the *Citrus medica*, used mainly as a flavouring agent.

Lenhossek's fibres (Lenhossek, J. von, Austrian anatomist, 1818–88). The formatio reticularis.

Lenhossek's processes (Lenhossek, M. von, Austrian anatomist, 1863–1937). The short processes of ganglion cells. **L.'s stria:** the stria alba tuberis of the corpora mamillaria.

lĕ·niceps (L. *lenis*, mild; *capere*, to seize). An obstetric forceps with short handles.

lĕ·nient, lĕ·nitive (L. *lenis*, mild). Emollient; demulcent.

Lennander's incision (Lennander, K. G., Swedish surgeon, 1857–1908). A paramedian abdominal incision, in which the rectus muscle is retracted laterally.

Lenoir's facet (Lenoir, C. A. H., French surgeon, born 1867). A facet on the medial surface of the patella.

lens (L., lentil). 1. A piece of transparent material with a regular curvature of one or both of its surfaces, used for conveying or diffusing light rays. 2. The crystalline lens of the eye, a biconvex transparent disc lying in its capsule behind the pupil.

lenticō·nus (L. *lens*, lentil; *conus*, cone). A congenital malformation of the lens, characterized by a conical prominence upon its anterior or posterior surface.

lenti·cula (L. dim. of *lens*, lentil). A freckle.

lenti·cular. 1. Relating to a lens. 2. Relating to the crystalline lens. 3. Shaped like a lentil. 4. Relating to the lenticular nucleus of the brain. **L. degeneration, progressive:** Hepatolenticular degeneration. **L. nucleus:** one of the basal ganglia of the brain, the lateral portion of the corpus striatum.

lenti·culo-op·tic (L. *lens*, lentil; G. *optikos*, of or for sight). Relating to the lenticular nucleus and the thalamus.

lenti·culostrī·ate (L. *lens*, lentil; *stria*, a furrow). Relating to the lenticular nucleus of the corpus striatum. **L.-s. artery:** one of the branches of the middle cerebral artery, the artery involved in vascular lesions of the internal capsule of the brain.

len·tiform (L. *lens*, lentil; *forma*, shape). 1. Shaped like a lentil. 2. Shaped like a lens.

lenti·go (L. *lentigo*, freckle). A freckle; a small circumscribed pigmented spot, occurring commonly on the face and the backs of the hands, caused by exposure to the sun, but rarely also of congenital origin.

Leonardo da Vinci (Italian artist, 1452–1519). The moderator band, structure first named by King in 1837, had been figured by Leonardo da Vinci.

leonti·asis (G. *leōn*, lion). A lion-like aspect of the face, as in 1. ossea and in the nodular form of leprosy. **L. ossea** or **L. ossium:** hyperostosis of the cranial bones (especially of the facial and maxillary bones) giving the face a lion-like appearance.

lĕ·per (G. *lepros*, scabby). A person affected with leprosy.

lepid·ic (G. *lepis*, scale (rind)). Relating to scales.

lĕ·pidoid (G. *lepis*, scale; *eidos*, form). Resembling a scale; squamous.

Lepidop·tera (G. *lepis*, scale; *ptĕron*, wing). A class of insects which includes moths and butterflies.

lepidō·sis (G. *lepis*, scale). Ichthyosis, *q.v.*

lĕ·pothrix (G. *lepos*, rind; *thrix*, hair). Fungus causing a mycotic affection in which the hairs, especially of the axillae or the pubic area, are surrounded by irregular masses of concretions. Syn. trichomycosis.

leprapho·bia (G. *lepros*, scabby; *phobos*, fear). A neurotic fear of becoming leprous.

leprosa·rium, lep·rosary (L. from G. *lepros*, scabby). A hospital or colony for lepers.

lep·rosy (G. *lepros*, scabby). An endemic, slowly progressing, systemic disease, characterized by granulomatous lesions in the skin and mucous membranes (nodular form) or in the peripheral nerves with pigmentary changes in the skin (anaesthetic form); caused by the *Bacillus leprae*.

lep·rous. Affected with or relating to leprosy.

leptan·dra (G. *leptos*, thin; *anēr*, man). The dried rhizome and roots of *Veronica virginica*. Cholagogue which is supposed to take effect without irritating the bowels.

leptā·zol. Synthetic substance $C_6H_{10}N_4$, used as a cardiac stimulant by virtue of its action in increasing coronary flow.

leptocĕ·phaly (G. *leptos*, slender; *kephalē*, head). Abnormal narrowness of the head; dolichocephaly with premature closure of the frontal and sphenoparietal sutures.

leptochrō·a (G. *leptos*, slender; *khroia*, skin). Abnormal sensitiveness of the skin.

leptochȳ·mia (G. *leptos*, slender; *khūmos*, juice). Condition characterized by abnormally diminished body fluids.

lep·tomenin·ges (G. *leptos*, narrow; *mēnigx*, membrane). The pia and the arachnoid.

lep·tomeningi·tis (G. *leptos*, narrow; *mēnigx*, membrane). Inflammation of the pia and arachnoid of the brain and/or the spinal cord.

leptŏ·prosope (G. *leptos*, narrow; *prosōpon*, face). A person with a long and narrow face.

lep·toprosŏ·pia (G. *leptos*, narrow; *prosōpon*, face). Narrowness of the face; the condition of having a facial index, *q.v.*, below 50.

lep·torrhĭ·nia (G. *leptos*, narrow; *rhis*, nose). Narrowness of the nasal bone; the condition of having a nasal index, *q.v.*, below 48.

lep·tosome (G. *leptos*, narrow; *soma*, body). 1. Asthenic physique. 2. An asthenic individual.

Leptospi·ra (G. *leptos*, narrow; *speira*, coil). A genus of spirochaetes. **L. icterohaemorrhagiae**: the spirochaete causing Weil's disease.

Lep·tothrix (G. *leptos*, narrow, *thrix*, hair). 1. A genus of bacteria. 2. A genus of fungi.

leptotri·chia (G. *leptos*, narrow; *thrix*, hair). 1. Abnormal fineness and delicacy of the hair. 2. Leptothrix, *q.v.*

Leptus (G. *leptos*, narrow). A genus of beetles. **L. autumnalis**: the harvest bug, a parasite which burrows under the skin, producing itching papules and wheals. A term often incorrectly used as the generic name of micro-organisms taking unbranched filamentous forms, the principle members of which are now grouped as Leptothricia.

lerē·sis (G.). Insane or senile loquacity.

les·bian love (Named from the island of *Lesbos*). Sexual relations between women.

lē·sion (L. *laesio*, a hurting) An injury, wound or morbid change in living tissue.

Lesser's triangle. A space bounded above by the hypoglossal nerve and below by the anterior and posterior bellies of the digastric muscle.

Lesshaft's muscle (Lesshaft, P. F., Russian anatomist, 1836–1909). 1. The levator ani proprius. 2. The subcutaneous m. perinei. **L.'s triangle**: the fascial triangle of Grynfelt.

lē·thal (L. *letum*, death). Fatal; relating to or producing death.

lethă·lity (L. *letum*, death). The ratio between those who have died from and those who have been affected by any particular disease.

lethar·gic (G. *lēthargia*, drowsiness). Relating to or affected with lethargy.

lĕ·thargy (G. *lēthargia*, drowsiness). Drowsiness; somnolence; stupor.

leucaē·mia (G. *leukos*, white; *haima*, blood). Leukaemia, *q.v.*

leucanae·mia (G. *leukos*, white; *an*, neg; *haima*, blood). Leukanaemia, *q.v.*

leu·cine (G. *leukos*, white). An amino-acid found in the urine in severe hepatic insufficiency.

Leuckart's canal (Leuckart, K. G. F. R., German anatomist, 1823–98). The uterovaginal canal, formed by the fusion of Müller's ducts in the embryo.

leuco-bases (G. *leukos*, white; *basis*, foundation). A group of colourless compounds, derived from triphenylmethane, produced by the reduction of certain dyes.

leū·cocyte (G. *leukos*, white; *kutos*, cell). The colourless or white blood corpuscles. The term comprises the cells of both the myeloid, and monocytic lymphatic series. **L., basophil**: a l. of the myeloid series possessing basophil granules scattered over the cytoplasm. **L., eosinophil**: a l. of the myeloid series possessing eosinophil granules scattered over the cytoplasm. **L., neutrophile, polymorphonuclear**: end product of the myeloid series of leucocytes, characterized by a nucleus subdivided into 2 to 5 (or more) lobes which are connected by fine filaments and having neutrophil granules scattered over the cytoplasm. See also lymphocyte, monocyte, myelocyte, metamyelocyte and stab-cell.

leu·cocythae·mia (G. *leukos*, white; *kutos*, cell; *haima*, blood). Leukaemia, *q.v.*

leucocȳt·ic. Relating to leucocytes.

leū·cocytogen·esis (G. *leukos*, white; *kutos*, cell; *genesis*, production). The formation of leucocytes.

leū·cocytŏ·lysis (G. *leukos*, white; *kutos*, cell; *lusis*, a loosening). The destruction of leucocytes.

leū·cocyto·meter (G. *leukos*, white; *kutos*, cell; *metron*, measure). A haemocytometer, *q.v.*, for counting leucocytes.

leū·cocytopē·nia. Leucopenia, *q.v.*

leū·cocytō·sis (G. *leukos*, white; *kutos*, cell). An increase in the number of white blood corpuscles in the bone-forming tissues and in the peripheral blood.

leū·cocytū·ria (G. *leukos*, white; *kutos*, cell; *ouron*, urine). Pyuria.

leucoder·ma, leucoder·mia (G. *leukos*, white; *derma*, skin). A chronic condition characterized by the loss or absence of normal pigmentation of patches of skin, surrounded by areas of increased pigmentation.

leuco·erythroblastō·sis (G. *leukos*, white; *eruthros*, red; *blastos*, germ). A clinical syndrome characterized by anaemia, the presence of immature red cells and of some immature white cells of the myeloid series in the peripheral blood, caused mainly by osseous metastases of carcinoma, by osteosclerosis due to marble-bone disease or by myelosclerosis. Syn. osteosclerotic anaemia; L.-e. anaemia.

leū·cokeratō·sis (G. *leukos*, white; *keras*, horn). Leucoplakia, *q.v.*

leucō·ma (G. *leukŏn*, white of egg). A white opacity of the cornea.

leū·comaine (G. *leukŏn*, white of an egg). Term applied to several toxic nitrogen compounds formed in animal tissues. See also ptomaine.

leū·comatō·sis (G. *leukos*, white). The development of opaque spots, e.g. in the cornea.

leucŏ·matous (G. *leukos*, white). Having the nature of or affected with leucoma.

Leuconos·toc. A genus of Streptococceae.

leuconū·clĕin (G. *leukos*, white; L. *nucula*, a small nut). A decomposition-product of nucleohiston.

leuconȳ·chia (G. *leukos*, white; *onux*, finger-nail). A whitish discoloration of the nails.

leucŏ·pathy (G. *leukos*, white; *pathos*, disease). Any deficiency of pigmentation; albinism. See also leucoderma.

leucopē·nia (G. *leukos*, white; *pĕnia*, poverty). An abnormal decrease in the number of leucocytes in the blood.

leucop·sin (G. *leukos*, white; *ōps*, eye). Visual white; the colourless material derived from rhodopsin by the action of light.

leucoplă·kia (G. *leukos*, white; *plax*, flat land). A chronic affection of the tongue, or of the buccal or genital mucous membrane, characterized by circumscribed, slightly raised patches of greyish-white colour, due to hypertrophy of the epidermis and papillae; sometimes leading to cancerous degeneration. L. of the tongue may be a manifestation of syphilis.

leucoplă·sia. Leucoplakia, *q.v.*

leu·coplast, leucoplas·tid (G. *leukos*, white; *plassein*, to form). A colourless cytoplasmic body, present especially in embryonic plant tissues.

leu·copoïe·sis (G. *leukos*, white; *poiein*, to make). Formation of white blood corpuscles.

leucorrhoe·a (G. *leukos*, white; *rhoia*, flow). A white-coloured mucopurulent discharge from the vagina and uterine canal.

leucŏ·sis (G. *leukos*, white). 1. Leukaemia. 2. Leucomatosis.

leucotac·tic (G. *leukos*, white; *taxis*, arrangement). Relating to leucotaxis.

leucotax·is (G. *leukos*, white; *taxis*, arrangement). Chemotaxis of leucocytes.

leucŏ·tomy (G. *leukos*, white; *tomē*, section). Division of some of the prefrontal fibres in the brain. Performed in certain mental conditions.

leucotrĭ·chia (G. *leukos*, white; *thrix*, hair). Greyness of the hair. Syn. canities.

Leudet's bruit (Leudet, T. E., French physician, 1825–87; Fr. *bruit*, noise). A delicate crackling snap in the ear which is audible in certain affections of the ear.

leukaē·mia (G. *leukos*, white; *haima*, blood). An acute or chronic progressive disease of the tissues forming leucocytes, characterized by the permanent presence of immature leucocytes in the peripheral blood, by excessive numbers of such cells in the bone-forming tissues, by the infiltration of other organs with these cells, by some degree of anaemia, by haemorrhages into the skin and mucous membranes; with or without considerable increase in the total number of leucocytes in the blood and bone-marrow. **L., aleukaemic:** a form or stage of l. in which the total number of white corpuscles in the peripheral blood is not increased or is below the normal. **L. cutis:** lesions of the skin associated with and due to leukaemia. **L., lymphoid** or **L., lymphatic:** the form of l. characterized by the proliferation of cells of the lymphatic series of leucocytes, by progressive enlargement of lymph glands and moderate enlargement of the spleen. Syn. L. lymphadenosis. **L., myeloid** or **L., myelogenic:** the form of l. characterized by proliferation of the myeloid series of leucocytes and by progressive enlargement of the spleen. Syn. L. myelosis. **L., monocytic:** the form of l. characterized by proliferation of the leucocytes derived from the monoblast.

leukaē·mic (G. *leukos*, white; *haima*, blood). Relating to leukaemia.

leukaē·moid (G. *leukos*, white; *haima*, blood; *eidos*, form). Resembling leukaemia.

leukanaē·mia (G. *leukos*, white; *an*, neg.; *haima*, blood). An obsolete term; it was mainly applied to conditions now classified as leuco-erythroblastosis or as aleukaemic leukaemia.

levā·tor (L. *levare*, to lift). 1. That which raises or elevates; term applied to certain muscles fulfilling such function. 2. An instrument used for lifting a depressed part.

lĕ·vel. Flat; in a straight line.

levigā·tion (L. *lēvigare*, to make smooth). The grinding of a substance in water followed by fractional sedimentation.

Lewin's erythema of the larynx. Syphilitic catarrh of the larynx.

Lexer's vessels (Lexer, E., German surgeon, 1867–1937). The juxta-epiphyseal vessels.

Leyden's ataxia (Leyden, E. V. von, German physician, 1832–1910). A disease which simulates tabes dorsalis.

Leyden-Charcot's crystals. Charcot's crystals, *q.v.*

Leyden-Moebius's type of progressive muscular atrophy (Leyden, E. V. von, German physician, 1832–1910; Moebius, P. J., German physician, 1853–1907). A variety of progressive muscular atrophy starting in the calves and often assuming the character of Duchenne's pseudo-hypertrophic paralysis.

Leydig's cells (Leydig, F. von, German anatomist, 1821–1908). The interstitial cells of the testis. **L.'s duct:** the Wolffian duct.

Li. The symbol for an atom of lithium.

libĭ·dinous (L. *libido*, desire). Characterized by sexual desire.

libĭ·do (L.). Sexual desire.

LiBr. Formula for one molecule of lithium bromide.

li·bra (L.). A pound. A weight of twelve troy ounces (5760 grammes). Also applied to the avoirdupois pound of 16 ounces (7000 grammes).

li·chen (G. *leikhēn*, lichen). A term applied to skin diseases characterized by the presence of papular or follicular eruptions. **L. acuminatus:** pityriasis rubra pilaris. A serious skin disease with a papulosquamous eruption. **L. annularis:** 1. planus characterized by an annular arrangement of the lesions. **L. atrophicus:** atrophic form of l. planus. **L. hypertrophicus:** hypertrophied form of l. planus. **L. nitidus:** a skin disease of perhaps tuberculous origin, characterized by numerous small flat-topped papules and nodules of granulomatous tissue, giving rise to little irritation. **L. obtusus corneus:** the same as prurigo. **L. pilaris:** a non-irritating skin disease, occurring especially in children characterized by patches of filiform spines projecting from small pinkish papules which originate from the hair follicles; a form of keratosis of the upper part of the hair follicles. **L. planus:** a skin disease characterized by small irregular, bluish-red, flat-topped, sometimes umbilicated papules giving rise to severe itching, occurring singly or arranged in groups, rings, etc., especially at the flexor aspects of the extremities, but often involving also other areas of the skin and the mucous membranes of the mouth, upper airways, rectum and vagina. At the latter parts they appear in whitish streaks and patches. **L. sclerosis:** a skin disease perhaps related to scleroderma, characterized by sharply defined white spots with follicular plugs and sometimes with thick scales. **L. scrofulosorum:** a tuberculide, characterized by minute reddish papules arranged in groups but tending to become generalized, occurring especially on the trunk. **L. simplex chronicus:** lichenification, *q.v.*, of itching affections of the skin. **L. spinosulus:** L. pilaris, *q.v.* **L. verrucosus:** warty form of l. planus. **L. urticatus:** Urticaria papulosa, *q.v.*

licheni·asis (G. *leikhēn*, lichen). 1. The formation of lichen. 2. The condition of a person suffering from lichen.

li·chenificā·tion (G. *leikhen*, lichen; L. *facere*, to make). The development of hyperkeratosis and infiltration of the papillary layer, producing thickening and roughening of the skin, from long-continued scratching of itching affections of the skin.

li·chenoid (G. *leikhēn*, lichen; *eidos*, form). Resembling lichen.

Lieberkühn's crypts (Lieberkühn, J. N., German anatomist, 1711–56). Intestinal glands which are found in large numbers over the whole of the mucous membrane of the small intestine, as well as that of the large bowel.

liēn (L.). The spleen.

li·enal. Relating to the spleen.

lienec·tomy (L. *liēn*, spleen; G. *ektomē*, excision). Excision of the spleen.

lieni·tis (L. *lien*, spleen). Inflammation of the spleen.

liē·nocle (L. *lien*, spleen; G. *kēlē*, hernia). Splenic hernia.

li·enun·culus (L. *lienunculus*, dim. of *lien*, spleen). An accessory spleen.

lientĕ·ric. Relating to lientery.

lī·entery (G. *leios*, smooth; *enteron*, intestine). A form of disturbed bowel function in which ingestion of food causes reflex bowel-movement. Syn. lienteric diarrhoea.

Lieutaud's sinus (Lieutaud, J., French physician, 1703–80). A connecting channel between the inferior longitudinal sinus and the lateral sinus. **L.'s triangle:** the trigonum vesicae.

life. 1. The totality of physico-chemical processes with which the maintenance of an individual as an organism is connected. 2. The period between birth and death.

lī·gament (L. *ligare*, to bind). 1. A structure mainly or entirely composed of connective tissue connecting skeletal or other parts. 2. Folds of the peritoneum. **Acromioclavicular:** a comparatively strong ligament which extends transversely from the superior surface of the acromium to the lateral extremity of the clavicle. **Annular:** (orbicular) is a strong fibrous band that forms four-fifths of a circle and surrounds the circumference of the head of the radius which it retains in contact with the radial notch. Its extremities are attached to the anterior and posterior margins of the radial notch. **Anterior atlanto-axial:** a broad, thin, membranous band which is attached superiorly along the inferior margin of the anterior arch of the atlas, and inferiorly to the anterior aspect of the body of the axis. **Anterior atlanto-occipital:** a thin membranous ligament attached inferiorly to the superior margin of the anterior arch of the atlas and superiorly to the inferior surface of the basilar part of the occipital bone. **Anterior longitudinal:** (anterior common ligament) is a dense band of white glistening fibres that extends over the anterior surfaces of the bodies of the vertebrae and intervertebral discs. It is continued from the axis to the first segment of the sacrum. **Anterior, of elbow joint:** a broad thin and weak ligament attached to the anterior aspect of the humerus above the coronoid and radial fossae and distally to the coronoid process of the ulna. **Anterior radiocarpal:** consists of two parts: the radial, a broad thick band of fibres that sweeps distally and to the ulnar side from the volar aspect of the distal end of the radius and its styloid process to the lunate, triquetral and capitate bones. The ulnar band is narrower, weaker, and more vertically disposed; it extends distally from the articular disc of the wrist to the triquetral and capitate bones. **Anterior radio-ulnar:** a loose and relatively weak ligament on the volar surfaces of the radius and ulna. **Anterior talo-fibular:** part of the lateral ligament of the ankle joint. It extends anteriorly and slightly towards the tibial side from the inferior part of the anterior border of the lateral malleolus to the fibular side of the neck of the talus. **Apical:** (middle odontoid ligament) is a narrow round cord attached inferiorly to the ridge of the head of the odontoid process, and superiorly to the anterior margin of the foramen magnum in the midline. **Arcuate:** (inferior pubic ligament or subpubic) is a strong, thick band of fibres, that lies at the antero-superior part of the pubic arch, where it fills up and rounds off the subpubic angle. It is attached superiorly to the lower part of the interpubic disc and laterally to the adjacent parts of the medial lips of the inferior pubic rami. **Bardinet's:** posterior part of the medial ligament of the elbow joint. It is attached proximally to the distal and posterior part of the medial epicondyle and distally to the medial margin of the olecranon process. **Bifurcated:** is situated in the foot. It is attached posteriorly to the superior surface of the neck of the calcaneum. It divides into two bands: of these, the fibular-sided band passes anteriorly to the cuboid, while the calcaneonavicular part passes anteriorly and towards the tibial side of the navicular bone. **Broad, uterine:** (alae vespertilionis) so called from their supposed resemblance to a bat's wings. Each is an extensive fold of peritoneum composed of two layers, anterior and posterior, which pass between the side of the uterus and the lateral wall of the pelvis. **Burns's:** the falciform border or free edge of the saphenous opening in the groin. **Caroticoclinoid:** a small band of fibres running between the middle and anterior clinoid processes of the sphenoid bone. **Calcaneofibular:** is the middle part of the lateral ligament of the ankle-joint. It is attached superiorly to the tip of the lateral malleolus, from which it passes inferiorly and with a posterior inclination to a tubercle on the fibular side of the calcaneum situated posterosuperiorly to the peroneal tubercle. **Cervical:** (ligamentum cervicis). The interosseous talocalcaneal ligament is a discrete and powerful band of union between the two bones. It is attached superiorly to a well-marked tubercle on the fibular side of the neck of the talus and inferiorly to a similar tubercle situated on the superior aspect of the neck of the calcaneum. **Cleland's:** (cutaneous ligaments of the digits) are the prolongations of the interdigital ligaments along the sides of the digits. **Conoid:** the medial and posterior part of the coracoclavicular ligament. It is attached inferiorly to the tubercle at the base of the coracoid process and, expanding in a fan-shaped manner, is attached above to the conoid tubercle on the inferior surface of the clavicle. **Cooper's:** (pectineal ligament) is a lateral extension of dense tendinous fibres from the base of the pectineal part of the inguinal ligament and passing along the pectineal line. **Coraco-acromial:** a triangular ligament attached by its apex to the tip of the acromion process and by its base to the postero-lateral border of the coracoid process. **Coracoclavicular:** consists of two parts: (a) the trapezoid ligament situated laterally and anterior to (b) the conoid ligament which lies medially and posterior. **Coracohumeral:** is a strong, thick band that strengthens the capsule of the shoulder joint in the interval between the tendons of the supraspinatus and infraspinatus. It is attached medially to the base of the coracoid process, inferior to the coraco-acromial ligament and passes laterally to the greater tuberosity of the humerus. **Cornuate:** see Burns's ligament; syn. Hey's ligament. **Coronary:** is part of the capsular ligament of the knee joint and extends from the semilunar cartilages to the tibia and serves to keep them in place. **Costocentral:** (radiate or stellate) the anterior costocentral ligament consists of strong white fibres that are attached to the anterior margin of the head of the rib. From this point the fibres radiate medially in three bands, one of which passes superiorly to be attached to the body of the superior vertebra, a second horizontally medially to be attached to the intervertebral disc, and a third inferiorly to be attached to the body of the inferior vertebra. **Costoclavicular:** (rhomboid) is attached inferiorly to the first costal cartilage and anterior extremity of the first rib. Superiorly it gains attachment to the rhomboid impression on the inferior surface of the medial end of the clavicle. **Costocoracoid:** is the upper part of the clavipectoral fascia extending from the sternal end of the first rib to the coracoid process. **Cricothyroid:** is the anterior portion of the cricovocal membrane, it is elastic and triangular and is attached by its base to the inferior border of the thyroid cartilage and by its apex to the superior border of the cricoid cartilage, close to the midline. **Cruciate:** is a composite ligament. The transverse portion is also known as the transverse ligament of the atlas and is attached on each side to the tubercle on the medial aspect of the lateral mass of the atlas.

It is arched posterior to the odontoid process and at the median line it is connected on the posterior aspect with the limbs of the vertical portion of the cruciate ligament. The vertical portion of the cruciate ligament consists of superior and inferior longitudinal bands. The superior band extends from the posterior surface of the transverse ligament at the midline to the posterior part of the basilar groove of the occipital bone. The inferior band extends from the posterior surface of the transverse ligament of the atlas at the midline to the posterior surface of the body of the axis. **Cutaneous:** of the digits. See Cleland's ligaments. **Deep gastric:** a fold of peritoneum extending from the base area of the liver to the lesser curvature of the stomach, it contains the left gastric artery and vein. **Deep transverse:** (foot) a band of fibres crossing the plantar aspect of the heads of all the metatarsal bones and connecting them together. It is adherent deeply to the capsular ligaments of the metatarsophalangeal joints. **Deep transverse:** (palm) ligaments connecting the heads of the four ulnar-sided metacarpals. These extend transversely across the palmar aspects of the heads and their fibres are attached to the fibrous plates on the palmar surfaces of the metacarpophalangeal joints. **Deltoid:** or medial ligament of the ankle joint. It is thick, flat and quadrangular. Superiorly it is attached to the inferior margin of the medial malleolus. The anterior fibres pass distally to the tuberosity of the navicular bone; the middle fibres are attached to the sustentaculum tali; the posterior fibres pass to the tubercle on the posterior aspect of the talus. **Dorsal calcaneocuboid:** is a flattened band that passes between the adjoining surfaces of the calcaneum and the cuboid bones of the foot. **Dorsal talonavicular:** is a thin fibrous sheet on the superior aspect of the joint. It is attached posteriorly to the superior surface of the head of the talus close to the edge of the articular surface, from which it sweeps antero-inferiorly to the superior surface of the navicular bone. **Epididymoscrotal:** the remains of the gubernaculum which extends from the tail of the epididymis and commencement of the vas deferens to the postero-inferior part of the scrotum. **Falciform, of liver:** (suspensory ligament) a peritoneal fold which extends between the inferior surface of the diaphragm and the posterior surface of the anterior abdominal wall on the one hand and the superior and anterior surfaces of the liver on the other. The base, which is free, extends from the umbilicus to the interlobar notch of the liver and contains its two layers the ligamentum teres. **Frondiform:** (Retzius). Part of the extensor retinaculi of the foot, the sling fibres which function as pulleys to preserve the position of the extensor tendons as they cross the ankle joint. **Funiculo-epididymal:** part of the tunica vaginalis which is attached to the head of the epididymis. **Gastrophrenic:** a reflection of peritoneum passing between the liver and the stomach. **Gastrosplenic:** peritoneal reflection attached by one extremity to the gastric impression of the spleen just in front of the hilum, the other extremity being connected with the cardiac end of the stomach on its posterior aspect. **Gimbernat's** (lacunar ligament): the pectineal part of the inguinal ligament is the reflection of the inguinal ligament from the pubic tubercle along the pectineal line. **Glenohumeral** ligaments are three bands of fibres, superior, middle, and inferior, that reinforce the capsule of the shoulder joint on its internal aspect. The superior glenohumeral ligament of Flood is attached medially to the superior part of the labrum glenoidale, laterally to the fovea capitis humeri. The middle glenohumeral ligament is attached medially to the anterior part of the labrum glenoidale and runs

downwards to be attached to the distal border of the lesser tuberosity of the humerus. The inferior glenohumeral ligament is the strongest of the three and reinforces the capsule inferiorly. It is attached medially to the anterior and inferior margins of the glenoid cavity and labrum glenoidale, it then runs transversely to be attached laterally to the medial side of the neck of the humerus. **Glenoid:** (labrum glenoidale) is a fibro-cartilaginous band attached to the periphery of the glenoid fossa which it helps to deepen. It is attached by its base to the margins of the glenoid fossa of the scapula. **Hesselbach's** (interfoveolar ligament): the semilunar expansion of the conjoint tendon which passes down to the deep femoral arch . **Hey's:** see Burns's ligament; syn. cornuate ligament. **Humphry's:** a small ligament which passes from the posterior part of the external semilunar cartilage to the anterior surface of the posterior cruciate ligament. **Hyo-epiglottic:** an elastic, semilunar membrane passing between the base of the epiglottis and the body of the hyoid bone. **Iliofemoral:** a very strong ligament which forms part of the capsule of the hip-joint. It is attached above to the lower part of the anterior inferior iliac spine. Distally it is attached to the upper and lower parts of the anterior intertrochanteric line of the femur. **Iliolumbar:** extends from the tip of the transverse process of the fifth lumbar vertebra to the medial lip of the iliac crest. It is triangular in shape, and its direction is laterally and slightly backward. **Iliotrochanteric** (band): part of the pubo-femoral ligament. **Inferior, of symphysis** (subpubic ligament): see arcuate ligament. **Inferior tibiofibular:** (anterior) is a thick and strong ligament which passes obliquely from the lower part of the anterior surface of the tibia to the fibula. **Inferior tibiofibular:** (posterior) is thicker and stronger than the anterior ligament. It also passes obliquely from the tibia to the fibula. **Infundibulopelvic:** (suspensory ligament of the ovary) a fold of peritoneum containing the ovarian vessels and nerves which passes from the broad ligament of the uterus to the peritoneum covering the psoas major muscle. **Inguinal:** (Poupart's) extends between the anterior superior iliac spine and the pubic tubercle. **Interclavicular:** is strong, acting as a tie ligament between the two clavicles. It is attached to the upper part of the posterior surface of both clavicles, near their medial extremities. **Intercornual:** passes between the sacral and coccygeal cornua on the posterior surface of the sacro-coccygeal articulation. **Interdigital:** these ligaments are a series of transverse fibres from the deep fascia and pass to the skin of the fingers. **Interfoveolar:** part of the conjoint tendon of the internal oblique and transversus abdominis muscles which passes down to the lower parts of the deep inguinal ring and is attached inferiorly to the deep femoral arch. **Interosseous naviculocuboid:** a very strong and thick ligament. It consists of short fibres, which, as a rule, completely fill the interval between the adjacent surfaces of the two bones. **Interosseous talocalcaneal:** see cervical ligament. **Interosseous tibiofibular:** consists of short fibres, that pass very obliquely from the rough triangular surface at the distal end of the tibia to the corresponding surface of the fibula. **Interspinous:** these ligaments which are thin and membranous, are situated between adjacent spinous processes, to the margins of which they are attached from root to tip. They are strongest in the lumbar region, and in the neck they are replaced by deep processes of the ligamentum nuchae. **Intertransverse:** these ligaments consist of scattered fibres, that pass between the extremities of the transverse processes in the thoracic and lumbar regions. In the neck they may be completely replaced by the intertransverse muscles. **Ischiofemoral:** is a triangular band on the posterior aspect of the hip joint. Its base is attached to the ischium close to the acetabular margin. The ligament passes across the posterior part of the capsule to be attached to the medial aspect of the greater trochanter of the femur. **Lacunar:** see Gimbernat's ligament. **Lateral arcuate:** is a thickening of the upper part of the anterior layer of the sheath of the quadratus lumborum muscle, and extends from the lower margin of the last rib to the front of the transverse process of the first lumbar vertebra. **Lateral, of elbow-joint:** consists of three bands attached proximally to the lateral epicondyle of the humerus. The *anterior* band passes distally to the coronoid process where it is attached immediately anterior to the radial notch. The *middle* band crosses the head of the radius and, inclining posteriorly, obtains attachment to the crest that forms the posterior limit of the radial notch. The *posterior* band, quadrilateral in shape, is attached distally to the radial border of the olecranon. **Lateral radiocarpal:** is a strong, flattened band that unites the tip of the styloid process of the radius to the tubercle of the scaphoid. **Lieno-phrenic:** (phrenicosplenic or suspensory ligament) is a fold of peritoneum which extends between the spleen, near its upper extremity and the adjacent part of the diaphragm. **Lienorenal:** a peritoneal ligament that extends from the hilum of the spleen to the front of the left kidney at its upper and lateral part. It contains the splenic branches of the splenic artery. **Lisfranc's:** (medial interosseous ligament of the medial tarsometatarsal joint). It extends anteriorly and towards the fibular side from the fibular side of the first cuneiform to the adjacent side of the base of the second metatarsal bone. **Lockwood's:** (suspensory ligament of the eyeball). A fascial shelf passing across the orbit beneath the globe of the eye. **Long lateral, of knee:** is a short rounded cord remarkably like a tendon in appearance. Attached proximally to the prominence on the lateral aspect of the lateral condyle of the femur it extends distally and posteriorly and is attached to the head of the fibula anterior to the styloid process. **Long medial, of knee:** is a long, broad, flattened band, about 4 inches long and $\frac{1}{2}$ an inch wide, attached proximally to a rough impression on the medial aspect of the medial condyle of the femur. It passes distally to be attached to the medial aspect of the shaft of the tibia. **Long plantar:** is the longest ligament in the foot. It clothes and is adherent to all the plantar surface of the calcaneum anterior to the two tubercles at the posterior part of the bone. From the calcaneum it passes to the plantar aspect of the cuboid, where it is adherent to the prominent ridge posterior to the peroneal groove. It passes anteriorly across the groove, and divides into slightly diverging bands that are attached to the bases of the second, third, and fourth metatarsal bones. **Lumbo-sacral:** extends from the lower aspect of the transverse process of the fifth lumbar vertebra anteriorly to the upper surface of the ala of the sacrum at its anterior and lateral part close to the sacro-iliac articulation. **Medial arcuate:** is a thickening of the upper part of the sheath of the psoas major muscle, and extends from the front of the transverse process of the first lumbar vertebra to the side of its body, and sometimes to that of the second vertebra. **Medial brachial:** (Struthers's) a fibrous band connected with the medial intermuscular septum of the arm, which extends from the humerus, distal to the tendon of attachment of the coracobrachialis, to the medial epicondyle. **Medial, of elbow joint:** is triangular with the apex proximal. It is attached at its proximal end to the medial epicondyle of the humerus and distally to the medial margin of the trochlear notch of the

ulna. **Medial radiocarpal:** is a rounded cord that extends from the tip of the styloid process of the ulna to the triquetral and pisiform bones. **Middle odontoid:** see apical. **Oblique, of Cooper:** the middle part of the medial ligament of the elbow joint, the fibres stretching from the olecranon process to the coronoid process. **Oblique posterior:** (Winslowii) of the knee joint is an expansion from the tendon of the semi-membranosus that extends proximally and towards the fibular side across the intercondylar notch and is attached to the lateral condyle of the femur. **Of Colles:** (triangular fascia); this is the reflected part of the inguinal ligament. Its fibres are derived from the external oblique aponeurosis of the opposite side; having crossed the linea alba they gain insertion into the pubic tubercle and crest. **Of Flood:** see gleno-humeral ligament. **Of head of femur:** (ligamentum teres) extends between the head of the femur and the acetabulum, and is, as regards its position, an intra-capsular structure. At one end it is attached by a relatively narrow flattened band to the small rough area interrupting the articular cartilage clothing the head of the femur. As it approaches the floor of the acetabulum it broadens into a triangular sheet, the margins of which are thickened bands attached on each side of the acetabular notch. **Of vena cava:** (vestigial fold of Marshall); a triangular fold of serous pericardium which is situated between the left pulmonary artery and the superior left pulmonary vein. Between its two layers there is a small fibrous cord, a vestige of the left duct of Cuvier. **Of Weit-brecht:** (chorda obliqua anterior); the oblique cord is a narrow band that inclines proximally and to the ulnar side from the distal and back part of the tuberosity of the radius to the tuberosity of the ulna. **Of Zinn:** is the inferior part of the common tendinous ring of the recti muscles in the orbit. It gives attachment to part of the rectus medialis, the rectus inferior, and the inferior head of the rectus lateralis. **Orbicular:** see annular. **Ovario-uterine:** (ligament of the ovary); a round cord containing plain muscle fibres extending from the ovary to the uterus. It represents the proximal portion of the gubernaculum testis of the male. **Peritoneal:** these are folds of peritoneum which connect viscera to the abdominal or pelvic parietes, or viscera of any kind to each other or to the diaphragm. **Petrosphenoidal:** a small ligament passing between the anterior part of the superior border of the temporal bone to the lateral border of the dorsum sellae of the sphenoid bone. **Phrenico-colic:** a fold of peritoneum passing from the region of the splenic flexure of the colon to the diaphragm opposite the tenth or eleventh left rib. It forms a platform upon which the colic surface of the spleen rests and is sometimes known as the sustentaculum lienis. **Phrenicosplenic:** see lienophrenic ligament. **Piso-hamate:** (pisometacarpal); a small ligament connecting the pisiform bone to the hook of the hamate bone. **Pisometacarpal:** see pisohamate. **Plantar calcaneo-navicular:** (spring) is attached posteriorly to the sustentaculum tali, and anteriorly to the plantar surface, to the tuberosity, and slightly to the dorsal surface of the navicular bone. **Posterior atlanto-axial:** is a broad, thin, membranous ligament which extends from the inferior aspect of the posterior arch of the atlas to the superior borders and adjacent portions of the lateral surfaces of the laminae of the axis. **Posterior, of elbow joint:** is thin and membranous. It is attached proximally to the margins of the olecranon fossa of the humerus and distally to the superior aspect of the olecranon process of the ulna and to the annular ligament of the radius. **Posterior longitudinal:** (posterior common ligament) is situated within the spinal canal, and extends over the posterior surfaces of the bodies of the vertebrae and intervertebral discs. It is broader superiorly, and consists of glistening fibres that extend from the axis to the first coccygeal vertebra. **Posterior occipito-axial:** (membrana tectoria) is a broad membranous band that is attached inferiorly to the posterior surface of the body of the axis, and superiorly to the posterior part of the basilar groove of the occipital bone. **Posterior radiocarpal:** is a broad thick ligament which consists of fibres that sweep distally and towards the ulnar side from the posterior border of the radius to the scaphoid, lunate and cuneiform bones. **Posterior radio-ulnar:** a loose and comparatively weak ligament attached to the adjacent portions of the radius and ulna in the region of the inferior radio-ulnar joint. **Posterior talofibular:** is the posterior bundle of the lateral ligament of the ankle joint. It is attached to the malleolar fossa of the fibula and passes backwards to the tubercle on the posterior aspect of the talus. **Poupart's:** see inguinal. **Pterygomandibular:** is a narrow band that extends from the hamulus of the medial pterygoid plate of the sphenoid bone to the posterior extremity of the mylohyoid line of the mandible close to the last molar socket. **Pterygospinous:** is a narrow band that extends from the sharp spine on the posterior border of the lateral pterygoid plate of the sphenoid bone, towards its upper part, to the spinous process of the sphenoid. This ligament is sometimes ossified. **Pubofemoral:** is a triangular band with its base attached to the ileopectineal eminence and to the superior pubic ramus. Its fibres converge towards and meet the ileofemoral ligament with which it is attached to the inferior tubercle of the neck of the femur. **Puboprostatic:** (medial) or anterior true ligaments of the bladder. Each is attached anteriorly to the posterior aspect of the body of the os pubis near the lower part of the symphysis and a little above the attachment of the anterior fibres of the levator ani. The fascial bands pass backwards to the sides of the prostate and bladder. **Pulmonary:** a fold of two layers of pleura in close apposition, which are continuous superiorly with the anterior and posterior pleural investments of the root of the lung. It extends, on the one hand, between the inferior border of the root of the lung and the diaphragm, to which it is attached, and, on the other hand, between the pericardium and the medial surface of the lung inferior to the level of the root. **Quadrate:** a loose fold of the capsule of the superior radio-ulnar joint extending from the medial side of the neck of the radius to the distal lip of the radial notch of the ulna. It contains some elastic fibres. **Radiate:** see costo-central, radiate or stellate. **Rhomboid:** see costo-clavicular. **Round:** (ligamentum teres) of the liver is a fibrous cord formed from the obliterated umbilical vein and is contained within the base of the falciform ligament between the umbilicus and the interlobar notch of the liver. **Round, uterine:** (ligamentum teres uteri) is a narrow, flat band, about 5 inches long, which is attached to the upper part of the side of the uterus in front of, and a little below, the medial end of the uterine tube. It is composed of fibrous tissue, which near the uterus has an admixture of plain muscular fibres continuous with those of the uterus. It lies in the anterior layer of the broad ligament, where it produces a slight prominence. It traverses the deep inguinal ring, the inguinal canal, the superficial inguinal ring and ends in the subcutaneous tissue of the labium majus. **Sacrosciatic, great:** (sacrotuberous) is attached by one extremity to the posterior inferior iliac spine, and the sides of the last three sacral and first coccygeal vertebrae, and by the other extremity to the medial border of the ischial tuberosity. **Sacrospinous:** (small sacro-sciatic ligament) is triangular in shape and is attached by its base to the sides of the last two sacral and first coccygeal vertebrae, where it is intimately connected with the more superficially placed sacrotuberous ligament. Its apex is attached to the spine of the ischium. **Sacrotuberous:** see great sacrosciatic ligament. **Short lateral, of knee:** (deep lateral) is attached proximally to the prominence on the lateral epicondyle of the femur that gives attachment to the long lateral ligament. Distally, it is attached to the styloid process of the fibula. **Short medial, of knee:** (deep medial) is attached proximally to the same rough impression on the medial epicondyle of the femur that furnishes attachment to the long or superficial ligament. Distally it is attached to the superior lip of the groove on the medial condyle of the tibia. **Short plantar:** is the shorter and thicker of the two plantar ligaments, and its fibres are more obliquely disposed. It extends anteriorly from the tubercle at the anterior extremity of the plantar surface of the calcaneum to the cuboid, where it is attached to the ridge forming the posterior limit of the peroneal groove. **Sphenomandibular:** (long internal lateral) is a triangular flat band that stands off from the mandibular joint and therefore has no direct relation to it. It is attached above to the spine of the sphenoid bone and below to the lingula and the inner margin of the mandibular foramen. **Spinoglenoid:** consists of a few fibres extending from the outer border of the spine of the scapula to the adjacent part of the margin of the glenoid cavity. It arches over the suprascapular vessels and nerve as they pass through the spinoglenoid notch. **Spiral:** is situated in the inner ear. It is a thickening of the periosteum of that part of the outer wall of the cochlea forming the outer wall of the scala media. It separates the ductus cochlearis from the scala tympani. **Spring:** see plantar calcaneonavicular. **Stellate:** see costo-central, radiate or stellate. **Struther's:** see medial brachial. **Stylohyoid:** is a narrow fibrous cord that is attached superiorly to the tip of the styloid process and inferiorly to the lesser horn of the hyoid bone. The ligament represents the usually unossified skeletal part of the second visceral arch, and ossification in it corresponds to the epihyal bone of lower mammals so well seen in the ruminants. **Stylomandibular:** extends from the styloid process of the temporal bone near its tip to the angle and adjacent part of the posterior border of the ramus of the mandible. **Subpubic:** see arcuate or inferior ligament of the symphysis. **Superficial transverse metatarsal:** part of the plantar aponeurosis. A distinct band of transverse fibres in the webs of the toes, it bridges over the intervals between the digital processes and covers the digital arteries and nerves and lumbrical muscles. **Suprascapular:** (transverse scapular) extends from the superior border of the scapula to the root of the coracoid process. It is thin and flat and bridges across the notch in the form of a double band. **Supraspinous:** consists of longitudinal fibres that connect the extremities of the spines. It extends from the spine of the seventh cervical vertebra to the spine of the fourth sacral segment and its fibres are arranged in a manner similar to those of the anterior longitudinal ligament. **Suspensory:** see phrenicosplenic or lienophrenic. **Suspensory, of eye:** see Lockwood's. **Suspensory, of Gerdy:** part of the clavipectoral fascia, which joins the axillary fascia. **Suspensory, of lens:** the anterior layer of the ciliary zonule, and is attached to the anterior wall of the capsule of the lens of the eye not far from the equator. **Suspensory, of liver:** see falciform. **Suspensory, of ovary:** a fold of peritoneum situated in the pelvis and containing the ovarian arteries. **Suspensory, of penis:** sometimes called the deep suspensory ligament, is strong and triangular in outline and is composed of fibrous and elastic tissue. It is attached superiorly to the front of the symphysis pubis where it is single, and inferiorly it divides into two laterally disposed, diverging laminae that blend with the fascial sheath of the penis. **Suspensory, of suprarenal:** a strand of fibrous tissue running from the fascia surrounding the suprarenal gland to the diaphragm. **Temporomandibular:** (external lateral ligament) is a short strong bundle of fibres, that is attached superiorly to the tubercle of root of the zygoma, and inferiorly to the condylar tubercle and the postero-lateral aspect of the neck of the mandible. **Thyro-epiglottic:** a band of fibro-elastic tissue joining the thyroid cartilage to the epiglottis. **Transverse, of hip joint:** bridges over the acetabular notch. It is composed of three bundles intimately blended with one another. The superficial bundle is formed by that part of the labrum acetabulare which stretches over the notch. The other two bundles are more deeply placed, and are arranged as two decussating bands extending between the margins of the notch. **Transverse, of knee joint:** is a narrow band towards the anterior aspect of the joint, and links the two semilunar cartilages together. Medially it is continuous with the anterior horn of the medial semilunar cartilage, from which it passes towards the fibular side to blend with the anterior aspect of the lateral semilunar cartilage. **Transverse atlas:** is the transverse portion of the cruciate ligament: see cruciate. **Transverse humeral:** a thick band of transverse fibres which are attached to the two tuberosities of the humerus and bridge the intertubercular sulcus. **Transverse metacarpal:** part of the anterior interosseous fascia of the fingers which is thickened in the region of the heads of the metacarpal bones. **Transverse palmar superficial:** part of the palmar aponeurosis which passes across the heads of the metacarpal bones in the region of the stasis point produced by the transverse palmar flexure lines. **Transverse pelvic:** (transverse ligament of the perineum) extends transversely between the inferior pubic rami immediately posterior to the inferior ligament of the symphysis. **Transverse, of perineum:** (transverse pelvic ligament) extends transversely between the inferior pubic rami immediately posterior to the inferior ligament of the symphysis. Posteriorly it is closely connected with the truncated apex of the perineal membrane. **Transverse scapular:** see suprascapular ligament. **Transverse tibiofibular:** (transverse ligament) fills in the interval between the distal ends of the tibia and the fibula. It is attached to the malleolar fossa of the fibula in common with the posterior talofibular ligament, whence it passes to the posterior surface of the tibia where it blends with the posterior tibiofibular ligament. **Trapezoid:** the lateral and anterior part of the coracoclavicular ligament. It is quadrilateral in shape and is attached inferiorly to the posterior part of the superior surface of the coracoid process. It passes upwards to be attached to the trapezoid ridge on the inferior aspect of the clavicle. **Triangular:** (perineal membrane) is triangular in shape and occupies the pubic arch, which it fills. Each lateral margin is attached along the medial border of the ischiopubic ramus, above the crus penis and ischiocavernosus muscle, as far back as the ischial tuberosity. **Triangular, of the liver:** the right triangular ligament is situated to the extreme right of the coronary ligament and consists of a double fold of peritoneum passing to the diaphragm. The left triangular ligament is a double fold of peritoneum passing from the postero-superior border of the left lobe of the liver to the diaphragm. **Winslow's:** see oblique posterior ligament of the knee joint. **Wrisberg's:** a well-marked band of fibres which runs from the posterior extremity of the external semilunar cartilage and is attached to the upper part of the posterior cruciate ligament. **Ligamenta alaria:** two fringes of the synovial membrane of the knee joint, attached to the anterior intercondylar area, and reaching to the patella. **L. arcuate:** thickened bands of fascia arching over the psoas and quadratus lumborum muscles. The diaphragm arises in part from these ligaments. **L., collateral:** ligaments on either side of the metacarpophalangeal articulations. **L., costotransverse:** three in number: *Superior* passing from the upper border of the neck of the rib to the lower border of the transverse process above; *Inferior* passing from the anterior surface of the transverse process to the posterior surface of neck of corresponding rib; *Lateral* passing from apex of transverse process to tubercle of rib. **L., cruciate:** interarticular ligaments of the knee joint. **L., denticulata:** narrow, fibrous ligaments on each side of the spinal cord, between the anterior and the posterior nerve roots. **L., digital vaginal:** small bands of synovial membrane, which convey minute blood vessels to the tendons. **L. flava:** thick ligaments situated within the vertebral canal connecting the laminae of adjacent vertebrae. **L. of Helvetius:** pyloric ligaments. **L., lateral cervical** (Mackenrodt): a band attached to the side of the cervix uteri and to the vault and lateral fornix of the vagina. **L. of Mackenrodt:** see lateral cervical ligaments. **L. of Malleus:** three in number: 1. Anterior: passing between the root of the anterior process and the edge of the squamo-tympanic fissure; 2. Lateral: passing between the lateral process and the posterior malleolar fold; 3. Superior: passing between the head of the malleus and the roof of the tympanum. **L., palpebral:** tendinous band attached to the upper part of the lacrimal crest and to the frontal process of the maxilla. **L., plantar:** see plantar ligaments. **L., pyloric:** thin striated band running from the muscular layer to the serous coat of the stomach in the region of the pylorus and causing a groove. **L., sacrococcygeal:** three ligaments which surround the sacrococcygeal joint in front, behind and laterally. **L., sacro-iliac:** two in number, anterior and posterior. Anterior sacro-iliac ligament is composed of short fibres and covers the sacro-iliac joint in front. Posterior sacro-iliac ligament is very strong and covers the joint behind. **L., sternocostal:** ligaments which pass from the superior and inferior borders of the costal cartilage to the side of the sternum. **L., sternopericardial:** two fibrous bands of the fibrous layer of the pericardium which pass to the deep surface of the manubrium sterni and the xiphoid process. **L., talocalcaneal:** four ligaments associated with the talocalcaneal articulation. The anterior, posterior and lateral ligaments surround the joint. The interosseous talocalcaneal ligament is the chief bond of union getween the talus and calcaneus and occupies the sinus tarsi. **L., thyro-arytenoid:** see l. vestibular and l. vocal. **L., thyrohyoid:** the thickened median and lateral parts of the thyrohyoid membrane. **L., vestibular:** (superior thyro-arytenoid ligaments) band of fibrous tissue occupying vestibular fold extending between the thyroid cartilage and the arytenoid cartilage. **L., vocal** (inferior thyro-arytenoid ligaments): a band of yellow fibrous tissue contained in the vocal fold. **Ligamentum arteriosum:** is a fibrous cord which is the remains of the ductus arteriosus in the heart. **L. nuchae:** is a band of fibrous tissue occupying the median line of the neck. It is attached superiorly to the external occipital protuberance and to the external occipital crest, inferiorly to the spine of the seventh cervical vertebra. **L. mucosum** (infrapatellar synovial fold): is part of the synovial membrane of the knee joint which extends from the upper part of the tibia to be attached to the anterior end of the intercondylar notch of the femur. **L. patellae** (infrapatellar tendon): is a thick broad band attached to the blunt apex and adjacent margins of the distal part of the patella and to a rough area occupying the distal part of the tubercle of the tibia. **L. pectinatum iridis:** the posterior fibres of the posterior elastic lamina of the eye which pass in a radiating manner into the iris. **L. suspensorium trochantii of Gunther:** the common tendon of the gluteus medius and minimus which may extend to the great trochanter of the femur. **L. teres:** see ligament of the head of the femur. **L. teres of the liver:** see round ligament of the liver. **L. teres uteri:** see round ligament of the uterus. **L. venosum:** a fibrous cord connecting the left branch of the portal vein to the ligamentum teres and represents the foetal ductus venosus.

ligamenta. See ligament.

ligamen·tal, ligamen·tary, ligamen·tous (L. *ligare*, to bind). Having the function of or pertaining to a ligament.

ligate (L. *ligare*, to bind). To apply a ligature.

ligā·tion (L. *ligare*, to bind). The operation of tying.

li·gator (L.). An instrument used in the fastening of ligatures.

li·gature (L. *ligatura*, a band). 1. A cord used for tying vessels. 2. Ligation.

light. Radiant energy of wave-lengths between 390 and 760 mμ; when rays fall upon the retina they give rise to the sensation of vision.

lig·neous (L. *lignum*, wood). Wooden. **L. thyroiditis:** Riedel's thyroiditis, *q.v.*

lignocēr·ic acid (L. *lignum*, wood; *cera*, wax). A fatty acid present in peanut oil and wood tar; also isolated from nerve tissue.

lig·num (L.). Wood.

li·gula (L., a shoe-strap). A tongue-shaped structure.

lily rash. Dermatitis due to handling daffodils.

limatū·ra (L. *limare*, to file). Filings.

limb. 1. An extremity attached to the trunk, used for grasping or locomotion. 2. A structure resembling a limb.

lim·bic (L. *limbus*, a hem). Relating to a border.

lim·bus (L.). A border; a margin.

lime¹ (Pers. *līmū*). The fruit of various citrus species.

lime². Calcium oxide, CaO; quicklime. Slaked lime, calcium hydroxide, $Ca(OH)_2$. **L., chlorinated:** A disinfectant made by passing chlorine over slaked lime

lime-water. A solution of calcium hydroxide in water.

li·men (L.). A threshold, border or boundary. **L. nasi:** the boundary between the bony and cartilaginous parts of the nasal cavity.

li·mic (G. *līmos*, hunger). Relating to hunger.

li·minal (L. *limen*, threshold). Relating to a threshold; e.g. relating to the lowest margin of perception.

li·miting (L. *līmes*, a boundary). Forming a boundary. **L. membrane, external:** the layer of the retina between the nuclear layer and that of the rods and cones. **L. membrane, internal:** in the eye, the innermost retinal layer.

Limnā·tis (G. *limnē*, a lake). The generic name of various water leeches.

li·mo (L.). Lemon.

limō·nis suc·cus (L.). Lemon juice.

limō·sis (G. *limos*, hunger). Abnormal hunger.

li·mosphere (L. *limus*, sidelong; G. *sphaira*, sphere). A spheroidal body of uncertain origin in sperm-cells.

limp. A halting gait. See also claudication.

limping. Walking with a limp.

linc·tus (L. *lingere*, to lick). A viscous, sweetened, liquid medicinal preparation.

Lindau's disease (Lindau, A., contemporary Swedish pathologist). Angioma, usually cystic, of the cerebellum.

line, li·nea (L. *linea*). 1. A narrow streak or stripe. 2. The twelfth part of an inch. 3. In anatomy, anything resembling a mathematical line; a guidemark or boundary. **L., absorption:** a dark line in the spectrum due to absorption of light on its passage through a gaseous, liquid or solid medium. **L., blue:** bluish discoloration of the dental margin of teeth-bearing gums, as present in chronic lead-poisoning.

li·neal. Relating to a line or lines.

li·neament (L. *lineamentum*, from *linea*, line). 1. The outline of the face. 2. The outline of the embryo.

li·near. Arranged in lines. **L. atrophy:** atrophic cutaneous striae.

Ling's system (Ling, P. H., Swedish gymnast, 1776–1839). A way of treating disease by gymnastic movements of the body; kinetotherapy; Lingism.

li·ngua (L.). The tongue. **L. geographica:** a condition of the tongue characterized by the transitory development at the dorsal surface in front of the circumvallate papillae of irregularly bounded smooth red patches with yellowish-white margins. Syn. geographical tongue; glossitis exfoliativa marginata.

li·ngual (L. *lingua*, tongue). 1. Relating to the tongue. 2. Shaped like a tongue.

linguā·lis muscle (L.). Muscle of the tongue.

li·nguiform (L. *lingua*, tongue; *forma*, shape). Resembling a tongue.

li·ngula (L. *lingua*, tongue). A structure resembling a tongue. **L. cerebelli:** a portion of the cerebellar vermis.

li·niment, linimen·tum (L. *linere*, to smear). A fluid preparation for application to the skin by friction. **Linimentum aconiti:** A.B.C. liniment, *q.v.*

li·nin (L. *linum*, thread). The oxyphilic substance of the framework of a cell-nucleus. Syn. parachromatin.

lini·tis plas·tica (L. from G. *linon*, flax; *plassein*, to form). A form of gastric cancer, characterized by considerable thickening of the stomach wall and reduction of the gastric cavity. Syn. leather-bottle stomach.

li·nkage. 1. In genetics, the mode of transmission of several characters in which either all characters are transmitted together or none of them. 2. In chemistry, the lines in a structural formula representing valency connections between the atoms.

linseed. The dried ripe seeds of *Linum usitatissimum*. **L. poultice:** a poultice made from crushed linseed and water.

lint (L. *linteum*, from *linum*, flax). A thick, loosely woven material used as an absorbent dressing for wounds.

li·num (L.). Flax.

Liouville's icterus (Liouville, H., French physician, 1837–87). Icterus neonatorum.

lip. 1. The fleshy upper or lower border of the mouth. 2. One of the labia majora or labia minora. 3. The margin of a wound.

lipae·mia (G. *lipos*, fat; *haima*, blood). Increase in the amount of fat in the blood, causing a milk-like appearance of the blood serum.

lipă·rocele (G. *liparos*, sleek; *kēlē*, hernia). A hernia the sac of which contains only some fatty tissue.

liparom·phalos (G. *liparos*, sleek; *omphalos*, navel). A fatty tumour of the umbilicus.

li·pase (G. *lipos*, fat). An enzyme present especially in pancreatic juice, decomposing by hydrolysis neutral fat into fatty acids and glycerol.

li·pid. Lipoid, *q.v.*

lip·iodol. Poppy seed oil containing 40 per cent iodine, used as contrast medium in radiography.

li·pocele (G. *lipos*, fat; *kēlē*, hernia). Liparocele, *q.v.*

lipochondrody·strophy (G. *lipos*, fat; *khondros*, cartilage; *dus*, ill; *trophē*, nourishment). See gargoylism.

li·pochrin (G. *lipos*, fat; *ōkhros*, sallow). A yellow pigment from retinal fat globules.

li·pochrome (G. *lipos*, fat; *khrōma*, colour). A fatty pigment found in various animal tissues, chemically related to the vegetable carotenes.

lipody·strophy (G. *lipos*, fat; *dus*, ill; *trophē*, nourishment). A disturbance of fat metabolism. **L., progressive:** a condition characterized by progressive symmetrical loss of subcutaneous fat-tissue at the upper part of the body, usually beginning in childhood and often disappearing in later life.

li·pofibro·ma (G. *lipos*, fat; L. *fibra*, fibre). A tumour composed of fatty and fibrous tissue.

lipofus·cin (G. *lipos*, fat; L. *fuscus*, dark). A fatty pigment found in various animal tissues, perhaps a compound of melanin and a lipoid substance.

lipoge·nesis (G. *lipos*, fat; *genesis*, production). The formation of fat.

lipogen·ic (G. *lipos*, fat; *gennan*, to produce). Relating to lipogenesis.

li·poid (G. *lipos*, fat; *eidos*, form). A term applied to a heterogeneous group of substances, characterized by their insolubility in water and their solubility in certain solvents, e.g. ether, chloroform, benzene. They are either esters of fatty acids or substances capable of forming such esters, and are found in all vegetable and animal matter. They may be classified into: (1) Simple lipoids, esters of fatty acids with various alcohols (fats, oils, waxes). (2) Compound lipoids; esters of fatty acids yielding other substances in addition to fatty acids and alcohol, e.g., phosphatides (lecithin, cephalin, sphingomyelin), and glycolipoids (cerebroside). (3) Derived lipoids: substances liberated during hydrolysis of simple and compound lipoids, e.g., sterols (e.g., cholesterol). **L. degeneration:** a form of fatty degeneration of tissue in which lipoid substances, mainly cholesterol and cholesterol ester, are involved. **L. nephrosis:** a type of nephrosis in which doubly refractile bodies are excreted in the urine. **L. histiocytosis:** see Gaucher's disease; Niemann's disease; gargoylism.

lipoido·sis (G. *lipos*, fat; *eidos*, form). A disturbance of the metabolism of the lipoids.

lipoidu·ria (G. *lipos*, fat; *eidos*, form; *ouron*, urine). A condition in which lipoids are found in the urine.

lipo·lysis (G. *lipos*, fat; *luein*, to loosen). Decomposition or splitting of fat.

lipolyt·ic. Relating to lipolysis.

lipo·ma (G. *lipos*, fat). A tumour composed of fatty tissue. **L. arborescens:** a hyperplasia of fatty tissue in a synovial membrane.

lipomato·sis (G. *lipos*, fat). Excessive formation of subcutaneous fat-tissue.

lipo·matous (G. *lipos*, fat). Relating to a lipoma.

lipome·ria (G. *leipein*, to leave; *meros*, part). Congenital absence of an extremity.

li·pometa·bolism (G. *lipos*, fat; *metabole*, change). The using of fat.

li·pomyxo·ma (G. *lipos*, fat; *muxa*, mucus). A myxolipoma, a tumour composed of lipomatous and myxomatous tissue.

lipopha·gic (G. *lipos*, fat; *phagein*, to eat). Absorbing fat.

lipo·phagy (G. *lipos*, fat; *phagein*, to eat). Lipolysis.

li·pophile (G. *lipos*, fat; *philein*, to love). Having an affinity for fat.

lipophre·nia (G. *leipein*, to leave; *phrēn*, mind). Loss of mental powers.

li·posarco·ma (G. *lipos*, fat; *sarx*, flesh). A tumour composed of sarcomatous and lipomatous tissue.

li·pose (G. *lipos*, fat). A blood lipase.

lipothy·mia (G. *leipein*, to leave; *thūmŏs*, mind). Loss of consciousness; fainting.

lipotri·chia (G. *leipein*, to leave; *thrix*, hair). Loss of hair.

lipoxan·thin (G. *lipos*, fat; *xanthos*, yellow). A yellow lipochrome.

lipŏ·xenous. Relating to lipoxeny.

lipŏ·xeny (G. *leipein*, to leave; *xenos*, stranger). Desertion of a host by a parasite after the latter has reached its developmental maturity.

Lipschütz's bodies (Lipschütz, B., Austrian dermatologist, 1878–1931). Intracellular and intranuclear eosinophilic inclusion bodies found in epidermal cells in herpes simplex, herpes zoster and varicella.

lipu·ria (G. *lipos*, fat; *ouron*, urine). The presence of fat droplets in the urine.

liq. Abbreviation for liquor.

liquefa·cient (L. *liquefacere*, to make liquid). Possessing the power to liquefy.

liquefac·tion (L. *liquefacere*, to make liquid). The process of becoming converted into a liquid form.

lique·scent (L. *liquescere*, to become liquid). Readily becoming liquid.

li·quid (L. *liquēre*, to be fluid). 1. Fluid. 2. Any readily flowing substance.

liquid paraffin. A colourless oily mixture of liquid hydrocarbons used in the treatment of chronic constipation.

li·quor (L.). 1. A liquid. 2. An aqueous solution. **L. amnii:** fluid contained in the amnion in which the foetus is enclosed.

Lisfranc's ligament (Lisfranc, J., French surgeon, 1790–1847). The interosseous ligament between the second metatarsal and the first cuneiform bone. **L.'s joint:** the tarsometatarsal articulations. **L.'s tubercle:** the tuberculum scaleni on the first rib.

lisp. Inability properly to pronounce sibilant letters.

Lissauer's tract (Lissauer, H., German neurologist, 1861–91). The postero-lateral ascending tract in the spinal cord. **L.'s zone:** constituting the marginal zone between the entering posterior root fibres and the margin of the cord.

lissencě·phaly (G. *lissos*, smooth; *egkephalos*, brain). Absence of convolutions of the cerebral cortex.

Lister's antiseptic (Lister, J. (Lord), English surgeon, 1827–1912). Perchloride of mercury. **L.'s dressing:** gauze impregnated with carbolic and other antiseptics. **L.'s tubercle:** the prominence on the posterior surface of the lower end of the radius adjacent to the groove for the tendon of the extensor pollicis longus.

Listing's plane (Listing, J. B., German physiologist, 1808–82). A transverse vertical plane, perpendicular to the anteroposterior axis of the eye. It contains the centre of motion of the eyes and in it lie the transverse and vertical axes of ocular rotation.

Liston's splint (Liston, R., Scottish surgeon, 1794–1847). Long straight splint formerly used in fractures of the hip bone. **L.'s knife:** large amputation knife.

liter. Litre, *q.v.*

li·thagogue (G. *lithos*, stone; *agōgos*, leading). Expelling calculi.

li·tharge (G. *lithos*, stone; *arguros*, silver). Yellow oxide of lead. PbO.

lithi·asis (G. *lithos*, stone). The formation of concretions in the body.

li·thic (G. *lithos*, stone). 1. Relating to calculi. 2. Relating to lithium.

li·thium (G. *lithos*, stone). A metal belonging to the group of alkalis. Symbol Li. Atomic weight 6·94.

li·thoceno·sis (G. *lithos*, stone; *kenōsis*, an emptying). The extraction of lithic fragments which have been crushed.

li·thoclast (G. *lithos*, stone; *klaein*, to break). See lithotrite.

lĭ·thoclasty (G. *lithos*, stone; *klaein*, to break). Lithotrity, *q.v.*

lithŏ·lapaxy (G. *lithos*, stone; *lapaxis*, evacuation of the bowels). The washing out of fragments of calculi by a catheter after lithotripsy.

lithomē·tra (G. *lithos*, stone; *mētra*, womb). Ossification of the uterus or within the uterus.

lithonĕ·phria (G. *lithos*, stone; *nephros*, kidney). Any disease caused by stones in the kidney.

lithonephrī·tis (G. *lithos*, stone; *nephros*, kidney). Kidney inflammation caused by the presence of renal calculi.

lithopae·dion (G. *lithos*, stone; *paidion*, child). A foetus, retained in the uterus, that has undergone calcification.

lĭ·thotome (G. *lithos*, stone; *tomē*, section). A knife used in lithotomy.

lithŏ·tomy (G. *lithos*, stone; *tomē*, section). Incision into the bladder for the removal of a calculus.

lĭ·thotripsy (G. *lithos*, stone; *tribein*, to rub). The operation of crushing calculi in the bladder by means of a lithotrite.

lĭ·thotrite (G. *lithos*, stone; L. *terere*, to crush). An instrument for crushing a calculus in the bladder.

lithŏ·trity. Lithotripsy, *q.v.*

lĭ·thous (G. *lithos*). Possessing the nature of a stone; relating to a stone.

lithurē·sis (G. *lithos*, stone; *ourēsis*, urination). The discharge of small calculi with the urine.

lit·mus. A blue pigment found in *Roccella tinctoria* and other lichen plants. **L. paper:** paper stained blue with l.; it turns red on contact with acid solutions. **Red l. paper:** obtained by staining with l. and sulphuric acid; this turns blue on contact with an alkaline solution.

litre (G. *litra*, a pound weight). The metric unit of capacity, equal to 0·88036 of an imperial quart. It is the volume of one kilogramme of water at 4° Centigrade.

Little's area (Little, J. L., American surgeon, 1836–85). On the nasal septum: the common site of nosebleeding.

Little's disease (Little, W. J., English physician, 1810–94). See diplegia, cerebral.

Littre's colostomy (Littre, A., French surgeon, 1658–1726). The establishing of an opening into the colon through the left iliac region. **L.'s glands:** the glands in the mucous membrane of the 'membranous' urethra. **L.'s hernia:** A hernial sac containing a Meckel's diverticulum. **L.'s sinus:** the transverse sinus.

live. Living; animate.

livē·do (L. from *livēre*, to be bluish). Lividity, *q.v.* **L. reticularis:** mottling of the skin, a bluish-red discoloration in a reticular pattern.

lĭ·vedoid (L. *livedo*; G. *eidos*, form). Livedo-like.

liver. The organ situated beneath the diaphragm in the right upper part of the abdominal cavity. It is the largest gland in the body forming 1/40th of the weight of the body. It secretes bile, forms and stores glycogen. It forms urea from waste products.

lĭ·vetin. One of the proteins of egg yolk.

lĭ·vid (L. *lividus*, bluish). Bluish discoloured; palebluish.

livi·dity (L. *lividus*, bluish). The condition of being livid. **L., cadaveric or post-mortem:** discoloration of the dependent parts of a corpse, caused by the gravitation of the non-oxygenated blood.

livor mortis (L.). See lividity, cadaveric.

Lizars's lines (Lizars, J., Scottish surgeon, 1783–1860). The surgical lines on the buttock.

Loa Loa. A species of the family Filariidae, one of the parasites causing filariasis. The larvae invade the blood, while the adult forms invade subcutaneous tissues and serous membranes.

lŏā·sis. The condition resulting from infestation with the Loa Loa.

lō·bar (G. *lobos*, lobe). Relating to a lobe. **L. pneumonia,** see under pneumonia, lobar.

lō·bate (G. *lobos*, lobe). Possessing lobes.

lobe (G. *lobos*). A part or process of an organ separated from the neighbouring parts by a fissure, sulcus or septum.

lobec·tomy (G. *lobos*, lobe; *ektomē*, excision). Excision of a lobe of an organ, e.g. of a lung.

lobē·lia. The dried aerial parts of *Lobelia inflata*; preparation used in the treatment of asthma.

loben·gulism. A disorder characterized by development of subcutaneous fat and with decrease of the sexual function.

lobī·tis (G. *lobos*, lobe). Inflammation of a lobe, usually a lobe of a lung.

Lobstein's cancer (Lobstein, J. G., German pathologist, 1777–1835). Retroperitoneal sarcoma. **L.'s disease:** osteogenesis imperfecta, osteopsathyrosis; constitutional fragility of bones. **L.'s ganglion:** an accessory ganglion of the great sympathetic in connection with the solar plexus.

lŏ·bular (L.L. *lobulus*, dim. of *lobus*, lobe). Relating to, resembling or composed of lobules. **L. pneumonia:** bronchopneumonia.

lŏ·bulated (L.L. *lobulus*). Consisting of lobes or lobules.

lŏ·bule (L.L. *lobulus*). A small lobe.

lŏ·bulet (L.L. *lobulus*, a small lobe). A sub-division of a lobule.

lŏ·bulus (L.L.). A small lobe.

lŏ·bus (L.L.). A lobe.

local (L. *locus*, place). Limited to a part; not generalized.

localizā·tion (L. *locus*, place). 1. The determination of the seat of a lesion or of an area associated with a certain function. 2. The limitation of a process to a particular area. 3. The power to locate sensory impressions.

lŏ·calized (L. *locus*, place). Limited to a particular area.

lŏ·cative (L. *locare*, to place). Denoting relative positions in a series.

lŏ·chia (G. *lokhos*, childbirth). The postpartum discharge from the genital organs.

lŏ·chial. Relating to the lochia.

lŏ·chiomē·tra (G. *lokhios*, of or belonging to childbirth; *mētra*, womb). An accumulation of lochia within the uterus.

lochiorrhā·gia (G. *lokhios*, of or belonging to childbirth; *rhēgnunai*, to break out). Excessive flow of lochia.

lŏ·chiorrhoe·a (G. *lokhios*, of or belonging to childbirth; *rhoia*, flow). Excessive flow of lochia.

lochiŏ·schesis (G. *lokhios*, of or belonging to childbirth; *skhesis*, retention). Retention or suppression of the lochia.

lŏ·chioperitonī·tis (G. *lokhios*, of childbirth; *peri*, around; *teinein*, to stretch). Puerperal peritonitis.

lockjaw. Trismus; tetanus.

Lockwood's ligament (Lockwood, C. B., English surgeon, 1858–1914). The suspensory ligament of the eyeball.

locomō·tion (L. *locus*, place; *movēre*, to move). Movement in space.

locomō·tive. Relating to locomotion.

locomō·tor (L. *locus*, place; *movēre*, to move). Relating to locomotion. **L. ataxia:** tabes dorsalis, *q.v.*

lŏ·cular (L. *loculus*, small place). Loculated; divided into loculi.

lŏ·culus (L.; pl. *loculi*). A small space.

locum tenens (L.). Keeping the place; i.e., a doctor replacing temporarily one who is absent.

lŏ·cus (L.). A place. **L. caeruleus:** a pigment-containing area situated caudal to the Sylvian aqueduct. **L. minoris resistantiae:** a place of diminished resistance.

Löffler's bacillus (Löffler, A. J., German bacteriologist, 1852–1915). See Klebs-Löffler bacillus. **L.'s blood-serum mixture:** blood-serum, 3; one per cent glucose bouillon, 2; coagulate at 70°C.: used in the cultivation of *C. diphtheriae.* **L.'s methylene blue:** an alkaline stain used in bacteriology.

logagnō·sia (G. *logos*, word; *a*, neg.; *gnosis*, knowledge). Aphasia, alogia, or other central word defect.

logagrã·phia (G. *logos*, word; *a*, neg.; *graphein*, to write). Inability to express ideas in writing.

logaphã·sia (G. *logos*, word; *a*, neg.; *phasis*, speech). Motor aphasia; inability to express ideas in speech.

logoclō·nia (G. *logos*, word; *klonos*, tumult). Repetition of syllables of a word or of meaningless verbal concoctions.

logomã·nia (G. *logos*, word; *mania*, madness). Psychotic talkativeness.

lŏ·goneurō·sis (G. *logos*, word; *neuron*, nerve). Any type of nervous disorder accompanied by speech disorders.

logorrhœ·a (G. *logos*, word; *rhoia*, flow). Excessive loquacity.

Löhlein's diameter (Löhlein, H., German gynaecologist, 1847–1901). The distance between the centre of the subpubic ligament and the antero-superior angle of the great sacrosciatic foramen.

loin. The lateral and posterior region of the trunk between the lower ribs and the iliac crest.

London paste. Sodium hydroxide, 5; slaked lime, 6; made into a paste with alcohol or glycerine. It is used as an escharotic.

longĕ·vity (L. *longus*, long; *aevum*, age). Long life.

longis·simus (L. superl. of *longus*, long). The longest. **L. dorsi muscle:** the intermediate column of the erector spinae mass of muscles on the back of the spinal column.

longitū·dinal (L. *longitudo*, length). In the direction of the long axis of a body.

longsightedness. Hypermetropia, *q.v.*

longus (L.). Long. **L. capitis:** a small prevertebral muscle, see muscle. **L. colli:** see muscle, longus cervicis.

loop. A turn or curve.

loose. Lax. **L. bowels:** diarrhoea. **L. body:** a body floating more or less freely in a joint cavity, representing a detached piece of cartilage, bone or synovial fringe, or a piece of organized blood-clot or exudate.

lor·doscoliō·sis (G. *lordos*, bent backward; *skolios*, curved). Lordosis accompanied by scoliosis.

lordō·sis (G. *lordos*, bent backward). An abnormal curvature of the lumbar spine with a forward convexity.

lordot·ic. Relating to lordosis.

Lorenz's operation (Lorenz, A., Austrian surgeon, 1854–1946). An operation used in disease of the hip. Subtrochanteric osteotomy performed and the upper end of lower fragment adducted to rest against the lower margin of the acetabulum.

Loreta's operation (Loreta, P., Italian surgeon, 1831–89). Forcible dilatation of the pylorus for the relief of stricture.

Lossen's rule (Lossen, H. F., German surgeon, 1842–1909). States that only women transmit haemophilia and only men suffer from it.

lotio (L., a washing). A lotion.

lotion (L. *lotio*, a washing). A medicinal solution for washing or bathing.

Louis's angle (Louis, A., French surgeon, 1723–92). Angulus Ludovici; a projection found in some persons at the point of junction of the manubrium and the sternum.

loupe (Fr.). A lens.

louping ill. A form of encephalitis in sheep, caused by a virus, and transmissible to man.

louse. See pediculus.

Löwe's ring (Löwe, K. F., German optician, born 1874). A ring in the visual field caused by the macula lutea. **L.'s test:** for acute pancreatitis. Dilatation of the pupil after instillation of adrenaline into conjunctival sac.

Lowenberg's canal (Lowenberg, B. B., German laryngologist, born 1836). The scala media of the cochlea.

Löwenthal's tract (Löwenthal, W., German physician, 1850–94). The descending anterolateral tract of the spinal cord.

Lower's tubercle (Lower, R., English anatomist, 1630–91). A small prominence in the right auricle between the openings of the superior and inferior venae cavae; tuberculum intervenosum.

Löwit's cells (Löwit, M., German physician, 1851–1918). The erythroblasts.

loxar·thron (G. *loxos*, oblique; *arthron*, joint). Any oblique deformity of a joint not due to luxation.

lŏ·zenge. Any medicated tablet with a basis of sugar.

Lubarsch's crystals (Lubarsch, O., German pathologist, 1863–1933). Crystals in the testis resembling sperm crystals.

lū·bricant (L. *lubricare*, to make smooth). 1. Making slippery. 2. Any agent, such as oil, by which a substance can be made slippery.

lubricã·tion. The process of making slippery by means of a lubricant.

Luc's operation (Luc, H., French laryngologist, 1855–1925). Drainage of the maxillary antrum.

Lucas's groove (Lucas, R. C., English physician, 1846–1915). The impression made at times on the spine of the sphenoid by the chorda tympani nerve; the 'stria spinosa' or 'sulcus spinosus'. **L.'s sign:** distension of the abdomen, an early symptom of rickets.

Lucas-Championnière's disease (Lucas-Championnière, J. M. M., French surgeon, 1843–1913). Chronic pseudo-membranous bronchitis.

Luciani's triad (Luciani, L., Italian physiologist, 1842–1919). Cerebellar asthenia, atonia and astasia.

lū·cid (L. *lucidus*). Clear. **L. interval:** the transitory return to a normal mental condition in psychotic states.

Lücke's operation (Lücke, G. A., German surgeon, 1829–94). Incision into the infraorbital nerve by way of the pterygoid process and the maxilla.

lückenschä·del (Ger., crannied skull). A skull characterized by defects on the inner surface in the form of depressions, especially in the frontal and parietal plates.

Ludwig's angina (Ludwig, W. F. von, German surgeon, 1790–1865). Angina Ludovici; phlegmonous cellulitis of the floor of the mouth, the pharynx and the upper part of the neck, seen in pyaemia, septicaemia, etc.

Ludwig's angle (Ludwig, D., German anatomist, 1625–80). See Louis's angle.

Ludwig's ganglia (Ludwig, K. F. W., German physiologist, 1816–95). The ganglionic masses; situated near the right auricle and connected with the cardiac plexus.

lū·es (L. plague). Syphilis.

lūĕt·ic (L. *lues*, plague). Syphilitic.

Lugol's caustic (Lugol, J. G. A., French physician, 1786–1851). Iodine and potassium iodide, of each 1 part, water 2 parts. **L.'s solution:** Iodine, 5; potassium iodide, 10; distilled water to 100.

lukewarm. Tepid.

lumbã·go (L. *lumbus*, loin). Fibrositis or muscular rheumatism affecting the lumbar muscles.

lum·bar (L. *lumbus*, loin). Relating to the loins. L. puncture: puncture of the dural membrane of the spinal cord below the third lumbar vertebra for the withdrawal of cerebrospinal fluid.

lumbocŏ·stal (L. *lumbus*, loin; *costa*, rib). Relating to the loins and ribs.

lumbocrū·ral (L. *lumbus*, loin; *crus*, leg). Relating to the lumbar and crural regions.

lumbodor·sal (L. *lumbus*, loin; *dorsum*, back). Relating to the lumbar and dorsal regions.

lumbo-in·guinal (L. *lumbus*, loin; *inguen*, the groin). Relating to the lumbar and inguinal regions.

lumbosā·cral (L. *lumbus*, loin; *sacer*, sacred). Relating to the lumbar vertebrae and the sacrum.

lumbricā·lis muscle (L. *lumbricus*, earthworm). Small muscles of hand and foot ; see muscles.

Lumbricus (L.). A genus of Annelid.

lumbus (L.). Loin.

lū·men (L., light). The bore of a tube, e.g. of an artery.

Luminal. A proprietary phenobarbitone preparation.

luminĭ·ferous (L. *lumen*, light; *ferre*, to bear). Conveying light.

lū·nacy (L. *luna*, moon). Insanity (formerly thought to be due to the influence of the moon).

lū·nar (L. *luna*, moon). Relating to the moon or to silver ('luna' of the alchemists). L. caustic: silver nitrate.

lū·natic (L. *luna*, moon). 1. Relating to or affected with insanity. 2. An insane person.

lung. The organ of the respiratory tract in which the blood becomes oxygenated. The lungs occupy the greater part of the thoracic cavity. Each lung is conical, the base being apposed to the diaphragm, the apex rising in the neck, and each has two surfaces and two borders.

lū·nula (L. dim. of *luna*, moon). 1. The white semilunar area at the base of a nail. 2. A structure resembling the crescent moon in shape.

lū·poid (L. *lupus*, wolf; G. *eidos*, form). Resembling lupus.

lūpō·ma (L. *lupus*, wolf). The primary nodule of lupus vulgaris.

lūpus (L. *lupus*, wolf). See l. vulgaris. L. erythematosus: a skin disease characterized by the eruption of macules with central scarlike depression and a reddish raised border, of usually symmetrical arrangement and mostly affecting the face. The disease is usually of a very chronic nature; the acute disseminated form may involve large areas of skin and include inflammatory lesions of the heart, kidneys, etc. L. hypertrophicus, L., papillomatous: forms of l. vulgaris. L. pernio: a form of sarcoidosis of Boeck, *q.v.*, affecting the nose, ears, hands and feet, resembling in naked-eye appearance the common chilblain. L. serpiginosus: 1. vulgaris, characterized by serpiginous distribution. L. verrucosus: the verrucous type of l. vulgaris. L. vulgaris: a chronic tuberculosis of the skin, characterized by the development of reddish translucent nodules in the corium, arranged singly or in groups, often leading to extensive atrophic scars or destruction of tissues, but only rarely affecting the general condition of the individual.

Luschka's bursa (Luschka, H. von, German anatomist, 1820–75). Pharyngeal bursa of infants. L.'s cartilage: a small cartilage in the anterior part of the true vocal cord. L.'s foramina: the lateral openings of the fourth ventricle at the ends of the lateral recesses. L.'s gland: the coccygeal body lying in front of and below the tip of the coccyx. Its function is unknown but it probably has a sympatho-chromaffin origin.

lust. Sexual desire.

lusus naturae (L.). A freak of nature; a monstrosity.

lū·teal. Relating to lutein.

lū·tein (L. *luteus*, yellow). 1. A yellow lipoid pigment, present, e.g., in the corpus luteum. 2. See progesterone.

luteinizā·tion (L. *luteus*, yellow). The development of Graafian follicles into corpora lutea.

lutĕō·ma (L. *luteus*, yellow). A tumour arising from corpus luteum cells, inhibiting full development of Graafian follicles and ovulation, producing amenorrhoea and sometimes masculinization. See also masculinoblastoma.

luxā·tio erecta (L.). A dislocation of the shoulder-joint in which the head of the humerus lies below the glenoid cavity and the shaft is held fixed above the patient's head.

luxā·tion (L. *luxare*, to dislocate). Dislocation, *q.v.*

lŭ·xus (L.). Excess.

Luys's body or nucleus (Luys, J. B., French physician, 1828-97). The nucleus hypothalamicus, a small ganglion beneath the optic layer, connected above with the corpus striatum and below with the superior cerebellar peduncle.

lycan·thropy (G. *lukos*, wolf; *anthrōpos*, man). Psychotic delusion in which the patient imagines that he is a wild beast.

lycomā·nia (G. *lukos*, wolf; *mania*, madness). Lycanthropy, *q.v.*

lye. 1. The alkaline solution obtained by leaching wood ashes. 2. A solution of sodium or potassium hydroxide.

lying-in. The puerperium, *q.v.*

lymph (L. *lympha*, water). 1. The fluid in the lymphatic vessels and lymph spaces. 2. The fluid material used for vaccination against smallpox; vaccine lymph. L. follicles: nodules of lymphatic tissue.

lymph·adenec·tasis (L. *lympha*, water; G. *adēn*, gland; *ektasis*, extension). Dilatation of lymph-gland sinuses.

lymphadē·nia (L. *lympha*, water; G. *adēn*, gland). A general hyperplasia of the lymphatic tissue.

lymph·adenī·tis (L. *lympha*, water; G. *adēn*, gland). Inflammation of a lymphatic gland.

lymphă·denoid (L. *lympha*, water; G. *adēn*, gland; *eidos*, form). Resembling or having the character of a lymph-gland or lymphatic tissue. L. goitre: diffuse lymphocytic infiltration of the thyroid gland resulting in myxoedema.

lymph·adenō·ma (L. *lympha*, water; G. *adēn*, gland). 1. A progressive disease affecting successively organs possessing lymphatic tissue, characterized by an enlargement of the lymph nodes and usually of the spleen, due to proliferation of reticulum and myeloid cells and of fibroblasts, by a progressive anaemia and by periods of undulant pyrexia. See also Sternberg-Reed giant cell. Syn. Hodgkin's disease; malignant lymphogranulomatosis. 2. An obsolete term for any hyperplasia of lymph glands.

lymph·agogue (L. *lympha*, water; G. *agōgos*, leading). Stimulating the flow of lymph.

lymph·angiĕc·tasis, lymph·angiĕctā·sia (L. *lympha*, water; G. *aggeion*, vessel; *ektasis*, extension). Dilatation of the lymphatic vessels.

lymph·angiō·ma (L. *lympha*, water; *aggeion*, vessel). A tumour composed of dilated lymph vessels.

lymphangī·tis (L. *lympha*, water; G. *aggeion*, vessel). Inflammation of a lymphatic gland.

lymphat·ic (L. *lympha*, water). Relating to or characterized by lymph. L. gland: an organ consisting of nodules of l. tissue, lying in the course of and being connected with l. vessels. L. leukaemia: see leukaemia, l. L. system: the system comprising the l. vessels, including the thoracic duct and the l. glands. L. vessel: a vessel conveying lymph.

lymphă·tics (L. *lympha*, water). The capillary lymph-conveying tubes.

lymph·atism (L. *lympha*, water). See status lymphaticus.

lymph·oblast (L. *lympha*, water; G. *blastos*, germ). The stem cell of lymphatic tissue, normally present only in the germinal centres of lymphatic tissue, having a diameter of 16–25μ, a usually roundish nucleus with fine chromatin structures and deeply basophilic cytoplasm; present in peripheral blood or bone marrow in cases of lymphatic leukaemia.

lymphoblastō·ma (L. *lympha*, water; G. *blastos*, germ). The form of lymphosarcoma characterized by proliferation of the lymphoblasts.

lymph·ocyte (L. *lympha*, water; G. *kutos*, cell). One of that group of leucocytes which are derived from the lymphoblast; having a diameter of 6–15μ, a usually roundish nucleus with coarse chromatin structure, relatively little amount of basophilic cytoplasm, containing azurophil granules.

lymphocythae·mia (L. *lympha*, water; G. *kutos*, cell; *haima*, blood). Lymphocytosis.

lymphocy̆·tic (L. *lympha*, water; G. *kutos*, cell). Consisting of or relating to lymphocytes.

lymphocytō·ma (L. *lympha*, water; G. *kutos*, cell). The form of lymphosarcoma characterized by proliferation of the lymphocytes.

lymph·ocytopē·nia (L. *lympha*, water; G. *kutos*, cell; *penia*, poverty). Lymphopenia, *q.v.*

lymphocytō·sis (L. *lympha*, water; G. *kutos*, cell). Absolute or relative increase of lymphocytes in the blood.

lymphoder·mia (L. *lympha*, water; G. *derma*, skin). An affection of the lymphatics of the skin. **L. perniciosa:** a condition now believed to be a form either of mycosis fungoides or of leukaemia, and not a disease *sui generis*.

lymphoede·ma (L. *lympha*, water; G. *oidēma*, swelling). Oedema due to blockage of the lymphatic vessels.

lympho·genous (L. *lympha*, water; G. *gennan*, to produce). Producing lymph.

lymphoglan·dula (L. *lympha*, water; *glandulae*, glands, dim. of *glans*, acorn). A lymphatic gland.

lymph·ogranulō·ma (L. *lympha*, water; *granulum*, dim. of *granum*, grain). Hodgkin's disease. **L. benign:** sarcoidosis of Boeck, *q.v.* **L. malign:** lymphadenoma, *q.v.* **L. inguinale:** a venereal disease, due to a filterable virus, characterized by the eruption of a small herpetiform vesicle or ulcer on the external genitals (primary sore) which is followed after an interval of 3 weeks to 2 months in the male by adenitis, especially of the inguinal glands, sometimes with suppuration and sinus-formation, and in the female by general lymphoedema of the labia and vagina, and in both cases by infiltration of the perirectal tissues leading to ulceration and stricture.

lymph·oid (L. *lympha*, water; G. *eidos*, form). Having the appearance or character of lymph or lymphatic cells. **L. leukaemia**, see leukaemia, lymphatic.

lymphō·ma (L. *lympha*, water). A tumour composed of lymphatic tissue.

lymphopē·nia (L. *lympha*, water; G. *penia*, poverty). Absolute or relative decrease below the usual number of lymphoctyes in the blood. Syn. lymphocytopenia.

lymphopoiē·sis (L. *lympha*, water; G. *poiēsis*, formation). The formation of lymphocytes.

lymphorrhā·gia (L. *lympha*, water; G. *rhegnunai*, to break out). Lymphorrhoea, *q.v.*

lymphorrhoe·a (L. *lympha*, water; G. *rhoia*, flow). A flow of lymph from a ruptured lymphatic vessel.

lymphosarcō·ma (L. *lympha*, water; G. *sarx*, flesh). A progressive neoplastic disease characterized by enlargement of the lymph nodes due to proliferation of lymphoblasts or lymphocytes and by the infiltration of parenchymatous organs by these cells. See also reticulosarcoma.

lymph scrotum (L. *lympha*, water; *scrotum*). Lymphangiectasis of the scrotum.

lymphū·ria (L. *lympha*, water; G. *ouron*, urine). Condition characterized by the presence of lymph in the urine.

ly̆·ra (G. *lura*, lyre). Longitudinal, transverse and oblique lines between the posterior limbs of the fornix and the corpus callosum, so called because of their lyre-like arrangement.

ly̆·sin (G. *luein*, to loosen). An antibody having the property of dissolving cells.

ly̆·sine. An essential amino-acid.

ly̆·sis (G. *luein*, to dissolve). 1. Gradual decline of a disease, especially of a fever. 2. The dissolving of a substance by the action of a lysin. 3. The decomposition of a substance or compound.

Lysol. A proprietary brand of compound solution of cresol; used as an antiseptic.

lysolē·cithin (G. *luein*, to dissolve; *lekithos*, vegetable pulse). A lecithin from which the unsaturated fatty acid radical has been removed as by the action of cobra venom. Has strongly haemolytic properties.

ly̆·sozyme (G. *luein*, to dissolve; *zumē*, leaven). A bactericide substance found in tears, leucocytes, nasal and other bodily secretions, egg albumin, turnips and various other plants, and in certain fish.

lyssa (G. *lussa*, frenzy). Hydrophobia or rabies.

lyssophō·bia (G. *lussa*, frenzy; *phobos*, fear). Morbid dread of rabies; pseudohydrophobia.

lytic (G. *luein*, to dissolve). 1. Relating to lysis. 2. Relating to a lysin.

R

M

M. Abbreviation of misce (mix); musculus (muscle); myopia.

m. Abbreviation of metre; minim.

μ. Abbreviation of micron (Gr.).

M+Am. Abbreviation of compound myopic astigmatism.

Macalister's muscle (Macalister, A., Irish anatomist, 1844–1919). The crico-trachealis muscle.

McBurney's point (McBurney, C., American surgeon, 1845–1914). A point one third of the way along a line drawn from the anterior superior iliac spine to the umbilicus. The point of maximal tenderness in cases of acute appendicitis.

McClintock's sign (McClintock, A. H., Irish physician, 1822–81). A pulse rate over 100 following parturition is indicative of commencing postpartum haemorrhage.

MacConkey's bouillon (MacConkey, A. T., English bacteriologist, 1861–1931). Selective medium for growth of coliform organisms. **M.'s stain:** for demonstration of bacterial capsules, containing methyl green, dahlia and fuchsin.

M'Dowel's fraenum (M'Dowel, B. G., Irish anatomist, 1829–85). The fraenum suspensorium of the pectoralis major tendon.

mace. The dried avillus of nutmeg.

macerā·tion (L. macerare, to soften). The process of softening a tissue by the action of a liquid.

Macewen's osteotomy (Macewen, Sir W., Scottish surgeon, 1848–1924). Supracondylar osteotomy of the femur for genu valgum. **M.'s triangle:** the suprameatal triangle; the surface marking of the mastoid antrum. Bounded above by the supramastoid crest, in front by the posterosuperior margin of the meatus and behind by a line drawn as a tangent to the posterior margin of the meatal orifice.

Mache unit (Mache, H., Austrian physicist, born 1876). A term formerly used to indicate the concentration of radium emanations.

ma·ciēs (L.). Leanness; wasting.

Mackenrodt's ligaments (Mackenrodt, A., German gynaecologist, 1859–1925). The ligamentum transversum colli of the uterus. **M.'s operation:** shortening the round ligaments of the uterus in backward displacements of the uterus.

McLeod's capsular rheumatism (McLeod, R., Scottish physician, 1795–1852). Rheumatoid arthritis with abundant effusion into the synovial sacs, sheaths and bursae.

MacMunn's test (MacMunn, C. A., English pathologist, 1852–1911). For indican. Boil urine in equal quantity of hydrochloric acid and a little nitric acid, cool and shake with chloroform which becomes violet and shows one absorption band due to indigo blue and one due to indigo red.

macrencephā·lia (G. makros, large; egkephalos, brain). A condition in which the brain is abnormally enlarged.

macro-aesthē·sia (G. makros, large; aisthēsis, perception). A disturbance of the stereognostic sense in consequence of which a touched object appears larger than it is.

macrobactē·rium (G. makros, large; baktron, a staff). A large bacterium.

macrobīō·sis (G. makros, long; bios, life). Longevity.

macrobīō·tic (G. makros, long; bios, life). Relating to long life; long-lived.

mac·roblast (G. makros, large; blastos, germ). A nucleated red blood cell, the precursor of the normoblast, normally present in blood-forming tissues, present in peripheral blood only in various abnormal conditions; characterized by its large size (10–20μ in diameter), a cytoplasm varying in the degree of basophilia and the amount of haemoglobin respectively, and a nucleus of fairly coarse chromatin structure. Syn. erythroblast.

macroblast·ic (G. makros, large; blastos, germ). Characterized by the presence of macroblasts.

macrobră·chia (G. makros, large; brakhiōn, arm). Arms of abnormal length or size generally.

macrocar·dius (G. makros, large; kardia, heart). A monster with an abnormally large heart.

macrocephā·lia, macrocĕ·phaly (G. makros, large; kephalē, head). Condition in which the head is abnormally large.

macrocĕ·phalous (G. makros, large; kephalē, head). Having an abnormally large-sized head.

macrochei·lia (G. makros, large; kheilos, lip). Excessive size of the lips.

macrochei·ria (G. makros, large; kheir, hand). Congenital over-development of the hands.

macrochĕ·mistry (G. makros, large; Arab. al-qimia, chemistry). Chemistry in which the reactions can be seen with the naked eye.

macrococ·cus (G. makros, large; kokkos, a grain). A coccus larger than average size.

macrocō·lon (G. makros, large; kŏlon, the colon). An abnormally long colon.

macrocor·nea (G. makros, large; L. cornu, horn). A cornea of abnormally large size.

mac·rocyst (G. makros, large; kustis, bladder). An exceptionally large cyst.

macrocȳ·tase (G. makros, large; kutos, cell). An enzyme that is found in leucocytes and is phagocytic in action.

mac·rocyte (G. makros, large; kutos, cell). An abnormally large erythrocyte, derived from a macroblast, and differing from a megalocyte by its circular form.

macrocȳ·tic (G. makros, large; kutos, cell). Characterized by the presence of macrocytes.

macrocytō·sis (G. makros, large; kutos, cell). Presence of macrocytes in the blood.

macrodactȳ·lia, macrodac·tylism, macrodac·tyly (G. makros, large; daktulos, finger). Congenital over-development of fingers or toes.

macrodŏn·tia (G. makros, large; odous, tooth). Abnormally large teeth.

macrodȳ·strophia (G. makros, large; dus-, ill-; trophein, to nourish). Progressive lipodystrophy.

macro-ĕ·rythroblast (G. makros, large; eruthros red; blastos germ). A large erythroblast.

macrogă·mete (G. makros, large; gamein, to marry). In certain lower organisms, one of a pair of gametes which is considerably larger than the other gamete (microgamete) and is regarded as the female sexual cell.

mac·rogamĕ·tocyte (G. makros, large; gamein, to marry; kutos, cell). The enlarged merozoite before it develops into the macrogamete in propagative reproduction of sporozoa.

macrŏ·gamy (G. makros, large; gamos, marriage). That type of conjugation in protozoa in which the fusing cells are of the same structural type as the original vegetative cells. Syn. hologamy.

macrogă·stria (G. *makros*, large; *gastēr*, belly). Abnormal distension of the stomach.

macrogĕ·nesy (G. *makros*, large; *genesis*, production). Gigantism, *q.v.*

mac·rogenitosŏ·mia prae·cox (G. *makros*, large; L. *genitalis*, generative; G. *sōma*, body; L. *praecox*, premature). Premature development or over-development of sexual characters, as found especially in male children suffering from a pineal tumour which is, however, probably not the direct cause of it.

macrō·glia (G. *makros*, large; *glia*, glue). A form of neuroglia, characterized by large multipolar cells. Syn. astroglia.

macroglos·sia (G. *makros*, large; *glōssa*, tongue). Enlargement of the tongue.

macrolymph·ocyte (G. *makros*, large; L. *lympha*, water; G. *kutos*, cell). A large lymphocyte with a diameter of 15–20μ, present especially in lymphatic nodules.

macromă·nia (G. *makros*, large; *mania*, madness). A mania in which the patient has delusions that objects are larger than they really are.

macromas·tia, macromā·zia (G. *makros*, large; *mastos*, or *mazos*, breast). Abnormal increase in the size of the breast.

macromē·lia (G. *makros*, large; *melos*, limb). Over-development of any member.

macrŏ·melus (G. *makros*, large; *melos*, limb). One having congenitally over-large limbs.

măc·romere (G. *makros*, large; *meros*, part). A large blastomere.

macronū·cleus (G. *makros*, large; L. *nucula*, dim. of *nux*, nut). 1. A large nucleus. 2. The principal nucleus of a cell.

macronŷ·chia (G. *makros*, large; *onux*, finger-nail). Congenital over-development of the size of the nails.

mă·cropathŏ·logy (G. *makros*, large; *pathology*). Pathology in which the microscope is not used.

mă·crophage (G. *makros*, large; *phagein*, to eat). A free (wandering) histiocyte found in zones of phagocytic activity, of large size, and rounded shape, containing one or several nuclei.

macrophă·gocyte (G. *makros*, large; *phagein*, to eat; *kutos*, cell). A large-sized phagocyte having a single nucleus and arising from a fixed connective tissue element.

macropō·dia (G. *makros*, large; *pous*, foot). Congenital over-development of the feet.

macropŏ·lycyte (G. *makros*, large; *polus*, many; *kutos*, cell). Unusually large polymorphonuclear cells with 6-10 lobes; found in the blood in pernicious anaemia.

mă·croprosŏ·pia (G. *makros*, large; *prōsōpŏn*, face). Congenitally over-large face.

macrop·sia (G. *makros*, large; *opsis*, vision). A perverted visual sensation in which objects seem larger than they are; usually due to disseminated choroiditis.

macrorhī·nia (G. *makros*, large; *rhis*, nose). Congenital over-development of the nose.

macroscĕ·lia (G. *makros*, large; *skelos*, leg). Congenital over-development of the legs.

macroscop·ic (G. *makros*, large; *skopein*, to view). Visible to the naked eye.

macrŏ·scopy (G. *makros*, large; *skopein*, to view). Naked eye inspection or examination.

macrō·sis (G. *makros*, large). Over-development.

macrosmat·ic (G. *makros*, large; *osme*, smell). Possessing an over-acute sense of smell.

macrosomā·tia, macrosŏ·mia (G. *makros*, large; *sōma*, body). Gigantism of the body.

mă·crosome (G. *makros*, large; *sōma*, body). A protoplasmic body differing from a microsome in its larger size and often in its staining reaction.

mă·crospore (G. *makros*, large; *spora*, seed). A spore of large type in some higher plants.

macrostŏ·ma, macrostŏ·mia (G. *makros*, large; *stoma*, mouth). Congenital malformation of the face, characterized by a cleft between the mandibular and maxillary processes, resulting in enlargement of the mouth.

macrō·tia (G. *makros*, large; *ous*, ear). Congenital over-development of the aural pinna.

mă·crotome (G. *makros*, large; *tome*, section). An instrument for cutting large anatomical sections.

mă·cula (L., pl. *maculae*). Spot; a circumscribed discoloration of the skin. **M. caeruleae:** bluish-grey spots on the skin caused by the action of the *Pediculus pubis*. **M. corneae:** corneal opacities. **M. lutea:** the yellow spot of the retina, the area of clearest vision.

mă·culate (L. *macula*, spot). Spotted.

maculā·tion (L. *macula*, spot). 1. The condition of being spotted. 2. The formation of maculae.

mă·cule. A macula.

mă·culopă·pular (L. *macula*, spot; *papula*, pimple). Applied to a rash which is characterized by the presence of both macules and papules.

mad. Insane.

madarō·sis (G. *madarōsis*, a falling off of the hair of the eyelids). Loss of the eyelashes and/or eyebrows.

madder. The *Rubia tinctoria*, from the root of which the dye alizarin is obtained.

Maddox's prism (Maddox, E. E., English ophthalmologist, 1860–1933). Two prisms with their bases together; a device for testing eyeball torsion. **M.'s rod:** optical device whereby a point of light before one eye is appreciated by the other eye as a line of light by passing it through a small glass rod or series of rods to prevent fusion of images from each eye.

Madelung's deformity (Madelung, O.W., German surgeon, 1846–1926). A forward bending of lower end of radius, with subluxation of inferior radioulnar joint. **M.'s disease:** Diffuse lipomata. **M.'s neck:** Diffuse lipomata in the neck. **M.'s operation:** lumbar colotomy. **M.'s sign:** Increasing difference between oral and rectal temperatures, indicating purulent peritonitis.

madē·scent (L. *madescere*, to become moist). Moist.

Madura foot (Madura, a district of India). A fungus disease, mycetoma, *q.v.*

maggot. A worm or grub.

Magendie's foramen (Magendie, F., French physiologist, 1783–1855). The median opening between 4th ventricle and subarachnoid space. **M.'s solution:** a solution of 16 grains of morphine sulphate in 1 fluid ounce of water used for hypodermic injection. **M.'s spaces:** spaces between the pia mater and arachnoid membrane corresponding to the sulci of the brain. The pia follows the cortex while the arachnoid bridges the sulci.

Magnan's sign (Magnan, V., French neurologist, 1835-1916). A hallucination of sensation which takes the form of a feeling of the presence of a round body beneath the skin; observed in chronic cocainism.

magnē·sia (Named from the district *Magnēsia*, in Thessaly). Magnesium oxide, MgO.

magnē·sic. Relating to or containing magnesia.

magnē·sium. A bluish-white metallic element, symbol Mg. **M. trisilicate:** a white, odourless, tasteless powder used for its adsorbent and anti-acid properties.

mag·net (G. *magnes* = coming from *Magnēsia*, in Thessaly). 1. Lodestone, magnetic iron oxide. 2. A body capable of attracting iron bodies.

magnet·ic. Pertaining to or having the properties of a magnet.

mag·netism. The phenomena of attraction or repulsion produced by magnetic forces.

mag·nificā·tion (L. *magnus*, great; *facere*, to make). Enlargement, especially of the image of an object by lenses.

mag·nify (L. *magnus*, large; *facere*, to make). To enlarge.

mag·nifying power. The power of a lens to enlarge the image of an object.

mag·num (L.). Large. M., os: the largest carpal bone, capitate. M., foramen: see foramen.

Mahler's sign (Mahler, R. A., contemporary German gynaecologist and obstetrician). In the puerperium an increase in pulse rate without rise of temperature is indicative of venous thrombosis.

maidenhead. The hymen.

Maier's sinus (Maier, R., German pathologist, 1824-88). The depression in the internal surface of the lacrimal sac.

maim. To cripple by injury or removal of a limb.

main-en-griffe (Fr.). Claw-hand; hyperextension of the metacarpophalangeal joints and flexion of the two interphalangeal joints; due to ulnar paresis.

Maisonneuve's bandage (Maisonneuve, J. G. F., French surgeon, 1809-97). A special type of plaster-of-paris bandage.

Maissiat's band (Maissiat, J. H., French anatomist, 1805-78). The iliotibial tract.

Majocchi's purpura (Majocchi, D., Italian physician, 1849-1929). Purpura annularis telangiectoides.

major (L.). Greater; larger.

Makins's murmur (Makins, Sir G. H., English surgeon, 1853-1933). The systolic murmur that may be heard over an aneurysm.

mal (Fr. from L. *malum*, an evil). Disease. M. de caderas: (Sp.), an infectious disease in horses, etc., caused by the *Trypanosoma equinum*. M. de mileda: a form of tylosis endemic in the island of Mileda off the Dalmatian coast. M. perforant: perforating ulcer of the foot due to a trophic lesion.

mā·la (L.). The cheek-bone or the cheek.

Malacarne's pyramid (Malacarne, M. V. G., Italian surgeon, 1744-1816). The posterior end of the pyramid of the cerebellum.

malā·cia (G. *malakia*, softness). A morbid softening of the tissues.

maladjust·ment. Inadequate adjustment. 1. Term used in the setting of fractures. 2. In psychology, defective adaptation to environment.

mă·lady (Fr. *malade*, ill). Disease.

malaise (Old Fr. *mal*, bad; *aise*, ease). A general feeling of being unwell.

malalign·ment. Poor position. Term used in the treatment of fractures.

mā·lar (L. *māla*, cheek-bone). Pertaining to the cheek-bones.

malăn·dria (L., blisters). A leprosy-like affection.

malā·ria (It. *mala aria*, bad air). An infectious disease caused by certain specific protozoa which are transmitted by the bite of mosquitoes of the genus Anopheles, and characterized by periodic fever, enlargement of the spleen and the presence of pathogenic protozoa in the blood. Syn. malarial fever. M., benign tertian: a form of m. caused by the *Plasmodium vivax* and characterised by fever paroxysms occurring in single infections at intervals of 48 hours. M., subtertian: a form of m. caused by *Plasmodium falciparum* and characterized by intermittent, continuous or irregular remittent fever. Syn. malign tertian fever; aestivo-autumnal fever. M., quartan: a form of m. caused by *Plasmodium malariae* and characterized by fever paroxysms at intervals of 72 hours.

malā·riaci·dal (Malaria; L. *caedere*, to kill). Destructive to malaria germs.

malā·rial. Relating to malaria. M. haemoglobinuria: blackwater fever, *q.v.* M. treatment: the treatment of general paralysis of the insane by artificial infection with benign tertian malaria.

Malassez's disease (Malassez, L. C., French physiologist, 1842-1911). Cystic disease of the testis.

Malassezi furfur. A fungus belonging to the Hyphomycetes, causing tinia versicolor. Syn. Microsporon furfur.

mal·assimilā·tion (L. *malus*, bad; *assimulare*, to make alike). Defective powers of assimilation.

malaxā·tion (G. *malassein*, to soften). Kneading; pétrissage, *q.v.*

male (L. *masculus*). 1. Pertaining to the sex that produces spermatozoa. 2. A member of the male sex.

male fern. The dried rhizome and leaf bases of *Dryopteris Filix-mas*, the extract of which is used as a remedy for tapeworm.

malformā·tion (L. *malus*, bad; *forma*, shape). A congenital abnormal development of a part of the body.

Malgaigne's fossa (Malgaigne, J. F., French surgeon, 1806-65). The fossa carotica. M.'s hernia: hernia of infancy, descent of the intestine into the open vaginal process of the peritoneum, prior to the descent of the testis. M.'s triangle: the superior carotid triangle.

malic acid (L. *malum*, apple). $C_4H_6O_5$, a dibasic acid found in unripe apples and grapes.

malig·nancy (L. *malignus*, evil). The property of being malignant.

malig·nant (L. *malignus*, evil). Threatening life. M. adenoma: adenocarcinoma. M. endocarditis: infective or ulcerative endocarditis. M. malaria: subtertian malaria. M. oedema: gas gangrene. M. pustule: anthrax. M. tumour: a tumour which is characterized by infiltrating growth, by dissemination in distant organs, by a tendency to recur after removal, and by causing a cachectic condition and ultimately destroying life.

malin·gerer (Fr. *malingre*). One who feigns illness or defect.

malin·gering. The feigning of illness or defect.

Mall's lobules (Mall, F. P., American anatomist, 1862-1917). The small areas of the splenic pulp outlined by the ultimate ramifications of the trabeculae.

mal·leal, mal·lear (L. *malleus*, hammer). Relating to the malleus (1).

malleā·tion (L. *malleare*, to hammer). Twitching of the hands.

mal·lĕŏlar (L. *malleolus*, dim. of *malleus*, hammer). Relating to a malleolus.

mal·lĕŏlus (L. *malleolus*, a small hammer). A part or process of bone shaped like a hammer, e.g. the tibial malleoli, two lateral processes at the distal end of the tibia.

mallĕŏ·tomy (L. *malleus*, hammer; G. *tomē*, section). Division of the malleolus.

mallĕoidō·sis. Usually called melioidosis, *q.v.*

mallet finger. A deformity of a finger characterized by flexion of the distal phalanx. Syn. hammer-finger.

mallet toe. A deformity of a toe, characterized by flexion of the distal phalanx. Syn. hammer-toe.

mal·leus (L. *malleus*, hammer). 1. One of the ossicles of the internal ear. 2. Glanders.

malnutri·tion (L. *malus*, bad; *nutrire*, to nourish). Imperfect nutrition; under-nourishment.

malocclū·sion (L. *malus*, bad; *occludere*, to shut upon). The occlusion of teeth not in their anatomical site.

Malpighi's bodies (Malpighi, M., Italian anatomist, 1628-94). Renal glomeruli and capsule. The glomerular capsule is the blind expanded end of the renal tubule and is indented by convoluted capillary blood vessels. M.'s capsule: see Bowman's capsule. M.'s corpuscles: see Malpighi's bodies. **M.'s pyramids:** pale, striated conical masses situated in series forming the renal medulla. **M.'s stigmata:** the points where the smaller veins enter the larger veins of the spleen. **M.'s stratum or layer:** rete mucosum of skin. Polyhedral cells with well marked cell bridges and fibrils.

malposi·tion (L. *malus*, bad; *positio*, position). An abnormal position of any part, especially of the foetus *in utero*, or of a tooth.

malprac·tice (L. *malus*, bad; L.L. *practicare*, to transact). Improper or injurious practice.

mal·presentä·tion (L. *malus*, bad; *praesentare*, to present). A position of the child during parturition which impedes delivery.

malrotä·tion (L. *malus*, bad; *rotare*, to turn). Insufficient rotation of an organ during foetal development.

malt. The seed of common barley which is caused to enter the incipient stage of germination by heat and then dried. *Extractum Malti* (B.P.), dose 60 to 480 mimims. *Extractum Malti cum Oleo Morrhuae* (B.P.) (extract of malt with cod liver oil), dose 60 to 480 minims.

Malta Fever. See fever, Mediterranean.

maltase. An enzyme, present in pancreatic juice, yeast, etc., decomposing maltose into glucose.

Malthus, doctrine of (Malthus, T. R., English political economist, 1766–1834). Malthusianism; the doctrine that the increase of population is proportionately greater than the increase of subsistence; and the teaching based thereon, that over-population should be prevented by sexual continence or late marriage.

maltose. A disaccharide which gives two molecules of glucose upon hydrolysis.

mal·toside. A glycoside of the sugar maltose.

maltosü·ria (*maltose*; G. *ouron*, urine). A condition in which maltose is present in the urine.

malt sugar. Maltose, *q.v.*

mä·lum (L. *mălum*, an evil). Disease.

malü·nion. Faulty joining of a fracture.

Maly's test (Maly, R. L., Austrian chemist, 1839–64). A test for hydrochloric acid in the stomach contents. Rarely used to-day.

mä·melon (Fr. from L. *mamilla*, dim. of *mamma*, nipple). A nipple.

mamelonne (Fr. from L. *mamilla*, dim. of *mamma*, nipple). Wart-like. See etat mamelonné.

mamil·la (L.). A nipple; a small prominence.

mam·illary (L. *mamilla*, dim. of *mamma*, breast). Pertaining to a nipple; nipple-shaped. **M. bodies:** the two small round structures situated in the floor of the third ventricle. Syn. corpora mamillaria.

mamillä·tion (L. *mamilla*, dim. of *mamma*, breast). Wart-like granulation, especially on a mucous membrane.

mam·ma (L.). The breast; the milk-secreting gland of the mother.

mammal·gia (L. *mamma*, breast; G. *algos*, pain). Pain in the breast.

Mammä·lia (L. *mamma*, breast). The order of vertebrates suckling their offspring.

mam·mary (L. *mamma*, breast). Pertaining to the mammae.

mammec·tomy (L. *mamma*, breast; G. *ektomē*, excision). Surgical removal of a breast.

mam·mate (L. *mamma*, breast). Having mammae, or breasts.

mammö·tomy (L. *mamma*, breast; G. *tomē*, section). Incision of a breast.

mandē·lic acid. $C_6H_5 \cdot CHOH \cdot COOH$ a white crystalline powder soluble in water. Dose 30–60 gr. four times a day. Used in the treatment of pyelitis and cystitis caused by *Bacterium coli*.

man·dible, mandĭ·bula (L. *mandibula*, from *mandere*, to chew). The inferior maxillary bone.

mandĭ·bula (L.). The mandible, or lower jawbone.

mandĭ·bular. Pertaining to the mandible.

Mandl's paint (Mandl, L., Hungarian physician, 1812–81). A solution used locally for inflamed throat. Consists of iodine $1\frac{1}{4}\%^w/_v$, with potassium iodide and oil of peppermint in a glycerin medium.

Mandrä·gora. A genus of solanaceous plants; the mandrake.

man·drin (Fr.). A firm stilet which can be inserted into a flexible catheter, to make introduction of the instrument possible.

manducä·tion (L.L. *manducatio*, a chewing). Mastication.

man·ganese. A brittle, hard, metallic element. Symbol Mn. Reputed to raise bodily resistance to the common pyogenic organisms. Various of its salts have been used in treating anaemia.

mange (Fr. *manger*, to eat). An infectious skin disease of horses, cattle, dogs, etc., caused by various species of acarus.

mango. The fruit of *Mangifera indica*.

mä·nia (G. *mania*, madness). 1. A psychosis characterized by considerable emotional excitement, flight of ideas, hallucinations, delusions, disturbance of orientation, extreme motor restlessness and incessant talking; usually a phase of manic-depressive insanity. 2. A syndrome due to an organic cause, such as chronic alcoholism (mania a potu) or dementia paralytica, with the main features of 1.

mä·niac (G. *mania*, madness). A person affected with mania.

mani·acal. Relating to mania.

mä·nic. Relating to mania. **M.-depressive insanity:** a psychosis occurring at intervals either as mania or as depression, not leading to a deterioration of the mental faculties during the intervening periods.

manipulä·tion (L. *manipulus*, a handful). Handling; the treatment of diseases or injuries of the joints, ligaments, bones, etc., mainly by the performance of certain passive movements of the injured part.

Mann's sign (Mann, J. D., English physician, 1840–1912). A disturbance of the normal balance of the muscles in the two orbits so that the two eyes appear not to be on the same level; observed in exophthalmic goitre and other affections characterized by tachycardia.

manna. The sugar-containing exudation of the flowering ash.

man·nerism. A characteristic mode of action.

Manning's exanthem. A septicaemic exanthem. It is a serious complication of scarlet fever and diphtheria.

man·nitol. $C_6H_{14}O_6$, an alcohol.

Mannkopf's sign (Mannkopf, E. W., German physician, 1836–1918). Increase in the frequency of the pulse following pressure over a painful spot.

man·nose. A monosaccharide produced by oxidation of mannitol.

manoeu·vre (Fr. from L. *manu operari*, to work by hand). A special movement of the hand or instrument.

manö·meter (G. *manos*, thin; *metron*, measure). An instrument for the estimation of the pressure of liquids and gases.

manomet·ric. Relating to manometry.

manö·metry. Estimation of liquid and gas pressures by means of the manometer.

Manson's disease (Manson, Sir P., British physician, 1844–1922). A skin disease or pyosis in which an eruption of vesicles takes place.

Mansonia. A genus of mosquitoes with characteristically broad scales on the wing veins. Syn. Taeniorhynchus. Implicated in the spread of filariasis, equinine encephalitis and yellow fever.

mantle. The cortex of the cerebrum.

Mantoux reaction (Mantoux, C., French physician, born 1877). An intradermal test for tuberculosis. An injection of 0.1 cc. of a dilution of old tuberculin which may vary in strength from $\frac{1}{10000}$ up to $\frac{1}{100}$. A positive reaction is shown by a red areola with some oedema and occasional vesication.

man·ual (L. *manus*, hand). 1. Relating to the hands. 2. Performed by the hands.

manū·brium (L. *manubrium*, handle). 1. A handle-shaped structure. 2. The upper portion of the sternum.

mă·nus (L.). The hand.

Manz's utricular glands (Manz, W., German ophthalmologist, 1833–1911). The epithelial utricles on the cornea.

Mapharsen. A proprietary anti-syphilitic preparation, the semi-alcoholate of *m*-amino-*p*-hydroxyphenylarsine oxide hydrochloride. It is a white amorphous, odourless powder, containing about 29 per cent of trivalent arsenic.

Mapharside. The same as Mapharsen, *q.v.*

Maragliano's endoglobular degeneration (Maragliano, E., Italian physician, 1849–1940). Large red blood corpuscles which exhibit irregular-shaped colourless areas.

maran·tic (G. *marasmos*, to decay). Relating to marasmus.

maras·mic. Relating to marasmus.

maras·mus (G. *marasmos*, a wasting). 1. A general wasting of the body. 2. See atrophy, infantile.

marble bone disease. A sometimes familial disease characterized by osteosclerosis, *q.v.*, affecting the entire skeleton, with increased fragility of the bones, and by that type of anaemia often associated with osteosclerotic conditions. See leuco-erythroblastosis. Syn. Albers-Schönberg's disease; osteopetrosis generalisata; osteosclerosis fragilis generalisata.

Marcacci's muscle (Marcacci, A., Italian physiologist, 1854–1915). The muscle fibres underlying the areola and nipple.

Marchand's glandules (Marchand, F., German pathologist, 1846–1928), The suprarenal glands situated in abnormal positions.

Marchant's zone (Marchant, G., French surgeon, 1850–1903). The 'zone decollable' of the dura mater.

Marchi's tract (Marchi, V., Italian anatomist, 1851–1908). Löwenthal's tract. The anterolateral descending tract of the spinal cord.

Marcille's triangle (Marcille, M., born 1871). The triangle bounded by the mesial margin of the psoas, the lateral margin of the vertebral column and below by the ilio-lumbar ligament.

Marey's law (Marey, E. J., French physiologist, 1830–1904). The pulse rate varies inversely as the arterial blood pressure.

mar·gin (L.). Relating to the margin or border.

mar·ginal. Relating to a margin.

margin·oplasty (L. *margo*, verge; G. *plassein*, to form). Plastic surgery of the margin of the eyelid.

mar·go (L., border). A margin or border.

margō·sa oil. Oil derived from the seeds of the margosa tree.

Marie's disease (Marie, P., French physician, 1853–1940). 1. Acromegaly. 2. Hereditary cerebellar ataxia. 3. Hypertrophic pulmonary osteoarthropathy. 4. Spondylosis rhizomelica; ankylosis of the spinal column and the hip-joint; also of the shoulder joint, but less often. The condition is also known as Strumpell's disease (2). **M.'s symptom:** tremor of the extremities or of the whole body in exophthalmic goitre.

Marie-Kahler's symptom (Marie, P.; Kahler, O., Austrian physician, 1849–93). Marie's symptom, *q.v.*

Marie-Robinson's syndrome. A type of diabetes associated with melancholia, insomnia, impotence and the presence of laevulose in the urine.

Mariotte's blind spot (Mariotte, E., French physicist, 1620–84). The 'blind spot' of the optic disc of the retina. **M.'s experiment:** a device for demonstrating the existence of the blind spot of the eye.

Marjolin's ulcer (Marjolin, R., French physician, 1812–95). A slowly progressing malignant ulcer with wart-like growths beginning on a cicatrix.

Marmorek's serum (Marmorek, A., Austrian physician, 1865–1923). Antistreptococcal serum; a polyvalent serum obtained by inoculating animals with varieties of streptococci.

marrow. The soft tissue filling the cavities or interstices of bones.

Marsden's paste (Marsden, A., English surgeon, 1832–1902). A paste consisting of gum arabic and white arsenic formerly used in the treatment of cancer.

Marsh's disease (Marsh, Sir H., Irish physician, 1790–1860). Exophthalmic goitre.

Marsh's test (Marsh, J., English chemist, 1789–1846). A test for arsenic.

Marshall Hall's disease (Marshall Hall, English physician, 1790–1857). Cerebral anaemia in infants, marked by symptoms simulating those of hydrocephalus. **M.H.'s facies:** the bulging forehead and small features seen in cases of hydrocephalus.

Marshall's oblique vein (Marshall, J., English anatomist, 1818–91). The oblique vein of the left atrium which joins the coronary sinus. A relic of the left duct of Cuvier. **M.'s vestigial fold:** the ligament of the left vena cava. A triangular fold of serous pericardium over the remains of the left duct of Cuvier lying between the left pulmonary artery and vein.

marsh-fever. Malaria.

marsh-gas. Methane.

marsū·pial (L. from, G. *marsippos*, pouch). A group of mammals possessing an abdominal pouch in which the young are carried.

marsū·pium (G. *marsippos*, pouch). A pouch.

marsū·pia patellā·ris (L.). The synovial alar ligaments of the knee joint.

Martegiani's area (Martegiani, J., Italian ophthalmologist. Observation published 1814). The dilatation at the posterior end of the vitreous-hyaloid canal.

Martin's bandage (Martin, H. A., American surgeon, 1824–84). An indiarubber bandage for making compression of a limb in treatment of varicose veins or ulcers. **M.'s haemostatic:** surgeon's agaric impregnated with ferric chloride.

Martinotti's cells (Martinotti, G., Italian physician, 1857–1928). A distinctive type of cell in the cortex cerebri.

mas·culine (L. *masculinus*, male). Male. **M. protest:** in individual psychology, a term applied to the efforts to overcome inferiority feelings, inferiority being identified with feminity.

masculi·nity (L. *masculinus*, male). The condition or character of male individuals.

mas·culizā·tion (L. *masculinus*, male). Loss of female and gain of male characteristics in a female or castrated individual.

mă·sculinoblastō·ma (L. *masculinus*, male; G. *blastos*, germ). An ovarian tumour of either benign or malignant character, arising probably either from adrenal rests or from corpus luteum cells, producing masculinization.

mask. 1. A covering for the lower parts of the face during surgical operations. 2. A bandage applied to the face in case of eczema, burns or scalds.

masked. Hidden.

mă·sochism (Named from Sacher-Masoch, L., American novelist, 1836–95). Sexual perversion in which libido is induced by receiving painful stimuli.

mă·sochist. A person addicted to masochism.

mass, massa (L. *massa*). 1. The quantity of matter contained in a body. 2. A cohesive substance that can be used in the preparation of pills. **M. action, law of:** the velocity of a chemical reaction is proportional to the product of the active masses of the reacting substances.

massage (Fr. from G. *massein*, to knead). Treatment by manual or instrumental rubbing, kneading or stroking parts of the body.

Masset's test (Masset, A. A., French physician, born 1870). A test for bile in the urine. To the urine some potassium nitrate and a few drops of sulphuric acid are added; a green colouration is indicative of bile.

massē·ter (G. *masētēr*, a chewer). A facial muscle lifting the lower jaw.

masseter·ic. Relating to the masseter muscle.

masseur (Fr.). A man who practises massage.

masseuse (Fr.). A woman who practises massage.

mas·sive. Heavy or bulky; complete.

Massol's bacillus (Massol, L., Swiss bacteriologist, 1837–1909). *B. bulgaricus.* An organism found in Bulgarian yoghurt. It ferments milk and produces considerable acidity. Also called *Lactobacillus bulgaricus.*

măst·adenī·tis (G. *mastos*, breast; *adēn*, gland). Inflammation of the breast.

măst·adenō·ma (G. *mastos*, breast; *adēn*, gland). Adenoma of the breast.

măstal·gia (G. *mastos*, breast; *algos*, pain). Pain in the breast.

mast-cell. A leucoctye containing coarse basophile granules. Syn. basophile cell.

mastec·tomy (G. *mastos*, breast; *ektomē*, excision). The surgical removal of the breast.

masthelcō·sis (G. *mastos*, breast; *helcōsis*, ulceration). Ulceration of the breast.

mas·tic (G. *mastax*, the jaws). A resin from a tree *Pistacia lentiscus.*

masticā·tion (Late L. *masticare*, to chew). The act of chewing.

mas·ticatory. Pertaining to mastication or to the muscles of mastication.

Mastigŏ·phora (G. *mastix*, whip; *pherein*, to bear). A class of protozoa, bearing flagella.

masti·tis (G. *mastos*, breast). Inflammation of the breast.

mas·tocarcinō·ma (G. *mastos*, breast; *karkinos*, cancer). Carcinoma of the breast.

mas·tochondrō·ma (G. *mastos*, breast; *khondros*, cartilage). A cartilaginous breast tumour.

mastodў·nia (G. *mastos*, breast; *odunē*, pain). Pain in the breast.

mas·toid (G. *mastos*, breast; *eidos*, form). 1. Nipple-shaped. 2. The processus mastoideus of the os temporale. 3. Pertaining to the mastoid process, e.g., m. antrum, m. operation.

mastoidal. Relating to the mastoid process.

mastoidal·gia (G. *mastos*, breast; *eidos*, form; *algos*, pain). Pain in the mastoid area.

mastoidec·tomy (G. *mastos*, breast; *eidos*, form; *ektomē*, excision). Excision of the mastoid cells. **M., radical:** an operation on the mastoid process in which the different spaces of the middle ear including the antrum and the cells of the mastoid process are converted into a single cavity and all inflamed tissues excised.

mastoi·deum (G. *mastos*, breast; *eidos*, form). The processus mastoideus of the temporal bone.

mastoidi·tis (G. *mastos*, breast; *eidos*, form). Inflammation of the mastoid process.

mastoidŏ·tomy (G. *mastos*, breast; *eidos*, form; *tomē*, section). Incision of the cells of the mastoid process.

mastomē·nia (G. *mastos*, breast; *mēn*, month). Menstruation from the breast.

mastŏ·pathy (G. *mastos*, breast; *pathos*, disease). Chronic cystic mastitis.

mas·topexy (G. *mastos*, breast; *pēxis*, fixation). Plastic operation on breast.

mastorrhā·gia (G. *mastos*, breast; *rhēgnunai*, to break out). Mammary haemorrhage.

masturbā·tion (L. *manus*, hand; *stuprare*, to defile). Production of the orgasm by manual stimulation of the genital organs.

Matas's operation (Matas, R., American surgeon, born 1860). Endo-aneurysmorrhaphy.

ma·té (Sp.). The dried leaves of *Ilex paraguayensis* which are used like tea. They possess diuretic properties.

materia medica (L.). The science of medicinal drugs.

mater·nal (L. *mater*, mother). Relating to the mother.

mā·trix (L.). A layer from which something is formed.

matter (L. *materia*). 1. Any substance occupying space. 2. Pus.

maturā·tion (L. *maturare*, to ripen). Ripening; attaining to full development.

mature (L. *maturus*). Ripe.

matū·rity (L. *maturus*, ripe). Ripeness, full development.

matū·tinal (L. *matutinus*, of the morning). Taking place in the morning.

Mauchart's ligaments (Mauchart, B. D., German anatomist, 1696–1751). The alar or check ligaments of the ocular muscles.

Maumené's test (Maumené, E. J., French chemist, born 1818). A test for sugar. Lint soaked with stannous chloride is dipped in the fluid; if sugar is present on heating the lint to 150°C., it will turn brownish black.

Maunoir's hydrocele (Maunoir, J. P., French surgeon, 1768–1861). A cystic swelling in the neck, occurring between the angle of the mandible and the mastoid process.

Mauriceau's method (Mauriceau, F., French obstetrician, 1637–1709). The after-coming head is delivered with the body of the foetus lying on the surgeon's forearm while his index finger in the foetus's mouth applies traction.

Mauthner's layer or sheath (Mauthner, L., Austrian ophthalmologist, 1840–94). The membrane surrounding the axis cylinder of a nerve within the sheath of Schwann.

mau·veine. Aniline purple dye.

maxil·la (L.). The jawbone; specifically the bone of the upper jaw.

max·illary. Relating to the maxilla.

max·imal (L. *maximus*, greatest). Relating to the maximum.

max·imum (L. *maximus*, greatest). The greatest or highest degree or value of a quantity; the highest point attainable. **M. dose:** the largest dose of a drug that may safely be given.

Maxwell's ring (Maxwell, P. W., Irish ophthalmologist, 1856–1917). Löwe's ring, *q.v.*

Mayer's ligament (Mayer, M. F., German anatomist, of 19th century). The 'suspensory ligament' of the carotid body.

Mayo's vein (Mayo, W. J., 1861–1939, and C. H., 1865–1939, American surgeons; brothers). The pyloric vein. This is an erroneous ascription, for the vein, if eponymously named, should be known as the 'Vein of Latarget'.

Mayo-Robson's point (Mayo-Robson, Sir A. W., English surgeon, 1853–1933). A point just above the umbilicus which causes pain if pressed upon in cases of pancreatic disease. **M.-R.'s position:** for operations on the biliary tract, a sand bag is placed under the loins so as to produce a definite lordosis and bring the liver forwards.

mazodȳ·nia (G. *mazos*, breast; *odunē*, pain). Pain in breast.

mazopathy. Mastopathy, *q.v.*

Mazzoni's corpuscles (Mazzoni, V., Italian physiologist). The tactile end organs; Golgi-Mazzoni bodies.

M & B (May and Baker, English chemists). M & B 693, see Sulphapyridine; M & B 760, see Sulphathiazole.

mean (Late L. *medianus*, from L. *medius*, middle). An average. **M., arithmetical:** the number obtained by dividing the sum of various factors by the number of these factors. **M., geometrical:** the nth root of the product of a number. **M. deviation:** the average amount by which an individual value in a statistical series differs from the arithmetical m. of that series. **M. corpuscular diameter:** the m. diameter of a single red blood cell of any sample of blood, estimated by statistical method from a large number of single measurements. **M. corpuscular volume:** the m. volume of a single red blood cell of any sample of blood, calculated by dividing the volume of packed cells in a unit of blood by the number of cells contained therein.

measles. An acute infectious disease characterized by high fever, by a catarrh of the conjunctiva and of the upper respiratory tract and by a papular eruption, usually appearing on the fourth day of the disease and rapidly spreading from behind the ears over the face, trunk and limbs. Syn. Morbilli. **German M.:** Rubella, *q.v.*

meā·tal (L. *meatus*, a passage). Relating to a meatus.

meătŏ·meter (L. *meatus*, a passage; G. *metron*, measure). An instrument used for the measurement of a meatus.

meā·totome (L. *meatus*, a passage; G. *tomē*, section). A knife used for meatotomy.

meătŏ·tomy (L. *meatus*, a passage; G. *tomē*, section). Surgical incision of a meatus from within, especially of the meatus urinarius.

meā·tus (L.). 1. A passage, a channel. 2. An orifice. **M., external auditory:** the passage extending from the concha to the tympanic membrane. **M., internal auditory:** the internal auditory canal. **M., nasal:** one of the passages into which the nasal cavity is divided by the turbinate bone. **M., urethral:** the orifice of the urethra.

mechă·nical (G. *mēkhanē*, machine). 1. Relating to the physical forces. 2. Machine-like.

mechă·nics (G. *mēkhanē*, machine). That part of physics which deals with the action of forces on bodies.

mĕ·chanism (G. *mēkhanē*, machine). 1. Any instrument or system transmitting or transforming force. 2. The manner in which this is accomplished.

Meckel's cartilage (Meckel, J. F., German surgeon, 1781–1833). The cartilage of the first branchial arch of the foetus.

mecŏ·nium (G. *mēcōn*, poppy). 1. The first dark-green-coloured faecal discharges of the newborn. 2. Opium.

mĕ·dia (L. *medius*, middle). 1. The middle coat of a vein, artery or lymph vessel. 2. The transparent parts of the eye: the cornea, aqueous humour, lens and vitreous humour.

mĕ·diad (L. *medius*, middle; *ad*, to). Towards the median line.

mĕ·dial (L. *medius*, middle). Situated in the middle; mesal or mesial.

mĕ·diăstĭ·nal. Relating to the mediastinum.

mĕ·diastinī·tis. Inflammation of the mediastinum.

mĕdiă·stīnopericardī·tis. Inflammation of the mediastinum and the pericardium.

mĕ·diăstī·num (L.). 1. The space in the centre of the chest between the two pleurae, consisting of the anterior, middle, posterior and superior m. 2. A partition, a fibrous membrane or septum separating parts.

mĕ·diate (L. *medius*, middle). 1. Indirect; interposed between two things. 2. To transmit; to interpose.

mĕ·diation (L. *mediare*, to be in the middle). The act of mediating.

mĕ·diător (L. *mediare*, to be in the middle). Applied to substances transmitting nerve impulses to muscle fibres.

mĕ·dicable (L. *mĕdēri*, to heal). Able to be cured.

mĕ·dical (L. *mĕdēri*, to heal). Relating to medicine. **M. diseases:** diseases treated by physicians. **M. ethics:** the principles regulating and guiding the conduct of physicians and surgeons.

medi·cament (L. *medicamentum*). A medicinal substance.

medicamentŏ·sus (L. *medicari*, to heal). 1. Relating to a drug. 2. Relating to a condition caused by a drug.

medicamen·tum (L.). A medicament. **M. arcanum:** a proprietary remedy.

mĕ·dicated. Impregnated with a medicament.

medicā·tion. 1. Impregnation with a medicament. 2. Treatment by means of medicine.

medi·cinal (L. *medicinalis*). 1. Pertaining to medical science. 2. Pertaining to a medicinal substance.

mĕ·dicine (L. *ars medicina*, the medical art). 1. The science of the treatment of disease, more especially that branch of it which deals with non-surgical diseases of internal organs. 2. Any substance given for the prevention or treatment of disease.

medico-chirur·gical (L. *medicus*, medical; G. *kheirourgia*, surgery). Relating to both medicine and surgery.

medico-lē·gal (L. *medicus*, medical; *legalis*, lawful). Relating both to medicine and to law. Syn. forensic medicine.

mĕ·dicus (L.). A physician.

Medinal. A proprietary preparation of barbitonum sodium, used as a sedative.

Medina-worm. Dracunculus medinensis.

Mediterranean fever. See under fever, Mediterranean.

mĕ·dium (L. *medius*, middle). 1. Any substance transmitting force. 2. Any substance used for the culture of micro-organisms. 3. A mean.

mĕ·dius (L.). Middle.

medul·la (L.). 1. Marrow, e.g. bone-marrow. 2. The medulla oblongata, the upper part of the spinal cord between the cerebral pons and the foramen magnum. 3. The inner portion of an organ, e.g. the adrenal m.

medul·lar, medul·lary (L. *medulla*, marrow). 1. Relating to the marrow or medulla. 2. Resembling marrow in consistency; e.g., m. cancer. 3. Relating to the medulla oblongata. 4. Myelin, e.g., m. sheath is the same as myelin sheath. 5. Neural, e.g., m. plate is the same as neural plate. **M. canal; M. groove; M. plate; M. ridge:** see neural canal, etc.

mĕ·dullated (L. *medulla*, marrow). Containing or surrounded by a medulla or marrow; especially applied to nerve fibres. See also myelinated.

medullā·tion (L. *medulla*, marrow). The process of acquiring a medulla.

medul·loblastŏ·ma (L. *medulla*; G. *blastos*, germ). A rapidly-growing tumour composed of embryonic cells of neuro-epithelial origin, occurring usually in the cerebellar midline in children, tending to spread throughout the subarachnoid spaces.

mĕ·gabactē·rium (G. *megas*, large; *bakterion*, a staff). A large bacterium.

mega·caecum (G. *megas*, large; L. *caecum*, blind). An abnormally large caecum.

megacar·dia (G. *megas*, large; *kardia*, heart). Distension of the heart.

megacĕ·phaly (G. *megas*, large; *kephalē*, head). Macrocephaly, *q.v.*

megacoc·cus (G. *megas*, large; *kokkos*, grain). A large coccus.

megacō·lon (G. *megas*, large; *kolon*, colon). Hirschsprung's disease, *q.v.*

mĕ·gadont (G. *megas*, large; *odous*, tooth). Having a dental index, *q.v.*, of over 44.

megaduodē·num (G. *megas*, large; L. *duodeni*, twelve each). Abnormal dilatation of the duodenum.

megakă·ryocyte (G. *megas*, large; *karuon*, nut; *kutos*, cell). The stem-cell of the blood platelets, normally present in blood-forming organs, characterized by a very large size (30– 60μ), a large irregularly shaped nucleus and a transparent, faintly basophil cytoplasm.

megakaryocytō·sis. Excessive number of megakaryocytes.

megalencephā·lia, megalencĕ·phaly (G. *megas*, large; *egkephalos*, brain). Any enlargement of the brain not due to a tumour or hydrocephalus.

mĕ·galoblast (G. *megas*, large; *blastos*, germ). A large dysplastic, immature, nucleated red blood corpuscle with non-granulated basophil cytoplasm, a nucleus with fine chromatin structure, often with a perinuclear halo indicating the beginning of haemoglobin formation; present in blood and blood-forming tissues in pernicious anaemia. The term is often incorrectly applied to macroblast, *q.v.*

megalocĕ·phaly (G. *megas*, large; *kephalē*, head). Macrocephaly, *q.v.*

megalocor·nea (G. *megas*, large; L. *corneus*, horny). See keratoglobus.

mĕ·galocyte (G. *megas*, large; *kutos*, cell). A large, dysplastic, ovoid erythrocyte, derived from the megaloblast, present in blood and blood-forming tissues in pernicious anaemia. The term is often applied for macrocyte, *q.v.*

megalodac·tylous (G. *megas*, large; *daktulos*, finger). Having abnormally large fingers and/or toes.

megalogă·stria (G. *megas*, large; *gastēr*, stomach). Abnormal distension of the abdomen.

megaloglos·sia (G. *megas*, large; *glōssa*, tongue). See macroglossia.

megalomā·nia (G. *megas*, large; *mania*, madness). Mental condition characterized by delusions of grandeur.

megalomē·lia (G. *megas*, large; *melos*, limb). Macromelia, *q.v.*

megalop·sia (G. *megas*, large; *opsis*, vision). Macropsia, *q.v.*

mĕ·gaphone (G. *megas*, large; *phōnē*, voice). An instrument for magnifying the sound of the voice.

mĕ·gaseme (G. *megas*, large; *sēma*, sign). Having an orbital index, *q.v.*, greater than 89, characteristic of the yellow races.

megasō·ma (G. *megas*, large; *sōma*, body). Unusually great stature, but not amounting to gigantism.

Méglin's palatine point (Méglin, J. A., French physician, 1756–1824). The point at which the descending palatine nerve emerges from the palatomaxillary canal.

Meibom's cyst (Meibom, H., German anatomist, 1638–1700). Retention cysts of Meibomian glands of the eyelids. **M.'s foramen:** see foramen caecum of tongue. **M.'s glands:** tarsal glands. Modified sebaceous glands each consisting of a straight tube with multiple diverticula lying in grooves on the inner surface of the tarsal plates of the eyelids. Their ducts open on the free margins of the lids. **M.'s stye:** inflammation of the tarsal glands.

meibomiani·tis. Inflammation of a meibomian gland.

Meigs's capillaries (Meigs, A. V., American physician, 1850–1912). The capillary blood vessels found between the muscular fibres of the heart.

Meinert's form of enteroptosis (Meinert, E., American physician; work published 1893). Enteroptosis in chlorotic patients.

Meinicke's reaction (Meinicke, E., German physician, born 1878). A precipitation test for the serodiagnosis of syphilis.

meiō·sis, miō·sis (G. *meiōn*, less). 1. The occurrence of two divisions of a nucleus accompanied by one division of its chromosomes, resulting in the production of four nuclei, each of which has half the number of chronosomes of the mother nucleus. 2. Contraction of pupil of the eye.

meiostag·min reaction. A serum reaction founded upon the lowered surface tension of a liquid when a specific antigen is added to a specific serum.

meiŏ·tic, miŏ·tic (G. *meiōn*, less). Characterized by or causing meiosis.

Meissner's corpuscles (Meissner, G., German histologist, 1829–1903). Tactile nerve endings, corpuscula tactus. **M.'s plexus:** a sympathetic plexus found in the submucous layer of the small intestine.

mel (L.). Honey.

melanae·mia (G. *melas*, black; *haima*, blood). Condition in which black pigment is found in the blood.

melae·na (G. *melas*, black). The discharge of stools stained black by altered blood, due to haemorrhage from the alimentary tract.

mela·gra (G. *melos*, limb; *agra*, seizure). Painful muscular affections of the extremities.

melal·gia (G. *melos*, limb; *algos*, pain). Pain in the limbs.

melanchō·lia, mĕ·lancholy (G. *melas*, black; *khŏlē*, bile). A psychotic condition characterized by emotional depression, delusions and motor and mental inhibition.

melanchol·ic (G. *melas*, black; *khŏlē*, bile). 1. Affected with melancholy. 2. A type of temperament characterized by a tendency to phases of depression.

melanĕ·mesis (G. *melas*, black; *emeein*, to vomit). Black vomit.

melanephidrō·sis (G. *melas*, black; *ephidrōsis*, superficial sweating). Secretion of dark-coloured sweat.

melanidrō·sis (G. *melas*, black; *hidros*, sweat). Melanephidrosis, *q.v.*

melani·ferous (G. *melas*, black; L. *ferre*, to carry). Containing melanin.

mĕ·lanin (G. *melas*, black). A black pigment, derived from tyrosin, occurring normally in the choroid coat of the eye, in the basal epithelial layer of the skin, the hair and the muscles, but in abnormal amounts in the skin and mucous membranes in Addison's disease and in melanotic tumours.

mĕ·lanism (G. *melas*, black). Abnormal deposition of melanin in an organ.

mĕ·lanoblast (G. *melas*, black; *blastos*, germ). A cell, present mainly in the basal epithelial layer of the skin, containing and probably producing a pigment and reacting positively with the dopa reagent.

melanoblastō·ma. A tumour composed of melanoblasts.

melanocarcinō·ma (G. *melas*, black; *karkinos*, an ulcer). See melanoma.

melanoder·ma (G. *melas*, black; *derma*, skin). Abnormal, usually localized hyperpigmentation of the skin.

melanodermati·tis tox·ica lichenoi·des (G. *melas*, black; *derma*, skin; *toxikon*, poison; *leikhēn*, scab; *eidos*, form). Tar-workers' dermatitis.

melă·nogen (G. *melas*, black; *gennan*, to produce). A precursor of melanin.

melanoglos·sia (G. *melas*, black; *glōssa*, tongue). See black tongue.

mĕ·lanoid (G. *melas*, black; *eidos*, form). Dark-coloured.

melanō·ma (G. *melas*, black). A variety of malignant neoplasm characterized by a black colour due to its content of melanin, arising sometimes from a pigmented mole or from the choroidea. Syn. melanotic carcinoma; melanotic sarcoma; melanosarcoma.

melanomatō·sis (G. *melas*, black). Multiple melanomata.

melanonў·chia (G. *melas*, black; *onux*, finger-nail). Blackening of a nail.

melanō·pathy (G. *melas*, black; *pathos*, disease). Any disease in which there is unusual darkening of the skin and/or tissues.

mĕ·lanophore (G. *melas*, black; *phoros*, bearing). A connective tissue cell having the function of taking up pigment by phagocytosis but not of producing it, and reacting negatively with the dopa reagent.

melanosarcō·ma (G. *melas*, black; *sarx*, flesh). Melanoma, *q.v.*

melanō·sis (G. *melas*, black). Melanoderma, *q.v.* **M. coli**: a condition characterized by pigmentation of the mucous membrane of the colon with melanin, probably caused by the action of certain aperients.

melanot·ic (G. *melas*, black). Containing melanin pigment.

melanotri·chia lin·guae (G. *melas*, black; *thrix*, hair; L. *lingua*, tongue). Black tongue, *q.v.*

melanū·ria (G. *melas*, black; *ouron*, urine). The excretion of urine containing melanin pigment.

melasic·terus (G. *melas*, black; *ikteros*, jaundice). Jaundice of especially dark tint, often present in obstruction of the common bile duct of long duration.

melas·ma (G. *melas*, black). Melanodermia.

melioidō·sis (G. *mēlis*, a distemper of asses; *eidos*, form). An infectious disease, resembling glanders, due to *Pfeiferella melioides*, occurring in rodents and transmissible to man.

Melissa. A genus of plants which includes the *M. officinalis*, or lemon-balm, yielding tannin and an essential oil.

melissophō·bia (G. *melissa*, bee; *phobos*, fear). A neurotic fear of bees.

meliten·sis (L., from Malta). Undulant fever.

mĕ·litose (L. *mel*, honey). A crystalline sugar from Australian manna, sugar beet and cotton seed. It is a trisaccharide $C_{18}H_{32}O_{16},5H_2O$. Syn. raffinose.

melomā·nia (G. *melos*, song; *mania*, madness). Excessive fondness for music.

melŏ·melus (G. *melos*, limb). A monster foetus with supernumerary limbs.

melon seed bodies. Small fibrous structures within a joint cavity or in a cyst of a tendon sheath.

melon·cus (G. *mēla*, cheeks; *ogkos*, bulk). A tumour of the cheek.

melorheostō·sis (G. *melos*, limb; *rheein*, to flow; *osteon*, bone). A condition, probably recessively transmitted, characterized by endosteal and periosteal osteosclerosis, resembling in its radiographic appearance candle drippings running along the periphery of the bone, usually affecting a single limb and accompanied by moderate pain, restriction of articular movement, and sometimes by disturbance of growth of the affected part.

melŏ·schisis (G. *mēla*, cheeks; *skhizein*, to cleave). Congenital cleft of the cheek between upper lip and lower lid.

melting-point. The temperature at which a solid changes into the liquid state at a given pressure.

Meltzer's sign (Meltzer, S. J., American physician, 1851–1920). Loss of the normal second sound, heard on auscultation of heart after swallowing. Indicative of occlusion or constriction of the lower oesophagus.

member (L. *membrum*). A part of the body, especially a limb.

membrā·na (L.). A membrane.

membranā·ceous (L. *membrana*). Membranous.

mem·brane (L. *membrana*). A thin layer of tissue surrounding a part or lining a cavity or interposed between two parts. **M., basement**: a thin layer beneath the epithelium of mucous surfaces. **M., basilar**: the m. separating the scala vestibuli from the scala tympani and supporting the organ of Corti. **M., croupous**: the fibrinous-purulent exudate forming on the laryngeal surface in croup. **M., diphtheritic**: the fibrinous-purulent exudate forming on a mucous or cutaneous surface of a diphtheritic lesion. **M., germinal**: the blastoderm. **M., hyaloid**: the m. surrounding the vitreous body of the eye. **M., limiting**: see limiting m. **M., mucous**: the m. containing mucous glands and lining the alimentary and respiratory tracts, the excretory passages of the urogenital tract, the conjunctiva and the middle ear. **M., nictitating**: the plica semilunaris of the eye. **M., pupillary**: a membrane closing the pupil in the foetus and disappearing normally during the 7th month of foetal life. **M., serous**: the m. covered with endothelial cells and lining the closed cavities of the body and the organs contained within the cavities. **M., synovial**: the m. lining the intra-articular parts of bones and ligaments. **M., vitelline**: the cell m. of the ovum.

mem·branoid (L. *membrana*; G. *eidos*, form). Like a membrane.

mem·branous (L. *membrana*). Relating to, having the nature of or being characterized by the formation or discharge of a membrane. **M. dysmenorrhoea**: a form of dysmenorrhoea characterized by the discharge of a membranous cast of the endometrium.

mem·brum (L.). Member. **M. muliebre**: the clitoris. **M. virile**: the penis.

mĕm·ory (L. *memoria*). The phenomenon of recall to consciousness of sensory impressions previously received.

mĕ·nagogue (G. *mēn*, month; *agōgos*, leading). Syn. of emmenagogue.

menaph·thone. $C_{11}H_8O_2$, 2-methyl-1:4-naphthaquinone, used to produce the physiological action of vitamin K.

menar·che (G. *mēn*, month; *arkhē*, beginning). The first appearance of menstruation.

men·delism (Mendel, J. G., Bohemian monk and naturalist, 1822–84). Theory of inheritance according to Mendel's observations; the basis of the modern theory of genetics.

mendō·sus (L.). False.

Ménière's disease or syndrome (Ménière, P., French physician, 1799–1862). Aural vertigo; characterized by nausea, vomiting, tinnitus and progressive deafness. **M.'s solution**: a dressing of alcohol, ether, balsam of Peru, guaiacol, eucalyptus and iodoform.

menin·gĕal (G. *mēnigx*, membrane). Relating to the meninges.

menin·geocor·tical (G. *mēnigx*, membrane; L. *cortex*, rind). Relating to the meninges and cortex of the brain.

menin·gēs (G. *mēniggĕs*, pl. of *mēnigx*, membrane.) The membranes of the brain and spinal cord: the dura, pia and arachnoid.

meningiō·ma (G. *mēnigx*, membrane). A tumour developing from the lepto-meningeal cells which line the arachnoid villi.

menin·gism (G. *mēnigx*, membrane). Signs of meningeal irritation, as headache with stiffness of the muscles of the dorsal aspect of the neck in the absence of meningitis.

meningi·tis (G. *mēnigx*, membrane). Inflammation of the meninges. See also pachy-m. **M., basal**: lepto-m. confined to the basal part of the brain, often of tuberculous origin. **M., cerebrospinal**: see fever, cerebrospinal. **M., serous:** a condition characterized by an increase in the amount of cerebrospinal fluid, but without very gross changes in the cellular and chemical composition of this fluid, with symptoms resembling either m. or cerebral tumour. See also choriomeningitis, lymphocytic and hydrocephalus. **M., tuberculous:** an often fatal meningitis, due to haematogenous spread of tubercle bacilli from a tuberculous lesion elsewhere. See also M., basal.

menin·gocele (G. *mēnigx*, membrane; *kēlē*, hernia). A protrusion of the cerebral or spinal meninges through a bony defect in the skull or vertebral column.

meningococ·cus (G. *mēnigx*, membrane; *kokkos*, grain). A bacterium, the cause of cerebrospinal fever.

menin·gocyte (G. *mēnigx*, membrane; *kutos*, cell). A meningeal histiocyte.

meningo-encephali·tis (G. *mēnigx*, membrane; *egkephalos*, brain). Inflammation of the brain and its membranes.

meningo-encě·phalocele (G. *mēnigx*, membrane; *egkephalos*, brain; *kēlē*, hernia). A protrusion of the brain and its meninges through a bony defect in the skull.

meningo-encě·phalomyelī·tis (G. *mēnigx*, membrane; *egkephalos*, brain; *muelos*, marrow). Inflammation of the meninges, brain and spinal cord.

meningo·myeli·tis (G. *mēnigx*, membrane; *muelos*, marrow). Inflammation of the spinal cord and its meninges.

meningomȳ·ělocele (G. *mēnigx*, membrane; *muelos*, marrow; *kēlē*, hernia). A protrusion of a portion of the spinal cord and its meninges through a bony defect of the vertebral column.

meningorě·cidive. Neurorecidive, *q.v.*

meningorhachī·dian (G. *mēnigx*, membrane; *rhakhis*, spine). Relating to the spinal meninges.

mě·ninx (G. *mēnigx*, membrane). A membrane, particularly one of the brain or of the spinal cord. See also meninges.

menischě·sis (G. *mēn*, month; *iskhanein*, to hinder). Holding in or retention of the menses.

menis·cocyte (G. *mēniskos*, crescent; *kutos*, cell). A sickle-shaped erythrocyte.

meniscŏ·tomy (G. *mēniskos*, a crescent; *temnein*, to cut). Surgical removal of a meniscus, especially of the knee joint.

meniscec·tomy (G. *mēniskos*, crescent; *ektome*, excision). Removal of intra-articular cartilaginous meniscus; usually applied to the knee joint.

menis·cus (G. *mēniskos*, crescent). 1. A crescentic structure. 2. An interarticular fibro-cartilaginous disc. 3. A concavo-convex (positive m.) or convexo-concave (negative m.) lens. 4. The crescentic surface of liquids in narrow tubes.

menolip·sis (G. *mēn*, month; *leipein*, to cease). Temporary interruption of menstruation.

mě·nopausal. Relating to the menopause.

mě·nopause (G. *mēn*, month; *pausis*, cessation). The physiological cessation of menstruation. See also climacteric.

menorrhā·gia (G. *mēn*, month; *rhēgnunai*, to break out). Excessive menstruation.

menorrhoē·a (G. *mēn*, month; *rhoia*, flow). 1. The normal flow of the menses. 2 (more usually). Excessive menstruation.

men·ses (L. *mensis*, month). The recurrent monthly discharge of blood from the uterus between puberty and menopause.

men·strual. Relating to menstruation.

menstruā·tion (L. *menstruus*, monthly). The periodic discharge of blood from the uterus between puberty and menopause.

men·struŭm (L. *menstruus*, monthly). In pharmacy, a solvent, so called because a drug to be extracted was formerly left in the solvent liquid for about a month.

mensurā·tion (L. *mensurare*, to measure). The act of measuring.

men·tal[1] (L. *mens*, mind). Pertaining to the mind.

men·tal[2] (L. *mentum*, chin). Relating to the chin.

mentā·lis muscle. See levator menti.

mentā·lity (L. *mens*, mind). The specific mental constitution of an individual.

Mentha. A genus of labiate plants, including *M. viridis*, the spearmint, yielding a carminative stimulant.

menthol. A white crystalline substance obtained from several species of *Mentha*. Externally applied it dilates the vessels causing a feeling of coldness; it is useful in headache and rheumatic pains. Given internally, it is a carminative, but it is liable to upset the digestion. Formula $CH_3.C_6H_9(OH)C_3H_7$.

men·thone (L. *mentha*, mint). A ketone obtained from oil of peppermint.

men·tism (L. *mens*, mind). A mental state in which mental images are formed involuntarily.

mentohȳ·oid (L. *mentum*, chin; G. *huoides*, y-shaped). Relating to both the chin and the hyoid bone.

mentolā·bial (L. *mentum*, chin; *labia*, lips). Relating conjointly to chin and lips.

men·tolabiā·lis (L.). The levator labii inferioris and the quadratus menti taken conjointly as one muscle.

mentulag·ra (L. *mentula*, penis; G. *agra*, seizure). Priapism.

men·tulate (L. *mentula*, penis). Having an unusually large penis.

men·tulomā·nia (L. *mentula*, penis; G. *mania*, madness). Masturbation.

men·tum (L.). The chin.

mepacrine. 2-chloro-5-(*w*-diethylamino-α-methylbutylamino)-7-methoxyacridine. Originally introduced as Atebrin, it is used for the suppression and treatment of malaria.

meral·gia (G. *mēros*, thigh; *algos*, pain). Neuralgic pain in the thigh. **M. paraesthetica:** anaesthesia, paraesthesia, hyperaesthesia, with or without pain, in an area on the anterior surface of the thigh, probably due to irritation of the nervus cutaneus femoris externus.

mercap·tans (L. *Mercurius*, the god Mercury; *captare*, to seize). Organic compounds possessing the –SH group attached directly to a carbon atom.

Mercier's bar (Mercier, L. A., French urologist, 1811–82). A transverse curved ridge joining the openings of the ureters on the inner surface of the bladder, forming the posterior boundary of the trigonum vesicae.

mercū·rial (L. *Mercurius*, the god Mercury. Alchemical symbol for the metal). 1. Relating to or caused by mercury. 2. Any preparation of mercury.

mercū·rialism (L. *Mercurius*, the god Mercury). Mercury-poisoning.

mercū·ric (L. *Mercurius*, the god Mercury). Relating to compounds of bivalent mercury.

mercuric chloride. $HgCl_2$. A heavy, white powder, slightly soluble in water and used as a powerful antiseptic and disinfectant. Syn. corrosive sublimate.

mer·curochrome. Consists chiefly of the disodium salt of 2:7-dibromo-4-hydroxy-mercurifluorescein and is used as an antiseptic.

mer·curous. Relating to compounds of univalent mercury.

mercurous chloride. Hg_2Cl_2. A dull, white, heavy powder used as a purgative and in ointments. Syn. calomel.

mer·cury (L. *Mercurius*, the god Mercury). A shining, silver-white, fluid, volatile, metallic element, with a sp. gr. of 13·55.

meri·dian (L. *meridies*, midday). A circle surrounding a globe and passing through the poles. **M. of the eye:** a line drawn through the poles of the vertical axis (vertical m.), or through those of the transverse axis (horizontal m.).

meridrō·sis (G. *meros*, part; *hidros*, sweat). Local perspiration.

mĕ·rispore (G. *meros*, part; *spora*, seed). A spore produced from another spore by fission.

mĕ·ristem (G. *merizein*, to divide). The undifferentiated embryonic tissue of plants.

meri·stic (G. *merismos*, division). Relating to the component parts of a structure.

Merizomў·ria. A genus of schizomycetes.

Merkel's corpuscles (Merkel, F. S., German anatomist, 1845–1919). One form of sensory 'tactile' nerve ending. M.'s corpuscles are sometimes wrongly ascribed to Merkel, K. L.

Merkel's fossa (Merkel, K. L., German anatomist, 1812–76). The central fossa between the two ventricles of the larynx. M.'s muscle: the keratocricoid muscle.

Mermith·idāē. A family of Nematoda.

meroăcrā·nia (G. *meros*, part; *a*, neg.; *kranion*, skull). Partial acrania.

meroănencĕ·phaly (G. *meros*, part; *a*, neg.; *egkephalos*, brain). Partial anencephaly.

mĕ·roblast (G. *meros*, part; *blastos*, germ). An ovum containing both formative and nutritive protoplasm.

meroblas·tic (G. *meros*, part; *blastos*, germ). Applied to an ovum the yolk of which contains nutritive material and which undergoes cleavage at one pole only.

mĕ·rocele (G. *mēros*, thigh; *kēlē*, hernia). Femoral hernia.

mĕ·rocrine (G. *meros*, part; *krinein*, to separate). That type of secretion in which the glandular cell remains intact throughout the cycles of formation and discharge.

mĕ·rocyte (G. *meros*, part; *kutos*, cell). Supernumerary sperm nucleus in the ovum in cases of polyspermy.

merŏ·gamy (G. *meros*, part; *gamos*, marriage). That type of conjugation in protozoa in which the gametes are structurally different from and much smaller than the original vegetable cells.

merogĕ·nesis (G. *meros*, part; *genesis*, production). Reproduction by segmentation.

merŏ·gony (G. *meros*, part; *gŏnē*, generation). The development of an egg fragment devoid of a nucleus fertilized by a normal sperm.

mĕ·rorhachi·schisis (G. *meros*, part; *rhakis*, spine; *skhizein*, to cleave). Partial or incomplete rhachischisis.

merŏ·tomy (G. *meros*, part; *temnein*, to cut). Division into segments.

merozō·ite (G. *meros*, part; *zōon*, animal). One of the spores resulting from the splitting up of the schizont in the asexual reproduction of protozoa.

mersalyl. The sodium salt of salicyl (ρ-hydroxymercuri-β-methoxypropyl) amido-acetic acid, a white deliquescent powder used as a diuretic.

Merseburg triad (From the German town of Merseburg). Goitre, exophthalmos and tachycardia; the three symptoms of exophthalmic goitre.

Merulius lacrimans. The dry-rot fungus.

Mery's glands (Mery, J., French anatomist, 1645–1722). The synonym for Cowper's glands.

mĕ·rycism (G. *mērukismos*, a chewing of the cud). Rumination.

mē·sad (G. *mesos*, middle; L. *ad*, to). Towards the median line.

mē·sal (G. *mesos*, middle). Relating to or lying in the median line or plane.

mē·saortī·tis (G. *mesos*, middle; *aortē*). Inflammation of the middle coat of the aorta; due to syphilis.

mesarā·ic (G. *mesos*, middle; *araia*, belly). Mesenteric.

mesarterī·tis (G. *mesos*, middle; *artēria*). Inflammation of the central coat of an artery.

mesencĕ·phalon (G. *mesos*, middle; *egkephalos*, brain). The midbrain; that section of the brain developed from the middle cerebral vesicle. It consists of the corpora quadrigemina, the tegmental region, the aqueduct of Sylvius, and the cerebral peduncles.

mesen·chyma (G. *mesos*, middle; *egkhuma*, infusion). The embryonic tissue developing from the mesoderm, after formation of the germ layers, and giving rise to the blood and to the various types of connective tissue.

mesen·chymal (G. *mesos*, middle; *egkhuma*, infusion). Pertaining to mesenchyma. M. cell, undifferentiated: a cell found especially in loose connective tissue near small blood-vessels, characterized by a faintly basophil protoplasm and an oval nucleus with scanty chromatin and a nucleolus.

mesenter·ic (G. *mesos*, middle; *enteron*, intestine). Relating to the mesentery.

mesenterī·olum. 1. A small mesenterium. 2. The mesoappendix.

mesenterī·tis (G. *mesos*, middle; *enteron*, intestine). Inflammation of the mesentery.

mesentē·rium (G. *mesos*, middle; *enteron*, intestine). Mesentery.

mesen·teron (G. *mesos*, middle; *enteron*, intestine). The middle part of the primitive digestive tract, giving rise to the section of the alimentary tract between the pharynx and the lower portion of the rectum.

mĕ·sentery (G. *mesos*, middle; *enteron*, intestine). A fold of the peritoneum connecting the small intestine with the posterior abdominal wall. See also mesoappendix; mesocaecum; mesocolon; mesorectum.

mē·siad (G. *mesos*, middle). Mesad, *q.v.*

mē·sial (G. *mesos*, middle). Mesal, *q.v.*

mē·sion (G. *mesos*, middle). Meson, *q.v.*

mes·merism (Mesmer, F. A., Austrian physician, 1734–1815). The teaching of Mesmer about so-called animal magnetism and its alleged importance in inducing hypnosis.

meso-appen·dix (G. *mesos*, middle; L. *appendix*, appendage). The mesentery of the vermiform appendix.

mesobactē·rium (G. *mesos*, middle; *bakterion*, little stick). A bacterium of middle size.

mesobilirū·bin (G. *mesos*, middle; L. *bilis*, bile; *ruber*, red). Reduced bilirubin.

mesobilirubin·ogen (G. *mesos*, middle; L. *bilis*, bile; *ruber*, red; G. *gennan*, to produce). Reduced mesobilirubin, identical with urobilinogen.

mē·soblast (G. *mesos*, middle; *blastos*, germ). See mesoderm.

mesocaē·cum (G. *mesos*, middle; L. *caecus*, blind). A peritoneal fold connecting the caecum with the right iliac fossa.

mesocar·dia (G. *mesos*, middle; *kardia*, heart). The position of the heart in the central and anterior part of the chest.

mesocephal·ic (G. *mesos*, middle; *kephalē*, head). 1. Possessing a skull of medium size, i.e. having a cephalic index, *q.v.*, between 75 and 80. 2. Relating to the mesocephalon.

mesocĕ·phalon (G. *mesos*, middle; *kephalē*, head). The middle cerebral vesicle in the embryo.

mē·sochord (G. *mesos*, middle; *khordē*, string). A fold of the amnion by which the umbilical cord sometimes adheres to the placenta.

mesochoroi·dea (G. *mesos*, middle; *khorion*, skin; *eidos*, form). The central coat of the choroid.

mesocoē·lia (G. *mesos*, middle; *koilos*, hollow). The mesocephalic cavity.

mesocol·ic (G. *mesos*, middle; *kolon*, colon). Relating to the mesocolon.

mesocŏ·lon (G. *mesos*, middle; *kolon*, colon). The peritoneal fold connecting the colon with the posterior abdominal wall.

mē·soderm (G. *mesos*, middle; *derma*, skin). The middle germinal layer of an embryo, giving rise to the epithelium of the urogenital organs, to striated muscle tissue, heart muscle and the mesenchyme.

mesoder·mal. Relating to the mesoderm.

mesodes·ma (G. *mesos*, middle; *desma*, band). The uterine broad ligament.

mesodiă·stolĕ (G. *mesos*, middle; *diastolē*, dilatation). Mid-diastole.

mē·sodont (G. *mesos*, middle; *odous*, tooth). Having a dental index, *q.v.*, between 42 and 44.

mesoduodē·num (G. *mesos*, middle; L. *duodeni*, twelve each). A mesentery of the duodenum, normally not present.

mesogas·ter (G. *mesos*, middle; *gastēr*, belly). That part of the primitive gut from which are derived the liver, pancreas and small intestine.

mesogă·stric (G. *mesos*, middle; *gastēr*, belly). Relating to the umbilical region.

mesogă·strium (G. *mesos*, middle; *gastēr*, belly). 1. The umbilical region of the abdomen. 2. A peritoneal fold connecting the stomach with the posterior abdominal wall in early foetal life.

mesoglutae͞·us (G. *mesos*, middle; *gloutos*, rump). The gluteus medius muscle.

mesognă·thion (G. *mesos*, middle; *gnathos*, jaw). The ossification centre in the os incisivum for the lateral incisor tooth.

meso-i·leum (G. *mesos*, middle; L. *ileum*). The mesentery of the ileum.

mesojejū·num (G. *mesos*, middle; L. *jejunus*, hungry). The mesentery of the jejunum.

mesŏ·lobus (G. *mesos*, middle; *lobos*, lobe). The corpus callosum.

mesolym·phocyte (G. *mesos*, middle; L. *lympha*, water; G. *kutos*, cell). A lymphocyte of medium size.

mē·somere (G. *mesos*, middle; *meros*, part). A medium-sized blastomere.

mesomē·trium (G. *mesos*, middle; *mētra*, uterus). Myometrium, *q.v.*

mē·son (G. *mesos*, middle). A plane dividing the body into right and left halves.

mesoneph·ric. Relating to the mesonephron.

mesoneph·ron (G. *mesos*, middle; *nephros*, kidney). The cranial part of the Wolffian body, *q.v.*

mesoŏ·phoron (G. *mesos*, middle; *ōon*, egg; *pherein*, to bear). A part of the parovarium.

mesŏ·phryon (G. *mesos*, middle; *ophrus*, eyebrow). The glabella.

mesoprosō·pic (G. *mesos*, middle; *prosōpon*, face). Having a face of moderate width.

mesor·chium (G. *mesos*, middle; *orkhis*, testis). A peritoneal fold containing the testes at about the fifth month of foetal life.

mesorec·tum (G. *mesos*, middle; L. *rectus*, straight). The peritoneal fold connecting the upper part of the rectum with the sacrum.

mē·sorrhine (G. *mesos*, middle; *rhis*, nose). Having a nasal index between 48° and 53°.

mesosal·pinx (G. *mesos*, middle; *salpigx*, tube). The upper part of the broad ligament enveloping the uterine tube.

mē·soseme (G. *mesos*, middle; *sēma*, sign). Having an orbital index between 84 and 89, characteristic of the white races.

mesosig·moid (G. *mesos*, middle; *sigma*, the letter S; *eidos*, form). The mesentery of the sigmoid colon.

mesosigmoidi·tis. Inflammation of the mesosigmoid.

mesosō·ma (G. *mesos*, middle; *sōma*, body). Medium physique.

mesoster·num (G. *mesos*, middle; *sternon*, breast). The gladiolus, or middle section of the sternum.

mesosy̆·philis (G. *mesos*, middle; L. L. *syphilis*). Secondary syphilis.

mesosystol·ic (G. *mesos*, middle; *sustolē*, contraction). Relating to the middle of a systole.

mesoten·don (G. *mesos*, middle; *teinein*, to stretch). Delicate connective tissue membrane surrounding a tendon.

mesothē·lial (G. *mesos*, middle; *thēlē*, nipple). Relating to the mesothelium.

mesotheliō·ma (G. *mesos*, middle; *thēlē*, nipple). A tumour composed of mesothelial tissue.

mesothē·lium (G. *mesos*, middle; *thēlē*, nipple). That part of the mesoderm which lines the wall of the primitive body-cavity; the precursor of the endothelium.

mesŏ·thenar (G. *mesos*, middle; *thĕnar*, palm of the hand). The adductor pollicis muscle.

mesovā·rium (G. *mesos*, middle; L. *ōvum*, egg). The peritoneal fold connecting the ovary and the broad ligament.

meta-arthrit·ic (G. *meta*, beyond; *arthron*, joint). Resulting from arthritis.

metabiō·sis (G. *meta*, beyond; *bios*, life). Obligatory dependence of one organism upon another.

metabol·ic (G. *metabolē*, change). Pertaining to metabolism.

metă·bolism (G. *metabolē*, change). The sum of physical and chemical changes in a living body. See also anabolism and catabolism. M., basal: the minimal production of heat in a resting individual 12 hours after intake of food.

metă·bolite (G. *metabolē*, change). Any product of metabolism.

metă·bolon (G. *metabolē*, change). An unstable intermediary product in the disintegration of radio-active substances.

metacercā·ria (G. *meta*, beyond; *kerkos*, tail). The encysted stage of trematodes.

metacar·pal (G. *meta*, beyond; *karpos*, wrist). Relating to the metacarpus or to any one of the bones constituting the metacarpus.

metacarpec·tomy (G. *meta*, beyond; *karpos*, wrist; *ektomē*, excision). Excision of any of the metacarpal bones.

metacar·pophalan·geal (G. *meta*, beyond; *karpos*, wrist; *phalagx*, the bone between two joints of fingers or toes). Relating to the metacarpus and the phalanges.

metacar·pus (G. *meta*, beyond; *karpos*, wrist). The portion of the hand situated between the carpus and the phalanges. It is composed of the five metacarpal bones.

mē·tacoele (G. *meta*, beyond; *koilia*, ventricle). The caudal part of the fourth ventricle.

metachromat·ic (G. *meta*, beyond; *khrōma*, colour). Relating to a change of colours; staining in a tint different from that of the other tissues, e.g. the Babes-Ernst bodies, spherical basophilic bodies found in the protoplasm of many lower organisms.

metachrō·matism (G. *meta*, beyond; *khrōma*, colour). The property of a tissue to become stained in different tints by the same stain.

metachrō·sis (G. *meta*, beyond; *khrōzein*, to colour). A change of colours.

metă·chysis (G. *meta*, beyond; *khusis*, effusion). Blood transfusion.

metacon·dyle (G. *meta*, beyond; *kondulos*, knuckle). The distal phalanx of a finger, or its bone.

metacrē·sol. A colourless liquid and strong antiseptic derived from coal-tar.

metacyē·sis (G. *meta*, beyond; *kuēsis*, conception). Extra-uterine pregnancy, especially one which is begun in the uterine tube and continued in the abdominal cavity.

metaduode·num (G. *meta*, beyond; L. *duodeni*, twelve each). That portion of the duodenum which develops from the midgut.

metagas·ter (G. *meta*, beyond; *gastēr*, belly). The permanent intestinal canal, derived from the primitive canal or protogaster.

metagĕ·nesis (G. *meta*, beyond; *genesis*, production). The alternation of asexual with sexual generation.

metakinē·sis (G. *meta*, beyond; *kinēsis*, movement). Movement of chromosomes into metaphase.

mĕ·tal (G. *metallon*, a mine). Any one of those elements which are characterized by ductility, malleability, lustre, the property of conducting heat and electricity and entering into chemical reactions as the positive ion.

metal·lic (G. *metallon*, a mine). Relating to a metal. **M. tinkling**: a tinkling metallic sound, somewhat resembling the faint tinkle of a bell, sometimes heard on auscultation during respiration over a pneumohydrothorax or a large pulmonary cavity.

mĕ·talloid (G. *metallon*, a mine; *eidos*, form). Any element with intermediate properties between typical metals and non-metals.

metallophō·bia (G. *metallon*, a mine; *phŏbos*, fear). Neurotic fear of touching a metallic object.

metallur·gy (G. *metallon*, a mine; *ergon*, work). The study of metals.

mĕ·tamere (G. *meta*, beyond; *meros*, part). A segment of the animal body.

metamer·ic. Relating to metamerism.

metă·merism (G. *meta*, beyond; *meros*, part). 1. Arrangement in metameres. 2. A class of isomerism.

mĕ·tamers (G. *meta*, beyond; *meros*, part). 1. Metameric compounds. 2. Arrangement in metameres.

metamitō·sis (G. *meta*, beyond; *mitos*, thread). A form of mitosis in which both nucleus and cytoplasm contribute to the formation of the mitotic figure.

metamor·phic, metamor·phous (G. *meta*, beyond; *morphē*, form). Relating to metamorphosis.

metamorphop·sia (G. *metamorphoun*, to transform; *opsis*, sight). A defect of vision in which objects appear distorted.

metamor·phosis (G. *metamorphōsis*, transformation from *meta*, beyond; *morphē*, form). 1. In pathology, a form of degeneration. 2. In biology, a form of development in which the individual animal undergoes a larval stage before attaining the adult form.

metamȳ·elocyte (G. *meta*, beyond; *muelos*, marrow; *kutos*, cell). A leucocyte transitional between the myelocyte and the polymorphonuclear leucocyte, present in the peripheral blood in cases of leucocytosis but in larger numbers only in myeloid leukaemia; characterized by a bean-shaped nucleus with coarse chromatin structure, and neutrophil, eosinophil or basophil granules in the cytoplasm.

metaneph·ron, metaneph·ros (G. *meta*, beyond; *nephros*, kidney). The caudal part of the Wolffian body, *q.v.*, forming at a later embryonal stage the permanent kidney.

mĕ·taphase (G. *meta*, after; *phasis*, phase). The middle stage of mitosis when the chromosomes lie nearly in a single plane at the equator of the spindle, forming thus the equatorial plate.

metaphosphor·ic acid. HPO_3, a phosphoric acid.

metaphrē·nia (G. *meta*, beyond; *phrēn*, mind). A mental state in which the interests of the patient are withdrawn from his family circle and directed to personal gain or aggrandisement.

metaphrē·non (G. *meta*, beyond; *phrēn*, diaphragm). The region between the shoulders.

metaphȳ·seal, metaphȳ·sial. Relating to a metaphysis.

metă·physis (G. *meta*, beyond; *phuesthai*, to grow). The distal, spongy part of the diaphysis.

metaphysī·tis. Inflammation of a metaphysis, especially of a long bone.

metaplā·sia (G. *meta*, beyond; *plassein*, to form). A transformation of a tissue into another tissue.

mĕ·taplasm (G. *meta*, beyond; *plasma*, something formed). Deutoplasm.

metaplā·stic (G. *meta*, beyond; *plassein*, to form). Relating to metaplasia.

metaplex·us (G. *meta*, beyond; L. *plexus*, a fold). The choroid plexus of the fourth ventricle.

metapneumon·ic (G. *meta*, beyond; *pneumon*, the lungs). Following pneumonia.

metapŏ·physis (G. *meta*, beyond; *apophusis*, offshoot). The mammillary process on the superior articular processes of certain vertebrae.

metă·stasis (G. *meta*, beyond; *stasis*, a placing). The transfer of particles from a primary focus of disease to another, distant, place by conveyance through the blood- or lymph-vessels.

metastat·ic. Characterized by or caused by or relating to metastasis.

metaster·num (G. *meta*, beyond; *sternon*, breast). The ensiform cartilage of the sternum.

metastruc·ture (G. *meta*, beyond; L. *structura*, arrangement). The assumed ultra-microscopical organization of protoplasm as distinguished from its chemical and molecular constitution.

met·asyphilit·ic (G. *meta*, beyond; syphilis). Following syphilis.

metatar·sal (G. *meta*, beyond; *tarsos*, flat of the foot). Relating to the metatarsus or to any one of the bones constituting the metatarsus.

metatarsal·gia (G. *meta*, beyond; *tarsos*, flat of the foot; *algos*, pain). A condition characterized by pain, burning or numbness of the heads of the metatarsal bones, or more especially of the 4th metatarsal bone, sometimes due to relaxation of the anterior arch of the foot. Syn. Morton's disease.

metatarsec·tomy (G. *meta*, beyond; *tarsos*, flat of the foot; *ektomē*, excision). Excision of any of the metatarsal bones.

metatar·sophalan·geal (G. *meta*, beyond; *tarsos*, flat of the foot; *phalagx*, bone between two joints of fingers or toes). Relating to the metatarsus and the phalanges.

metatar·sus (G. *meta*, beyond; *tarsos*, flat of the foot). That portion of the foot between the tarsus and the phalanges. It consists of the five metatarsal bones.

metatē·la (G. *meta*, beyond; L. *tēla*, web). The tela choroidea of the 4th ventricle.

metathă·lamus (G. *meta*, beyond; *thalamos*, an inner chamber). The medial and lateral geniculate bodies.

Metazō·a (G. *meta*, beyond; *zōon*, animal). A division of the animal kingdom including all species composed of more than one cell.

Metchnikoff's larva (Metchnikoff, E., Russian biologist, 1845–1916). The parenchymula; the embryonic stage of which the closed blastula is the precursor. **M.'s theory**: the phagocytic theory, that the body is protected against infection by the leucocytes and other cells which englobe and destroy the invading micro-organisms.

metencĕ·phalon (G. *meta*, beyond; *egkephalos*, brain). 1. The after-brain; the part from which the medulla oblongata is developed. Syn. myelencephalon. 2. Formerly applied to that part of the brain from which the pons and the cerebellum are developed; the hind-brain.

mĕ·teorism (G. *mĕteōrizein*, to raise up). Gaseous distension of the abdomen. Syn. tympanites.

meteorŏ·logy (G. *meteōros*, high in the air; *logos*, a discourse). The science dealing with the causes and phenomena of climatic conditions.

methaemal·bumin (G. *meta*, beyond; *haima*, blood; L. *albumen*, white of egg). An extracorpuscular pigment found in the plasma in haemoglobinurias and certain haemolytic anaemias, forming with concentrated, ammonium sulphide a haemochromogen. Syn. pseudo-methaemoglobin.

mĕt·haēme (G. *meta*, beyond; *haima*, blood). Haematin.

met·haēmoglō·bin (G. *meta*, beyond; *haima*, blood; L. *globus*, globe). An isomere of haemoglobin, but having its oxygen more firmly united with it. It is formed in the blood in poisoning with chlorates, the nitrites, etc. See also methaemalbumin.

met·haemoglobinae·mia (G. *meta*, beyond; *haima*, blood; L. *globus*, globe; G. *haima*, blood). The presence of methaemoglobin in the blood.

met·haemoglobinū·ria (G. *meta*, beyond; *haima*, blood; L. *globus*, globe; G. *ouron*, urine). The excretion of methaemoglobin in the urine.

mĕ·thane. Marsh gas, CH_4, the simplest saturated hydrocarbon.

methet·ic (G. *methexis*, participation). Applied to communications between the different strata of a man's personality, e.g. exhibited in automatic writing.

methionine. An essential amino acid containing sulphur.

mĕ·thod. The way in which any act is performed or operation carried out.

methomā·nia (G. *methu*, wine; *mania*, madness). 1. Dipsomania. 2. Mania a potu.

mĕ·thyl (G. *meta*, after; *hulē*, wood). The univalent hydrocarbon radicle—CH_3. **M. alcohol:** CH_3OH, a substance formed in the dry distillation of wood. **M. testosterone:** methyl derivative of testosterone.

mĕ·thylated spirit. Four varieties are recognized. They consist of ethyl alcohol denatured by the addition of wood spirit.

mĕ·thylene (G. *meta*, after; *hulē*, wood). A bivalent hydrocarbon radical. **M. blue:** a blue aniline dye of alkaline reaction used as a stain in microscopy.

mĕ·thylglyŏx·al (G. *meta*, after; *hulē*, wood; *glukus*, sweet; *oxus*, sharp). $CH_3CO\text{-}CHO$, a substance formed in the intermediary metabolism of carbohydrate.

methylsul·phonal. $(CH_3)(C_2H_5)C(SO_2.C_2H_5)_2$, a hypnotic.

metŏ·pagus (G. *metōpon*, forehead; *pagos*, a fixture). A double monster with two heads united at the foreheads.

metop·ic (G. *metōpon*, forehead). 1. Relating to the forehead; frontal. 2. Relating to metopism.

mĕ·topism (G. *metōpon*, forehead). Continuance of the frontal suture in adult life.

mĕ·tra (G. *mētra*). The uterus.

metral·gia (G. *mētra*, uterus; *algos*, pain). Pain in the uterus.

metranŏik·ter (G. *mētra*, uterus; *anoigein*, to open). A uterine dilator with two or four blades.

metre (G. *metron*, measure). The unit of linear measure of the metric system, 39·37 inches.

metrechŏ·scopy (G. *metron*, measure; *ēkhō*, sound; *skopein*, to view). Conjoined measuring, auscultation and visual examination.

metrecta·sia (G. *mētra*, uterus; *ektasis*, extension). Dilatation of the uterus in a non-pregnant woman.

metrec·tomy (G. *mētra*, womb; *ektomē*, excision). Hysterectomy, *q.v.*

metrectō·pia, metrec·topy (G. *mētra*, uterus; *ektopos*, displaced). Displacement of the uterus.

met·ric (G. *metron*, measure). 1. Relating to the system of weights and measures, the basis of which is the metre. 2. Relating to measurement.

metri·tis (G. *mētra*, uterus). Inflammation of the uterus.

metrocarcinō·ma (G. *mētra*, uterus; *karkinos*, crab). Carcinoma of the uterus.

mĕ·trocele (G. *mētra*, uterus; *kēlē*, hernia). Hernia of the uterus.

mĕ·troclyst (G. *mētra*, uterus; *kluzein*, to wash). Apparatus for performing uterine douching.

mĕtrocol·pocele (G. *mētra*, uterus; *kolpos*, womb; *kēlē*, hernia). Prolapse of the uterus into the vagina.

mĕtrodў·nia (G. *mētra*, uterus; *odunē*, pain). Pain in the uterus.

met·ronome (G. *metron*, measure; *nomos*, law). An instrument recording short periods of time by audible sounds.

mĕ·tropară·lysis (G. *mētra*, uterus; *para*, beside; *lusis*, a loosening). Paralysis of the uterus.

mĕtropă·thia, metrŏ·pathy (G. *mētra*, uterus; *pathos*, disease). A disease of the uterus. **M. haemorrhagica:** a disease characterized by hyperplasia of the uterine endometrium with cystic dilatation of its glands, painless menorrhagia with or without preceding amenorrhoea, associated with atrophic ovaries bearing follicular cysts, and probably due to a lack of luteinizing hormone.

mĕtropath·ic (G. *mētra*, uterus; *pathos*, disease). Relating to affections of the uterus.

mĕ·troperitonī·tis (G. *mētra*, uterus; *peri*, around; *teinein*, to stretch). 1. Inflammation of the uterus and peritoneum. 2. Peritonitis secondary to uterine inflammation. 3. Inflammation of the peritoneal covering of the uterus.

mĕ·trophlebī·tis (G. *mētra*, uterus; *phleps*, vein). Inflammation of the uterine veins.

mĕtroptō·sis (G. *mētra*, uterus; *ptōsis*, a fall). Prolapse of the uterus.

mĕtrorrhā·gia (G. *mētra*, uterus; *rhēgnunai*, to break out). Uterine haemorrhage not connected with menstruation.

mĕtrorrhoē·a (G. *mētra*, uterus; *rhoia*, flow). Any morbid uterine discharge.

mĕtrorrhex·is (G. *mētra*, uterus; *rhēxis*, rupture). Rupture of the uterus.

mĕ·trosalpingi·tis (G. *mētra*, uterus; *salpigx*, tube). Inflammation of the uterus and uterine tube.

mĕtrosal·pinx (G. *mētra*, uterus; *salpigx*, tube). The uterine (Fallopian) tube.

mĕtrostax·is (G. *mētra*, uterus; *staxis*, a dripping). Slight but continuous haemorrhage from the uterus.

mĕ·trostenō·sis (G. *mētra*, uterus; *stēnōsis*, contraction). Contraction of the uterine cavity.

mĕ·trosterē·sis (G. *mētra*, uterus; *sterēsis*, deprivation). Excision of the uterus.

Mett's test (Mett, E. L. P., German physician of the 19th century). A test for the estimation of pepsin using digestion of coagulated albumin.

Meyer's cartilages (Meyer, E. V., German laryngologist, 1864–1931). The anterior sesamoid cartilages situated in the anterior extremities of the inferior thyroarytenoid ligaments.

Meyer's disease (Meyer, H. W., Danish physician, 1824–98). Hypertrophy of the pharyngeal tonsil; adenoid growths on the pharynx.

Meyer's organ (Meyer, G. H. von, German anatomist, 1815–92). The aggregation of glands beneath the tongue, situated on the hyoglossus muscle. **M.'s rings:** the faint rings seen to surround a candle-flame placed against a dark background; they appear more distinct when the eyes are briefly exposed to osmic acid fumes. **M.'s sinus:** the depression in the floor of the external auditory meatus.

Meyerholtz's muscle (Meyerholtz, of Göttingen, 19th century German anatomist). The radially disposed muscle fibres underlying the areola of the nipple.

Meynert's bundle (Meynert, T., Austrian anatomist, 1833–92). Fasciculus retroflexus. A small bundle of nerve fibres running between the habenula, centre for co-ordination of smell, to the interpedunculated space. **M.'s commissure:** nerve fibres which extend from the floor of the 3rd ventricle through the optic tracts to the subthalamic body. **M.'s dorsal tegmental decussation:** found in the midbrain at the level of the superior colliculus and between the nuclei in the dorsal part of the median raphe. **M.'s fibres:** nerve fibres conveying light sensation from the anterior corpora quadrigemina to the oculomotor nerve. **M.'s layer:** the third layer of the cerebral cortex. The layer of large pyramidal cells. **M.'s solitary cells:** cells of the ganglionic layer of the cerebral cortex.

Meynet's nodosities (Meynet, P. C. H., French physician, 1831–92). Growths of nodular type connected with joint, tendon and tendon-sheath capsules and sometimes formed in the neighbourhood of the affected joints in acute rheumatism.

Mg. The symbol of magnesium.

mg. The abbreviation of milligramme.

MgO. Magnesium oxide.

MgSO$_4$. Magnesium sulphate.

MgSO$_4$.7H$_2$O. Epsom's salts.

mi·asm, miăs·ma (G. *miainein*, to stain.) An obsolete term formerly used to denote any pathogenic particles or emanations which were thought to invade the body from without; (soil, air, water).

miăsmat·ic (G. *miainein*, to stain). Relating to, caused by or having the nature of miasm.

Mibelli's disease (Mibelli, V., Italian dermatologist, 1860–1910). A rare hereditary skin disease characterized by irregular horny epidermal ridges which slowly spread eccentrically leaving a dry atrophic central area.

mi·ca (L.). 1. A crumb. 2. A laminated silica mineral.

micā·ceous (L. *mica*, a crumb). Friable.

micā·tion (L. *micare*, to move quickly). Rapid motion.

micel·le (L.L. *micella*, dim. of *mica*, crumb). 1. A colloidal ion. 2. An aggregation of molecules held loosely together.

Michel's clips (Michel, G., French surgeon, 1875–1937). Small metal clips used in closing the skin after operation.

micracous·tic (G. *mikros*, small; *akoustikos*, of or for hearing). Assisting in hearing faint sounds.

micrencĕ·phalon (G. *mikros*, small; *egkephalos*, brain). An abnormally small brain.

micrencĕ·phalous (G. *mikros*, small; *egkephalos*, brain). Relating to micrencephalon.

micrencĕ·phalus (G. *mikros*, small; *egkephalos*, brain). An individual with an abnormally small brain.

Microbactē·ria (G. *mikros*, small; *baktron*, staff). A species of bacteria.

mi·crobalance (G. *mikros*, small; L. *bis*, double; *lanx*, disc). A balance for the weighing of minute quantities.

mi·crobe (G. *mikros*, small; *bios*, life). A living organism of minute size, e.g. a bacterium.

micrŏ·bial, micrŏ·bic (G. *mikros*, small; *bios*, life). Relating to or of the nature of a microbe.

mi·crobiŏ·logy (G. *mikros*, small; *bios*, life; *logos*, a discourse). The science relating to micro-organisms.

mi·crobiophŏ·bia (G. *mikros*, small; *bios*, life; *phŏbos*, fear). Neurotic fear of microbes.

mi·croblast (G. *mikros*, small; *blastos*, germ). An abnormally small erythrocyte.

mi·croblephă·ria, mi·croblĕ·pharon (G. *mikros*, small; *blepharon*, eyelid). Abnormal congenital smallness of the eyelids.

microbrā·chia (G. *mikros*, small; *brakhiōn*, arm). Abnormal congenital smallness of the arms.

microcar·dia (G. *mikros*, small; *kardia*, heart). Abnormal congenital smallness of the heart.

microcen·trum (G. *mikros*, small; *kentron*, centre). A structure of the cytoplasm comprising the centrosome and the asters.

microcephă·lia (G. *mikros*, small; *kephalē*, head). Abnormal congenital smallness of the head.

microcephal·ic (G. *mikros*, small; *kephalē*, head). Having an abnormally small head.

microcĕ·phalism (G. *mikros*, small; *kephalē*, head). Microcephaly.

microcĕ·phalous (G. *mikros*, small; *kephalē*, head). Relating to microcephaly.

microcĕ·phalus (G. *mikros*, small; *kephalē*, head). A person with an abnormally small head.

microcĕ·phaly (G. *mikros*, small; *kephalē*, head). Abnormal congenital smallness of the head.

microchĕ·mistry (G. *mikros*, small; Arab. *al kimia*, chemistry). 1. Chemical reactions obtained with small quantities of a substance. 2. The study of chemical reactions with a microscope.

Mĭ·crococcā·cea. A family belonging to the order Eubacteriales and including the Micrococcus, Staphylococcus, Gaffkya and Sarcina.

Micrococ·cus (G. *mikros*, small; *kokkos*, grain). A genus of the family Coccaceae.

microcor·nea (G. *mikros*, small; L. *cornea*, from *cornu*, horn). Abnormal congenital smallness of the cornea.

microcos·mic (G. *mikros*, small; *kosmos*, world). Relating to the human body.

microcou·lomb (G. *mikros*, small; C. A. de Coulomb, French physicist, 1736–1806). One-millionth part of a coulomb, *q.v.*

mi·crocyst (G. *mikros*, small; *kustis*, bladder). A very small cyst.

mi·crocyte (G. *mikros*, small; *kutos*, cell). A red blood-corpuscle of less than the normal average diameter.

mic·rocythae·mia (G. *mikros*, small; *kutos*, cell; *haima*, blood). A blood condition in which the erythrocytes are smaller than the normal average size.

mi·crocytŏ·sis (G. *mikros*, small; *kutos*, cell). The condition in which microcytes are the prevalent or only type of red corpuscles in the blood.

mi·crodactÿ·lia (G. *mikros*, small; *daktulos*, finger). Abnormal congenital smallness of the fingers.

mi·crodont (G. *mikros*, small; *odous*, tooth). Having a dental index, *q.v.*, under 42.

microdon·tism (G. *mikros*, small; *odous*, tooth). Abnormal congenital smallness of the teeth.

mi·crofilā·ria (G. *mikros*, small; L. *filum*, thread). A non-generic term applied to filariidae known only in the larval stage.

mi·crofilm (G. *mikros*, small). A photographic film used for copying books, documents, etc., on a much reduced scale.

microgă·mete (G. *mikros*, small; *gamein*, to marry). In certain lower organisms, one of a pair of gametes which is considerably smaller than the other gamete (macro-gamete) and is regarded as the male sexual cell.

micrŏ·gamy (G. *mikros*, small; *gamos*, marriage). Merogamy, *q.v.*

microgă·stria (G. *mikros*, small; *gastēr*, belly). Abnormal congenital smallness of the stomach.

micrŏ·glia (G. *mikros*, small; *glia*, glue). A form of neuroglia, of probably mesodermal origin, characterized by small cells possessing a deeply staining nucleus and twisted processes. Syn. Hortega's cells.

micrŏ·gliacyte (G. *mikros*, small; *glia*, glue; *kutos*, cell). A primitive cell, the precursor of the microglia.

microglos·sia (G. *mikros*, small; *glōssa*, tongue). Abnormal congenital smallness of the tongue.

micrognā·thia (G. *mikros*, small; *gnathos*, jaw). Abnormal congenital smallness of the jaw, more especially of the lower jaw; the condition of having a gnathic index, *q.v.*, under 98.

mi·crogramme (G. *mikros*, small; *gramma*, small weight). A millionth part of a gramme; symbol μg or γ.

micro·graphy (G. *mikros*, small; *graphein*, to write). Writing in letters of minute size.

microgy̆·ria (G. *mikros*, small; *guros*, circle). Abnormal smallness and narrowness of the cerebral convolutions, due either to malformation or as a sequel to scar-formation.

microhepă·tia (G. *mikros*, small; *hēpar*, liver). Abnormal congenital smallness of the liver.

microlym·phoblast (G. *mikros*, small; L. *lympha*, water; G. *blastos*, germ). A lymphoblast of a size smaller than usually seen.

micromā·nia (G. *mikros*, small; *mania*, madness). The delusion of being a very small size.

micromā·zia (G. *mikros*, small; *mazos*, breast). Abnormal smallness of the breasts.

micromē·lia (G. *mikros*, small; *melos*, limb). Abnormal congenital smallness of the extremities.

micro·melus (G. *mikros*, small; *melos*, limb). An autosite monster characterized by having abnormally small extremities.

micrŏ·meter (G. *mikros*, small; *metron*, measure). An instrument for the measurement of the length of objects seen through a microscope.

micro-method (G. *mikros*, small; *methodos*, method). Any chemical method in which the estimation is made from a very small amount of substance.

mi·crometre (G. *mikros*, small; *metron*, measure). The one-millionth part of a metre, or 1/25400 of an inch. Syn. A micron. Symbol μ.

micrŏ·metry (G. *mikros*, small; *metron*, measure). The measurement of objects by means of a micrometer.

micromi·cron (G. *mikros*, small). The one-millionth part of a micron, *q.v.* Symbol $\mu\mu$.

micromil·limetre (G. *mikros*, small; L. *mille*, thousand; G. *metron*, measure). The one-millionth part of a millimetre. Syn. millimicron. Symbol mμ. Also used to denote a micrometre, *q.v.*

mi·cromō·toscope (G. *mikros*, small; L. *movēre*, to move; G. *skopein*, to view). An apparatus for photographing and exhibiting the movements of microscopic objects.

mi·cromy̆e·lia (G. *mikros*, small; *muelos.*, marrow). Abnormal congenital smallness of the spinal cord.

mi·cromy̆·eloblast (G. *mikros*, small; *muelos*, marrow; *blastos*, germ). A myeloblast of a size smaller than usually seen.

mi·cromy̆·elocyte (G. *mikros*, small; *muelos*, marrow; *kutos*, cell). A myelocyte of a size smaller than usually seen.

mi·cron[1] (G. *mikros*, small). One-thousandth part of a millimetre. Symbol μ. See also micrometre.

mi·cron[2] (G. *mikros*, small). A colloid particle which can be observed under the microscope.

micronū·cleus (G. *mikros*, small; L. *nucula*, dim. of *nux*, nut). 1. A small nucleus. 2. A nucleolus.

micro-or·ganism (G. *mikros*, small; *organon*, instrument). An organism of the animal or vegetable kingdom which, owing to its minute size, can be observed only under the microscope.

micropathŏ·logy (G. *mikros*, small; *pathos*, disease; *logos*, a discourse). 1. Morbid histology. 2. The study of micro-organisms in relation to disease.

mi·crophage (G. *mikros*, small; *phagein*, to eat). A minute phagocyte.

microphŏ·bia (G. *mikros*, small; *phŏbos*, fear). A neurotic fear of small things.

mi·crophone (G. *mikros*, small; *phōnē*, voice). An instrument that amplifies sounds.

microphŏ·tograph (G. *mikros*, small; *phōs*, light; *graphein*, to write). 1. A photograph of an object which has been enlarged through a microscope. 2. A photograph of minute size.

microphthal·mus (G. *mikros*, small; *ophthalmos*, eye). Abnormal congenital smallness of the ocular bulbus.

mi·crophyte (G. *mikros*, small; *phuton*, plant). Any vegetable micro-organism, especially one that is parasitic.

microp·sia (G. *mikros*, small; *opsis*, vision). A disturbance of vision in which objects appear smaller than they are.

micrō·pus (G. *mikros*, small; *pous*, foot). An individual with abnormal congenitally small feet.

mi·cropyle (G. *mikros*, small; *pulē*, gate). The small opening in the membrane enveloping the ovum through which a spermatozoon may penetrate.

mi·croscope (G. *mikros*, small; *skopein*, to view). An instrument with magnifying lenses used for the observation of objects not visible to the naked eye.

microscop·ic (G. *mikros*, small; *skopein*, to view). 1. Relating to the microscope. 2. Visible only when a microscope is used.

micro·scopy (G. *mikros*, small; *skopein*, to view). Examination under a microscope.

mi·croseme (G. *mikros*, small; *sēma*, sign). Having wide orbits, or an orbital index, *q.v.*, under 84; characteristic of the black races.

microsō·mia (G. *mikros*, small; *sōma*, body). Abnormal congenital smallness of the whole body, but not amounting to dwarfism. Syn. nanism.

mi·crospore (G. *mikros*, small; *sporos*, seed). A spore of small type, in some higher plants.

mi·crospori·dēs (G. *mikros*, small; *sporos*, seed). A group of acute generalized eruptions, due to ringworm fungi.

Micrŏ·sporon (G. *mikros*, small; *sporos*, seed). One of several species belonging to the hyphal fungi, e.g., *M. Audouini*, the parasite causing juvenile ringworm; *M. minutissimum*, the parasite causing erythema; *M. furfur*, the parasite causing pityriasis versicolor.

mi·crostat (G. *mikros*, small; *statos*, standing). The stage and finder of the microscope.

microstō·mia (G. *mikros*, small; *stoma*, mouth). Abnormal congenital smallness of the mouth.

micrō·tia (G. *mikros*, small; *ous*, ear). Abnormal congenital smallness of the external ear.

mi·crotome (G. *mikros*, small; *tomē*, a cutting). An instrument for cutting tissues into sections thin enough for microscopic examination.

micrŏ·tomy (G. *mikros*, small; *tomē*, a cutting) The cutting of sections.

mi·crovolt (G. *mikros*, small; Volta, A., Italian physicist, 1745–1827). One-millionth part of a volt.

mic·tion (L. *micturire*, to urinate). Micturition, *q.v.*

mic·turate (L. *micturire*, to urinate). To pass urine.

mic·turition (L. *micturire*, to urinate). The act of passing urine.

mid-axil·lary line. A line drawn perpendicularly downwards from the apex of the axilla.

mid-body. The deeply staining thickenings in the equatorial plane in mitotic division. Syn. cell-plate.

midbrain. The mesencephalon.

mid-clavĭ·cular line. A line drawn perpendicularly from the mid-point of the clavicle.

midgut. The part of the primitive gut which extends from the second part of the duodenum to the middle of the transverse colon.

midsternal line. A line drawn perpendicularly from the incisura of the manubrium sterni.

midwife. A nurse attending women in childbirth.

midwifery. Obstetrics.

Mierjejevsky's foramen (Mierjejevsky, J. L., Russian neurologist, 1839–1908). The foramen of Key and Retzius. See foramen of Luschka.

Miescher's tubes (Miescher, J. F., Swiss pathologist, 1811–87). Cysts in muscles infested with Sarcosporidia.

migraine (Fr.). A condition characterized by paroxysmal attacks of, usually unilateral, headache often

s

associated with nausea, vomiting and sometimes with visual disturbances. **M. ophthalmic**: a form of m. characterized by the prevalence of visual disturbances such as scotomata, hemianopsia, etc. **M., ophthalmoplegic**: a form characterized by periodic paresis of the third cranial nerve, sometimes due to a leakage of a cerebral aneurysm.

mi·grans (L. *migrare*, to depart). Wandering.

migrā·tion (L. *migrare*, to depart). A wandering; a passage of an object.

migrā·tory (L. *migrare*, to depart). Wandering.

mĭ·kron (G. *mikros*, small). See micron.

Mikulicz's cells (Mikulicz, J. von, Polish surgeon, 1850–1905). Round clear cells filled with a gelatinous material which may give the cytoplasm a foamy and reticulated appearance. Seen histologically in rhinoscleroma, an infective granuloma of Eastern origin. **M.'s disease**: a slowly developing bilateral enlargement of the lacrimal and salivary glands. The aetiology is unknown.

mil (L. *mille*, thousand). 1. The one-thousandth part of an inch. 2. The one-thousandth part of a litre; one cubic centimetre.

miliā·ria (L. *milium*, millet). A severe inflammatory affection of the sweat glands. **M. rubra**: an eruption of reddish papules arranged in clusters and of some vesicles, preceded by profuse perspiration and accompanied by a pricking or tingling sensation, due to an acute inflammation of the sweat glands with obstruction of their ducts. Syn. prickly heat.

mĭ·liary (L. *milium*, millet). 1. Resembling a millet-seed. 2. Marked by the formation of many lesions resembling a millet-seed in size.

milieu (Fr.). Environment.

mĭ·lium (L. *milium*, millet). A small, pearly, cyst-like structure of about millet-seed size, containing horny material, situated just under the epidermis, mainly on the face. **M., colloid**: a small, yellow, translucent cyst-like structure, containing gelatinous material, situated in the skin, mainly on the face.

milk. 1. The opaque white secretion of the mammary glands of female mammalia. 2. Milk-like juice of plants. **M., certified**: cow's m. obtained and bottled according to certain sanitary prescriptions, designed to minimize the danger of carrying infection. **M., condensed**: cow's m. from which part of the water has been evaporated. **M. crust**: see crusta lactea. **M., homogenized**: milk treated so as to reduce all fat globules to a uniformly small size, thus ensuring even distribution of fat in milk kept in bulk. **M. pasteurized**: milk in which pathogenic bacteria have been destroyed by heating the milk to a definite temperature for a definite time. **M., skimmed**: m. from which the cream has been removed. Syn. separated m. See also buttermilk; lactic acid; lactic acid milk.

milk-tooth. One of the first set of deciduous teeth.

Milkman's syndrome (Milkman, L. A., contemporary U.S. radiologist). Condition characterized by bizarre rarefaction of long and flat bones.

Millar's disease (Millar, J., Scottish surgeon, 1735–1801). Laryngismus stridulus; Kopp's thymic asthma.

Millard-Gubler's syndrome (Millard, A. L. J., French surgeon, 1830–1916; Gubler, A., French physician, 1821–79). See hemiplegia, crossed.

Miller-Abbott tube (Miller, T. G., contemporary, Abbot, W. O., 1902–43, U.S. physicians). Double-bore intestinal tube for relieving obstructions of upper intestinal tract.

mil·liampere (L. *mille*, thousand; Ampère, A. M., French physicist, 1775–1836). One-thousandth of an ampère.

mil·ligramme (L. *mille*, thousand; G. *gramma*, gramme). A thousandth part of a gramme. Symbol mgm.

mil·lilitre (L. *mille*, thousand; G. *litra*, a pound weight). A thousandth part of a litre; one cubic centimetre. Symbol cc. or ml.

mil·limetre (L. *mille*, thousand; G. *metron*, measure). A thousandth part of a metre. Symbol mm.

millimĭ·cron (L. *mille*, thousand; G. *mikros*, small). A thousandth part of a micron. Symbol mμ. Syn. micromillimetre.

mimet·ic (G. *mimētikos*). Imitative, especially in animals as a behaviour serving to protect against enemies.

mind-blindness. A condition characterized by absence or loss of memory of optic images, in which the patient, while capable of seeing, is not able to recognize an object, commonly due to a lesion in the occipital area.

mind-deafness. A condition characterized by absence or loss of memory of acoustic impressions, in which the patient, while capable of hearing, is not able to understand what he has heard; commonly due to a lesion in the intermediate temporal cortex.

mĭ·neral (Fr. *miner*, to mine, from L. *minare*, to drive). Any inorganic or fossilized organic compound found in nature.

miner's elbow. Inflammation of the bursa over the olecranon. **M.'s nystagmus**: (G. *nustazein*, to nod). Nystagmus occurring in miners. **M.'s phthisis**: a chronic lung disease. Syn. silicosis. **M.'s spit**: sputum of miners containing particles of coal dust.

mĭ·nim (L. *minimus*, least). One-sixtieth part of a fluid drachm. Symbol ♏.

mĭ·nimal (L. *minimus*, least). Least; lowest. Of dose, the least effective quantity.

mĭ·nimum (L. *minimus*, least). The least; the lowest.

mĭ·nor (L.). 1. Less, smaller. 2. An individual who has not yet attained legal age.

miocar·dia (G. *meion*, less; *kardia*, heart). Heart contraction; systole.

miodĭ·dymus, mĭo·dymus, (G. *meiōn*, less; *didumos*, twin). A monster with two heads joined by the occiputs.

miō·pus (G. *meiōn*, less; *ōps*, face). A double-headed monster with one rudimentary face.

miō·sis. See meiosis.

miŏt·ic. See meiotic.

mirror-speech. Speech in which the word-letters are spoken backwards.

mirror-writing. Writing in which the words are written backwards, as they appear in a mirror.

misan·dry (G. *mīsein*, to hate; *anēr*, male). Aversion from or hatred of men.

mĭ·santhrope (G. *misein*, to hate; *anthrōpos*, man). A person averse from or hating the society of other people.

miscar·riage. Abortion.

mis·cē (L. *miscere*, to mix). 'Mix', a direction placed on prescriptions. Symbol M.

mis·cible (L. *miscere*, to mix). Said of a substance which can be mixed with another substance.

Mises's marginal plexus (Mises, F. von, pseudonym of G. T. Fechner, German physician, 1801–87). The marginal plexus of nerves in the eyelid.

misŏ·gamy (G. *misein*, to hate; *gamōs*, marriage). A neurotic hatred of marriage.

misŏ·gyny (G. *misein*, to hate; *gunē*, woman). Aversion from or hatred of women.

missed abortion. The retention of a dead foetus in the uterus after the appearance of uterine bleeding.

missed labour. The retention of a foetus in the uterus after the occurrence of ineffectual labour-pains.

mistū·ra (L. *mixtura*). A mixture; a pharmaceutical preparation.

Mitchell's disease. Erythromelalgia: syn. Weir Mitchell's disease.

mite. A name applied to several species of the order Acarina.

mithrĭ·datism (From Mithridates, King of Pontus). Immunity to a poison acquired by administration of the drug in increasing doses.

mĭ·tigate (L. mitigare, to soften). To ameliorate.

mĭ·tis (L.). Mild.

mĭtochon·dria (G. mitos, thread; khondros, cartilage). Minute granules scattered through cell-protoplasm, capable of multiplication, belonging to the category of chondriosomes.

mĭtō·ma, mĭ·tome (G. mitos, thread). One of the many terms used to designate the fibrillar network of protoplasm.

mĭtō·sis (G. mitos, thread). Karyokinesis, q.v.

mĭ·tosome (G. mitos, thread; sōma, body). The remainder of the spindle after chromosomal division.

mĭtot·ic (G. mitos, thread). Characterized by mitosis.

mĭ·tral (G. mitra, head-dress). 1. Resembling a mitre. 2. Relating to the auriculo-ventricular valve of the left side of the heart.

mit·telschmerz (German, middle pain). Intermenstrual pain, a condition characterized by pelvic pain, coming on regularly midway between the periods, due perhaps to the changes in Graafian follicles occurring at that particular time.

mix·ture (L. mixtura). The result of mixing any number of substances which do not chemically combine.

m.l.d. Abbreviation for minimum lethal dose.

Mn. The symbol for manganese.

mnē·mē (G. memory). A term used to denote the basis of memory.

mnemon·ics (G. mnēmon, mindful). Devices to improve the ability to memorize.

Mo. The symbol for Molybdenum.

mō·bile (L. movere, to move). Movable.

mobi·lity (L. movere, to move). The property of being movable.

mobilizā·tion (L. movere, to move). The act of re-establishing mobility in an ankylosed part.

Möbius's disease (Möbius, P. J., German physician, 1853–1907). Periodic migraine with paralysis of the eye muscles. M.'s sign: a weakness in the power of convergence in exophthalmos.

mō·diolus (L. modiolus, hub). 1. The central axis of the labyrinthine cochlea. 2. The crown of a trephine.

mogiphō·nia (G. mogis, with difficulty; phōnē, voice). Difficulty in maintaining the tension of the vocal cords while singing or during accentuated speaking.

M.O.H. Abbreviation for Medical Officer of Health.

Mohrenheim's fossa (Mohrenheim, J., Freiherr von, Austrian surgeon, died 1799). The infra-clavicular fossa bounded by the clavicle, pectoralis major, deltoid, and laterally and deeper by pectoralis minor; trigonum deltoideopectorale.

moi·ety. One half.

moist. Damp.

mō·lar¹ (L. moles, mass). 1. Relating to a mole. 2. Relating to the molecular weight of a substance in grammes.

mō·lar² (L. mola, a mill). 1. Grinding. 2. A grinding tooth, one of posterior teeth (three each side of each jaw).

molă·riform (L. mola, mill; forma, shape). Resembling a molar tooth.

mole (L. moles, mass). 1. Naevus. 2. A mass formed in the uterus by a degenerated ovum. M., carneous: a haemorrhagic mole (2) that has become more solid and lost some of its blood-pigment. M., haemorrhagic: the early stage of a uterine mass consisting of an ovum which has become destroyed by haemorrhage into the chorio-decidual space. M., hydatidiform: a disease, probably of the ovum itself, characterized by proliferative and cystic degeneration of the chorionic villi, leading to undue enlargement of the pregnant uterus, sanguineous discharge, and often to spontaneous abortion. M., vesicular: a hydatidiform mole.

molĕ·cular (L. molecula, dim. of moles, mass). Relating to a molecule. M. concentration: the number of gram molecular weights of a substance in solution. M. weight: the sum of the atomic weights of all the atoms constituting the molecule.

mō·lecule (L. molecula, dim. of moles, mass). The chemical combination of any number of atoms; the smallest quantity in which a substance can exist in the free state and retain its specific characteristics.

mō·limen (L. molimen). An effort.

Moll's glands (Moll, J. A., Dutch ophthalmologist, 1832–1914). The glandulae ciliares.

mollĭ·tiēs (L.). Softness. M. ossium: osteomalacia.

Mollus·ca (L. molluscus, soft). A large branch of the animal kingdom comprising the slugs, snails, mussels, clams, oysters, whelks and limpets.

mollus·cum (L. molluscus, soft). An obsolete term for any soft tumour of the skin. M. contagiosum: an infectious skin disease, probably of viral origin, characterized by the formation of small, pearly, round, flat-topped tumours with a central depression, containing cheesy epithelial detritus, originating in the prickle-cell layer. M. fibrosum: the peripheral, often pedunculated, tumour in neurofibromatosis.

mollus·cus (L. soft). 1. Pertaining to the disease molluscum. 2. Pertaining to the mollusca.

molybdē·num (G. molubdos, lead). A metallic element. Symbol Mo.

momen·tum (L.). 1. Quantity of motion. 2. The product of the mass of a moving body and its velocity.

Monă·didae (G. monas, unity). A family of the class Mastigophora.

Monakow's bundle (Monakow, C. von, Swiss neurologist, 1853–1930). The tractus rubro-spinalis. M.'s nucleus: the funiculus cuneatus externus.

monă·mide (G. monos, alone). An amide produced by the replacement of the hydrogen in one molecule of ammonia by an acid radicle.

monă·mine (G. monos, alone). The amine produced by the replacement of one of the hydrogen atoms of the molecule of ammonia by a hydrocarbon radicle.

monaminū·ria (G. monos, alone; ouron, urine). A condition in which monamines are present in the urine.

monar·thric (G. monos, single; arthron, joint). Monarticular, q.v.

monarthri·tis (G. monos, single; arthron, joint). Inflammation in one joint.

monartĭ·cular (G. monos, single; L. articulus, joint). Pertaining to a single joint.

monă·ster (G. monos, single; astēr, star). The figure formed in that type of mitosis which proceeds without division of the central body.

monatom·ic (G. monos, single; atomos, indivisible). A molecule consisting of one atom.

monau·ral (G. monos, single; L. auris, ear). Relating to one ear.

Mönckeberg's arteriosclerosis (Mönckeberg, J. G., German pathologist, 1878–1925). A form of arteriosclerosis seen in medium and small arteries as an extensive degeneration of the media, with atrophy of the muscular elements and calcareous deposits in the atrophied muscle cells.

monĕ·rula (G. monērēs, single). The impregnated ovum at a stage when it has no nucleus.

Mongolian idiocy. See idiocy, Mongolian.

Mongolian spot. A small darkly pigmented area of the skin over the sacral region, present in Mongolians and occasionally in children of European descent.

mon·golism. See idiocy, Mongolian.

monĭ·lethrix (L. monile, necklace; thrix, hair). An affection of the hair characterized by more or less regularly arranged spindle-shaped enlargements of the hair-shaft, the intervening portions being devoid of pigment. Syn. beaded hair.

Moni·lia (L. *monile*, necklace). A genus of budding fungi.

monili·asis. See monoliasis.

moni·liform (L. *monile*, necklace; *forma*, shape). Shaped like a necklace; beaded; resembling a string of beads.

Monneret's pulse (Monneret, J. E. A., French physician, 1810–68). The soft, slow pulse characterizing icterus.

mono-anaesthē·sia (G. *monos*, single; *aisthēsis*, perception). Anaesthesia of one single part or organ.

monobā·sic (G. *monos*, single; *basis*, base). A term applied to an acid containing only one atom of hydrogen replaceable by a metal or radicle to form a salt.

mŏ·noblast (G. *monos*, single; *blastos*, germ). A cell perhaps normally present in bone marrow and possibly in the spleen, closely resembling the myeloblast, but giving rise to the monocyte; present in the bone marrow in monocytic leukaemia.

monoblep·sis (G. *monos*, single; *blepsis*, sight). 1. A condition in which each individual eye has better vision than both together. 2. Colour-blindness in which only a single colour can be perceived.

monobrā·chius (G. *monos*, single; *brakhion*, arm). Congenital absence of one arm.

monocar·dian (G. *monos*, single; *kardia*, heart). Having a single-chambered heart.

monocĕ·phalus (G. *monos*, single; *kephalē*, head). A monster consisting of a single head with two bodies, which may be wholly or partly fused.

mŏ·nochord (G. *monos*, single; *khordē*, string). An instrument for testing upper tone audition. Consists of a long steel or silver wire fastened at the ends. A movable clamp produces tone by friction.

mŏ·nochromat·ic (G. *monos*, single; *khrōma*, colour). Having only one colour.

mŏ·nocle (G. *monos*, single; L. *oculus*, eye). A lens for one eye.

monŏ·cranus (G. *monos*, single; *kranion*, skull). A double monster with a single cranium.

monŏ·cular (G. *monos*, single; L. *oculus*, eye). 1. Relating to, or performed with, or affecting only one eye. 2. Having a single eyepiece, as a m. microscope.

monŏ·culus (G. *monos*, single; L. *oculus*, eye). 1. A monster with only one eye. 2. In surgery, a bandage to cover one eye.

mŏ·nocyte (G. *monos*, single; *kutos*, cell). One group of the white cells present in blood and blood-forming organs; in size larger than a neutrophil leucocyte ($15-20\mu$) and further characterized by the relatively large amount of cytoplasm, containing azurophil granules, and a nucleus of irregular, often horseshoe, shape and a loose-meshed chromatin structure. It is not yet ascertained from which cell the monocyte normally arises; perhaps it is formed from undifferentiated mesenchymal cells in the medulla of lymph nodes.

monocyt·ic (G. *monos*, single; *kutos*, cell). Pertaining to the monocyte. M. leukaemia: see leukaemia, m.

mŏ·nocytopē·nia (G. *monos*, single; *kutos*, cell; *pēnia*, poverty). Decrease in the monocyte count in the blood.

mŏ·nocytopoiē·sis (G. *monos*, single; *kutos*, cell; *poiein*, to make). The process whereby monocytes are formed.

monocytō·sis (G. *monos*, single; *kutos*, cell). Abnormal increase in the number of monocytes in the blood.

monodac·tylism (G. *monos*, single; *daktulos*, finger). A congenital malformation characterized by the presence of only one finger or toe on the hand or foot.

monodac·tylous (G. *monos*, single; *daktulos*, finger). Having only one finger or toe.

monogĕ·nesis (G. *monos*, single; *genesis*, production). Non-sexual reproduction.

monoger·minal (G. *monos*, single; L. *germen*, sprig). Originating from one ovum; applied to twins enclosed in one chorionic sac.

monogō·nium (G. *monos*, single; *gonos*, seed). The asexual form of the malarial parasite. Occurring in blood, it produces febrile attacks.

monŏ·gony (G. *monos*, single; *gonos*, seed). Monogenesis, q.v.

monohȳ·brid (G. *monos*, single; L. *hybrida*, mongrel). Hybrid in one characteristic only; said of the young whose progenitors differ in a single characteristic.

monohȳ·drated (G. *monos*, single; *hūdor*, water). Combined with a single molecule of water.

monohȳ·dric (G. *monos*, single; *hudōr*, water). Containing one hydroxyl group.

monoli·asis (L. *monile*, necklace). A localized or systemic disease caused by infection with virulent fungi of the genus Monilia; it may affect the skin and its appendages, mucous membrane, the gastro-intestinal tract or the lungs. Syn. moniliasis.

monolŏ·cular (G. *monos*, single; L. *loculus*, dim. of *locus*, place). Unilocular.

monomā·nia (G. *monos*, single; *mania*, madness). A term used to denote a neurosis characterized by fixed ideas.

momomā·niac. A person suffering from monomania.

monomer·ic (G. *monos*, single; *meros*, part). Composed of single molecules.

monom·phalus (G. *monos*, single; *omphalos*, navel). A double monster united by a single umbilicus.

mononū·clear (G. *monos*, single; L. *nucula*, dim. of *nux*, nut). Having a single nucleus.

mŏ·nonucleō·sis (G. *monos*, single; L. *nucula*, dim. of *nux*, nut). A condition characterized by the presence of an abnormally large number of mononuclear leucocytes in the blood. M., infective: an acute infectious disease of mostly mild, but especially in adults, protracted course; characterized by fever, glandular enlargement, the presence of large numbers of (usually atypical) lymphocytes in the blood, and sometimes by a pharyngitis and/or a maculo-papular rash. Syn. glandular fever.

monoparaesthē·sia (G. *monos*, single; *para*, beside; *aisthēsis*, perception). Paraesthesia of a single limb.

monoparē·sis (G. *monos*, single; *paresis*, a slackening). Paresis of a single limb.

monŏ·pathy (G. *monos*, single; *pathos*, disease). A disease affecting a single organ or part.

monophā·sia (G. *monos*, single; *phasis*, a statement). A form of aphasia characterized by limitation of speech to a single syllable, word or phrase.

monophō·bia (G. *monos*, single; *phŏbos*, fear). Neurotic fear of being alone.

monophthal·mia (G. *monos*, single; *ophthalmos*, eye). The congenital condition of having a single eye.

monophthal·mous (G. *monos*, single; *ophthalmos*, eye). Single-eyed.

monophylet·ic (G. *monos*, single; *phulē*, race). Having a phylogenetically common origin.

monoplē·gia (G. *monos*, single; *plēgē*, stroke). 1. Paralysis of one limb. 2. Paralysis of one group of muscles.

mŏ·nops (G. *monos*, single; *ōps*, eye). An individual with congenital absence of one eye.

mŏ·nopus (G. *monos*, single; *pous*, foot). An individual with congenital absence of one foot.

monor·chid (G. *monos*, single; *orkhis*, testicle). An individual with congenital absence of one testicle.

monosac·charide (G. *monos*, single; *sakkharon*, sugar). Sugars with the formula $C_nH_{2n}O_n$, which cannot be hydrolysed into simpler sugars.

monosō·mus (G. *monos*, single; *sōma*, body). A double monster with a single body and two more or less separated heads.

mŏ·nospasm (G. *monos*, single; *spasmos*, contraction). Spasm limited to a single muscle or group of muscles.

monosymptomat·ic (G. *monos*, single; *sun*, with; *ptōma*, a fall). Having only one dominant symptom or sign.

monotō·nia (G. *monos*, single; *tonos*, tone). Uniformity of voice; absence of modulation.

Mŏ·notremes. The lowest order of mammals. They lay large-yolked eggs, similar to those of reptiles.

monŏ·trichous (G. *monos*, single; *thrix*, hair). Applied to bacteria possessing a single flagellum.

monova·lent (G. *monos*, single; L. *valere*, to be strong). Univalent.

monox·ide (G. *monos*, single; *oxus*, sharp). An oxide containing only one oxygen atom.

Monro's fissure (Monro, A., primus, Scottish anatomist, 1737–1817). The hypothalamic sulcus. **M.'s foramen:** the interventricular foramen between lateral and third ventricle. **M.'s line:** an imaginary line drawn from the umbilicus to the anterior iliac spine.

mons (L.). A mountain. **M. pubis:** A rounded eminence lying in front of the symphysis pubis formed by fatty tissue beneath the skin. Becomes covered with hair at time of puberty. **M. veneris:** syn. M. pubis.

Monsel's salt. Ferric subsulphate; used mainly in solution as a styptic.

mon·ster (L. *monstrum*). 1. An individual who, owing to foetal maldevelopment, differs in a marked degree from the normal type of the species. Syn. teratism. **M., double:** a pair of twin monsters, one of which is by some part or parts conjoined to the other or wholly included within the other.

monstrō·sity (L. *monstrositas*, from *monstrum*). 1. The condition of being a monster. 2. A monster.

Monteggia's dislocation (Monteggia, G. B., Italian surgeon, 1762–1815). That dislocation of the hip-joint in which the head of the femur is towards the anterior superior spine of the ilium, the limb being rotated outwards.

Montgomery's tubercles or glands (Montgomery, W. F., Irish obstetrician, 1797–1859). Secondary areola of the nipple. Sebaceous glands of the areola previously described by, and known as, tubercles of Morgagni.

monthly courses, monthly sickness. The menses.

montĭ·culus (L. *monticulus*, dim. of *mons*, mount). A small elevation.

mood. State of mind characterized by some particular emotion, latent but readily evoked.

Moon's teeth (Moon, H., English surgeon, 1845–1892). Dome-shaped permanent first molar teeth which may be found in congenital syphilitics.

Moore's fracture (Moore, E. M., American surgeon, 1814–1902). A fracture of the lower end of the radius with dislocation of the head of the ulna.

Moore's test (Moore, J., English physician, born 1879). Test for glucose. Add to some urine in a test tube some potassium hydroxide and warm. The colour passes from yellow to orange and then brown according to the amount of glucose present.

Mooren's ulcer (Mooren, A., German oculist, 1828–99). A chronic ulcer of the cornea occurring in aged people.

Morand's disease (Morand, S. F., French surgeon, 1697–1773). A localized paralysis affecting one or more of the lower extremities. **M.'s foot:** a deformity of the foot consisting of the presence of eight toes. **M.'s spur:** the calcar avis (hippocampus minor).

Morax-Axenfeld conjunctivitis (Morax, V., French ophthalmologist, 1866–1935; Axenfeld, T., German ophthalmologist, 1867–1930). A mild form of conjunctivitis. **M.-A.'s diplococcus:** a bacillus causing conjunctivitis.

moral imbecile. Person with inherent criminal tendencies, with or without mental defect.

moral insanity. An obsolete term formerly used to denote a syndrome characterized by impairment of moral values.

mor·bid (L. *morbidus*, from *morbus*, disease). Relating to disease or diseased parts.

morbĭ·dity (L. *morbidus*, from *morbus*, disease). 1. The ratio of the number of individuals affected by a particular disease, or diseases, to the total population of a locality. 2. The quality of being diseased.

morbil·li (L.L.). Measles, *q.v.*

morbil·liform (L.L. *morbilli*, measles; *forma*, shape). Resembling measles, more especially resembling the skin eruption of measles.

mor·bus (L.). Disease.

morcellā·tion (Fr. *morceler*, ult. from L. *mordere*, to bite). Piecemeal removal, e.g. of a foetus or tumour.

morcellement (Fr.). See morcellation.

mor·dant (L. *mordere*, to bite). A substance, such as chromic salts, aniline or oil, which makes possible the staining of such tissues or bacteria as are difficult to stain.

Morgagni's cataract (Morgagni, G. B., Italian anatomist, 1682–1771). A soft cataract with a hard nucleus. **M.'s concha:** the ethmoid superior turbinated bone. **M.'s foramen:** the Meibomian foramen. **M.'s fossa:** the fossa navicularis of the urethra. **M.'s fraenum or retinaculum:** a fold around the cavity of the caecum formed by prolongation of the folds of the iliocaecal valve. **M.'s glands:** Littre's glands. **M.'s globules:** small hyaline spheres sometimes appearing between the crystalline lens and its capsule in cases of cataract. **M.'s hydatid:** the remnant of the Müllerian duct attached to the oviduct in the female and the testicle in the male. **M.'s lacunae:** small pits in the urethral mucosa into which the glands of Littre open. **M.'s liquor:** a clear fluid found post-mortem in the crystalline lens between the epithelium and fibres. **M.'s nodules:** corpora arantii, *q.v.* **M.'s sinuses:** small pouches opening in an upward direction and formed above the anus by the rectal mucosa. **M.'s tubercles:** Montgomery's tubercles. **M.'s valves:** M.'s sinuses, *q.v.* **M.'s ventricle:** the sacculus laryngis, situated between the superior vocal chords and the inner portion of the thyroid cartilage.

morgue (Fr.). A place in which unknown dead are laid to await identification.

mō·ria (G. folly). Morbid obsession to make remarks meant as witty, sometimes caused by tumours of the frontal lobes of the brain.

mŏ·ribund (L. *moribundus*, dying). In a dying state.

Morison's pouch (Morison, J. R., British surgeon, 1853–1939). A deep recess above the upper pole of the kidney, lined by peritoneum.

morning sickness. The nausea of pregnant women, occurring mainly in the morning during the early months of pregnancy.

Moro's reaction (Moro, E., German paediatrician, born 1874). A test for tuberculosis. 'Old' tuberculin in lanolin is rubbed into the skin of the abdomen. If an area of hyperaemia occurs within 24 to 48 hours the reaction is positive.

mo·ron (G. *mōros*, stupid). An individual with the slightest degree of feeble-mindedness.

mor·phinans. A name applied to a number of synthetic substances, chemically related to morphine, some of which possess pronounced analgesic action.

mor·phine. $C_{17}H_{19}O_3N_7H_2O$; an important alkaloid with analgesic properties found in opium. Dose $\frac{1}{8}-\frac{1}{3}$ gr.

mor·phinism. Morphine addiction.

morphœ·a (G. *morphē*, form). Circumscribed patches of sclerodermia, *q.v.* **M. guttata:** a form of m. affecting mainly the neck and the upper part of the trunk. Syn. white-spot disease.

morphogĕ·nesis (G. *morphē*, shape; *genesis*, production). See morphogeny.

morphŏ·geny (G. *morphē*, shape; *gennan*, to produce). Development of form and structure.

morpholŏ·gical (G. *morphē*, form; *logos*, a treatise). Relating to the form and structure of organisms.

morphŏ·logy (G. *morphē* form; *logos*, treatise). The part of biology dealing with the form and structure of organisms.

morphŏ·lysis (G. *morphē*, form; *lusis*, dissolution). The destruction of form.

morphŏ·metry (G. *morphē*, form; *metron*, measure). The measurement of the forms of organisms.

morphō·sis (G. *morphē*, form). Process of formation, e.g. of a tissue or organ.

morphot·ic (G. *morphē*, form). Relating to morphosis.

Morrant-Baker's cysts (Morrant-Baker, W., English surgeon, 1839–96). Hernial protrusions of the synovial membrane through the fibrous capsule of joints seen in connection with osteo-arthritis.

Morris's kidney box (Morris, Sir H., English surgeon, 1844–1926). The surface marking for the kidney in the loin.

mors (L.). Death.

mor·sus (L.). A bite. **M. diaboli:** devil's bite; the fimbriated end of the uterine tube.

mor·tal (L. *mortalis*). 1. Causing death. 2. Liable to death.

mortă·lity (L. *mortalis*, mortal). 1. The ratio of the number of deaths to the total population or to a class of the population. 2. The quality of being mortal.

Morton's cough (Morton, R., English physician, 1637–98). A cough succeeded by the vomiting of blood, often occurring in pulmonary tuberculosis.

Morton's disease (Morton, T. G., American surgeon, 1835–1903). Metatarsalgia, *q.v.*

mor·tuary (L. *mortuarius*, from *mortuus*, dead). 1. A morgue, *q.v.* 2. Relating to death or burial.

mo·rula (L. *morus*, mulberry). That stage in the development of a fertilized ovum in which it consists of a mass of small blastomeres, somewhat resembling a mulberry in appearance. Syn. blastula.

Morus (L.). A genus of the family of Urticaceae, which includes the Mulberry.

Morvan's chorea (Morvan, A. M., French physician, 1819–97). Fibrillary chorea; fibrillary contractions of the calf muscles or those of the posterior parts of the thighs, often reaching the trunk and upper extremities but not the face and neck. **M.'s disease:** analgesic paresis, a progressive paralysis and atrophy of the forearms and hands and the formation of painless whitlows.

Mosher's cells (Mosher, M. P., American laryngologist, born 1867). The ethmoidal sinus extensions beneath the bulla ethmoidalis.

mosqui·to (Sp. *mosquito*, dim. of *mosca*, fly). A nongeneris name applied to several stinging insects of the order Diptera. See also Anophelini, Culex, Aedes, Phlebotomus.

moss. A plant of the order Musci. **Sphagnum m.:** a marsh-growing moss which is used in the preparation of absorbent surgical dressings.

Moss's blood grouping (Moss, W. L., American haematologist, born 1876). A system of blood typing (see blood) under which serum from persons of Group I will not agglutinate cells from other persons; Group II serum will agglutinate cells of Groups I and III. Group III serum will agglutinate cells of Groups I and II. Group IV serum will agglutinate the cells of all other groups.

moth. A night-flying insect belonging to the order Lepidoptera. **M.-patches:** chloasma.

mother. The female parent.

mō·tile (L. *movere*, to move). Capable of spontaneous motion.

moti·lity (L. *movere*, to move). 1. Voluntary or spontaneous movements. 2. Ability to perform voluntary movements.

mō·tion (L. *motio*, from *movere*, to move). 1. Continuous change of position. 2. An evacuation of the bowels. 3. Evacuated matter from the bowels.

mō·tor (L. *movere*, to move). Pertaining to or causing motion, e.g., m. nerve. **M. aphasia:** See aphasia, m. **M. area:** that part of the cerebral cortex which is involved in the central regulation of voluntary movements. **M. points:** those points on the surface of the body from which stimulation of single muscles or motor nerves by electric current can best be obtained.

motō·rial (L. *movere*, to move). Relating to motion.

motō·rium (L. *movere*, to move). The motor apparatus of the body.

mouches (Fr.). Flies. **M. volantes:** Muscae volitantes, *q.v.*

mountain sickness. A syndrome characterized by dyspnoea, tachycardia, vomiting, headache and impairment of mental functions, due to anoxic anoxia, which is caused by rarefied air.

mounting. Preparation of anatomical or histological specimens on a support and in the appropriate medium, i.e., for macroscopic specimens usually glycerine, for microscopic specimens Canada balsam.

mouth. 1. The first part of the alimentary canal; the cavity in which food is masticated. 2. The entrance to any canal or cavity; an orifice.

movement (L. *movere*, to move). The act of moving. **M., amoeboid:** m., e.g. of leucocytes, resembling that of amoebae. **M., associated:** involuntary m. of one part consequent upon voluntary movement of another part or parts.

moxa (Japanese). Combustible mixture applied to the skin in order to produce an eschar.

M.P.S. Member of the Pharmaceutical Society.

M.R.C.P. Member of the Royal College of Physicians.

M.R.C.P.E. Member of the Royal College of Physicians of Edinburgh.

M.R.C.P.I. Member of the Royal College of Physicians of Ireland.

M.R.C.S. Member of the Royal College of Surgeons.

M.S. Master of Surgery.

Much's bacillus (Much, H. C. R., German physician, 1880–1932). *Mycobacterium tuberculosis.* **M.'s granules:** non-acid-fast rods found in tuberculous sputum. Regarded as modified tubercle bacilli, they stain by Gram method. **M.'s reaction:** one seen in dementia praecox and manic-depressive states, in which cobra venom fails to haemolyse the red blood cells. **M.'s stain:** a method of staining tubercle bacilli in methyl violet, alcohol and phenol.

mucic acid. $C_6H_{10}O_8$. A dibasic acid obtained by the oxidation of lactose with nitric acid.

muci·ferous (L. *mucus*; *ferre*, to bear). Secreting mucus.

mū·ciform (L. *mucus*; *forma*, shape). Like mucus.

mū·cigen (L. *mucus*; G. *gennan*, to produce). The specific product of any cell producing mucus; the antecedent of mucin.

muci·genous (L. *mucus*; G. *gennan*, to produce). Producing mucus.

mū·cilage (L.L. *mucilago*). In pharmacy, an aqueous solution of a gum or of starch.

mucilă·ginous (L.L. *mucilago*). Relating to or of the nature of mucilage.

mucila·go (L.L.). See mucilage.

mū·cin (L. *mucus*). One of those glyco-proteins which occur in the secretions of the fluids of the body; the characteristic constituent of mucus. It is insoluble in water but soluble in dilute alkali, and is precipitated by alcohol and acetic acid.

mucinae·mia (L. *mucus*; G. *haima*, blood). A condition characterized by the presence of mucin in the blood.

mū·cinase (L. *mucus*). An enzyme, produced by the intestinal mucosa, which coagulates mucin.

mū·cinoid (L. *mucus*, mucus; G. *eidos*, form). Resembling mucin.

mucinū·ria (L. *mucus*; G. *ouron*, urine). The presence of mucin in the urine.

mucĭ·parous (L. *mucus*; *parere*, to produce). Secreting mucin.

mucĭ·tis (L. *mucus*). Inflammation of mucous membrane.

mū·cocele (L. *mucus*; *kēlē*, hernia). Accumulation of mucus in a cavity.

mū·cocutā·neous (L. *mucus*; *cutis*, skin). Relating to the mucous membrane and the skin.

mū·coid (L. *mucus*; G. *eidos*, form). 1. Resembling mucus. 2. One of those glyco-proteins occurring in tissues such as ligaments and cartilage; differing from mucins mainly in solubility.

mucolyt·ic (L. *mucus*; G. *luein*, to dissolve). Destroying mucus.

mucomem·branous (L. *mucus*; *membrana*, membrane). Relating to mucous membranes.

mū·coperiŏ·steal. Relating to mucoperiosteum.

mu·coperiŏ·steum (L. *mucus*; G. *peri*, around; *osteon*, bone). Periosteum having a mucous surface, occurring in the auditory apparatus.

mucopū·rulent (L. *mucus*, mucus; *pus*, pus). Consisting of mucus and pus.

mū·copus (L. *mucus*; *pus*). A combination of mucus and pus.

Mucor (L.). A genus of hyphomycetes.

mucō·sa (L. *mucosus*, of mucus). A mucous membrane; membrana mucosa.

mucō·sal. Relating to mucous membrane.

mū·cosangui·neous (L. *mucus*; *sanguis*, blood). Composed of mucus and blood.

mucŏ·sity (L. *mucus*). Sliminess.

mū·cous (L. *mucus*). Containing or relating to mucus, e.g., m. membrane. **M. colitis**: see colitis, m.

mū·cus (L.). The viscid fluid secreted by mucous membranes, containing as its specific substance a mucin.

Muir's tract (Muir, J. C., contemporary Scottish neurologist). The septo-marginal tract of Bruce and Muir.

Mules's operation (Mules, P. H., English ophthalmologist, 1843–1905). Evisceration of the eye.

mulespinner's disease. Warts or ulcers of the skin, especially of the scrotum, with a strong tendency to become malignant. Found chiefly among operators of spinning mules.

muliĕ·bris (L.). Relating to a woman.

Müller's duct (Müller, J., German pathologist, 1801–58). The paramesonephric duct which in the female forms the uterine tubes and uterovaginal canal. In the male it atrophies but remains as the appendix testis and prostatic sinus. **M.'s eminence**: an elevation on the dorsal wall of the urogenital sinus caused by the Müllerian ducts. **M.'s experiment**: a deep inspiration is made with the glottis closed. As no air can enter the lungs the pressure is lowered and the pulmonary capillaries dilate. Cerebral anaemia may result. Possibly the cause of laryngeal vertigo. **M.'s tubercle**: see M.'s eminence.

Müller's fibres (Müller, H., German anatomist, 1820–64). Long neuroglia cells which pass through several retinal layers. Beginning on the inner surface with expanded bases and extending through all the layers to the outer granule layer. **M.'s muscle**: the circular ciliary muscle of the eye. **M.'s ring**: a muscular ring surrounding the junction of the body and cervix of the uterus in the later stages of pregnancy.

Müller's fluid (Müller, H. F., German histologist, 1866–98). A fluid containing potassium bichromate and sodium sulphate and used for hardening microscopical specimens.

Müller's sign (Müller, F. von, Hungarian physician, 1858–1941). Rhythmical pulsation of the uvula with swelling and redness of the velum palati and tonsils in aortic insufficiency.

multan·gulum (L. *multus*, much; *angulus*, angle). A bone with several angles, e.g. os multangulum majus.

multicap·sular (L. *multus*, much; *capsula*, small box). Composed of many capsules.

multicel·lular (L. *multus*, much; *cellula*, dim. of *cella*, cell). Having many cells.

multicus·pid, multicus·pidate (L. *multus*, much; *cuspis*, point). Having a number of cusps. **M. teeth**: the molar teeth.

multiden·tate (L. *multus*, much; *dentatus*, toothed). Said of parts armed with many teeth or tooth-like processes.

multidi·gitate (L. *multus*, much; *digitus*, finger). Having many fingers or finger-like processes.

multifoetā·tion (L. *multus*, much; *fetus*, progeny). Pregnancy with three or more foetuses.

multiflagel·late (L. *multus*, much; *flagellum*, whip). Having a number of flagella.

multigrā·vida (L. *multus*, much; *gravidus*, pregnant). A pregnant woman who has had two or more previous pregnancies. Syn. pluripara.

multilŏ·bular (L. *multus*, much; G. *lobos*, lobe). Having many lobes.

multilŏ·cular (L. *multus*, much; *loculus*, dim of *locus*, place). Containing many cavities; polycystic.

multinū·clear, multinū·cleated (L. *multus*, much; *nucula*, dim. of *nux*, nut). Having more than one nucleus. Syn. polynuclear.

multĭ·para (L. *multus*, much; *parĕre*, to produce). A pregnant woman who has previously had one or more children. Syn. pluripara.

multipă·rity (L. *multus*, much; *parĕre*, to produce). The state of being multiparous. Syn. pluriparity.

multi·parous. Having produced several children. Syn. pluriparous.

mul·tiple (L. *multus*, much; *plērĕ*, to fill). Manifold; affecting or relating to more than one thing. **M., myeloma**: see myeloma, m. **M. neuritis**: see under neuritis. **M. sclerosis**: see sclerosis, disseminated.

multipŏ·lar (L. *multus*, much; G. *polos*, pole). Having more than one pole. **M. nerve-cells**: nerve-cells possessing more than one process.

multivā·lent (L. *multus*, much; *valere*, to be worth). Having a valency of three or more.

Mummery's fibres (Mummery, J. H., English dentist, 1847–1926). The fibrillar structures in developing dentine.

mummificā·tion (Arabic *mum*, wax; L. *facere*, to make). 1. Shrivelling in utero of a dead foetus. 2. Dry gangrene.

mumps. An acute infectious disease characterized by inflammatory swelling of the salivary glands, especially of the parotids; sometimes involving the testicle or the pancreatic gland. Syn. epidemic parotitis.

Munzer's bundle or **tract** (Munzer, E., Austrian physician, 1865–1924). A fibre tract from the internal geniculate body to the formatio reticularis of the lateral part of the pons; tractus tectopontinus.

mū·ral (L. *murus*, wall). Relating to a wall. **M. fibroid**: a fibroid situated within the uterine wall. **M. pregnancy**: pregnancy in the uterine end of a uterine tube.

murmur (L.). A blowing, whistling or rolling sound heard on auscultation over the heart or a bloodvessel. **M., cardiac**: any adventitious sound heard over the heart and produced within the heart. **M., cardiopulmonary** or **cardiorespiratory**: a m. produced in a portion of the lung which is being compressed by the action of the heart.

Murphy's button (Murphy, J. B., American surgeon, 1857–1916). An appliance formerly used for bringing together the visceral surfaces of the intestine in intestinal anastomosis. **M.'s treatment**: 1. Of pulmonary tuberculosis, by causing collapse of the affected lung through intrapleural injection of nitrogen. 2. Of peritonitis, by drainage from the lower part of the abdomen or pelvis and continuous low-pressure proctoclysis, the patient being placed in Fowler's position.

muscae (L. *musca*, fly; pl. *muscae*). Flies. **M. hispaniolae**: cantharides. **M. volitantes**: 'flying flies', a type of entoptic phenomena due to the presence of small particles in the vitreous humour which are perceived as usually floating spots which appear to fly away when an attempt is made to look at them directly.

mus·carine. $Me_3N.CH_2CHO$, the poisonous base present in the fungus *Amanita muscaria*, which simulates the action of acetylcholine on the effective organs, muscles and glands.

muscle (L. *musculus*). A structure composed of fibres having the property of contraction, their combined contraction producing movement of the structure. Muscles are of two kinds: the striped or striated, or voluntary, which is innervated by the peripheral nerves and is subject to the will; and the smooth or unstriated, or involuntary muscle, which is innervated by the autonomic nervous system and not subject to the will. **Abductor digiti minimi**: (hand) a small muscle of the hand which abducts the little finger. **Abductor digiti minimi**: (foot) a small muscle of the foot which abducts the little toe. **Abductor hallucis**: a muscle on the inner side of the foot which abducts the great toe. **Abductor ossis metatarsi digiti quinti pedis**: (Wood's muscle) is part of the abductor digiti minimi muscle. **Abductor pollicis brevis**: a small muscle of the hand which abducts the thumb. **Abductor pollicis longus**: a muscle of the front of the forearm which abducts the thumb and hand. **Accelerator urinae**: (bulbospongiosus) arises from the central perineal tendon and is inserted on the under surface of the perineal membrane and the sides of the corpus cavernosum. Supplied by pudendal nerve. **Accessorius**: (quadratus plantae) a muscle on the sole of the foot, which is inserted into the long flexor tendons. It flexes the toes, correcting the obliquity of the pull of the long flexor tendons. **Adductor brevis**: arises from body and ramus of pubis and is inserted into a line leading from lesser trochanter to linea aspera of femur. It adducts thigh, flexes hip, and rotates thigh outwards. Supplied by the obturator nerve. **Adductor hallucis**: a muscle on the sole of the foot having two heads. It adducts the big toe and binds the toes together. **Adductor longus**: a muscle on the inner side of the thigh which adducts the thigh, flexes the hip, and rotates the thigh outwards. **Adductor magnus**: a large muscle on the inner side of the thigh, which adducts the thigh and rotates the thigh outwards. **Adductor pollicis**: a muscle on the palmar surface of the hand which adducts and flexes the thumb. **Anconeus**: a muscle on the back of the elbow, it extends the elbow joint. **Antitragicus**: a small muscle of the ear which extends from the lateral surface of the

antitragus postero-superiorly, to be attached to the tail of the helix. **Articularis genu**: deep distal part of the vastus intermedius muscle. **Ary-epiglotticus**: part of the arytenoideus obliquus muscle which passes forwards within the ary-epiglottic fold to be inserted into the side of the epiglottis. **Arytenoideus**: lies across the posterior surfaces of the arytenoid cartilages. It consists of two parts, superficial (arytenoideus obliquus) and deep (arytenoideus transversus). **Arytenoideus obliquus**: a small muscle which is attached to the muscular process of the arytenoid cartilage on one side and to the summit of the arytenoid cartilage of the opposite side. The two muscles close the inlet of the larynx. It is supplied by the recurrent laryngeal nerve. **Arytenoideus transversus**: extends transversely from the posterior surface of the lateral border of the arytenoid cartilage to those of the other. It draws the arytenoid cartilages together and thus approximates the vocal cords. It is supplied by the recurrent laryngeal nerve. **Attolens aurem**: see auricularis superior. **Attrahens aurem**: see auricularis anterior. **Auricular**: the intrinsic muscles of the auricle are six in number, four being situated on the lateral surface and two on the cranial surface. **Auricularis anterior**: (attrahens aurem) arises from the lateral part of the epicranial aponeurosis and is inserted into the anterior part of the helix of the auricle. It draws the auricle forwards. It is supplied by the facial nerve. **Auricularis posterior**: (retrahens aurem) arises from the lateral part of the mastoid process and is inserted into the cranial surface of the auricle. It draws the auricle backwards. It is supplied by the facial nerve. **Auricularis superior**: (attollens aurem) arises from the lateral part of the epicranial aponeurosis and is inserted into the cranial surface of the auricle. It raises the auricle. It is supplied by the facial nerve. **Azygos uvulae**: (musculus uvulae) arises from the side of the posterior nasal spine and is inserted into the submucous tissue of the uvula. It elevates and shortens the uvula. It is supplied by the pharyngeal plexus. **Biceps brachii**: a muscle with two heads which extends from the shoulder joint to the elbow joint. It flexes the shoulder and elbow joints and supinates the forearm. **Biceps femoris**: a muscle on the back of the thigh which flexes the knee, and extends the thigh and rotates the leg outwards. **Biventer cervicis**: the tendinous intersection of the lower part of the semispinalis capitis muscle. **Brachialis**: a muscle on the anterior surface of the arm. It flexes the elbow joint. **Brachioradialis**: a muscle on the anterior and lateral surface of the forearm. It flexes the elbow joint and pronates or supinates the forearm from extreme position to midway between pronation and supination. **Buccinator**: a facial muscle which closes the mouth, also prevents food collecting between teeth and lips; it also maintains the tone of the cheeks, as in whistling. **Bulbospongiosus**: see accelerator or ejaculator urinae muscle. **Cervicalis ascendens**: (costocervicalis) is the continuation of the costalis muscle upward in the neck. **Chondroglossus**: an inconsistent muscle. It usually consists of the fibres of the hyoglossus muscle which are attached to the lesser horn of the hyoid bone. **Ciliary**: is the muscle of accommodation. It is composed of unstriped fibres which are arranged in two sets—radial and circular. It is supplied by the short ciliary nerves. **Circumflexus palati**: part of the tensor palati muscle. **Coccygeus**: a small muscle situated within the bony pelvis. It extends from the spine of the ischium to the coccyx and last piece of the sacrum. It supports the pelvic floor. **Complexus**: (semispinalis capitis) arises from the transverse processes of the upper six thoracic and last cervical vertebrae and is inserted into an

SUPERFICIAL MUSCLES

ANTERIOR

1. EPICRANIAL APONEUROSIS
2. FRONTALIS
3. TEMPORALIS
4. CORRUGATOR SUPERCILII
5. ORBICULARIS OCULI
6. LEVATOR LABII SUP. ALAEQUE NASI
7. LEVATOR LABII SUP.
8. ZYGOMATICUS (maj. and min.)
9. MASSETER
10. BUCCINATOR
11. DEPRESSOR ANGULI ORIS
12. ORBICULARIS ORIS
13. DEPRESSOR LABII INF.
14. STERNOMASTOID
15. OMOHYOID (sup. belly)
16. STERNOHYOID
17. OMOHYOID (inf. belly)
18. TRAPEZIUS
19. DELTOID
20. PECTORALIS MAJ.
21. CORACOBRACHIALIS
22. TRICEPS (lateral head)
23. BICEPS
24. LATISSIMUS DORSI
25. TRICEPS (medial head)
26. BRACHIALIS
27. PRONATOR TERES (sup. head)
28. RADIAL EXTENSOR
29. BICIPITAL APONEUROSIS
30. PRONATOR RADII TERES
31. BRACHIORADIALIS
32. FLEXOR CARPI RADIALIS
33. PALMARIS LONGUS
34. FLEXOR DIG. SUBLIMIS
35. FLEXOR CARPI ULNARIS
36. AB. AND FLEX. POLLICIS BREVIS
37. PALMARIS BREVIS
38. FLEXOR BREVIS DIG. MIN.
39. SERRATUS MAGNUS
40. EXT. OBLIQUE ABDOMINAL
41. RECTUS ABDOMINIS
42. LINEA ALBA
43. ANT. SUP. ILIAC SPINE
44. CUT EDGE OF RECTUS FASCIA
45. APONEUROSIS OF EXT. OBLIQUE
46. ILIO-INGUINAL LIGT. (Poupart's)
47. PYRAMIDALIS
48. PUBIC TUBERCLE
49. GLUTEUS MEDIUS
50. TENSOR FASCIAE LATAE
51. SARTORIUS
52. ILIACUS
53. PSOAS MAJ.
54. PECTINEUS
55. ADDUCTOR LONGUS
56. GRACILIS
57. RECTUS FEMORIS
58. VASTUS LATERALIS
59. FASCIA LATA
60. VASTUS MEDIALIS
61. MED. CONDYLE FEMUR
62. BICEPS FEMORIS
63. HEAD OF FIBULA
64. PERONEI
65. GASTROCNEMIUS (med. head)
66. EXT. DIGITORUM LONGUS
67. TIBIA (ant. border of crest)
68. TIBIALIS ANTERIOR
69. SOLEUS
70. EXT. HALLUCIS LONGUS
71. SUP. EXT. RETINACULUM
72. PERONEUS TERTIUS
73. INFERIOR EXT. RETINACULUM
74. EXTENSOR DIGITUS BREVIS

impression on the external aspect of the occipital bone between the superior and inferior nuchal lines. It inclines the head to the same side and rotates it to the opposite side. It is supplied by the posterior divisions of the cervical nerves. **Compressor glandulae cowperi:** part of the sphincter urethrae muscle. **Compressor naris:** arises from the maxilla between the canine fossa and the nasal notch and is inserted by means of an aponeurosis into the cartilaginous portion of the nose. It is supplied by the facial nerve. **Compressor sacculi laryngis:** a few muscular fibres on the medial aspect of the larynx which surround the saccule. **Compressor urethrae:** (Sphincter urethrae) a muscle consisting of a series of fibres which arise from the pubic arch, ischio-pubic junction and perineal membrane and converge round the urethra. The muscle assists in emptying the urethral canal. The dorsal nerve of the penis supplies the muscle. **Compressor venae dorsalis penis:** (levator penis) the inferior fibres of the ischiocavernosus muscle. **Constrictor radicis penis:** see Houston. **Coracobrachialis:** a muscle on the inner side of the arm. It flexes the shoulder-joint and adducts the arm. **Corrugator cutis ani:** (subcutaneous external sphincter of Ellis) part of the sphincter ani externus. **Corrugator supercilii:** arises from the medial extremity of the superciliary arch of the frontal bone and is inserted into the deep surface of the skin of the eyebrow. Produces the act of frowning. Supplied by the facial nerve. **Costalis:** a deep muscle of the back attached to the ribs. **Costocervicalis:** a deep muscle of the back attached to the upper ribs. **Cremaster:** (peculiar to male) arises from the middle of inguinal ligament and internal oblique and is inserted into the crest of the pubis. Supports and raises testis. Supplied by the genitofemoral nerve. **Crico-arytenoideus lateralis:** arises from the lateral portion of the cricoid cartilage and is inserted into the anterior aspect of the muscular process of the arytenoid cartilage. The muscles approximate the vocal cords and narrow the rima glottidis. Supplied by recurrent laryngeal nerve. **Crico-arytenoideus posterior:** arises from the posterior surface of the cricoid cartilage and is inserted into the posterior surface of the muscular process of the arytenoid cartilage. The muscle opens the rima glottidis. Supplied by the recurrent laryngeal nerve. **Cricothyroideus:** a small muscle situated on the outer side of larynx. It is a tensor of the vocal cords. **Crureus:** (vastus intermedius) a muscle on the front of the thigh. It acts as an extensor to the knee joint. **Cucullaris:** the two trapezius muscles present a four-sided appearance like a monk's hood or cowl (L. *cucullus*). **Dartos:** is part of the skin musculature, the panniculus carnosus, and has a brick-red colour. It is situated in the scrotum. **Deep transverse perineal:** see Henle's muscle. **Deltoid:** a large muscle covering the shoulder and giving it a rounded contour. It abducts the arm. **Depressor alae nasi:** (depressor septi) arises from the incisive fossa of maxilla and is inserted into posterior part of ala and septum of nose. Depresses ala of nose. Supplied by facial nerve. **Depressor anguli oris:** (triangularis menti) arises from the oblique line of the mandible and is inserted into the angle of the mouth where some of the fibres are attached to the skin. It depresses the angle of the mouth. Supplied by the facial nerve. **Depressor labii inferioris:** a small muscle arising from the oblique line of the mandible from symphysis to mental foramen. It is inserted into the orbicularis oris. Draws down lower lip, everting it. Supplied by facial nerve. **Depressor septi:** (depressor alae nasi) arises from incisive fossa of maxilla and is inserted into the posterior part of the ala and adjacent part of septum of nose. Depresses the ala of the nose. Supplied by

facial nerve. **Detrusor urinae:** the longitudinal stratum of external longitudinal fibres of the urinary bladder in the region of the base of the organ. So called from its supposed function in expelling the urine from the bladder. **Digastric:** has two bellies joined by an intermediate tendon. Posterior belly arises from groove on medial surface of mastoid process. Anterior belly from inner surface of mandible by side of symphysis. The intervening tendon is bound down to hyoid bone by a process of cervical fascia. Action: with posterior belly fixed and hyoid bone depressed, it depresses mandible; with the mandible fixed, it raises hyoid. Anterior belly supplied by mylo-hyoid branch of inferior dental nerve. Posterior belly by the facial nerve. **Dilator naris anterior:** arises from the cartilage of the aperture of the nose and is inserted into the deep surface of the skin over the ala of the nose. Dilates the nostril. Supplied by facial nerve. **Dilator naris posterior:** arises from the margin of the nasal notch of the maxilla. It is inserted into the skin over the posterior part of the ala of the nose. Dilates the nostril. Supplied by the facial nerve. **Dilator pupillae:** the radiating fibres of the iris in the eye. They dilate the pupil. The nerve supply comes from the sympathetic via the ciliary ganglion. **Dorsal interosseous:** (foot) four in number. Each arises by two heads from adjacent sides of metatarsal bones and are inserted into the side of and dorsal extensor expansion of proximal phalanx. The two medial go to second toe, one on each side, lateral two to lateral sides of third and fourth toes. They abduct from middle line of second toe. All supplied by lateral plantar nerve. **Dorsal interosseous:** (hand) four in number. They occupy the four intermetacarpal spaces. Each is attached to the adjoining sides of the shafts of the two metacarpal bones between which it is placed. Each is inserted into the base of proximal phalanx and partly into extensor expansion. They abduct fingers from middle line of hand. Supplied by ulnar nerve. **Ejaculator urinae:** (Bulbospongiosus) is composed in the male of two lateral parts that are united by a sagittal tendinous raphe. Each half consists of layers of muscular fibres surrounding the bulb of the penis, the posterior part of the corpus spongiosum, and in many cases, by a narrow band of the most anterior fibres, the body of the penis as well. It compresses the bulb of the urethra. It is supplied by the perineal branch of the pudendal nerve. **Ellis's:** see subcutaneous external sphincter ani or corrugator cutis ani. **Erector clitoridis:** see ischiocavernosus. Replaces the ischiocavernosus of the penis and is of small size. **Erector penis:** see ischiocavernosus muscle. **Erector spinae:** (sacrospinalis) a composite muscle which is single below in the region between the last rib and iliac crest, where it is tendinous medially and fleshy laterally. Extending upwards, it divides into three longitudinal columns—medial, intermediate and lateral. **Extensor carpi radialis brevis:** a muscle of the forearm which extends from the elbow to the wrist. It extends the elbow and wrist joints and abducts the hand. **Extensor carpi radialis longus:** a muscle of the forearm extending from the elbow to the wrist. It extends the elbow joint and extends and abducts the hand. **Extensor carpi ulnaris:** a muscle of the forearm extending from the elbow to the base of the little finger. It extends the wrist and carpal joints and the metacarpophalangeal joint of the little finger. It abducts the hand. **Extensor digiti minimi:** a small muscle on the back of the forearm extending from the elbow to the little finger. It extends the wrist and all the joints of the little finger. **Extensor digitorum brevis:** a small muscle on the dorsum of the foot extending from the calcaneum to the four inner toes. It extends the toes and flexes the

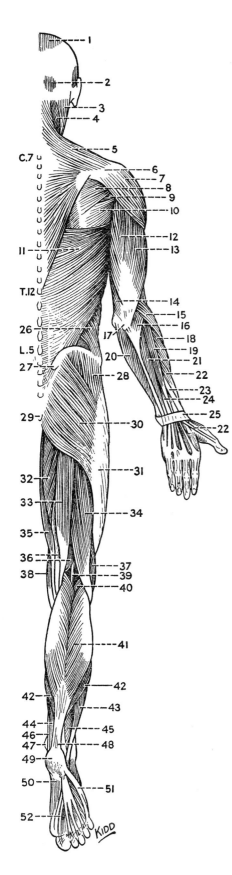

SUPERFICIAL MUSCLES

POSTERIOR

1. Epicranial Aponeurosis
2. Occipitalis
3. Sternomastoid
4. Splenius Capitis
5. Trapezius
6. Spine of Scapula
7. Deltoid
8. Infraspinatus
9. Teres Minor
10. Teres Major
11. Latissimus Dorsi
12. Triceps (long head)
13. Triceps (lateral head)
14. Triceps (medial head)
15. Ext. Carpi Radialis Longus
16. Anconeus
17. Olecranon Process (of ulna)
18. Ext. Carpi Radialis Brevis
19. Ext. Digitorum
20. Flex. Carpi Ulnaris
21. Ext. Carpi Ulnaris
22. Abd. Pollicis Longus
23. Ext. Pollicis Brevis
24. Ext. Digiti Minimi
25. Ext. Retinaculum
26. External Oblique
27. Ilium Post. Sup. Spine
28. Gluteus Medius
29. Coccyx
30. Gluteus Maximus
31. Fascia Lata
32. Adductor Magnus
33. Semitendinosus
34. Biceps Femoris (long head)
35. Gracilis
36. Semimembranosus
37. Biceps Femoris (short head)
38. Sartorius
39. Popliteal Nerve in Popliteal Fossa
40. Plantaris
41. Gastrocnemius
42. Soleus
43. Peroneus Longus
44. Flex. Digitorum Longus
45. Peroneus Brevis
46. Tibialis Posterior
47. Medial Malleolus
48. Tendo Calcaneus
49. Os Calcis (calcaneum)
50. Adductor Hallucis
51. Abductor Digiti Minimi
52. Flex. Hallucis Brevis

275

tarsal joints. **Extensor digitorum communis:** a muscle on the back of the forearm extending from the elbow to the back of the four fingers. It extends the wrist and all joints of the carpus and fingers. **Extensor digitorum longus:** a muscle on the front of the leg extending from just below the knee to the toes. It flexes the ankle and extends the joints of the tarsus and toes. **Extensor hallucis brevis:** is the innermost tendon of the extensor digitorum brevis of the foot. **Extensor hallucis longus:** a muscle on the outer side of the leg. It extends from the fibula to the great toe. It flexes the ankle joint and the tarsal joints and the great toe. **Extensor indicis:** a muscle on the back of the forearm. It extends the wrist joint and all the joints of the index finger. **Extensor pollicis brevis:** a muscle on the back of the forearm extending to the thumb. Abducts the hand and extends the first metacarpophalangeal joint of the thumb. **Extensor pollicis longus:** a muscle on the back of the forearm extending to the thumb. It abducts the thumb and hand. **External intercostals:** a series of muscles attached to the ribs and filling in the intercostal spaces. They elevate the ribs and aid respiration. **External oblique abdominal:** a muscle of the anterior abdominal wall extending from the lower ribs to the crest of the bony pelvis. It supports and compresses the viscera, draws down the lower ribs and laterally flexes the thorax. **Flexor accessorius:** a muscle on the sole of the foot extending from the calcaneum to the toes. It flexes the toes and corrects the obliquity of the pull of the long flexor tendons. **Flexor carpi radialis:** arises from the medial epicondyle of the humerus, the aponeurosis of forearm and intermuscular septa. Inserted into bases of palmar aspect of second and third metacarpal bones. Flexes elbow and wrist. Supplied by median nerve. **Flexor carpi ulnaris:** a muscle of the forearm extending from the elbow to the wrist. It flexes the elbow and wrist and adducts the hand. **Flexor digiti minimi brevis:** (foot) arises from the base of the fifth metatarsal and sheath of peroneus longus and is inserted into the lateral side of base of proximal phalanx of little toe. Flexes metatarsophalangeal joint of the little toe. Supplied by the lateral plantar nerve. **Flexor digiti minimi:** (hand) arises from the tip of hook of hamate and flexor retinaculum, and is inserted into the medial side of the base of the proximal phalanx of the little finger. Flexes little finger. Supplied by ulnar nerve. **Flexor digitorum brevis:** a small muscle on the sole of the foot extending from the calcaneum to the four lateral toes. It flexes the tarsal joints and the first interphalangeal joints of the toes. **Flexor digitorum sublimis:** a large muscle arising from the medial condyle of humerus, the medial border of the coronoid process of the ulna, and the oblique line of the radius. It is inserted by four tendons into the middle phalanges of the fingers. It flexes the elbow, wrist, carpal, metacarpal and first interphalangeal joints. It is supplied by the median nerve. **Flexor hallucis brevis:** arises from the medial border of cuboid and lateral cuneiform and the tendon of the tibialis posterior. It is inserted into the lateral and medial sides of base of proximal phalanx of great toe. It flexes the great toe and adducts it to middle line of foot. Supplied by medial plantar nerve. **Flexor hallucis longus:** arises from lower two-thirds of posterior surface of shaft of fibula and is inserted into the base of distal phalanx of great toe. Extends ankle, flexes tarsal joints and joints of great toe. Supplied by posterior tibial nerve. **Flexor indicis brevis:** arises from the palmar surface of the base of the index metacarpal bone, it is inserted into the radial side of the proximal phalanx of the index finger. **Flexor pollicis brevis:** arises by two heads. Lateral from lower border of retinaculum trapezii

and is inserted into the lateral margin of the base of the proximal phalanx of the thumb. Supplied by median nerve. Medial from medial side of base of first metacarpal and inserted into medial border of base of proximal phalanx of thumb. Supplied by ulnar nerve. It flexes metacarpophalangeal and first interphalangeal joint of thumb. **Flexor pollicis longus:** arises from middle half of anterior surface of shaft of radius and base of coronoid process of ulna and is inserted into base of distal phalanx of thumb. Flexes wrist and all joints of thumb. Supplied by anterior interosseous nerve. **Flexor profundus digitorum:** arises from upper three-quarters of anterior and medial surfaces of shaft of ulna, upper three-quarters of medial half of interosseous membrane and aponeurosis from posterior border of ulna. Inserted into palmar surfaces of bases of distal phalanges. Flexes wrist, metacarpal, phalangeal and all the interphalangeal joints. Medial half of muscle supplied by ulnar nerve, lateral half by anterior interosseous nerve. **Gastrocnemius:** arises by two heads. Medial head from impression on posterior part of medial surface of medial condyle and medial supracondylar line of femur. Lateral head from impression on lateral surface of lateral condyle. The two heads unite with the tendon of soleus to form tendo calcaneus which is inserted into the lower half of the posterior surface of calcaneum. Flexes knee and extends ankle. Supplied by medial popliteal nerve. **Gemellus inferior:** arises from the superior and lateral border of tuberosity of ischium and is inserted into superior border of great trochanter with the obturator internus tendon. Rotates thigh outwards. Supplied by the sacral plexus. **Gemellus superior:** arises from the lateral surface of ischial spine and is inserted into superior border of great trochanter of femur with obturator internus tendon. Rotates thigh outwards. Supplied by sacral plexus. **Genioglossus:** arises from the superior genial tubercle on inner surface of mandible near symphysis and is inserted into body of hyoid bone and inferior surface of tongue from root to tip. Raises tongue and hyoid bone, draws tongue forwards and protrudes it to opposite side. Supplied by hypoglossal nerve. **Geniohyoid:** arises from the inferior genial tubercle on the inner surface of mandible near symphysis and is inserted into the middle of the body of the hyoid bone. Raises and draws forward hyoid bone. Supplied by first and second cervical nerves. **Gluteus maximus:** arises from the lateral surface of the ilium between posterior gluteal line and posterior one-third of lateral lip of crest of ilium, from the posterior surface of the coccyx and of last two pieces of sacrum and sacro-tuberous ligament. It is inserted into fascia lata and gluteal tuberosity of the femur. It is an extensor and rotator outwards of thigh. Supplied by inferior gluteal nerve. **Gluteus medius:** arises from the bone between iliac crest and posterior gluteal line above, and middle gluteal line below. It is inserted into the lateral surface of great trochanter of femur. Extends and abducts thigh. Supplied by superior gluteal nerve. **Gluteus mininus:** arises from the posterior surface of ilium between middle and inferior gluteal lines; inserted on anterior part of great trochanter. Abducts and rotates thigh inwards. Supplied by superior gluteal nerve. **Gracilis:** arises from medial margin of anterior surface of inferior pubic ramus and is inserted into medial side of tibia in its upper one-fifth. It adducts thigh and flexes knee. Supplied by obturator nerve. **Hamstring:** the muscles in the posterior compartment of the thigh. They are biceps femoris, semitendinosus and semimembranosus. **Helicis major:** a muscle of the external ear. It extends from the spine of the helix along the anterior part of the helix as high as the level at which it curves backwards. **Helicis minor:** a small muscle of the external ear; it lies on the crus helicis. **Henle's:** the transversus perinei profundus muscle, a part of the sphincter urethrae. **Horner's:** (tensor tarsi) lacrimal portion of orbicularis oculi. **Houston's:** constrictor radicis penis, the anterior band of fibres of the bulbospongiosus muscle. **Hyoglossus:** arises from the side of the body and the greater horn and lesser horn of the hyoid bone. It is inserted into the back and sides of the tongue. It depresses sides of tongue, making surface convex transversely. Supplied by hypoglossal nerve. **Iliacus:** arises from the upper half of iliac fossa, iliolumbar ligament, lateral mass of sacrum and capsule of hip-joint. Inserted into tendon of psoas muscle and into triangular surface anterior to and below the lesser trochanter of femur. It flexes hip-joint and rotates femur laterally. Supplied by the femoral nerve. **Iliacus minor:** (iliocapsularis) is a detached slip of the iliacus which is attached proximally to the anterior inferior iliac spine and by its distal extremity to the medial part of the intertrochanteric line of the femur. **Iliocapsularis:** see iliacus minor. **Iliococcygeus:** is part of the levator ani muscle and is attached to a thickening of the fascia covering the obturator internus. **Iliocostalis:** is the direct continuation of the lateral part of the sacrospinalis and is attached superiorly to the inferior border of the twelfth rib, and by fleshy and tendinous bundles to the angles of the ribs from the seventh to the eleventh. **Iliopsoas:** the composite muscle made up of the psoas and iliacus muscles. **Inferior constrictor:** arises from the side of the cricoid cartilage, the inferior horn of the thyroid cartilage and the outer surface of the lamina of the thyroid cartilage. It is inserted into the median raphe on the posterior wall of the pharynx. Supplied by the pharyngeal plexus. **Infraspinatus:** arises from the infraspinous fossa of the scapula and is inserted on to the middle impression on the greater tuberosity of the humerus. Supplied by the subscapular nerve. **Intercostales intimi, Internal intercostal:** eleven in number on each side. They arise from the medial lip of the groove on inferior border of rib extending from angle to sternum and are inserted on to the medial ridge of superior border of rib below. Supplied by intercostal nerve. **Internal oblique abdominal:** arises from the lateral half of inguinal ligament, anterior two-thirds of middle lip of iliac crest and lumbar fascia between iliac crest and twelfth rib. It is inserted into the inferior edges of the cartilages of lower three ribs and aponeurosis blending with its fellow at linea alba. Supplied by the lower intercostal nerves. **Interosseous** (foot): seven in number, and are arranged in two groups —three plantar and four dorsal. See plantar and dorsal. **Interosseous** (hand): eight in number, occupy the intermetacarpal spaces and are arranged in two groups, four palmar and four dorsal. See palmar and dorsal interosseous muscles. **Interspinales:** muscles placed in pairs, one on each side of the interspinous ligament between the spinous processes of the vertebrae. They help to extend the spine and are supplied by branches of cervical, thoracic and lumbar nerves. **Intertransversales:** lie between transverse processes in cervical, thoracic and lumbar regions of the spine. Laterally flex spine. Supplied by medial posterior branches of cervical, thoracic and lumbar nerves. **Intracostals:** (intercostales) are confined to the dorsal portion of each intercostal space. Each muscle is attached superiorly to the internal lip and to the floor of the subcostal groove of the rib above and inferiorly to the internal margin of the superior border of the rib below. **Ischiobulbosus:** (Cuvier) part of the bulbo-spongiosus muscle. **Ischio-**

cavernosus: (Erector penis) arises from the medial surface of the tuberosity of the ischium and inserted into medial and lateral surfaces of crus penis. Compresses crus and produces erection of penis. Supplied by the pudendal nerve. **Ischiococcygeus:** see coccygeus muscle. **Laryngeal:** are the muscles by which the cartilages are moved and the condition of the vocal cords determined. They are cricothyroideus, cricothyroideus posterior, cricothyroideus lateralis, thyroarytenoideus, arytenoideus, and ary-epiglotticus, **Lateral pterygoid:** arises from the infratemporal crest and lateral surface of lateral pterygoid plate and is inserted into pterygoid depression in front of neck of mandible and articular disc of mandible. Is a muscle of mastication and protrudes the jaw. Supplied by mandibular nerve. **Latissimus dorsi:** arises from the spinous processes of lower six thoracic vertebrae, supraspinous ligaments, lateral edge of iliac crest, and lower three or four ribs. It is inserted into the floor of the bicipital groove of the humerus. Draws arm down and backwards. Supplied by long scapular nerve. **Laxator tympani:** (band of Meckel) in the temporal bone of the skull. **Levator anguli oris:** arises from the superior part of the canine fossa of the maxilla and is inserted into the angle of the mouth. Raises the angle of the mouth. Supplied by the facial nerve. **Levator ani:** arises from the posterior surface of pubis near symphysis, spine of ischium, from rectovesical fascia. Inserted into central perineal tendon, sides of rectum and coccyx. Supports pelvic viscera, compresses and raises lower part of rectum in defaecation. Supplied by fourth sacral and pudendal nerves. **Levator glandulae thyroidae:** a fibrous band which sometimes contains muscular fibres, which extends from the isthmus of the thyroid gland to the body of the hyoid bone. **Levator labii superioris:** arises from the maxilla and zygomatic bone above the infra-orbital foramen and inserted into the orbicularis oris. Raises upper lip. Supplied by facial nerve. **Levator labii superioris alaeque nasi:** arises from root of frontal process of maxilla and is inserted into cartilage of ala and orbicularis oris. Raises ala of nose and upper lip. Supplied by facial nerve. **Levator menti:** (mentalis) arises from the incisive fossa of the mandible and is inserted into the skin of the chin. It is supplied by the facial nerve. **Levator palati:** arises from the inferior aspect of the petrous part of the temporal bone and the inferoposterior part of the cartilage of the pharyngotympanic tube. It is inserted into the aponeurosis of the soft palate. It is supplied by the pharyngeal plexus. **Levator palpebrae superioris:** arises from the inferior surface of the lesser wing of the sphenoid anterior to the optic foramen. It is inserted into the upper border of the superior tarsus. It is supplied by the oculomotor nerve. **Levator penis:** (compressor venae dorsalis penis). Part of the ischiocavernosus muscle which passes on to the corpus cavernosum of the penis. **Levator prostatae:** part of the anterior fibres of the levator ani muscle. **Levator scapulae:** arises by four tendinous slips from the posterior tubercles of the transverse processes of the upper four cervical vertebrae. It is inserted to the medial border of the scapula immediately above the triangular surface at the root of the spine. It is supplied by branches of the third, fourth and fifth cervical nerves. **Levatores costarum:** are twelve small muscles on each side. The highest muscle is attached to the tip of the transverse process of the seventh cervical vertebra and the succeeding eleven are attached to the tips of the transverse processes of the thoracic vertebrae from the first to the eleventh inclusively. Each muscle is attached to the external surface of the rib below, extending from the tubercle to the angle. They are supplied by the intercostal nerves. **Longissimus:** the intermediate column of the erector spinae muscle, consisting of three muscles, the longissimus thoracis, the longissimus cervicis, and the longissimus capitis, in order from below upwards. **Longitudinalis linguae inferior:** the inferior bundle of intrinsic muscle fibres of the tongue. **Longitudinalis linguae superior:** the superior sheet of intrinsic muscle of the tongue situated immediately beneath the mucous membrane. Supplied by the hypoglossal nerve. **Longus capitis:** (rectus capitis anticus major). Arises by four short tendons from the anterior tubercles of the transverse processes of the third, fourth, fifth and sixth cervical vertebrae. It is inserted into the inferior surface of the basilar process of the occipital bone. It is supplied by the first and second cervical nerves. **Longus cervicis:** (longus colli) consists of three portions: superior oblique, vertical and inferior oblique. The superior oblique portion arises from the anterior tubercles of the transverse processes of the third, fourth, fifth and sixth cervical vertebrae. It is inserted into the lateral aspect of the tubercle of the anterior arch of the atlas. The vertical portion arises from the anterior aspect of the bodies of the last two cervical and the first three thoracic vertebrae. It is inserted into the anterior aspects of the bodies of the second, third and fourth cervical vertebrae. Inferior oblique portion arises from the anterior aspect of the bodies of the first three thoracic vertebrae in common with the inferior portion of the vertical part. It is inserted into the anterior tubercles of the transverse processes of the fifth and sixth cervical vertebrae. It is supplied by the adjacent spinal nerves. **Longus colli:** see longus cervicis. **Lumbrical** (foot): four in number. They arise from the long flexor tendons, from adjacent sides of two tendons, except innermost, which arises from medial side of first flexor tendon. They are inserted into the medial sides of the bases of the proximal phalanx of four lateral toes. The first muscle is supplied by the medial plantar nerve and the rest by the lateral plantar nerve. **Lumbrical:** (hand) four tapering muscles connected with deep flexor tendons in the palm. They arise from the lateral sides of the deep flexor tendons and are inserted into the lateral sides of the tendinous expansion on the dorsal surface of the proximal phalanges. The two lateral muscles are supplied by the median nerve and the two medial by the ulnar nerve. **Masseter:** arises from the anterior two thirds of the inferior border of the zygomatic arch and from the medial surface of the same arch. It is inserted into the lower part of the lateral surface of the ramus of the mandible. Supplied by the mandibular division of the trigeminal nerve. **Medial pterygoid** (internal pterygoid): arises from the medial surface of the lateral pterygoid plate of the sphenoid, the tuberosity of the palate bone and tuberosity of the superior maxilla. It is inserted into the medial aspect of the angle of the mandible. Supplied by the mandibular nerve. **Mentalis:** see levator menti. **Middle constrictor of the pharynx:** arises from the superior border of the greater horn of the hyoid bone, the posterior border of the lesser horn, and the hyoid attachment of the stylohyoid ligament. It is inserted into the median raphe on the posterior wall of the pharynx. It is supplied by the pharyngeal plexus. **Multifidus:** a big mass of muscle arising from the back of the sacrum, the medial surface of the posterior superior iliac spine, posterior sacro-iliac ligament, transverse processes of the thoracic and the articular processes of the lower five cervical vertebrae. It is inserted into the spines and neural arches of the vertebrae from the third sacral to the second cervical. Supplied by the spinal nerves. **Mylohyoid:** arises from the mylo-hyoid line of the mandible and is inserted into the anterior surface of the hyoid bone, the central fibrous raphe that extends from the symphysis menti to the body of the hyoid bone. Supplied by the mylohyoid branch of the inferior dental nerve. **Obliqui, of eyeball:** two in number. Obliquus inferior arises from a small depression at the anterior and medial part of the floor of the orbit, and is inserted into the lateral surface of the sclera under cover of the rectus lateralis. Supplied by the oculomotor nerve. Obliquus superior arises from the wall of the orbit directly anterior to the optic foramen. It is inserted by an expanded tendon into the superior and lateral aspect of the sclera. It is supplied by the trochlear nerve. **Obliquus abdominis internus:** arises from the lateral half of inguinal ligament, anterior two-thirds of middle lip of iliac crest and lumbar fascia. It is inserted into the inferior edges of the cartilages of the last three ribs, aponeurosis blending with its fellow at linea alba. Supplied by lower intercostal nerves. **Obliquus abdominis externus:** arises by eight digitations from inferior borders and lateral surfaces of eight lower ribs, upper five interdigitating with serratus anterior, lower three with latissimus dorsi. It is inserted into the anterior half of the lateral lip of the iliac crest, and aponeurosis in front of abdomen which is attached to pubic tubercle and symphysis below. Supplied by lower intercostal nerves. **Obliquus auriculae:** a small muscle which extends over the depression corresponding to the inferior crus of the antihelix on the lateral surface of the ear. **Obliquus capitis inferior:** arises from the lateral aspect of the spine of the axis and is inserted into the inferior and posterior surface of the transverse process of the atlas. Supplied by the suboccipital nerve. **Obliquus capitis superior:** arises from the superior and posterior surface of the transverse process of the atlas and is inserted into the occipital bone between the lateral portions of the superior and inferior nuchal lines. Supplied by suboccipital nerve. **Obliquus inferior:** see obliqui of eyeball. **Obliquus superior:** see obliqui of eyeball. **Obturator externus:** arises from the medial two-thirds of the external aspect of the obturator membrane and the adjacent parts of the body of the os pubis. It is inserted into the digital fossa of the femur. Supplied by the obturator nerve. **Obturator internus:** arises from the intrapelvic surface of the obturator membrane, and from the os innominatum. It is inserted into a depression on the medial surface of the greater trochanter of the femur. Supplied by the fifth lumbar and first and second sacral nerves. **Occipitofrontalis:** consists of two occipital bellies, two frontal bellies and the epicranial aponeurosis. Each occipital belly is attached to the highest nuchal line of the occipital bone and is inserted into the aponeurosis. Each frontal belly is attached to the subcutaneous tissue of the eyebrow and root of nose and is inserted into the aponeurosis. It is supplied by the facial nerve. **Of Bell:** the bundle of muscular fibres situated within the urethro-ureteric ridge in the bladder. **Of Treitz:** (suspensory muscle of the duodenum) a fibro-muscular band which extends from the right crus of the diaphragm to the duodenojejunal junction. **Of uterus:** is composed of plain muscle which is disposed in three strata—outer, middle, and inner. The outer stratum is thin and its fibres are disposed longitudinally. The middle stratum is very thick and is composed of interlacing fibres. The inner stratum is very thick with longitudinally disposed fibres. **Omohyoid:** consists of two bellies, superior (anterior) and inferior (posterior), and an intermediate tendon. The superior belly is attached to the lateral third of the inferior border of the body of the hyoid bone. The inferior belly is attached to the superior border of the scapula, and to the suprascapular ligament. The intermediate tendon which unites the two bellies is encased in deep cervical fascia which is attached to the posterior aspect of the medial end of the clavicle. The two bellies are supplied by the first, second and third cervical nerves. **Opponens digiti minimi:** (foot) some fibres of the flexor digiti minimi brevis which are attached to the fifth metatarsal bone. **Opponens digiti minimi:** (hand) arises from the lumbar surface of the hook of the hamate and is inserted into the ulnar aspect of the shaft of the fifth metacarpal bone. It is supplied by the ulnar nerve. **Opponens pollicis:** arises from the superficial surface of the flexor retinaculum and the crest of the trapezium, and is inserted into the radial border of the shaft of the metacarpal bone of the thumb. It is supplied by the median nerve. **Orbicularis oculi:** (Orbicularis palpebrarum) sphincter of eyelids, arises from the nasal part of the frontal bone, frontal process of maxilla, the medial palpebral ligament and is inserted into the lateral palpebral ligament. It is supplied by the facial nerve. **Orbicularis oris:** sphincter of mouth. The labial part is free from attachment to bone, and forms red part of lips. The facial part is connected with the muscles which converge to the angles of the mouth, and is attached in the upper lip to septum of nasi and incisive fossa of maxilla. It is supplied by the facial nerve. **Orbicularis palpebrarum:** see orbicularis oculi. **Palatoglossus:** arises from the surface of the palatine aponeurosis and is inserted into the posterior part of the side of the tongue. It is supplied by the pharyngeal plexus. **Palatopharyngeus:** arises from the palatine aponeurosis and posterior margin of the hard palate and is inserted into the superior and posterior borders of the lamina of the thyroid cartilage and the lateral and posterior wall of the pharynx. It is supplied by the pharyngeal plexus. **Palmar interosseous:** three in number; originating at sides of metacarpal bones and inserted at aponeurosis of extensor tendons and neighbouring parts of first phalanges. These muscles adduct fingers, flex first and extend second and third phalanges. Supplied by the ulnar nerve. **Palmaris brevis:** a small muscle arising from the flexor retinaculum and palmar fascia and inserted into the skin on the medial side of the palm. Supplied by the ulnar nerve. **Palmaris longus:** arises from the medial epicondyle of the humerus and is inserted into the palmar fascia. It is supplied by the median nerve. **Papillary:** small conical muscles attached to the walls of the ventricles of the heart. Their free extremities are connected with a number of filiform processes, named chordae tendineae, which pass to the margins and ventricular surfaces of the segments of the atrioventricular valve. **Pectineus:** arises from the pectineal part of the ileopectineal line and the posterior half of the superior surface of the superior pubic ramus. It is inserted into the posterior aspect of the femur below the lesser trochanter. It is supplied by the femoral nerve. **Pectoralis major:** arises from the sternal half of the clavicle, the front of the sternum and the cartilages of the upper six ribs. It is inserted into the lateral ridge of the bicipital groove of humerus. Supplied by the lateral and medial pectoral nerves. **Pectoralis minor:** arises from third, fourth and fifth ribs lateral to their costal cartilages. It is inserted into the anterior half of the superior surface and medial border of the coracoid process of the scapula. It is supplied by the medial pectoral nerve. **Peripenic** (Sappey): part of the dartos muscle the fibres of which form a fine interlacement extending from the root of the penis into the prepuce. **Peroneus brevis:** arises from the lower two-thirds of the lateral surfaces of the shaft of the fibula and is inserted into the base of the fifth metatarsal bone. It is supplied by the musculocutaneous nerve. **Peroneus longus:** arises from the upper two-thirds of the lateral surface of the shaft of the fibula and is inserted into the lateral part of the plantar surface of the medial cuneiform and base of first metatarsal. It is supplied by the musculocutaneous nerve. **Peroneus tertius:** arises from the lower quarter of the anterior surface of the shaft of the fibula and is inserted into the base of the fifth metatarsal bone. Supplied by the anterior tibial nerve. **Plantar interosseous:** three in number; originating at inner and outer surfaces of three outer metatarsal bones and inserted at inner sides of first phalanges of corresponding toes. They adduct first phalanges of three outer toes; flex phalanges of first row and extend the others. Supplied by external plantar nerve. **Plantaris:** arises from a line above the lateral condyle of the femur and from the posterior ligament of the knee joint. It is inserted into the medial tubercle of the calcaneum. It is supplied by the medial popliteal nerve. **Platysma:** (platysma myoides) is attached to the superficial fascia that covers the clavicular parts of the pectoralis major and deltoid muscles, the lateral part of the body of the mandible, and the angle of the mouth where the fibres blend with those of the depressor anguli oris and orbicularis oris. Supplied by facial nerve. **Popliteus:** arises from the anterior half of an impression on the lateral surface of lateral condyle of femur and the posterior ligament of the knee joint. It is inserted into the triangular space on posterior surface of shaft of tibia above soleal line. Supplied by medial popliteal nerve. **Prevertebral:** in front of vertebral column. They are longus capitis, rectus capitis anterior, rectus capitis lateralis, and longus cervicis (longus colli). **Procerus:** the medial fibres of the frontal belly of the occipitofrontalis muscle. **Recto-urethralis:** some of the longitudinal fibres of the muscular coat of the anal canal which pass towards the membranous urethra. **Rectovesical:** some fibres of the external longitudinal muscle of the bladder which blend posteriorly with the anterior longitudinal coat of the rectum. **Rectus abdominis:** arises from the pubic crest and symphysis and is inserted into the xiphoid process and costal cartilages of the fifth, sixth and seventh ribs. It is supplied by the lower intercostal and subcostal nerves. **Rectus capitis anticus major:** see longus capitis. **Rectus capitis anticus minor:** (rectus capitis anterior) arises from the anterior aspect of the lateral mass of the atlas and is inserted into the inferior surface of the basilar part of the occipital bone. It is supplied by the first cervical nerve. **Rectus capitis lateralis:** arises from the superior border of the extremity of the transverse process of the atlas and is inserted on to the inferior surface of the jugular process of the occipital bone. Supplied by the first cervical nerve. **Rectus capitis posterior major:** arises from the spine of the axis and is inserted into the lateral part of the inferior nuchal line of the occipital bone. It is supplied by the suboccipital nerve. **Rectus capitis posterior minor:** arises from the posterior tubercle of the atlas and is inserted into the medial third of the inferior nuchal line of the occipital bone. It is supplied by the suboccipital nerve. **Rectus femoris:** arises by two heads. The *straight head* is attached to the anterior inferior iliac spine. The *reflected head* is attached to a groove on the gluteal surface of the ilium immediately superior to the margin of the acetabulum. It is inserted into the proximal edge of the patella. Supplied by the femoral nerve. **Retrahens aurem:** see auricularis posterior. **Rhomboideus major:** arises from the spines and supraspinous ligaments of the thoracic vertebrae from the second to fifth. It is inserted into the medial border of the scapula from the triangular surface at the root of the spine to the inferior angle. Supplied by fifth cervical nerve. **Rhomboideus minor:** arises from the lower part of the ligamentum nuchae and the spines of, and the supraspinous ligament between, the seventh cervical and the first thoracic vertebrae. It is inserted into the medial border of the scapula as far down as the triangular surface at the root of the spine. Supplied by the fifth cervical nerve. **Risorius:** arises from the deep fascia that covers the masseter muscle and parotid gland and is inserted into the skin at the angle of the mouth. It is supplied by the facial nerve. It gives rise to the 'risus sardonicus'. **Rotatores:** small muscles confined to the thoracic region, eleven in number. They are attached to the postero-superior aspects of the transverse processes and to the lower borders of the laminae of the vertebrae immediately above. Supplied by the spinal nerves. **Sacrospinalis:** see erector spinae. **Sartorius:** arises from the anterior superior iliac spine and the upper part of the notch immediately inferior to it. It is inserted into the proximal end of the medial surface of the shaft of the tibia. Supplied by the femoral nerve. **Scalenus anterior** (scalenus anticus): arises by four short tendons from the anterior tubercles of the transverse processes of the third, fourth, fifth and sixth cervical vertebrae. Inserted into the scalene tubercle of the first rib. Supplied by the fifth and sixth cervical nerves. **Scalenus medius:** arises by six short tendons from the anterior tubercles of the transverse processes of the lower six cervical vertebrae. Inserted into the superior surface of the first rib from the groove for the subclavian artery posteriorly as far as the tubercle. Supplied by third, fourth, fifth, sixth, seventh and eight cervical nerves. **Scalenus pleuralis** (scalenus minimus or scalenus quartus): an inconstant muscle and only present in 35 per cent of cases. It is attached above to the anterior tubercle of the transverse process of the seventh cervical vertebra and below to the medial borders of the first rib. Supplied by the cervical nerves. **Scalenus posterior:** (scalenus posticus) arises by two or three short tendons from the posterior tubercles of the transverse processes of the lower two or three cervical vertebrae. It is inserted into the upper part of the outer surface of the second rib. Supplied by the sixth, seventh and eighth cervical nerves. **Semimembranosus:** arises by a broad flat tendon from the superolateral impression on the posterior surface of the ischial tuberosity. Inserted into the distal lip of the horizontal groove on the medial condyle of the tibia; it is also inserted into the posterior ligament of the knee joint and the fascia over the popliteus muscle. Supplied by the sciatic nerve. **Semispinalis capitis:** see complexus. **Semitendinosus:** arises from the inferior and medial impression on the posterior surface of the ischial tuberosity and is inserted into the proximal part of the medial surface of the shaft of the tibia. Supplied by the sciatic nerve. **Serratus anterior:** arises from the external surfaces of the upper eight or nine ribs at their anterior angles. It is inserted into medial border of the scapula. Supplied by the long respiratory nerve of Bell from the fifth, sixth and seventh cervical nerves. **Serratus posticus inferior:** arises from the posterior lamina of the lumbar fascia and is inserted by four fleshy slips to the lower borders of the last four ribs. Supplied by ninth, tenth and eleventh intercostal nerves. **Serratus posticus superior:** arises from the lower part of the ligamentum nuchae and the spines and supraspinous ligaments of the last cervical and first two thoracic vertebrae. It is inserted

into the superior borders of the second, third, fourth and fifth ribs, lateral to their angles. Supplied by second, third and fourth intercostal nerves. **Soleus:** arises from the posterior surface of the head and the proximal third of the lateral surface and the proximal quarter of the posterior surface of the shaft of the fibula and the soleal line of tibia. Inserted into back of os calcis. Supplied by medial popliteal nerve. **Sphincter ani externus:** arises from the tip and back of coccyx and subcutaneous fatty layer on either side; it is inserted into the central perineal tendon. Closes anus. Supplied by the fourth sacral and inferior rectal nerves. **Sphincter ani internus:** is the involuntary musculature of the large intestine thickened about half inch deep. Closes anus. **Sphincter ani tertius:** (sphincter of Nelaton). The rectal muscular fibres contained in the first horizontal fold of the rectum (Houston's folds). **Sphincter of Nelaton:** see Sphincter ani tertius. **Sphincter pupillae:** the unstriped circular muscular fibres of the iris. They are nearer the posterior surface than the anterior. Supplied by the oculo-motor nerve by means of the motor root of the ciliary ganglion. **Sphincter urethrae:** see compressor urethrae. **Sphincter vaginae:** (bulbospongiosus) arises from the perineal body and passes forwards and divides into two parts,which surround the vaginal orifice and vestibule, and blends with the fibrous sheath of the corpus spongiosum. Supplied by pudendal nerve. **Sphincter vesicae:** is part of the middle circular fibres of the muscular coat of the bladder. **Spinalis:** the medial column of the erector spinae muscle. **Splenius:** is so named because it holds down the muscles beneath it. It arises from the lower two-thirds of the ligamentum nuchae and the spines of the last cervical and first six thoracic vertebrae. It divides into two parts: the splenius capitis which is inserted into the posterior and inferior part of the lateral surface of the mastoid process and lateral one-third of the superior nuchal line of the occipital bone; and splenius cervicis which is inserted into the posterior tubercles of the transverse processes of the first two or three cervical vertebrae. **Stapedius:** arises from the wall of the canal within the pyramid of the middle ear and is inserted into the posterior aspect of the neck of the stapes. It is supplied by the facial nerve. **Sternalis:** an inconstant variable muscle situated superficial to the pectoralis major muscle. **Sternocostalis:** (triangularis sterni) is a bilateral fan-shaped muscle, the fibres of which pass superiorly and laterally from the inferior part of the posterior aspect of the sternum and xiphisternum to the costal cartilages and ribs. Supplied by the intercostal nerves. **Sternohyoid:** arises from the posterior surface of the manubrium sterni, the sternoclavicular ligament and the posterior surface of the clavicle at its medial end. It is inserted into the medial two-thirds of the inferior border of the body of the hyoid bone. Supplied by the ansa hypoglossi nerve. **Sternomastoid:** arises by two heads. The sternal head is attached to the superior and lateral part of the anterior surface of the manubrium sterni. The clavicular head is attached to the superior surface of the clavicle at its medial end. It is inserted into the lateral surface of the mastoid process of the temporal bone and the superior nuchal line of the occipital bone along its lateral half or two-thirds. Supplied by the accessory nerve and the second cervical nerve. **Sternothyroid:** arises from the posterior surface of the manubrium sterni and the posterior surface of the first costal cartilage. It is inserted into the oblique line on the outer surface of the lamina of the thyroid cartilage. Supplied by ansa hypoglossi nerve. **Styloglossus:** arises from the anterior aspect of the styloid process of the temporal bone and the stylomandibular ligament. It is inserted into the inferior surface of the tongue close to its lateral border. Supplied by the hypoglossal nerve. **Stylohyoid:** arises from the posterior and lateral aspect of the styloid process of the temporal bone near its base. It is inserted into the anterior surface of the hyoid bone at the junction of the body and greater horn. Supplied by facial nerve. **Stylopharyngeus:** arises from the base of the styloid process of the temporal bone and is inserted into the posterior border of the lamina of the thyroid cartilage and lateral wall of the pharynx. Supplied by the glossopharyngeal nerve. **Subanconeus:** part of the medial head of the triceps which gains attachment to the posterior ligament of the elbow-joint. **Subclavius:** arises from the upper surface of the first rib at its junction with its cartilage and is inserted into the subclavian groove on the inferior surface of the clavicle. Supplied by fifth and sixth cervical nerves. **Subcostal:** consists of a series of muscles that appears continuous from the first to the twelfth rib. The muscle fibres are continuous anteriorly with the intercostals and are attached by tendinous fibres to the inner surfaces of the ribs. Supplied by intercostal nerves. **Subcrureus** (articularis genu): is a deep lamination of the distal part of the vastus intermedius. **Subscapularis:** arises from the ventral surface of the scapula and is inserted on to the lesser tuberosity of the humerus. Supplied by the upper and lower subscapular nerves. **Subscapularis minor of Gruber** (subscapulohumeralis of Macalister): the lower fibres of the subscapularis muscle which may form a separate bundle and are inserted into the neck of the humerus below the lesser tuberosity. **Superficial transverse perineal** (Transversus perinei superficialis): arises from the inferior ramus of the ischium and adjacent perineal membrane, and is inserted into the perineal body. Supplied by the pudendal nerve. **Superior constrictor:** arises from the inferior third of the posterior border of the medial pterygoid plate, posterior aspect of the pterygomandibular raphe, posterior extremity of the mylohyoid line, the mucous membrane of the mouth and the side of the tongue. It is inserted into the median raphe in the posterior wall of the pharynx, where it meets its fellow of the opposite side. Supplied by the pharyngeal plexus. **Supinator:** arises from the lateral epicondyle of humerus, lateral ligament of elbow joint, annular ligament of radius, depression below radial notch and the lateral border of the ulna for two inches. It is inserted into the proximal third of the shaft of the radius on its volar, radial and extensor aspects. Supplied by the posterior interosseous nerve. **Supraspinatus:** arises from the supraspinous fossa of the scapula and is inserted on the upper of the three facets upon greater tuberosity of humerus. Supplied by suprascapular nerve. **Suspensory, of duodenum** (of Treitz): a fibro-muscular bundle passing from the right crus of the diaphragm to the duodenojejunal flexure. **Temporalis:** arises from the temporal fascia and temporal fossa and is inserted into the medial surface and forepart of the coronoid process of the mandible. Supplied by the mandibular nerve. **Tensor fasciae latae:** arises from the lateral edge of iliac crest for one inch, anterior superior iliac spine and half notch below it; it is inserted into the fascia lata about one-third down the thigh, anterior to greater trochanter. Supplied by superior gluteal nerve. **Tensor palati:** arises from the scaphoid fossa at the root of the medial pterygoid plate of the sphenoid; it is inserted into the transverse ridge on the inferior surface of the horizontal plate of the palatine bone and into the aponeurosis of the soft palate. Supplied by the otic ganglion. **Tensor tarsi** or **muscle of Horner:** see orbicularis oculi. **Tensor tympani:** arises from

T

the cartilaginous part of the pharyngotympanic tube, the apex of the petrous part of the temporal bone and the wall of the osseous canal through which the muscle passes. It is inserted into the medial aspect of the handle of the malleus. Supplied by the otic ganglion. **Teres major:** arises from an oval impression on the dorsal surface of the scapula near its inferior angle; it is inserted into the medial lip of the bicipital groove of the humerus. Supplied by the lower scapular nerve. **Teres minimus:** (Gruber) a separate bundle of the fibres of the teres minor which is attached to the humerus below the greater tuberosity. **Teres minor:** arises from superior two-thirds of lateral border of dorsum of scapula and its investing fascia; it is inserted into the lowest of the three facets upon greater tuberosity of humerus. Supplied by circumflex nerve. **Thyro-arytenoideus:** arises from the lower half of the receding angle of the thyroid cartilage and is inserted into the edge of vocal process and lateral surface of the arytenoid cartilage. Supplied by the recurrent laryngeal nerve. The superior fibres of the muscle are known as the thyro-epiglotticus. The most medial part of the muscle is known as the vocalis muscle. **Thyro-epiglotticus:** see thyroarytenoideus. **Thyrohyoid:** arises from the oblique line of the thyroid cartilage and is inserted into the medial half of greater horn and lateral part of body of hyoid bone. Supplied by the first and second cervical nerves. **Tibialis anterior:** arises from the lateral condyle and upper two-thirds of lateral surface of shaft of tibia and is inserted into the medial surface of medial cuneiform and base of metatarsal bone of great toe. Supplied by anterior tibial nerve. **Tibialis posterior:** arises from the posterior surface of interosseous membrane, lateral part of posterior surface of tibia and medial surface of shaft of fibula. It is inserted into the tuberosity of navicular and slips to cuneiforms, cuboid, bases of second, third and fourth metatarsal bones and sustentaculum tali. Supplied by posterior tibial nerve. **Tragicus:** a small muscle which lies upon the lateral surface of the tragus of the ear; its fibres being almost vertical. **Transversus abdominis:** arises from the lateral one-third inguinal ligament, anterior three-quarter medial lip of iliac crest, medial surfaces of cartilages of lower six ribs and from lumbar fascia. Its lower fibres end in the conjoint tendon, inserted into pubis and pectineal line; rest of fibres terminate in an aponeurosis attached to linea alba. Supplied by lower intercostal nerves. **Transversus auriculae:** is a small muscle on the back of the ear which extends over the depression that corresponds to the antihelix on the lateral surface, its attachments being to the convexity of the concha on the one hand, and the convexity of the fossa of the helix on the other. **Transversus cervicis:** (longissimus cervicis) is the continuation of the longissimus thoracis into the neck. Its thoracic attachment is to the transverse processes of the upper five or six thoracic vertebrae and the cervical attachment is to the posterior tubercles of the transverse processes of cervical vertebrae from the second to sixth inclusive. **Transversus linguae:** the transverse fibres of the intrinsic muscles of the tongue. **Transversus nuchae:** a small muscle which extends from the external occipital protuberance to the superior attachment of the sterno-mastoid. **Transversus pedis:** arises by three slips from the inferior tarsal, metatarsal and transverse metatarsal ligaments and is inserted at the base of the first phalanx of the great toe, which it adducts. Supplied by the external plantar nerve. **Trapezius:** arises from the spinous processes of all thoracic and seventh cervical vertebrae, with supraspinous ligamentum nuchae and medial one-third of superior nuchal line of occipital bone. It is inserted into lateral one-third of posterior border of clavicle, superior edge of acromion, superior lip of posterior border of spine of scapula, and rough impression on spine about one inch from root. Supplied by accessory and third and fourth cervical nerves. **Triangularis menti:** see depressor anguli oris. **Triangularis sterni:** see sternocostalis. **Triceps:** arises by three heads, long, lateral and medial. Long head arises from the depression on lateral border of scapula, close beneath glenoid cavity. Lateral head from root of greater tuberosity to groove for radial nerve on posterior surface of humerus. Medial head from posterior surface of shaft of humerus by side of and below radial groove. It is inserted into the posterior surface of olecranon process of ulna. Supplied by the radial nerve. **Vastus intermedius:** arises from the upper two-thirds anterior and lateral surfaces of shaft of femur and lower half intermuscular septum. Inserted into common extensor tendon into patella. Supplied by the femoral nerve. **Vastus lateralis:** arises from the upper half of shaft of femur and is inserted into the common extensor tendon into patella. Supplied by femoral nerve. **Vastus medialis:** arises from the medial lip of the linea aspera, lower part of spiral line and from the tendons of the adductores longus and magnus. It is inserted into common extensor tendon into patella. Supplied by femoral nerve. **Verticalis linguae:** part of the intrinsic musculature of the tongue which extends from the mucosa of the dorsum to that of the inferior surface. **Vocalis:** see thyro-arytenoideus. **Wood's:** see abductor ossis metatarsi digiti quinti pedis. **Zygomaticus major:** arises from the zygomatic bone in front of temporal process and is inserted into the angle of the mouth. Supplied by the facial nerve. **Zygomaticus minor:** arises from the zygomatic bone near maxillary suture and is inserted into the angle of the mouth. Supplied by the facial nerve.

mus·cular (L. *musculus*, muscle). 1. Relating to muscles. 2. Possessing well-developed muscles. **M. dystrophy:** see dystrophy, m. **M. rheumatism:** see fibrositis; myalgia. **M. sense:** see kinaesthesia.

musculă·ris mucō·sae (L.). The layer of unstriped muscular tissue in mucous membranes, situated between the mucosa and the submucosa.

mus·culature (L. *musculus*, muscle). The muscular system of the body, or of one of its parts.

mus·culocută·neous (L. *musculus*, muscle; *cutis*, skin). Relating to or supplying the muscles and skin.

mus·culomem·branous (L. *musculus*, muscle; *membrana*, membrane). Relating to or consisting of both muscles and membrane.

mus·culospī·ral. Supplying the muscles and having a spiral course; the m. nerve.

mus·culus (L.). Muscle.

Musset's sign (Musset, L. C. A. de, French poet, 1810–57, who exhibited the sign). Movements of the head synchronous with the radial pulse, generally observed in people with aortic disease.

mussitā·tion (L. *mussitare*, to mumble). Murmuring words without the production of articulate speech.

Mussy. See Guéneau de Mussy.

must. Unfermented grape juice.

mustard gas. B′B′-dichlorodiethyl sulphide, a poisonous gas causing blistering of the skin.

mū·tacism (G. *mutakismos*, fondness of the letter m). The substitution of the m. sound for other sounds.

mū·tarotā·tion (L. *mutare*, to change; *rotare*, to turn round). The spontaneous change in optical activity of an optically active substance in solution, e.g. glucose.

mū·tase. A preparation made from leguminous plants and used as a food.

mutā·tion (L. *mutare*, to change). 1. Change. 2. A transmissible change in the germ-plasm, occurring in a single gene, or due to loss of one or more genes or of chromosomes, producing a detectable change in the characteristics of the individual.

mute (L. *mutus*). Dumb; unable to utter articulate speech.

mutilā·tion (L. *mutilare*, to maim). 1. The act of disfiguring or maiming. 2. The state thus produced.

mū·tism (L. *mutus*, dumb). Dumbness.

mū·tualism (L. *mutuus*, reciprocal). The relation between organisms living in symbiosis.

My. Abbreviation for myopia.

Mya's disease (Myà, G., Italian physician, 1857–1911). see Hirschsprung's disease.

mўăl·gia (G. *mus*, muscle; *algos*, pain). A condition characterized by pain in voluntary muscles, supposed to be due to inflammation of the fibrous tissue of muscle sheaths, ligaments, etc. Syn. fibrositis; muscular rheumatism.

mўamoe·ba (G. *mus*, muscle). A muscle cell.

mўanē·sin. α:β-dihydroxy-γ-(2-methylphenoxy) propane, used to increase the relaxation of abdominal muscles in anaesthesia.

mўasthē·nia (G. *mus*, muscle; *a*, neg.; *sthenos*, strength). Muscular debility. **M. gravis:** a disease characterized by rapid exhaustion of voluntary muscles, leading to transient paresis, affecting especially the external ocular muscles and associated with, if not primarily caused by, a failure in equilibrium between the rate of liberation of acetylcholine at the neuromyal junction and the rate of its destruction by the esterase locally present. Syn. Erb's disease, Hoppe-Goldflam's symptom complex.

mўasthē·nic reaction (G. *mus*, muscle; *a*, neg.; *sthenos*, strength). A muscular reaction to faradic current, found in myasthenia gravis, characterized by a gradual decrease of muscular contractibility; after a period of rest the fibres again become excitable.

mўatō·nia (G. *mus*, muscle; *a*, neg.; *tonos*, tone). Absence of muscular tone. **M. congenita:** a congenital disease, characterized by muscular flaccidity, affecting especially the limbs, and absence of deep reflexes, not leading to muscular atrophy or galvanic excitability. Syn. Oppenheim's disease; amyotonia congenita.

mўă·trophy (G. *mus*, muscle; *a*, neg.; *trophia*, nourishment). Muscular atrophy.

mycē·lium (G. *mukēs*, mushroom; *hēlos*, nail). The vegetative filaments of fungi, generally forming an interwoven network.

mycē·tēs (G. *mukēs*, mushroom). The fungi.

mў·cetism (G. *mukēs*, mushroom). Mushroom-poisoning.

mycetō·ma (G. *mukēs*, mushroom). A fungus disease endemic in parts of India, characterized by pinkish or black granulomata of the skin tending to form large nodular masses discharging granules and by swelling and induration of the involved parts; affecting mainly the foot. Syn. Madura foot.

Mў·cobacteriā·ceae (G. *mukēs*, mushroom; *baktērion*, a stick). A family of Schizomycetes, including the genera Mycobacterium and Corynebacterium.

Mў·cobactē·rium. A genus of bacteria belonging to the Mycobacteriaceae. *M. leprae:* the bacillus of leprosy. *M. tuberculosis:* the tubercle bacillus.

mў·codermati·tis (G. *mukēs*, mushroom; *derma*, skin). Inflammation of a mucous membrane.

mўcohae·mia (G. *mukēs*, mushroom; *haima*, blood). The presence of fungi in the blood.

mycŏ·logy (G. *mukēs*, mushroom; *logos*, treatise). The sum of what is known of fungi.

mўcoprō·tein (G. *mukēs*, mushroom; *prōton*, first). General term for the protein of bacterial cells.

mycŏ·sis (G. *mukēs*, mushroom). 1. Any disease caused by fungus. 2. Sometimes used also to denote a disease caused by micro-organisms other than fungi. **M. fungoides:** a systemic disease of granulomatous or perhaps neoplastic character. The first (premycotic) stage is characterized by intense pruritus, a polymorph eruption or erythrodermia, and followed after a variable interval (up to ten years) by the development of soft tumours in the form of infiltrated plaques on the trunk, the upper part of the limbs, and the face. Although spontaneous remissions are not rare, it ultimately causes death. **M. f. à tumeurs d'emblée:** m. f. beginning, with tumour formation, not preceded by a premycotic stage. **M. intestinalis:** gastro-intestinal anthrax.

mȳ·costat (G. *mukēs*, mushroom; *statikos*, stopping). Any agent inhibiting the growth of fungi.

mycot·ic (G. *mukēs*, mushroom). Relating to mycosis; caused by micro-organisms, more especially by fungi.

mycotox·in (G. *mukēs*, mushroom; *toxikon*, poison). A toxin from fungus.

myctĕ·ric (G. *muktēr*, nose). Relating to the cavities of the nose.

mydrī·asis (G. *mudriasis*). Extreme dilatation of the pupil of the eye.

mydriăt·ic. Relating to or causing midriasis.

mȳĕc·tomy (G. *mus*, muscle; *ektomē*, excision). Surgical removal of a portion of any muscle.

mȳ·el (G. *muelos*, marrow). The spinal cord.

mȳ·elencephalī·tis (G. *muelos*, marrow; *egkephalos*, brain). Inflammation conjointly of the brain and spinal cord.

mȳ·elencĕ·phalon (G. *muelos*, marrow; *egkephalos*, brain). The caudal part of the after-brain.

mȳ·elin (G. *muelos*, marrow). The substance of Schwann; the white sheath enveloping medullated nerve fibres.

mȳ·elinā·tion (G. *muelos*, marrow). Formation of a myelin sheath.

mȳelin·ic (G. *muelos*, marrow). 1. Relating to myelin or to m. nerve fibres. 2. Medullated.

mȳĕliniză·tion (G. *muelos*, marrow). The process of obtaining a myelin sheath.

mȳĕli·tis (G. *muelos*, marrow). Inflammation of the spinal cord. **M., acute ascending:** a febrile disease of rapid progress, characterized by progressively ascending paralysis and anaesthesia, affecting also the sphincter muscles, and by trophic changes. **M., disseminated:** encephalomyelitis. **M., transverse:** an acute or chronic disease caused by a lesion extending wholly across the spinal cord, characterized by paralysis and anaesthesia up to a certain level, paralysis of the sphincters, flaccidity and later spasticity of deep reflexes.

mȳ·elo-architecton·ics (G. *muelos*, marrow; *arkhitektōn*, architect). The structure and arrangement of myelinated fibres in the brain.

mȳ·eloblast (G. *muelos*, marrow; *blastos*, germ). The stem cell of the myeloid series of the leucocytes; normally present in small numbers in blood-forming organs, in larger numbers and also in the peripheral blood in myeloid leukaemia; characterized by a large size (15–25μ), a round or oval nucleus with fine chromatin structure containing nucleoli and a clear basophil cytoplasm.

mȳ·eloblastāe·mia (G. *muelos*, marrow; *blastos*, germ; *haima*, blood). A condition characterized by the presence of myeloblasts in the blood.

mȳ·eloblastic. Characterized by the presence of myeloblasts.

mȳ·elocele (G. *muelos*, marrow; *kēlē*, hernia). Protrusion of a portion of the spinal cord through a vertebral cleft.

mȳ·elocoele (G. *muelos*, marrow; *koilia*, cavity). The central canal of the spinal cord.

mȳ·elocys·tocele (G. *muelos*, marrow; *kustis*, bladder; *kēlē*, hernia). A myelocele associated with a cyst-like enlargement of the central spinal canal.

mȳ·elocys·tomenin·gocele (G. *muelos*, marrow; *kustis*, bladder; *mēnigx*, membrane; *kēlē*, hernia). Myelocystocele associated with a meningocele.

mȳ·elocyte (G. *muelos*, marrow; *kutos*, cell). The cell arising from the myeloblast, normally present in blood-forming organs; present in the peripheral blood sometimes in severe infections, in large numbers only in myeloid leukaemia; in size somewhat smaller than the myeloblast, with a round or oval nucleus of coarser chromatin structure and with a faintly basophil cytoplasm containing either neutrophil, eosinophil or basophil granules.

mȳ·elocyt·ic (G. *muelos*, marrow; *kutos*, cell). Characterized by the presence of myelocytes.

mȳ·elocytō·sis (G. *muelos*, marrow; *kutos*, cell). Presence of myelocytes in peripheral blood.

mȳ·elodysplā·sia (G. *muelos*, marrow; *dus-*, ill-; *plassein*, to form). A congenital, often familial, malformation of the spinal cord, usually of its lower portion, failure in closure of the sacral part of the medullary canal and abnormalities of the central grey substance, characterized clinically by sensory, trophic and motor disturbances in the lower extremities and by sphincter weakness; sometimes associated with syndactyly.

mȳ·elo-encephal·ic (G. *muelos*, marrow; *egkephalos*, brain). Relating to both the spinal cord and the brain.

mȳ·elo-encephalī·tis (G. *muelos*, marrow; *egkephalos*, brain). Inflammation of spinal cord and brain.

mȳ·elogen·ic, mȳelŏ·genous (G. *muelos*, marrow; *gennan*, to produce). Produced by myeloid (3) cells of the blood-forming tissues.

mȳelŏ·graphy (G. *muelos*, marrow; *graphein*, to write). Radiological examination of the spinal cord after introduction of an X-ray opaque substance, or of air, in the subarachnoidal space by lumbar puncture or cisternal puncture.

mȳ·eloid (G. *muelos*, marrow; *eidos*, form). 1. Resembling marrow. 2. Derived from bone-marrow cells. 3. Relating to those leucocytes which derive from the myeloblast. **M. leukaemia:** see leukaemia, m.

mȳeloi·din (G. *muelos*, marrow; *eidos*, form). A nitrogenous material, containing phosphorus, found in brain-matter.

mȳelŏ·ma (G. *muelos*, marrow). A tumour arising from bone marrow cells. **M., multiple** or **myelomatosis, multiple:** a chronic progressive disease characterized by the development of tumours from bone-marrow cells, mostly from plasma cells, but probably also from myelocytes, especially in vertebral, costal and cranial bones, often effecting compression of spinal cord or peripheral nerves, and further characterized by the presence of Bence-Jones protein in the urine, by an amyloidosis and an increase in the globulin portion of the plasma-protein. Syn. Kahler's disease.

mȳ·elomalā·cia (G. *muelos*, marrow; *malakia*, softness). Morbid softening of the spinal cord.

mȳ·elomeningi·tis (G. *muelos*, marrow; *mēnigx*, membrane). Spinal meningitis.

mȳ·elomenin·gocele (G. *muelos*, marrow; *mēnigx*, membrane; *kēlē*, hernia). Protrusion of a portion of the spinal cord with its meningeal membranes, through a vertebral cleft. Syn. myelocele.

mȳ·elomere (G. *muelos*, marrow; *meros*, part). An embryonic segment of the spinal cord; the unconstricted portion of the spinal cord.

mȳ·elon (G. *muelos*, marrow). The spinal cord.

mȳelon·ic. Relating to the spinal cord.

mȳ·elopară·lysis (G. *muelos*, marrow; *paralusis*, paralysis). Paralysis of the spine.

mȳ·elopath·ic (G. *muelos*, marrow; *pathos*, disease). Relating to myelopathy. **M. muscular atrophy:** a disease characterized by progressive muscular atrophy due to degeneration of cells of the anterior horns of the spinal cord or of the motor nuclei of cranial nerves.

mȳelŏ·pathy (G. *muelos*, marrow; *pathos*, disease). Any disease of the spinal cord.

mȳelŏph·thisic (G. *muelos*, marrow; *phthinein*, to waste). Caused by exhaustion of bone-marrow function.

mȳ·eloplasm (G. *muelos*, marrow; *plassein*, to form). A protoplasmic network as the basis of the neural wall at an early stage of embryonic development.

mȳ·eloplē·gia (G. *muelos*, marrow; *plēgē*, stroke). Paralysis of the spine.

mȳ·elopoiĕ·sis (G. *muelos*, marrow; *poiein*, to form). The formation of bone marrow.

mȳ·elorrhā·gia (G. *muelos*, marrow; *rhēgnunai*, to burst forth). Haemorrhage into the spinal cord.

mȳelor·rhaphy (G. *muelos*, marrow; *rhaphē*, suture). Repair by suturing of a severed spinal cord.

mȳ·elosc_lerŏ·sis (G. *muelos*, marrow; *sklēros*, hard). 1. Sclerosis of the spinal cord. 2. Osteosclerosis.

mȳelŏ·sis (G. *muelos*, marrow). Myeloid leukaemia.

mȳ·elospon·gium (G. *muelos*, marrow; *spoggos*, sponge). The structure arising from myeloplasm during embryonic development of the neural canal.

mȳe·lotome (G. *muelos*, marrow; *tomē*, section). Instrument for cutting the spinal cord.

mȳelŏ·tomy (G. *muelos*, marrow; *tomē*, section). Operation of cutting the spinal cord.

mȳelotox·ic (G. *muelos*, marrow; *toxikon*, poison). Relating to toxic action on bone-marrow cells.

mȳentĕ·ric (G. *mus*, muscle; *enteron*, intestine). 1. Relating to the muscular layer of stomach and intestines. 2. Relating to a plexus of postganglionic parasympathetic neurons situated in the muscular layer of the intestines.

mȳī·asis (G. *muia*, fly). Any morbid condition caused by the presence of flies or their larvae within the body. **M. linearis:** see creeping disease.

mȳ·iodesop·sia (G. *muiōdēs*, like flies; *opsis*, vision). The subjective appearance of muscae volitantes.

mylohȳ·oid (G. *mulē*, mill; *huoeidēs*, shaped like the letter y). Relating to the region of the lower molar teeth and the hyoid bone.

mȳ·oblast (G. *mus*, muscle; *blastos*, germ). A cell which develops into a muscle-fibre.

myoblastō·ma (G. *mus*, muscle; *blastos*, germ). A tumour of muscle made up of cells which resemble the primitive myoblasts.

myocardī·tis (G. *mus*, muscle; *kardia*, heart). Inflammation of the myocardium.

myocar·dium (G. *mus*, muscle; *kardia*, heart). The muscular tissue of the heart.

mȳ·ocele (G. *mus*, muscle; *kēlē*, hernia). The protrusion of a muscle through a tear in its sheath.

myoclon·ic epilep·sy (G. *mus*, muscle; *klonos*, a turmoil; *epilepsis*, seizure). A chronic familial disease characterized by epileptic fits associated with myoclonus, and usually in later stages by progressive dementia.

myoclŏ·nus (G. *mus*, muscle; *klonos*, turmoil). Sudden clonic spasm, recurring in various muscles. See paramyoclonus multiplex.

mȳocom·ma (G. *mus*, muscle; *komma*, a piece). A remnant of the intervals between the muscle segments in the embryo.

myocris·mus (G. *mus*, muscle; *krizein*, to creak). Sound heard on auscultation over a contracting muscle.

mȳ·odegenerā·tion (G. *mus*, muscle; L. *degenerare*). Degeneration of muscular tissue.

mȳ·odesop·sia. Myiodesopsia, *q.v.*

mȳodȳ·nia (G. *mus*, muscle; *odunē*, pain). Muscular pain.

mȳ·ofibrō·ma (G. *mus*, muscle; L. *fibra*, fibre). A tumour composed of muscular and fibrous tissue.

mȳ·ogen·esis (G. *mus*, muscle; *genesis*, production). The growth of muscular tissue.

mȳ·odynamŏ·meter (G. *mus*, muscle; *dunamis*, power; *metron*, measure). Device for testing the power of muscles.

mȳ·ogenet·ic, myogen·ic (G. *mus*, muscle; *gennan*, to produce). Originating in muscular tissues.

myŏ·glia (G. *mus*, muscle; *glia*, glue). A fibrillar substance formed by muscle cells.

myoglŏ·bulin (G. *mus*, muscle; L. *globulus*, dim. of *globus*, globe). Myosin, *q.v.*

mȳ·ogram (G. *mus*, muscle; *gramma*, writing). The tracing made by the myograph.

mȳ·ograph (G. *mus*, muscle; *graphein*, to write). An instrument for recording muscular contractions.

myograph·ic. Relating to myography.

myŏ·graphy (G. *mus*, muscle; *graphein*, to write). 1. A description of the muscles. 2. Examination with the myograph.

mȳohaemoglŏ·bin (G. *mus*, muscle; *haima*, blood; L. *globus*, globe). The red pigment of muscle, a substance related to blood-haemoglobin.

mȳoidē·ma (G. *mus*, muscle; *oidein*, to swell). A phenomenon seen in wasting conditions on percussion of the flat muscles of the chest, consisting of a wave contraction moving along the muscle fibres in opposite directions from the point of percussion and immediately followed by a small muscular swelling at this point.

myokȳ·mia (G. *mus*, muscle; *kuma*, wave). Transient fibrillary or fascicular tremor of muscle.

myolem·ma (G. *mus*, muscle; *lemma*, husk). The sarcolemma.

mȳ·olipō·ma (G. *mus*, muscle; *lipos*, fat). A myoma containing fatty tissue.

myŏ·logy (G. *mus*, muscle; *logos*, treatise). The part of anatomy dealing with muscles.

myŏ·lysis (G. *mus*, muscle; *lusis*, dissolution). Destruction of muscle tissues.

myŏ·ma (G. *mus*, muscle). A tumour composed of muscular tissues. See also leiomyoma and rhabdomyoma.

mȳ·omalā·cia (G. *mus*, muscle; *malakia*, softness). Softening of the muscular tissue of the heart following coronary occlusion and due to ischaemia.

myŏ·matous (G. *mus*, muscle). Resembling a myoma.

myomec·tomy (G. *mus*, muscle; *ektomē*, excision). Excision of a myoma, especially from the uterine wall.

mȳ·omere (G. *mus*, muscle; *meros*, part). A muscular segment, composed of myoblasts, of the mesenchymal layer at an early stage.

mȳ·ometrī·tis (G. *mus*, muscle; *mētra*, womb). Inflammation of the muscular tissue of the uterus.

myomē·trium (G. *mus*, muscle; *mētra*, womb). The uterine muscular tissue.

mȳ·on (G. *muōn*, a cluster of muscles). A group of muscles regarded as a unit.

myoneu·ral (G. *mus*, muscle; *neuron*, nerve). Relating to both muscle and nerve. **M. junction:** the end-plates of nerve fibrils in muscular tissue. Syn. neuromyal junction.

myopä·thia, myŏ·pathy (G. *mus*, muscle; *pathos*, disease) 1. Any disease of the muscles. 2. A group of disorders, often familial, characterized by progressive muscular weakness with atrophy or pseudo-hypertrophy of the muscles, and absence of any anatomical changes in neural structure. Syn. muscular dystrophies.

myopath·ic (G. *mus*, muscle; *pathos*, disease). 1. Relating to any disease of the muscles. 2. Relating to any disease belonging to the group of muscular dystrophies, *q.v.*

mȳ·ope (G. *muein*, to shut; *ōps*, eye). A person with myopia.

mȳ·opericardī·tis (G. *mus*, muscle; *peri*, around; *kardia*, heart). Inflammation of both the myocardium and the pericardium.

myō·pia (G. *muein*, to shut; *ōps*, eye). Short-sightedness, an anomaly of optical refraction in which focal images from parallel rays are formed in front of the retina either owing to too great a length of the visual axis or to an increase in curvature or refractory power of the ocular media.

myō·pic. Affected with myopia.

mȳ·oplasm (G. *mus*, muscle; *plasma*, something formed). The contractile part of a muscle fibre. See also sarcoplasm.

myoplas·tic. Relating to myoplasty.

mȳ·oplasty (G. *mus*, muscle; *plassein*, to form). Plastic operation on muscle.

mȳ·oprō·tein (G. *mus*, muscle; *prōton*, first). A protein contained in muscle tissue.

myor·rhaphy (G. *mus*, muscle; *rhaphē*, suture). Suture of a muscle.

myorrhex·is (G. *mus*, muscle; *rhēxis*, rupture). Rupture of a muscle.

mȳ·osarcō·ma (G. *mus*, muscle; *sarx*, flesh). Sarcoma arising in a muscle.

mȳ·osclerō·sis (G. *mus*, muscle; *skleros*, hard). Abnormal hardening of a muscle.

mȳ·osēism (G. *mus*, muscle; *seismos*, a shaking). Jerky muscular contraction.

myosep·tum (G. *mus*, muscle; L. *septum*, fence). The intermuscular septum between the metameres of muscles of certain animals.

mȳ·osin (G. *mus*, muscle). A globulin derived from myosinogen, present in muscle plasma after coagulation.

myosi·nogen (G. *mus*, muscle; *gennan*, to produce). A pseudo-globulin, one of the two chief proteins of muscle; the antecedent of myosin.

myō·sis. Meiosis, *q.v.*

myosit·ic. Relating to myositis.

myosi·tis (G. *mus*, muscle). Inflammation of the muscles. M. ossificans: a condition characterized by formation of osseous tissue in striped muscles.

mȳ·ospasm (G. *mus*, muscle; *spasmos*, spasm). Muscular spasm, cramp.

myostěō·ma (G. *mus*, muscle; *osteon*, bone). The development of an osseous tumour in muscle tissue.

myotac·tic (G. *mus*, muscle; L. *tangere*, to touch). Relating to muscle sense.

mȳ·otenŏ·tomy (G. *mus*, muscle; *tenōn*, a tendon; *tomē*, section). Incision into muscles or tendons.

myot·ic. Meiotic, *q.v.*

mȳ·otome (G. *mus*, muscle; *tomē*, section). 1. The lateral and ventral portion of mesenchymal somites in the embryo, giving rise to segmental muscular structures. 2. An instrument used for myotomy.

myō·tomy (G. *mus*, muscle; *tomē*, section). Surgical division of a muscle.

myotŏ·nia, myotŏ·nus (G. *mus*, muscle; *tonos*, tone). 1. Tonic muscular spasm. 2. Muscular tone or tension. M. acquisita: tonic muscular spasm following injury or disease. Syn. Talma's disease. M. atrophica: see dystrophic m. M. congenita: a congenital developmental disease, transmitted by dominant inheritance, characterized by difficulty in relaxing voluntary muscles after contraction. This disease is closely related to, if not a partial syndrome of, dystrophia myotonica, *q.v.* Syn. Thomsen's disease.

myoton·ic pupillary reaction. A condition characterized by extremely sluggish reaction of one pupil, or more rarely both pupils, especially to light, not associated with a systemic disorder of the nervous system.

myozȳ·mase (G. *mus*, muscle; *zumē*, leaven). One of the enzyme systems involved in muscular contraction.

mȳrin·ga (L.L.). The tympanic membrane.

myringi·tis (L.L. *myringa*). Inflammation of the tympanic membrane.

myrin·godec·tomy (L.L. *myringa*, the tympanic membrane; G. *ektomē*, excision). Excision of the membrana tympani, or of a part of it.

myrin·gomycō·sis (L.L. *myringa*, the tympanic membrane; G. *mukēs*, mushroom). Fungus infection of the tympanic membrane, especially by Aspergillus.

myrin·goplasty (L.L. *myringa*, the tympanic membrane; G. *plassein*, to form). A plastic operation on the tympanic membrane.

myrin·goscope (L.L. *myringa*, the tympanic membrane; G. *skopein*, to view). An instrument for examining the interior of the ear.

myrin·gotome (L.L. *myringa*, the tympanic membrane; G. *tomē*, section). An instrument for incising the tympanic membrane.

myringŏ·tomy (L.L. *myringa*, the tympanic membrane; G. *tomē*, section). Incision of the tympanic membrane.

mȳ·rinx (L.L.). The tympanic membrane.

myrrh. The oleo-gum-resin from the stem of *Commiphora molmol* (Engl.).

myr·tiform (L. *myrtus*, myrtle; *forma*, shape). Shaped like a myrtle leaf.

mysophō·bia (G. *musos*, filth; *phobos*, fear). Neurotic fear of soiling or contamination.

mȳ·tilotox·in (G. *mutilos*, mussel; *toxikon*, poison). A leucomaine, *q.v.*, a toxic metabolic product of mussels, formerly believed to be the cause of mussel-poisoning. See also ptomaines.

myxă·deni·tis labiā·lis (G. *muxa*, slime; *adēn*, gland; L. *labium*, lip). A disease characterized by painless papules on the mucous membrane of the lips. Syn. Baelz's disease.

Myx·obacteriā·lēs (G. *muxa*, slime; *baktērion*, a stick). An order of the class of Schizomycetes; not pathogenic.

myx·ochondrō·ma (G. *muxa*, slime; *khondros*, cartilage). A tumour composed of cartilagenous and myxomatous tissue.

myxoedē·ma (G. *muxa*, slime; *oidein*, to swell). A chronic disease characterized by peculiar, not pitting, subcutaneous generalized oedema with dryness of skin and by slowness of mental and bodily functions, including especially a lowering of the metabolic rate, due to insufficiency of thyroid function. M., congenital: m. present at birth and especially characterized by failure in development of mental functions, marked retardation in osseous development resulting in stunted growth, macroglossia, and coarse physiognomic features. See also cretinism.

myx·ofibrō·ma (G. *muxa*, slime; L. *fibra*, fibre). A tumour composed of fibrous and myxomatous tissue.

myx·oid (G. *muxa*, slime; *eidos*, form). Resembling mucus.

myx·olipō·ma (G. *muxa*, slime; *lipos*, fat). A tumour composed of lipomatous and myxomatous tissue.

myxō·ma (G. *muxa*, slime). 1. Connective tissue tumour containing an abundance of spaces filled with mucoid material. 2. Any connective tissue tumour of which the tissue has largely undergone mucoid or myxomatous degeneration.

myxomatō·sis (G. *muxa*, slime). 1. Development of multiple myxomas. 2. Myxomatous degeneration.

myxŏ·matous (G. *muxa*, slime). Relating to myxoma.

Myx·omycē·tēs (G. *muxa*, slime; *mukēs*, mushroom). A class of non-pathogenic moulds.

myxorrhoē·a (G. *muxa*, slime; *rhoia*, a flow). A severe mucous discharge.

myxosarcō·ma (G. *muxa*, slime; *sarx*, flesh). A sarcoma containing myxomatous tissue.

N

N. Symbol for Nitrogen.

Na. Symbol for Sodium.

$Na_2B_4O_7 10H_2O$. Borax.

Nabothian cysts or **ovules** (Naboth, M., German anatomist, 1675–1721). Small cysts formed by the N. follicles. **N. follicles:** the mucous follicles of the cervix uteri in the region of the external os. **N. menorrhagia:** (hydrorrhoea gravidarum), a mucous discharge from the pregnant uterus which accumulates as the result of excessive secretion of the uterine glands.

NaBr. Sodium bromide.

NaCl. Sodium chloride.

NaClO. Sodium hypochlorite.

$NaClO_3$. Sodium chlorate.

Na_2CO_3. Sodium carbonate.

nae·vocarcino·ma (L. *naevus*, mole; G. *karkinos*, ulcer). Carcinoma developing from a mole.

nae·void (L. *naevus*, mole; G. *eidos*, form). Resembling a naevus.

nae·vous (L. *naevus*, mole). Spotted with moles.

nae·vus (L.). A mole. **N. cavernosus:** venous angioma of the skin. **N. pigmentosus:** a pigmented spot on the skin. **N. vascularis:** angioma of the skin, usually congenital. **N. vinosus:** 'port wine' mark or strawberry mark on the skin.

naga·na (African). An infectious tropical disease of horses and cattle, caused by *Trypanosoma brucei*, transmitted by mosquitoes of the genus Glossina.

Nagel's test (Nagel, W., German physiologist, 1870–1911). A test for colour vision performed by means of cards with the colours printed in concentric circles.

$NaHCO_3$. Sodium bicarbonate.

nail. Horny dorsal plate on the distal phalanx of a finger or toe. **N.-bed:** the part of the cutis in which the n. rests. **N. fold:** the portion of the epidermis covering the proximal and lateral margins of a n. **N., ingrowing:** the growth of a lateral portion of a n. into soft tissues. **N. matrix:** the proximal portion of the n.-bed. **N., spoon:** see koilonychia.

nā·nism (G. *nanos*, dwarf). Nanosomia, *q.v.*

nanocĕ·phalous (G. *nanos*, dwarf; *kephalē*, head). Having a dwarfed head.

nanocĕ·phaly (G. *nanos*, dwarf; *kephalē*, head). Abnormal congenital smallness of the head.

nanocor·mia (G. *nanos*, dwarf; *kormos*, trunk). Dwarfism of the body or trunk.

nā·noid (G. *nanos*, dwarf; *eidos*, form). Resembling a dwarf.

nanomĕ·lia (G. *nanos*, dwarf; *melos*, limb). Abnormal congenital smallness of a limb.

nanophthal·mus (G. *nanos*, dwarf; *ophthalmos*, eye). Microphthalmia without any other ocular deformity.

nanosō·mia (G. *nanos*, dwarf; *sōma*, body). Dwarfism. Syn. nanism. **N., pituitary:** dwarfism characterized by normal proportions between head, trunk and limbs, due to hypofunction of the growth-hormone-secreting (eosinophil) cells of the anterior pituitary. Syn. ateleiosis.

nā·nous. Dwarfish; stunted.

nā·nus (G. *nanos*, dwarf). A dwarf.

NaOH. Sodium hydroxide.

nape. Back or scruff of the neck; the nucha.

nā·pex. Portion of the scalp lying below the occipital protuberance.

naph·tha. Inflammable oils obtained by the distillation of coal tar. **N., wood:** methyl alcohol.

naph·thol. $C_{10}H_8O$. Exists as α and β isomers; antiseptic substances obtained from coal tar.

naph·tholism. Naphthol poisoning.

Napier's aldehyde test (Napier, L. E., English physician, born 1888). A drop of 40 per cent formaldehyde is added to 1 c.c. of blood serum. If the serum becomes white and opalescent, kala-azar is present.

napkin erythē·ma. E. of the napkin area in infants, caused by the irritation of soiled napkins. Syn. Jacquet's erythema.

Narath's operation (Narath, A., Austrian surgeon, 1864–1924). Fixation of omentum to the abdominal wall to establish collateral circulation in cases of portal obstruction.

nar·ceine (G. *narkē*, numbness). An opium alkaloid, soluble in water but almost insoluble in alcohol. A sedative of doubtful value.

nar·cism, narcis·sism (G. *Narkissos*, character in Greek mythology, who fell in love with his own image reflected in water). 1. Self-love. 2. In psychoanalysis, the normal stage in infantile psychosexual development in which the love-object of the child is its own person, and more especially the neurotic persistence of this stage in the adult.

narco·analysis (G. *narkē*, numbness; *analuein*, to dissolve). Psycho-analysis while patient is under the influence of narcotics.

nar·colepsy (G. *narkē*, numbness; *lēpsis*, a seizing). A condition characterized by short, irresistible paroxysms of sleep, occurring repeatedly during the day, and by sudden attacks of loss of postural tone following any emotional stimulus.

narcolep·tic (G. *narkē*, numbness; *lēpsis*, a seizing). Related to or characterized by narcolepsy.

narcō·sis (G. *narkē*, numbness). General anaesthesia.

narcot·ic (G. *narkōtikos*, benumbing). Producing or relating to general anaesthesia.

nar·cotism. Narcosis, *q.v.*

nar·cotize (G. *narkōtikos*, benumbing). Anaesthetize.

nā·rēs (L.). Nostrils.

nā·sal (L. *nasus*, nose). Relating to the nose.

nā·scent (L. *nasci*, to be born). 1. Just born; in process of coming into existence. 2. Just liberated from a chemical combination.

nā·siform (L. *nasus*, nose; *forma*, shape). Resembling a nose in shape.

nā·sion (L. *nasus*, nose). The middle point of the frontonasal suture.

Nasmyth's membrane or cuticle (Nasmyth, A., Scottish dentist, died 1847). The delicate cuticle covering the free surface of young teeth.

nasoci·liary (L. *nasus*, nose; *cilium*, eyelid). Relating to the nose and the ciliary body.

nasolā·bial (L. *nasus*, nose; *labia*, lips). Relating to both nose and lips.

nasolā·crimal (L. *nasus*, nose; *lacrima*, a tear). Relating to both nose and lacrimal apparatus.

naso-occĭ·pital (L. *nasus*, nose; *ob*, at; *caput*, head). Relating to both nose and occiput.

nasopă·latine (L. *nasus*, nose; *palatum*, palate). Pertaining to both nose and palate.

nā·sopharyn·geal (L. *nasus*, nose; G. *pharugx*, throat). Pertaining to both nose and pharynx or to the nasopharynx.

nā·sopharyngi·tis (L. *nasus*, nose; G. *pharugx*, throat). Inflammation of the nasopharynx.

nasophă·rynx (L. *nasus*, nose; G. *pharugx*, throat). The part of the pharynx above the soft palate.

na·soscope (L. *nasus*, nose; G. *skopein*, to view). An instrument used for examining the nasal cavity.

nā·sus (L.). The nose.

nā·tal¹ (L. *natalis*, from *nasci*, to be born). Pertaining to birth.

nā·tal² (L. *nates*, buttocks). Pertaining to the buttocks.

nată·lity (L. *natalis*, from *nasci*, to be born). The birth-rate.

nā·tēs (L.). The buttocks.

nā·tive (L. *nativus*, from *nasci*, to be born). 1. Inborn. 2. A pure substance occurring in nature.

nā·trium (L.). Sodium.

nă·tural (L. *natura*). Not artificial; produced by nature.

naupă·thia (G. *naus*, ship; *pathos*, disease). Sea-sickness.

nau·sĕa (G. *nausia*, sea-sickness). Sensation of sickness; feeling of imminent vomiting.

nau·sĕănt (G. *nausia*, sea-sickness). Inducing nausea.

nau·sĕous (G. *nausia*, sea-sickness). Producing nausea.

nā·vel. The umbilicus.

navi·cular (L. *navicula*, dim. of *navis*, ship). Boat-shaped.

near-point. The nearest point of clear vision on maximal accommodation.

near-sighted. Myopic, *q.v.*

nēarthrō·sis (G. *neos*, new; *arthron*, joint). The formation or presence of a joint at an abnormal place, e.g. between fragments of a fractured bone.

nebenkern (Ger., near nucleus). 1. The chondriosome-body cf the spermatid. Syn. paranucleus. 2. A structure appearing during functional activity in the basal cells of the pancreatic acinus.

nĕ·bula (L., mist). 1. Opacity; cloudiness. 2. Slight corneal opacity.

nĕ·bulae (L., mists). Sprays. These are solutions of medicaments in aqueous, alcoholic, glycerinated or oily media, for application to the nose or throat by means of an atomiser.

nĕ·bulizer (L. *nebula*, mist). An instrument for spraying.

Necā·tor (L. *necator*, murderer). A genus of nematodes. N. americanus: a hookworm of the genus Necator.

neck. 1. The part between the head and the thorax. 2. A constricted part near the extremity of an organ.

nec·robiŏ·sis (G. *nekros*, corpse; *bios*, life). Degeneration of tissue, followed by gradually progressing necrosis. N. lipoidica diabetica: a chronic affection of the skin, often but not invariably associated with diabetes mellitus, characterized by violet and yellow coloured plaques, particularly on the lower limbs, showing, microscopically, n., deposition of lipoid substances and haemosiderin, and vascular changes.

necrŏ·phagous (G. *nekros*, corpse; *phagein*, to eat). Living on dead bodies.

necrŏ·phily (G. *nekros*, corpse; *philein*, to love). A form of sexual perversion in which the love-object is a dead body.

necrophō·bia (G. *nekros*, corpse; *phobos*, fear). Neurotic fear of dead bodies or of death.

nĕ·cropsy (G. *nekros*, corpse; *opsis*, vision). Autopsy.

necrŏ·sis (G. *nekrōsis*, deadness). Death of a circumscribed portion of tissue. N., coagulative: n. associated with coagulation of intra- and extracellular protein and with formation of fibrin. N., colliquative: n. associated with softening and liquefaction of the dead tissue, owing to the action of autolytic enzymes. N., liquefactive: colliquative n.

N., fat: formation of opaque yellowish-white necrotic areas, scattered through otherwise normal fatty tissue, in the pancreas or subperitoneal fat, due to action of liberated lipolytic enzyme.

necrosper·mia (G. *nekros*, corpse; *sperma*, seed). Spermal ejaculate containing only dead spermatozoa.

necrot·ic (G. *nekros*, corpse). Relating to necrosis.

necrŏ·tomy (G. *nekros*, corpse; *tomē*, section). 1. Autopsy. 2. Excision of a sequestrum.

needle. A sharp instrument for sewing or puncturing.

needling. Puncture, especially of a cataract, with a needle.

Neef's hammer (Neef, C. E., German physician, 1782–1849). A device used for the rapid making and breaking of a galvanic circuit.

Neftel's disease (Neftel, W. B., American neurologist, 1830–1906). Atremia; hysterical inability to sit or walk without discomfort and paraesthesia of the head and back. When the patient is recumbent all movements are possible.

nĕ·gative (L. *negare*, to deny). 1. Absence of a re-action. 2. Charged with electrons. N. ion: an anion.

nĕ·gativism (L. *negare*, to deny). Impulsive resistance to suggestions coming from others, resulting in not doing what has been asked, or doing the opposite.

Negri bodies (Negri, L., Italian physician, 1876–1912). Oval or round inclusion bodies seen in the protoplasm and sometimes in the processes of nerve cells of animals dead of hydrophobia, their presence is considered conclusive proof of rabies.

Neisser-Wechsberg's phenomenon (Neisser, M., German bacteriologist, 1869-1938; Wechsberg, F., German physician). See complement, deviation of.

Neissĕ·ria (Neisser, A. L. S., German dermatologist, 1855–1916). A genus of diplococci, including the gonococcus and the meningococcus.

Nélaton's catheter (Nélaton, A., French surgeon, 1807–73). A soft-rubber catheter. N.'s dislocation: fracture dislocation of the ankle, the astragalus being forced between the tibia and fibula. N.'s fold: a transverse mucosal fold at the junction of the middle and lower thirds of the rectum. N.'s haematocele: haematoma of the Fallopian tube. N.'s line: a line drawn from the anterior superior iliac spine to the tuberosity of the ischium.

nĕ·lavan. African sleeping-sickness.

Nematelmin·thēs (G. *nēma*, thread; *helmins*, worm). Nematoda, *q.v.*

nĕ·matocide (G. *nēma*, thread; *eidos*, form; L. *caedere*, to kill). An agent destructive to nematode worms.

Nematō·da (G. *nēma*, thread; *eidos*, form). A class of worms, containing the families Ascaridae, Oxyuridae, Ankylostomidae, Filariidae, Trichinellidae, etc.

nĕ·matode (G. *nēma*, thread; *eidos*, form). 1. Like a thread. 2. Any worm belonging to the Nematoda.

nematō·sis (G. *nēma*, thread; *eidos*, form). Infestation with nematode worms.

Nembutal. A proprietary pentobarbitol sodium preparation.

neoarsphenă·mine. An arsenic compound used in the treatment of syphilis and protozoal infections.

neo-arthrō·sis. Nearthrosis, *q.v.*

neoblas·tic (G. *neos*, new; *blastos*, germ). Relating to new tissue.

Nē·ocaine. A proprietary preparation of procaine hydrochloride. A powerful local anaesthetic, but transient in its effect unless adrenaline is also given.

nĕ·ocyte (G. *neos*, new; *kutos*, cell). An immature leucocyte.

nĕ·o-encĕ·phalon (G. *neos*, new; *egkephalos*, brain). The new brain—referring to cerebral cortex.

neolă·lia (G. *neos*, new; *lalia*, speech). Speech characterized by the frequent use of neologisms.

nĕŏ·logism (G. *neos*, new; *logos*, discourse). A newly constructed word.

neonā·tal (G. *neos*, new; L. *natalis*, from *nasci*, to be born). Relating to the newborn.

neonā·tus (G. *neos*, new; L. *natus*, born). The newborn.

neopal·lium (G. *neos*, new; L. *pallium*, cloak). The cerebral cortex exclusive of the olfactory portion, the latter being of less recent phylogenetic origin.

neoplā·sia (G. *neos*, new; *plassein*, to form). The formation of a neoplasm.

nĕ·oplasm (G, *neos*, new; *plassein*, to form). A circumscribed autonomous new formation of tissue, reproducing to some extent the tissue from which it arises and serving no useful function.

neoplas·tic (G. *neos*, new; *plassein*, to form). Relating to neoplasm.

nĕ·oplasty (G, *neos*, new; *plassein*, to form). Plastic restoration of lost tissue.

Neosalvarsan. A proprietary preparation of neoarsphenamine.

neostig·mine. A synthetic substitute for physostigmine for the treatment of myasthenia gravis. Syn. Prostigmine.

neostrīā·tum (G. *neos*, new; L. *stria*, a furrow). The phylogenetically more recent portion of the corpus striatum, the caudate nucleus and the putamen; present in animals from the reptiles onwards.

neothă·lamus (G. *neos*, new; *thalamos*, inner chamber). The phylogenetically younger portion of the thalamus, present only in mammals.

nephelŏ·meter (G. *nephele*, cloud; *metron*, measure). An instrument for measuring the amount of particles in a suspension by comparing the degree of light reflected by the particles with that reflected by a standard suspension.

nephelŏ·metry (G. *nephele*, cloud; *metron*, measure). The method of quantitative analysis by means of a nephelometer.

nephral·gia (G. *nephros*, kidney; *algos*, pain). Any kidney pain.

nephrectā·sia (G. *nephros*, kidney; *ektasis*, extension). Dilatation of a kidney.

nephrec·tomy (G. *nephros*, kidney; *ektome*, excision). Excision of a kidney.

neph·ric (G. *nephros*, kidney). Relating to the kidney.

nephri·dium (G. *nephridion*, dim. of *nephros*, kidney). The embryonic tube from which the kidney is developed.

nephrĭt·ic (G. *nephritikos*, affected with kidney disease). Relating to nephritis.

nephri·tis (G. *nephros*, kidney). Inflammation of the parenchymatous part of the kidney. See also nephrosis, nephrosclerosis and neuroretinopathy. **N., acute interstitial:** a condition complicating septic states, especially secondary streptococcal invasions in acute infectious disease of childhood, usually producing no manifestations in life; characterized by exudation in the interstitial tissue, accompanied by, but not dependent on, epithelial degeneration. **N., embolic focal:** n. affecting only small localized portions of the glomerular apparatus, leading to haematuria but not to other general or renal manifestations, due to the arrest of bacterial emboli in the glomeruli, occurring especially in the course of subacute bacterial endocarditis. **N., glomerulo-, acute:** acute inflammation of the kidney, limited to but affecting all the glomeruli and leading to oliguria, albuminuria, haematuria, cylindruria, rise in blood-pressure and renal oedema; in its aetiology often related to an infection with haemolytic streptococci of some other part of the body. Syn. acute n.; acute parenchymatous (or diffuse) n.; acute Bright's disease. **N., glomerulo-, chronic:** a condition either following an acute glomerulo-n., or of more insidious origin, due to progressive fibrotic contraction of both kidneys characterized by progressive renal insufficiency with variable degrees of oedema, albuminuria, haematuria, cylindruria, but invariably with rise of blood-pressure and eventually by azotaemia and uraemia and/or cardiac failure. Syn. chronic n.; chronic parenchymatous n.; chronic Bright's disease. See also neuroretinopathy.

neph·rocapsulec·tomy (G. *nephros*, kidney; L. *capsula*, small box; G. *ektome*, excision). Excision of the renal capsule.

neph·rocapsulŏ·tomy (G. *nephros*, kidney; L. *capsula*, small box; *tome*, a cutting). Incision of the renal capsule.

nephrocar·diac (G. *nephros*, kidney; *kardia*, heart). Relating conjointly to kidney and heart.

neph·rocele (G. *nephros*, kidney; *kele*, hernia). Hernia-like protrusion cf a kidney.

nephrogen·ic (G. *nephros*, kidney; *gennan*, to produce). Arising from or in a kidney; forming kidney tissue.

neph·rolith (G. *nephros*, kidney; *lithos*, stone). Stone in the kidney.

neph·rolithī·asis (G. *nephros*, kidney; *lithos*, stone). The condition caused by the presence of one or more calculi in the kidney or in the renal pelvis.

nephrolithŏ·tomy (G. *nephros*, kidney; *lithos*, stone; *tome*, section). An operation for the removal of a renal calculus; the kidney is incised.

nephrŏ·logist (G. *nephros*, kidney; *logos*, treatise). A specialist in kidney diseases.

nephrŏ·ma (G. *nephros*, kidney). Any kidney tumour.

nephromalā·cia (G. *nephros*, kidney; *malakia*, softness). Softening of the kidney.

nephromegā·lia, nephromĕ·galy (G. *nephros*, kidney; *megas*, large). Enlargement of the kidney, e.g. in glycogen disease.

neph·ron (G. *nephros*, kidney). The functional unit of the kidney, consisting of a glomerulus with the secreting segment of its appertaining tubule; an adult human kidney contains about one million such units.

neph·ropară·lysis (G. *nephros*, kidney; *paralusis*). Paralysis of the kidney.

nephrŏ·pathy (G. *nephros*, kidney; *pathos*, disease). Any disease of the kidney.

neph·ropexy (G. *nephros*, kidney; *pexis*, fixation). Surgical fixation of a displaced kidney.

nephroph·thisis (G. *nephros*, kidney; *phthisis*, decay). Renal tuberculosis.

nephroptō·sis (G. *nephros*, kidney; *ptosis*, a falling). Downward displacement of the kidney.

nephror·rhaphy (G. *nephros*, kidney; *rhaphe*, suture). Suturing of a kidney.

neph·ros (G.). The kidney.

neph·rosclerŏ·sis (G. *nephros*, kidney; *skleros*, hard). A vascular disease associated either with renal arteriosclerosis or with arteriolosclerosis, but always with high blood-pressure, producing variable degrees of renal contraction; in the first case starting in more advanced age and of more protracted course, in the second affecting especially middle-aged individuals and progressing rapidly to renal insufficiency with azotaemia, uraemia and/or cardiac failure. The former group is also called Arteriosclerotic kidney; ischaemic nephritis; the latter, malignant hypertension; chronic interstitial nephritis; red granular kidney. See also neuroretinopathy.

nephrŏ·sis (G. *nephros*, kidney). A chronic disease characterized by degenerative lesions of the tubular apparatus of both kidneys, by gross oedema and albuminuria, by hypoproteinaemia and hypercholesterolaemia, not progressing to renal insufficiency, uraemia and cardiac failure unless associated with glomerulo-nephritic changes of the kidney. See also lipoid nephrosis.

nephrostō·ma, neph·rostome (G. *nephros*, kidney; *stoma*, mouth). The coelomic orifice of a pronephric tubule.

nephrŏ·stomy (G. *nephros*, kidney; *stoma*, mouth). Surgical formation of a fistula from the renal pelvis.

nephrot·ic (G. *nephros*, kidney). Relating to nephrosis.

neph·rotome (G. *nephros*, kidney; *tomos*, a slice). A segment of the mesodermal intermediate cell structure which itself gives rise to the pronephros.

nephrŏ·tomy (G. *nephros*, kidney; *tomē*, section). A surgical incision into the kidney. **N., abdominal:** n. performed after a laparotomy. **N., lumbar:** n. performed through an incision in the loin.

neph·rotuberculō·sis (G. *nephros*, kidney; L. *tuberculum*, dim. of *tuber*, a swelling). Tuberculous disease of the kidney.

nephrotȳ·phoid (G. *nephros*, kidney; *tuphos*, stupor; *eidos*, form). A form of typhoid fever in which nephritic signs are dominant; they are nearly always due to a concomitant focal nephritis.

neph·ro-ur·ēterec·tomy (G. *nephros*, kidney; *ourētēr*, urinal duct; *ektomē*, excision). Excision of a kidney and the whole or part of the ureter.

Nernst's theory (Nernst, W. H., German physicist, born 1864). That electrical stimulus to tissues acts by causing dissociation of ions, thus charging the concentration of salts at cell membrane.

nerve (L. *nervus*). A collection of bundles of nerve fibres which conveys either motor or sensory impulses from one part of the body to another. **N.-block:** suspension of the passage of impulses through a nerve, caused, e.g., by the local application of a paralysing drug. **N.-cell:** 1. A neuron. 2. The cell-body of a neuron without its processes. **N.-conduction:** the transmission of an excitatory wave along nerve fibres. **N. deafness:** deafness due to an affection of the acoustic n. or of its nucleus. **N. end-plate:** the terminal structure of motor nerve fibrils in muscle tissue. **N. fibre:** the axis cylinder of a neuron, the fibre projecting from the n.-cell (2). **N., mixed:** a n. composed of both motor and sensory fibres. **N. plexus:** a network of peripheral n. fibres. **N. root:** the first portion of a spinal n. at its emergence from the spinal cord. The nerves are: **Abducent:** sixth cranial nerve, arises from the floor of the fourth ventricle of the brain and emerges from the sulcus between the pons and medulla and passes through the cavernous sinus to the orbit. It supplies the lateral rectus muscle. **Accessory:** the eleventh cranial nerve arises from two roots. The cranial root from the lateral tract of the medulla below the vagus, the cervical root from the side of the cord as low down as the fifth cervical root. The cranial root passes out of the jugular foramen close to the vagus, and sends one or two branches to the superior ganglion. It does not blend with the inferior ganglion but joins the vagus below. The principal part joins the pharyngeal and superior laryngeal branches, but offsets are sent to the cardiac and recurrent laryngeal branches. The cervical root enters the skull through the foramen magnum and passes to the jugular foramen; it is enclosed in the same sheath of dura mater as the vagus. Issuing from the foramen, it passes downwards between the internal carotid artery and internal jugular vein, and then backwards superficial to the internal jugular vein to upper part of sternomastoid, which it pierces, at the same time communicating with the branch to the muscle from the second cervical nerve. Crossing the occipital part of the posterior triangle, it enters the under surface of the trapezius, where it joins with branches of the third and fourth cervical nerves to form a plexus in the substance of the muscle. The nerve supplies the sternomastoid and trapezius muscles. **Accessory obturator:** an inconstant nerve. When present it arises from the third and fourth lumbar nerves from the trunk of the obturator nerve. It passes down on medial side of psoas muscle, under pectineus muscle and supplies the pectineus muscle and hip-joint. **Accessory phrenic:** inconstant. Occasionally the fibres from the anterior ramus of the fifth cervical nerve run separately and join the phrenic nerve in the upper part of the thorax. **Anterior crural:** see femoral. **Anterior cutaneous, of the neck** (superficial cervical nerve) ; arises by two roots from the anterior primary rami of the second and third cervical nerves, and turning round the posterior border of the sternomastoid muscle, it passes to the anterior triangle of the neck; it divides into two branches, ascending and descending, which are distributed to the integument over the anterior triangle. **Anterior ethmoidal:** a branch of the nasal branch of the first division of the trigeminal nerve. The nerve passes through the anterior ethmoidal foramen and divides into two branches, septal and lateral. The septal is distributed to the mucous membrane over the anterior and superior part of the septum, and the lateral branch to that over the anterior portions of the middle and inferior conchae. **Anterior interosseous:** a branch of the median nerve of the arm, it is given off just below the elbow joint. It passes down lateral to the anterior interosseous artery on the membrane, between the flexor profundus and flexor pollicis longus, to end in the deep surface of the pronator quadratus. It supplies flexor longus pollicis, pronator quadratus and lateral half of flexor digitorum profundus. **Anterior tibial:** a branch of the lateral popliteal nerve of the leg. It is given off in the substance of the peroneus longus muscle and passes to the front of the interosseous membrane by piercing extensor digitorum longus to reach the lateral side of the anterior tibial artery, with which it descends to the ankle-joint, where it divides into a medial and lateral branch. It supplies a branch to the knee joint and muscular branches to tibialis anterior, extensor digitorum longus, peroneus tertius, extensor hallucis longus and extensor digitorum brevis. The internal terminal branch supplies the skin on the adjacent sides of the first and second toes. **Arnold's** (auricular branch of the vagus): is a branch of the superior ganglion of vagus nerve. Having traversed the mastoid canaliculus in the petrous part of the temporal bone, which it reaches through a minute opening in the lateral wall of the jugular fossa, it emerges through the tympanomastoid fissure between the mastoid process and tympanic plate and then divides into two branches. One branch takes part in the supply of the cranial surface of the auricle, and also supplies the postero-inferior part of the external auditory meatus. The other branch joins the posterior auricular nerve. **Auditory:** eighth cranial nerve. It has two parts, the cochlear part concerned with hearing and the vestibular with balance. They appear together immediately behind and lateral to the facial nerve between the lower border of the pons and the restiform body. The nerve passes into the internal auditory meatus and divides into two branches which enter the foramina at the bottom of the meatus. The posterior or vestibular branch supplies the utricle, saccule and ampullae of the semicircular canals. The inferior or cochlear branch is distributed to the cochlea. **Auricular, great:** a cutaneous nerve arising from the second and third cervical nerves in the neck, it winds round the posterior margin of the sternomastoid muscle to reach the parotid gland. It supplies the skin over the parotid, and the back part of the pinna and mastoid process. **Auricular, posterior:** a branch of the facial nerve, it passes up behind and between mastoid process and meatus, dividing into auricular to supply auricularis posterior, and occipital to posterior belly of occipito-frontalis. **Auricular, of vagus:** see Arnold's nerve. **Auriculotemporal:** is a branch of the mandibular division of the trigeminal nerve. It arises by two roots, between which the middle meningeal nerve passes, runs backwards under lateral pterygoid muscle, round mandibular capsule, then upwards, with superficial temporal artery, beneath parotid gland to temporal fossa, it supplies the skin of tragus, pinna, meatus and the membrana tympani. **Buccal:** a branch of the mandibular division of the trigeminal nerve, it comes out between heads of lateral pterygoid to reach buccinator, and is frequently joined to the anterior temporal and lateral pterygoid nerves; it communicates with the facial, and is distributed to mucous membrane and skin of cheek. **Cardiac, great** (middle): is a branch of the middle cervical ganglion of the sympathetic. On the right side it passes in front of or behind the subclavian artery to the front of the trachea, and joins the deep cardiac plexus. Communicates in the neck with the superior cardiac and recurrent laryngeal nerves. On the left sides it lies between the left carotid and left subclavian arteries, and joins the deep cardiac plexus. **Cardiac, inferior:** a small branch of the inferior cervical ganglion of the sympathetic, it passes behind the subclavian artery, joins the recurrent laryngeal and enters the deep cardiac plexus. **Cardiac, superior:** the right superior cardiac nerve comes off by two roots from the superior cervical ganglion. It passes down behind the carotid sheath and ends in the deep cardiac plexus. The left superior cardiac nerve passes along the left common carotid artery and, crossing the arch of the aorta, joins the superficial cardiac plexus. **Caroticotympanic:** a small nerve which arises from the carotid plexus and passes backwards in a small canal in the processus cochleariformis, to join the tympanic plexus. **Cervical:** a branch of the facial nerve which perforates the cervical fascia beneath the mandible, to supply the platysma, and joins the anterior cutaneous nerve of the neck. **Chorda tympani:** a branch of the facial nerve, which is given off just before the facial nerve passes out of the stylomastoid foramen. It ascends to the tympanum through posterior canaliculus and courses between the membrana tympani and the base of the pyramid; it emerges at the medial end of the squamotympanic fissure to join the lingual nerve. It forms the sensory root of the submandibular ganglion, and supplies the mucous membrane of the anterior two-thirds of the tongue with taste fibres. **Circumflex:** a branch of the posterior cord of the brachial plexus from the fifth and sixth cervical. It passes backwards with posterior circumflex vessels at the lower border of the subscapularis through the quadrilateral space and supplies the deltoid and teres minor muscles. It also supplies the shoulder joint and the skin over the lower part of the deltoid muscle. **Coccygeal:** last nerve to be given off from the spinal cord. It divides into an anterior branch, which pierces the sacrotuberous ligament and coccygeus, supplies skin over coccyx, and communicates with the fifth sacral, forming part of the anococcygeal plexus; and a posterior branch which supplies the coccygeal skin. **Cochlear:** a branch of the auditory nerve, it is given off in the internal auditory meatus and its branches perforate a number of foramina at the bottom of a spiral groove and are supplied to the various parts of the cochlea. **Common peroneal:** (Lateral popliteal) a terminal branch of the great sciatic nerve. It passes along the popliteal space under cover of and medial to biceps tendon, then over lateral head of gastrocnemius to the fibula; one inch below the head of that bone it pierces the peroneus longus, and in that muscle divides into anterior tibial and musculocutaneous nerves. **Cranial:** the cranial nerves are arranged in twelve pairs, and as they leave the cranial cavity they receive sheath from the meninges of the brain. 1. Olfactory nerve of smell. 2. Optic nerve of sight. 3. Oculomotor to muscles of eyeball. 4. Trochlear to muscle of eyeball. 5. Trigeminal sensory to face, motor to muscles of mastication. 6. Abducent to muscle of eyeball. 7. Facial supplies muscles of facial expression. 8. Auditory nerve of hearing and balance. 9. Glossopharyngeal sensory nerve to back of tongue and pharynx. 10. Vagus sensory to larynx, oesophagus and stomach. 11. Accessory motor nerve to sternomastoid and trapezius muscles. 12. Hypoglossal. Motor nerve to muscles of the tongue. **Cutaneous, of thigh** (lateral): a branch of the lumbar plexus coming from the second and third lumbar; perforates middle of lateral border of psoas muscle, and enters the thigh just below anterior superior iliac spine, where it divides into: Anterior branch which supplies lateral part of anterior surface of thigh; Posterior branch which supplies the lateral surface of thigh to the middle. **Deep petrosal:** a branch of the nerve of the pterygoid canal, it joins the sympathetic on the carotid artery. **Deep temporal:** three branches anterior, middle and posterior from the mandibular nerve all of which supply the temporal muscle. **Dental, inferior:** is a branch of the mandibular nerve which passes through the mandibular foramen on the inner surface of the lower jaw. It supplies the molar and bicuspid teeth and emerges at the mental foramen. **Dental, posterior superior:** is a branch of the maxillary nerve which comes off just before the nerve enters the infra-orbital canal. It supplies the gums, the molar teeth and the mucous membrane of the maxillary antrum. Middle and anterior superior dental arise from the maxillary nerve as it is in the infra-orbital canal. The middle supplies the bicuspid teeth and the anterior supplies the incisor and canine teeth. **Digastric:** a branch of the facial nerve given off at exit from stylomastoid foramen, it divides in the parotid gland forming the parotid plexus. **Digital:** Median: five small nerves supplying lateral three and a half fingers. First or second supply the thumb, third to radial side of index finger also supplies first lumbrical; fourth supplies second lumbrical and adjacent sides of index and middle fingers; fifth supplies adjacent sides of ring and middle fingers. Plantar: four in number. First supplies medial border of first toe and the flexor hallucis brevis, the second supplies the adjacent sides of the first and second toes and the first lumbrical, the third supplies the adjacent sides of the second and third toes, and the fourth supplies the adjacent sides of the third and fourth toes. Radial: four dorsal digital nerves. First to medial side of thumb, second to lateral side of index, third to adjacent sides of index and middle, fourth to adjacent sides of middle and ring fingers. Ulnar: two in number, which supply the skin of the medial one and a half fingers. **Dorsal, of penis:** a sensory branch of the pudendal nerve which supplies the penis. **Dorsalis pedis:** the medial terminal branch of the anterior tibial nerve. It supplies the skin of the adjacent sides of the first and second toes. **Dorsolumbar:** a small communicating branch of the subcostal nerve which joins the first lumbar nerve. **External laryngeal:** a branch of the superior laryngeal branch of the vagus. The nerve communicates with the pharyngeal plexus and upper cardiac of sympathetic, supplies the cricothyroid and inferior constrictor muscle. **External petrosal:** a communicating nerve which runs from the ganglion on the facial nerve to

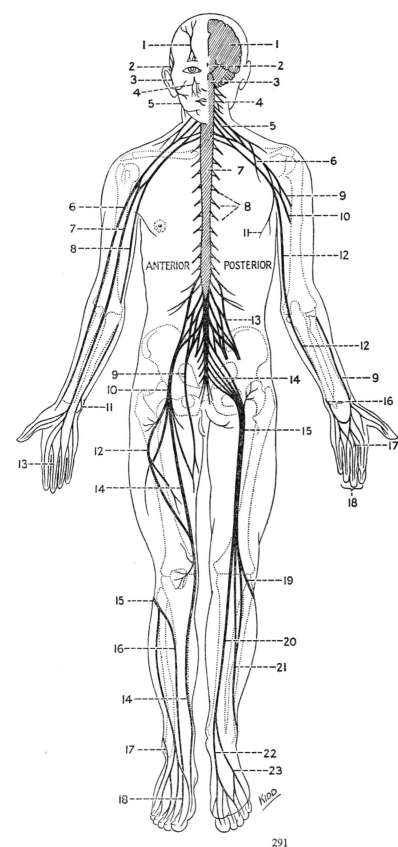

NERVES

ANTERIOR

1. SUPRA-ORBITAL
2. TEMPORAL BRANCH OF FACIAL
3. UPPER TERMINAL BRANCH OF FACIAL
4. INFRA-ORBITAL
5. LOWER TERMINAL OF FACIAL
6. RADIAL
7. MEDIAN
8. ULNAR
9. OBTURATOR
10. FEMORAL
11. DORSAL CUTANEOUS BRANCH OF ULNAR
12. MEDIAL CUTANEOUS
13. BRANCHES OF MEDIAN AND ULNAR
14. SAPHENOUS
15. LATERAL POPLITEAL
16. ANTERIOR TIBIAL
17. SURAL
18. MID TERMINAL BRANCH OF ANTERIOR TIBIAL

POSTERIOR

1. CEREBRUM
2. PONS
3. MEDULLA OBLONGATA
4. CERVICAL PLEXUS
5. BRACHIAL PLEXUS
6. SUPRASCAPULAR
7. SPINAL CORD (canal— medulla)
8. INTERCOSTALS
9. RADIAL
10. MEDIAN
11. N. SUPPLYING LATISSIMUS DORSI
12. ULNAR
13. LUMBAR PLEXUS
14. SACRAL PLEXUS
15. SCIATIC
16. DORSAL CUTANEOUS BRANCH OF ULNAR
17. DORSAL CUTANEOUS (Branches of)
18. BRANCHES DERIVED FROM MEDIAN AND ULNAR
19. LATERAL POPLITEAL
20. POSTERIOR TIBIAL
21. SURAL
22. MEDIAL PLANTAR
23. LATERAL PLANTAR

the plexus on the middle meningeal artery. **Facial:** the seventh cranial nerve. It arises from the floor of the fourth ventricle and emerges from the side of the pons and enters the internal auditory meatus, traverses the tympanum and emerges from the temporal bone at the stylomastoid foramen, it passes forwards into the parotid gland and supplies the muscles of facial expression. **Femoral:** arises from the second, third and fourth lumbar nerves and passes down beneath the inguinal ligament to the thigh. It supplies the knee and hip joints, the pectineus, sartorius and quadriceps muscles and gives cutaneous branches to the inner and middle surfaces of the thigh. Its saphenous branch supplies the inner side of the leg. **Frontal:** the largest branch of the ophthalmic nerve, it enters orbit just lateral to the trochlear nerve, passes forwards on levator palpebrae and divides into supratrochlear and supra-orbital nerves. **Genicular:** are two or three in number all arising from the medial popliteal nerve. They accompany the genicular arteries and supply the knee joint. **Genicular obturator:** a small branch from the posterior division of the oburator nerve which supplies the knee joint. **Genitocrural:** see genitofemoral nerve. **Genitofemoral** (genitocrural nerve): is made up of fibres from the first and second lumbar nerves, it passes on the psoas muscle to the inguinal ligament and divides into genital branch which supplies the cremaster muscle and a femoral branch which supplies the skin of upper part and front of thigh. **Glossopharyngeal:** the ninth cranial nerve. Arises from floor of fourth ventricle of brain and issues from the upper part of the medulla and leaves the skull through the jugular foramen and is distributed to the pharynx and tongue. It is the nerve of sensation to the mucous membrane of pharynx, oropharyngeal isthmus and tonsil; of motion to stylopharyngeus muscle; and of taste to the posterior one-third of the tongue. **Greater occipital:** comes from the posterior primary ramus of the second cervical nerve. It passes through the semispinalis capitis and trapezius, and ascends with the occipital artery to the back of the scalp which it supplies. **Greater palatine:** a descending branch of the maxillary nerve, it passes through the greater palatine canal to hard palate, there dividing into branches which run forward in grooves in the bone nearly to the incisor teeth. Joining the long sphenopalatine nerve it supplies the gums and mucous membrane of the hard palate. **Greater splanchnic:** arises from the thoracic part of the sympathetic trunk. It is formed by the union of branches from the sixth, seventh, eighth, ninth and tenth ganglia. It passes medially over the bodies of the vertebrae, perforates the crus of the diaphragm, and ends in the coeliac ganglion. **Greater superficial petrosal:** a branch of the maxillary nerve which comes off in the foramen lacerum and passes along the petrous bone to the canal for the facial nerve, it joins the ganglion on the facial nerve. **Hypoglossal:** the twelfth cranial nerve. Arises from the hypoglossal triangle in floor of fourth ventricle of the brain. The nerve passes in two bundles through the anterior condylar foramen to the lower border of the digastric muscle and ends in the muscles of the tongue. **Iliohypogastric:** arises from the first lumbar nerve and appears at upper part of lateral border of psoas, crosses quadratus lumborum to iliac crest, and, piercing the transversus abdominis, divides into lateral branch which supplies the skin of the buttock, and an anterior branch which supplies the skin of hypogastric region. **Ilioinguinal:** arises from the first lumbar nerve; passes over quadratus lumborum and iliacus to iliac crest, pierces the transversus abdominis and internal oblique; it then accompanies the spermatic cord through the canal

and superficial ring, and is distributed to the skin of the groin and the scrotum. **Incisive:** is the termination of the inferior dental nerve and supplies the pulps of the lower canine and incisor teeth. **Inferior dental:** see dental nerve. **Inferior gluteal:** arises from the fifth lumbar, first and second sacral nerves; passes out of pelvis below the piriformis at the lower border of which it runs backwards, and dividing into numerous branches it supplies the deep aspect of gluteus maximus. **Inferior haemorrhoidal:** may have an independent origin from the sacral plexus or be a branch of the perineal or of the main trunk of the pudendal nerve. It passes across the ischiorectal fossa to the anus and is distributed to the deep and subcutaneous portions of the external sphincter and to the skin between the anus and ischial tuberosity. **Inferior nasal:** are branches of the greater palatine branch of the sphenopalatine ganglion and are distributed to the mucous membrane over the greater part of the inferior concha and middle and inferior meatus. **Infra-orbital:** is the terminal part of the maxillary division of the trigeminal nerve. It leaves the infra-orbital canal through the infra-orbital foramen, where it is deep to the levator labii superioris. It divides into three sets of branches—palpebral, nasal and labial. The palpebral branches ascend to supply the skin and conjunctiva of the lower lid. The nasal branches supply the skin of the side of the nose and the labial the upper lip. **Infratrochlear:** is a branch of the nasociliary nerve. It is given off as the nerve enters the anterior ethmoidal foramen; it passes to medial angle of orbit, and supplies lacrimal sac, skin of eyelids and root of nose. **Intercostal:** are the anterior primary rami of the thoracic nerves, these are twelve on each side; each communicates with the corresponding ganglion of the sympathetic trunk. The upper six pass forwards in the intercostal spaces, supply the intercostal muscles and skin of the thoracic wall. The lower six supply the musculature and skin of the abdominal wall. **Intercostobrachial:** is the lateral cutaneous branch of the second thoracic nerve; it joins the medial cutaneous nerve of arm and supplies the skin of the medial side of the arm. **Internal carotid:** is a branch of the superior cervical ganglion of the sympathetic trunk and it enters the carotid canal in the petrous part of the temporal bone in company with the internal carotid artery and divides into two parts: Lateral division, which forms the carotid plexus; Medial division, which forms the cavernous plexus. **Internal laryngeal:** a branch of the superior laryngeal branch of the vagus nerve. It passes through the thyrohyoid membrane and is distributed to the mucous membrane of the larynx above the vocal cords. **Jacobson's nerve** (tympanic nerve): arises from the inferior ganglion of the glossopharyngeal nerve. It enters a minute canal in the bone between the jugular foramen and carotid canal to reach the medial wall of the tympanum; runs in a groove over the promontory, giving off several branches, and, after communicating with the facial, is continued forwards as the lesser superficial petrosal nerve. This nerve pierces the petrous portion of the temporal to reach the middle fossa, and passing through the sphenopetrosal suture ends in the otic ganglion. **Lacrimal:** a branch of the ophthalmic nerve, it passes along the lateral wall of orbit to under surface of lacrimal gland, pierces orbital fascia, and supplies skin of upper eyelid. **Laryngeal** (superior): is principally a sensory nerve, it arises from the inferior ganglion of the vagus and contains fibres of the cranial root of the accessory nerve. It passes deep to the internal carotid artery and divides into two branches, internal and external. The internal laryngeal is sensory to the larynx and the external supplies the cricothyroid muscle. **Lateral cutaneous** (external cutaneous): of forearm is a branch of the radial nerve. It pierces the deep fascia on the radial side of the biceps and descends posterior to the median cephalic vein, giving one or two twigs to the skin in the neighbourhood and then divides into two branches. One supplies the skin on the radial side of the front of the forearm and the other gives branches to the skin on the posterior surface of the forearm. **Lateral cutaneous, of thigh:** is formed from a loop between the second and third lumbar nerves. It perforates the middle of lateral border of psoas, and enters thigh just below anterior superior iliac spine; it divides into two branches which supply the lateral part of the thigh. **Lateral pectoral:** arises from the fifth, sixth and seventh cervical nerves, from the lateral cord of the brachial plexus; crosses over axillary artery and pierces the clavipectoral fascia to reach the under-surface of pectoralis major muscle which it supplies. **Lateral plantar:** a terminal branch of the posterior tibial nerve. It passes across the foot to the lateral side supplying abductor digiti minimi and flexor accessorius; it divides into two branches: Superficial: which divides into two plantar digital nerves, one supplying the lateral side of the little toe, the flexor digiti minimi brevis, and the two interossei of the fourth space, the other supplies the adjacent sides of the fourth and fifth toes; Deep: supplies adductor hallucis, three lateral lumbricals and interossei of three medial spaces. **Lateral popliteal** (common peroneal nerve): one of the terminal branches of the great sciatic nerve. It passes along the popliteal space under cover of and medial to biceps tendon, then over lateral head of gastrocnemius to the fibula; one inch below head of fibula it pierces the peroneus longus and in that muscle divides into anterior tibial and musculocutaneous nerves. It supplies the knee joint and the skin over the back and lateral side of the leg. **Least splanchnic** (lowest): arises from the twelfth thoracic ganglion of the sympathetic trunk. It enters the abdomen under the medial arcuate ligament to join the aorticorenal ganglion. **Lesser occipital:** is a branch of the second cervical nerve, it ascends along posterior border of sternomastoid to scalp, lying between ear and occipital artery. Supplies skin of scalp and cranial surface of auricle. **Lesser palatine:** small nerves which descend from the sphenopalatine ganglion. They are distributed to the mucous membrane of the soft palate and tonsil. **Lesser splanchnic:** arises by two roots from the ninth and tenth thoracic ganglia of the sympathetic trunk. It enters the abdomen by piercing the corresponding crus of the diaphragm lateral to the greater splanchnic and gives branches to the coeliac and superior mesenteric ganglia. **Lesser superficial petrosal:** see Jacobson's nerve. **Lingual:** a branch of the mandibular nerve and lies at first medial to the lateral pterygoid muscle; it then passes downwards in front of the inferior dental nerve, and is joined at an acute angle by the chorda tympani from the facial. It then passes down to the tip of the tongue. It is distributed to the anterior two-thirds of the mucous membrane of the dorsum of the tongue. **Long ciliary:** usually two in number, arise from the nasociliary immediately it has crossed the optic nerve, and they communicate with the short ciliary nerves from the ciliary ganglion, which they accompany to the posterior part of the sclera. Here they pierce the sclera and are distributed along with the short ciliary nerves. **Long pudendal** (of Soemmering): is a branch of the posterior cutaneous nerve of the thigh. It supplies the skin of the scrotum. **Long sphenopalatine** (nasopalatine nerve): is a medial branch of the sphenopalatine ganglion. It enters the nasal cavity

along with the short sphenopalatine nerves. It crosses the roof of the cavity, and then passes anteroinferiorly upon the septum, lying in the groove on the lateral surface of the vomer. Having arrived at the incisor crest, the left nerve descends through the anterior incisive canal and the right through the posterior. The nerves then form a plexus giving filaments to the mucous membrane of the hard palate. **Lowest splanchnic:** see least splanchnic nerve. **Mandibular:** is the largest of the three divisions of the trigeminal nerve. The large sensory root comes from the inferior angle of the Gasserian ganglion and is joined on its deep aspect by the small motor root which lies under the sensory root. The united nerve leaves the skull by the foramen ovale, and immediately breaks up into anterior and posterior divisions. **Masseteric:** a branch of the mandibular nerve which passes laterally with nerve to internal pterygoid above the lateral pterygoid, then over mandibular notch, to deep surface of masseter and gives twigs to mandibular joint. **Maxillary:** the second division of the trigeminal nerve. It is a sensory nerve. It passes from the middle of the trigeminal ganglion through foramen rotundum, then across pterygopalatine fossa to enter the infraorbital canal, and here receives the name of infraorbital. **Medial calcanean:** a branch of the posterior tibial nerve which is given off at the ankle and pierces flexor retinaculum, to supply skin of heel and medial side of sole of foot. **Medial cutaneous, of arm** (lesser internal cutaneous of Wrisberg): arises from the first thoracic from the medial cord of the brachial plexus. It descends along the inner side of the brachial vessels to the middle of the arm and is distributed to the skin of the ulnar side of the arm. **Medial cutaneous, of forearm** (internal cutaneous): arises from the eighth cervical and first thoracic nerves from the medial cord of the brachial plexus. It lies in front of the third part of the axillary artery and becomes cutaneous about the middle of the arm. It supplies the medial side of the forearm as low as the wrist, and the back of medial side of forearm to about the middle. **Medial pectoral:** arises from the eighth cervical and first thoracic from medial cord of the brachial plexus; it passes between the axillary artery and vein to supply the two pectoral muscles. **Medial plantar:** the larger terminal branch of the posterior tibial nerve. It passes between the abductor hallucis and flexor digitorum brevis to divide opposite the bases of the metatarsal bones into four branches. It is cutaneous to the sole of the foot, muscular to abductor hallucis and flexor digitorum brevis and four digital arteries. **Medial popliteal** (tibial nerve): is the larger terminal branch of the sciatic nerve. It passes along the middle of the popliteal space to the lower border of the popliteus, where it gets the name of posterior tibial nerve. It gives branches to the knee joint, gastrocnemius and plantaris muscles. **Median:** from the fifth, sixth, seventh, eighth cervical and first thoracic nerves. It arises by two roots, one from the lateral cord, the other from the medial cord of the brachial plexus. At first the nerve lies lateral to the axillary artery, but about the middle of the arm it crosses the brachial artery to reach its medial side. It enters the forearm between the two heads of the pronator teres; it passes down the forearm; beneath the flexor retinaculum it becomes flattened and divides into two parts to supply the lateral three and a half fingers. **Meningeal:** a small branch from the superior ganglion of the vagus nerve which passes backwards to the dura mater of the posterior fossa of the skull. **Mental:** one of the terminal branches of the inferior dental nerve. It passes out of the mental foramen in the mandible and divides into branches which supply the skin of the chin and lower lip. **Musculocutaneous** (of arm): from the fifth and sixth cervical, from the lateral cord of the brachial plexus; perforates coracobrachialis, passing to lateral side of arm between biceps and brachialis, supplying the three named muscles; filaments also given to elbow joint; becomes cutaneous as lateral cutaneous nerve of forearm just below elbow. **Musculospiral** (radial): from the fifth, sixth, seventh and eighth cervical nerves from the posterior cord of the brachial plexus; winds round between lateral and medial heads of triceps in the spiral groove to the lateral side of arm. Piercing the lateral intermuscular septum, it passes to the front of the lateral epicondyle between the brachioradialis and brachialis, where it gives off the posterior interosseous branch. It gives branches to the three heads of the triceps, to the anconeus, brachioradialis, extensor carpi radialis longus and brachialis muscles. **Mylohyoid**: a branch of the inferior dental nerve, it descends in a groove on the medial side of the ramus of the jaw to lower surface of mylohyoid muscle, supplying it, and giving a branch to the anterior belly of the digastric muscle. **Nasal**: a small branch of maxillary nerve given off on the face and supplying the skin of the side of the nose. **Nasociliary**: a branch of the ophthalmic nerve, it enters the orbit between the two heads of the lateral rectus muscle, passes forwards and medially over optic nerve along the medial side of the orbit, through the anterior ethmoidal foramen; re-entering cranium, it passes down nasal slit by the side of the crista galli, and supplies mucous membrane of septum and skin of ala and tip of nose. **Nasopalatine**: see long sphenopalatine nerve. **Obturator**: arises from the second, third and fourth lumbar nerves; passes from medial border of psoas, near brim of pelvis to canal in upper part of obturator foramen. Divides into two branches: Anterior, which descends in front of adductor brevis, behind pectineus and adductor longus; it supplies the hip joint, gracilis, adductor longus and adductor brevis; and Posterior, which passes through obturator externus and behind adductor brevis, supplies adductor magnus, obturator externus and adductor brevis and knee joint. **Obturator internus**: a branch from the sacral plexus from the fifth lumbar and first and second sacral nerves; it emerges from the pelvis through the greater sciatic foramen, winds over the ischial spine and supplies the medial surface of the muscle. **Oculomotor**: third cranial nerve. Arises from the front of the pons and pierces dura mater near posterior clinoid process and enters orbit through superior orbital fissure. It divides into two branches. Superior branch supplies superior rectus and levator palpebrae superioris. Inferior branch supplies medial rectus, inferior rectus and inferior oblique. It also supplies ciliary muscle and sphincter fibres of the iris. **Oesophageal**: a branch of the vagus nerve given off in the thorax to form oesophageal plexus. **Of Bell** (long respiratory): the nerve to serratus anterior from the fifth, sixth and seventh cervical nerves of the brachial plexus, it descends on the lateral surface of the muscle through the axillary space and supplies the muscle at its lower border. **Of heart**: see cardiac nerves. **Of quadratus femoris**: from the lumbosacral trunk and first sacral nerve; passes anterior to obturator internus tendon to anterior surface of quadratus femoris, giving on its way a branch to gemellus inferior and an articular branch to the hip-joint. **Of Sapolini**: the nervus intermedius of Wrisberg or sensory root of the seventh cranial nerve. This name was employed by Guiseppe Sapolini in 1881, and the nervus intermedius is therefore sometimes spoken of as the thirteenth cranial nerve of Sapolini.

Of serratus anterior: see Of Bell. **Of tongue**: the sensory nerves are: 1. Lingual branch of the mandibular, it supplies the mucous membrane over the anterior two-thirds. 2. Chorda tympani to the taste buds of the anterior two-thirds. 3. Lingual branch of glossopharyngeal to posterior one-third. 4. Internal branch of superior laryngeal to the root of the tongue. 5. Lingual branch of facial to taste buds in the region of the pillars of the fauces. Motor nerve is hypoglossal which supplies the lingual muscles. **Of Wrisberg**: the lesser internal cutaneous of arm, arising in the brachial plexus. **Olfactory**: first cranial nerve. Nerve of smell. The olfactory tract passes forwards in the olfactory sulcus on the under surface of the frontal lobe of the brain, resting on cribriform plate and expanding into olfactory bulb. From the bulb about twenty nerve filaments pass downwards through foramina in the cribriform plate of the ethmoid and supply the mucous membrane of the olfactory area of the nose. **Ophthalmic**: is the smallest branch of the trigeminal nerve, it is entirely sensory. It courses along the lateral wall of the cavernous sinus and enters the orbit through the superior orbital fissure and divides into three branches, frontal, lacrimal and nasociliary. **Optic**: second cranial nerve. Nerve of sight. It arises from the optic tract which comes from two roots: Lateral, from the lateral geniculate body, thalamus and brachium of superior quadrigeminal body; Medial, from medial geniculate body. The nerve winds across lateral and anterior surfaces of cerebral peduncle, uniting with fellow to form optic chiasma; the nerves separate at forepart of chiasma and pass into orbit, each pierces the sclerotic and choroid coats of the eyeball and expands to form innermost layer of retina. **Orbital**: two or three in number from the sphenopalatine ganglion they enter the orbit through the inferior orbital fissure to be distributed to the periosteum. **Palatine**: see greater and lesser palatine nerves. **Palmar cutaneous**: a branch of the median nerve which is given off just proximal to the wrist and pierces the fascia just above the flexor retinaculum, and ends in the skin of the palm. **Palmar**: cutaneous of ulnar nerve arises about the middle of the forearm and descends for some distance anterior to the ulnar artery. At the wrist it pierces the deep fascia and supplies the skin of forearm and hand. **Pathetic** (trochlear): fourth cranial nerve. Arises from superior medullary velum of the brain and winds round the lateral surface of cerebral peduncle and passes forwards in the lateral wall of the cavernous sinus and enters orbit through superior orbital fissure, it is distributed to superior oblique muscle. **Pelvic splanchnic** (nervi erigentes): the parasympathetic fibres from the anterior primary divisions of the second, third and fourth sacral nerves. **Perineal**: a small branch of the posterior cutaneous nerve of thigh, it supplies the skin on the upper and medial side of the thigh and scrotum. **Perforating cutaneous**: arises from the back of the second and third sacral nerves; perforates sacrotuberous ligament, and winding round lower border of gluteus maximus, supplies skin over lower part of buttock. **Petrosal**: there are four petrosal nerves: greater superficial, lesser superficial, external and deep. **Pharyngeal**: three or four in number, are branches of the glossopharyngeal; cross the internal carotid artery, join branches of vagus and sympathetic to form pharyngeal plexus, supplying the mucous membrane of the pharynx. **Phrenic**: arises from the third, fourth and fifth cervical nerves; lies in front of scalenus anticus, descends medially on it in front of subclavian artery to enter chest. Descends in front of root of lung, pierces the diaphragm and is distributed on its abdominal surface. **Plantar:** two in number, medial and lateral, are the terminal branches into which the posterior tibial nerve divides on the posterior aspect of the medial malleolus of the tibia. **Posterior auricular:** a branch of the facial nerve, it passes up behind and between mastoid process and meatus, dividing into auricular to supply auricularis posterior, and occipital to posterior belly of occipito-frontalis muscle. **Posterior cutaneous of arm:** is a branch of the radial nerve which comes off near the axilla, and supplies the skin on the back of the arm to near the olecranon. **Posterior cutaneous of thigh:** small sciatic nerve comes off from the second and third sacral nerves and supplies the skin of the lower part of the buttock and back of thigh. **Posterior ethmoid:** a small branch of the nasociliary nerve which passes through the posterior ethmoidal canal to supply the mucous membrane of the ethmoidal and sphenoidal sinuses. **Posterior interosseous:** a branch of the radial nerve which reaches the back of the forearm by piercing the supinator muscle, it passes between the superficial and deep muscles of the forearm to about the middle of the forearm, where it passes deep to reach interosseous membrane, on which it lies as far as the wrist; there it ends in a gangliform enlargement. It supplies the muscles on the back of the forearm. **Posterior scapular** (rhomboid): arises from the posterior aspect of the fifth cervical nerve, it passes backwards through the scalenus, medius muscle to supply the rhomboid muscles. **Posterior thoracic:** see nerve Of Bell or Of serratus anterior. **Posterior tibial:** is the direct continuation of the medial popliteal and it begins at the lower border of the popliteus muscle, and runs with the posterior tibial vessels to the interval between the medial malleolus and heel where it divides into lateral and medial plantar. It supplies the soleus, tibialis posterior, flexor digitorum longus, and flexor hallucis longus muscles. **Presacral:** branches of the hypogastric plexus of nerves which divide on the fifth lumbar vertebra to form the right and left pelvic plexuses. The common surgical name 'the presacral nerve' is a misnomer since the structure is not a nerve nor is it presacral in position. **Pudendal:** comes off the second, third and fourth sacral nerves, passes out of the greater sciatic foramen, winds over ischial spine and re-enters pelvis through lesser foramen and passes along a canal in the obturator fascia on the lateral wall of the ischio-rectal fossa, it supplies branches to the skin of anus and scrotum or labium. **Pudic:** see pudendal nerve. **Pulmonary:** branches from the vagus in the thorax to the posterior part of the root of the lung. These join branches from the second, third and fourth thoracic ganglia of sympathetic, forming the posterior pulmonary plexus. **Radial:** see musculospiral nerve. **Ramus descendens hypoglossi:** a small branch of the hypoglossal nerve given off as the nerve hooks round the occipital artery, passes down carotid sheath, joining in a loop from the second and third cervical nerves to supply branches to sternohyoid, sternothyroid and both bellies of the omohyoid. **Recurrent laryngeal:** branch of the vagus. The *right* nerve arises in front of subclavian artery, winds back round it and passes up behind common carotid and inferior thyroid arteries to right side of trachea. The *left* nerve arises in front of the arch of aorta, round which it winds to the left of the ligamentum arteriosum and passes up by left side of trachea. Each nerve ascends in a groove between the trachea and oesophagus, and enters larynx by passing under lower border of inferior constrictor muscle. The nerve supplies all the muscles of the larynx except the cricothyroid. **Rhomboid:** see posterior scapular nerve. **Sacral:** the sacral

plexus is formed by the lumbo-sacral trunk (fourth and fifth lumbar) anterior primary rami of the first and part of the second and third sacral nerves. It lies on the anterior surface of the pyriformis, behind the inferior gluteal and pudendal arteries. **Saphenous:** a branch of the posterior branch of the femoral nerve, it accompanies the femoral vessels as far as subsartorial canal, becomes cutaneous on the inner side of the knee and is distributed to inner side of leg and medial side of foot as far as ball of great toe. **Sciatic:** the largest nerve in the body. It is derived from the lumbosacral trunk, the first, second and third sacral nerves. It passes out of the pelvis below the pyriformis, and about the middle of the back of the thigh the nerve bifurcates into medial and lateral popliteal. It supplies branches to biceps, semimembranous, semitendinosus and medial part of adductor magnus. **Scrotal:** two small nerves given off from the pudendal nerve, they supply the skin of the scrotum. **Short ciliary:** small branches from the ciliary ganglion of the ophthalmic nerve, they are distributed to the ciliary muscle, the iris, and the cornea. **Sixth cranial:** see abducent nerve. **Small sciatic:** see posterior cutaneous nerve of thigh. **Soemmering's nerve:** the perineal branch of the posterior cutaneous nerve of the thigh. **Sphenopalatine:** a medial branch of the sphenopalatine ganglion of the maxillary nerve. It passes inwards through the sphenopalatine foramen, crosses roof of nasal fossa to the septum and gives branches to the mucous membrane over the septum. **Spinal:** there are thirty-one pairs of spinal nerves: eight cervical, twelve thoracic, five lumbar, five sacral and one coccygeal. Each nerve arises from the spinal cord by an anterior (motor) and a posterior (sensory) root, the latter having a ganglion developed upon it. **Splanchnic:** see greater, lesser and least splanchnic nerves. **Stylohyoid:** a small muscular branch of the facial nerve given off at the exit from the stylomastoid foramen, it supplies stylohyoid muscle. **Subcostal:** is the anterior primary division of the twelfth thoracic nerve. It is in series with the eleventh intercostal nerve, but is not ranked as an intercostal nerve, since it lies along the lower border of the twelfth rib. It is commonly known as the last thoracic nerve. **Suboccipital:** is the posterior primary ramus of the first cervical nerve; it only occasionally supplies the skin of the lateral side of the greater occipital area. **Subscapular:** three in number, all arise from the posterior cord of the brachial plexus. Upper is a small nerve from the fifth and sixth cervical nerves and it supplies the subscapularis muscle. Middle (nerve to latissimus dorsi) arises chiefly from the seventh cervical, but also from the sixth and eighth. It descends with the subscapular artery to the latissimus dorsi which it supplies. Lower from the fifth and sixth cervical and supplies the teres major and subscapularis muscles. **Superficial cervical** (anterior cutaneous nerve of neck): arises from loop between second and third cervical nerves, passes forwards over the middle of the sternomastoid muscle, perforates the cervical fascia, and divides beneath platysma into: ascending branch which supplies the skin of the front of the upper part of neck; descending branch which supplies the skin as low as the sternum. **Superior dental:** three in number. Anterior from the infra-orbital nerve near the anterior end of the infra-orbital canal; supplies the mucous membrane of the maxillary antrum and the pulps of the upper canine and incisor teeth. Middle, an inconstant branch of the maxillary nerve; supplies pulps of the upper two molars and the gum. Posterior arises from the maxillary nerve as it passes through the inferior orbital fissure; supplies the pulps of the three upper molar teeth and mucous membrane of the maxillary antrum. **Superior gluteal:** a branch of the sacral plexus from the lumbosacral trunk and first sacral nerve, passes out of greater sciatic foramen, above the pyriformis and divides into two branches: superior branch supplies gluteus medius and inferior branch supplies gluteus minimus and tensor fasciae latae. **Superior laryngeal:** see laryngeal nerve. **Superior nasal:** small branches of the anterior superior dental nerve, they are distributed to the mucous membrane over the anterior part of the inferior meatus of the nose. **Supraclavicular:** branches of the cervical plexus, they arise from the third and fourth cervical nerves and supply the skin as far as the middle line, the skin over the pectoral muscle and to the skin of shoulder. **Supraorbital:** a branch of the frontal nerve, it passes through the supra-orbital notch to supply the scalp as far as the coronal suture of the skull. **Suprascapular:** is formed by the union of the fifth and sixth cervical nerves, passes beneath trapezius to upper border of scapula, enters supraspinous fossa through suprascapular notch, supplies the supraspinatus and infraspinatus and shoulder joint. **Supratrochlear :** a branch of the frontal nerve which is distributed to the forehead. **Sural:** a branch of the medial popliteal nerve, it passes down the leg superficially between the two heads of the gastrocnemius, pierces the deep fascia about the middle of the leg, there being joined by the sural communicating branch of the lateral popliteal; it then follows the course of the short saphenous vein round the lateral malleolus, and supplies the skin of lateral side of foot and little toe. **Sural communicating:** a branch of the lateral popliteal which joins with the sural branch of the medial popliteal. See sural nerve. **Sural cutaneous:** are small terminal branches of the femoral cutaneous nerve. They supply the skin of the proximal part of the posterior aspect of the leg. **Temporal deep:** three in number. Anterior, from the buccal nerve to supply front of temporal muscle. Middle, to deep aspect of temporal muscle. Posterior, often united with masseteric nerve, to back part of temporal muscle. **Third cranial:** see oculomotor nerve. **Third occipital:** a branch of the third cervical nerve which supplies the skin at the base of the occiput. **Thirteenth cranial:** see Of Sapolini. **Tibial:** see medial popliteal. **To popliteus:** a small slender nerve from the medial popliteal which supplies the popliteus muscle on its anterior surface. **To rhomboids:** a branch from the fifth cervical nerve. **To subclavius:** from the trunk formed by the fifth and sixth cervical nerves, it passes downwards in front of the third part of the subclavian artery to the deep surface of the subclavius muscle. **To thyrohyoid:** a branch of the hypoglossal nerve, it passes round the greater horn of hyoid bone to supply the thyrohyoid muscle. **Transverse cervical:** see superficial cervical nerve. **Trigeminal:** fifth cranial nerve. Arises from the side of the pons, by a small motor and a large sensory root, the latter having a ganglion on it. The two roots pass forwards through oval opening in dura mater near apex of petrous bone, the sensory root entering the trigeminal (Gasserian) ganglion. The motor root passes under ganglion and is not connected with it, but goes through foramen ovale, uniting with the mandibular division. The trigeminal ganglion gives off from its anterior edge the ophthalmic, maxillary and mandibular trunks. **Trochlear:** see pathetic or fourth cranial nerve. **Tympanic:** see Jacobson's nerve. **Ulnar:** arises from eighth cervical and first thoracic nerves from the posterior cord of the brachial plexus: passes down the medial side of the axillary and brachial arteries to middle of arm; it then runs

through the medial intermuscular septum to behind epicondyle. It then runs down ulnar side of forearm as far as pisiform bone, passes over flexor retinaculum and divides into superficial and deep branches. **Ulnar, collateral:** a branch of the radial nerve which runs down the arm to supply the lower part of the triceps muscle. **Vagus:** tenth cranial nerve. Arises from the sulcus between the inferior cerebellar peduncle and olive. It passes through the jugular foramen into carotid sheath and so to the thorax; forms a plexus on the wall of the oesophagus and stomach. Gives branches to larynx, pharynx, heart, lung, oesophagus and stomach. **Vestibular:** a branch of the auditory nerve, it supplies the utricle, saccule, and semicircular canals of the inner ear. **Zygomatic:** a branch of the maxillary nerve, it enters orbit by pterygomaxillary fissure and divides into zygomaticotemporal and zygomaticofacial nerves. **Zygomaticofacial:** a branch of the zygomatic nerve, it passes to lower and lateral angle of orbit, goes through the zygomatic foramen and supplies skin over the side of the face. **Zygomaticotemporal:** A branch of the zygomatic nerve, it passes along groove in lateral wall of orbit, and through a foramen in zygomatic zone and enters temporal fossa and supplies the skin in that region.

ner·vi (L., pl. of *nervus*, nerve). N. nervorum: nerve filaments in the epineurium, innervating the bloodvessels of n.

ner·vone. A cerebroside, $C_{48}H_{91}O_8N$, present in nerve tissue.

ner·vous (L. *nervosus*). 1. Relating to a nerve or nerves. 2. Relating to nervousness. **N. dyspepsia:** a gastric manifestation of nervous instability.

ner·vousness (L. *nervosus*, nervous). A state of restlessness and increased irritability.

ner·vus (L.). Nerve. (Pl. *nervi*).

nettlerash. Urticaria.

Nettleship's dots (Nettleship, E., English ophthalmologist, 1845–1913). Small white dots dispersed in rather large numbers between the macula and periphery of the retina. They are associated with pigment changes and night-blindness, and are often familial.

Neubauer's artery (Neubauer, J. E., German anatomist, 1742–77). The deep thyroid artery; an inconstant artery arising from the aorta and supplying the thyroid gland. **N.'s ganglion:** the large ganglion formed by the junction of the lower cervical and first thoracic ganglion.

Neumann's corpuscles (Neumann, E., German pathologist, 1834–1918). Nucleated erythrocytes, sometimes found in the blood when a regenerative process is going on. **N.'s crystals:** Charcot's crystals, *q.v.* **N.'s sheaths:** those forming the walls of the dentinal tubules.

Neumann's disease (Neumann, I., Austrian dermatologist, 1832–1906). Pemphigus vegetans.

neū·rad (G. *neuron*, nerve; L. *ad*, to). Towards a neural axis.

neurag·mia (G. *neuron*, nerve; *agmos*, fracture, from *agnunai*, to break). Avulsion of nerve fibre from ganglion.

neū·ral (G. *neuron*, nerve). Relating to a nerve or to the nervous system. **N. canal:** the structure formed by union of the two neural ridges. **N. fold:** n. ridge. **N. groove:** a longitudinal groove formed on the neural plate. **N. hiatus:** caudal openings between the neural folds. **N. plate:** a cellular layer in a gastrula from which the central nervous system is formed in later stages of embryonic development. **N. ridge:** one of the two margins of the n. groove. **N. sheath:** the myelin sheath of a nerve. **N. tube:** n. canal.

neural·gia (G. *neuron*, nerve; *algos*, pain). A condition characterized by intermittent pain in a nerve or nerves.

neural·gic (G. *neuron*, nerve; *algos*, pain). Relating to neuralgia.

neurasthē·nia (G. *neuron*, nerve; *a*, neg.; *sthenos*, strength). A vague term, becoming obsolete, applied to a condition characterized by lack of mental and bodily vigour.

neură·xis (G. *neuron* nerve; L. *axis*). 1. An axis-cylinder. 2. The cerebrospinal part of the nervous system.

neură·xon (G. *neuron*, nerve; *axōn*, axis). An axis-cylinder process of a nerve-cell.

neure (G. *neuron*, nerve). See neuron.

neurec·tasis (G. *neuron*, nerve; *ektasis*, extension). The surgical stretching of a nerve.

neurec·tomy (G. *neuron*, nerve; *ektomē*, excision). The excision of a portion of a nerve.

neurectō·pia (G. *neuron*, nerve; *ektopos*, out of place). Abnormal situation of a nerve.

neurentĕ·ric (G. *neuron*, nerve; *enteron*, intestine). Relating to the embryonic neural tube and the primitive digestive tube. N. canal: the canal connecting the n. tube with the primitive digestive tube.

neurilem·ma (G. *neuron*, nerve; *lemma*, husk). The thin membranous outer covering surrounding the myelin sheath of a nerve fibre or the axis-cylinder of a non-medullated nerve fibre.

neu·rilemmī·tis (G. *neuron*, nerve; *lemma*, husk). Inflammation of a neurilemma.

neu·rin, neu·rine (G. *neuron*, nerve). A toxic product from putrefaction, probably derived from choline.

neurinō·ma (G. *neuron*, nerve). A tumour arising from sheath-cells of nerves, especially at the spinal nerve roots or at the cerebello-pontine angle (acoustic n.).

neu·rit, neu·rite (G. *neuron*, nerve). An axis-cylinder process of a nerve-cell.

neurit·ic (G. *neuron*, nerve). Relating to neuritis.

neuri·tis (G. *neuron*, nerve). A lesion of a peripheral nerve, characterized by inflammation of its fibrous tissue, with or without degeneration of axis-cylinder and myelin sheath, by pain and loss of its normal function in variable degrees. N., multiple: n. affecting simultaneously several peripheral nerves, especially of the limbs, often symmetrically; usually producing flaccid paralysis with loss of deep reflexes and muscular atrophy, sensory disturbances and quantitative and qualitative changes in electric excitability. Its more common causes are alcohol, lead, arsenic, diabetes, beri-beri, the so-called idiopathic form is perhaps due to a virus infection. Syn. polyneuritis; peripheral n. N., multiple, diphtheritic: m.n. affecting especially the palate, pharynx, larynx and/or external ocular muscles, occurring in second or third week of convalescence from diphtheria. N., interstitial: n. limited to the interstitial fibrous tissue of a nerve. N., parenchymatous: n. involving degeneration of axis-cylinder and myelin-sheath. N., optic: see papilloedema. N., retrobulbar: inflammation or lesion of other origin (e.g. disseminated sclerosis) of the optic nerve proximal to the nerve head.

neuro-ană·tomy (G. *neuron*, nerve; *anatomē*, dissection). The anatomy of the nervous system.

neu·robiotax·is (G. *neuron*, nerve; *bios*, life; *taxis*, arrangement). A term for the physico-chemical phenomena influencing the growth and direction of neural elements.

neu·roblast (G. *neuron*, nerve; *blastos*, germ). 1. An embryonic cell which develops into a ganglion cell. 2. An embryonic cell which develops into a sympathetic neuron.

neu·roblastō·ma (G. *neuron*, nerve; *blastos*, germ). A malignant neoplasm in children, arising from neuroblasts in the adrenal medulla, leading to metastases in the skull (when primary tumour in left adrenal gland) or in the liver and lungs (when tumour in the right adrenal gland).

neurocar·diac (G. *neuron*, nerve; *kardia*, heart). Relating to the heart and its autonomic nerve supply.

neu·rocyte (G. *neuron*, nerve; *kutos*, cell). A neuron.

neu·rodermatī·tis (G. *neuron*, nerve; *derma*, skin). Lichenification, *q.v.*, provoked by scratching severely itching dermatoses, such as chronic eczema, prurigo, etc.

neu·rodermatō·sis (G. *neuron*, nerve; *derma*, skin). Any affection of the skin characterized by abnormal sensibility of the skin and absence of a visible primary lesion.

neuro-en·docrine (G. *neuron*, nerve; *endon*, within; *krinein*, to separate). Relating to the nervous and endocrine systems.

neuro-epider·mal (G. *neuron*, nerve; *epi*, upon; *derma*, skin). Relating to the nervous and epidermal tissues.

neuro-epithē·lial layer (G. *neuron*, nerve; *epi*, upon; *thēlē*, nipple). The layer of rods and cones and the outer nuclear layer of the retina, taken together.

neuro-epithelĭō·ma (G. *neuron*, nerve; *epi*, upon; *thēlē*, nipple). A malignant tumour of the brain, the least differentiated of all cerebral tumours.

neuro-epithē·lium (G. *neuron*, nerve; *epi*, upon; *thēlē*, nipple). 1. Epithelium forming the perceptive elements of the sense-organs, e.g. the cells of Corti or the neuro-epithelial layer of the retina. 2. The epithelium of the epiblast, the origin of the cerebrospinal axis in the embryo.

neu·rofibril·lae, neurofi·brils (G. *neuron*, nerve; L. *fibrilla*, dim. of *fibra*, fibre). The fibrillar structures within an axis-cylinder or cell-body of a neuron.

neu·rofibrō·ma (G. *neuron*, nerve; L. *fibra*, fibre). A tumour arising from the fibrous tissue of a nerve.

neu·rofibromatō·sis (G. *neuron*, nerve; L. *fibra*, fibre). A congenital dysplastic disease, characterized by the development of central (auditory nerve, spinal roots) and/or peripheral neurofibromata, producing divers nervous syndromes and skeletal changes, and by pigmentary changes of the skin, especially by so-called café-au-lait spots. Syn. von Recklinghausen's disease.

neu·rofil (G. *neuron*, nerve; L. *filum*, thread). A network of processes springing from the beginning of the axis-cylinder and surrounding the cell.

neurogĕ·nesis (G. *neuron*, nerve; *genesis*, production). The development of nervous tissue; the formation of nerves.

neurŏ·genous (G. *neuron*, nerve; *gennan*, to produce). 1. Arising in the nervous system. 2. Arising from some lesion of the nervous system.

neurŏ·glia (G. *neuron*, nerve; *glia*, glue). The supporting tissue of the central nervous system. Syn. glia. See also macroglia, oligodendroglia and microglia.

neu·roglĭō·ma (G. *neuron*, nerve; *glia*, glue). A glioma, a tumour composed of neuroglial tissue.

neu·rohistŏ·logy (G. *neuron* nerve; *histos*, web; *logos*, treatise). Histology of the nervous system.

neurohū·moral (G. *neuron*, nerve; L. *humor*, moisture). Neuro-endocrine.

neu·roid (G. *neuron*, nerve; *eidos*, form). Like a nerve.

neurokĕ·ratin (G. *neuron*, nerve; *keras*, horn). The type of keratin occurring in nerve-sheaths; the supporting framework of the myelin sheath.

neurolŏ·gic. Relating to neurology.

neurŏ·logist. A physician specializing in neurology.

neurŏ·logy (G. *neuron*, nerve; *logos*, treatise). That part of medical science dealing with the nervous system.

U

neū·rolymph (L. *neuron*, nerve; *lympha*, water). Cerebrospinal fluid.

neurolȳ·sin. A cytolysin which has a specific destructive action upon nerve cells.

neurŏ·lysis (G. *neuron*, nerve; *lusis*, dissolution). 1. Freeing of a nerve from adhesions. 2. Disintegration of nerve-tissue.

neurō·ma (G. *neuron*, nerve). A tumour arising from a peripheral nerve. N., amputation: a n. arising at the distal end of a limb shortened by amputation. N., ganglionic: a tumour composed of ganglionic and nerve fibres.

neuromalā·cia (G. *neuron*, nerve; *malakia*, softness). Softening of the nerves.

neū·romere (G. *neuron*, nerve; *meros*, part). A segment of the neural tube, corresponding in position to a primary somatic segment.

neuromus·cular (G. *neuron*, nerve; *mus*, muscle). Relating to both nerve and muscle. (See also neuromyal). N. spindle: a form of sensory nerve ending in striated muscle.

neuromȳ·al (G. *neuron*, nerve; *mus*, muscle). Relating to the structure between nerve fibre terminal and muscle. Syn. myoneural.

neū·ron, neū·rone (G. *neuron*, nerve). A nerve-cell with all its processes. N., lower motor: a n. originating in central grey columns of the cord and terminating in the skeletal muscle. N., upper motor: a n. originating in the motor area of the cerebral cortex and terminating in the motor nuclei of a cerebral nerve or in the central grey column of the cord.

neū·ronal, neuron·ic. Relating to a neuron.

neū·ronophā·gia (G. *neuron*, nerve; *phagein*, to eat). The destruction of nerve cells by phagocytes.

neuronō·sis (G. *neuron*, nerve). Any nervous disease.

neuronyx·is (G. *neuron*, nerve; *nuxis*, puncture). The surgical puncturing of a nerve.

neuro-ophthalmŏ·logy (G. *neuron*, nerve; *ophthalmos*, eye; *logos*, a discourse). The part of medicine dealing with the neurological significance of ophthalmological lesions.

neū·ropară·lysis (G. *neuron*, nerve; *paralusis*, paralysis). Paralysis due to an affection of the nervous system.

neuropă·thic (G. *neuron*, nerve; *pathos*, disease). Relating to neuropathy.

neuropathŏ·logy (G. *neuron*, nerve; *pathos*, disease; *logos*, treatise). The pathology of the nervous system.

neurŏ·pathy (G. *neuron*, nerve; *pathos*, disease). 1. Any disease of the nervous system. 2. Neurotic diathesis.

neurophō·nia (G. *neuron*, nerve; *phōnē*, voice). Psychogenic respiratory spasm, characterized by the uttering of loud barking cries.

neū·rophysiŏ·logy (G. *neuron*, nerve; *phusis*, nature; *logos*, treatise). The physiology of the nervous system.

neū·ropile (G. *neuron*, nerve; *pilos*, felt). A network of non-medullated fibres in the central nervous system.

neū·roplasm (G. *neuron*, nerve; *plassein*, to form). The protoplasm of nervous tissue.

neū·roplasty (G. *neuron*, nerve; *plassein*, to form). A plastic operation on a nerve; nerve-grafting.

neū·ropŏ·dia (G. *neuron*, nerve; *pous*, foot). The terminal knobs or plates of a telodendrion.

neū·ropore (G. *neuron*, nerve; *poros*, pore). The small opening at the anterior end of the neural tube.

neū·ropsychī·atry (G. *neuron*, nerve; *psukhē*, soul; *iatros*, physician). The part of medicine dealing with the psychiatric aspects of nervous diseases.

neū·rorĕ·cidive (G. *neuron*, nerve; L. *recīdere*, to cut away). Nervous lesions, especially lesions of the cranial nerves and subacute meningitis, appearing during, or after, insufficient antisyphilitic treatment.

neū·roretini·tis (G. *neuron*, nerve; L. *rētē*, a net). See neuroretinopathy.

neū·roretinŏ·pathy (G. *neuron*, nerve; L. *rētē*, a net; G. *pathos*, disease). The combination of papilloedema, oedema, fatty changes and haemorrhages of the retina and narrowing of retinal arteries with dilatation of retinal veins; present in malignant hypertension and in the end-stages of glomerulonephritis.

neurorhex·is (G. *neuron*, nerve; *rhēxis*, a rent). The tearing out of a nerve.

neuror·rhaphy (G. *neuron*, nerve; *rhaphe*, suture). The suturing of a divided nerve.

neurō·sis (G. *neuron*, nerve). A condition at least partly due to unconscious repression of ideas and wishes connected with important problems of the emotional life, and characterized by abnormal mental and/or bodily reactions to significant or seemingly insignificant events. N., actual: n. characterized by bodily disturbances resulting from a more or less immediate mental or physical trauma. N., anxiety: a n. characterized by overwhelming anxiety for not immediately obvious reasons. N., cardiac: a condition characterized mainly by the perception of pain in the cardiac region and palpitations, not due to a disease of the heart but to psychogenic factors. N., conversion: see n., transference. N., obsessional: a n. characterized by compulsive ideas, which dominate the conduct of the patient. N., transference: a n. which is mainly determined by an abnormal substitution of the libido. N., traumatic: a n. brought about by a trauma in a person disposed to react in such a way. N., war: a n. brought about by some experience connected with warfare in a person disposed to react in such a way.

neuroskĕ·leton (G. *neuron*, nerve; *skeleton*, skeleton). The vertebrate or true skeleton. Syn. endoskeleton.

neū·rosomes (G. *neuron*, nerve; *sōma*, body). Minute acidophile granules found at nodal points of the protoplasm of axis-cylinders and in the cytoplasm of the nerve-cell body.

neurospon·gium (G. *neuron*, nerve; *spoggia*, sponge). The network formed by the processes of ependymal cells and spongioblasts within the nuclear and marginal zones of the foetal spinal cord.

neurosur·geon (G. *neuron*, nerve; *kheirourgia*, surgery). A specialist in neurosurgery.

neurosur·gery (G. *neuron*, nerve; *kheirourgia*, surgery). The surgery of the central and peripheral nervous system.

neū·rosuture (G. *neuron*, nerve; L. *suture*, stitch). The suture of a divided nerve.

neū·rosȳ·philis. (G. *neuron*, nerve; L.L. *syphilis*). Syphilis involving the central nervous system.

neuroten·dinal (G. *neuron*, nerve; L. *tendĕre*, to stretch). Relating to both nerve and tendon. N. spindle: a form of sensory nerve ending in tendons.

neū·rothele (G. *neuron*, nerve; *thēlē*, nipple). A nerve-papilla.

neurot·ic (G. *neuron*, nerve). 1. Relating to neurosis. 2. Suffering from a neurosis.

neurotmē·sis (G. *neuron*, nerve; *tmēsis*, a cutting). Term introduced by Seddon in classification of peripheral nerve injuries. Indicates the state of a nerve that has been completely severed; the injury produces a lesion in every sense complete.

neu·rotome (G. *neuron*, nerve; *tomē*, section). 1. A needle-like knife used in neurotomy. 2. The nerve-tissues of an embryonic metamere; a neural segment.

neurŏ·tomy (G. *neuron*, nerve; *tomē*, section). The division of a nerve.

neuroton·ic reaction (G. *neuron*, nerve; *tonos*, tone). A type of pupillary reaction to light in which light stimulus causes a tonic slow contraction, the pupil remaining contracted for some considerable time.

neurotox·in (G. *neuron*, nerve; *toxikon*, poison). A toxin destructive to nervous tissue.

neurotrip·sy (G. *neuron*, nerve; *tribein*, to crush). The crushing of a nerve.

neurotrŏ·phic (G. *neuron*, nerve; *trophē*, nourishment). Relating to the influence exercised by nerves on cellular metabolism of the innervated area.

neū·rotrope, neurotrop·ic (G. *neuron*, nerve; *trĕpein*, to turn). Relating to neurotropism.

neurŏ·tropism (G. *neuron*, nerve; *trĕpein*, to turn). 1. The attraction or repulsion exercised upon regenerating nerve-fibres. 2. The property of an infective agent to act only upon nervous tissue.

neurovas·cular (G. *neuron*, nerve; L. *vasculum*, dim. of *vas*, vessel). Relating to both nervous and vascular structures.

Neusser's granules (Neusser, E. von, Austrian dermatologist, 1852–1912). Basophilic granules occasionally found in the white blood cells, near the nuclei. According to N. they are closely connected with the uric acid diathesis, but they have been seen also in other conditions.

neu·tral (L. *neutralis*, from *neuter*, neither). 1. Possessing neither acid nor alkali property. 2. In electricity, neither positive nor negative. 3. Inactive. 4. Bland. N. solution: a solution in which the number of H-ions equals that of the OH-ions.

neutră·lity (L. *neuter*, neither). The condition of being neutral.

neu·tralize (L. *neuter*, neither). 1. To render neutral. 2. To counter-balance an action, to nullify a quality.

neutropē·nia. Granulopenia, *q.v.*

neū·trophil, neū·trophile (L. *neuter*, neither; G. *philein*, to love). 1. Readily stained by neutral aniline dyes. 2. A leucocyte possessing cytoplasmic granules which stain with neutral dyes.

neutrophi·lia (L. *neuter*, neither; G. *philein*, to love). Absolute or relative increase in neutrophil leucocytes in the blood.

newborn. A child during the first fortnight after birth.

new-growth. Neoplasm, *q.v.*

Newton's colour rings (Newton, Sir I., English physicist, 1642–1726). The colour-rings produced by chromatic aberration when a cover glass is pressed upon a slide.

NH₃. Ammonia.

NH₄Br. Ammonium bromide.

NH₄Cl. Ammonium chloride.

(NH₂)₂CO. Urea.

NH₄NO₃. Ammonium nitrate.

(NH₄)₂SO₄. Ammonium sulphate.

Ni. Symbol for Nickel.

ni·acin. Nicotinic acid.

nickel (Swedish *nickel* from *nick*, an evil spirit). A metallic element. Symbol Ni.

Nicklès's test (Nicklès, F. J. J., French chemist, 1821–69). To distinguish glucose from cane sugar. The solution is heated to 100°C with carbon tetrachloride; if cane sugar is present the solution turns black; there is no colour change with glucose.

Nicol prism (Nicol, W., English physicist, 1768–1851). A prism of Iceland spar, cut diagonally across the principal axis, which reflects the ordinary ray of light out of the field, while the so-called polarized ray is transmitted.

nicotină·mide. The amide of nicotinic acid used in the treatment of pellagra. Formula C₆H₆ON₂.

ni·cotine. C₁₀H₁₄N₂. A poisonous liquid alkaloid which is found in the leaves of the tobacco plant.

nicotinic acid. C₅H₅N.COOH. A component, in the form of its amide, of a co-enzyme concerned in the oxidation-reduction mechanisms of cells. It is an essential component of mammalian diet.

ni·cotinism (Nicot, J., 1530–1600, introducer of tobacco into France). Morbid effects from excessive use of tobacco; nicotine poisoning.

nictā·ting, nic·titating (L. *nictare*, to wink). Winking. N. membrane: a membrane present in many vertebrates, forming a third eyelid. In man it is represented by the plica semilunaris.

nictitā·tion (L. *nictare*, to wink). The act of blinking or winking.

ni·dal (L. *nidus*, nest). Relating to a nidus.

nidā·tion (L. *nidus*, nest). Implantation, e.g., that of a fertilized ovum in the uterus.

ni·dus (L.). 1. A nest; a cluster. 2. A focus. 3. A nucleus.

Niemann's disease (Niemann, A., German paediatrician, 1880–1921). A disease occurring in childhood in which there is gross enlargement of the liver and spleen associated with some pigmentation of the skin.

Niemeyer's pill (Niemeyer, F. von, German physician, 1820–71). A pill composed of powdered digitalis ½ gr., ipecacuanha ¼ gr., powdered opium ¼ gr., extract of helenium ½ gr. It is used in combating the fever of phthisis.

night-blindness. Sub-normal acuity of vision in dim light. Syn. hemeralopia.

nightmare. A dream producing anxiety. Syn. incubus.

night-screaming, night-terrors. A state of deep anxiety due to a disturbing dream, from which the patient does not awake and for which he has later complete amnesia.

night-sweat. Excessive sweating during the night.

night-walking. Somnambulism, *q.v.*

nigres·cent (L. *niger*, black). Turning black.

nigri·tiēs lin·guae (L.). Black tongue.

ni·kethamide. The diethylamide of nicotinic acid, used as a respiratory stimulant.

nil nocēre (L.). 'You should not do any harm', the primary principle of therapeutics.

ninth nerve. The glossopharyngeal nerve.

niphablep·sia (G. *niphas*, snow; *ablepsia*, blindness). Snow-blindness.

nipple. The conical elevation in the centre of the mammary areola containing the outlets of the milk ducts.

Nisbet's chancre (Nisbet, W., English physician, 1759–1822). Abscesses appearing on the penis as a sequel of lymphangitis from soft chancre.

Nissl's bodies (Nissl, F., German neurologist, 1860–1919). Tigroid or chromophile corpuscles; the chromophilic portions of a nerve-cell, finely granular bodies of different sizes and shapes, brought out between the cytoreticulum by staining with N.'s stain (methylene-blue). N.'s degeneration: degeneration of the cell-body occurring after division of a nerve-fibre.

ni·sus (L.). An impulse; an effort; a striving.

nit. Popular name for the egg or larva of a louse.

Nitabuch's stria or fibrin stria (Nitabuch, R., Swiss anatomist, work published 1887). The layer of fibrin in the intervillous spaces of the placenta.

Nithsdale neck (Nithsdale, in Scotland). Goitre.

nitrae·mia (G. *nitron*, a carbonate of soda; *haima*, blood). The presence of an abnormal amount of nitrogen in the blood.

nitrae·mia (G. *nitron*, a carbonate of soda; *haima*, blood). Nitric acid, or any compound containing the NO₃ radical.

ni·trated. Term applied to organic substances produced by the entry of a -NO₂ group into the molecule.

nitrā·tion (G. *nitron*, a carbonate of soda). The introduction of the -NO₂ group into an organic compound.

nitre (G. *nitron*, a carbonate of soda). Saltpetre; potassium nitrate.

ni'tric (G. *nitron*, a carbonate of soda). Containing nitric acid. **N. acid**: (B.P.) a colourless, fuming very acid liquid made from sodium nitrate by distilling with sulphuric acid. It contains 70 per cent of hydrogen nitrate and 30 per cent water. HNO₃.

ni'tride (G. *nitron*, a carbonate of soda). A compound of a metal with nitrogen.

ni·trificā·tion (G. *nitron*, a carbonate of soda; L. *facere*, to make). The formation of nitrites or nitrates, especially that due to the action of nitrobacteria.

ni·trile (G. *nitron*, a carbonate of soda). Any organic compound containing the -CN group.

ni·trite (G. *nitron*, a carbonate of soda). Any salt of nitrous acid, or any compound containing the NO₂ radical.

Ni·trobacter (G. *nitron*, a carbonate of soda; *bakterion*, little stick). A genus of the tribe Nitrobacterieae. Rod-shaped cells, non-motile, not growing readily on organic media or in the presence of ammonia, but capable of securing growth energy by the oxidation of nitrites to nitrates.

ni·trobactē·ria (G. *nitron*, a carbonate of soda; *baktērion*, a stick). Micro-organisms present in the soil which oxidize ammonia and its derivatives or atmospheric nitrogen to nitrites or nitrates.

Ni·trobacteriā·cēae. A systematic family of the order Eubacteriales. Usually rod-shaped; capable of metabolising carbon, hydrogen, nitrogen or sulphur or simple compounds of these. Tribes: (1) Nitrobacterieae. (2) Azotobacterieae.

Ni·trobacteriĕ·ae. A tribe of the family Nitrobacteriaceae. Oxidize simple inorganic compounds of carbon, hydrogen, nitrogen or sulphur. Genera: (1) Hydrogenomonas. (2) Methanomonas. (3) Carbacidomonas. (4) Nitrosomonas. (5) Nitrosococcus. (6) Nitrobacter. (7) Acetobacter. (8) Thiobacillus.

nitro·erythrite (G. *nitron*, a carbonate of soda; *eruthros*, red). A vaso-dilator, erythrityl tetranitrate.

ni·trogen (G. *nitron*, a carbonate of soda). A gaseous element, forming 80 per cent of the atmospheric air and present in combination in animal and vegetable tissues. Symbol N.

nitrŏ·genous (G. *nitron*, a carbonate of soda; *gennan*, to produce). Containing nitrogen.

nitrŏ·meter (G. *nitron*, a carbonate of soda; *metron*, measure). An apparatus for measuring nitrogen gas set free during a chemical reaction.

ni·trous (G. *nitron*, a carbonate of soda). Any compound containing nitrogen as a univalent or trivalent element. **N. acid**: an acid, HNO₂, with one atom of oxygen less than nitric acid. **N. oxide**: N₂O, laughing gas, used as a general anaesthetic.

N.N.N. medium. Novy, MacNeal, Nicolle—medium used for culture of Leishmaniae and Trypanosomes.

Nocar·dia (Nocard, E. I. E., French veterinary surgeon, 1850–1903). Actinomycosis.

noci·association (L. *nocēre*, to harm; *associare*, to join to). The releases of nervous activity seen in shock and exhaustion, caused by trauma or surgical operation.

nocicep·tive (L. *nocēre*, to injure; *capere*, to take). 1. Applied to any stimulus which gives rise to pain and tissue disintegration. 2. Applied to any reflex produced by a painful stimulus.

nocicep·tor (L. *nocēre*, to injure; *capere*, to take). A receptor-organ whose stimuli are harmful to the body.

noctambulā·tion (L. *nox*, night; *ambulare*, to walk). Sleep-walking.

noctū·ria (L. *nox*, night; G. *ouron*, urine). The passing of abnormal amounts of urine during the night.

noctur·nal (L. *nocturnus*, from *nox*, night). Relating to the night.N.haemoglobinuria: see Haemoglobinurian.

nŏ·cuous (L. *nocuus*, harmful). Noxious.

nod. 1. To let the head fall forward with a quick involuntary movement. 2. The movement so made.

nō·dal (L. *nodus*, knot). Relating to a node. **N. point**: the point in the eye through which all lines pass joining points in the visual field with their retinal images.

nodding spasm. See spasmus nutans.

node (L. *nodus*, knot). 1. A knot, swelling or excrescence. 2. A lymph gland. 3. A point of narrowing or constriction. **N., Aschoff's**: auriculoventricular n. **N., auriculoventricular**: the structure situated at the base of the interauricular septum, belonging to the conducting system of the heart. **N., Heberden's**: see under Heberden. **N., Parrot's**: see under Parrot. **N., Ranvier's**: see under Ranvier. **N., Singer's**: small nodules at the free margin of the vocal cords due to chronic inflammation. **N., sino-auricular**: the structure situated at the orifice of the right vena cava superior into the right auricle, the starting point of the cardiac conducting system. Syn. Keith's sino-atrial node.

nō·dose (L. *nodosus*, knotty). Relating to or characterized by nodes.

nodŏ·sity (L. *nodus*, knot). 1. The condition of having nodes. 2. A node.

nō·dular (L. *nodus*, knot). Composed of or characterized by the presence of nodules.

nō·dule (L. *nodulus*, dim. of *nodus*, knot). A small node. **N., rheumatic**: a n. developing from fibrous tissue, especially near the wrist or elbow, palpable through the skin; occurring in limited numbers in graver cases of rheumatic fever in childhood, nearly always pathognomonic of cardiac involvement.

nō·dulus (L.). A nodule. **N. vermis**: a lobule at the anterior end of the vermis inferior.

nō·dus (L.). A node.

nŏĕmat·ic (G. *noēma*, a thought). Pertaining to thought or to any mental process.

nŏĕ·sis (G., thought). The process of thinking; the working of the intellect.

Nogū·chia (Noguchi, H., American physician of Japanese birth, 1876–1928). *Bacterium* (or *Noguchia*) *granulosis*, a small gram-negative bacillus isolated by Noguchi from cases of trachoma. Injection of *B. granulosis* into monkeys produces a granular conjunctivitis—but not trachoma.

noli me tangere (L., touch me not). Malignant ulcer.

nō·ma (G. *nomē*, a spreading). A rapidly spreading gangrenous stomatitis, cheilitis or vulvo-vaginitis, occurring in severely debilitated children, especially after measles, or very rarely in adults. Syn. cancrum oris; gangrenous stomatitis.

nomen·clature (L. *nomen*, name; *calatio*, a calling). A system of technical terms.

nō·mogram (G. *nomos*, law; *gramma*, mark). The representation of correlations by graphs or charts.

non-adhe·rent (L. *non*, not; *ad*, to; *haerere*, to stick). Not attached. A clinical term used in surgery.

nō·nan (L. *nonus*, ninth). Recurring every ninth day.

non compos mentis (L.). Of unsound mind.

non-conductor (L. *non*, not; *conducere*, to lead together). A substance not transmitting a particular form of energy.

nonigrā·vida (L. *nonus*, ninth; *gravidus*, pregnant). A woman in her ninth pregnancy.

noni·para (L. *nonus*, ninth; *parere*, to bear). A woman who has borne nine children.

Nonne-Apelt reaction. (Nonne, M., born 1861; Apelt, F., 1877–1911, German physicians). A test for globulin in the cerebrospinal fluid.

non-nū·cleated (L. *non*, not; *nucleus*, kernel). Having no nucleus.

nŏn·ose (L. *nonus*, ninth). A carbohydrate with a molecule containing nine atoms.

nonpā·rous (L. *non*, not; *parere*, to bear). Nulliparous, *q.v.*

non-protein nitrogen (L. *non*, not; G. *prōtos*, first). 1. Any compound containing nitrogen but of simpler composition than a protein, e.g. creatinine, urea, etc. 2. The total amount of all such compounds present in the blood.

non repetatur (L.). Do not repeat.

non-union (L. *non*, not; *unus*, one). The failure of broken bones to join correctly.

nō·nus (L. ninth). The hypoglossal nerve.

non-viable (L. *non*, not; *vita*, life). Unable to live.

norm (L. *norma*, rule). A standard or type.

nor·ma (L., rule). 1. Norm; model. 2. Rule; line. 3. In anatomy, an aspect or view, especially of the skull.

nor·mal (L. *norma*, rule). According to or conforming to any empirical or conventional rule, division or unit. **N. solution:** a solution of a substance containing 1 gramme equivalent of the substance in 1 litre of solution. See also decinormal solution. **N. saline:** isotonic solution of sodium chloride. Syn. physiological saline solution.

nor·mative (L. *norma*, rule). Relating to the norm.

nor·moblast (L. *norma*, rule; G. *blastos*, germ). A nucleated red blood corpuscle of the size of an erythrocyte; the precursor of the erythrocyte.

normoblas·tic. Relating to normoblasts.

nor·moblastō·sis (L. *norma*, rule; G. *blastos*, germ). A condition characterized by the presence of normoblasts.

nor·mocyte (L. *norma*, rule; G. *kutos*, cell). An erythrocyte of normal size.

normocyt·ic. Relating to normocytes.

nor·mocytō·sis (L. *norma*, rule; *kutos*, cell). A condition characterized by the presence of normocytes in the peripheral blood.

Norris's colourless corpuscles (Norris, R., English physiologist, 1831–1916). Decolourized red blood corpuscles, invisible in the blood plasma.

nose. The structure serving as first part of the respiratory tract and as the peripheral organ of olfactory perception.

nosē·ma (G. *nosos*, a sickness). 1. Disease; illness. 2. A genus of parasitic protozoa.

nosocō·mium (G. *nosos*, a sickness; *komein*, to attend to). A hospital.

nosō·geny (G. *nosos*, a sickness; *gennan*, to produce). Producing illness.

nosohae·mia (G. *nosos*, a sickness; *haima*, blood). Any disease of the blood.

nosō·logy (G. *nosos*, a sickness; *logos*, treatise). An old term denoting the science of disease.

nosomā·nia (G. *nosos*, a sickness; *mania*, madness). The delusion of being ill.

nŏ·somycō·sis (G. *nosos*, disease; *mukēs*, mushroom). Any fungus disease.

nosophi·lia (G. *nosos*, a sickness; *philein*, to love). A neurotic desire to be ill.

nosophō·bia (G. *nosos*, a sickness; *phobos*, fear). Neurotic fear of some disease.

nŏ·sotoxicō·sis (G. *nosos*, a disease; *toxikon*, poison). Any disease caused by poisoning.

nostal·gia (G. *nostos*, a return; *algos*, pain). Homesickness.

nostrils. The anterior nares; the external orifices of the nose.

nos·trum (L. *noster*, our). A secret or quack medicine.

nō·tal (G. *nōton*, back). Relating to the back.

nō·tancephā·lia (G. *nōton*, back; *an*, neg.; *kephalē*, head). Congenital absence of the back of the head.

nō·tanencephā·lia (G. *nōton*, back; *an*, neg.; *egkephalos*, brain). Congenital absence of the cerebellum.

notch. A deep indentation.

notched. Indented.

note-blindness. A form of alexia, characterized by inability to read musical notes.

nō·tencephā·locele (G. *nōton*, back; *egkephalos*, brain; *kēlē*, hernia). Occipital encephalocele.

notencē·phalus (G. *nōton*, back; *egkephalos*, brain). A monster with an encephalocele through a defective occiput.

Nothnagel's symptom (Nothnagel, C. W. H., German physician, 1841–1905). 1. Dizziness, staggering and rolling gait, with irregular forms of oculomotor paralysis and frequent nystagmus, seen in tumour of the corpora quadrigemina. 2. Paralysis of the muscles of the face, less marked on voluntary movements than on movements connected with emotions. This type of paralysis has been noted in tumour of the optic thalamus. **N.'s type of facial paralysis:** see N.'s symptom.

nō·tifiable (L. *notificare*, to make known). Term applied to a disease cases of which must be made known to the health authorities.

nō·tochord (G. *nōton*, back; *khordē*, gut-string). The embryonic tissue from which the vertebral spine develops.

notŏ·melus (G. *nōton*, back; *melos*, limb). A double monster with rudimentary limbs attached to the back.

Novarsan. A proprietary brand of neoarsphenamine.

Novarsenobenzol. A proprietary brand of neoarsphenamine.

Novarsenobillon. A proprietary brand of neoarsphenamine.

Nō·vocain. A proprietary local anaesthetic.

noxa (L., harm). An injurious substance or organism.

noxious (L. *noxius*, harmful). Harmful; damaging.

nubē·cula (L. *nubecula*, dim. of *nubes*, cloud). A cloudiness, especially of the cornea.

nū·bile (L. *nubilis*, from *nubere*, to marry). Marriageable; of an age at which there is the possibility of procreation or child-bearing.

nubi·lity (L. *nubilis*, from *nubere*, to marry). The condition of sexual development when marriage may be consummated.

nū·cha (Mediaeval L. *nucha*, nape). The nape of the neck.

nū·cis. Genitive of L. *nux*, nut.

Nuck's canal (Nuck, A., Dutch anatomist, 1650–1692). The prolongation into the female inguinal canal of the processus vaginalis. **N.'s diverticulum:** N.'s canal, *q.v.*

nū·clear (L. *nucula*, dim. of *nux*, nut). Relating to a nucleus. **N. agenesis; N. aplasia:** congenital absence of the nucleus of a cranial nerve. **N. jaundice:** kernicterus, *q.v.* **N. paralysis:** p. due to a nuclear lesion of a cranial nerve. **N. sap:** karyolymph. **N. stain:** a dye staining a cell-nucleus.

nū·cleāses (L. *nucleus*, kernel). Enzymes acting upon nucleic acids.

nū·cleated. Having a nucleus.

nuclē·ic acids. The non-protein portion of nucleoprotein, consisting of organic compounds composed from phosphoric acid, purines, pyrimidines and carbohydrates.

nū·cleiform (L. *nucleus*, kernel; *forma*, shape). Like a nucleus.

nū·cleins. Compounds of protein with nucleic acids.

nū·cleo-albū·min. A term formerly used for a phosphoprotein, *q.v.*

nū·cleohī·ston. A protein found in the nuclei of leucocytes.

nū·cleolar (L. *nucleus*, kernel). Relating to the nucleolus.

nuclē·olus (L. *nucleus*, kernel). A small more or less spherical structure within a cell-nucleus.

nū·cleomicrosō·ma (L. *nucleus* kernel; G. *mikros*, small; *sōma*, body). An intranuclear chromatin granule.

nu·cleoplasm (L. *nucleus*, kernel; G. *plassein*, to form). The protoplasm of a cell-nucleus. Syn. karyoplasm.

nū·cleoplas·mic ratio (L. *nucleus*, kernel; G. *plassein*, to form). The ratio of nuclear to cytoplasmic volume.

nu·cleoprō·teins (L. *nucleus*, kernel; G. *prōtos*, first). Compounds containing protein and nucleic acid; the constituents of animal and vegetable cell nuclei.

nū·cleosidases (L. *nucleus*, kernel). Enzymes acting upon nucleosides.

nū·cleosides (L. *nucleus*, kernel). Glycoside derivatives of nucleic acids.

nuclěō·tidases (L. *nucleus*, kernel). Enzymes acting upon nucleotides.

nū·cleotides (L. *nucleus*, kernel). Nucleosides in combination with phosphoric acid.

nu·cleotox·in (L. *nucleus*, kernel; G. *toxikon*, poison). 1. A poison derived from cell-nuclei. 2. A toxin affecting the nuclei of cells.

nu·cleus (L., kernel). 1. A central part or element. 2. A structure of specialized substance and function within a cell, staining darker than the surrounding cytoplasm. 3. A circumscribed accumulation of ganglion-cells associated with a particular function. N. pulposus: the semi-fluid structure situated in the centre of an intervertebral disc; the only remnant of the notochord in postfoetal life.

Nuel's space (Nuel, J. P., Belgian ophthalmologist, 1847–1920). A space between the outer rods of Corti and the neighbouring row of hair cells.

Nuhn's gland (Nuhn, A., German anatomist, 1814–89). The glandula lingualis anterior.

nulli·para (L. *nullus*, none; *parēre*, to bear). A woman who has never borne a child.

nullipā·rity. The condition of being nulliparous.

nulli·parous (L. *nullus*, none; *parēre*, to bear). Never having given birth to a child.

numb. Having defective sensibility.

number. Symbol of figure; count or sum.

numbness. Local anaesthesia.

num·miform (L. *nummus*, coin; *forma*, shape). Nummular.

num·mular (L. *nummulus*, dim. of *nummus*, coin). 1. Coin-shaped. 2. Resembling rouleaux or rolls of coins.

nummulā·tion (L. *nummulus*, dim. of *nummus*, coin). 1. The formation of nummular structures. 2. Rouleaux-formation of red blood corpuscles.

nun's murmur. A humming sound heard over the large veins at the root of the neck in anaemia, and sometimes in healthy persons; bruit de diable.

nunnā·tion (Arab. *nun* = the letter n). The too frequent or abnormal use of the *n*-sound.

nurse. 1. To care for the sick or for an infant. 2. A person doing so. Wet n.: one who suckles an infant not her own.

Nussbaum's cellules (Nussbaum, M., German histologist, 1850–1915). The cells in the pyloric gastric glands.

nutans (L. *nutare*, to nod). Nodding.

nutā·tion (L. *nutare*, to nod). Nodding of the head.

nutmeg-liver. Term describing the macroscopic appearance of a section of a congested liver in cases of circulatory insufficiency; it is characterized by a mottled surface, each lobule having a dark centre (congested intralobular vein) and a brownish-yellow periphery (bile-stained, atrophic or fatty degenerated liver cells).

nū·trient (L. *nutrire*, to nourish). 1. Nourishing; supplying nutrition. 2. Any nourishing substance.

nū·triment (L. *nutrimentum*, from *nutrire*, to nourish). Any nourishing substance.

nutri·tion (L. *nutrire*, to nourish). 1. The process of the assimilation of food. 2. The science of feeding.

nutri·tional (L. *nutrire*, to nourish). Relating to nutrition.

nutri·tious (L. *nutrire*, to nourish). Nutritive.

nū·tritive (L. *nutrire*, to nourish). Nourishing; affording nutrition.

nux vomica (L.). Seeds of *Strychnos nuxvomica*, from which strychnine is obtained.

nyctal·gia (G. *nux*, night; *algos*, pain). Pain occurring chiefly at night.

nyc·talope (G. *nux*, night; *alaos*, blind; *ōps*, eye). One who sees better at night or in dim light than by daylight.

nyctalō·pia (G. *nux*, night; *alaos*, blind; *ōps*, eye). This properly means night blindness, but the term is sometimes used with the opposite sense to mean day blindness, when a person sees better in a dim light than by daylight.

nyctophi·lia (G. *nux*, night; *philein*, to love). The neurotic preference of night to day.

nyctophō·bia (G. *nux*, night; *phobos*, fear). Neurotic fear of the dark.

nyctū·ria (G. *nux*, night; *ouron*, urine). The passing of urine during night or during the time of sleep.

nȳ·lon. A proprietary artificial silk; it is sometimes used for sutures.

nympha (G. *numphē*, maiden). A labium minus of the vulva.

nymphec·tomy (G. *numphē*, maiden; *ektomē*, excision). Excision of one or both the nymphae.

nymphi·tis (G. *numphē*, maiden). Inflammation of the nymphae.

nymphomā·nia (G. *numphē*, maiden; *mania*, madness). Excessive sexual desire in women.

nymphŏ·tomy (G. *numphē*, maiden; *tomē*, section). Incision of one or both nymphae.

nystag·mic (G. *nustazein*, to nod in sleep). Relating to nystagmus.

nystag·miform (G. *nustazein*, to nod in sleep; L. *forma*, shape). Like nystagmus.

nystag·mograph (G. *nustazein*, to nod in sleep; *graphein*, to write). An instrument for recording nystagmic movements of the eyeballs.

nystag·mus (G. *nustazein*, to nod in sleep). An involuntary rhythmic movement of the eyeballs. N., amblyopic: n. due to ocular lesions preventing fixation. N., amaurotic: n. occurring in a blind individual. N., caloric: n. produced by irrigating the ear with a warm or cold fluid. N., central: n. caused by a central lesion of the vestibular nerve. N., conjugate: n. characterized by rhythmic regularity and symmetrical distribution. N., disjunctive: n. in which the eyes describe rhythmic and symmetrical opposite movements. N., dissociated: n. in which the movements are unrelated in the two eyes. N., galvanic: n.

produced by electrical stimulation of the labyrinth. **N., jerky:** n. in which a slow lateral movement is followed by a rapid return to the original position. **N., miner's:** see miner's n. **N., ocular:** n. due to impairment of fixation. **N., optico-kinetic:** n. occurring when successive moving objects pass into the visual field. **N. of eccentric fixation:** n. occurring when the eyes are deviated beyond the binocular field. **N., pendular:** n. in which the movement is of equal speed in each direction. **N., rotatory:** n. characterized by rotary movements. **N., undulatory:** n. both phases of which are equally rapid. **N., vestibular:** n. due to stimulation or paralysis of the labyrinthine organ.

O

O. The symbol for oxygen.

oak. A tree of the genus *Quercus*. The dried bark of the British oaks contains a considerable amount of tannin and is used as an astringent in the treatment of haemorrhoids and other conditions.

oā·sis. A healthy area in diseased tissue.

obduc·tion (L. *obducere*, to bring forward). A postmortem examination; a necropsy.

O'Beirne's sphincter (O'Beirne, J., Irish surgeon, 1786–1862). The sphincter superior of the rectum.

obĕ·lion (G. *obĕlos*, a cooking spit). Juncture of the sagittal suture and a line joining the parietal foramina.

Obermayer's test (Obermayer, F., Austrian chemist, 1861–1925). A test for indican in urine.

Obermeier's spirillum (Obermeier, O. H. F., German physician, 1843–73). *Treponema recurrentis*, the causal agent of European relapsing fever, first observed by Obermeier in 1873.

obese (L. *obesus*, fat). Excessively fat; stout.

obē·sity (L. *obesus*, fat). Fatness; corpulence.

ō·bex (L., barrier). A band of white matter at the calamus scriptorius between the clava and the tela chorioidea of the fourth ventricle.

obfuscā·tion (L. *obfuscare*, to darken). Darkening or cloudiness, as of the cornea.

obĭ·tuary (L. *obitus*, death). 1. Pertaining to death. 2. Death notice.

object-blindness. Inability to apprehend visual perceptions as objects.

objec·tive (Mediaeval L. *objectivus*, from *objicere*, to present). 1. Relating to an object. 2. Physical. 3. Verifiable by any investigator. 4. Relating to those conditions of the body that may be observed by another (o. signs of disease). 5. In optical instruments, the lens nearest to the object under examination.

ob·ligate (L. *obligare*, to put under obligation). Compelled to act in a given manner; conditional; bound. **O. aerobe:** a micro-organism which can live only as an aerobe. **O. parasite:** a parasite which cannot live without a host.

oblique (L. *obliquus*). Slanting; inclined; not direct. In anatomy, applied to various muscles which have a course other than vertical or horizontal.

obliquī·meter (L. *obliquus*, slanting; G. *metron*, measure). An instrument for measuring the degree of obliquity of the pelvic brim.

oblĭ·quity (L. *obliquus*, slanting). The condition of being slanted or inclined.

oblī·quus (L.). Term applied to various muscles. See oblique.

obliterā·tion (L. *oblitterare*, to erase). Entire closure of a lumen or cavity.

oblonga·ta (L.). The medulla oblongata.

obmutes·cence (L. *obmutescere*, to be dumb). Loss of voice; aphonia.

observā·tion (L. *observatio*). The systematic examination of phenomena.

obses·sion (L. *obsidēre*, to besiege). An irresistible idea or urge.

ob·solete (L. *obsoletus*, worn out). No longer in use.

obstet·ric, obstet·rical (L. *obstetrix*, from *obstare*, to stand against). Pertaining to obstetrics. **O. paralysis:** partial paralysis of the brachial plexus due to a lesion occurring during delivery of the child. Syn. birth palsy; Erb-Duchenne paralysis.

obstetrĭ·cian. One skilled in obstetrics.

obstet·rics (L. *obstetrix*, from *obstare*, to stand against). The part of medicine dealing with pregnancy, childbirth and the puerperium.

obstipā·tion (L. *ob*, against; *stipare*, to press). Constipation.

obstruc·tion (L. *obstruere*, to obstruct). 1. The state of being blocked up. 2. The act of impeding or blocking, e.g. an opening or passage. 3. An impediment or obstacle.

obstruc·tive (L. *obstruere*, to obstruct). 1. Stopping or blocking. 2. Due to an obstruction.

ob·struent (L. *obstruere*, to obstruct). Obstructive; said, e.g., of an agent which closes the lumen or orifice of a vessel or duct.

obtund (L. *obtundere*). To blunt, dull or lessen.

obtun·dent (L. *obtundere*, to blunt). Soothing; quieting.

obturā·tion (L. *obturare*, to close). The closing or blocking of an opening or passage.

obturator (L. *obturare*, to close). 1. That which closes or blocks an opening. 2. Relating to the o. foramen, membrane, muscles, nerves or vessel. **O. canal:** a gap in the o. membrane through which the o. nerve and vessels pass. **O. foramen:** a foramen in the anterior section of the innominate bone. **O. hernia:** a hernia through the o. canal. **O. membrane:** the membrane closing the o. foramen.

obtuse (L. *obtundere*, to blunt). Blunt.

obtū·sion (L. *obtundere*, to blunt). The condition of being blunt; a weakening of normal sensation.

occĭ·pital (L. *ob*, at; *caput*, head). Regarding or in relation with the occiput. **O. lobe:** the part of a cerebral hemisphere posterior to the parieto-occipital fissure. **O. protuberance:** the prominences on the internal and external surfaces of the o. bone. **O. sinus:** the venous vessel running along the margin of the foramen magnum and opening into the lateral sinus.

occipito-anterior. See position, o-a.

occi·pito-cervĭ·cal (L. *occiput*; *cervix*, neck). Relating to the occiput and the neck.

occi·pito-fron·tal (L. *occiput*; *frons*, forehead). Relating to the occiput and the forehead, or to the occiput and frontal lobes.

occi·pito-fā·cial (L. *occiput*; *facies*, face). Relating to the occiput and the face.

occi·pito-men·tal (L. *occiput*; *mentum*, chin). Relating to the occiput and the chin.

occi·pito-parĭ·etal (L. *occiput*; *paries*, wall). Relating to the occiput and the parietal bones, or to the occipital and parietal lobes.

occi·pito-postē·rior. See position, o-p.

occi·pito-tem·poral (L. *occiput*; *tempora*, temples). Relating to the occiput and the temporal bones, or to the occipital and temporal lobes.

occi·pito-thalam·ic (L. *occiput*; G. *thalamos*, chamber). Relating to the occipital lobe and the optic thalamus.

oc·ciput (L. *ob*, at; *caput*, head). The back part of the head.

occlū·ding (L. *occludere*, to shut). Closing.

occlū·sio (L. *occludere*, to shut). Occlusion. **O. pupillae:** (L.) blocked pupil due to the formation of a pseudo-membrane in iritis.

occlū·sion (L. *occludere*, to shut). 1. The blocking up of an opening. 2. The state of being closed or shut. 3. The adhesion of a gas or liquid on or within a solid mass. 4. The full contact of the masticating surfaces of the upper and lower teeth.

occlū·sive (L. *occludere*, to shut). Closing; shutting up. **O. pessary:** a pessary occluding either the uterine cervix or part of the vaginal vault, used for contraception.

occult (L. *occultus*, obscure). Hidden; secret. **O. blood:** blood the presence of which cannot be recognized without chemical or microscopical examination.

occupational disease. One produced by the occupation of the patient. **O. neurosis:** a neurosis affecting specifically the patient's ability to perform his work, e.g. writer's cramp, pianist's cramp.

occupational therapy. Treatment of a disorder by occupational work.

ocel·lus (L. *ocellus*, dim. of *oculus*, eye). The simple eye of invertebrate animals, composed either of a single epithelial cell or of many epithelial cells acting without functional association.

ochlophō·bia (G. *ŏkhlos*, crowd; *phobos*, fear). Neurotic fear of crowds.

ōchroder·mia (G. *ōkhros*, pale yellow; *derma*, skin). Yellow skin.

ochronō·sis (G. *ōkhros*, pale yellow). A brownish or blackish discoloration of cartilage or fibrous tissue due to alkaptonuria or to derivatives of carbolic acid.

Ochsner's solution (Ochsner, A. J., American surgeon, 1858–1925) Phenol, 0·5 per cent; aqueous solution of boric acid, 66 per cent; alcohol 33 per cent. **O.'s sphincter:** a sphincter described in the duodenum below the opening of the bile duct.

oc·tan (L. *octo*, eight). Recurring every eight days, as an o. fever.

oc·tane (L. *octo*, eight). The eighth member of the paraffin series.

octä·valent (L. *octo*, eight; *valere*, to be strong). Possessing a valency of eight.

octā·vus (L. *octavus*, from *octo*, eight). The eighth cranial nerve.

octigrā·vida (L. *octo*, eight; *gravidus*, pregnant). A woman in her eighth pregnancy.

octi·para (L. *octo*, eight; *parere*, to bear). A woman who has had eight children.

oc·tose (L. *octo*, eight). A sugar with eight carbon atoms to the molecule.

ŏ·cular (L. *oculus*, eye). 1. Relating to the eye. 2. The eye-piece of an optical instrument.

oculen·ta (L. *oculus*, eye). Ointments for the eye.

ŏ·culist (L. *oculus*, eye). An ophthalmologist.

oculo-cardiac (L. *oculus*, eye; G. *kardia*, heart). Relating to the eye and the heart. **O.-c. reflex:** reflex bradycardia following pressure upon the ocular bulbus. Syn. Aschner's reflex.

oculogȳ·ral, oculogyr·ic (L. *oculus*, eye; G. *guros*, a circle). Causing movements of the eye. **O. attacks** or **spasms:** spasmodic attacks of conjugate ocular deviation, e.g. in epidemic encephalitis.

oculomō·tor (L. *oculus*, eye; *movere*, to move). 1. Relating to the movement of the eye, as the o. nerve. 2. Relating to the third cranial or o. nerve.

ŏ·culomotor·ius (L. *oculus*, eye; *movere*, to move). The third cranial nerve.

ŏ·culomycō·sis (L. *oculus*, eye; G. *mukēs*, mushroom). Any disease of the eye or its appendages caused by infection with a fungus.

ŏ·culozygomat·ic (L. *oculus*, eye; G. *zugōma*, a bolt). Relating to the eye and the zygoma.

ŏ·culus (L.). An eye.

o.d. Abbreviation for L. *oculus dexter*, right eye.

Oddi's sphincter (Oddi, R., Italian physician, work published 1887). The sphincteric fibres around the termination of the common bile duct.

odontal·gia (G. *odous*, tooth; *algos*, pain). Toothache.

odontat·rophy (G. *odous*, tooth; *atrophia*). Atrophy of the teeth.

odontex·esis (G. *odous*, tooth; *exĕsis*, dismissal). Removal of deposits and concretion of the teeth.

odon·tia (G. *odous*, tooth). 1. Odontalgia. 2. Any abnormality of the teeth.

odonti·asis (G. *odous*, tooth). Dentition.

odon·tinoid (G. *odous*, tooth; *eidos*, form). Resembling teeth.

odonti·tis (G. *odous*, tooth). Inflammation of a tooth.

odon·toblast (G. *odous*, tooth; *blastos*, germ). A cell of the peripheral layer of dental papilla, forming the dentine.

odon·toboth·rion (G. *odous*, tooth; *bothriŏn*, a small trench). A tooth socket.

odon·tobothri·tis (G. *odous*, tooth; *bothriŏn*, a small trench). Inflammation of the socket of a tooth.

odontŏ·clasis (G. *odous*, tooth; *klaein*, to break). Fracture of a tooth.

odon·toclast (G. *odous*, tooth; *klaein*, to break). A cell of the peripheral layer of the root portion of the dental sac, absorbing the roots of the deciduous teeth.

odon·togen (G. *odous*, tooth; *gennan*, to produce). A substance producing dentine.

odon·togĕ·nesis, odontŏ·geny (G. *odous*, tooth; *gennan*, to produce). The origin and development of teeth.

odon·toglyph (G. *odous*, tooth; *gluphein*, to carve). An instrument for scraping the teeth.

odon·tograph (G. *odous*, tooth; *graphein*, to write). An instrument for recording the inequalities of the surface of the enamel.

odon·toid (G. *odous*, tooth; *eidos*, form). Resembling a tooth.

odon·tolith (G. *odous*, tooth; *lithos*, a stone). A calcareous deposit on the teeth.

odontŏ·logy (G. *odous*, tooth; *logos*, treatise). The part of medicine dealing with the teeth. Syn. dentistry.

odontolox·ia, odontŏ·loxy (G. *odous*, tooth; *loxos*, slanting). Irregularity of the teeth.

odontŏ·ma (G. *odous*, tooth). A tumour derived from tooth-forming tissue.

odon·tome (G. *odous*, tooth). Odontoma, *q.v.* **Complex o.:** a composite odontoma composed of enamel, dentine and cementum. **Composite o.:** a tumour derived from both dental epithelium and mesoblastic dental tissues. **Compound o.:** term applied to a complex odontoma when multiple.

odon·tonecrō·sis (G. *odous*, tooth; *nekrōsis*, mortification). Dental necrosis.

odontŏ·pathy (G. *odous*, tooth; *pathos*, disease). Any disease of the teeth.

odontŏ·sis (G. *odous*, tooth). Odontogenesis.

odontotrip·sis (G. *odous*, tooth; *tribein*, to wear away). The wearing away of teeth.

odontŏ·tripy (G. *odous*, tooth; *trupan*, to bore). Drilling of a tooth.

odori·ferous (L. *odor*, a smell; *ferre*, to bear). Emitting an odour.

odour (L. *odor*, a smell). 1. A sensation due to stimulation of the end-organs of the olfactory or first cranial nerve. 2. A scent.

O'Dwyer's tubes (O'Dwyer, J. P., American physician, 1841–98). Tubes of various sizes for laryngeal intubation.

oecŏ·logy, ecŏ·logy (G. *oikos*, a dwelling; *logos*, treatise). The part of biology dealing with the interrelations between organisms and their environment.

oedē·ma (G. *oidema*, a swelling). Abnormal accumulation of a serous fluid in the tissues. **Oe., angioneurotic:** a condition characterized by the sudden transient occurrence of localized oedematous swellings of the skin, mucous membrane or joints. **Oe., cardiac:** oe. due to circulatory insufficiency. **Oe., cerebral:** oe. of the cerebral tissue. **Oe., collateral:** oe. in the neighbourhood of an inflamed part. **Oe., hereditary:** a hereditary condition characterized by chronic oe. of the legs, usually appearing at or after adolescence, without obvious cause. Syn. Milroy-Meige-Nonne's disease. **Oe., hunger:** Oe., nutritional, *q.v.* **Oe., malignant:** gangrenous inflammation due to the presence of Clostridium oedematis maligni. **Oe., nutritional:** oe. due to nutritional protein deficiency. **Oe., pulmonary:** oe. of the lungs, due to insufficiency of the left heart. **Oe., renal:** oe. due to renal disease.

Oedipus complex (*Oidipous*, G. mythological hero, who killed his father and married his mother). A group of more or less repressed, emotionally charged ideas, originating in the erotic attachment of a male child to his mother.

Oehl's layer (Oehl, E., Italian anatomist, 1827–1903). The stratum lucidum of the epidermis. **O.'s muscles:** the muscle bundles in the chordae tendinae of the left auriculoventricular valve.

Oertel's treatment (Oertel, M. J., German physician, 1835–97). The treatment of chronic cardiac disease by: 1. Reduction of the amount of fluid ingested and increase in the excretion of fluids; by frequent small meals, with avoidance of taking fluids and solids at the same time; also by graduated hill-climbing and other measured exercise. 2. Reduction of obesity, largely by abstaining as much as possible from fluids and by taking graduated exercise.

oesophă·geal (G. *oisophagos*, gullet). Relating to the oesophagus.

oesophagec·tasis (G. *oisophagos*, gullet; *ektasis*, extension). Dilatation of the oesophagus.

oesophagec·tomy (G. *oisophagos*, gullet; *ektomē*, excision). Resection of the oesophagus.

oesophagis·mus (G. *oisophagos*, gullet). Spasmodic contraction of the oesophagus.

oesophagī·tis (G. *oisophagos*, gullet). Inflammation of the oesophagus.

oesophă·gocele (G. *oisophagos*, gullet; *kēlē*, hernia). Diverticulum of the oesophagus.

oesŏ·phagoduodenŏ·stomy (G. *oisophagos*, gullet; L. *duodeni*, twelve each; G. *stoma*, mouth). The surgical formation of a passage between the oesophagus and the duodenum.

oesŏ·phago-enterŏ·stomy (G. *oisophagos*, gullet; *enteron*, intestine; *stoma*, mouth). The surgical formation of a passage between the oesophagus and a portion of the small intestine.

oesŏ·phagogastrŏ·stomy (G. *oisophagos*, gullet; *gastēr*, belly; *stoma*, mouth). The surgical formation of a passage between oesophagus and stomach.

oesŏ·phagojejunŏ·stomy. An anastomosis between the oesophagus and the jejunum.

oesophagomală·cia (G. *oisophagos*, gullet; *malakia*, softness). Morbid softening of the oesophagus.

oesophagŏ·meter (G. *oisophagos*, gullet; *metron*, measure). An instrument for measuring the length of the oesophagus.

oesŏ·phagomycō·sis (G. *oisophagos*, gullet; *mukēs*, mushroom). Disease of the oesophagus due to fungi.

oesophă·goplasty (G. *oisophagos*, gullet; *plassein*, to form). Plastic surgery of the oesophagus.

oesophă·goscope (G. *oisophagos*, gullet; *skopein*, to view). An instrument for the endoscopic examination of the oesophagus.

oesophă·gospasm (G. *oisophagos*, gullet; *spasmos*, spasm). Oesophagismus, *q.v.*

oesŏ·phagostenō·sis (G. *oisophagos*, gullet; *stenōsis*, constriction). Constriction of the oesophagus.

oesophagŏ·stoma (G. *oisophagos*, gullet; *stoma*, mouth). An abnormal opening into the oesophagus.

oesŏ·phagostomi·asis. Infestation with the oesophagostomum.

Oesophagŏ·stomum (G. *oisophagos*, gullet; *stoma*, mouth). A genus of nematode worms of the Strongylidae family.

oesophagŏ·stomy (G. *oisophagos*, gullet; *stoma*, mouth). The formation of an artificial opening in the oesophagus.

oesophagŏ·tomy (G. *oisophagos*, gullet; *tomē*, section). Opening of the oesophagus by an incision.

oesŏ·phagus (G. *oisophagos*). The gullet; the musculomembranous canal, some nine inches in length, reaching from the pharynx to the stomach.

oestradi·ol (G. *oistros*, gadfly, orgasm). The hormone contained in the Graafian follicles. **Oe. benzoate:** benzoate salt of oestradiol. **Oe. dipropionate:** the double ester of oestradiol and propionic acid.

oe·strin (G. *oistros*, gadfly, orgasm). The name originally given to the active principles present in alcoholic extracts from the ovary.

oe·striol (G. *oistros*, gadfly, orgasm). A substance obtained from placental tissue and pregnancy urine. Syn. trihydroxyoestrin.

oes·trone (G. *oistros*, gadfly, orgasm). Female sex hormones, secreted by the Graafian follicle, inducing the development of secondary female sex characters, endometrial proliferation and changes in the vaginal mucosa.

oes·trum, oes·trus (G. *oistros*, gadfly, orgasm). Sexual desire, especially the periodic sexual desire in female animals.

offi·cial (L. *officium*, duty). Of medicines, those described in the national pharmacopoeia.

offi·cinal (L. *officina*, shop). For sale in shops; kept on sale in a pharmacy.

Ogston's line (Ogston, A., Scottish surgeon, 1844–1929). An imaginary line from the tuberosity of the ischium to the intercondyloid notch of the femur. **O.'s operation:** (1) Removal of inner condyle of femur for knock-knee. (2) Excision of wedge of tarsus to restore arch in flat foot.

Ogston-Luc operation (Ogston, A., Scottish surgeon, 1844–1929; Luc, H., French laryngologist, 1855–1925). An operation for frontal sinus disease through an incision over the edge of the orbit.

ohm (Ohm, G. S., German physicist, 1787–1854). The unit of electrical resistance; the resistance of a mercury column of 106·3 cm. length, of 14·45 grm. mass and constant cross section to electric current.

Ohm's law. The intensity of an electric current is directly proportional to the electromotive force and inversely proportional to the resistance of the circuit.

Oïd·iomycē·tes (G. *oidion*, dim. of *ōon*, egg; *mukēs*, mushroom). A genus of fungi.

oïd·iomycō·sia (G. *oidion*, dim. of *ōon*, egg; *mukēs*, mushroom). A disease produced by yeast-fungi of the genus Oidium.

Oïd·ium (G. *oidion*, dim. of *ōon*, egg). A genus of fungi. *O. albicans*; the common cause of thrush. Syn. *Monilia albicans. Candida albicans.*

oils (L. *oleum*, oil, from *olea*, an olive). Liquid esters of various fatty acids with glycerol.

ointment (L. *unguentum*). A fatty material, usually impregnated with some medicinal substance, for external use.

Oken's body (Oken, L., German physiologist, 1779–1851). The Wolffian body.

o.l. Abbreviation for L. *oculus laevus*, the left eye.

Ol. Abbreviation for L. *oleum*, oil.

ō·lea (L.). 1. Olive. 2. Plural of *oleum*, oil.

olĕa·ginous (L. *oleum*, oil). Oily.

ō·leate (L. *oleum*, oil). 1. Any compound of an alkaloid or a metal with oleic acid. 2. A suspension of a drug in oleic acid.

olĕ·cranal (G. *ōlenē*, elbow; *kranion*, skull). Relating to the olecranon.

olĕ·cranoid (G. *ōlenē*, elbow; *kranion*, skull; *eidos*, form). Resembling the olecranon.

olĕ·cranon (G. *ōlenē*, elbow; *kranion*, skull). The point at the upper end of the ulna.

olĕ·fiant (L. *oleum*, oil; *facere*, to make). Making oil. **O. gas:** ethylene.

ō·lefine (L. *oleum*, oil). Any unsaturated hydrocarbon of the formula C_nH_{2n}.

olĕ·ic acid. $C_{18}H_{34}O_2$; an unsaturated fatty acid present as the glyceride in many oils and fats.

ō·lĕin (L. *oleum*, oil). Glyceryl trioleate, a neutral fat, occurring in olive oil, butter and other animal and vegetable fats.

oleo-infusion (L. *oleum*, oil; *infusio*, a watering). An oily infusion of a drug.

olĕō·meter (L. *oleum*, oil; G. *metron*, measure). An instrument used in estimating the purity of oils.

oleorĕ·sin (L. *oleum*, oil; *rēsīna*, resin). A combination of resinous substances and essential oils.

olĕō·sus (L. *oleum*, oil). Oily.

oleothō·rax (L. *oleum*, oil; G. *thōrax*, chest). Introduction of an oily liquid into the pleural cavity for obtaining pulmonary collapse.

ō·leum (L.). Oil.

olfac·tion (L. *olfacere*, to smell). The sense or function of smelling.

olfactō·meter (L. *olfacere*, to smell; G. *metron*, measure). An instrument for measuring the threshold of olfactory stimuli.

olfactō·metry (L. *olfacere*, to smell; G. *metron*, measure). Estimation of olfactory sensibility.

olfac·tory (L. *olfacere*, to smell). Relating to the sense of smell. **O. area:** the cerebral area containing the nuclei of the o. nerve. Also called o. centre. **O. bulb:** the anterior end of the o. tract. **O. bundle:** a bundle of fibres in the fornix dividing at the locus perforatus anterior and passing to the o. tract and the uncus. **O. cells:** the peripheral end-organ of the o. nerve. **O. centre:** see o. area. **O. lobe:** the cerebral region beneath the frontal lobe. **O. nerve:** the nerve transmitting the perception of odour; the first cranial nerve. **O. tract:** a bundle of fibres in the lower surface of the frontal lobe, terminating in the o. bulb and in the o. trigone. **O. trigone:** an area above the optic nerve near the chiasma.

oligae·mia (G. *oligos*, few; *haima*, blood). A condition in which the quantity of the blood is diminished.

olighi·dria, oligi·dria (G. *oligos*, few; *hidrōs*, sweat). Deficiency of perspiration.

ŏ·ligochō·lia (G. *oligos*, few; *khŏlē*, bile). Deficiency of bile.

ŏ·ligocythae·mia (G. *oligos*, few; *kutos*, cell; *haima*, blood). A deficiency of erythrocytes in the blood.

ŏ·ligodactȳ·lia, oligodac·tyly (G. *oligos*, few; *daktulos*, finger). Congenital absence of one or more fingers or toes.

ŏ·ligoden·drocyte (G. *oligos*, few; *dendron*, tree; *kutos*, cell). Non-nervous cells of supporting type believed to take part in the formation of myelin material which sheaths the nerve fibres.

ŏ·ligodendro·glia (G. *oligos*, few; *dendron*, tree; *glia*, glue). A type of glial cells, characterized by roundish shape, small nucleus and long and often ramified processes.

ŏ·ligodendroglīō·ma (G. *oligos*, few; *dendron*, tree; *glia*, glue). A type of cerebral tumour, arising from oligodendroglia, occurring in the white matter of the cerebral hemispheres.

ŏ·ligodynam·ic (G. *oligos*, few; *dunamis*, power). Active in minute quantity; applied to the property of extremely dilute solutions of heavy metals to inhibit fermentation and bacterial growth.

ŏ·ligogalac·tia (G. *oligos*, few; *gala*, milk). Deficiency in the secretion of milk.

ŏ·ligohae·mia (G. *oligos*, few; *haima*, blood). Oligaemia, *q.v.*

ŏ·ligohydram·nios (G. *oligos*, few; *hudōr*, water; *amnion*, the membrane round the foetus). A deficiency in the quantity of amniotic fluid.

ŏ·ligŏ·melus (G. *oligos*, few; *melos*, limb). Congenital absence of a limb.

ŏ·ligomenorrhoe·a (G. *oligos*, few; *mēn*, month; *rhoia*, flow). Insufficiency of the menstrual flow.

ŏ·ligopnoe·a (G. *oligos*, few; *pnŏē*, breath). Diminished frequency of respiration.

ŏ·ligopy·rene (G. *oligos*, few; *purēn*, fruit-stone). Applied to abnormal spermatozoa in which only a part of the chromosome group enters the nucleus.

ŏ·ligosper·mia (G. *oligos*, few; *sperma*, sperm). Deficiency in the secretion of semen or in the number of sperms in the semen.

ŏ·ligotrĭ·chia (G. *oligos*, few; *thrix*, hair). Scantiness of hair.

oligū·ria (G. *oligos*, few; *ouron*, urine). A diminution in urinary secretion.

olī·va (L., olive). The olivary body.

ŏ·livary (L. *oliva*, olive). 1. Like an olive in shape. 2. The olivary body, an oval mass of grey matter behind the anterior pyramid of the medulla.

olive. The fruit of the tree *Olea europaea*.

Ollier's disease (Ollier, L. L. X. E., French surgeon, 1830–1901). Achondroplasia. **O.'s layer:** the osteogenetic layer of the periosteum.

Ollier-Thiersch's method of skin-grafting (Ollier, L. L. X. E., French surgeon, 1830–1901; Thiersch, K., German surgeon, 1822–95). See under Thiersch.

Ol. oliv. Abbreviation for L. *oleum olivae*, olive oil.

olophō·nia (G. *ŏloos*, destructive; *phŏnē*, voice). Abnormal speech caused by malformation of the vocal organs.

o.m. Abbreviation for L. *omni mane*, each morning.

-oma. A concrete suffix indicating a material feature produced by a certain condition; in particular, a tumour.

omacĕ·phalus (G. *ōmos*, shoulder; *a*, neg.; *kephalē*, head). A monster characterized by absence of head and upper extremities.

omă·gra (G. *ōmos*, shoulder; *agra*, seizure). Gout of the shoulder-joint.

omal·gia (G. *ōmos*, shoulder; *algos*, pain). Pain in the shoulder.

omarthrī·tis (G. *ōmos*, shoulder; *arthron*, joint). Inflammation of the shoulder-joint.

omen·tal (L. *omentum*, caul). Relating to the omentum.

omentec·tomy (L. *omentum*; G. *ektomē*, excision). Removal of the omentum.

omenti·tis (L. *omentum*). Inflammation of the omentum.

omen·topexy (L. *omentum*; G. *pēxis*, fixation). Surgical fixation of the omentum to some other part, e.g. to the abdominal wall or to the pericardium, made to establish a new collateral circulation.

omen·tum (L.). Peritoneal folds extending between the stomach and other abdominal organs. 1. Greater (gastro-colic) omentum which is the fold extending from the greater curvature of the stomach to envelop the transverse colon. 2. Lesser (gastro-hepatic) omentum; the fold joining the lesser curvature of the stomach to the transverse fissure of the liver. 3. Gastro-splenic omentum: fold of peritoneum connecting stomach and spleen.

omentumec·tomy (L. *omentum*, G. *ektomē*, excision). Surgical removal of the omentum.

omi·tis (G. *ōmos*, shoulder). Inflammation of the shoulder.

ommati·dium (G. *omma*, eye). The functionally associated group of cells, the functional unit of the compound eye of invertebrate animals.

omn. hor. Abbreviation for L. *omni hora*, each hour.

omni·vorous (L. *omnis*, all; *vorare*, to eat). Subsisting on both animal and vegetable food.

omn. noct. Abbreviation for L. *omni nocte*, each night.

omocĕ·phalus (G. *ōmos*, shoulder; *kephalē*, head). A monster without arms and with an incomplete head.

omodў·nia (G. *ōmos*, shoulder; *odunē*, pain). Pain in the shoulder.

omohў·oid (G. *ōmos*, shoulder; *huoeidēs*, shaped like the letter y). Relating both to the scapula and the hyoid bone.

ō·moplate (G. *ōmos*, shoulder; *platē*, flat surface). The scapula.

omphalec·tomy (G. *omphalos*, navel; *ektomē*, excision). Excision of the umbilicus.

omphal·ic (G. *omphalos*, navel). Relating to the umbilicus.

omphali·tis (G. *omphalos*, navel). Inflammation of the umbilicus.

omphă·locele (G. *omphalos*, navel; *kēlē*, hernia). Umbilical hernia.

omphă·locyte (G. *omphalos*, navel; *sitos*, food). A monster characterized by absence of the heart, receiving its blood-supply through the umbilical vessels. Death occurs when the navel cord is severed.

om·phalomesentĕ·ric (G. *omphalos*, navel; *mesos*, middle; *enteron*, intestine). Relating both to the umbilicus and to the mesentery.

omphalo·pagus (G. *omphalos*, navel; *pēgnunai*, to make fast). A double monster joined at the umbilicus.

om·phalophlebi·tis (G. *omphalos*, navel; *phleps*, vein). Inflammation of the umbilical vein.

om·phalorrhă·gia (G. *omphalos*, navel; *rhēgnunai*, to break out). Haemorrhage from the umbilicus.

om·phalorrhœ·a (G. *omphalos*, navel; *rhoia*, flow). An effusion of lymph at the umbilicus.

om·phalos (G). The umbilicus.

omphalŏ·tomy (G. *omphalos*, navel; *tomē*, section). The cutting of the navel cord.

om. quar. hor. Abbreviation for L. *omni quadranti hora*, each quarter of an hour.

o.n. Abbreviation for L. *omni nocte*, each night.

ō·nanism (From Onan, son of Judah). Masturbation.

Onanoff's reflex (Onanoff, J., French physician, born 1859). Contraction of the bulbocavernous muscle on pressure of the glans penis.

Onchocer·ca (G. *ogkos*, mass; *kerkos*, tail). A genus of filariidae.

on·chocerci·asis, on·chocercŏ·sis (G. *ogkos*, mass; *kerkos*, tail). The condition produced by infestation with Onchocerca.

on·cocyte (G. *ogkos*, mass; *kutos*, cell). Any tumour cell.

oncŏ·graphy (G. *ogkos*, mass; *graphein*, to write). The recording of measurements by an oncometer.

oncŏ·logy (G. *ogkos*, mass; *logos*, discourse). The part of pathology dealing with tumours.

oncŏ·lysis (G. *ogkos*, mass; *lusis*, dissolution). The destroying of tumour cells.

oncŏ·ma (G. *ogkōma*, a swelling). A swelling or tumour.

oncŏ·meter (G. *ogkos*, mass; *metron*, measure). An instrument for determining variations in the volume of an organ.

oncŏ·sis (G. *ogkos*, mass). 1. A state characterized by the growth of tumours. 2. Tumefaction.

on·cosphere (G. *ogkos*, mass; *sphaira*, a ball). The embryo of a tapeworm.

oncŏ·tomy (G. *ogkos*, mass; *tomē*, section). The incision of an abscess or other swelling.

ondŏ·meter (Fr. *onde*, wave; G. *metron*, measure). Apparatus used for estimation of wavelength of electro-magnetic radiations associated with oscillating currents particularly of high frequency. English equivalent is wavemeter.

onei·ric (G. *oneiros*, dream). Relating to dreams.

onei·rism (G. *oneiros*, dream). A waking dream state.

o·neirodў·nia (G. *oneiros*, dream; *odunē*, pain). Nightmare.

oneirŏ·logy (G. *oneiros*, dream; *logos*, a discourse). The study of dreams.

ō·niomā·nia (G. *ōnios*, for sale; *mania*, madness). Neurotic or psychotic desire to make unnecessary purchases.

onion. The bulb of the *Allium cepa*.

onomatomā·nia (G. *onoma*, name; *mania*, madness). An obsession relating to words.

ontogĕ·nesis (G. *ōn*, existing; *gennan*, to produce). The development of the individual organism or of an organ or function in an individual.

on·togenet·ic (G. *ōn*, existing; *gennan*, to produce). Relating to ontogenesis.

ontŏ·geny (G. *ōn*, existing; *gennan*, to produce). The development of an individual from the fertilized egg to maturity.

onychă·trophy (G. *onux*, finger-nail; *atrophia*, atrophy). Atrophy of the nails.

onychaux·is (G. *onux*, finger-nail; *auxein*, to increase). Hypertrophy of the nail-plate.

onychec·tomy (G. *onux*, finger-nail; *ektomē*, excision). Surgical removal of a nail.

onў·chia (G. *onux*, finger-nail). Inflammation of the matrix of a nail.

onychi·tis (G. *onux*, finger-nail). Onychia, *q.v.*

ō·nychocryptŏ·sis (G. *onux*, finger-nail; *kruptos*, concealed). Ingrowing nails.

ō·nychogryphŏ·sis, ō·nychogrypŏ·sis (the latter is the correct form). (G. *onux*, finger-nail; *grupōsis*, a hooking). Hypertrophy resulting in a claw-like deformation of the nails.

ō·nychoid (G. *onux*, finger-nails; *eidos*, form). Resembling a nail.

onychŏ·lysis (G. *onux*, finger-nail; *lusis*, dissolution). Loosening of the nail from its bed.

ō·nychomadē·sis (G. *onux*, finger-nail; *madesis*, a becoming bald). A disorder of nail-growth characterized by periodic or intermittent shedding of one or more nails.

ō·nychomalā·cia (G. *onux*, finger-nail; *malakia*, softness). Abnormal softening of the nails.

ō·nychomycŏ·sis (G. *onux*, finger-nails; *mukēs*, mushroom). Disease of the nails due to parisitic fungi, such as trichophyton. Syn. tinea unguium.

onychŏ·phagy (G. *onux*, finger-nail; *phagein*, to eat). The neurotic habit of biting the nails.

ō·nychorhex·is (G. *onux*, finger-nails; *rhēxis*, a breaking). Abnormal brittleness of the nails.

onychŏ·schisis (G. *onux*, fingernail; *skhizein*, to separate). Partial or complete separation of the nails at the free end or matrix.

onychŏ·sis (G. *onux*, finger-nail). Any disease of the nails.

ō·nyx (G. *onux*, finger-nail). 1. A nail of the fingers or toes. 2. An obsolete term for hypopyon, which was formerly thought to lie between the corneal lamellae at the most dependent part.

onyx·is (G. *onux*, finger-nail). A condition of congenital ingrowing nails.

ō·oblast (G. *ōon*, egg; *blastos*, germ). A cell of the germinal epithelium of the ovarium.

ōocȳē·sis (G. *ōon*, egg; *kuēsis*, conception). Ovarian pregnancy.

ō·ocyst (G. *ōon*, egg; *kustis*, bladder). The encysted fertilized cell in sporozoa.

ō·ocyte (G. *ōon*, egg; *kutos*, cell). The egg-cell prior to completion of the maturation process. O., **primary**: the egg-cell containing chromatic material in the cytoplasm, prior to mitotic division. O., **secondary**: the larger of the two cells formed after mitotic division of the primary o.

ōō·deocele (G. *ōon*, egg; *eidos*, form; *kēlē*, hernia). Obturator hernia.

ōō·gamous (G. *ōon*, egg; *gamos*, marriage). Relating to oogamy.

ōō·gamy (G. *ōon*, egg; *gamos*, marriage). The conjugation of two gametes, dissimilar in size.

ōōgē·nesis (G. *ōon*, egg; *genesis*, reproduction). The development of the egg.

ōōgō·nium (G. *ōon*, egg; *gonē*, generation). A cell of the ovarian germinal epithelium, derived from the primordial germ-cell and giving rise to the primary oocyte.

ō·okinē·sis (G. *ōon*, egg; *kinein*, to move). The changes which take place in the egg during the processes of maturation, fertilization and segmentation.

ō·ōkinete (G. *ōon*, egg; *kinein*, to move). In sporozoa, the motile body into which the zygote develops prior to the oocyst stage.

ōōlem·ma (G. *ōon*, egg; *lemma*, sheath). The membrane surrounding the ovum. Syn. zona pellucida.

ōō·phagy (G. *ōon*, egg; *phagein*, to eat). Egg-eating.

ōōphorec·tomy (G. *ōon*, egg; *pherein*, to bear; *ektomē*, excision). Ovarectomy.

ōōphori·tis (G. *ōon*, egg; *pherein*, to bear). Inflammation of the ovary.

ōō·phorohysterec·tomy (G. *ōon*, egg; *pherein*, to bear; *hustera*, womb; *ektomē*, excision). Excision of the uterus and the ovaries.

ōō·phoromalā·cia (G. *ōon*, egg; *pherein*, to bear; *malakia*, softness). Softening of an ovary.

ōō·phoron (G. *ōon*, egg; *pherein*, to bear). The ovary.

ōō·phorŏ·pathy (G. *ōon*, egg; *pherein*, to bear; *pathos*, disease). Any ovarian disease.

ōō·phoropexy (G. *ōon*, egg; *pherein*, to bear; *pēxis*, fixation). Operation whereby ovary is fixed higher in the pelvis than it is found lying.

ōō·phoroplasty (G. *ōon*, egg; *pherein*, to bear; *plassein*, to form). Plastic surgery of the ovaries.

ōō·phorosalpingec·tomy (G. *ōon*, egg; *pherein*, to bear; *salpigx*, tube; *ektomē*, excision). Excision of the ovary and oviduct.

ōō·phorosalpingi·tis. Salpingo-oophoritis, *q.v.*

ō·ōplasm (G. *ōon*, egg; *plassein*, to form). The cytoplasm of the oocyte.

ō·ōtid (G. *ōon*, egg). The egg subsequent to meiosis.

ōōxan·thine (G. *ōon*, egg; *xanthos*, yellow). The yellow pigment of egg-shells.

opā·city (L. *opacitas*, shadiness). 1. The state of being impervious to light. 2. An opaque spot, e.g., o. of the cornea.

opales·cence (G. *opallios*, an opal). An iridescent reflection of light, e.g. from a solution.

opaque (L. *opacus*, shady). Impervious to light; not transparent.

open. 1. Exposed to the air. 2. Interrupted.

ŏ·perable (L. *operari*, to work). Capable of being operated upon with some prospect of improvement.

operā·tion (L. *operari*, to work). 1. Anything done or performed. 2. A method of doing anything. 3. A surgical procedure.

ŏ·perative (L. *operari*, to work). 1. Effective. 2. Relating to operations.

ŏ·perator (L. from *opus*, work). A surgeon.

oper·cular (L. *operculum*, from *operire*, to cover). 1. Relating to an operculum. 2. Designed for closure of a cavity.

oper·culum (L.). 1. A cover or lid. 2. The cerebral convolutions covering the island of Reil.

ophi·asis (G. *ophis*, snake). The type of alopecia areata involving the margin of the scalp.

ophĭ·diophō·bia (G. *ophis*, snake; *phobos*, fear). A neurotic fear of snakes.

ō·phiotoxae̅·mia (G. *ophis*, snake; *toxikon*, poison; *haima*, blood). Poisoning caused by the venom of serpents.

ō·phryon (G. *ophrus*, eyebrow). The centre of the glabella.

ophthalmal·gia (G. *ophthalmos*, eye; *algos*, pain). Eye pain.

oph·thalmă·trophy (G. *ophthalmos*, eye; *atrophia*, atrophy). Atrophy of the eyeball.

ophthalmec·tomy (G. *ophthalmos*, eye; *ektomē*, excision). Surgical removal of the eye.

ophthalmencĕ·phalon (G. *ophthalmos*, eye; *egkephalos*, brain). The whole visual apparatus from retina to visual centres in the brain.

ophthal·mia (G. *ophthalmos*, eye). Inflammation of the eye, especially that form in which the conjunctiva is involved. O. **neonatorum**: purulent, especially gonorrhoeal, conjunctivitis of the newborn.

ophthal·mic (G. *ophthalmos*, eye). Relating to the eye.

ophthalmī·tis (G. *ophthalmos*, eye). Inflammation of the eye. **Sympathetic o.**: that which follows inflammation of or injury to the fellow-eye.

ophthal·moblenorrhoe̅·a (G. *ophthalmos*, eye; *blenna*, mucus; *rhoia*, flow). Conjunctivitis.

ophthal·mocarcinō·ma (G. *ophthalmos*, eye; *karkinos*, crab). Cancer of the eye.

ophthal·modiaphan·oscope (G. *ophthalmos*, eye; *dia*, through; *phainein*, to show; *skopein*, to view). An instrument devised for the examination of the fundus of the eye, by means of illumination through the mouth.

ophthal·modynamŏ·meter (G. *ophthalmos*, eye; *dunamis*, power; *metron*, measure). An instrument which is used to measure the power of convergence of the eyes.

ophthalmofun·doscope (G. *ophthalmos*, eye; L. *fundus*, bottom; G. *skopein*, to view). An instrument used for examining the fundus of the eye.

ophthal·mograph (G. *ophthalmos*, eye; *graphein*, to write). An instrument for photographing eye movements during reading.

ophthalmŏ·logist (G. *ophthalmos*, eye; *logos*, a discourse). A specialist in ophthalmology.

ophthalmŏ·logy (G. *ophthalmos*, eye; *logos*, discourse). The part of medicine relating to the eye.

ophthal·momalā·cia (G. *ophthalmos*, eye; *malakia*, softness). Abnormal softness and shrinkage of the eye with less than normal tension; essential phthisis of the eye.

ophthalmŏ·meter (G. *ophthalmos*, eye; *metron*, measure). 1. An instrument for measuring the corneal curvatures. 2. An instrument for measuring the capacity of the chambers of the eye.

ophthal·momĕ·troscope (G. *ophthalmos*, eye; *metron*, measure; *skopein*, to view). An ophthalmoscope with an attachment for measuring the refraction of the eye.

ophthalmŏ·metry (G. *ophthalmos*, eye; *metron*, measure). The determination of errors of refraction by means of the ophthalmometer (1).

ophthal·momyŏ·tomy (G. *ophthalmos*, eye; *mus*, muscle; *tomē*, section). Division of the eye muscles.

ophthalmŏ·pathy (G. *ophthalmos*, eye; *pathos*, disease). Any disease of the eye.

ophthal·mophakŏ·meter (G. *ophthalmos*, eye; *phakos*, a lentil; *metron*, measure). An apparatus for measuring the curvature radius of the crystalline lens.

ophthalmoph·tl.is'is (G. *ophthalmos*, eye; *phthisis*, a wasting). Ophthalmomalacia, *q.v.*

ophthal·moplasty (G. *ophthalmos*, eye; *plassein*, to form). Plastic surgery of the eye.

ophthalmoplē·gia (G. *ophthalmos*, eye; *plēgē*, stroke). Paralysis of the eye muscles. O. externa: paralysis of the external muscles of the eye. O. interna: paralysis of the internal eye muscles.

ophthal·mo-reaction. The reaction of the conjunctiva to a tuberculin test, performed by instillation of one drop of a certain tuberculin solution into the eye.

ophthalmorrhā·gia (G. *ophthalmos*, eye; *rhēgnunai*, to burst out). Haemorrhage of the eye.

ophthalmorrhex·is (G. *ophthalmos*, eye; *rhēxis*, rupture). Rupture of the eyeball.

ophthal·moscope (G. *ophthalmos*, eye; *skopein*, to view). An instrument for illumination and inspection of the interior of the eye. It consists of a perforated mirror reflecting light through the pupil of the eye; the light is reflected back from the ocular background through the hole of the mirror into the observer's eye.

ophthalmŏ·scopy (G. *ophthalmos*, eye; *skopein*, to view). The examination of the interior of the eye by means of the ophthalmoscope. **Direct o.**: the method by which the observer closely approaches the patient's eye, obtaining an erect, magnified image of the fundus. **Indirect o.**: in which the observer is placed about one yard from the patient and, placing a strong convex lens between observer and patient, obtains an inverted, magnified image of the fundus.

ophthalmŏ·stasis (G. *ophthalmos*, eye; *stasis*, a standing). Fixation of the eye during an ophthalmic operation.

ophthal·mostatŏ·meter (G. *ophthalmos*, eye; *statos*, standing; *metron*, measure). An apparatus for determining the position of the eyes.

ophthal·mothermŏ·meter (G. *ophthalmos*, eye; *thermē*, heat; *metron*, measure). An instrument for measuring the temperature of the eye.

ophthal·motonŏ·meter (G. *ophthalmos*, eye; *tonos*, tone; *metron*, measure). An instrument for measuring intra-ocular tension.

ophthal·motonŏ·metry (G. *ophthalmos*, eye; *tonos*, tone; *metron*, measure). Measurement of intra-ocular tension.

ophthal·motrope (G. *ophthalmos*, eye; *trepein*, to turn). An apparatus for demonstrating the action of the individual ocular muscles.

ophthal·motropŏ·meter (G. *ophthalmos*, eye; *trepein*, to turn; *metron*, measure). An instrument used in measuring the movements of the eyeballs.

ophthal·motropŏ·metry (G. *ophthalmos*, eye; *trepein*, to turn; *metron*, measure). Measurement of the movements of the eyeballs.

ō·piate (G. *ŏpion*, opium). A preparation of opium.

ō·piomā·nia (G. *ŏpion*, opium). Addiction to opium.

opiŏ·phagism (G. *ŏpion*, opium; *phagein*, to eat). Opium-eating.

opis·thion (G. *opisthen*, in the rear). The middle point of the posterior edge of the foramen magnum.

opisthŏ·gnathism (G. *opisthen*, in the rear; *gnathos*, jaw). Recession of the lower jaw.

opisthorchī·asis (G. *opisthen*, in the rear; *orkhis*, testicle). The condition resulting from infestation with Opisthorchis.

Opisthor·chis (G. *opisthen*, in the rear; *orkhis*, testicle). A genus of the class of Trematoda; its usual habitat is liver and bile-duct.

opisthŏ·tonoid (G. *opisthen*, in the rear; *tonos*, tone; *eidos*, form). Resembling opisthotonos.

opisthŏ·tonos (G. *opisthen*, in the rear; *tonos*, tone). Tetanic spasm of the muscles of the back, resulting in backward retraction of the head and lower limbs.

ō·pium (G. *ŏpion*, opium). The inspissated juice of the poppy, *Papaver somniferum*. It is obtained by incision of the unripe capsules.

opium habit. Addiction to opium; the habitual taking of opium.

ō·piumism (G. *ŏpion*, opium). 1. The opium habit. 2. Chronic opium-poisoning.

opocĕ·phalus (G. *ōps*, eye; *kephalē*, head). A monster characterized by fusion of both ears and eyes and absence of nose and mouth.

opodi·dymus (G. *ōps*, eye; *didumos*, twin). A double monster with a single body and two heads which are fused at the posterior part but separated at the front.

opotherapeu·tic (G. *opos*, juice; *therapeia*, treatment). Organotherapeutic, *q.v.*

Oppenheim's disease (Oppenheim, H., German neurologist, 1858–1919). Syn. amyotonia congenita, myatonia congenita.

Oppenheim's gait (Oppenheim, H., German neurologist, 1858–1919). A modification of the spastic gait of disseminated sclerosis, in which there are large and irregular oscillations of the head, trunk and extremities.

oppō·nens (L. *opponere*, to oppose). Opposite.

opsi·nogens (G. *opsōnion*, victuals; *gennan*, to produce). Substances producing opsonin.

opsomā·nia (G. *opson*, cooked food; *mania*, madness). Craving for some special food.

opson·ic (G. *opsōnion*, victuals). Relating to opsonins. O. index: the ratio of the number of bacteria devoured by the white blood cells of a healthy person compared with that consumed by those of the patient. O. negative phase: the decrease in o. power that follows inoculation of dead bacteria. O. positive phase: the increase of o. power following the negative phase.

op·sonin (G. *opson*, victuals). A thermolabile substance present in serum, promoting phagocytosis of bacteria.

opsonothē·rapy (G. *opsōnion*, victuals; *therapeia*, treatment). The treatment of bacterial diseases by injecting vaccine of the particular micro-organism in order to increase the content of opsonin in the blood.

op·tic (G. *optikos*, of or for vision). Relating to vision or to optics. O. atrophy: atrophy of the o. nerve. O. axis: the line joining the centres of curvature of the refracting surfaces of an optical system. O. chiasma: the junction and partial decussation of the two o. nerves, situated behind the tuberculum sellae and in front of the tuber cinereum. O. cup: the secondary o. vesicle. O. disc: the eminence formed on the retina by nerve-fibres which from here onwards form in their centripetal course the o. nerve. O. foramen: the oval opening at the apex of the orbital roof. O. nerve: the second cranial nerve. O. neuritis: inflammation of the o. nerve. O. pit: one of the two lateral pouches of the anterior end of the neural tube. O. plate: the embryonic structure at the anterior end of the neural fold from which the retina develops. O. thalamus: the two large nuclei of grey matter situated at the base of the brain upon either side of the third ventricle, caudal and medial to the corpus striatum. O. tract: the band-like structure containing mainly the fibres of the o. nerves, starting at the o. chiasma and splitting into its two roots at the o. thalamus. O. vesicle, primary: the embryonic structure from which the eye develops. O. vesicle, secondary: the embryonic structure following invagination of the primary o. vesicle.

op·tical (G. *optikos*, of or for vision). Optic, *q.v.* **O. activity**: the property of a substance or solution to rotate the plane of polarized light to the left or to the right.

opti·cian (G. *optikos*, of or for vision). A maker of optical instruments.

op·tics (G. *optikos*, of or for vision). The branch of physics relating to light.

op·timum (L. *optimus*, best). The most favourable condition, e.g. the temperature most suitable for a particular function.

op·togram (G. *optos*, seen; *gramma*, mark). A photographic image on the retina after death, due to the bleaching effect of light rays on the visual purple.

optŏ·meter (G. *optos*, seen; *metron*, measure). An instrument for determining the visual acuity, especially the degree of refractive power.

optŏ·metry (G. *optos*, seen; *metron*, measure). The measurement of visual powers.

optostri·ate (G. *optos*, seen; L. *striatus*, from *stria*, a furrow). Relating to the optic thalamus and the corpus striatum.

or·a (L. border). Margin. **O. serrata**: the serrated anterior margin of the retina.

or·al (L. *os*, mouth). Relating to the mouth.

orange. The fruit of the tree *Citrus aurantium*.

orbi·cular (L. *orbiculus*, dim. of *orbis*, circle). Circular; a term applied to circular muscles, e.g. the o. muscle of the mouth.

or·biculā·ris (L.). Circular muscles. See orbicularis oris and orbicularis palpebrarum, under muscle.

orbi·culus ciliā·ris (L.). Ciliary ring, a narrow zone lying anterior to the choroid of the eye.

or·bit (L. *orbita*, from *orbis*, sphere). The bony cavity containing the eyeball, with the ocular muscles, nerves and blood vessels, the lacrimal gland, and a large amount of fat. It presents an apex, a base, and four sides or walls.

or·bita (L.). The orbit.

or·bital (L. *orbita*, a circular track). Relating to the orbit.

or·cëin. A brown colouring matter $C_{28}H_{24}N_2O_7$ from lichens and by treatment of orcinol. Used as a stain.

or·cin, or·cinol. An antiseptic principle $CH_3C_6H_3$. $(OH)_2$ obtained synthetically and from lichens. It is a cardiac poison and an antiseptic and is used like resorcinol in skin diseases.

orchec·tomy (G. *orkhis*, testicle; *ektomē*, excision). Orchidectomy, *q.v.*

or·cheoplasty (G. *orkhis*, testicle; *plassein*, to form). Orchioplasty, *q.v.*

orchial·gia (G. *orkhis*, testicle; *algos*, pain). Pain in the testicle.

orchidec·tomy (G. *orkhis*, testicle; *ektomē*, excision). Orchiectomy, *q.v.*

orchidopex·ia, orchi·dopexy (G. *orkhis*, testicle; *pēxis*, fixation). Orchiorrhaphy, *q.v.*

orchidor·rhaphy (G. *orkhis*, testicle; *rhaphē*, suture). Orchiorrhaphy, *q.v.*

orchidŏ·tomy (G. *orkhis*, testicle; *tomē*, section). Orchiotomy, *q.v.*

orchiëc·tomy (G. *orkhis*, testicle; *ektomē*, excision). Excision of a testicle.

or·chiĕpididymi·tis (G. *orkhis*, testicle; *epi*, upon; *didumos*, twin). Inflammation of both testis and epididymis.

or·chiocele (G. *orkhis*, testicle; *kēlē*, hernia). Scrotal hernia.

or·chiody·nia (G. *orkhis*, testicle; *odunē*, pain). Pain in the testicles.

or·chiopexy (G. *orkhis*, testicle; *pēxis*, fixation). Orchiorrhaphy, *q.v.*

or·chioplasty (G. *orkhis*, testicle; *plassein*, to form). Any plastic operation on the scrotum.

orchiŏr·rhaphy (G. *orkhis*, testicle; *rhaphē*, suture). Surgical fixation of the testicle to the scrotum.

orchiŏ·tomy (G. *orkhis*, testicle; *tomē*, section). Incision of the testicle.

or·chis (G. *orkhis*, testicle). The testicle.

orchit·ic (G. *orkhis*, testicle). Relating to orchitis.

orchi·tis (G. *orkhis*, testicle). Inflammation of the testicle.

orchŏ·tomy (G. *orkhis*, testicle; *tomē*, section). Castration.

order (L. *ordo*). In the classification of species, a group higher than family and lower than class.

or·dinate (L. *ordinare*, to dispose). The vertical axis in a chart.

orf. A popular name in Scotland for an infectious pustular dermatitis of sheep, transmissible to man and caused by a filtrable virus.

or·gan (G. *organon*, implement). Any part of the body characterized by a particular function.

organelle (G. *organon*, implement). Any one of those parts of a unicellular organism possessing a special function.

organ·ic (G. *organon*, implement). 1. Relating to an organ or substance derived from an organism. 2. Relating to the animal and vegetable worlds. 3. Affecting the structure of organs. **O. chemistry**: that part of chemistry relating to carbon compounds.

or·ganism (G. *organon*, implement). A structure composed of one or more cells.

organizā·tion (G. *organon*, implement). Any structure characterized by differentiated functions.

or·ganizer (G. *organon*, implement). A group of cells within the ovum characterized by the property of being able to influence the development of neighbouring parts in a certain way.

or·ganogĕ·nesis (G. *organon*, implement; *gennan*, to produce). The process of development of an organ.

or·ganon (G.). 1. An organ, *q.v.* 2. A code of principles.

organŏ·pathy (G. *organon*, implement; *pathos*, disease). Any organic disease.

or·ganotherapeu·tic (G. *organon*, implement; *therapeuein*, to treat). Relating to organotherapy.

or·ganothĕ·rapy (G. *organon*, implement; *therapeia*, treatment). The administration of preparations of animal organs for the treatment of diseases, especially of those believed to be due to diminished function of the analogous organ.

or·gasm (G. *organ*, to swell). The height of libidinous feeling, forming the culmination of the sexual act.

oriĕn·tal (L. *oriens*, east). Relating to the Orient or East. **O. sore**: Delhi Boil, Bagdad Boil, Aleppo Boil, or Lahore Sore. An indolent, ulcerating granuloma due to *Leishmania tropica*.

orientā·tion (L. *oriens*, east). 1. The act of determining the spatial or temporal relations of objects. 2. The ability to judge one's own spatial or temporal relations. 3. The relative position of the substitution elements or radicals in the benzene ring.

ŏ·rifice (L. L. *orificium*, from *os*, mouth; *facere*, to make). An opening.

orifi·cial. Relating to an orifice.

ŏ·rigin (L. *origo*, beginning). The starting-point of anything.

orinā·sal (L. *os*, mouth; *nasus*, nose). Oronasal *q.v.*

or·nithine (G. *ornis*, bird). A diamino acid, derived from arginine, one of the end-products of metabolism.

Or·nithodo·rus (G. *ornis*, bird; *dōron*, gift). A genus of ticks, transmitting the causal organism of relapsing fever.

orolin·gual (L. *os*, mouth; *lingua*, tongue). Relating to the mouth and the tongue.

oronā·sal (L. *os*, mouth; *nasus*, nose). Relating to the mouth and the nose.

oropharyn·geal (L. *os*, mouth; G. *pharugx*, throat). Relating to or situated in the oropharynx.

orophā·rynx (L. *os*, mouth; *pharugx*, throat). The pharynx proper, which lies below the lower border of the soft palate; see also nasopharynx.

Oroya fever. See fever, Oroya.

or·thobīō·sis (G. *orthos*, straight; *bios*, life). Healthy living.

or·thocaine. A white crystalline powder, methyl *m*-amino-*p*-hydroxybenzoate, having local analgesic and antiseptic properties.

or·thocephal·ic (G. *orthos*, straight; *kephalē*, head). Relating to orthocephaly.

orthoce·phaly (G. *orthos*, straight; *kephalē*, head). The state of having a cephalic height index, *q.v.*, between 70 and 75.

orthocre·sol. One of the three isomeric types of cresol, a deliquescent solid which melts at about 30° and boils at 191°. It is a valuable disinfectant.

or·thodi·agram (G. *orthos*, straight; *dia*, through; *gramma*, mark). The record made by an orthodiagraph.

orthodiā·graphy (G. *orthos*, straight; *dia*, through; *graphein*, to write). A method for determining size and shape of the heart by drawing its silhouette as visible on the fluorescent screen. The instrument used is the orthodiagraph, a radiographic apparatus.

orthodon·tia (G. *orthos*, straight; *odous*, tooth). The correction of irregularities in the teeth.

orthodon·tic. Relating to orthodontia.

orthodon·tics. The science or practice of orthodontia.

orthodon·tist. One skilled in orthodontia.

ortho·gnathism (G. *orthos*, straight; *gnathos*, jaw). The state of being orthognathous, i.e. having jaws with little or no forward projection.

orthŏ·gnathous (G. *orthos*, straight; *gnathos*, jaw). Having a gnathic index, *q.v.*, between 98 and 103.

orthŏ·meter (G. *orthos*, straight; *metron*, measure). An instrument for measuring the degree of exophthalmus.

orthopae·dic (G. *orthos*, straight; *pais*, child). Relating to the correction of deformities. **O. surgery:** that branch of surgery relating to the correction of deformities.

orthopae·dist (G. *orthos*, straight; *pais*, child). A specialist in orthopaedic surgery.

orthophor·ia (G. *orthos*, straight; *phoros*, bearing). Normal parallelism of the visual lines dependent on bifocal vision.

orthopnoē·a (G. *orthos*, straight; *pnoē*, breath). The highest degree of dyspnoea, *q.v.* in which relief is obtained only by maintaining an upright position.

Orthop·tera (G. *orthos*, straight; *pteron*, wing). An order of insects which includes locusts, grasshoppers, etc.

orthop·tic (G. *orthos*, straight; *optikos*, of or for sight). Relating to normal binocular vision. **O. training:** a method of correcting defective vision in strabismus or muscular imbalance by stereoscopic and other ocular exercises.

orthop·tist. One skilled in orthoptic training.

or·thoscope (G. *orthos*, straight; *skopein*, to view). 1. An instrument consisting of a box with glass sides filled with water, used to illuminate corneal refraction in ocular examination. 2. An instrument used in drawing the projections of skulls.

orthoscŏ·pic (G. *orthos*, straight; *skopein*, to view). 1. Relating to an orthoscope. 2. Term applied to lenses cut from the periphery of a large lens.

orthō·sis (G. *orthos*, straight). The correcting of a crooked part.

orthostā·tic (G. *orthos*, straight; *statos*, standing). Relating to or caused by standing upright. **O. albuminuria:** albuminuria occurring when the patient is in an upright position and disappearing when a horizontal position is taken; possibly related to the degree of lordosis appearing in the upright position. Syn. cyclic albuminuria.

orthŏ·tonus (G. *orthos*, straight; *tonos*, tone). A form of tetanic cramp, in which the patient lies rigid and stretched out.

Ory·za (G. *oruza*). Rice.

o.s. Abbreviation for oculus sinister, the left eye.

Os. The symbol for Osmium.

os¹. (L. *os*, bone; gen. *ossis*; pl. *ossa*). A bone.

ōs². (L. *os*, mouth; gen. *oris*; pl. *ora*). The mouth.

ō·sazone. A compound formed on heating a solution containing sugar with phenylhydrazine and dilute acetic acid.

oscē·do (L. *oscitare*, to yawn). 1. Yawning. 2. Aphthae.

os·cheal (G. *oskheon*, scrotum). Relating to the scrotum.

oschĕi·tis (G. *oskheon*, scrotum). Inflammation of the scrotum.

os·cheocele (G. *oskheon*, scrotum; *kēlē*, hernia). Scrotal hernia.

os·cheohȳ·drocele (G. *oskheon*, scrotum; *hudōr*, water; *kēlē*, hernia). A hydrocele occupying the sac of a scrotal hernia after the return of the bowel to the peritoneal cavity and the seclusion of the sac from the peritoneal cavity.

os·cheolith (G. *oskheon*, scrotum; *lithos*, stone). A concretion in the sebaceous glands of the scrotum.

oschĕō·ma (G. *oskheon*, scrotum). A scrotal tumour.

os·cheoplasty (G. *oskheon*, scrotum; *plassein*, to form). A plastic operation on the scrotum.

Oscilla·ria. A genus of Algae.

oscillā·tion (L. *oscillatio*, swinging). A swinging or vibration.

oscil·lograph (L. *oscillare*, to swing; G. *graphein*, to write). Any instrument recording wave-like motions.

oscillŏ·meter (L. *oscillare*, to swing; G. *metron*, measure). An instrument for measuring the amount of pulsation transmitted to a pneumatic cuff applied to a segment of a limb.

Os·cinis pal·lipes. A genus of flies. They are transmitters of yaws.

oscitā·tion (L. *oscitatio*, a yawn). The act of yawning.

os·culum (L. *osculum*, dim. of *os*, mouth). A small aperture.

-osis. An abstract suffix indicating a prolonged or continuous condition.

Osler's disease (Osler, Sir W., Canadian physician, 1849–1919). Polycythaemia cyanotica. **O.'s nodes:** small painful nodules found in the pulp of the finger-tips in subacute infectious endocarditis. **O.'s phenomenon:** Agglutination of the blood-platelets which is observed in blood immediately after its withdrawal from the body.

os·mate. Salt of osmic acid.

osmē·sis (G., a smelling). The act of smelling.

osmic acid. OsO_4. The oxide of osmium used in histology as a stain for fat.

osmidrō·sis (G. *osmē*, smell; *hidrōs*, sweat). Sweat secretion of an offensive odour. Syn. bromidrosis.

os·mium (G. *osmē*, smell). A heavy metallic element in the platinum group. Specific gravity 22·48; atomic weight 190·2. Symbol Os.

osmō·sis (G. *osmos*, a thrusting). The passage of solvent molecules through a semi-permeable membrane from a weaker to a stronger solution.

osmot·ic (G. *ōsmos*, a thrusting). Relating to osmosis. **O. pressure**: the pressure produced when a solvent is separated from a solution by a semi-permeable membrane.

osphrē·sis (G.). The sense of smell.

ossa (L. pl. of *os*, bone). Bones.

os·sĕin (L. *os*, bone). A protein, closely related to collagen, forming the chief constituent of bone tissue.

os·seo-al·bumoid (L. *os*, bone; *albumen*, albumin; G. *eidos*, form). A protein, closely resembling elastin, probably derived from the Haversian canals.

os·seocartilă·ginous (L. *os*, bone; *cartilago*). Relating to bone and cartilage.

osseomū·coid (L. *os*, bone; *mucus*, mucus; G. *eidos*, form). A glucoprotein, present in bone tissue.

os·seous (L. *os*, bone). Bony.

os·sicle (L. *ossiculum*, dim. of *os*, bone). A small bone, especially one of the chain of bones in the middle ear.

ossi·cula (L. pl. of *ossiculum*, a small bone). **O. auditus**: the auditory ossicles.

ossiculec·tomy (L. *ossiculum*, a small bone; G. *ektomē*, excision). The surgical removal of an ossicle or of the auditory ossicles.

ossi·ferous (L. *os*, bone; *ferre*, to bear). Producing or containing bone tissue.

ossi·fic, ossi·ficans (L. *os*, bone; *facere*, to make). Producing bone; undergoing ossification.

ossificā·tion (L. *os*, bone; *facere*, to make). The formation of bone.

os·siform (L. *os*, bone; *forma*, shape). Bone-like.

os·sify (L. *os*, bone; *facere*, to make). To transform into bone.

os·teal (G. *osteon*, bone). Bony.

ostĕál·gia (G. *osteon*, bone; *algos*, pain). Skeletal pains.

ostec·tomy (G. *osteon*, bone; *ektomē*, excision). See osteo-ectomy.

ostec·topy (G. *osteon*, bone; *ektopos*, displaced). See osteo-ectopy.

os·tĕin, os·tĕine (G. *osteon*, bone). Ossein.

ostĕi·tis (G. *osteon*, bone). Inflammation of bone. **O. deformans**: a chronic disease, characterized by resorption of bone and later by excessive deposition of osteoid tissue subperiosteally and within the marrow which finally calcifies, leading to curving and enlargement of the affected parts (chiefly skull, spine, pelvis, tibia). Syn. Paget's disease. **O. fibrosa**: a systemic disease, most probably due, but certainly related, to parathyroid hyperfunction with hyperglycaemia, hypophosphataemia and excessive urinary excretion of calcium and phosphorus; characterized by resorption of bone which is replaced by fibrous and to a small extent by osteoid tissue, leading to formation of cysts and tumour-like masses in the affected bone. Syn. von Recklinghausen's disease.

osteo-arthrī·tis (G. *osteon*, bone; *arthron*, joint). A subchronic disease affecting one or, more commonly, several joints; characterized by thickening of peri-articular tissue and osteophytic outgrowths from cartilage, leading to deformity of joints, limitation of movement, pain especially at night (owing to muscular relaxation on rest). See also Heberden's nodes.

osteo-arthrŏ·pathy (G. *osteon*, bone; *arthron*, joint; *pathos*, disease). Any disease of the joints. **O.-a., pulmonary, hypertrophic**: a condition characterized by symmetrical enlargement of the distal bones of limbs and by clubbing of the terminal phalanges, caused by chronic diseases of the lungs or by congenital diseases of the heart.

osteo-arthrŏ·tomy (G. *osteon*, bone; *arthron*, joint; *tomē*, section). Excision of the articular end of a bone.

os·teoblast (G. *osteon*, bone; *blastos*, germ). A cell of mesoblastic origin, the precursor of the osteocyte.

os·teochondrī·tis (G. *osteon*, bone; *khondros*, cartilage). Inflammation involving both bone and cartilage. **O. dissecans**: a condition characterized by a septic necrosis of cartilage and pericartilaginous bone, affecting especially the medial condyle of the femur and the lateral condyle of the humerus, and giving rise to 'loose bodies' within the joint.

os·teochondrō·ma (G. *osteon*, bone; *khondros*, cartilage). A tumour composed of osseous and cartilaginous tissue.

os·teochondromatō·sis (G. *osteon*, bone; *khondros*, cartilage). A congenital dysplasia characterized by multiple development of osteochondromata.

os·teochon·drosarcō·ma (G. *osteon*, bone; *khondros*, cartilage; *sarx*, flesh). A sarcoma derived from osseous and cartilaginous cells.

os·teochondrō·sis (G. *osteon*, bone; *khondros*, cartilage). A disease of one or more of the growth or ossification centres in children, which begins as a degeneration or necrosis followed by regeneration or recalcification.

os·teoclā·sia (G. *osteon*, bone; *klasis*, a breaking). See osteoclasis.

ostĕŏ·clasis (G. *osteon*, bone; *klasis*, a breaking). 1. The absorption of bony tissue by osteoblasts. 2. Fracture of bones in order to correct deformity. Syn. brisement forcé.

os·teoclast (G. *osteon*, bone; *klastos*, broken). 1. A multinuclear giant cell absorbing newly-formed bone, and thus forming Howship's lacunae. 2. An instrument for the performance of osteoclasis.

os·teoclastō·ma (G. *osteon*, bone; *klastos*, broken). Giant cell tumour arising in, and locally invading, bone; regarded as benign though recurrence may occur after removal.

os·teoclasty (G. *osteon*, bone; *klastos*, broken). Osteoclasis (2).

os·teocope, osteocop·ic pain (G. *osteon*, bone; *kŏpos*, pain). Pain in a bone, generally worse at night.

os·teocrā·nium (G. *osteon*, bone; *kranion*, skull). The ossified, as distinguished from the cartilaginous, part of the cranium.

os·teocyte (G. *osteon*, bone; *kutos*, cell). A bone cell.

os·teoder·mia (G. *osteon*, bone; *derma*, skin). Ossification in a portion of the skin.

os·teodiă·stasis (G. *osteon*, bone; *diastasis*, separation). Separation of the epiphysis from the metaphysis.

os·teodystrō·phia (G. *osteon*, bone; *dus-*, ill-; *trŏphe*, nourishment). Defective bone formation.

osteo-ec·tomy (G. *osteon*, bone; *ektomē*, excision). Excision of a bone or of part of a bone.

osteo-ec·topy (G. *osteon*, bone; *ektopos*, displaced). Displacement of a bone.

osteo-epi·physis (G. *osteon*, bone; *epi*, upon; *phuesthai*, to grow). A bony epiphysis.

os·teofibrō·ma (G. *osteon*, bone; L. *fibra*, fibre). A tumour composed of osseous and fibrous tissue.

os·teogĕ·nesis (G. *osteon*, bone; *gennan*, to produce). The development of bony tissue. **O. imperfecta**: a hereditary condition characterized by enchondral and periosteal o., causing abnormal fragility of the bones ('spontaneous' fractures), associated with blue sclerae and often otosclerosis. Syn. osteopsathyrosis; Lobstein's disease; fragilitas ossium.

osteogenet·ic (G. *osteon*, bone; *gennan*, to produce). Relating to osteogenesis.

osteogen·ic (G. *osteon*, bone; *gennan*, to produce). osteogenetic, *q.v.* **O. sarcoma**: a sarcoma derived from osteoblasts.

os·tĕoid (G. *osteon*, bone; *eidos*, form). 1. Non-calcified osseous tissue. 2. Resembling bone. **O. chondroma**: a form of chondroma arising beneath the periosteum of long bones and composed of cells from

x

which true bone may be formed. **O. sarcoma:** a sarcoma composed of non-calcified bony tissue.

ostĕŏ·logy (G. *osteon*, bone; *logos*, a discourse). The part of anatomy relating to the bones.

ostĕŏ·lysis (G. *osteon*, bone; *lusis*, a loosening). Absorption of bone; a local defect characterized by destruction of the cortical, compact and spongy parts of the bone.

ostĕŏ·ma (G. *osteon*, bone). A tumour composed of osseous tissue. **O., cancellous:** a spongy exostosis, derived from cancellous bone. **O., compact:** an ivory exostosis, derived from compact bone.

os·teomalā·cia (G. *osteon*, bone; *malakia*, softness). A disease characterized by softening of bones, hypocalcaemia, hypophosphataemia, hypercaluria and hyperphosphaturia, leading to curving, deformities and liability to 'spontaneous' fractures, due to vitamin D deficiency in adult life.

ostĕŏ·metry (G. *osteon*, bone; *metron*, measure). Measurement of bones.

os·teomȳelit·ic (G. *osteon*, bone; *muelos*, marrow). Relating to osteomyelitis.

os·teomȳeli·tis (G. *osteon*, bone; *muelos*, marrow). Inflammation of the medullary cavity of a bone.

os·teonecrō·sis (G. *osteon*, bone; *nekros*, corpse). Necrosis of a bone.

ostĕŏ·nosus (G. *osteon*, bone; *nosos*, sickness). Any bone disease.

os·teopae·dion (G. *osteon*, bone; *pais*, child). Lithopaedion, *q.v.*

os·teopath, ostĕŏ·pathist (G. *osteon*, bone; *pathos*, disease). One skilled in osteopathy.

osteopă·thic (G. *osteon*, bone; *pathos*, disease). Relating to osteopathy.

ostĕŏ·pathy (G. *osteon*, bone; *pathos*, disease). 1. Any disease of bone. 2. A system of treating diseases by manual manipulation of bones, based on the assumption that a structural derangement of skeletal parts is the most significant factor in disease.

os·teoperiosti·tis (G. *osteon*, bone; *peri*, around; *osteon*, bone). Inflammation of both bone and periosteum.

os·teopetrō·sis (G. *osteon*, bone; *petra*, a rock). Marble bone disease, *q.v.*

os·teophā·gia (G. *osteon*, bone; *phagein*, to eat). A perversion marked by the eating of bones.

ostĕŏ·phony (G. *osteon*, bone; *phōnē*, voice). Sound transmission through bone.

os·teophore (G. *osteon*, bone; *pherein*, to carry). A strong forceps used in the crushing of bone.

ostĕŏph·thisis (G. *osteon*, bone; *phthisis*, a wasting). Wasting of the bones.

os·teophȳ·ma (G. *osteon*, bone; *phuma*, a growth). Any tumour of bone.

os·teophyte (G. *osteon*, bone; *phuton*, plant). A small localized cortical or subcortical deposit of bone from the periosteum.

os·teoplas·tic (G. *osteon*, bone; *plassein*, to form). 1. Relating to the formation of bone. 2. Relating to osteoplasty.

os·teoplasty (G. *osteon*, bone; *plassein*, to form). Plastic operation on bone.

os·teopoi·kily (G. *osteon*, bone; *poikilos*, mottled). A congenital developmental dysplasia, inherited by dominant transmission, not giving rise to any discomfort; characterized by circumscribed roundish foci or osteosclerosis of pin-point to lentil size, usually in the spongy part of carpal, tarsal and phalangeal bones, in the pelvis and in epiphyseal and metaphyseal parts of long bones.

os·teoporō·sis (G. *osteon*, bone; *poros*, passage). That form of local or generalized bone atrophy which is characterized by loss of osseous tissue without any changes in the shape of the affected bone.

os·teopsathyrō·sis (G. *osteon*, bone; *psathuros*, crumbling). Osteogenesis imperfecta, *q.v.*

osteorrhā·gia (G. *osteon*, bone; *rhegnunai*, to burst forth). Bone haemorrhage.

ostĕor·rhaphy (G. *osteon*, bone; *rhaphē*, suture). The suturing of bones.

os·teosarcō·ma (G. *osteon*, bone; *sarx*, flesh). A sarcoma composed of bony tissue.

os·teosclerō·sis (G. *osteon*, bone; *sklēros*, hard). A local or generalized condition characterized by increased formation of osseous tissue within the bone, by which the spongy portion becomes compact bone, thus leading to encroachment on the bone marrow. Syn. eburnation of bone.

os·teosep·tum (G. *osteon*, bone; L. *septum*, barrier). The bony nasal septum.

ostĕŏ·sis (G. *osteon*, bone). The formation of bone.

os·teostĕātō·ma (G. *osteon*, bone; *steatōma*, sebaceous tumour). Fatty tumour of bone.

os·teostix·is (G. *osteon*, bone; *stixis*, a pricking). Puncture of a bone.

os·teosū·ture (G. *osteon*, bone; L. *suture*, suture). Osteorrhaphy, *q.v.*

os·teotome (G. *osteon*, bone; *tomē*, section). 1. An instrument for cutting bone. 2. An instrument for cutting the bones of the foetal head in embryotomy.

ostĕŏ·tomy (G. *osteon*, bone; *tomē*, section). 1. The division of a bone. 2. Excision of a section (e.g., wedge-shaped) of a bone.

os·teotrite (G. *osteon*, bone; L. *terĕre*, to rub). An instrument for scraping away diseased bone.

os·tial (L. *ostium*, an entrance). Relating to an opening.

osti·tis (G. *osteon*, bone). Osteitis, *q.v.*

os·tium (L.). A mouth or opening; an aperture.

os·tid (G. *osteon*, bone; *eidos*, form). Osteoid, *q.v.*

os·treotoxis·mus (G. *ostreon*, oyster; *toxikon*, poison). Poisoning from oysters.

otal·gia (G. *ous*, ear; *algos*, pain). Earache.

otec·tomy (G. *ous*, ear; *tomē*, section). Removal of the ossicles from the middle ear.

othaematō·ma (G. *ous*, ear; *haima*, blood). Haematoma of the external ear, especially the pinna.

othaemorrhā·gia (G. *ous*, ear; *haima*, blood; *rhēgnunai*, to burst forth). Haemorrhage from the ear.

othaemorrhoē·a (G. *ous*, ear; *haima*, blood; *rhoia*, flow). A blood-containing discharge from the ear.

ō·tic (G. *ōtikos*, from *ous*, ear). Relating to the ear.

otit·ic (G. *ous*, ear). Relating to otitis.

oti·tis (G. *ous*, ear). Inflammation of the ear. **O. externa:** inflammation of the external ear. **O. media:** that affecting the middle ear. **O. interna:** labyrinthitis.

otocĕ·phalus (G. *ous*, ear; *kephalē*, head). A monster characterized by the union or juxtaposition of the ears, and usually by the absence of one ocular bulbus and of the nose.

otoclei·tis (G. *ous*, ear; *kleisis*, closure). Occlusion of the ear.

otocŏ·nia (G. *ous*, ear; *kŏnia*, dust). Otolith.

otocrā·nium (G. *ous*, ear; *kranion*, skull). The cavity of the petrous part of the skull, the seat of the organ of hearing.

ō·tocyst (G. *ous*, ear; *kustis*, bladder). 1. A hollow sac between ectoderm and neural tube, giving rise to the internal ear. 2. The otolithic sac in invertebrates.

otŏ·genous (G. *ous*, ear; *gennan*, to produce). Originating in the ear.

ō·tolith (G. *ous*, ear; *lithos*, stone). One of the calcareous concretions in the membranous labyrinth of the ear.

otŏ·logist (G. *ous*, ear; *logos*, a discourse). A specialist in otology.

otŏ·logy (G. *ous*, ear; *logos*, a discourse). The part of medicine relating to the ear.

otomycō·sis (G. *ous*, ear; *mukēs*, mushroom). The condition due to aural infection with fungi.

ō·topharyn·geal (G. *ous*, ear; *pharugx*, throat). Relating to the ear and the pharynx. **O. tube**: the pharyngotympanic or Eustachian tube.

ō·tophone (G. *ous*, ear; *phōnē*, voice). 1. An ear-trumpet, or some other device for collecting and intensifying sound-waves. 2. An auscultating tube used in diseases of the ear.

otopi·esis (G. *ous*, ear; *piesis*, pressure). Abnormal pressure on the labyrinth, causing deafness.

ō·toplasty (G. *ous*, ear; *plassein*, to form). Plastic surgery of the external ear.

ō·topyorrhoe·a (G. *ous*, ear; *puon*, pus; *rhoia*, flow) A discharge of pus from the external auditory meatus.

ōtorhi·nolaryngŏ·logy (G. *ous* ear; *rhis*, nose; *larugx*, larynx; *logos*, a discourse). That part of medicine dealing with the ear, nose and throat.

otorrhā·gia (G. *ous*, ear; *rhēgnunai*, to burst out). A discharge of blood from the external auditory meatus.

otorrhoe·a (G. *ous*, ear; *rhoia*, flow). A discharge from the external auditory meatus.

otosal·pinx (G. *ous*, ear; *salpigx*, trumpet). The pharyngotympanic or Eustachian tube.

ō·toscleronec·tomy (G. *ous*, ear; *sklēros*, hard; *ektomē*, excision). Excision of sclerosed or ankylosed sound conductors in chronic otitis media.

ō·tosclerō·sis (G. *ous*, ear; *sklēros*, hard). A usually hereditary, chronic condition characterized by gradually progressive deafness due to abnormal ossification of the otic capsule and degeneration of Corti's organ.

ō·toscope (G. *ous*, ear; *skopein*, to view). 1. An instrument for auscultating the ear. 2. An instrument for examining the tympanic membrane. Syn. auriscope.

otŏ·tomy (G. *ous*, ear; *tomē*, section). Dissection of the ear.

ou·abain. A glycoside obtained from the seeds of *strophanthus gratus*, used as a heart stimulant.

ounce (L. *uncia*). A unit of weight. **O. avoirdupois**: the 16th part of the avoirdupois pound or 437·5 gr. (28·35 gm.). **O. troy** or **apothecaries**: the 12th part of the troy pound or 480 gr. (31·10 gm.).

outlet. The lower opening of the pelvic canal.

out-patient. A hospital patient who is not treated in the wards; an ambulatory patient.

oval (L. *ovum*, egg). 1. Egg-shaped. 2. Relating to an ovum.

ovā·rian (L. *ovum*, egg). Relating to the ovary. **O. pregnancy**: the development of the fertilized ovum within the ovary.

ovariĕc·tomy (L. *ovum*, egg; G. *ektomē*, excision). Excision of an ovary; oophorectomy.

ovā·riocele (L. *ovum*, egg; *kēlē*, hernia). Hernia of the ovary.

ovā·riocentē·sis (L. *ovum*, egg; G. *kentēsis*, puncture). Surgical puncture of the ovary or of an ovarian cyst.

ovā·riocyē·sis (L. *ovum*, egg; *kuēsis*, conception). Ovarian pregnancy.

ovā·riohysterec·tomy (L. *ovum*, egg; G. *hustera*, uterus; *ektomē*, excision). Excision of the ovaries and uterus.

ovariŏ·tomy (L. *ovum*, egg; *tomē*, section). Oophorectomy.

ovari·tis (L. *ovum*, egg). Oophoritis, *q.v.*

ovā·rium (L. *ovum*, egg). An ovary or oophoron. **O. masculinum**: Morgagni's hydatid.

ō·vary (L. *ovum*, egg). The female sex-gland.

over-determination. A psychoanalytical term. The mechanism by which a symptom is produced by a number of converging, mainly unconscious, mental processes.

over-extension. Excessive extension; extension beyond the normal limit.

overflow. A continuous escape of fluid.

Overlach's spines (Overlach, M., German histologist, of the 19th century). The protoplasmic prolongations of cells of the epithelium of the cervix uteri.

overlying of children. The lying of one of the parents upon an infant child causing the death of the child from suffocation.

over-riding. The slipping of a fractured bone end over the other fragment.

over-strain. Extreme fatigue produced by exertion, but not amounting to exhaustion.

over-weight. Obesity.

ovicap·sule (L. *ovum*, egg; *capsula*, small box). The internal coat of a Graafian follicle.

ō·viduct (L. *ovum*, egg; *ductus*, a conducting). The uterine or Fallopian tube; the tube connecting the ovary and uterus.

ovi·ferous (L. *ovum*, egg; *ferre*, to bear). Producing ova.

ovificā·tion (L. *ovum*, egg; *facere*, to make). The production of ova.

ō·viform (L. *ovum*, egg; *forma*, shape). Egg-shaped.

ovi·genous (L. *ovum*, egg; G. *gennan*, to produce). Producing ova.

ō·vigerm (L. *ovum*, egg; *germen*, germ). A cell producing an ovum or developing into an ovum.

ovi·gerous (L. *ovum*, egg; *gerere*, to bear). Producing or carrying ova.

ovi·parous (L. *ovum*, egg; *parere*, to produce). Laying eggs; producing young in the egg-state of development.

ō·visac (L. *ovum*, egg; *saccus*, bag). The membrane enclosing the ovum within the ovary.

ovites·tis (L. *ovum*, egg; *testis*, testicle). See ovotestis.

ovo-al·bumin (L. *ovum*, egg; *albumen*). The albumin of egg white.

ovoge·nesis (L. *ovum*, egg; G. *genesis*, production). The development or production of the ovum.

ovoglō·bin (L. *ovum*, egg; *globus*, globe). The globulin of egg-white.

ō·void (L. *ovum*, egg; G. *eidos*, form). Egg-shaped.

ovolĕ·cithin (L. *ovum*, egg; G. *lekithos*, yolk). A lecithin obtained from eggs.

ovomū·cin (L. *ovum*, egg; *mucus*). A glycoprotein comprising about 7 per cent of the protein matter of egg-white.

ovomū·coid (L. *ovum*, egg; *mucus*; G. *eidos*, form). A glycoprotein present in white of egg.

ō·voplasm (L. *ovum*, egg; G. *plasma*, something formed). The substance or protoplasm of an unimpregnated egg-cell.

ovotes·tis (L. *ovum*, egg; *testis*, testicle). A gland containing both ovarian and testicular tissue.

ovovitel·lin (L. *ovum*, egg; *vitellus*, yolk of egg). A phosphoprotein present in egg-yolk.

ō·vovivi·parous (L. *ovum*, egg; *vivere*, to live; *parĕre*, to bear). Reproducing by means of eggs hatched within the body.

ō·vular (L. *ovum*, egg). Relating to an ovulum or ovum.

ō·vulase (L. *ovum*, egg). An enzyme thought to be present in living eggs and to stimulate karyokinesis.

ovulā·tion (L. *ovum*, egg). The escape of an ovum from the Graafian follicle.

ō·vule (L. *ovulum* dim. of *ovum*, egg). A small egg, particularly a small egg-like body. **O. of Naboth**: a small cyst at the uterine cervix due to obstruction of a glandular duct.

ovulum (L. dim. of *ovum*, egg). An ovule.

ōvum (L. *ovum*, egg; pl. *ova*). The reproductive cell of an animal or plant; an egg.

Owen's line (Owen, Sir R., English anatomist, 1804–92). The lines across the dentine caused by irregularities in the axis of the dental tubes.

ox·alate (G. *oxălis*, sorrel). A salt of oxalic acid.

oxalae·mia (G. *oxălis*, sorrel; *haima*, blood). The presence of an excessive amount of calcium oxalate in the blood.

oxalic acid. $C_2H_2O_4$ a crystalline solid which is prepared by treating sawdust with caustic soda and potash.

oxalū·ria (G. *oxălis*, sorrel; *ouron*, urine). The presence of an excessive quantity of calcium oxalate in the urine.

oxaluric acid. $C_3H_4N_2O_4$ an oxidation product from uric acid.

oxgall. Fresh bile of the ox.

ox·idase (G. *oxus*, sharp). Any one of a group of widely distributed enzymes which take up molecular oxygen and transfer it to a substance which is thus oxidized. See also catalase; peroxidase.

oxidā·tion (G. *oxus*, sharp). 1. The act of combining with oxygen. 2. The introducing or increasing the proportion of an electro-negative element in a compound.

oxide (G. *oxus*, sharp). A binary compound of oxygen and another element or radical.

ox·idize (G. *oxus*, sharp). To combine or cause to combine with oxygen.

oxido-reduction (G. *oxus*, sharp; *reducere*, to lead back). A reaction between two substances in which the one is oxidized, the other reduced.

oxyphenar·sine. 3-amino-4-hydroxyphenylarsine oxide, the hydrochloride and tartrate of which are used in the treatment of syphilis.

ox·y̆acō·a, ox·y̆akoi·a (G. *oxus*, sharp; *akoē*, hearing). Increased acuteness of hearing.

oxyblep·sia (G. *oxus*, sharp; *blepsis*, vision). Increased visual perception.

oxyce·phaly (G. *oxus*, sharp; *kephalē*, head). The condition characterized by a high and pointed skull; turricephaly.

oxychlor·ide (G. *oxus*, sharp; *khlōros*, greenish-yellow). A compound of a basic element or radical with both oxygen and chlorine.

oxychrō·matin (G. *oxus*, sharp; *khrōma*, colour). Nuclear granules which are readily stained by acid dyes.

ox·ydum. Oxide, *q.v.*

ox·y̆ecoi·a (G. *oxus*, sharp; *akoē*, hearing). Oxyakoia, *q.v.*

oxygen (G. *oxus*, sharp; *gennan*, to produce). A colourless, odourless gas, essential to the respiration of animals and constituting about one-fifth of the atmosphere; it is combined with hydrogen in water, and is one of the main constituents of organized bodies and of the earth's crust. It combines with most elements its combination with the non-metallic substances giving acidic anhydrides. Symbol O.

ox·ygenase (G. *oxus*, sharp). An enzyme present in plant tissues, taking up oxygen from the air and forming the peroxides.

oxygenā·tion (G. *oxus*, sharp; *gennan*, to produce). The saturation of a substance with oxygen.

oxygeu·sia (G. *oxus*, sharp; *geusis*, taste). Abnormally acute sense of taste.

ox·yhaemoglō·bin (G. *oxus*, sharp; *haima*, blood; L. *globus*, globe). Oxidized haemoglobin; a loose chemical combination by which oxygen is carried from the lungs to the tissues, giving the brighter red colour to arterial as compared with venous blood.

oxyhy̅·drogen (G. *oxus*, sharp; *hudōr*, water; *gennan*, to produce). A gaseous mixture of hydrogen and oxygen.

oxy̆ō·pia (G. *oxus*, sharp; *ōps*, eye). Increased visual perception.

ox·yphil, ox·yphile (G. *oxus*, sharp; *philein*, to love). Applied to tissues easily stained by acid dyes.

oxypū·rine. Any compound derived from purines by the addition of one or more atoms of oxygen.

oxytō·cia (G. *oxus*, sharp; *tokos*, birth). Rapid childbirth.

oxytō·cic (G. *oxus*, sharp; *tokos*, birth). 1. Hastening parturition. 2. Applied to that hormone of the posterior part of the pituitary gland which stimulates contractions of the uterus in the last stage of pregnancy; it has also a stimulating effect on smooth muscle of intestines and bladder.

oxytō·cin. The oxytocic hormone secreted by the posterior lobe of the pituitary gland.

oxyuri·asis (G. *oxus*, sharp; *oura*, tail). Harbouring Oxyures.

Oxyū·ris (G. *oxus*, sharp; *oura*, tail). A genus of nematodes, the pinworms. *O. vermicularis:* the common seatworm or pinworm.

oz. Abbreviation for ounce.

ozae·na (G. *ozein*, to have a smell). A form of atrophic rhinitis, characterized by foetid discharge and loss of olfactory sense.

ozochrō·tia (G. *ozein*, to have a smell; *khrōs*, skin). An offensive odour from the skin.

ō·zone (G. *ozein*, to have a smell). A modification of oxygen, its molecule consisting of three atoms of oxygen.

ozostō·mia (G. *ozein*, to have a smell; *stoma*, mouth). Offensive breath.

P

P. Symbol for Phosphorus.

p. Abbreviation for para-.

P₂. Abbreviation for pulmonary second sound.

P wave. In the electrocardiogram, the deflection (1–3 mm. in height) representing the spread of excitation over the auricles, normally of 0·1 sec. duration (about one-third of the duration of the auricular systole).

păˑbular (L. *pabulum*, food). Relating to pabulum.

păˑbulum (L.). Food; anything nutritive.

Pacchioni's bodies (Pacchioni, A., Italian anatomist, 1665–1726). Small vegetations occupying the convex surface of the meninges, chiefly along the superior longitudinal sinus and over the convexity of the cerebrum. **P.'s depressions:** the depressions produced by P.'s bodies on the inner surface of the skull. **P.'s foramen:** the opening in the tentorium for the passage of the encephalic isthmus.

pacemaker. The site from which the stimulus for the heart-beat originates. See node, sino-auricular.

pachyblěˑpharon (G. *pakhus*, thick; *blepharon*, eyelid). Thickening of the free margin of the eyelids.

pachycěˑphalous (G. *pakhus*, thick; *kephalē*, head). Having a thick skull.

pachycěˑphaly (G. *pakhus*, thick; *kephalē*, head). An abnormal thickness of the bones of the cranial vault.

pachychīˑlia (G. *pakhus*, thick; *cheilos*, lip). Abnormal thickness of the lips.

păˑchyderm (G. *pakhus*, thick; *derma*, skin). Thick-skinned animal.

pachyderˑma, pachyderˑmia (G. *pakhus*, thick; *derma*, skin). Thickening of the skin. **P. laryngis:** thickening of the mucous membrane of the larynx, usually confined to the posterior part of the vocal cords, due to chronic laryngitis.

păˑchydermăˑtocele (G. *pakhus*, thick; *derma*, skin; *kēlē*, hernia). A form of neurofibromatous growth, giving rise to irregular nodulated masses of soft tissue hanging around the neck or in other regions. Syn. elephantiasis nervosum.

pachyderˑmatous (G. *pakhus*, thick; *derma*, skin). Thick-skinned.

pachyglosˑsia (G. *pakhus*, thick; *glōssa*, tongue). Abnormal thickness of the tongue.

pachygyˑria (G. *pakhus*, thick; *guros*, a circle). Broadness and thickness of the gyri of the whole or of a part of the brain, usually associated with anomalies of cortical structure.

pachylōˑsis (G. *pakhus*, thick). Condition of dryness and thickening of the skin.

pachyměˑnia (G. *pakhus*, thick; *humēn*, membrane). Thickening of a membrane.

păˑchymeningīˑtis (G. *pakhus*, thick; *mēnigx*, membrane). Inflammation of the dura mater. **P. externa:** p. of the external layer of the dura. **P. interna:** p. of the internal layer of the dura. **P. haemorrhagica interna:** Syn. subdural haematoma. **P. spinalis hypertrophica:** p. leading to fibrosis, commonly in the cervical region of the cord, producing compression of anterior and posterior nerve-roots of the cord.

pachyměˑninx (G. *pakhus*, thick; *mēnigx*, membrane). The dura mater.

pachyněˑma (G. *pakhus*, thick; *nēma*, thread). Thick threads, forming the post-synaptic spireme, *q.v.*, in meiosis, *q.v.*

pachyonyˑchia (G. *pakhus*, thick; *onux*, finger-nail). Abnormal thickening of the nails.

păˑchytene (G. *pakhus*, thick; *tainia*, a riband). Pachynema, *q.v.*

pachyˑtrichous (G. *pakhus*, thick; *thrix*, hair). Thick-haired.

pachyˑtic (G. *pakhutēs*, thickness). Thick; fat.

păˑchyvaginīˑtis (G. *pakhus*, thick; L. *vagina*, sheath). Chronic vaginitis with thickening of the vaginal wall.

Pacini's corpuscles or bodies (Pacini, F., Italian anatomist, 1812–83). Oval corpuscles forming the peripheral endings of sensory nerves. They consist of medullated nerve-fibres enclosed in concentric capsules. **P.'s fluid:** a conserving and diluting fluid used in counting the red blood corpuscles. Corrosive sublimate, 1; sodium chloride, 2; glycerol, 13; distilled water, 113; allow this to stand two months. For use, mix one part of solution to three parts of water and filter.

pack. A blanket or sheet wrapped around the patient's body.

pad. A small cushion placed to protect or support a part of the body.

p. ae. Abbreviation for L. *partes aequales*, equal parts.

paēˑderast (G. *pais*, boy; *erastēs*, lover). One who practises paederasty.

paēˑderasty (G. *pais*, boy; *erastēs*, lover). Sexual intercourse with boys through the anus.

paēˑdiatriˑcian, paēˑdiatrist (G. *pais*, child; *iatros*, physician). A specialist in paediatrics.

paediăˑtrics (G. *pais*, child; *iatros*, physician). That part of medicine relating to the diseases of children.

paedicˑterus (G. *pais*, child; *iktěros*, jaundice). Icterus neonatorum.

paedophīˑlia (G. *pais*, child; *philein*, to love). Sexual love for children.

Page's disease (Page, H. W., English surgeon, 1845–1926). Railway spine, a traumatic neurasthenia; psychosomatic syndrome following an accident for which compensation is being claimed. Syn. Erichsen's disease.

Pagenstecher's ointment (Pagenstecher, A., German ophthalmologist, 1828–79). An ointment of yellow oxide of mercury, used in ophthalmic practice.

Paget's disease (Paget, Sir J., English surgeon, 1814–99). Osteitis deformans; hypertrophic deforming osteitis. **P.'s disease of the nipple:** malignant papillary dermatitis; psorospermosis of the nipple and areola. **P.'s recurrent fibroid:** spindle-celled sarcoma of subcutaneous tissues.

pain (L. *poena*, punishment). 1. A specific sensation transmitted by a sensory nerve. 2. One of the regular uterine contractions during parturition.

painter's colic. Lead poisoning in painters.

Pajot's hook (Pajot, C., French obstetrician, 1816–96). A hook for decapitating the foetus. **P.'s law:** that a solid body contained within another body having smooth walls will tend to conform to the shape of those walls. Governs rotating movements of the child during labour.

păˑlatal (L. *palatum*). Relating to the palate.

păˑlate (L. *palatum*). The roof of the mouth. **P., cleft:** cleft palate, *q.v.* **P., hard:** the anterior osseous part of the p. **P., soft:** the posterior, muscle part of the p. Syn. velum palatinum.

pală·tiform (L. *palatum*; *forma*, shape). Shaped like a palate.

pă·latine (L. *palatum*). Relating to the palate. **P. arches:** the two anterior (arcus glosso-palatinus) and posterior (arcus pharyngo-palatinus) arches running from the soft palate to the root of the tongue and the pharynx respectively. **P. paresis:** paresis of the soft palate.

palatī·tis (L. *palatum*). Inflammation of the palate.

pă·latoglos·sal (L. *palatum*, G. *glōssa*, tongue). Relating to both palate and tongue.

pă·latoglos·sus muscle (L. *palatum*; G. *glōssa*, tongue). A small muscle which constricts the fauces. It arises from the soft palate and is inserted into the side and dorsum of the tongue.

palatŏ·gnathus (L. *palatum*; G. *gnathos*, jaw). Cleft palate, *q.v.*

pă·latograph (L. *palatum*; G. *graphein*, to write). An instrument used to make recordings of the movements of the soft palate.

pă·latomax·illary (L. *palatum*; *maxilla*, maxilla). Relating to both the palate and the maxillary bones.

pă·latonā·sal (L. *palatum*; *nasus*, nose). Relating to the palate and the nose.

pă·latopharyn·geal (L. *palatum*; G. *pharugx*, throat). Relating to both palate and pharynx.

pă·latopharyn·geus muscle (L. *palatum*; G. *pharugx*, throat). Arises in the soft palate, inserted into posterior border of thyroid cartilage and aponeurosis of pharynx. Narrows fauces and closes off the nasopharynx.

pă·latoplasty (L. *palatum*; G. *plassein*, to form). Plastic surgery of the palate.

pă·latoplē·gia (L. *palatum*; G. *plēgē*, a stroke). Paralysis of the soft palate.

palator·rhaphy (L. *palatum*; G. *rhaphē*, suture). Operative suture of the palate. Syn. staphylorrhaphy.

palatŏ·schisis (L. *palatum*; G. *skhisis*, a cleaving). Cleft palate, *q.v.*

pă·latum (L.). The palate.

pa·le-encĕ·phalon (G. *palaios*, old; *egkephalos*, brain). The phylogenetically old brain; all the brain except the cerebral cortex and its dependencies.

pa·leocerebel·lum (G. *palaios*, old; L. *cerebellum*, dim. of *cerebrum*, brain). Vermis, flocculus and paraflocculus, forming the phylogenetically older part of the cerebellum.

pa·leostriā·tum (G. *palaios*, old; L. *stria*, a furrow). The globus pallidum, the phylogenetically older part of the striatum.

pa·leothā·lamus (G. *palaios*, old; *thalamos*, an inner chamber). The phylogenetically older part of the thalamus, a centre for correlation of sensory impressions, primitive emotions and emotive expression.

Palfyn's sinus (Palfyn, J., Belgian anatomist, 1650–1730). A space described within the crista galli of the ethmoid, said to communicate with the frontal and ethmoidal cells.

palilă·lia (G. *palin*, backward; *lalia*, babble). Form of perseveration in which the last word(s) of a phrase is or are repeated several times.

palindrō·mia (G. *palin*, backward; *dromos*, a running). The recurrence of a disease.

palingĕ·nesis (G. *palin*, backward; *gennan*, to produce). The repetition in the embryonic development of an organism of the various stages which occurred in the evolution of its species.

palingră·phia (G. *palin*, backward; *graphein*, to write). Form of perseveration in which the last word(s) is/ are repeated when writing.

palinphră·sia (G. *palin*, backward; *phrasis*, speech). Form of perseveration in which words or phrases are repeated in speech.

palirrhoe·a (G. *palin*, backward; *rhoia*, flow). 1. The recurrence of a discharge. 2. Regurgitation.

palisade cells. Cells which are elongated at right angles to the surface, as those of the basal layer of the stratum mucosum.

pallă·dium (G. *Pallas*, the goddess of wisdom). A rare metallic element. Symbol Pd.

pallaesthē·sia (G. *pallein*, to brandish; *aisthēsis*, perception). Sensation of vibration.

pal·liate (L. *pallium*, cloak). To soothe.

pal·liative (L. *pallium*, cloak). Effecting some temporary relief, but not the cure, to a disease.

pal·lid, pal·lidus, pal·lida (L. *pallidus*). Pale.

pal·lidum (L. *pallidus*, pale). See globus pallidus.

pal·lium (L. *pallium*, cloak). 1. The cerebral cortex together with the underlying white matter. 2. Globus pallidus.

pal·lor (L. *pallidus*, pale). Paleness.

palm (L. *palma*). The flexor surface of the hand. Syn. vola manus.

palma (L.). The palm.

palmar (L. *palma*, palm). Relating to the palm of the hand.

palmă·ris muscles (L. *palma*, palm). Palmaris longus muscle which renders the palmar fascia tense; and the palmaris brevis which corrugates the skin of the palm.

pal·mature (L. *palma*, palm). Webbing or adhesion of the fingers. This may be congenital or be caused by injuries such as burns.

pal·mic (G. *palmos*, a pulsation). Relating to palmus.

pal·miped (L. *palma*, palm; *pes*, foot). Web-footed.

pal·mitate (L. *palma*, palm). A salt of palmitic acid.

palmit·ic (L. *palma*, palm). 1. Relating to palm-oil. 2. Relating to palmitin. P. acid: $C_{16}H_{32}O_2$ an acid which is found in solid fats.

pal·mitin (L. *palma*, palm). The glycerin ester of palmitic acid.

pal·mityl (L. *palma*, palm). The radical of palmitic acid.

pal·mus (G. *palmos*, pulsation). 1. A pulsation. 2. A tic. 3. Rhythmical fibrillary contractions in a muscle. 4. Lâtah, jumpers' disease.

pă·lograph (G. *pallein*, to oscillate; *graphein*, to write). An instrument for recording oscillations of arterial pulse, by means of a lever floating on column of fluid in a U-tube and a smoked drum.

pal·pable (L. *palpare*, to stroke). Capable of being felt.

palpate (L. *palpare*, to stroke). 1. To examine by touch. 2. Having tactile organs.

palpā·tion (L. *palpare*, to stroke). Examination by touch.

pal·pebra (L.). The eyelid. **P. inferior:** the lower eyelid. **P. superior:** the upper eyelid.

pal·pebral (L. *palpebra*, eyelid). Relating to the eyelid.

palpebrā·tion (L. *palpebra*, eyelid). Winking.

palpitā·te (L. *palpitare*, to throb). To flutter or beat abnormally fast, as of the heart.

palpitā·tion (L. *palpitare*, to flutter), Fluttering or beating fast; especially applied to the sensation of throbbing and fast heart-beats.

palsy (G. *paralusis*). Paralysis.

pă·ludal (L. *pălus*, marsh). Relating to or originating in marshes.

pă·ludism (L. *pălus*, marsh). Malaria.

Paludrine. A synthetic antimalarial product, $Cl.C_6H_4.NH.C(:NH)NH.C(:NH).CH(CH_3)_2$. Syn. Proguanil.

Pamaquin. A synthetic antimalarial. A salt of 6-methoxy-8-(1-methyl-4-diethylamino)butylamino-quinoline. It destroys gametocytes of all forms of malaria. Syn. Plasmochin.

p-aminosalicylic acid. See aminosalicylic acid.

pampĭ·niform (L. *pampinus*, tendril; *forma*, shape). Like a tendril.

pamplē·gia (G. *pas*, all; *plēgē*, a stroke). Generalized paralysis.

pan. A low, flat-bottomed vessel. Bed-p.: a pan used as a receptacle for the faecal or urinary excretions of patients in bed.

panacē·a (G. *panakeia*, all-healing). A remedy alleged to cure every disease.

panagglutinā·tion (G. *pas*, all; L. *agglutinare*, to glue). Agglutination of blood corpuscles with serum of the same (or ordinarily compatible) blood group due to the presence of cold agglutinogen or to bacterial contamination (Thomson's phenomenon).

panari·tium (Probably corrupted from G. *parōnychia*, a whitlow, from *para*, beside; *onux*, nail). Acute purulent inflammation of finger or toe; whitlow. See also paronychia.

panarthrī·tis (G. *pas*, all; *arthron*, joint). 1. Inflammation of all structures of a joint. 2. Inflammation of all joints.

Panas's solution (Panas, P., French ophthalmologist, 1832–1903). A mild antiseptic eye lotion, consisting of mercuric iodide, 1; absolute alcohol, 400; distilled water to make 20,000 parts.

panblas·tic (G. *pas*, all; *blastos*, germ). Connected with all the layers of the blastoderm.

pancardī·tis (G. *pas*, all; *kardia*, heart). Inflammation of the endocardium, myocardium and pericardium. Syn. carditis.

pan·creas (G. *pagkreas*, sweetbread, lit. 'all flesh'). A gland lying behind the stomach transversely across the posterior wall of the abdomen; having both an external and an internal secretion. The former contains enzymes acting upon proteins (trypsin), fat (lipase) and carbohydrate (diastase), and is conveyed to the duodenum by the duct of Wirsung (pancreatic duct) and the accessory duct of Santorini. The internal secretion (insulin) regulates carbohydrate metabolism and is developed in the beta-cells of the islands of Langerhans, *q.v.*

pan·crĕatal·gia (G. *pagkreas*, sweetbread; *algos*, pain). Pancreatic pain.

pan·crĕatec·tomy (G. *pagkreas*, sweetbread; *ektomē*, excision). Excision of the pancreas.

pancrĕat·ic (G. *pagkreas*, sweetbread). 1. Relating to the pancreas. 2. Due to disease of the pancreas; e.g., p. diabetes, p. infantilism.

pancrĕat·ico-duodē·nal (G. *pagkreas*, sweetbread; L. *duodeni*, twelve each). Pertaining to both pancreas and duodenum.

pancrĕa·ticoduodenec·tomy (G. *pagkreas*, sweetbread; L. *duodeni*, twelve each; G. *ektomē*, excision). An operation involving resection of first, second and third parts of the duodenum and head and neck of the pancreas, performed for malignant disease involving the head of the pancreas.

pan·crĕa·tico-entero·stomy (G. *pagkreas*, sweetbread; *enteron*, intestine; *stoma*, mouth). Operative procedure in which the pancreatic duct, or the divided body of the pancreas, is implanted in the wall of the small intestine. It is usually performed during pancreaticoduodenectomy for malignant disease of the head of the pancreas.

pancrĕa·ticojejunŏ·stomy (G. *pagkreas*, sweetbread; L. *jejunus*, hungry; G. *stoma*, mouth). The surgical creation of an anastomosis between the pancreas and the jejunum.

pan·creatin. A preparation obtained from the pancreas, containing the enzymes trypsin, diastase and lipase. Used to assist the digestion of starch and protein.

pan·crĕatī·tis (G. *pagkreas*, sweetbread). Inflammation of the pancreas. P., acute: a haemorrhagic

necrosis, developing sometimes into gangrene or abscess of the pancreas, with necrosis of intra-abdominal fatty tissue (owing to liberation of lipase), clinically characterized by excruciating epigastric pain of acute onset, radiating to the left side and back, by circulatory collapse, vomiting, abdominal distension, tenderness and rigidity of the abdominal wall, and by a considerable increase in the diastase content of the urine; due to an escape of trypsin into the interstitial tissues of the pancreas, which may be caused by reflux of bile or by infection or obstruction of the pancreatic duct or a proliferative metaplasia of the duct epithelium, or by an acute oedema of the pancreas.

pancrĕătŏ·genous (G. *pagkreas*, sweetbread; *gennan*, to produce). Originating in the pancreas.

pan·creatolīp·ase. The fat-splitting enzyme, lipase, found in pancreatic juice.

pancrĕa·tolith (G. *pagkreas*, sweetbread; *lithos*, stone). A pancreatic calculus.

pan·crĕatŏ·tomy (G. *pagkreas*, sweetbread; *tomē*, section). Incision of the pancreas.

pancrĕolyt·ic (G. *pagkreas*, sweetbread; *lusis*, dissolution). Destructive to pancreatic tissue.

pancrĕŏ·pathy (G. *pagkreas*, sweetbread; *pathos*, disease). Any pancreatic disease.

pandem·ic (G. *pas*, all; *dēmos*, people). A widespread epidemic.

Pander's cells, nucleus (Pander, H. C. von, German anatomist, 1794–1865). The nerve cells in the subthalamic nucleus. P.'s false amnion: the membrana serosa of von Baer; chorionic membrane.

Paneth's cells (Paneth, J., German physician, 1857–90). The 'cellules étroites' of the mucosa of the small intestine.

pan·gen (G. *pas*, all; *gennan*, to produce). The hypothetical ultimate unit of the cell, conceived as primary bearer of the individual characters of the cell. Syn. biophore; plasome.

pangĕ·nesis (G. *pas*, all; *gennan*, to produce). Darwin's theory of heredity: the evolution of an organism from hypothetical germs assumed to be segregated from all the parental somatic cells, stored in the germ-cells, and to determine the transmission of hereditary characters.

panhidro·sis (G. *pas*, all; *hidrōs*, sweat). See panidrosis.

panhydrŏ·meter (G. *pas*, all; *hudōr*, water; *metron*, measure). An instrument for determining the specific gravity of liquids.

panhȳ·grous (G. *pas*, all; *hygros*, moist). Overall surface dampness.

pan·hysterec·tomy (G. *pan*, all; *hustera*, uterus; *ektomē*, excision). Extirpation of the uterus.

pani·cula (L. *panicula*, dim. of *pānus*, a swelling). A swelling.

panidrō·sis (G. *pas*, all; *hidrōs*, sweat). Prolonged perspiration of the whole body.

panis (L.). Bread.

Panizza's foramen (Panizza, B., Italian anatomist, 1785–1867). The interventricular foramen of the heart, abnormal in mammals but normal in lower vertebrates. P.'s plexuses: two lymphatic plexuses lying in the outer fossa of the preputial frenum.

panmyeloph·thisis (G. *pas*, all; *muelos*, marrow; *phthisis*, a wasting). Aplastic anaemia.

panniculi·tis (L. *panniculus*, dim. of *pannus*, a cloth). Inflammation of the superficial fascial tissue.

panni·culus (L. dim. of *pannus*, a cloth). A layer. P. adiposus: the subcutaneous fat-tissue.

pan·nus (L. a cloth). Abnormal vascular granulation-tissue, growing from the conjunctiva into the cornea.

panophthal·mia, pan·ophthalmī·tis (G. *pas*, all; *ophthalmos*, eye). Inflammation of all the eyeball tissues.

panop·tic (G. *pas*, all; *optikos*, of or for sight). Applied to a method of differential staining of blood cells, rendering them all visible.

panoptō·sis (G. *pas*, all; *ptosis*, a falling). Downward displacement of all abdominal organs.

Pansch's sulcus (Pansch, A., German anatomist, 1841–87). The sulcus intraparietalis.

pan·sinusī·tis (G. *pas*, all; L. *sinus*, a hollow). Inflammation of all the sinuses of the facial bones.

pansphyg·mograph (G. *pas*, all; *sphugmos*, a throbbing; *graphein*, to write). An instrument for recording simultaneously cardiac movements, arterial pulse and respiration.

Panstron·gylus. A genus of bugs, certain species of which transmit Trypanosoma.

pant. To breathe hard or rapidly.

pantal·gia (G. *pas*, all; *algos*, pain). Pain through the entire body.

Pan·topon. A purified mixture of the natural alkaloids of opium, suitable for injection.

pantothē·nic acid. The antidermatitis factor essential for the development of chicks and rats. It is one of the vitamin B complex. $CH_2OH·C(CH_3)_2.$ $CHOH–CO.NH.CH_2·CH_2.COOH.$

papā·in. An impure proteolytic enzyme or mixture of enzymes, prepared from the juice of the unripe fruit of *Carica papaya*. Used to assist protein digestion.

papā·ver (L. poppy). A genus of papaveraceous plants. *P. somniferum* affords opium.

papaverē·tum. Consists of the hydrochlorides of the alkaloids of opium.

papa·verine (L. *papaver*, poppy). One of the alkaloids of opium. Used as an antispasmodic.

papil·la (L. *papilla*, nipple; dim. of *papula*, pimple). 1. The nipple. 2. A small nipple-shaped eminence. 3. The optic disc. **P. circumvallata:** one of the papillae at the root of the tongue, which are surrounded by a circular wall. **P. duodeni:** the eminence in the duodenal mucous membrane containing the orifice of the pancreatic and/or common bile duct. Syn. P. of Vater. **P. filiformis:** one of the common papillae of the tongue. **P. fungiformis:** one of the low, broad papillae of the tongue. **P. lacrimalis:** the small eminence at the inner canthus of an eyelid containing the punctum lacrimalis. **P., renal:** the summit of one of the renal pyramids.

pap·illary (L. *papilla*, nipple). 1. Pertaining to the nipple. 2. Formed of or containing papillae. 3. Like a papilla.

papillec·tomy (L. *papilla*, nipple; G. *ektomē*, excision). Excision of a papilla.

papilli·ferous (L. *papilla*, nipple; *ferre*, to bear). Bearing papillae.

papil·liform (L. *papilla*, nipple; *forma*, shape). Formed like a papilla.

papillī·tis (L. *papilla*, nipple). See papilloedema.

papilloedē·ma (L. *papilla*, nipple; G. *oidēma*, swelling). Oedematous swelling of the optic disc, rendering its outlines more or less indistinct, with narrowing of the arteries and dilation of the veins. Syn. choked disc; papillitis; optic neuritis.

papillō·ma (L. *papilla*, nipple). A branching, or lobulated, benign tumour derived from epithelium.

papillomatō·sis (L. *papilla*, nipple). The condition characterized by the formation of multiple papillomata.

papilloretinī·tis (L. *papilla*, nipple; *rete*, net). Neuroretinopathy, *q.v.*

papil·lose (L. *papilla*, nipple). Bearing papillae.

papil·lous (L. *papilla*, nipple). Characterized by the presence or formation of papillae.

Pappataci fever. See fever, phlebotomus.

Pappenheim's staining (Pappenheim, A., German physician, 1870–1917). A method of staining tub-

ercle bacilli in which the specimen is stained with hot carbol-fuchsin solution rinsed with an alcoholic solution of rosolic acid and methylene blue. The bacilli are stained bright red.

pap·rika. A condiment and source of vitamin C from the *Capsicum annuum*.

pă·pular (L. *papula*, pimple). Characterized by the presence or formation of papules.

papulā·tion (L. *papula*, pimple). Formation of papules in certain exanthematous diseases.

pă·pule (L. *papula*, pimple). A small nodular elevation of the skin.

pă·pulonecrot·ic tuber·culide (L. *papula*, pimple; G. *nekros*, corpse; L. *tuberculum*, dim. of *tuber*, a protuberance). A group of skin affections of tuberculous origin, comprising acnitis, *q.v.*, disseminated facial lupus, and the p. t. of the limbs (acne scrofulosorum) characterized by a usually symmetrical eruption of nodules in the corium showing perivascular infiltration of epitheloid and mononuclear cells, giant cells and vascular lesions, usually progressing to necrosis of the central part of the lesion.

pă·pulopus·tular (L. *papula*, pimple; *pustula*, pustule). Characterized by the presence of papulopustules or of both papules and pustules.

pă·pulopus·tule (L. *papula*, pimple; *pustula*, pustule). A papule surmounted by a pustule.

pă·pulovesī·cular (L. *papula*, pimple; *vesicula*, dim. of *vesica*, bladder). Characterized by the presence of papulovesicles or of both papules and vesicles.

pă·pulovē·sicle (L. *papula*, pimple; *vesica*, bladder). A papule surmounted by a vesicle.

papyrā·ceous (G. *papuros*, papyrus). Resembling paper; as thin as paper.

Paquelin's cautery (Paquelin, C. A., French surgeon, 1836–1905). A thermocautery; a hollow platinum point kept at an even temperature by a benzene vapour current.

para-amino-benzene-sulphonamide. Sulphanilamide, *q.v.*

para-aminobenzō·ic acid. See *p*-aminobenzoic acid.

para-aminosalicy̆·lic acid. See *p*-aminosalicylic acid.

para-anaesthē·sia (G. *para*, beside; *an*, neg.; *aisthēsis*, feeling). Anaesthesia of both arms or both legs.

paraban·ic acid. Oxalylurea. A product obtained by oxidizing uric acid with nitric acid.

parabiō·sis (G. *para*, beside; *bios*, life). 1. Partial union of two individuals causing a mutual physiological influence. 2. Temporary suppression of excitability and conductivity in a nerve.

parablep·sis (G. *para*, beside; *blepsis*, vision). False or incorrect vision.

parabū·lia (G. *para*, beside; *boulē*, will). Abnormality of volition.

paracanthō·ma (G. *para*, beside; *akantha*, prickle). A tumour derived from the prickle-cell layer of the skin.

paracar·diac (G. *para*, beside; *kardia*, heart). Near the heart.

paracā·sein (G. *para*, beside; L. *caseus*, cheese). The product of action of rennin upon milk-casein.

paracele (G. *para*, beside; *koilia*, cavity). Old term for the lateral ventricle of the brain.

paracentē·sis (G. *para*, beside; *kentēsis*, puncture). Puncture, e.g. of the tympanic membrane, or of the thoracic or abdominal wall.

paracen·tral (G. *para*, beside; *kentron*, point). Near the centre.

paracĕ·phalus (G. *para*, beside; *kephalē*, head). A monster with rudimentary head, trunk and limbs.

parachor·dal (G. *para*, beside; *khordē*, string). Relating to one of the two cartilages situated at either side of the cranial part of the foetal notochord from which part of the cranial base takes origin.

parachroi·a (G. *para*, beside; *khroia*, colour). Abnormal coloration.

parachrō·matin (G. *para*, beside; *khrōma*, colour). The achromatic parts of the nucleoplasm which during mitosis form the spindle figures. Syn. linin.

parachrō·matism (G. *para*, beside; *khrōma*, colour). Incorrect perception of colour.

parachromŏ·phorous (G. *para*, beside; *khrōma*, colour; *pherein*, to bear). Secreting a pigment which does not diffuse away from the cell wall.

Pa·racoccidĭoi·dĕs (G. *para*, beside; *kokkos*, berry; *eidos*, form). A genus of fungi which reproduce by extrusion of multiple gemmae through the capsule.

pă·racoele (G. *para*, beside; *koilia*, cavity). Lateral ventricle of the brain. Syn. paracele.

pă·racolpī·tis (G. *para*, beside; *kolpos*, womb). Inflammation of the connective tissue surrounding the vagina.

paracrē·sol. A disinfectant, one of the three isomeric forms of cresol, and is a solid melting at 36° F. and boiling at about 201° F.

paracrÿ·stals. Syn. mesomorphic state and 'liquid crystals'—a turbid liquid which is doubly refracting and gives interference patterns in polarised light, obtained by melting crystals of certain substances.

paracū·sia, paracū·sis (G. *para*, beside; *akouein*, to hear). Defect of hearing, characterized by increase in auditory acuity in the presence of noise.

paracyē·sis (G. *para*, beside; *kuēsis*, conception). Extra-uterine pregnancy.

paracystī·tis (G. *para*, beside; *kustis*, bladder). Inflammation of the tissues adjacent to the bladder.

paracys·tium (G. *para*, beside; *kustis*, bladder). The connective tissue which is found surrounding the urinary bladder.

paradichlor·obenzene. $C_6H_4Cl_2$. An insecticide particularly useful against moths and beetles.

paradi·dymis (G. *para*, beside; *didumos*, testicle). The atrophic remains of the secretory part of the Wolffian body in the male, situated within the spermatic cord between the head of the epididymis and the pampiniform plexus. Syn. Giraldès's organ.

paradox (G. *para*, beyond; *doxa*, opinion). A statement that appears to be ridiculous, although it may not actually be so.

paraesthē·sis (G. *para*, beside; *aisthēsis*, feeling). An abnormal sensation, such as tingling or pricking, on the skin.

paraffins (L. *parum*, little; *affinis*, akin). Aliphatic hydrocarbons of general formula C_nH_{2n+2}, obtained principally from petroleum. The lower members are gases, the higher members are liquids, e.g. liquid p., and those above $C_{16}H_{34}$ are waxy solids, e.g. soft p., hard p.

paraffinō·ma (L. *parum*, little; *affinis*, akin). A tumour caused by tissue reaction to subcutaneously injected paraffin.

parafloc·culus (G. *para*, beside; L. *floccus*, a lock of wool). A small lobe near the flocculus.

paraformal·dehyde. $(CH_2O)_n$. A solid polymer of formaldehyde used as a disinfectant.

paragammacis·mus (G. *para*, beside; *gamma*, the Greek letter G). Abnormality of speech in which the sounds *d* or *t* are substituted for *g* and *k*.

par·aganglĭō·ma (G. *para*, beside; *gagglion*, subcutaneous tumour). Phaeochromocytoma, *q.v.*

paragang·lion (G. *para*, beside; *gagglion*, subcutaneous tumour). A nodular collection of phaeochromocytes, *q.v.*, along the aorta, at the bifurcation of the common carotid, along the inferior mesenterial artery, etc.

parageu·sis, paragēu·sia (G. *para*, beside; *geusis*, taste). Distortion of the sense of taste.

paragglutinā·tion (G. *para*, beside; L. *agglutinare*, to glue). Agglutination by an immune serum of microorganisms which are biologically related to the organism against which the immunity has been developed.

paraglŏ·bulin (G. *para*, beside; L. *globulus*, dim. of *globus*, globe). A serum-globulin.

pară·gnathus (G. *para*, beside; *gnathos*, jaw). A double monster the parasite of which is connected to the mandible of the autosite.

paragomphō·sis (G. *para*, beside; *gomphoein*, to fasten). Impaction of the foetal head in the pelvic cavity.

paragonimi·asis (G. *para*, beside; *gonimos*, productive). The condition caused by infestation with the Paragonimus.

Parago·nimus (G. *para*, beside; *gonimos*, productive). One of the trematode worms. **P. Westermanii**: the *Distoma pulmonale*.

paragram·matism (G. *para*, against; *gramma*, letter). Errors in grammatical form and word-order, related to sensory aphasia, *q.v.*

paragră·phia (G. *para*, against; *graphein*, to write). Disturbance of the ability to write characterized by the use of wrong and misplaced words.

pă·rahaemoglō·bin (G. *para*, beside; *haima*, blood; L. *globus*, globe). An artificial preparation of blood containing 5 per cent of iron.

parahepat·ic (G. *para*, beside; *hēpar*, liver). Near the liver.

pă·rahydrŏ·xyphē·nylĕ·thylă·mine. Tyramine.

pa·rakeratō·sis (G. *para*, beside; *keras*, horn). A condition characterized by the formation of imperfectly keratinized corneous cells which form friable masses and scales. **P. variegata**: retiform or lichenoid type of parapsoriasis, *q.v.* Syn. lichen variegatus.

paralac·tic acid. Sarcolactic acid.

paralā·lia (G. *para*, beside; *lalia*, speech). Disturbance of the ability to utter certain sounds.

paralamb·dacism (G. *para*, beside; *lambda*, the Greek letter L). Disturbance of speech in which other consonants are substituted for the sound *l*.

paralbū·min (G. *para*, beside; L. *albumen*, white of egg). Pseudomucin.

paral·dehyde. A colourless liquid, soluble in water, alcohol and ether, obtained by treating aldehyde with sulphuric acid. It is used as a hypnotic and anodyne.

paral·dehydism. The condition resulting from overuse of paraldehyde.

paralex·ia (G. *para*, beside; *lexis*, phrasing). Disturbance of the ability to read, the patient making use of substitution of words or syllables.

paralgē·sia (G. *para*, beside; *algos*, pain). Disturbance of sensibility in which normally painful stimuli are experienced as comfortable.

pă·rallax. The apparent displacement of an object as seen from two different points.

paralō·gia (G. *para*, beside; *logos*, reason). False reasoning.

pară·lysis (G. *para*, beside; *luein*, to dissolve). Loss of nervous function, especially of the function of a motor efferent nerve. **P., acute ascending**: a syndrome characterized by flaccid p. of the lower limbs or lower trunk, progressing rapidly in cranial direction; usually due to anterior poliomyelitis, post-vaccinal myelitis or diphtheritic polyneuritis. **P.-agitans**: a chronic disease characterized by rigidity of voluntary muscles, muscular weakness, poverty and slowness of movements, tremor, an attitude of flexion of head, trunk and limbs; due to involutional lesions of the corpus striatum and subthalamic region. Syn. Parkinson's disease. **P., bulbar**: a condition affecting speech, mastication, swallowing and respiration, due to lesions of the motor nuclei of the related cranial nerves in the medulla oblongata. **P., crutch:** p. of axillary nerves due to pressure by a crutch. **P., familial periodic:** a familial disease, starting early in life, characterized by periodic transitory attacks of flaccid paralysis with paraesthesia associated with a disturbance of potassium metabolism. **P., general, of the insane:** a metasyphilitic disease of the brain, characterized when fully developed by progressive dementia, maniac delusions, dysarthria, transient seizures, tremor, absence of pupillary light-reflex, syphilitic reactions of blood and cerebrospinal fluid, and pathologically by widespread cerebral atrophy with loss of cortical neurons, glial overgrowth, perivascular infiltrates, meningeal thickening and the intracerebral presence of spirochaetes. **P., obstetrical:** paralysis of the brachial plexus or of its upper cord, due to trauma to the infant during birth. **P., pseudobulbar:** a syndrome characterized by disorders of speech, mastication and swallowing, due to bilateral lesions of corticobulbar pathways.

paralyt·ic (G. *para*, beside; *luein*, to dissolve). 1. Pertaining to paralysis. 2. A person affected with paralysis.

paramam·mary (G. *para*, beside; L. *mamma*, breast). Relating to structures about a mamma.

paramasti·tis (G. *para*, beside; *mastos*, breast). Inflammation of the connective tissue around the mamma.

paramas·toid (G. *para*, beside; *mastos*, breast; *eidos*, form). Situated near the mastoid process.

paramē·dian (G. *para*, beside; L. *medius*, middle). Close to the median plane.

paramē·nia (G. *para*, beside; *mēn*, month). Dysmenorrhoea, *q.v.*

paramet·ric (G. *para*, beside; *mētra*, womb). Relating to tissues around the uterus.

parametri·tis (G. *para*, beside; *mētra*, womb). Inflammation of the cellular tissue around the uterus. Syn. pelvic cellulitis.

paramē·trium (G. *para*, beside; *mētra*, womb). The connective tissue around the uterus.

parami·mia (G. *para*, against; *mīmēsis*, imitation). Facial expression not corresponding to actual emotion.

parami·tome (G. *para*, beside; *mitos*, thread). The clear substance of the cytoplasm contained in the meshes of the mitome. Syn. cell-sap.

paramnē·sia (G. *para*, beside; *amnēsia*, forgetfulness). Illusion of memory, especially the phenomenon of *déjà vu, q.v.*

Paramoe·cium (G. *para*, beside; *mēkos*, length). A small ciliated protozoa. **P. coli:** a species found in normal and loose stools.

paramor·phine. See the baine.

paramū·sia (G. *para*, beside; *mousa*, music). Disturbance of musical understanding, in which notes and intervals are wrongly used.

pă·ramyoclō·nus mul·tiplex (G. *para*, beside; *mus*, muscle; *klonos*, disturbance; L. *multus*, many; *plicare*, to fold). A disease of still obscure pathogenesis, characterized by sudden clonic spasms of individual voluntary muscles, affecting usually the corresponding muscles on both sides of the body, especially of the proximal parts of the limbs.

pa·ramyotō·nia congen·ita (G. *para*, beside; *mus*, muscle; *tonos*, tone: L. *congenitus*, congenital). A form of myotonia congenita, *q.v.*, characterized by tonic spasm, especially of the face, neck and throat, aggravated by cold, formerly believed to be a disease sui generis, but since observed in families affected with myotonia congenita.

paranaethē·sia (G. *para*, beside; *an*, neg.; *aisthēsis* feeling). Para-anaesthesia, *q.v.*

paranĕ·phric (G. *para*, beside; *nephros*, kidney). Near the kidney.

paranephrī·tis (G. *para*, beside; *nephros*, kidney). Inflammation of tissues near the kidney.

paranĕ·phros, paranĕ·phrus (G. *para*, beside; *nephros*, kidney). The adrenal gland.

paraneu·ral (G. *para*, beside; *neuron*, nerve). Close to a nerve.

paranoi·a (G. *para*, beside; *nous*, mind). A psychosis characterized by systematized and fixed delusions, in the absence of any other signs of mental impairment.

paranoi·ac (G. *para*, beside; *nous*, mind). One affected with paranoia.

paranoi·ic (G. *para*, beside; *nous*, mind). Relating to paranoia.

pă·ranoid (G. *para*, beside; *nous*, mind). Relating to p. dementia, that type of schizophrenic psychosis which is mainly characterized by the presence of delusions and hallucinations.

paranū·clear (G. *para*, beside; L. *nucleus*, kernel). Relating to a paranucleus.

paranū·cleāte. A salt of paranucleic acid.

paranū·clein (G. *para*, beside; L. *nucleus*, kernel). A compound of albumin with metaphosphoric acid, derived from nucleo-albumin.

paranū·cleŭs (G. *para*, beside; L. *nucleus*, kernel). An irregular body occasionally seen in cell-protoplasm near the nucleus. See also nebenkern.

para-omphal·ic (G. *para*, beside; *omphalos*, navel). Situated near the umbilicus.

paraparē·sis (G. *para*, beside; *parēsis*, paralysis). Paresis of both the upper or both the lower limbs; usually the term denotes paresis of the lower limbs.

paraparet·ic (G. *para*, beside; *parēsis*, paralysis). Relating to paraparesis.

paraphā·sia (G. *para*, beside; *phasis*, statement). A form of aphasia characterized by the use of wrong words in voluntary speech. Syn. jargon aphasia.

paraphimō·sis (G. *para*, beside; *phimoun*, to muzzle). Constriction of the penis by a retracted and too narrow prepuce.

paraphō·nia (G. *para*, beside; *phōnē*, voice). Abnormal condition of the voice.

paraphrā·sia (G. *para*, beside; *phrasis*, speech). Paraphasia.

paraphrē·nia (G. *para*, beside; *phrēn*, mind). A psychosis formerly believed to be a disease sui generis, intermediate between paranoia and schizophrenia; now regarded as a form of schizophrenia.

pă·raplasm (G. *para*, beside; *plasma*, a formation). 1. The paramitome. 2. Inert or relatively passive inclusions in protoplasm.

paraplas·tic (G. *para*, beside; *plassein*, to form). See ergastic.

paraplec·tic (G. *para*, beside; *plēgē*, a stroke). Affected with paraplegia.

paraplē·gia (G. *para*, beside; *plēgē*, a stroke). Paralysis of both upper or both lower limbs; usually the term denotes paralysis of the lower limbs.

paraplē·gic (G. *para*, beside; *plēgē*, a stroke). Relating to or affected with paraplegia.

parapneumŏn·ic (G. *para*, beside; *pneumōn*, lung). Relating to a morbid condition co-existent with a lobar pneumonia, e.g. pleurisy.

parap·sis (G. *para*, beside; *hapsis*, touch). Any disorder of the tactile sense.

parapsori·asis (G. *para*, beside; *psōra*, skin-disease). A group of skin diseases resembling in various respects both psoriasis and lichen planus, characterized by macular or maculopapular, smooth or scaly, superficial, scarcely infiltrating eruptions. The group is classified according to spread and coalescence of the initial lesion into P. en gouttes, P. lichenoides and P. en plaques.

parapylor·ic (G. *para*, beside; *pulōros*, pylorus). Around the pylorus.

para·queduct (G. *para*, beside; L. *aqua*, water; *ductus* from *ducerc*, to lead). Lateral extension of the aqueduct of Sylvius.

pararec·tal (G. *para*, beside; L. *rectus*, straight). Around the rectum.

pararē·nal (G. *para*, beside; L. *ren*, kidney). Around the kidney.

pararhō·tacism (G. *para*, beside; *rho*, the Greek letter R). Use of other sounds in place of the *r* sound. See also rhotacism.

parar·thria (G. *para*, beside; *arthron*, joint). Imperfect articulation of speech.

parasā·cral (G. *para*, beside; L. *sacer*, sacred). Near the sacrum.

pă·rasalpingi·tis (G. *para*, beside; *salpigx*, trumpet). Inflammation of the tissue around the uterine (Fallopian) tube.

parasig·matism (G. *para*, beside; *sigma*, the Greek letter S). Use of other sounds instead of the *s* or *sh* sounds.

pă·rasinoi·dal (G. *para*, beside; L. *sinus*, a hollow; G. *eidos*, form). Beside a cerebral sinus.

pă·rasite (G. *para*, beside; *sitos*, food). An organism (plant or animal) living more or less continuously upon or within and at the expense of another organism.

parasit·ic (G. *para*, beside; *sitos*, food). 1. Pertaining to parasites; of the nature of a parasite. 2. Caused by parasites.

parasi·ticide (G. *para*, beside; *sitos*, food; L. *caedere*, to kill). Destructive to parasites.

pă·rasitism (G. *para*, beside; *sitos*, food). 1. Any association in which an organism lives on or within the body of an organism of another species. 2. More especially, such an association involving an obvious injury by the parasite to its host.

parasitŏ·logy (G. *para*, beside; *sitos*, food; *logos*, treatise). The science of parasites.

parasi·totrope, parasitrop·ic (G. *para*, beside; *sitos*, food; *trepein*, to turn). Acting upon parasites.

paraspā·dia (G. *para*, beside; *spaein*, to draw forth). An opening of the urethra on the side of the penis.

paraster·nal (G. *para*, beside; *sternon*, the chest). 1. Beside the sternum. 2. Relating to a line parallel to and midway between sternal and clavicular lines.

parastru·ma (G. *para*, beside; *struma*, a scrofulous tumour). Enlargement of the parathyroid gland or glands.

pă·rasympathet·ic nerves or system (G. *para*, beside; *sun*, with; *pathos*, suffering). The cranial and sacral divisions of the autonomous nervous system.

parasynap·sis (G. *para*, beside; *sun*, with; *haptein*, to grasp). Side-by-side conjugation of chromosomes in synapsis. Syn. parasyndesis.

parasyndē·sis (G. *para*, beside; *sundein*, to bind together). Parasynapsis, *q.v.*

parasynovi·tis (G. *para*, beside; *sun*, with; L. *ovum*, egg). Inflammation of the connective tissue around a joint.

parasyphilit·ic (G. *para*, beside; *syphilis*). An obsolescent term applied to those forms of neurosyphilis which do not affect primarily the meninges or arteries.

parathor·mone (G. *para*, beside; *thureos*, a shield; *hormē*, onset). The hormone secreted by the parathyroid gland.

parathȳ·roid (G. *para*, beside; *thureos*, a shield; *eidos*, form). One of the four endocrine glands situated usually on the dorsal aspect of the thyroid gland. **P. hormone:** the hormone secreted by the parathyroid gland; promoting urinary excretion of phosphates, decrease of inorganic phosphates of blood plasma, and increase in blood calcium.

pa·rathyroi·dal (G. *para*, beside; *thureos*, a shield; *eidos*, form). Relating to the parathyroid glands.

pa·rathyroidec·tomy (G. *para*, beside; *thureos*, a shield; *eidos*, form; *ektomē*, excision). The surgical removal of the parathyroid gland(s).

parathyropriv·ic (G. *para*, beside; *thureos*, a shield; *eidos*, shape; L. *privus*, deprived of). Pertaining to the condition due to removal of the parathyroid glands.

paratrichō·sis (G. *para*, beside; *thrix*, hair). Growth of hair at abnormal places.

paratȳ·phoid bacilli (G. *para*, beside; *tuphos*, stupor; *eidos*, form). The organisms belonging to the group of *Bacterium paratyphosum* A, B and C.

paratȳ·phoid fever (G. *para*, beside; *tuphos*, stupor; *eidos*, form). An acute disease due to infection with one of the p. bacilli, resembling in its clinical course either typhoid fever or acute gastro-enteritis.

paraver·tebral (G. *para*, beside; L. *vertebra*). Beside the spinal column.

paravesi·cal (G. *para*, beside; L. *vesica*, bladder). Beside the urinary bladder.

parax·ial (G. *para*, beside; L. *axis*). Beside the axis of the body.

Paré's suture (Paré, A., French surgeon, 1510–90). Strips of cloth pasted along wound edges and then stitched together to approximate the margins of the wound.

paregŏ·ric (G. *parēgorikos*, consoling). 1. Soothing. 2. The camphorated tincture of opium; used as an anodyne.

parencephali·tis (G. *para*, beside; *egkephalos*, brain). Inflammation of the cerebellum.

parencē·phalocele (G. *para*, beside; *egkephalos*, brain; *kēlē*, hernia). Hernia of the cerebellum.

parencē·phalon (G. *para*, against; *egkephalos*, brain). The cerebellum.

parencē·phalus (G. *para*, against; *egkephalos*, brain). One with congenital malformation of the brain.

paren·chyma (G. *para*, beside; *egkhein*, to pour in). The essential tissue of an organ as distinguished from the supporting connective tissue, vessels, nerves, etc.

parenchȳ·matous (G. *para*, beside; *egkhein*, to pour in). Pertaining to the parenchyma.

parenchymi·tis (G. *para*, against; *egkhein*, to pour in). Inflammation of a parenchyma.

parenchȳ·mula (G. *para*, against; *egkhein*, to pour in). Embryonic stage following that of the closed blastula.

paren·teral (G. *para*, beside; *enteron*, intestine). 1. Outside the intestinal tract. 2. Relating to administration of a substance by a way other than that of the alimentary tract, e.g. by subcutaneous, intramuscular or intravenous injection. **P. diarrhoea:** diarrhoea in infants when caused by a disease outside the alimentary tract, e.g. by a respiratory infection.

parĕ·picele (G. *para*, beside; *epi*, upon; *koilos*, hollow). The lateral recess of the fourth ventricle of the brain.

parepidi·dymis (G. *para*, beside; *epi*, upon; *didumos*, twin). Paradidymis, *q.v.*

parē·sis (G. *paresis*, paralysis). Slight paralysis.

pă·reso-analgē·sia (G. *paresis*, paralysis; *an*, neg.; *algos*, pain). Paresis with analgesia.

paret·ic (G. *paresis*, paralysis). Pertaining to or affected with paresis.

pareu·nia (G. *pareunos*, a bedfellow). Coitus.

paridrō·sis (G. *para*, beside; *hidrōs*, perspiration). Any abnormal condition of sweat secretion.

pă·riēs (L. *paries*, wall). An enveloping structure or outer wall.

pari·etal (L. *paries*, wall). 1. Forming or situated on a wall: e.g., p. layer of the pleura. 2. Relating to or in relation with the p. bone of the skull (p. foramen, p. lobe of the brain). **P. bone:** one of the two bones in the middle region of the roof of the skull. **P. cells:** one of the types of cells of the gastric glands, situated between zymogenic cells and the basement membrane. **P. lobe:** that cerebral lobe which is bounded in front by the Rolandic fissure, behind by the parieto-occipital fissure and on the side and below by the Sylvian fissure.

parī·etēs (L., pl. of *paries*, wall). The walls of any cavity.

pari·etofron·tal (L. *paries*, walls; *frons*, forehead). Relating to the parietal and frontal bones.

pari·eto-occip·ital (L. *paries*, wall; *ob*, against; *caput*, head). Relating to the parietal and occipital bones or lobes.

pari·eto-tem·poral (L. *paries*, wall; *tempora*, pl. of *tempus*, temple). Relating to the parietal and temporal bones.

Parinaud's conjunctivitis (Parinaud, H., French ophthalmologist, 1844–1905). A serious type of mucopurulent conjunctivitis supposed to be caused by infection from animals. **P.'s ophthalmoplegia:** paralysis of the external rectus of the one side; peripheral in origin.

Paris green. Copper acetoarsenite, used for spraying fruit trees.

Park's aneurysm (Park, H., English surgeon, 1744–1831). Arterio-venous aneurysm.

Parker's arches (Parker, W. K., English anatomist, 1823–90). The 'occipital arches' of the developing skull that complete the occipital portion of the primitive cranium.

Parkinson's disease (Parkinson, J., English physician, 1755–1824). Paralysis agitans. **P.'s facies** or **mask:** the immobile and expressionless facies of paralysis agitans.

Parkinsonism (Parkinson, J., English physician, 1755–1824). The condition of suffering from Parkinson's disease, *q.v.*

paroccip·ital (G. *para*, beside; L. *ob*, against; *caput*, head). Around or beside the occipital region.

parodontī·tis (G. *para*, beside; *odous*, tooth). Inflammation of the socket of a tooth.

parŏ·livary (G. *para*, beside; L. *oliva*, an olive). Around or beside the olivary body.

paromphă·locele (G. *para*, beside; *omphalos*, navel; *kēlē*, hernia). A hernia near the navel.

Parona's space (Parona, F., Italian surgeon). The deep forearm (intermuscular) space.

paronŷ·chia (G. *para*, beside; *onux*, nail). Inflammation about the nail. Syn. whitlow; felon.

parŏŏ·phoron (G. *para*, beside; *ōon*, egg; *pherein*, to bear). A group of tubules in the ligamentum latum in the female, remnants of the Wolffian body.

parŏ·pion (G. *para*, beside; *ōps*, eye). An eye-shade.

parop·sis (G. *para*, beside; *opsis*, vision). Disordered vision.

parorchī·dium (G. *para*, beside; *orkhis*, testicle). Misplacement of the testicle.

parorex·ia (G. *para*, beside; *orĕxis*, appetite). Perversion of appetite.

paros·mia (G. *para*, beside; *osmē*, smell). Perversion of the sense of smell; a hallucination of smell.

parostŏ·sis (G. *para*, beside; *osteon*, bone). Formation of osseous tissue outside the periosteum.

parot·ic (G. *para*, beside; *ous*, ear). Situated near the ear.

parŏ·tid (G. *para*, beside; *ous*, ear). Relating to or affecting the p. gland. **P. gland:** one of the salivary glands, situated below and in front of the external ear.

parotidec·tomy (G. *para*, beside; *ous*, ear; *ektomē*, excision). Surgical removal of the parotid gland.

parŏ·tis (G. *para*, beside; *ous*, ear). The parotid gland.

parotī·tis (G. *para*, beside; *ous*, ear). Inflammation of the parotis. **P., epidemic:** an acute infectious disease, characterized by swelling of the salivary glands, especially of the parotid glands. Syn. mumps.

pa·rous (L. *parĕre*, to bear). 1. Bringing forth; bearing. 2. Having borne one or more children.

parovā·rian (G. *para*, beside; L. *ovum*, egg). 1. Near the ovary. 2. Relating to the parovarium.

parovā·rium (G. *para*, beside; L. *ovum*, egg). The remnant of the Wolffian body of the female, situated between the layers of the broad ligament between the ovarium and the lateral end of the uterine tube. Syn. the organ of Rosenmüller; epoophoron.

pă·roxysm (G. *para*, beside; *oxus*, sharp). A sudden attack; a sudden increase in the severity of existing symptoms.

paroxys·mal (G. *para*, beside; *oxus*, sharp). Of the nature of or occurring in paroxysms. **P. hypertension:** p. attacks of hypertension due to sudden secretions of adrenaline from a phaeochromocytoma. **P. rhinorrhoea:** 1. Vasomotor rhinitis, *q.v.* 2. Hay fever, *q.v.* **P. tachycardia, auricular:** the more common type of p. tachycardia, due to new impulses arising in the auricle producing sudden acceleration of the heart rate, the latter being of about 160–180 per minute, of regular rhythm, and unaffected by exertion or atropine; usually characterized in the electrocardiogram by inversion of the P wave in leads 1 and 2, diphasic P wave in lead 3, and upright P wave in lead 4. **P. tachycardia, ventricular:** p. tachycardia of ventricular origin, usually a serious disturbance of rhythm which tends to be less regular than in auricular p. t., characterized electrocardiographically by ventricular complexes in the shape of ventricular premature beats, sometimes with an alternate reversal of direction and of true intervals.

Parrish's Chemical Food. A compound syrup of ferrous phosphate; used as a tonic.

Parrot's atrophy of the new-born (Parrot, J. M., French physician, 1829–83). Athrepsia; primary infantile atrophy. **P.'s disease:** pseudo-paralysis of the extremities due to the separation of the epiphyses, which prevents spontaneous movements, seen in hereditary syphilis of the new-born. **P.'s nodes:** nodular osteophytes of the frontal and parietal bones around the anterior fontanelle in hereditary syphilis. **P.'s sign:** dilatation of the pupil when the skin is pinched; observed in meningitis. **P.'s ulcers:** the whitish or yellowish patches seen in cases of thrush.

parrot disease. Psittacosis, *q.v.*

Parry's disease (Parry, C. H., English physician, 1755–1822). Exophthalmic goitre.

pars (L.). A part.

parsley. The *Petroselinum sativum*. Sometimes used in renal disease.

Parsons's disease (Parsons, J., English physician, 1705–70). Exophthalmic goitre.

part. aeq. Abbreviation for L. *partes aequales*, equal parts.

par·thenogĕ·nesis (G. *parthenos*, virgin; *genesis*, reproduction). The more or less complete development of an organism from an unfertilized ovum.

partial pressure. The pressure exerted by one constituent of a mixture of gases.

particle (L. *particula*, dim. of *pars*, part). A minute part of a solid body, incapable of mechanical division.

partū·rient (L. *parturire*, to be in labour). Being in labour; the act of giving birth.

par·turifā·cient (L. *parturire*, to be in labour; *facere*, to cause). Promoting parturition.

parturī·tion (L. *parturire*, to be in labour). The act of giving birth.

partus (L.). The producing of offspring.

part. vic. Abbreviation for L. *partibus vicibus*, in alternate doses.

parū·lis (G. *para*, beside; *oulon*, gum). Abscess beneath the periosteum of an alveolar process.

P.A.S. See *p*-aminosalicylic acid.

Paschen bodies (Paschen, E., German pathologist, 1860–1936). Bodies supposed to contain the virus of smallpox. They can be differentiated by fixing with sublimate alcohol at 37°C. and by staining with Giemsa's solution.

passage. 1. A channel. 2. The act of passing.

Passavant's bar (Passavant, P. G., German surgeon, 1815–93). The projecting ridge on the posterior wall of the pharynx produced by contraction of the upper fibres of the palatopharyngeus muscle. **P.'s cushion:** the bulging of the posterior pharyngeal wall produced during the act of swallowing by the upper fibres of the superior constrictor muscle of the pharynx.

passive (L. *passivus*, from *pati*, to suffer). Not active. **P. congestion:** congestion due to obstruction of venous outflow. **P. immunity:** see immunity, p. **P. movements:** movements produced with the help of another person.

paste. A medical preparation for external application of soft but sticky consistency, usually compounded with a base of paraffin, starch and glycerine.

Pasteur's fluid (Pasteur, L., French chemist and bacteriologist, 1822–95). A liquid prepared from sugar, ammonium carbonate and ashes of yeast, used in the cultivation of bacteria.

Pasteurella (Pasteur, L.). A group of short non-motile, non-spore-bearing bacilli, including *P. boviseptica, P. oviseptica* and *P. suipestifer*.

pasteurellō·sis (Pasteur, L.). Any infection with one of the organisms of the Pasteurella group; a haemorrhagic septicaemia in cattle, deer, rodents, wild hog and other animals.

pasteurizā·tion (Pasteur, L.). Method of preserving organic fluids, such as milk, by destruction of ferments and micro-organisms by heating to 60°—70°C.

pastille (L. *pastillus*, lozenge). 1. A soft mass of medicated glyco-gelatine used for application to mouth and throat. 2. A coated paper disc which changes colour on being exposed to X-rays; an obsolescent measure of X-ray dosage.

past-pointing. The physiological inability to touch a given object correctly with the extended arm and finger and with closed eyes after artificial stimulation of the labyrinth (by cold or warm water or by galvanic stimulation or rotary movements).

patch. An irregular spot. **Mucous p.:** a whitish papule on mucous membranes and at muco-cutaneous junctions, one of the characterized lesions of secondary syphilis.

pate. The crown of the head.

patefac·tion (L. *patefacere*, to lay open). The act of opening.

patel·la (L. *patella*, dim. of *patina*, pan). The kneecap; the sesamoid bone in front of the knee.

patel·lapexy (L. *patella*; G. *pēxis*, fixation). An operation in which the patella is fixed to the lower end of the femur in order to stabilize the knee.

patel·lar (L. *patella*). Relating to the patella. **P. reflex:** see knee-jerk. **P. clonus:** persistent knee-jerks, elicited by drawing the patella downwards and keeping it in this position; a sign of muscular hypertonus (usually due to a lesion of the pyramidal tracts).

pā·tency (L. *patēre*, to be open). The condition of being open.

patent (L. *patēre*, to be open). Open.

Paterson's corpuscles (Paterson, R., Scottish physician, 1814–89). The molluscum corpuscles; oval, shining bodies found in the contents of the tubercles of molluscum contagiosum.

path. A tract. Used in neurology to denote the course of nerve fibres.

pathet·ic (G. *pathētikos*, impassioned). 1. Arousing emotions. 2. Applied to the fourth cranial nerve

which innervates the muscle rolling the eye outward and downward.

pathě·ticus (G. *pathētikos*, impassioned). The fourth cranial nerve.

pathfinder. A small filiform bougie used for discovering the opening of an urethral stricture.

pā·thic (G. *pathikos*, passive). Diseased; pathological.

pathŏ·clisis (G. *pathos*, disease; *klisis*, inclination). Vogt's conception of an abnormal vulnerability of systems of ganglion cells or nerve fibres, determined by the physiochemical constitution of definite anatomically definable, neuronal units, which may result in an active disease process in later stages of life.

pă·thogen, pathogě·nic (G. *pathos*, disease; *gennan*, to produce). Producing disease.

pathogě·nesis (G. *pathos*, disease; *genesis*, reproduction). The mode of development of a disease.

pă·thogenet·ic (G. *pathos*, disease; *genesis*, reproduction). Relating to pathogenesis.

pă·thogenĭ·city (G. *pathos*, disease; *gennan*, to produce). The state of being pathogenic.

pathŏ·geny (G. *pathos*, disease; *gennan*, to produce). Pathogenesis, *q.v.*

pathognomon·ic (G. *pathos*, disease; *gnōmōn*, indicator). Characteristic of a disease; distinguishing it from others.

pathŏ·gnomy (G. *pathos*, disease; *gnōmē*, opinion). The science of the distinguishing signs and symptoms of diseases.

pathŏ·gical (G. *pathos*, disease; *logos*, treatise). Relating to pathology; relating to disease.

pathŏ·logist (G. *pathos*, disease; *logos*, treatise). One skilled in pathology.

pathŏ·logy (G. *pathos*, disease; *logos*, treatise). That branch of medical science dealing with structural or functional changes caused by disease. **Clinical p.:** the study of pathology in the living being.

pathophō·bia (G. *pathos*, disease; *phobos*, fear). Neurotic fear of disease.

pathopoiē·sis (G. *pathos*, disease; *poisēsis*, a making). The cause of disease.

patient (L. *pati*, to suffer). A sick person.

patten (Fr. *patin*, skate). A support placed under one foot to extend a diseased limb or to equalize the length of the two legs.

pă·tulous (L. *patēre*, to be open). Open; distended.

Paul's sign (Paul, C. C. T., French physician, 1833–96). Feeble apex-beat with forcible impulse over the heart observed in cases of adherent pericardium.

Paul's tube (Paul, F. T., English surgeon, 1851–1941). A glass drainage tube with a flange on one end used in cases of intestinal obstruction to drain the bowel.

Paul-Bragg's apparatus. A mechanical device for producing artificial respiration which can be operated by a motor, or by water, for indefinitely long periods. It consists of a rubber air-bag wrapped round the chest and rhythmically inflated and deflated.

Paul-Bunnell test (Paul, J. R., born 1893; Bunnell, W. W., born 1902, American physicians). A test used in the diagnosis of infective mononucleosis. The blood of patients suffering from this disease contains agglutinins which act specifically on the red blood cells of sheep.

paulocar·dia (G. *paula*, pause; *kardia*, heart). A sensation of intermission of the heart-beat.

paunch. The abdominal cavity and what it contains.

pavement epithelium. Epithelium consisting of scalelike cells resembling in arrangement the tiles of a pavement.

Pavlov's method (Pavlov, I. P., Russian physiologist, 1849–1936). A study of the influence of the mind on the salivary reflex. **P's stomach:** part of a dog's stomach which was isolated from the rest of it and made to open on to the abdominal wall; Pavlov used it to study gastric secretion

Pavlov's tract (Pavlov, V. A., Russian histologist, born 1863). The tractus reto-reticularis.

pa·vor (L. *pavor*, dread). Fright; fear. **P. nocturnus**: night terrors. See also nightmare.

Pavy's disease (Pavy, F. W., English physician, 1829–1911). Cyclic albuminuria.

Pawlik's folds (Pawlik, K., Austrian surgeon, 1849–1914). The anterior columns of the vagina, which form the lateral boundary of P.'s triangle. **P.'s triangle**: the triangular space formed by the divergent columns of the vagina and the transverse ridge below the external orifice of the neck of the bladder.

Paxton's disease (Paxton, F. V., English physician, died 1924). Tinea nodosa.

Payr's clamp (Payr, E., German surgeon, born 1871). Intestinal crushing clamp. **P.'s disease**: kinking and adhesion between transverse and descending colon, producing chronic intestinal stenosis. **P.'s sign**: pain on pressure over the inner side of the foot in early post-operative thrombosis.

Pb. The symbol for lead. (L. *plumbum*).

Pb(CH₃.COO)₂. Lead acetate.

$Pb(CH_3.COO)_2$. Lead acetate.

$PbCO_3$. Lead carbonate.

PbI_2. Lead iodide.

$Pb(NO_3)_2$. Lead nitrate.

PbO. Lead monoxide.

PbO_2. Lead dioxide.

PbS. Lead sulphide.

$PbSO_4$. Lead sulphate.

p.c. Abbreviation for L. *post cibum*, after food.

Pd. The symbol for Palladium.

Péan's forceps (Péan, J., French surgeon, 1830–98). Metal forceps for the removal of small pieces of tissue. **P.'s operation**: the removal of tumours in small pieces in cases where the growth is too large for removal through the incision.

pearl disease. Tuberculosis of the serous membrane in animals, especially in cattle, characterized by small translucent nodules ('pearls') on the affected membranes. **Pearls, epithelial**: spheroidal concentric masses of epithelial cells, as seen in, e.g., cholesteatoma or in squamous epithelioma.

pearly bodies. Pearls, epithelial, *q.v.*

peau de chagrin (Fr.). A shagreen patch, an irregular thickened area of the skin, especially over the trunk, often present in epiloia, *q.v.*

pebrine (Provençal *pebrino*, from *pebre*, pepper). An infectious disease of silkworms.

pec·cant (L. *peccare*, to sin). Morbid; pathogenic; unhealthy.

Pechlin's glands (Pechlin, J. N., Dutch anatomist, 1644–1706). Peyer's patches, *q.v.*

Pecquet's cistern (Pecquet, J., French anatomist, 1622–74). The receptaculum chyli. **P.'s duct**: the thoracic duct.

pec·tase. A nitrogenous enzyme which acts on venous pectins and is found in fruits.

pecten (L. comb). 1. A comb-like structure. 2. The zone between the skin lining the lower portion of the anal canal and the rectal mucosa above.

pecteni·tis (L. *pecten*, comb). Inflammation of the anal pecten.

pectenō·sis (L. *pecten*, comb). Fibrous infiltration of the pecten (2), usually caused by chronic passive congestion of the anal canal.

pectenō·tomy (L. *pecten*, comb; G. *tomē*, section). Incision of the pecten.

pectic acid. $C_{16}H_{22}O_{15}$ prepared from pectin.

pectin (G. *pēktos*, congealed). A polysaccharide contained in ripe fruit (e.g. apple); absorbs water to form stable gels.

pec·tinase (G. *pēktos*, congealed). An enzyme which is capable of transforming pectin.

pec·tinate (L. *pecten*, comb). Disposed like the teeth of a comb. **P. ligament**: connective tissue fibres at the angle of the interior chamber of the eye, between iris and cornea. **P. muscles**: the musculi pectinati, parallel muscular ridges in the auricles of the heart.

pecti·neal (L. *pecten*, comb). 1. Comb-shaped. 2. Relating to the pecten ossis pubis.

pecti·neus muscle. A small muscle in the upper part of the thigh. It arises from the pectineal line of the hip-bone and is inserted into the upper part of the posterior surface of the femur.

pecti·niform (L. *pecten*, comb; *forma*, shape). Comb-shaped.

pec·toral (L. *pectus*, male breast). 1. Concerning the chest, as the p. muscles. 2. Any remedy for diseases of the chest.

pectorā·lis muscle (L. *pectus*, male breast). A muscle situated on the anterior surface of the chest.

pectori·loquy (L. *pectus*, male breast; *loqui*, speak). The transmission of articulate speech to the ear on auscultation.

pec·tose (G. *pēktos*, congealed). Progenitor of pectin, found in unripe fruits and plants.

pectō·sinase (G. *pēktos*, congealed). Enzyme which changes pectose into pectin and pectin into various sugars.

pec·tus (L.). The chest or breast. **P. carinatum**: a chest projecting in the region of the sternum. Syn. pigeon-breast.

pē·dal (L. *pes*, foot). 1. Pertaining to the foot. 2. Pertaining to the pes of the crus cerebri.

pedē·sis (G., a leaping). The quick, darting motion of fine particles of a substance suspended in a translucent liquid. Syn. Brown's phenomenon.

pediăl·gia (L. *pes*, foot; G. *algos*, pain). Pain in the foot.

pě·dicle (L. *pediculus*, dim. of *pes*, foot). A slender process, serving as a stem.

pedi·cular¹ (L. *pediculus*, dim. of *pes*, foot). Relating to a pedicle.

pedic·ular² (L. *pediculus*, louse). Relating to pediculosis.

pediculā·tion (L. *pediculus*, dim. of *pes*, foot). The process of developing a pedicle.

Pediculoi·des ventricō·sus (L. *pediculus*, louse; G. *eidos*, form). A species of acarus living in the stalks of cereals, the organism causing 'grain itch' in man.

pedi·culophō·bia (L. *pediculus*, louse; G. *phobos*, fear). Neurotic fear of becoming louse infested.

pediculō·sis (L. *pediculus*, louse). Infestation with lice.

pedi·culus (L.). The louse; a small parasitic insect. **P. capitis**: the head louse. **P. corporis**: the body louse. **P. pubis**: the *Phthirus pubis*.

pě·dicure (L. *pes*, foot; *cura*, solicitude). Care of the feet.

pedŏ·meter (L. *pes*, foot; G. *metron*, measure). An instrument for the automatic measurement of distances travelled.

pedun·cle (L. *pedunculus*, dim. of *pes*, foot). A narrow process serving as a support; a stalk. **P., cerebellar, inferior**: a structure of white matter (afferent fibres) connecting the corpus restiforme with the cerebellum. **P., cerebellar, middle**: a structure of white matter connecting the pons and the cerebellum. **P., cerebellar, superior**: a structure of white matter (efferent fibres) connecting the nucleus dentatus and other cerebellar nuclei with nucleus ruber and optic thalamus of the opposite side.

pedun·cular (L. *pedunculus*, dim. of *pes*, foot). Relating to a peduncle.

pedun·culated (L. *pedunculus*, dim. of *pes*, foot). Having a peduncle.

peg. 1. A pointed wooden or metal pin. 2. A wooden leg. **P.-teeth:** a term applied to the molar (permanent) teeth of subjects with congenital syphilis, from the peg-like aspect of the crowns.

pē·jorative (L. *pejor*, worse). Worsening.

pē·lage (Old Fr. *pel*, from L. *pilus*, hair). The hairy portion of the body.

Pel-Ebstein's disease (Pel, P. K., Dutch physician, 1852–1919; Ebstein, W., German physician, 1836–1912). Lymphadenoma marked by pyrexia which rises over three days, stays raised for three days, falls to normal for three days and then repeats the cycle.

peliŏ·sis rheumă·tica (G. *peliosis*, a livid spot). See purpura rheumatica.

pellă·gra (G. *pella*, skin; G. *agra*, seizure). A disease, probably due to deficiency in vitamin-B_2-containing food, characterized by lesions of the skin (pigmented erythema or dermatitis, especially at exposed parts), alimentary tract (glossitis, stomatitis, sialorrhoea, diarrhoea) and nervous system (peripheral neuritis or atactic paraplegia), by anaemia and by mental changes. The anti-pellagra factor is vitamin B_6; nicotinic acid, nicotinic acid amide.

pel·lagrin (G. *pella*, skin; *agra*, seizure). One affected with pellagra.

pella·grous (G. *pella*, skin; *agra*, seizure). Relating to pellagra.

pellet. A small pill.

pellet·ierine (Pelletier, J., French chemist, 1782–1842). A water-soluble alkaloid, optically inactive, a derivative of coniine, from the root-bark of pomegranate. Used in the form of pelletierine tannate to destroy tapeworms.

pel·licle (L. *pellicula*, dim. of *pellis*, skin). 1. A small thin transparent membrane or cuticle. 2. A delicate film on the surface of a liquid.

pellū·cid (L. *pellucidus*, from *per*, through; *lucere*, to shine). Transparent.

pel·ma (G.). The sole of the foot.

pelohāē·mia (G. *pēlos*, mud; *haima*, blood). Abnormal thickness of the blood.

pelother·apy (G. *pēlos*, mud; *therapeia*, treatment). The use of mud in treatment of disorders.

pel·veoperitonī·tis (L. *pelvis*, basin; G. *peritonaion*, membrane containing the lower viscera). Pelvioperitonitis, *q.v.*

pelvic (L. *pelvis*, basin). Relating to the pelvis. **P. abscess:** a collection of pus in the pelvic cavity, usually due to appendicitis, or gonorrhoeal infection in women. **P. cellulitis:** inflammation of the connective tissue in the pelvis. **P. index:** the ratio of the anteroposterior to the transverse diameter of the pelvis.

pelvĭ·meter (L. *pelvis*, basin; G. *metron*, measure). An instrument for measuring the pelvic dimensions.

pelvĭ·metry (L. *pelvis*, basin; G. *metron*, measure). The measurement of the pelvic dimensions.

pel·vioperitonī·tis (L. *pelvis*, basin; G. *peritonaion*, membrane containing the lower viscera). Pelvic peritonitis.

pelvirec·tal. Having relation to the pelvis and the rectum.

pelvis (L.). 1. A basin-shaped cavity, as the p. of the kidney. 2. The structure formed by the two innominate bones with the sacrum coccyx. 3. The cavity encircled by the bony pelvis.

pem·phigoid (G. *pemphix*, bubble; *eidos*, form). Resembling pemphigus.

pem·phigus (G. *pemphix*, bubble). An acute or chronic disease of the skin characterized by irregularly distributed bullae arising on normal or slightly inflamed skin, sometimes associated with severe systemic symptoms. **P. foliaceus:** a chronic affection of the skin characterized by the eruption of flattened bullae followed by universal redness and epidermal exfoliation, leaving denuded discharging areas. **P. neonatorum:** acute p. in newborn infants, usually due to streptococcal infection of the skin. **P. syphiliticus:** p. in newborn infants affected with congenital syphilis, occurring on the palms of the hands and soles of the feet. **P. vegetans:** a form of p. characterized by the eruption of bullae followed by the development of papillary vegetations, often leading to ulceration and gangrene of the skin, occurring mainly about the axillae and perineum. **P. vulgaris:** a form of p. not leading to any final loss of epidermal tissue.

pencil (L. *penicillum*, a painter's brush). A medicated cylindrical stick for external application.

pen·dulous (L. *pendēre*, to hang). Hanging down.

pē·netrance (L. *penetrare*, to enter). Manifestation of the effects of a gene.

penetrā·tion (L. *penetrare*, to enter). 1. The act of entering beneath a surface. 2. The focal depths of a microscope. 3. The entry of the penis into the vagina.

penicil·late (L. *penicillum*, a painter's brush). Shaped like a painters' brush.

penicil·lin. An antibiotic from *Pencillium notatum*; effectively inhibits growth of gram-positive organisms, especially staphylococci, haemolytic streptococci and gonococci. **P. (calcium salt) eye ointment:** Aseptically prepared to contain 1,000 units per g. in a sterile base of yellow soft paraffin (90 parts) and wool fat (10 parts). Used in the treatment of ophthalmic infection, styes, etc. **P. (calcium salt) ointment:** aseptically prepared ointment containing 500 units per g. in a paraffin base (Ointment of Wool Alcohols B.P.). Used in the treatment of pyogenic infections. **P. cream:** a sterile soft cream incorporating penicillin 500 units per g. **P. injection:** a sterile solution of the sodium or the calcium salt in water. **P. injection, oily:** a sterile suspension of penicillin in an oily base prepared from arachis oil and white beeswax.

pē·nile (L. *penis*). Relating to the penis.

pē·nis (L.). The male organ of copulation.

pen·niform (L. *penna*, feather; *forma*, shape). Shaped like a feather.

pennyroyal. Popular name for the herb *Mentha pulegium*, which produces an oil, oleum pulegii, which acts as a mild irritant to the kidneys and bladder and by reflex action produces uterine contractions. It is used as an emmenagogue.

pennyweight. A troy weight, equalling twenty-four grains.

penŏ·logy (G. *poinē*, penalty; *logos*, treatise). The scientific investigation of the punishment and prevention of crime.

pentamethō·nium iodide. $((CH_3)_4\overset{+}{N}.(CH_2)_5\overset{+}{N}(CH_3)_4)2I$. See hexamethonium.

pen·tane (G. *pente*, five). A liquid hydrocarbon, (C_5H_{12}). It is a constituent of petroleum ether.

pentă·valent (G. *pente*, five; *valere*, to be worth). Possessing a valence of five.

pentobar·bital sō·dium. The monosodium derivative of 5.ethyl-5-(1-methylbutyl)-barbituric acid. A white crystalline powder. Soluble in water and alcohol, insoluble in ether. Hypnotic.

pentosāē·mia (G. *pente*, five; *haima*, blood). The presence of pentose in the blood.

pen·tosan. A polysaccharide derived from pentoses.

pen·tose (G. *pente*, five). A monosaccharide of general formula, $C_5H_{10}O_5$, e.g. arabinose, ribose and xylose.

pentosī·dase (G. *pente*, five). An enzyme hydrolysing a pentoside.

pen·toside (G. *pente*, five). A compound formed from a pentose and an alcohol by the elimination of the element of water.

pentosū·ria (G. *pente*, five; *ouron*, urine). The presence of pentose in the urine.

pen·tothal sō·dium. The monosodium derivative of 5-ethyl-5-(1-methylbutyl)-thiobarbituric acid. An ultra-short-acting barbiturate anaesthetic. May be administered rectally.

pentox·ide. Any oxide with five atoms of oxygen.

pĕŏ·tomy (G. *peos*, penis; *tomē*, section). Surgical removal of the penis.

pepper. The dried seeds of *Piper nigrum*; they are carminative and stimulant.

peppermint. The herb *Mentha piperita* from the leaves of which peppermint oil is obtained. Used as a carminative. *Mentha piperita* also yields menthol.

pep·sin (G. *peptein*, to digest). A proteolytic enzyme secreted by the chief cells of the gastric glands.

pepsi·nogen (G. *peptein*, to digest; *gennan*, to produce). The inactive or precursor form of pepsin.

pepsinū·ria (G. *peptein*, to digest; *ouron*, urine). The presence of pepsin in the urine.

pep·tic (G. *peptein*, to digest). 1. Relating to pepsin. 2. Relating to digestion. **P. ulcer:** round ulcer of the stomach or duodenum.

pep·tidase. An enzyme which hydrolyses peptides.

peptide (G. *peptein*, to digest). A compound of several amino acids linked through their amino and carboxyl groups (-CONH-), but of structure less complete than that of peptones.

peptŏ·genous (G. *peptein*, to digest; *gennan*, to produce). Producing pepsin or peptones.

peptonae·mia (G. *peptein*, to digest; *haima*, blood). The presence of peptones in the blood.

pep·tone (G. *peptein*, to digest). Compounds formed by partial enzymatic breakdown of proteins, consisting of numerous amino acid residues.

peptonizā·tion (G. *peptein*, to produce). Conversion of proteins into peptones.

pep·tonize (G. *peptein*, to digest). To convert into peptones; to digest with pepsin; to pre-digest.

peptonū·ria (G. *peptein*, to digest; *ouron*, urine). The presence of peptones in the urine.

peracě·phalus (G. *peri*, exceedingly; *akephalos*, headless). A monster characterized by acephaly, absence of the upper extremities and malformation of the thorax.

peraci·dity (L. *per*, exceedingly; *acidus*, acid). A considerable degree of hyperacidity.

peracute (L. *per*, exceedingly; *acutus*, sharp). Very sharp.

per anum (L.). Through the anus.

perarticulā·tion (L. *per*, through; *articulare*, to articulate). Diarthrosis.

percaine. The hydrochloride of α-butyloxycinchoninic acid diethylethylenediamide. Soluble in water. Used as a local anaesthetic and for spinal anaesthesia. Syn. Nupercain.

percep·tion (L. *percipere*, to perceive). 1. The act of receiving impressions through any one of the sense organs. 2. A mental complex based upon sensory experiences.

percepti·vity (L. *percipere*, to perceive). The capability of receiving impressions.

per·colate (L. *per*, through; *colare*, to filter). 1. To subject to percolation. 2. The solution obtained by percolation.

percolā·tion (L. *per*, through; *colare*, to filter). The process of extracting the soluble constituents of a substance placed in a percolator by slow passage of a solvent through the substance.

per·colator (L. *per*, through; *colare*, to filter). A conical or cylindrical vessel used for extracting the soluble constituents of a substance.

Percorten. A proprietary preparation of desoxycorticosterone acetate, used in the treatment of Addison's disease.

percuss (L. *percutere*, to beat). To perform percussion.

percus·sion (L. *percutere*, to beat). Tapping the surface of a part with a finger or a percussor, in order to determine the condition of the underlying organ from the character of the sounds elicited.

percus·sor (L. *percutere*, to beat). A hammer for performing percussion.

percutā·neous (L. *per*, through; *cutis*, skin). Through the skin, e.g. as applied to tests performed by rubbing a substance into the skin.

Perez's sign (Perez, F., Spanish physician, 1863–1935). A distinct friction murmur audible over the sternum when the patient lifts his arms above his head and then lets them fall; noted in aneurysm of the arch of the aorta and in fibrous mediastinitis.

perflā·tion (L. *perflare*, to blow through). Blowing of air into or through a cavity in order to expel its contents.

per·forans (L. *perforare*, to pierce). Perforating.

per·forate (L. *perforare*). To pierce; pierced.

perforā·tion (L. *perforare*, to pierce). 1. The act of piercing a part. 2. A hole made through a part.

per·forator (L. *perforare*, to pierce). An instrument for perforation of the foetal skull or for perforating other bones.

perforatō·rium (L. *perforare*, to pierce). Perforator; cephalotome.

perfricā·tion (L. *perfricare*, to rub). Inunction.

perfū·sion (L. *perfundere*, to pour over). 1. A pouring of fluid into or through. 2. The forcing of a liquid through organs by way of the blood-vessels.

periă·cinous (G. *peri*, around; L. *ăcinus*, berry). Around an acinus.

periădeni·tis (G. *peri*, around; *adēn*, gland). Inflammation of the connective tissue around a lymph gland.

periă·nal (G. *peri*, around; L. *anus*, anus). Around the anus.

periăngii·tis (G. *peri*, around; *aggeion*, vessels). Inflammation of the tissues surrounding an artery.

periăngiocholi·tis (G. *peri*, around; *aggeion*, vessel; *kholē*, bile). Inflammation of the tissues around the intrahepatic bile ducts.

periă·pical (G. *peri*, through; L. *apex*, summit). Around the apex, e.g., of a tooth.

periappendici·tis (G. *peri*, around; L. *appendix*, appendage). Inflammation of the tissues surrounding the appendix vermiformis.

periarteri·tis (G. *peri*, around; *artēria*, artery). Inflammation of the outer sheath of an artery. **P. nodosa:** a usually progressive chronic disease characterized by inflammatory lesions of the arteries and arterioles in various parts of the body, beginning at the outer coat but later involving commonly all coats of the vessel, and clinically by fever, emaciation and signs according to the site of the lesions, e.g. haematuria, melaena, neuritis.

periarthri·tis (G. *peri*, around; *arthron*, joint). Inflammation of the tissues around a joint.

periarti·cular (G. *peri*, around; L. *articulus*, joint). Around a joint.

periax·ial (G. *peri*, around; L. *axis*). 1. Around an axis. 2. Periaxonal.

periăx·illary (G. *peri*, around; L. *axilla*, armpit). Around an axilla.

periăx·onal (G. *peri*, around; *axōn*, axone). Surrounding an axone.

pĕ·riblast (G. *peri*, around; *blastos*, germ). The protoplasm around the cell-nucleus.

periblep·sis (G. *peri*, around; *blepsis*, sight). The staring expression of an insane person.

peribron·chial (G. *peri*, around; *brogkhos*, bronchus). Around a bronchus.

peribronchī·tis (G. *peri*, around; *brogkhos*, bronchus). Inflammation of the tissues around the bronchi.

pericae·cal (G. *peri*, around; L. *caecus*, blind). Around the caecum.

pericanali·cular (G. *peri*, around; L. *canalis*, canal). Occurring around small ducts.

pericap·sular (G. *peri*, around; L. *capsula*, small box). Surrounding a capsule.

pericar·diac, pericar·dial (G. *peri*, around; *kardia*, heart). Relating to the pericardium.

pericardiĕc·tomy (G. *peri*, around; *kardia*, heart; *ektomē*, excision). Excision of part of the pericardium.

pericar·diocentē·sis (G. *peri*, around; *kardia*, heart; *kentēsis*, puncture). Puncture of the pericardium and the withdrawal of fluid from the pericardial sac.

pericardiŏ·lysis (G. *peri*, around; *kardia*, heart; *lusis*, a loosening). Cardiolysis, *q.v.*

pericardiŏ·tomy (G. *peri*, around; *kardia*, heart; *tomē*, section). Opening the pericardium.

pericardī·tis (G. *peri*, around; *kardia*, heart). Inflammation of the pericardium. **P., adhesive:** adhesions between the two layers of the pericardium, with or without adhesions between the external pericardial layer and surrounding structures, such as mediastinal structures, sternum, etc., resulting from p., clinically characterized by cardiac failure (low arterial pressure), impeding of venous return to the heart (high venous pressure), leading to ascites, engorgement of liver and peripheral veins, etc. **P., fibrinous:** acute p. with fibrinous exudation, characterized by fever, dyspnoea, pain (usually) and a superficial grating 'to-and-fro', murmur due to friction of the membrane (if the anterior wall of the heart is involved). **P., haemorrhagic:** p. with sanguineous effusion. **P. with effusion:** p. with sero-fibrinous, purulent or haemorrhagic effusion, characterized by dyspnoea, absence of palpable apex beat, increase in area and character of cardiac dullness on percussion, muffled heart sounds, low blood pressure, by signs of pulmonary collapse at the left axilla or at the angle of the left scapula, with or without pyrexia.

pericar·dium (G. *peri*, around; *kardia*, heart). The membranous sac around the heart. **P., parietal:** the layer external to the visceral layer. **P., visceral:** the layer adjacent to the heart.

pericel·lular (G. *peri*, around; L. *cellula*, dim. of *cella*, chamber). Tissue surrounding a cell.

pericementi·tis (G. *peri*, around; L. *caementum*, quarry-stone). Periodontitis, *q.v.*

pericholangi·tis (G. *peri*, around; *kholē*, bile; *aggeion*, vessel). Inflammation of the tissue around the bile ducts.

pericholecystī·tis (G. *peri*, around; *kholē*, bile; *kustis*, bladder). Inflammation of the tissue surrounding the gall-bladder. leading to adhesions between the gall-bladder and the surrounding structures.

perichon·dral (G. *peri*, around; *khondros*, cartilage). Relating to or affecting the perichondrium.

perichondrī·tis (G. *peri*, around; *khondros*, cartilage). Inflammation of the perichondrium.

perichon·drium (G. *peri*, around; *khondros*, cartilage). The connective tissue covering cartilage surfaces.

pĕ·richord (G. *peri*, around; *khordē*, string). The notochordal sheath.

perichor·dal. Relating to the perichord.

perichŏ·roid, perichoroi·dal (G. *peri*, around; *khorion*, membrane enclosing the foetus; *eidos*, form). Around the choroid.

pĕ·richrome (G. *peri*, around; *khroma*, colour). Applied to a type of Nissl bodies, *q.v.*, arranged in rows immediately below the cell membrane.

periclā·sis (G. *peri*, around; *klasis*, a fracture). A comminuted fracture.

pericon·chal (G. *peri*, around; *kogkhē*, mussel-shell). Around the cavity of the ear.

periconchi·tis (G. *peri*, around; *kogkhē*, mussel-shell). Inflammation of the orbital periosteum.

pericor·neal (G. *peri*, around; L. *corneus*, horny). Around the cornea.

pericoxī·tis (G. *peri*, around; L. *coxa*, the hip). Inflammation of the hip-joint tissues.

pericrā·nium (G. *peri*, around; *kranion*, skull). The external periosteum of the cranial bones.

pericystī·tis (G. *peri*, around; *kustis*, bladder). Inflammation of the tissues around the urinary bladder.

pericys·teum (G. *peri*, around; *kustis*, bladder). 1. The outer vascular wall of a cyst. 2. The tissues which surround the urinary bladder.

periden·tal (G. *peri*, around; L. *dens*, tooth). Around a tooth or its roots; periodontal.

periden·tine (G. *peri*, around; L. *dens*, tooth). Cementum, *q.v.*

peridentī·tis (G. *peri*, around; L. *dens*, tooth). Periodontitis, *q.v.*

peridesmī·tis (G. *peri*, around; *desmos*, bond). Inflammation of the peridesmium.

perides·mium (G. *peri*, around; *desmos*, bond). The membranes investing a ligament.

peridiă·stolĕ (G. *peri*, around; *diastolē*, expansion). The interval between systole and diastole.

peridĭ·dymis (G. *peri*, around; *didumos*, twin). The tunica albuginea testis, the serous coat investing the testis.

peridŭc·tal (G. *peri*, around; L. *ductus*, duct). Surrounding a duct. Usually applied to conditions in the mammary gland.

periduodenī·tis (G. *peri*, around; L. *duodeni*, twelve each). Inflammation of the tissues around the duodenum, leading to duodenal adhesions.

perifolliculī·tis (G. *peri*, around; L. *folliculus*, dim. of *follis*, an inflated bag or ball). Inflammation about a hair follicle.

perigas·tric (G. *peri*, around; *gastēr*, belly). Around the stomach.

perigastrī·tis (G. *peri*, around; *gastēr*, belly). Inflammation of the tissues surrounding the stomach and stomach bed.

perihepat·ic (G. *peri*, around; *hēpar*, liver). Around the liver.

perihepatī·tis (G. *peri*, around; *hēpar*, liver). Inflammation of the serous covering of the liver.

perilaryngī·tis (G. *peri*, around; *larugx*, larynx). Inflammation of the tissue around the larynx.

pĕ·rilymph (G. *peri*, around; L. *lympha*, water). The fluid between the membranous and the osseous labyrinth of the ear.

pĕ·rilymphadenī·tis (G. *peri*, around; *lympha*, water; *adēn*, gland). Inflammation of the connective tissue surrounding lymphatic glands.

pĕ·rilymphangi·tis (G. *peri*, around; *lympha*, water; *aggeion*, vessel). Inflammation of the tissues surrounding a lymphatic vessel.

perilymphat·ic (G. *peri*, around; L. *lympha*, water). 1. Pertaining to the perilymph. 2. Around a lymph vessel.

perimastī·tis (G. *peri*, around; *mastos*, breast). Inflammation of the tissue around the breast.

perimedul·lary (G. *peri*, around; L. *medulla*, marrow). The tissue around the medulla oblongata.

peri·meter (G. *peri*, around; *metron*, measure). 1. Circumference. 2. An instrument for determining the field of vision.

perimetrī·tis (G. *peri*, around; *mētra*, womb). Inflammation of the uterine peritoneum.

perimē·trium (G. *peri*, around; *mētra*, womb). The peritoneal covering of the uterus.

Y

peri·metry (G. *peri*, around; *metron*, measure). Measurement of the visual field.

perimyosi·tis (G. *peri*, around; *mus*, muscle). Inflammation of the connective tissue around a muscle.

perimysii·tis (G. *peri*, around; *mus*, muscle). Inflammation of the perimysium.

perimy·sium (G. *peri*, around; *mus*, muscle). The membranous sheath of a muscle and its fascicles.

peri·neal (G. *perinaion*, space between anus and scrotum). Relating to the perineum.

perinē·ocele (G. *perinaion*, space between anus and scrotum; *kēlē*, hernia). Perineal hernia.

perinē·oplasty (G. *perinaion*, space between anus and scrotum; *plassein*, to form). Any plastic operation on the perineum.

perinēor·rhaphy (G. *perinaion*, space between anus and scrotum; *rhaphē*, suture). Suture of the perineum.

perinēŏ·tomy (G. *perinaion*, space between anus and scrotum; *tomē*, section). Incision into the perineum.

perinĕph·ric (G. *peri*, around; *nephros*, kidney). Around the kidney.

perinephri·tis (G. *peri*, around; *nephros*, kidney). Inflammation, usually purulent, of the tissues around the kidneys.

perinĕph·rium (G. *peri*, around; *nephros*, kidney). The connective and fatty tissue surrounding the kidney.

perinē·um (G. *perinaion*). The region between the anus and scrotum or vulva.

perineū·ral (G. *peri*, around; *neuron*, nerve). Around a nerve.

perineurī·tis (G. *peri*, around; *neuron*, nerve). Inflammation of the perineurium.

perineū·rium (G. *peri*, around; *neuron*, nerve). 1. The connective tissue sheath of the secondary nerve fibre bundles. 2. The epineurium, *q.v.*

perinū·clear (G. *peri*, around; L. *nucula*, dim. of *nux*, nut). Around the nucleus.

periŏ·cular (G. *peri*, around; L. *oculus*, eye). Surrounding the eye.

period (G. *periodos*, period). Menstruation.

peri·odate. A salt of periodic acid.

period·ic (G. *periodos*, period). Recurring at more or less regular intervals.

periodic acids. Acids related to HIO$_4$, of varying degrees of hydration. Powerful oxidising agents.

periodi·city (G. *periodos*, period). Recurrence at regular definite intervals.

periodon·tal (G. *peri*, around; *odous*, tooth). 1. Surrounding a tooth. 2. Relating to the periodontium.

periodonti·tis (G. *peri*, around; *odous*, tooth). Inflammation of the periodontal tissues.

periodon·tium (G. *peri*, around; *odous*, tooth). The membrane lining the cement of a tooth; the periodontal membrane.

periodontoclā·sia (G. *peri*, around; *odous*, tooth; *klaein*, to break). Any degenerative or destructive disease of the periodontium.

periodontŏ·logy (G. *peri*, around; *odous*, tooth; *logos*, discourse). Science and study of periodontium and periodontal disease.

periŏnў·chia (G. *peri*, around; *onux*, nail). Inflammation around a nail.

periŏnў·chium (G. *peri*, around; *onux*, nail). The epidermal border at the root of the nail.

periŏŏphori·tis (G. *peri*, around; *ōon*, egg; *pherein*, to bear). Inflammation of the peritoneal covering of the ovary.

periŏptŏ·metry (G. *peri*, around; *optos*, visible; *metron*, measure). Perimetry.

perior·bit, perior·bita (G. *peri*, around; L. *orbita*, from *orbis*, sphere). The periosteum of the orbit.

perior·bital (G. *peri*, around; L. *orbita*, from *orbis*, sphere). 1. Surrounding the orbit. 2. Relating to the periorbita.

periŏrchi·tis (G. *peri*, around; *orkhis*, testis). Inflammation of the tunica vaginalis of a testis.

pĕ·riŏst (G. *peri*, around; *osteon*, bone). Periosteum.

periŏ·steal (G. *peri*, around; *osteon*, bone). Pertaining to the periosteum.

periŏstēi·tis. Periostitis, *q.v.*

periŏstēŏ·tomy (G. *peri*, around; *osteon*, bone; *tomē*, section). Incision of the periosteum.

periŏ·steum (G. *peri*, around; *osteon*, bone). The fibrous membrane investing the surfaces of bones, except at articular surfaces.

periŏsti·tis (G. *peri*, around; *osteon*, bone). Inflammation of the periosteum.

periŏ·tic (G. *peri*, around; *ous*, ear). Around the ear.

peripachmeningi·tis (G. *peri*, around; *pakhus*, thick; *menigx*, membrane). Pachymeningitis externa.

peripancreati·tis (G. *peri*, around; *pagkreas*, pancreas). Inflammation of the connective tissue around the pancreas.

peripă·pillary (G. *peri*, around; L. *apilla*, dim. of *papula*, pimple). Around a papilla.

peripatet·ic (G. *peri*, around; *patein*, to walk). Moving about.

periphaci·tis (G. *peri*, around; *phakos*, lentil). Inflammation of the capsule surrounding the crystalline lens.

periphā·cus (G. *peri*, around; *phakos*, lentil). The capsule enclosing the crystalline lens.

peri·pherad (G. *periphereia*, periphery; L. *ad*, to). Towards the periphery.

peri·pheral, peri·pheric (G. *periphereia*, from *peri*, around; *pherein*, to carry). Pertaining to or situated near the periphery. **P. nerve:** any (motor, sensory, or mixed) nerve connecting the end-organs (receptor or effector) with the spinal cord or brain, excluding the autonomic nerve and usually excluding the cranial nerves. **P. neuritis:** see neuritis, multiple.

peri·phery (G. *periphereia*, periphery). Circumference.

periphlebī·tis (G. *peri*, around; *phleps*, vein). Inflammation of the external coat of a vein and of the tissues surrounding the vein.

peripor·tal (G. *peri*, around; L. *porta*, gate). Around the portal vein.

periprocti·tis (G. *peri*, around; *prōktos*, anus). Inflammation of the connective tissue around the rectum or anus.

pĕ·riprostati·tis (G. *peri*, around; *prostatēs*, protector). Inflammation of the connective tissue around the prostate.

perirec·tal (G. *peri*, around; L. *rectus*, straight). Around the rectum.

perirē·nal (G. *peri*, around; L. *ren*, kidney). Around the kidney.

perirhi·nal (G. *peri*, around; *rhis*, nose). Around the nose.

perisalpingi·tis (G. *peri*, around; *salpigx*, trumpet). Inflammation of the peritoneal surface of the uterine (Fallopian) tube.

perisigmoidi·tis (G. *peri*, around; *sigma*, the letter S; *eidos*, form). Inflammation of the tissues surrounding the sigmoid colon.

perisīnusi·tis (G. *peri*, around; L. *sinus*, cavity). Inflammation of the tissues surrounding a sinus.

perisplanch·nic (G. *peri*, around; *splagkhna*, the viscera). Around a viscus.

perisplanchni·tis (G. *peri*, around; *splagkhna*, viscera). Inflammation of the tissues around a viscus.

perispleni·tis (G. *peri*, around; *splēn*, spleen). Inflammation of the peritoneal surface of the spleen.

peristal·sis (G. *peri*, around; *stalsis*, compression). The wave-like movement of the alimentary tract and other hollow tubes having longitudinal and transverse muscular fibres, by which the contents of the tubes are propelled.

peristal·tic. Relating to or resembling peristalsis.

peristă·phyline (G. *peri*, around; *staphulē*, uvula). Around the uvula.

peristaphylī·tis (G. *peri*, around; *staphulē*, uvula). Inflammation of the connective tissues surrounding the uvula.

peri·stolē (G. *peri*, around; *stellein*, to place). 1. Peristalsis. 2. An individual peristaltic movement.

peri·stoma (G. *peri*, around; *stoma*, mouth). Peristome, *q.v.*

pĕ·ristome (G. *peri*, around; *stoma*, mouth). In lower animals, the parietal region surrounding the mouth.

perisys·tolē (G. *peri*, around; *sustolē*, contraction). The interval between two systoles.

peritendi·neum (G. *peri*, around; L. *tendere*, to stretch). The fibrous covering of a tendon.

peritendini·tis (G. *peri*, around; L. *tendere*, to stretch). Inflammation of a peritendineum.

per·itenoni·tis (G. *peri*, around; L. *tendere*, to stretch). Inflammation of the covering of a tendon.

perithē·cium (G. *peri*, around; *thēkion*, a small box). A cup- or flask-shaped envelope which encloses the fruits of certain fungi and moulds.

perithē·lial (G. *peri*, around; *thēlē*, nipple). Relating to the perithelium.

peritheliŏ·ma (G. *peri*, around; *thēlē*, nipple). A tumour of sarcomatous character originating in the perithelium of a vessel.

perithē·lium (G. *peri*, around; *thēlē*, nipple). The cell-layer surrounding the capillaries and smaller vessels.

perithyroidī·tis (G. *peri*, around; *thureos*, a shield; *eidos*, form). Inflammation of the outer covering of the thyroid gland.

peri·tomy (G. *peri*, around; *tomē*, section). 1. The removal of a small area around the cornea, a treatment of pannus. 2. Circumcision.

peritonē·al (G. *peritonaion*, peritoneum). Relating to the peritoneum.

peritonĕŏ·tomy (G. *peritonaion*, peritoneum; *tomē*, section). A cutting into the peritoneum.

peritonē·um (G. *peritonaion*, peritoneum). The serous, membranous lining of the interior of the abdominal cavity and its contained viscera.

peritoniŏ·scopy (G. *peritonaion*, peritoneum; *skopein*, to view). Examination of the peritoneal cavity by means of an instrument passed through the abdominal wall.

peritonit·ic. Relating to peritonitis.

per·itoni·tis (G. *peritonaion*, peritoneum). Inflammation of the peritoneum. **P., acute:** p. of sudden onset, characterized by fever, leucocytosis, intense abdominal pain, tenderness and rigidity, by vomiting and initially by tachycardia. **P., chronic adhesive:** more or less localized p. with fibrous adhesions between intra-abdominal organs. **P., pneumococcal:** p. due to pneumococcal infection, occurring usually in girls between 5 and 10 years, characterized by diarrhoea, high fever, signs of acute peritonitis and a severe general condition already at the onset of the disease. **P., tuberculous:** p. due to tuberculous infection, characterized either by ascites or, more commonly, by ulceration and caseation or by fibrotic proliferation of the peritoneal tubercles. **P., gonococcal:** p. due to gonococcal infection, more common in females, from extension of gonorrhoeal salpingitis. **P., puerperal:** p. following parturition, usually due to streptococcal infection of the uterus.

periton·sillar (G. *peri*, around; L. *tonsillae*, tonsils). Around the tonsil.

peritonsillī·tis (G. *peri*, around; L. *tonsillae*, tonsils). Inflammation of the connective tissues surrounding the tonsil.

Perĭ·tricha (G. *peri*, around; *thrix*, hair). A group of bacteria having flagella at the poles and sides.

perityphlī·tis (G. *peri*, around; *tuphlos*, blind). Inflammation of the peritoneal covering of the appendix and caecum.

periŭ·reteri·tis (G. *peri*, around; *ourēter*, ureter). Inflammation of the tissues about the ureter.

periŭrethrī·tis (G. *peri*, around; *ourēthra*, urethra). Inflammation of the tissues around the urethra.

periŭ·terine (G. *peri*, around; L. *uterus*). Around the uterus.

perivas·cular (G. *peri*, around; L. *vasculum*, dim. of *vas*, vessel). Around a vessel.

perlèche (Fr.). A type of pityriasic streptococcal infection of the skin, characterized by dry, scaly, more or less symmetrical lesions about labial commisures which are the site of streptococcal fissures.

Perlia's nucleus (Perlia, R., 19th century German ophthalmologist). The medial group of cells in the the nucleus of origin of the oculomotor nerve.

perman·ganate. A salt of permanganic acid.

permangan·ic acid. $HMnO_4$. A monobasic acid. A powerful oxidising agent.

per·meable (L. *per*, through; *meare*, to pass). Pervious; capable of being penetrated.

perni·cious (L. *perniciosus*). Deadly; fatal. **P. anaemia:** see anaemia, p. **P. malaria:** see malaria, subtertian. **P. vomiting:** see vomiting-sickness of Jamaica.

per·nio (L.). Chilblain.

perobrā·chius (G. *pēros*, maimed; *brakhion*, arm). One with congenital malformation of the arms.

perocĕ·phalus (G. *pēros*, maimed; *kephalē*, head). A monster with a rudimentary head.

perochei·rus (G. *pēros*, maimed; *kheir*, hand). One with congenital malformation of the hands.

perodac·tylus (G. *pēros*, maimed; *daktulos*, finger). One with congenital malformation of the fingers or toes.

peromē·lia (G. *pēros*, maimed; *melos*, limb). A congenital malformation of the limbs.

perŏ·melus (G. *pēros*, maimed; *melos*, limb). A monster with rudimentary limbs.

peronae·us muscle. See peroneus.

per·ŏnē (G., brooch). The fibula.

peronē·al (G. *perŏnē*, brooch). Relating to the fibula.

peroneal muscular atrophy. See Charcot-Marie-Tooth disease.

peronē·um (G. *perŏnē*, brooch). Perone.

peronē·us muscle (G. *perŏnē*, brooch). A muscle on the outer side of the leg arising from the fibula.

pĕ·ropus (G. *pēros*, maimed; *pous*, foot). One with congenital malformation of the feet.

peror·al (L. *per*, through; *os*, mouth). Through the mouth.

per os (L.). Peroral; through the mouth.

perŏ·sis (G. *pēros*, maimed). The condition of defective formation.

perosō·mus (G. *pēros*, maimed; *sōma*, body). A monster with malformation of the entire body.

peros·seous (L. *per*, through; *os*, bone). Through bone.

perox·idase. An enzyme that splits organic peroxides.

perox·ide (L. *per*, through; G. *oxus*, sharp). A dioxide in which two oxygen atoms are linked directly to each other, as H-O-O-H (hydrogen peroxide).

per primam intentionem (L.). By first intention.

per rectum (L.). Through the rectum.

perseverā·tion (L. *perseverare*, to persist). A useless and senseless repetition of plainly spoken words.

per·sonal (L. *persona*, person). Relating to a person. **P. equation:** the individual difference between observers in recording the same perception.

personă·lity (L. *persona*, person). Comprises those features of mental make-up of a human being that characterize his relations with other persons and with his environment.

perspirā·tion (L. *per*, through; *spirare*, to breathe). 1. The secretion of sweat. 2. Sweat. **P., insensible:** (*a*) The loss of water through skin and respiratory tract. (*b*) More correctly, the loss of body weight due to loss of water through skin and respiratory tract, plus the positive or negative amount representing the difference of CO_2 output and O_2 intake.

Perthes's disease (Perthes, G. C., German surgeon, 1869–1927). Pseudocoxalgia, or coxa plana. A disease affecting the upper femoral epiphysis in young people.

Pertick's diverticulum (Pertick, O., Hungarian histologist, 1852–1913). An inconstant lateral outpouching of the fossa of Rosenmüller.

per tubam (L.). Through a tube.

pertus·sis (L. *per*, through; *tussis*, cough). Whooping-cough, *q.v.*

Peru balsam. A balsam obtained from the trunk of *Myroxylon pereirae*. It is used for inhalation in cases of pharyngitis and also as a dressing for wounds.

perver·sion (L. *per*, through; *vertere*, to turn). A turning away from the normal. **P., sexual:** preference for obtaining sexual gratification by some other act than coitus.

pervert, sexual. A person obtaining sexual gratification by some other act than coitus.

per vias naturales (L.). By natural ways.

per·vious (L. *per*, through; *via*, way). Capable of being passed through.

pes (L.). A foot or foot-like process. **P. anserinus:** 'goose's foot', a term applied to the terminal branches of the facial nerve. **P. cavus:** a foot with increased curvature of the arch. **P. planus:** flat-foot. See also talipes.

pes·sary (G. *pessos*). 1. An instrument placed in the vagina to hold the uterus in proper position. 2. An instrument placed in the vagina or placed to cover the uterine orifice so as to prevent conception. 3. A vaginal suppository.

pes·simism (L. *pessimus*, worst). A neurotic disposition always to see and to expect the worst.

pest (L. *pestis*). Plague, *q.v.*

pesti·ferous (L. *pestis*, pest; *ferre*, to bear). Causing pestilence.

pě·stilence (L. *pestilentia*). Any deadly disease of epidemic origin, i.e., the plague.

pestle (L. *pistillum*, pestle). Instrument for pounding substances in a mortar.

petē·chia (It. *petecchie*, purple-spots). A small effusion of blood beneath the epidermis.

petē·chial (It. *petecchie*, purple-spots). Characterized by the formation of petechiae.

pě·thidine.

C. (C_6H_5) $(CO.OC_2H_5)$ $CH_2CH_2.N$ $(CH_3).$ CH_2CH_2 HCl. The hydrochloride of ethyl 1-methyl-4-phenyl-piperidine-4-carboxylate. An analgesic.

Petit's aponeurosis (Petit, P., French anatomist, born 1889). The posterior aponeurosis of the broad ligament of the uterus; 'pelvirecto-genital aponeurosis of Petit'.

Petit's canal (Petit, F. P. du, French anatomist, 1664–1741). The space between the zonule of Zinn and the vitreous.

Petit's ligaments (Petit, J. L., French anatomist, 1664–1750). The 'posterior round ligaments of the uterus'; uterosacral ligaments. **P.'s triangle:** a 'triangle of lumbar hernia' between the crest of the ilium and the margins of the external oblique and latissimus dorsi muscles.

petit mal (Fr. little ill). A minor attack of epilepsy, consisting in a momentary more or less partial loss of

consciousness, often presenting itself only by cessation of talk, a fixed, vacant expression of the face, or transient mental confusion.

Petri dishes (Petri, J., German bacteriologist, 1852–1921). Shallow glass dishes used for cultivating organisms.

petrifac·tion (L. *petra*, stone; *facere*, to make). Change to stony hardness.

petrissage (Fr.). A manipulation used in massage in which the soft tissues are carefully lifted away from the deeper structures and gently squeezed.

Petrolā·gar. A proprietary emulsion of paraffin and agar.

pě·trolate. Soft paraffin.

petrolā·tum. Soft paraffin.

petrō·leum. Natural mineral oil.

petromas·toid (G. *petra*, stone; *mastos*, breast; *eidos*, form). Pertaining conjointly to the petrous and mastoid portions of the temporal bone.

pet·rosphē·noid (G. *petra*, stone; *sphēn*, wedge; *eidos*, form). That part of the skull which pertains to the petrous portions of the temporal bone and the sphenoid bone.

pet·rous (G. *petra*, stone). As hard as stone. **P. ganglion:** the inferior ganglion of the glosso-pharyngeal nerve.

pex·is (G. *pēxis*, fixation). Surgical fixation of a part.

Peyer's nodules (Peyer, J. K., Swiss anatomist, 1653–1712). The noduli lymphatici solitarii. **P.'s patches:** the noduli lymphatici aggregati of the small intestine.

Peyerian fever (Peyer, J. K.). Typhoid fever.

Pfannenstiel's incision (Pfannenstiel, J., German gynaecologist, 1862–1909). A transverse incision in the cleavage line of the skin above the symphysis pubis and within the pubic hair line.

Pf. Abbreviation for Pfeifferella.

Pfeiffer's glandular fever (Pfeiffer, E., German physician, 1846–1921). An acute infectious disease marked by inflammatory swelling of the lymph glands.

Pfeifferella (Pfeiffer, R. F. J., German bacteriologist, born 1858). The former name of the genus of bacteria, Malleomyces.

Pflüger's tubes (Pflüger, E. F. W., German physiologist, 1829–1910). Ovarian tubes from the germ epithelium of the Wolffian body, ultimately forming the cortex of the ovary. **P.'s laws:** (1) In respect of physiological electronics, where he stated that the threshold of excitability of a nerve could be lowered or raised by the passage of a constant polarizing current in one or the other direction. (2) In respect of the relative nerve-stimulating properties of the positive and negative electrode at make and break of the current. This is epitomized as follows: KCC > ACC > KOC.

pH. Scale of values from 1–14 used to denote the hydrogen ion concentration of solutions. pH is the common logarithm of the reciprocal of the hydrogen ion concentration.

phace, phacē·a (G. *phakos*, lentil). The crystalline lens.

phǎ·coid (G. *phakos*, lentil; *eidos*, form). Lens-shaped.

phacoi·doscope (G. *phakos*, lentil; *eidos*, form; *skopein*, to view). Phacoscope, *q.v.*

phacō·ma (G. *phakos*, lentil). 1. A tumour of the lens. 2. Flat oval tumour, especially of the retina as found in tuberous sclerosis.

phǎ·coscope (G. *phakos*, lentil; *skopein*, to view). An instrument testing the accommodative changes of the lens of the eye.

phaeochrō·moblast (G. *phaios*, dusky; *khrōma*, colour; *blastos*, germ). The embryonic precursor of the phaeochromocyte, *q.v.*

phaeochrō·mocyte (G. *phaios*, dusky; *khrōma*, colour; *kutos*, cell). One of the two cell-types present in the sympathetic ganglia and in the adrenal medulla—that which is characterized by the property of staining brown with chromic salts.

phaeochrōmocytō·ma (G. *phaios*, dusky; *khrōma*, colour; *kutos*, cell). A non-invasive tumour composed of phaeochromocytes, *q.v.*, arising usually in an adrenal gland, producing a syndrome of paroxysmal hypertension (sometimes resulting in oedema of the lungs), hyperglycaemia and changes in cardiac rhythm and rate, owing to sudden release of adrenalin formed by the tumour cells. Syn. paraganglioma.

phagedae·na (G. *phagedaina*, a canker). Gangrenous ulceration.

phă·gocyte (G. *phagein* to eat; *kutos*, cell). A cell characterized by the property of surrounding and digesting micro-organisms, foreign bodies or cells.

phagocyt·ic (G. *phagein*, to eat; *kutos*, cell). Pertaining to phagocytosis.

phagocytō·sis (G. *phagein*, to eat; *kutos*, cell). Destruction by phagocytes.

phă·gokarўō·sis (G. *phagein*, to eat; *karuon*, nut). Phagocytosis by the cell nucleus.

phagomā·nia (G. *phagein*, to eat; *mania*, madness). Uncontrollable craving for food.

phagophō·bia (G. *phagein*, to eat; *phŏbos*, fear). A neurotic fear of eating.

phalan·geal (G. *phalagx*, phalange). Pertaining to the phalanges.

phalangī·tis (G. *phalagx*, phalange). Phalangeal inflammation.

phă·lanx (G. *phalagx*, phalange, pl. phalanges). One of the finger-bones or toe-bones.

phallec·tomy (G. *phallos*, penis; *ektomē*, excision). Surgical removal of the penis.

phal·lic (G. *phallos*, penis). Pertaining to the penis.

phallī·tis (G. *phallos*, penis). Inflammation of the penis.

phal·lus (G. *phallos*). The penis.

phanerŏ·scopy (G. *phaneros*, evident; *skopein*, to view). A method of examining the skin, especially for lupus nodules, by illumination through a plane convex lens.

phan·tom (G. *phantazein*, to make visible). 1. An apparition. 2. A dummy used for practising operative procedures. **P. tumour**: a pseudo-tumour.

pharmaceu·tic, pharmaceu·tical (G. *pharmakeutēs*, from *pharmakon*, a drug). Relating to pharmacy.

pharmaceutical chemistry. The chemistry of substances used in and related to the practise of pharmacy.

pharmacist (G. *pharmakon*, a drug). A person qualified by examination, registered and authorized by the Pharmacy and Poisons Act of 1933 to keep open shop for the sale of poisons and the dispensing of medicines.

pharmaco-dynam·ics (G. *pharmakon*, a drug; *dunamis*, power). The science of the action of drugs.

pharmacognō·sis, pharmacog·nosy (G. *pharmakon*, a drug; *gnosis*, knowledge). The science dealing with the source, preparation, dosage, etc., of drugs.

pharmacŏ·logy (G. *pharmakon*, a drug; *logos*, a treatise). The science of the properties of drugs.

pharmacomā·nia (G. *pharmakon*, a drug; *mania*, madness). Neurotic preoccupation with taking or giving medicines.

phar·macopoe·ia (G. *pharmakon*, a drug; *poiein*, to make). A collection of methods and formulae for the preparation of drugs, especially a book of such formulae edited by an authorized body, such as the British Pharmacopoeia, produced by the General Medical Council.

phar·macy (G. *pharmakeia*, from *pharmakon*, a drug). 1. The art of preparing and dispensing medicines. 2. Premises kept open for the sale of poisons and dispensing of medicines and registered under the Pharmacy and Poisons Act, 1933.

pharyn·geal (G. *pharugx*, throat). Relating to the pharynx.

pharyngec·tomy (G. *pharugx*, throat; *ektomē*, excisions). Excision of the pharynx.

pharyngis·mus (G. *pharugx*, throat). Spasm of the muscles of the pharynx.

pharyngī·tis (G. *pharugx*, throat). Inflammation of the pharynx.

pharyngo-amygdalītis (G. *pharugx*, throat; *amugdala*, almond). Inflammation conjointly of the pharynx and the tonsils.

pharyn·gocele (G. *pharugx*, throat; *kēlē*, hernia). A pouch of the pharynx projecting through a gap in the pharyngeal wall.

pharyngoglos·sus (G. *pharugx*, throat; *glōssa*, tongue). Glossopharyngeus; that part of the superior constrictor of the pharynx arising from the mucous membrane of the mouth and side of the tongue.

pharyn·gokeratō·sis (G. *pharugx*, throat; *keras*, horn). Irregular thickening of the mucous lining of the pharynx.

pharyn·golaryngī·tis (G. *pharugx*, throat; *larugx*, larynx). Inflammation of the pharynx and larynx.

pharyn·golith (G. *pharugx*, throat; *lithos*, stone). A calculus in the pharynx.

pharyn·gomycō·sis (G. *pharugx*, throat; *mukēs*, mushroom). Mycotic disease of the pharynx (disease due to the action of fungi).

pharyn·gopară·lysis (G. *pharugx*, throat; *paralusis*, paralysis). Paralysis of the pharynx.

pharyngŏ·pathy (G. *pharugx*, throat; *pathos*, disease). Any pharyngeal disease.

pharyn·gostaphyli·nus muscle. Palatopharyngeus muscle.

phase (electrical). The angular displacement between two semilunar oscillations of the same frequency.

phē·mitone. Methylphenobarbitone, N-methyl-5-phenyl-5-ethylbarbituric acid. A hypnotic.

phenacetin. p-$C_2H_5O.C_6H_4.NHCOCH_3$, aceto-p-phenetidin, an antipyretic substance.

phē·nazone. 1-phenyl-2:3-dimethyl-5-pyrazolene. An antiseptic substance. Syn. Antipyrin.

phenobar·bitone. 5-phenyl-5-ethylbarbituric acid. A hypnotic.

phenolphthā·lein. A condensation product of phenol and phthalic anhydride. It is used as an indicator, pH range 8·3–10. Also as a purge, dose 1–5 gr.

phenylmercu·ric nitrate. C_6H_5HgOH, $C_6H_5HgNO_3$, obtained by the action of a solution of N_2O_4 in ice-cold chloroform with dyphenylmercury in ice-cold chloroform. Antibacterial agent and preservative.

pheny·toin. The sodium salt of 5:5-diphenyl-hydrantoin. A hypnotic.

phlebŏ·clysis (G. *phleps*, vein; *klusis*, a drenching). Injection of fluid into a vein.

phleborrhā·gia (G. *phleps*, vein; *rhēgnunai*, to burst out). Haemorrhage from a vein.

phlebor·rhaphy (G. *phleps*, vein; *rhaphē*, suture). Suture of a vein.

phleborrhex·is (G. *phleps*, vein; *rhēxis*, rupture). Rupture of a vein.

phlebothrombō·sis (G. *phleps*, vein; *thrombos*, clot). Formation of a venous thrombos.

Phlebŏ·tomus. A genus of dipterous insects.

phlebŏ·tomy (G. *phleps*, vein; *tomē*, section). Opening of a vein for the purpose of blood-letting. Venesection.

phlegm (G. *phlegmasia*, inflammation). A viscid, stringy mucus secreted by the mucosa of the upper respiratory tract. 2. One of the four humours of the old writers; apathy.

phlegmā·sia (G. *phlegmasia*, inflammation). Inflammation. **P. alba dolens:** white leg, a painful swelling of the leg, beginning either at the ankle and ascending, or at the groin and extending down the thigh. The usual cause is septic infection following childbirth.

phlegmat·ic (G. *phlegmasia*, inflammation). Full of phlegm; hence indifferent, apathetic.

phleg·mon (G. *phlegmŏnē*, inflammation). An inflammation characterized by a spreading cellulitis of the tissues.

phleg·monous (G. *phlegmonē*, inflammation). Like, or relating to, phlegmon.

phlŏ·gogen (G. *phlox*, flame; *gennan*, to produce). Any substance capable of producing inflammation in a tissue with which it is brought into contact.

phlogogen·ic (G. *phlox*, flame; *gennan*, to produce). Causing inflammation.

phlogō·sis (G. *phlogōsis*, inflammation). 1. Inflammation. 2. Erysipelas.

phlor·etin (G. *phloios*, bark of trees; *rhiza*, root). A substance produced by treating phloridzin by dilute acids. On administration to animals it produces glycosuria in a manner similar to phloridzin.

phlorid·zin, phlori·zin (G. *phloios*, bark; *rhiza*, root). A glycoside found in the trunk of some fruit trees, including the apple and the pear. **P.-diabetes:** the glycosuria induced by the administration of the glycoside p., which inhibits reabsorption of glucose in the renal tubules.

phlyctē·na (G. *phluktaina*, blister). A vesicle.

phlyc·tenoid (G. *phluktaina*, blister; *eidos*, form). Phlyctenular, *q.v.*

phlyctē·nula (G. *phlŭktaina*, blister). A small vesicle.

phlyctē·nular. Relating to a phlyctenula. **P. conjunctivitis:** see conjunctivitis, p. **P. keratitis:** see keratitis, p.

phlyc·tenule (G. *phluktaina*, blister). A small vesicle.

phlyză·cion, phlyză·cium (G. *phluzein*, to boil). A boil.

phō·bia (G. *phŏbos*, fear). Any irrational fear.

phocŏ·melus (G. *phŏkē*, seal; *melos*, limb). A monster with incomplete limbs, the hands and feet being attached almost directly to the trunk.

phonasthē·nia (G. *phōnē*, voice; *a*, neg.; *sthenos*, strength). Voice failure due to extreme fatigue.

phonā·tion (G. *phōnē*, voice). 1. The production of vocal sounds. 2. Speech.

phō·natory (G. *phōnē*, voice). Relating to phonation.

phonen·doscope (G. *phōnē*, voice; *endon*, inside; *skopein*, to view). A special type of stethoscope which intensifies the auscultatory sounds.

phonet·ic (G. *phōnē*, voice). 1. Relating to or representing sounds. 2. Relating to the voice.

phō·nic (G. *phōnē*, voice). Relating to the voice. **P. spasm:** a spasm of the laryngeal muscles occurring on the attempt to speak.

phō·nica (G. *phōnē*, voice). Diseases of the vocal organs.

phonŏ·meter (G. *phōnē*, voice; *metron*, measure). 1. An instrument which measures the intensity of the voice. 2. An instrument used for studying the arterial blood pressure when taken by the auscultatory method.

phonophō·bia (G. *phōnē*, voice; *phŏbos*, fear). 1. A fear of speaking. 2. Morbid dread of any noise or sound.

phō·nophore (G. *phōnē*, voice; *pherein*, to bear). An auditory ossicle, regarded as a transmitter of sound.

phonop·sia (G. *phōnē*, voice; *opsis*, vision). The perception of colour sensations by auditory stimuli.

phō·norecep·tor (G. *phōnē*, voice; L. *recipere*, to receive). A cell responding to sound.

phor·ēsis (G. *pherein*, to bear). A suffix suggesting migration, e.g., iontophoresis, implying migration of ions usually in electric fields, or electrophoresis, meaning movement of a fluid (usually water) adsorbed on a charged colloid particle.

phorŏ·logy (G. *pherein*, to bear; *logos*, a treatise). The science relating to disease carriers.

phorŏ·meter (G. *pherein*, to bear; *metron*, measure). An instrument devised for measuring the relative strength of the ocular muscles.

phos·gen, phos·gene (G. *phōs*, light; *gennan*, to produce). 1. Producing light. 2. $COCl_2$, carboxyl chloride; a poisonous gas formed from carbon monoxide and chlorine.

phosphagen·ic (G. *phōs*, light; *gennan*, to produce). Producing phosphates.

phosphatae·mia (G. *phōs*, light; *pherein*, to bear; *haima*, blood). The presence of phosphates in the blood.

phos·phatase (G. *phōs*, light; *pherein*, to bear). An enzyme which splits the phosphoric acid esters of carbohydrates.

phos·phate (G. *phōs*, light; *pherein*, to bear). A salt of phosphoric acid.

phosphat·ic (G. *phōs*, light; *pherein*, to bear). 1. Containing phosphates. 2. Marked by the excretion of considerable quantities of phosphates.

phos·phatide (G. *phōs*, light; *pherein*, to bear). Lipoid substances, being triglycerides, usually containing two long-chain fatty acids, phosphoric acid and an organic base.

phos·phatine (G. *phōs*, light; *pherein*, to bear). A member of a group of phosphorus compounds which resemble phosphates and which are found in brain substance.

phosphatŏ·meter (G. *phōs*, light; *pherein*, to bear; *metron*, measure). An instrument used for the estimation of phosphates in urine.

phosphatū·ria (G. *phōs*, light; *pherein*, to bear; *ouron*, urine). The passing of an excess of phosphates in the urine.

phos·phene (G. *phōs*, light; *phainein*, to show). The production of a subjective luminous sensation by pressure on the eyeball.

phos·phide (G. *phōs*, light; *pherein*, to bear.) Compounds of phosphorus and another element (usually a metal).

phos·phite (G. *phōs*, light; *pherein*, to bear). A salt of phosphorous acid.

phosphocrĕă·tinase (G. *phōs*, light; *pherein*, to bear; *kreas*, meat). The enzyme which splits phosphocreatine into creatine and phosphoric acid, in the presence of adenosine triphosphate.

phosphocrē·atine (G. *phōs*, light; *pherein*, to bear; *kreas*, meat). A compound consisting of creatinine and phosphoric acid, the breakdown of which supplies energy for muscular contraction and which is resynthesized during recovery.

phospholĭ·pids, phospholĭ·poids (G. *phōs*, light; *pherein*, to bear; *lipos*, fat; *eidos*, form). Lipoids containing phosphorus.

phosphoprō·tein (G. *phōs*, light; *pherein*, to bear; *prōtos*, first). A protein compound of a protein molecule in combination with some as yet undefined phosphorus-containing substance other than nucleic acid or lecithin.

phos·phorated (G. *phōs*, light; *pherein*, to bear). Containing phosphorus.

phosphores·cence (G. *phōs*, light; *pherein*, to bear). The luminous properties exhibited by phosphorus and certain other substances in the dark.

phosphores·cent (G. *phōs*, light; *pherein*, to bear). Having the quality of phosphorescence.

phos·phoretted (G. *phōs*, light; *pherein*, to bear). Combined with phosphorus.

phosphor·ic acid. H_3PO_4 obtained by the oxidation of phosphorus.

phos·phorism (G. *phōs*, light; *pherein*, to bear). Chronic phosphorus poisoning.

phosphorous acid. H_3PO_3 a dibasic oxyacid of phosphorus.

phosphorū·ria (G. *phōs*, light; *pherein*, to bear; *ouron*, urine). 1. Phosphorescent urine. 2. Urine containing an excess of phosphorus.

phos·phorus (G. *phōs*, light; *pherein*, to bear). A nonmetallic element, symbol P., which is poisonous and very inflammable.

phosphosū·cride (G. *phōs*, light; *pherein*, to bear; Fr. *sucre*, sugar). A substance containing phosphoric acid, sugar and fatty acids.

photal·gia (G. *phōs*, light; *algos*, pain). Pain caused by exposure to great intensity of light.

phō·tic (G. *phōs*, light). Relating to light.

photo-actin·ic (G. *phōs*, light; *aktis*, ray). Giving off both luminous and actinic rays.

photobactē·rium (G. *phōs*, light; *baktērion*, dim. of *baktron*, staff). A type of bacteria the cultures of which are phosphorescent.

photobiŏ·tic (G. *phōs*, light; *bios*, life). Living exclusively in the light.

photochĕ·mistry (G. *phōs*, light; *khumeia*, alchemy). That branch of chemistry which treats of the chemical action of light.

photoder·mia (G. *phōs*, light; *derma*, skin). Skin affections caused by exposure to light.

photŏ·dromy (G. *phōs*, light; *drŏmos*, a running). Irresistible movement towards (positive) or away from (negative) light.

photodў·nia (G. *phōs*, light; *odunē*, pain). Pain caused by great intensity of light; severe photophobia.

phŏtodysphor·ia (G. *phōs*, light; *dusphoria*, distress). Intolerance of light; photophobia.

phŏto-electri·city (G. *phōs*, light; *ēlektron*, amber). Electricity produced by light influences.

phō·togen (G. *phōs*, light; *gennan*, to produce). A micro-organism producing phosphorescence or light.

photŏ·graphy (G. *phōs*, light; *graphein*, to write). The production of an image of an object by throwing the rays of light reflected from it upon a surface coated with a film of a material such as silver salt, which is easily decomposed by light; subsequently treating the film with developing agents which bring out the image and then dissolving the salt not acted upon by the light.

phō·tolyte (G. *phōs*, light; *luein*, to dissolve). A substance which the action of light decomposes.

photŏ·meter (G. *phōs*, light; *metron*, measure). An instrument used to measure the intensity of light.

photŏ·metry (G. *phōs*, light; *metron*, measure). Measurement of intensity.

photomi·crograph (G. *phōs*, light; *mikros*, small; *graphein*, to write). A photograph of a small object, made with the help of a microscope. See also microphotograph.

photomicrŏ·graphy (G. *phōs*, light; *mikros*, small; *graphein*, to write). The art of making photomicrographs.

phō·ton (G. *phōs*, light). A particle of light; it is analogous to the electron, being a mass of cosmic ray energy.

photŏ·nosus (G. *phōs*, light; *nosos*, disease). A diseased condition, such as snowblindness, caused by prolonged exposure to glaring light.

photo-ophthal·mia (G. *phōs*, light; *ophthalmos*, eye). Ophthalmia caused by intense light.

phō·toparaesthē·sia (G. *phōs*, light; *para*, amiss; *aisthēsis*, feeling). Defective retinal sensibility.

photŏ·pathy (G. *phōs*, light; *pathos*, disease). Any disease or disorder arising from exposure to light.

photophō·bia (G. *phōs*, light; *phŏbos*, fear). Abnormal intolerance of light.

photop·sia (G. *phōs*, light; *opsis*, vision). Abnormal subjective sensations of flashes of light occurring in certain morbid conditions of tne optic nerve, the retina or the brain.

photoptŏ·metry (G. *phōs*, light; *ōps*, eye; *metron*, measure). Measurement of light perception.

phŏ·toradiŏ·meter (G. *phōs*, light; L. *radius*, ray; G. *metron*, measure). An instrument devised for the measurement of the quantity of X-rays passing through a given surface.

phŏ·torecep·tor (G. *phōs*, light; L. *recipere*, to receive). A cell responding to light.

photosen·sitive (G. *phōs*, light; L. *sentire*, to feel). Having sensitivity to light.

photosyn·tax (G. *phōs*, light; *sustassein*, to arrange). The process whereby plants produce carbohydrates.

photosyn·thesis (G. *phōs*, light; *sunthĕsis*, combination). A chemical reaction brought about by the action of light. Usually applied to building up of carbohydrates, in plants, from carbon dioxide and water.

phototax·is (G. *phōs*, light; *tassein*, to arrange). Phototropism. See tropism.

photothĕ·rapy (G. *phōs*, light; *therapeia*, treatment). 1. The treatment of disease by light. 2. Finsen's light treatment. 3. The application of ultra-violet light to the skin surfaces of the body.

photŏ·tropism (G. *phōs*, light; *trepein*, to turn). See under tropism.

photox·ylin, photox·ylon (G. *phōs*, light; *xulon*, wood). A substance derived from wood pulp by the action of sulphuric acid and potassium nitrate.

phrēn (G.). 1. The diaphragm. 2. Mind.

phrenal·gia (G. *phrēn*; *algos*, pain). 1. Melancholia. 2. Diaphragmatic neuralgia.

phrenasthē·nia (G. *phrēn*; *a*, neg.; *sthenos*, strength). 1. Paralysis of the diaphragm. 2. Feebleness of mind.

phrenasthen·ic. 1. Relating to phrenasthenia; imbecile. 2. One who is feeble-minded.

phrenasthē·sia (G. *phrēn*; *asthenēs*, weak). Idiocy.

phrenē·sis (G., inflammation of the brain). Delirium; insanity.

phrenet·ic (G. *phrēn*, midriff). Maniacal.

phren·ic (G. *phrēn*, midriff). 1. Relating to the diaphragm, as the p. nerve or p. artery. 2. Relating to the mind.

phrenicec·tomy (G. *phrēn*, midriff; *ektomē*, excision). Removal of a portion of the phrenic nerve.

phrenicŏ·tomy (G. *phrēn*, midriff; *tomē*, section). Division of the phrenic nerve.

phreni·tis (G. *phrēn*, midriff or mind). 1. Inflammation of the brain. 2. Inflammation of the diaphragm. 3. Delirium.

phren·ograph (G. *phrēn*, midriff; *graphein*, to write). An instrument for recording the diaphragmatic movements.

phrenohepat·ic (G. *phrēn*, midriff; *hepar*, liver). Relating to the diaphragm and the liver.

phrenŏ·logy (G. *phrēn*, mind; *logos*, a treatise). The discredited theory that the various mental qualities are situated at certain distinct areas in the brain, and that the possession of such faculties can be predicted from the contours of those parts of the skull situated over the areas where these faculties are supposed to be found.

phrenŏ·pathy (G. *phrēn*, mind; *pathos*, disease). Mental disease.

phrenoplē·gia (G. *phrēn*, mind; *plēgē*, stroke). 1. Failure of mental power. 2. Paralysis of the diaphragm.

phrenoptŏ·sis (G. *phrēn*, midriff; *ptosis*, a falling). Prolapse of the diaphragm.

phrenosin. A galactoside obtained from brain substance.

phrenosin·ic acid. $C_{25}H_{50}O_3$—an acid which is obtained by hydrolysis of phrenosin.

phrĕ·nospasm (G. *phrēn*, midriff; *spasmos*, spasm). Spasm of the diaphragm.

phruno·lysin (G. *phrunē*, toad; *lusis*, solution). The toxin of the fire-toad, *Bombinator igneus*.

phthā·late. Any salt of phthalic acid.

phthā·lic acid. $C_6H_4(COOH)_2$, benzene decarboxylic acid, a dibasic acid formed by the oxidation of naphthalene.

phtheirī·asis, phthirī·asis (G. *phtheir*, louse). Pediculosis, *q.v.*

phtheirophō·bia (G. *phtheir*, louse; *phŏbos*, fear). Morbid dread of being infested with lice.

phthī·noid (G. *phthiein*, to decay; *eidos*, form). Possessing tuberculous characteristics.

phthī·sic (G. *phthiein*, to decay). 1. Affected with or resembling phthisis or asthma. 2. Pertaining to phthisis or asthma. 3. One who is affected with phthisis or asthma.

phthī·sical (G. *phthiein*, to decay). Relating to or suffering from phthisis or tuberculosis.

phthī·siophō·bia (G. *phthiein*, to decay; *phŏbos*, fear). A neurotic fear of tuberculosis.

phthī·sis (G. *phthiein*, to decay). Pulmonary tuberculosis.

phȳ·gogalac·tic (G. *phŭgē*, flight; *gala*, milk). 1. Checking milk secretion. 2. Any agent that inhibits the secretion of milk.

phylac·tic. Relating to phylaxis.

phylax·is (G. *phulax*, a guard). The activity exhibited by the body in defending itself against infection.

phyl·lode (G. *phullon*, leaf; *eidos*, form). Shaped like a leaf.

phylogen·esis, phylŏ·geny (G. *phulon*, tribe; *gennan*, to produce). The evolution of the species.

phȳ·lum (G. *phulon*, tribe). In biology, a primary division or stem of the animal or vegetable kingdom.

Physep·tone. Proprietary brand of amidone.

physiăt·rics (G. *phusis*, nature; *iatreia*, healing). The curative power of nature in certain diseases.

physic (G. *phusis*, nature). 1. The science of medicine. 2. A medicine. 3. To administer medicine. 4. To purge.

physical (G. *phusis*, nature). 1. Relating to nature. 2. Relating to the body or to material things. 3. Relating to physics. **P. diagnosis:** the investigation of disease by direct aid of the senses, sight, touch and hearing. **P. examination:** examination of the patient's body to determine the state of the various organs. **P. signs:** the phenomena observed in inspection, palpation, percussion, or auscultation.

physī·cian (G. *phusis*, nature). A qualified medical practitioner.

Physick's encysted rectum (Physick, P. S., American surgeon, 1768–1837). A condition in which the rectal pouches are dilated and thickened.

phȳ·sicist (G. *phusis*, nature). One skilled in physics.

physics (G. *phusis*, nature). The branch of science that deals with the qualities of matter and the dynamics governing it.

physiŏ·gnomy (G. *phusis*, nature; *gnōmōn*, interpreter). The countenance; the facial expression.

physiolŏ·gical (G. *phusis*, nature; *logos*, treatise). 1. Relating to physiology. 2. Relating to natural processes, as distinct from pathological ones.

physiŏ·logist (G. *phusis*, nature; *logos*, treatise). One skilled in physiology.

physiŏ·logy (G. *phusis*, nature; *logos*, treatise). The science of the functions of a living organism and its parts.

physiothĕ·rapy (G. *phusis*, nature; *therapeia*, treatment). The use of physical agents, such as heat and electricity, in the treatment of disease.

physique. The structure of the body.

physocĕ·phaly (G. *phusa*, a blowing; *kephalē*, head). Emphysema of the head.

physohae·matomē·tra (G. *phusa*, a blowing; *haima*, blood; *mētra*, womb). An accumulation of gas, or air, and blood in the uterus, as in decomposition of retained menses or placental tissue.

physomē·tra (G. *phusa*, a blowing; *mētra*, womb). Distension of the uterus with gas.

physopyosal·pinx (G. *phusa*, a blowing; *puon*, pus; *salpigx*, trumpet). Pyosalpinx containing gas.

physostig·mine (G. *phusa*, a blowing; *stigma*, mark). An alkaloid found in the seed of *Physostigma venenosum* (the Calabar bean). It is used locally as a miotic. Syn. Eserine.

phytal·bumin (G. *phuton*, plant; L. *albus*, white). A vegetable albumin.

phytal·bumose (G. *phuton*, plant; L. *albus*, white). A vegetable albumose.

phȳ·tase. An enzyme capable of splitting phytic acid, a phosphoric acid ester of inositol.

phy·tate. Any salt of phytic acid.

phȳ·tic acid. A compound of inositol and phosphoric acid.

phytobezō·ar (G. *phuton*, plant; Persian *padzahr*, dispelling poison). A hair-ball.

phytochĕ·mistry (G. *phuton*, plant; *khumeia*, alchemy). Plant chemistry.

phytogen·esis (G. *phuton*, plant; *gennan*, to produce). The science dealing with the origin and development of plants.

phytŏ·genous (G. *phuton*, plant; *gennan*, to produce). Produced by plants.

phȳ·toid (G. *phuton*, plant; *eidos*, form). Plant-like.

phytō·melin (G. *phuton*, plant; *meli*, honey). See rutin.

Phytō·monas. A genus of plant-destroying bacteria.

phȳtopathogĕ·nic (G. *phuton*, plant; *pathos*, disease; *gennan*, to produce). Producing plant diseases.

phytopathŏ·logy (G. *phuton*, plant; *pathos*, disease; *logos*, treatise). The science dealing with the diseases of plants.

phȳ·toplasm (G. *phuton*, plant; *plasma*, from *plassein*, to form). Plant protoplasm.

phytŏ·sis (G. *phuton*, plant). Any disease caused by vegetable parasites.

phytotox·in (G. *phuton*, plant; *toxikon*, poison). A plant toxin; e.g. abrin, crotin and ricin.

phytozō·on (G. *phuton*, plant; *zōon*, animal). An animal-resembling plant.

pia, pia mater (L. *pia*, tender; *mater*, mother). The outer of three investing membranes of the brain and spinal cord.

pī·al (L. *pius*, tender). Relating to the pia.

pī·alyn (G. *piar*, fat; *luein*, to loosen). See steapsin.

pian (Fr.). See framboesia.

pianist's cramp. An occupational disorder, characterized by painful spasm of the fingers or hand.

piarachnī·tis (L. *pius*, tender; G. *arakhnē*, spider). Inflammation of the pia mater and arachnoid; also called leptomeningitis.

pī·ca (L. *pīca*, magpie). A desire for unnatural articles of food; a symptom encountered in some forms of insanity and hysteria, sometimes also in pregnancy.

Pick's bundle (Pick, A., Prague psychiatrist, 1857–1924). An occasional bundle of nerve fibres in the medulla oblongata connected with the pyramidal tract.

Pick's disease (Pick, F., Prague physician, 1867–1926). A disease marked by general inflammation of serous membranes leading to adherent pericardium and cirrhosis of the liver.

picotement (Fr. *picoter*, to prick). A pricking sensation; tingling.

picram·ic acid. 2-amino-4:6-dinitrophenol.

picrate. A salt of picric acid.

picric acid. 2:4:6-trinitrophenol.

picrocar·mine. A solution of carmine and picric acid, used for staining specimens for the microscope.

pǐ·crotoxin. A glycoside from the seed of *Anamiota paniculata*.

piē·dra (Sp. stone). South American name for Trichosporosis tropica, *q.v.*

piěsǐ·meter, pǐēzǒ·meter (G. *piezein*, to press; *metron*, measure). 1. An instrument for measuring the degree of sensitiveness of the skin to pressure. 2. An upright tube for measuring the pressure in a horizontal pipe through which water is flowing. 3. An instrument for measuring the displacement of the globe in the orbit.

pig·ment (L. *pigmentum*, paint). A dye; a colouring agent.

pig·mentary (L. *pigmentum*, paint). Relating to or forming pigment.

pigmentā·tion (L. *pigmentum*, paint). 1. Deposition of pigment. 2. Colouring or discolouring caused by pigments.

pigmented. Having a deposit of pigment.

pǐ·lary (L. *pilus*, hair). Relating to the hair.

pilǎ·stered (L. *pila*, pillar). Flanged so as to look fluted; arranged in columns. **P. femur:** undue prominence of the linea aspera of the femur.

pǐ·leous (L. *pilus*, hair). Hairy.

piles (L. *pila*, pillar). Haemorrhoids, *q.v.*

pǐ·leum (L. *pileum*, hat). One of the cerebellar hemispheres.

piliā·tion (L. *pilus*, hair). The growth of hair.

pill (L. *pilula*). A small round ball, containing one or more medicaments administered orally.

pillar (L. *pila*, pillar). A column-like structure serving as a support. **P. of the fauces:** one of the folds of mucous membrane situated on either side of the fauces.

pilocar·pine. An alkaloid derived from pilocarpus and used locally as a miotic. It is a powerful sudorific and sialogogue.

Pilocar·pus. A genus of shrubs found in tropical parts of America. See also jaborandi.

pilomo·tor (L. *pilus*, hair; *movere*, to move). Causing the hair to move.

piloni·dal (L. *pilus*, hair; *nidus*, nest). Containing hair; said of certain types of cyst, especially in sacrococcygeal region.

pǐ·lose, pǐ·lous (L. *pilus*, hair). Hairy; covered with soft hairs.

pilō·sis (L. *pilus*, hair). Abnormal growth of hair.

pil·ula (L.). A pill.

pil·ular (L. *pilula*, pill). Like, or relating to, a pill.

pimelō·ma (G. *pimelē*, fat). Lipoma, *q.v.*

pim·elorrhoē·a (G. *pimelē*, fat; *rhoia*, a flow). Diarrhoea characterized by the presence of fat.

pimelō·sis (G. *pimelē*, fat). 1. Conversion into fat. 2. Fatty degeneration of tissues. 3. Obesity.

pimelū·ria (G. *pimelē*, fat; *ouron*, urine). The presence of fat in the urine; lipuria.

pimple. A small pustule.

pin. A delicate metal rod used to fix the fractured ends of bones.

Pinard's sign (Pinard, A., French obstetrician, 1844–1934). Tenderness of fundus uteri at six month's pregnancy indicates breech presentation.

pince-ciseaux (Fr.). Cutting forceps used in iridectomy.

pincement (Fr.). A pinching of the tissues in massage.

pincers (Fr. *pincer*, to pinch). Forceps.

pincet, pincette. A small forceps.

pine (L. *pinus*). A genus of trees belonging to the order Coniferae; they yield turpentine and allied substances.

pin·eal (L. *pinea*, pine-cone). Relating to or resembling a pine-cone. **P. body, P. gland:** the epiphysis cerebri, a structure situated behind the third ventricle, of unknown function; it was formerly believed to secrete a hormone.

pingǔe·cula (L. *pinguis*, fat). A small yellowish three-cornered patch seen on the conjunctiva between the cornea and canthus of the eye. It is composed of connective tissue and occurs in old age.

pinhole. A very small perforation such as might be made by pricking with a pin. **P. os:** an abnormal degree of contraction of the os uteri seen in some young women.

pi·niform (L. *pinea*, pine-cone). Shaped like a cone.

pink disease. A form of infantile erythroedema. Syn. acrodynia.

pink-eye. A loose term covering any epidemic conjunctivitis.

pinna (L., feather). That part of the ear external to the head; the auricle.

pinnal (L. *pinna*, feather). Relating to the pinna.

pint. The eighth part of a gallon, or 16 fluid ounces. The imperial pint is equal to 20 fluid ounces.

pinta (Sp. spot). A tropical skin disease characterized by eruption of coloured patches due to various species of chromogenic fungi.

pinworm. See Oxyuris and Ascaris.

Piorkowski's stain (Piorkowski, M., German bacteriologist, born 1859). For metachromatic granules. Stain alkaline methylene blue, decolorise 3 per cent hydrochloric acid in alcohol, stain 1 per cent aqueous eosin.

pipette (Fr., little pipe). A graduated glass vessel designed to deliver a stated volume of liquid under certain specified conditions.

piqûre (Fr.). Puncture.

Pirie's bone (Pirie, G. A., contemporary British anatomist). The dorsal astragalo-scaphoid bone.

pǐ·riform (L. *pirum*, pear; *forma*, shape). Pyriform, *q.v.*

Pirogoff's amputation (Pirogoff, N. I., Russian surgeon, 1810–81). An amputation through the ankle joint, the os calcis being fixed to the cut surface of the tibia. Not used to-day. **P.'s angle:** the angle formed by the internal jugular and subclavian veins. **P.'s triangle:** the area bounded by the intermediate tendon of the digastric muscle, the posterior border of the mylohyoid and the hypoglossal nerve.

Piroplas·ma (L. *pirum*, pear; *plasma*, from *plassein*, to form). A genus of haematozoa. **P. hominis:** the species causing Rocky Mountain spotted fever in man.

pi·roplasmō·sis. Infection with Piroplasma.

Pirquet's reaction (Pirquet, C., Freiherr von, Austrian paediatrician, 1874–1929). Local inflammatory reaction produced by tuberculin.

pi·siform (L. *pisum*, pea; *forma*, shape). Pea-shaped. **P. bone:** a small bone situated on the anterior and inner portion of the carpus.

pit. 1. A depression, e.g. the p. of the stomach. 2. To indent by means of pressure.

pitch (1). (L. *pix*, pitch). The height of a sound; the quality depending upon the frequency of the vibrations producing the sound.

pitch (2). Dark-coloured resinous substance, hard when cold and semi-liquid when hot. It is obtained from various species of pine and from tar.

pitchblende. The mineral substance from which radium is obtained.

pith. 1. The tissue situated in the middle of plant stems. 2. Bone marrow. 3. Spinal marrow. 4. To pierce the brain and spinal cord.

pithǐǎt·ric (G. *peithein*, to persuade; *iatrike*, medicine). Capable of being controlled or abated by means of suggestion or persuasion; term applied to hysteria.

pi·thing. Destruction of the central nervous system by piercing the brain and spinal cord; decerebration.

pi·tocin (L. *pituita*, phlegm). A hormone of the posterior lobe of the pituitary gland, stimulating contraction of smooth muscles.

Pitres's areas (Pitres, A., French physician, 1848–1927). The areas of the cerebral cortex. **P.'s sign:** hyperaesthesia of the scrotum and the testes in cases of tabes dorsalis.

pitres·sin. A hormone of the posterior lobe of the pituitary gland, of anti-diuretic activity.

pitted. Marked by pits, as from smallpox.

pitting. The formation of pits.

pitu·ita (L. *phlegm*). Phlegm; mucus.

pitu·itary (L., *phlegm*). 1. Secreting or containing mucus. 2. Relating to the p. gland. **P. basophilism:** a condition characterized by obesity, plethoric appearance, osteoporosis, hypertension, purple striae distensae, especially of the skin of abdomen and thighs, hirsutism, amenorrhoea, hyperglycaemia, sometimes by polyuria, due to hyperplasia, or an adenoma, of the basophilic cells of the anterior lobe of the p. gland. Syn. Cushing's syndrome. **P. body** or **P. gland:** a small structure situated within the sella turcica of the skull, consisting of a larger anterior lobe (pars glandularis) and a smaller posterior lobe (pars neuralis), of a pars intermedia and a pars tuberalis. The first two secrete hormones, regulating growth, function of all other endocrine glands, lactation, metabolism of carbohydrates and fat (anterior lobe) and stimulating contraction of smooth muscles and controlling diuresis (posterior lobe). The function of the posterior lobe is especially intimately connected with that of the hypothalamus. Syn. hypophysis cerebri. **P. stalk:** the connection between hypothalamus and pituitary gland, containing nonmyelinated nerve fibres.

pituitary gonadotrophine. Gonadotrophic fraction of anterior pituitary hormones.

Pitū·itrin. A proprietary preparation made from the posterior lobe of the pituitary gland.

pityri·asis (G. *pituron*, bran). Term applied to various skin diseases, characterized by delicate, branny desquamations and the absence of obvious signs of inflammation. **P. rosea:** a disease of the skin characterized by initial eruption of a scaly, rose-coloured, oval or circular patch (herald-patch) with well-defined slightly raised border, followed from 1–2 weeks later by the eruption of widely disseminated, irregularly outlined, scaly, usually itching, macules or papules, which by peripheral spread tend to form irregular patches, and by spontaneous disappearance after 4–6 weeks' time. **P. rubra pilaris:** see lichen acuminatus. **P. versicolor:** syn. tinea versicolor.

placē·bo (L., I will please). A treatment or, especially, a medicine given to humour the patient.

placen·ta (L., a flat cake). The structure on the uterine wall to which the embryo is attached and from which it receives its nourishment. The placenta develops at about the third month of gestation. At term it weighs about one pound. **P. praevia:** placenta developing in the lower uterine segment so that it covers, or partially covers, the internal os.

placen·tal (L. *placenta*, a flat cake). Relating to the placenta.

Placentã·lia. A subclass of mammals including all except the monotremes and marsupials.

placentã·tion (L. *placenta*, a flat cake). Formation and mode of attachment of the placenta.

placenti·tis (L. *placenta*, a flat cake). Inflammation of the placenta.

placen·toid (L. *placenta*, a flat cake; G. *eidos*, form). Like a placenta.

Placido's disc (Placido, G., Portuguese ophthalmologist). A disc marked with alternate black and white circles, used as a keratoscope.

placing reflexes. A group of postural reflexes serving to maintain normal standing.

plă·code (G. *plax*, a plain; *eidos*, form). A thickening of the ectoderm in the head of the embryo which takes part in the formation of the ganglia of the cranial nerves.

plă·giocephă·lic (G. *plagios*, oblique; *kephalē*, head). Having a skull showing plagiocephaly.

plă·giocě·phaly (G. *plagios*, oblique; *kephalē*, head). Malformation of the skull due to closure of part of the coronal suture.

plague (L. *plaga*, a blow). 1. A contagious disease with a high mortality rate endemic in Eastern and Central Asia and caused by the *Bacillus pestis*. Incubation 3–8 days; begins with fever, pain, swelling of the lymph nodes. Delirium, vomiting and/or diarrhoea may be present. 2. Any contagious malignant epidemic disease.

Planck's constant (Planck, M., German physicist, 1858–1947). Quantum constant. The universal constant $h = 6.557 \times 10^{-27}$ erg seconds. Symbol, h.

plane (L. *planus*). 1. Any flat, smooth surface. 2. A hypothetical flat surface, whether tangent to or dividing the body.

plani·meter (L. *planus*, flat; G. *metron*, measure). 1. See perimeter. 2. An instrument for the measuring of planes.

planocel·lular (L. *planus*, plane; *cellula*, a small chamber). Flat-celled.

planocon·cave. Term used to describe a lens plane on one side, concave on the other.

planocon·vex. Term used to describe a lens plane on one side, convex on the other.

planomã·nia (G. *planos*, a wandering; *mania*, madness). A morbid tendency to wander.

plan·ta (L.). The sole of the foot.

plan·tar (L. *planta*, sole). Relating to the sole of the foot.

plantă·ris muscle. A small muscle at the back of the calf of the leg.

plă·nula. Name given to embryo in stage of two layers, ectoderm and entoderm.

plă·num (L. *planus*, flat). A plane or surface. **P. occipitale:** occipital plane.

plaque (Fr.). A patch. **Blood-p.:** see blood-platelet. **Opaline p.:** scattered white spots appearing on the fauces, hard palate, cheeks and lips; an early lesion in syphilis.

plas·ma (G. *plasma*, from *plassein*, to form). 1. The fluid portion of unclotted blood and lymph. 2. Protoplasm.

plasmat·ic, plas·mic (G. *plasma*, anything formed). 1. Relating to plasma. 2. Plastic.

plasmodes·mus (G. *plasma*, anything formed; *desmos*, band). Cytoplasmic filament connecting adjoining cells.

plasmō·diblast (G. *plasma*, anything formed; *eidos*, form; *blastos*, germ). Trophoblast, *q.v.*

plasmō·dium (G. *plasma*, anything formed; *eidos*, form). 1. The structure formed by the fusion of two or more amoebiform bodies scattered in a common cytoplasmic mass, especially in protista. 2. A genus of Haemosporidiidea. **P. falciparum:** the organism causing subtertian, malignant or tropical malaria. **P. malariae:** the organism causing quartan malaria. **P. vivax:** the organism causing benign tertian malaria.

plasmō·gamy (G. *plasma*, anything formed; *gamos*, marriage). Cytoplasmic fusion.

plas·mogen (G. *plasma*, anything formed; *gennan*, to produce). Formative protoplasm.

plasmō·lysis (G. *plasma*, anything formed; *luein*, to dissolve). The escape of fluid from a cell by altered osmotic pressure.

plasmorrhex·is (G. *plasma*, anything formed; *rhēxis*, a bursting). The rupture of a cell and consequent escape of plasma.

plasmŏ·schisis (G. *plasma*, anything formed; *skhizein*, to split). The spontaneous splitting of a cell.

plas·mosome (G. *plasma*, anything formed; *sōma*, body). 1. One of the minute cytoplasmic granules. 2. An acidophilic nucleolus.

plasmŏ·tropism (G. *plasma*, anything formed; *trepein*, to turn). Protoplasmic degeneration.

pla·some (G. *plassein*, to form). See pangen.

plasson (G. *plassein*, to form). Primitive protoplasm; the protoplasm of the cytode.

plaster (G. *emplastron*, a plaster). 1. An adhesive substance spread upon flexible material such as fine cloth for application as strapping with or without medicament to the surface of the body. 2. Calcined gypsum or calcium sulphate; used for the immobilization of a limb, etc.

plastic (G. *plassein*, to form). 1. Formative; repairing blemishes or defects, as in plastic surgery. 2. Capable of being moulded.

plasti·city (G. *plassein*, to form). The quality of being plastic.

plas·ticule (G. *plassein*, to form). A molecule of plastic substance.

plas·tid (G. *plassein*, to form). 1. An elementary organism; a cytode. 2. A cytoplasmic body having the quality of independent growth and division.

plas·tin (G. *plassein*, to form). Linin, *q.v.*

plastŏ·gamy (G. *plasma*, anything formed; *gamos*, marriage). Plasmogamy, *q.v.*

plas·tomere (G. *plassein*, to form; *meros*, a part). 1. One of the bodies formed in coccidian reproduction by division of the trophozoite, each plastomere becoming the centre of merozoite formation. 2. The portion of the sperm formed of cytoplasm.

plate (G. *platus*, broad). 1. Any flattened part, especially a flattened bone surface. 2. A thin piece of metal or other substance to which dentures are attached. 3. A thin metal plate used in internal fixation of fractures.

platelet. See blood platelet.

plă·ticulture (G. *platus*, broad; L. *cultura*, cultivation). The cultivation of bacteria on plates.

plating. 1. See platiculture. 2. Internal fixation of fractures by means of metal plates.

platinum. A silver-white metal occurring native or alloyed with other metals. At. wt. 195.2. Symbol Pt. Sp. g. 21.4. Melting point 1755°C. Insoluble in mineral acids, except aqua regia; extensively used for chemical apparatus such as crucibles. In a finely divided state platinum absorbs large volumes of gases at its surface, hence used as a catalyst in hydrogenation reactions.

platybasia. See basilar impression.

platycephă·lic, platycĕ·phalous (G. *platus*, wide; *kephalē*, head). Having a skull of considerable width with a vertical index of less than 70.

Platyhelmin·thēs (G. *platus*, wide; *helmins*, worm). Flat-bodied, more or less elongated worms, usually bisexual.

platyhiĕ·ric (G. *platus*, wide; *hieros*, sacred). Having a broad sacrum; with a sacral index of more than 100.

platypel·lic (G. *platus*, wide; *pellis*, a bowl). Having a broad pelvis.

platypŏ·dia (G. *platus*, wide; *pous*, foot). Flat-footedness.

plă·tyrrhīne (G. *platus*, wide; *rhis*, nose). Having a broad, flat nose.

platys·ma (G. *platus*, wide). 1. Anything possessing considerable superficial dimensions. 2. A thin flat muscle extending from the clavicle to the angle of the mouth.

Plaut's angina (Plaut, H. K., German physician, 1858–1928). Vincent's angina. An infection by Fusobacterium plauti-vincenti which affects the tonsils.

Playfair's treatment (Playfair, W. S., English physician, 1836–1903). Rest cure. Absolute rest in bed.

pledget. A small, flattened compress of wool.

plegaphō·nia (G. *plēgē*, a stroke; *a*, neg.; *phōnē*, voice). The sound produced when the larynx is percussed.

Plehn's granules (Plehn, A., German physician, 1861–1935). Basophile granules which are found in the parasite of malaria.

plei·ocholū·ria (G. *pleōn*, more; *chloros*, green; *ouron*, urine). A condition marked by an excess of chlorides in the urine.

pleochrō·ic (G. *pleōn*, more; *khroia*, colour). Pleochromatic, *q.v.*

pleochrō·ism (G. *pleōn*, more; *khroia*, colour). The quality possessed by some bodies (especially crystalline bodies) of showing different colours when examined in the direction of different axes.

pleochromat·ic (G. *pleōn*, more; *khrōma*, colour). Relating to pleochroism.

pleocytō·sis (G. *pleōn*, more; *kutos*, a container). Increase of lymphocytes in the cerebrospinal fluid.

pleomă·stia, pleomă·zia (G. *pleōn*, more; *mastos* or *mazos*, breast). The condition of having more than two breasts. Cf. polymastia.

pleomor·phism (G. *pleōn*, more; *morphē*, shape). Pleomorphic state.

pleonec·tic (G. *pleonexia*, greed). Pertaining to pleonexia.

pleonex·ia (G., greed). Undue desire to possess.

plĕ·thora (G. *plēthōrē*, fullness). The state of being over full.

plethor·ic (G. *plēthōrē*, fullness). Overloaded.

plethȳs·mograph (G. *plēthunein*, to increase; *graphein*, to record). An apparatus for ascertaining and registering the variations in the size of a limb or organ; and hence the variations in the amount of blood passing through the limb or organ.

plethysmŏ·meter (G. *plethunein*, to increase; *metron*, measure). The recording apparatus attached to a plethysmograph.

pleū·ra (G., rib). The serous membrane covering the lungs and lining the thorax.

pleū·ral. Relating to the pleura.

pleural·gia (G. *pleura*, rib; *algos*, pain). Pain in the pleura or the side.

pleurapŏ·physis (G. *pleura*, rib; *apo*, away; *phusis*, a growing). A lateral process of a vertebra which has the morphological valence of a rib.

pleū·rapostē·ma (G. *pleura*, rib; *apostēma*, an abscess). The presence of pus in the pleural cavity.

pleurec·tomy (G. *pleura*, rib; *ektomē*, excision). Excision of one or more ribs.

pleū·risy (G. *pleura*, rib). Pleuritis; inflammation of the pleura, which may be acute or chronic. The three chief types, varying according to the character of the exudates, are: (a) fibrinous or plastic; (b) serofibrinous; (c) purulent.

pleurit·ic. Relating to or affected with pleurisy.

pleuri·tis. Pleurisy, *q.v.*

pleurobronchi·tis (G. *pleura*, rib; *brogkhos*, windpipe). Pleurisy accompanied by bronchitis.

pleū·rocele (G. *pleura*, rib; *kēlē*, hernia). 1. Hernia of the lung. 2. An effusion of serum into the pleural cavity.

pleurocentē·sis (G. *pleura*, rib; *kentesis*, puncture). Puncture of the pleura.

pleurodȳ·nia (G. *pleura*, rib; *odunē*, pain). A severe pain affecting the intercostal muscles and caused by rheumatism.

pleū·rolith (G. *pleura*, rib; *lithos*, stone). A stone or calculus occurring in the pleura.

pleuropericardi·tis. Pleurisy associated with pericarditis.

pleūroperitonē·al (G. *pleura*, rib; *peritonaion*, peritoneum). Relating to the pleura and the peritoneum.

pleūropneumō·nia (G. *plēūra*, rib; *pneumōn*, the lungs). Inflammation of the pleura and of the lung; applied especially to a variety found in cattle.

pleūropnēūmonŏ·lysis (G. *pleura*, rib; *pneumōn*, the lungs; *lusis*, dissolution). Excision of ribs on one side of the chest so as to bring about collapse of the lung.

pleuropul·monary (G. *pleura*, rib; L. *pulmo*, lung). Relating to the pleura and the lungs.

pleurosō·ma (G. *pleura*, rib; *sōma*, body). A monster with lateral eventration and atrophy of upper extremity on same side.

pleurothŏ·tonos (G. *pleura*, rib; *ōthein*, to push; *tonos*, tension). Tetanic muscular spasm, bending the body to one side.

pleurŏ·tomy (G. *pleura*, rib; *tomē*, a cutting). An incision into the pleura.

plex·iform (L. *plexus*, a plait; *forma*, shape). Like a plexus or network.

plexor. A hammer used for percussion.

plexus (L., a plait). A network, especially an intricate interweaving of a collection of vessels or nerves. **Aortic p.:** is found on the abdominal aorta, it derives its fibres from the coeliac ganglia and the coeliac plexus. **Auerbach's p.** (myenteric p.): a ganglionic plexus situated between the longitudinal and circular fibres of the external muscular coat of the small intestine. **Brachial p.:** is situated in the lower part of the posterior triangle of the neck, it is a complicated network of nerves which are distributed to the upper extremity. **Buccal p.:** a plexus of nerves situated on the superficial surface of the buccinator muscle. **Cardiac p.:** is one of the three large prevertebral plexuses. It is situated partly in the concavity of the arch of the aorta and partly upon the trachea. **Cavernous p.:** a sympathetic plexus on the walls of the internal carotid artery while that vessel is in the cavernous sinus. **Cervical p.:** situated in the upper part of the neck. It is formed by the anterior primary rami of the first three cervical nerves and the greater part of the fourth. **Choroid p.:** a plexus of veins within the ventricles of the brain. Cerebrospinal fluid is secreted by this plexus. **Coccygeal p.:** is formed by the lower branch of the anterior primary division of the fourth sacral, the anterior primary division of the fifth sacral, and the anterior primary division of the coccygeal nerve. **Coeliac p.** (solar p.): of the sympathetic system is of large size and is situated deeply in the epigastric region, behind the stomach and in front of the aorta. **Coronary p.:** two in number, right and left. These nerve plexuses accompany the right and left coronary arteries. **Diaphragmatic p.** (phrenic p.): a nerve plexus from the upper part of the coeliac ganglion, it accompanies the phrenic artery to the diaphragm. **Extraperitoneal p.** (of Turner): an arterial plexus of the lumbar arteries which anastomose on the posterior abdominal wall. **Hepatic p.:** part of the coeliac plexus which accompanies the hepatic artery and receives branches from the left vagus nerve. **Hypogastric p.:** is formed by the fusion of the two halves of the aortic plexus. It is a large flat nerve plexus. **Inferior mesenteric p.:** is part of the aortic plexus, it accompanies the inferior mesenteric artery and gives off superior left colic, inferior left colic and superior rectal plexuses. **Infraorbital p.:** the terminal branches of the superior buccal branches of the facial nerve which form a plexus under cover of the levator labii superioris muscle on the face. **Internal carotid p.:** an interlacement of sympathetic nerve fibres from the superior cervical ganglion which are found on the internal carotid artery. **Left gastric p.:** a plexus on the left gastric artery which is derived from fibres from the coeliac plexus. **Lumbar p.:** a large plexus situated in the substance of the psoas muscle. It is formed by the anterior primary divisions of the first three lumbar nerves and the greater part of the fourth. **Meissner's p.** (submucous p.): a small and delicate nerve plexus situated in the submucous coat of the small bowel. **Myenteric p.:** see Auerbach's plexus. **Ovarian p.:** an offshoot from the renal and aortic plexuses which accompanies the ovarian artery to the ovary. **Pampiniform p.:** a venous plexus made up of the testicular veins, it forms a network around the vas deferens in the spermatic cord. **Parotid p.** (pes anserinus): terminal branches of the facial nerve which are distributed over the parotid gland. **Patellar p.:** is a network of fine nerves on the anterior aspect of the patella. **Pelvic p.:** two in number, right and left; derived from the hypogastric sympathetic plexus, they pass down on the medial side of the internal iliac artery to the rectum and bladder. **Pharyngeal p.:** situated upon the middle constrictor of the pharynx. It is formed from branches of the vagus, glossopharyngeal and superior cervical ganglion of the sympathetic. **Phrenic p.:** see diaphragmatic plexus. **Prostatic venous p.:** a dense venous plexus situated between the capsule and the fascial sheath of the prostate gland. **Pterygoid venous p.:** a large plexus that surrounds the lateral pterygoid muscle. **Pudendal p.:** the lower part of the sacral nerve plexus. **Pulmonary p.:** plexiform fibres of the right vagus nerve which are distributed to the root of the lung and posterior mediastinum. **Rectal venous p.:** a plexus of rectal veins situated in the rectum. **Renal p.:** an offshoot of the coeliac plexus going to the kidney via the renal artery. **Sacral p.:** a large flattened mass of nerves lying on the pyriformis muscle, formed from the anterior primary divisions of the fourth and fifth lumbar nerves and the first, second and third sacral nerves. **Solar p.:** see coeliac plexus. **Spermatic p.** (testicular p.): derives its fibres from the renal and aortic plexuses and accompanies the testicular artery to the testis. **Splenic p.:** part of the coeliac plexus which runs with the splenic artery and receives branches from the left vagus nerve. **Submucous p.:** see Meissner's plexus. **Subsartorial p.:** a nerve plexus situated about the middle third of the thigh, deep to sartorius muscle. **Superior mesenteric p.:** a sympathetic nerve plexus derived from the solar plexus and containing obvious ganglia embedded in it. **Suprarenal p.:** a sympathetic nerve plexus which receives its fibres from the coeliac ganglion and coeliac plexus. It is distributed to the suprarenal gland. **Testicular p.:** see spermatic plexus. **Turner's p.:** see extraperitoneal arterial plexus. **Tympanic p.:** a small delicate nerve plexus on the promontory of the middle ear.

plī·ca (L. *plicare*, to fold). A fold. **P. fimbriata:** an indistinct fringed fold on the lateral part of the frenulum linguae. **P. semilunaris:** a vertical, semilunar fold of conjunctiva situated on the lateral side of the caruncle. It corresponds to the membrana nictitans, or third eyelid, of some animals. **P. sublingualis:** a mucous fold in the floor of the mouth caused by the sublingual gland. **P. transversalis recti:** horizontal fold of the rectum or the lowest Houston's valve.

pli·cate (L. *plicare*, to fold). Folded.

plicŏ·tomy (L. *plicare*, to fold; *tomē*, a cutting). The dividing of the posterior fold of the tympanic membrane.

pli·ers (F. *plier*, to fold). Pincers.

Plugge's test (Plugge, P. C., Dutch biochemist, 1847–97). A test for phenol. A red colour is produced when mercuric nitrate containing a trace of nitrous acid is added to phenol.

plum·bage. Term used to denote the filling of a cavity with paraffin wax. Syn. plombage.

plumbā·go (L. *plumbum*, lead). Graphite, *q.v.*

plum·bic (L. *plumbum*, lead). Relating to or containing lead.

plum·bism (L. *plumbum*, lead). Lead-poisoning.

plumbum (L.). Lead, an element. Symbol Pb.

Plummer's pill (Plummer, A., Scottish physician, 1698–1756). A pill composed of antimony and calomel.

pluriglan·dular (L. *plus*, more; *glans*, acorn). Relating to two or more glands, or to the secretions of several glands; e.g., p. extract.

pluri·para (L. *plus*, more; *parere*, to bring forth). Multipara, *q.v.*

plutomā·nia (G. *ploutos*, riches; *mania*, madness). Morbid delusion of possessing great wealth.

pnēodynam·ics (G. *pnein*, to breathe; *dunamis*, power). The dynamics of respiration.

pnē·ogaster (G. *pnein*, to breathe; *gastēr*, belly). The air passages.

pnē·ograph (G. *pnein*, to breathe; *graphein*, to write). An apparatus for recording respiratory movements.

pnēŏ·meter (G. *pnein*, to breathe; *metron*, measure). Spirometer, *q.v.*

pneumarthrō·sis (G. *pneuma*, air; *arthron*, joint). The presence of gas or air in a joint.

pneu·ma (G.). 1. Air; a breath. 2. (Obsolete). The vital principle.

pneumat·ic (G. *pneuma*, air). Relating to air or respiration.

pneumat·ics (G. *pneuma*, air). The branch of physics dealing with the physical properties of air and gases.

pneumă·tocele (G. *pneuma*, air; *kēlē*, hernia). 1. A swelling which contains air or gas. 2. Pneumonocele, *q.v.* 3. A scrotal swelling caused by the presence of gas.

pneumă·togram (G. *pneuma*, air; *gramma*, writing). A tracing showing the character of the respiratory movements.

pneumatŏ·meter (G. *pneuma*, air; *metron*, measure). An instrument for measuring the pressure of respiratory movements.

pneumatŏ·metry (G. *pneuma*, air; *metron*, measure). 1. The measurement of respiratory force; used in diagnosis. 2. The treatment of pulmonary diseases by means of a pneumatic apparatus, such as the 'iron lung'.

pneumatŏ·sis (G. *pneuma*, air). The presence of air or gas in abnormal places in the body.

pneumatothĕ·rapy (G. *pneuma*, air; *therapeia*, treatment). Treatment by means of compressed or rarefied air.

pneumatothor·ax. Pneumothorax, *q.v.*

pneumatū·ria (G. *pneuma*, air; *ouron*, urine). The presence of gas or air in the urine.

pneumec·tomy (G. *pneumōn*, lung; *tomē*, a cutting). Pneumonectomy, *q.v.*

pneu·mocele (G. *pneuma*, air; *kēlē*, hernia). Pneumatocele, *q.v.*

pneu·mococcaē·mia (G. *pneumōn*, lungs; *kokkos*, berry; *haima*, blood). A condition in which pneumococci are present in the blood.

pneumococ·cal. Relating to pneumococci.

pneumococ·cus, pl. **pneumococci** (G. *pneumōn*, the lungs; *kokkos*, berry). The *Micrococcus lanceolatus.* Syn. *Diplococcus pneumoniae.*

pneumoconĭō·sis. Pneumokoniosis, *q.v.*

pneumocrā·nia, pneumocrā·nium (G. *pneuma*, air; *kranion*, skull). Presence of air or gas under the dura mater.

pneumoder·ma (G. *pneuma*, air; *derma*, skin). Subcutaneous emphysema.

pneumo-enteri·tis (G. *pneumōn*, the lungs; *enteron*, intestine). Combined inflammation of the lungs and intestines.

pneumogas·tric (G. *pneumōn*, the lungs; *gastēr*, belly). 1. Relating to the lungs and stomach. 2. Relating to the pneumogastric or vagus nerve.

pneu·mogram (G. *pneumōn*, the lungs; *gramma*, a mark). A pneumographic tracing.

pneu·mograph (G. *pneumōn*, the lungs; *graphein*, to write). An instrument for recording the chest movements in respiration.

pneumohae·mopericar·dium (G. *pneuma*, air; *haima*, blood; *perikardion*, the pericardium). Condition in which air and blood are present in the pericardium.

pneumohaēmothor·ax (G. *pneuma*, air; *haima*, blood; *thōrax*, the chest). The presence of gas or air and blood in the pleural cavity.

pneumohydromē·tra (G. *pneuma*, air; *hudōr*, water; *metra*, uterus). Condition in which air and fluid is present in uterus.

pneumohȳdropericar·dium (G. *pneuma*, air; *hudōr*, water; *peri*, around; *kardia*, heart). The presence of air and fluid in the pericardial sac.

pneumohydrothor·ax (G. *pneuma*, air; *hudōr*, water; *thōrax*, chest). The presence of air or gas and fluid in the pleural cavity.

pneumokonĭō·sis (G. *pneumōn*, the lungs; *konis*, dust). Chronic induration or inflammation of the lung fibres, caused by the inhalation of dust.

pneu·molith (G. *pneumōn*, the lungs; *lithos*, stone). A lung calculus.

pneumolithī·asis (G. *pneumōn*, the lungs; *lithos*, stone). A condition characterized by the presence of calculi in the lungs.

pneumomas·sage (G. *pneuma*, air; Fr. *masser*, to rub). Pneumatic massage of the tympanum.

pneumŏ·meter, pneumonŏ·meter (G. *pneuma*, air; *metron*, measure). Spirometer, *q.v.* Also called pneumatometer.

pneumomycō·sis (G. *pneumōn*, the lungs; *mukēs*, mushroom). A lung disease due to fungus.

pneumomȳĕlŏ·graphy (G. *pneuma*, air; *muelos*, marrow; *graphein*, to write). X-ray examination after the injection of air or oxygen into the spinal canal.

pneumonectā·sia, pneumonec·tasis (G. *pneumōn*, the lungs; *ektasis*, extension). Emphysema of the lungs.

pneumonec·tomy (G. *pneumōn*, the lungs; *ektomē*, excision). Excision of a part of the lung.

pneumō·nia (G. *pneumōn*, the lungs). Inflammation of the lungs; pneumonitis.

pneumon·ic (G. *pneumōn*, the lungs). Relating to the lungs or to pneumonia.

pneumoni·tis. The same as pneumonia.

pneumŏ·nocele (G. *pneumōn*, the lungs; *kēlē*, hernia). A lung hernia.

pneumonokoni·osis. Pneumokoniosis, *q.v.*

pneumonŏ·lysis (G. *pneumōn*, lung; *lusis*, loosening). The operation of stripping the parietal pleura from the chest wall, to allow the lung to collapse. **Intrapleural p.:** the visceral pleura is stripped from the parietal pleura.

pneumonomelanō·sis (G. *pneumōn*, the lungs; *melas*, black). Melanosis or anthracosis of the lung.

pneumonŏ·meter. Spirometer, *q.v.*

pneumonŏ·pathy (G. *pneumōn*, the lungs; *pathos*, disease). Any lung disease.

pneumonor·rhaphy (G. *pneumōn*, the lungs; *rhaphē*, suture). Suture of the lung.

pneumonosep·sis (G. *pneumōn*, the lungs; *sepsis*, putrefaction). Inflammation of the lung characterized by sepsis.

pneumonō·sis (G. *pneumōn*, the lungs). Any lung disease.

pneumonŏ·tomy (G. *pneumōn*, the lungs; *tomē*, a cutting). Incision into the lung.

pneumopă·ludism (G. *pneumōn*, the lungs; L. *palus*, a swamp). Malarial disease of the lungs.

pneumopericar·dium (G. *pneuma*, air; *peri*, around; *kardia*, heart). The presence of air in the pericardial sac.

pneumoperitonē·um (G. *pneuma*, air; *peritonaion*, peritoneum). Gas in the peritoneal cavity.

pneumophō·nia (G. *pneuma*, air; *phōnē*, voice). A manner of speaking characterized by breathiness.

pneumopyopericar·dium (G. *pneuma*, air; *puon*, pus; *peri*, around; *kardia*, heart). Air or gas and pus in the pericardium.

pneumopȳothor·ax (G. *pneuma*, air; *puon*, pus; *thōrax*, chest). An accumulation of air and pus in the cavity of the thorax, expecially the pleural cavity.

pneumorrhā·gia (G. *pneumōn*, the lungs; *rhēgnunai*, to burst forth). Pulmonary apoplexy; haemorrhage into the air-cells and tissue of the lung. See also haemoptysis.

pneumothĕ·rapy[1] (G. *pneuma*, air; *therapeia*, treatment). The use of air as a therapeutic agent.

pneumothĕ·rapy[2] (G. *pneumōn*, the lungs; *therapeia*, treatment). The treatment of diseases of the lung.

pneumothō·rax (G. *pneuma*, air; *thōrax*, chest). Gas or air in the pleural cavity. **Artificial p.** is induced in the treatment of tuberculosis. **Spontaneous p.** is seen in disease.

pneumŏ·tomy (G. *pneumōn*, the lungs; *tomē*, a cutting). Incision into the lung.

pneumotym·panum (G. *pneuma*, air; *tumpanon*, drum). The presence of air in the tympanic cavity.

pneumotȳ·phus (G. *pneumōn*, the lungs; *tuphos*, stupor). Pneumonia occurring together with typhoid fever.

pneumoū·ria (G. *pneuma*, air; *ouron*, urine). Pneumaturia, *q.v.*

pneū·sis (G.). Respiration.

pock. A pustule seen in eruptive diseases, especially smallpox; the scar left by such a pustule.

pocket. A sac.

pocketing. The tracking of pus into blind cavities.

pock-marked. Marked with the scars of smallpox.

pŏ·culum (L.). Cup. **P. diogenis:** the hollow of the hand.

podă·gra (G. *pous*, foot; *agra*, seizure). Gout, especially of the feet.

podal·gia (G. *pous*, foot; *algos*, pain). Any pain in the feet.

podal·ic (G. *pous*, foot). Relating to the feet. **P. version:** the manipulation of the foetus *in utero*, in order to bring the feet to the outlet.

podarthri·tis (G. *pous*, foot; *arthron*, joint). Inflammation of all or any of the joints of the feet.

podelcō·ma (G. *pous*, foot; *helkos*, an ulcer). Madura foot, *q.v.*

podencĕ·phalus (G. *pous*, foot; *egkephalos*, brain). A monster with a protrusion of the cranial contents from the top of the head.

podī·atrist (G. *pous*, foot; *iatros*, a physician). One who treats diseases of the foot.

podobromidrō·sis (G. *pous*, foot; *brōmos*, a stench; *hidrōs*, perspiration). Offensive perspiration of the feet.

pododȳ·nia (G. *pous*, foot; *odunē*, pain). Pain in the foot; applied especially to non-inflammatory pain in the heel.

podoedē·ma (G. *pous*, foot; *oidēma*, swelling). Swelling of the foot.

podophyl·lin. The resin of the *Podophyllum peltatum*.

Podophyl·lum (G. *pous*, foot; *phullon*, leaf). The dried rhizome of *P. peltatum*, of the family Berberidaceae. Its resin, podophyllin, contains podophyllotoxin and is used as a laxative and as a cathartic.

pogoni·asis (G. *pōgōn*, beard). 1. Excessive growth of the beard. 2. Growth of the beard in a woman.

pogō·nion (G.). The anterior middle point of the chin.

poi·kiloblast (G. *poikilos*, variegated; *blastos*, germ). A large nucleated erythrocyte of irregular shape and varying in size.

poikilocyte (G. *poikilos*, variegated; *kutos*, a container). An irregularly shaped erythrocyte.

poikilocytō·sis (G. *poikilos*, variegated: *kutos*, a container). A blood condition in which poikilocytes are present; variation in form of the red blood cells.

poikiloder·matomyosī·tis (G. *poikilos*, variegated; *derma*, skin; *mus*, muscle). Poikiloderma associated with myositis.

poi·kiloder·mia (G. *poikilos*, variegated; *derma*, skin). A condition of the skin characterized by atrophy, pigmentation and telangiectasia. **P. atrophicans vascularis** (Jacobi): a condition characterized by multiple small more or less symmetrically arranged atrophic patches, surrounded by telangiectases and darkly pigmented rings.

poikilŏ·nymy (G. *poikilos*, variegated; *onuma*, name). The mingling of names from different terminologies.

poi·kilotherm·ism (G. *poikilos*, variegated; *thermē*, heat). The power possessed by cold-blooded animals of adapting themselves to the temperature of their habitat.

poi·kilothrom·bocyte (G. *poikilos*, variegated; *thrombos*, clot; *kutos*, cell). A blood platelet of abnormal formation.

point. 1. The sharp apex of an object; a minute area. 2. The limit at which an event or condition occurs, e.g., melting-p.

pointillage (Fr.). Use of the finger-tips in massage.

Poirier's gland (Poirier, P., French surgeon, 1853–1907). The lymphatic gland situated on the uterine artery where it crosses the ureter. **P.'s line:** from the nasion to the lambda.

poison. A noxious biological or chemical substance.

Poisson's fossa (Poisson, F., French surgeon, born 1871). The infraduodenal peritoneal recess.

poker back. Spondylitis deformans.

polar (G. *polos*, axis). Relating to or lying near a pole. **P. body:** Polocyte, *q.v.* **P. caps:** accumulation of fibrillar cytoplasm at opposite poles of the nucleus, giving rise to the spindle, in certain forms of mitosis.

polari·meter (G. *polos*, axis; *metron*, measure). An instrument for measuring the degree of rotation of a polarized ray of light.

polari·metry (G. *polos*, axis; *metron*, measure). The use of the polarimeter.

polă·riscope (G. *polos*, axis; *skopein*, to view). Polarimeter, *q.v.*

polar·ity (G. *polos*, axis). 1. Having two poles. 2. Showing opposite effects at two extremities. 3. The property whereby a nerve shows anelectrotonus and catelectrotonus.

polarizā·tion (G. *polos*, axis). 1. The production of vibration of light waves in one plane only. 2. Fall in flow of current due to the slowness of one or more of the processes occurring at the electrode during the discharge or the formation of an ion.

pō·larizer (G. *polos*, axis). An instrument or apparatus for the polarization of light.

pole. 1. The extremity of any axis. 2. Either of two points which have opposite physical qualities, electrical or other.

pollen. Mass of spores which are the male germ cells of plants.

polio-encephali·tis (G. *polios*, grey; *egkephalos*, brain). Inflammation of the grey matter of the brain. **P. haemorrhagica superior:** a condition, usually associated with either pregnancy or chronic alcoholism, characterized by endarteritis of the vessels of the periventricular and aquaeductus Sylvii areas and of the corpora mammillaria, leading to necroses and glial proliferation in the diencephalon, metencephalon and medulla oblongata, producing ophthalmoplegia, nystagmus, ataxia, tremor, dysarthria, optic neuritis, disorders of consciousness, delirium, hallucinations. Syn. Wernicke's disease.

poliomyelencephali·tis (G. *polios*, grey; *muelos*, marrow; *egkephalos*, brain). Combined poliomyelitis and polio-encephalitis.

poliomyeli·tis (G. *polios*, grey; *muelos*, marrow). Inflammation of the grey matter of the spinal cord. **Acute anterior p.**: infantile paralysis, severe inflammation of the anterior horns of the spinal cord grey matter; most usually seen in children and young persons. Caused by a transmissible virus.

poliomyelo-encephali·tis (G. *polios*, grey; *muelos*, marrow; *egkephalos*, brain). Inflammation of the grey matter of the spinal cord and brain, which occurs in infantile paralysis.

polioplasm (G. *polios*, grey; *plasma*, something formed). The granular protoplasm of a cell.

poliō·sis (G. *polios*, grey). Early greying of the hair.

Politzer's bag (Politzer, A., Austrian otologist, 1835–1920). A pear-shaped rubber bag for inflating the pharyngotympanic tube. **P.'s cone of light**: the 'luminous triangle' on the membrana tympani. **P.'s method**: inflation of the pharyngotympanic tube and tympanum by forcing air into the nasal cavity at the instant the patient swallows.

pŏlitzerizā·tion. Inflation of the middle ear by means of Politzer's bag, *q.v.*

poll. The posterior portion of the head.

pol·lex (L.). The thumb. **P. pedis**: the big toe.

pollinō·sis (L. *pollen*, fine dust). Hay fever.

pollū·tion (L. *polluere*, to pollute). 1. The act of rendering impure. 2. The producing of a sexual orgasm by a stimulus other than coitus. **Nocturnal p.**: a nocturnal involuntary discharge of semen. **Self-p.**: masturbation.

pŏ·locyte (G. *polos*, axis; *kutos*, a container). Each of the two small cells formed after mitotic division of the primary oocyte and situated near the upper pole of the oocyte.

polō·nium. A rare radio-active metal discovered by M. and Mme. Curie in 1898 in pitchblende.

Polya's operation (Polya, E., contemporary Hungarian surgeon). An operation for peptic ulcer or gastric carcinoma. Subtotal gastrectomy and excision of the first part of the duodenum is performed; the stump of the stomach is then anastomosed to a loop of the first part of the jejunum posterior to the transverse colon.

polyāe·mia (G. *polus*, many; *haima*, blood). Abnormal increase in the total volume of blood; plethora.

polyalgē·sia (G. *polus*, many; *algēsis*, sense of pain). A condition in which the patient feels a single pinprick in several places.

polyăn·drous (G. *polus*, many; *anēr*, man). Having more than one husband.

polyar·thric (G. *polus*, many; *arthron*, joint). Relating to several joints.

polyarthrī·tis (G. *polus*, many; *arthron*, joint). Inflammation of many joints.

polyartī·cular (G. *polus*, many; L. *articulus*, dim. of *artus*, joint). Affecting a number of joints. (The term **multi-articular** is to be preferred.)

polyatom·ic (G. *polus*, many; *a*, neg.; *temnein*, to cut). Containing a number of atoms.

polyaxon. A nerve cell with four or more axons.

polyaxon·ic (G. *polus*, many; *axōn*, axle). Relating to a polyaxon.

polybā·sic (G. *polus*, many; *basis*, base). Any acidic substance which has more than two hydrogen atoms replaceable by bases to form salts.

polychēı·ria (G. *polus*, many ; *kheir*, hand). Having a supernumerary hand.

polychromat·ic (G. *polus*, many; *khrōma*, colour). Many-coloured.

polychromatophil·ic (G. *polus*, many; *khrōma*, colour; *philein*, to love). Capable of being stained with more than one dye.

polychrō·mia (G. *polus*, many; *khrōma*, colour). Abnormal formation of pigment.

polycō·ria (G. *polus*, many; *korē*, pupil). The presence of more than one pupil in the iris.

polycrot·ic (G. *polus*, many; *krotos*, a beat). Having several secondary waves to each pulse.

polycȳē·sia, polycȳē·sis (G. *polus*, many; *kuēsis*, conception). Multiple pregnancy.

polycys·tic (G. *polus*, many; *kustis*, bladder). Composed of or containing many cysts.

polycythāe·mia (G. *polus*, many; *kutos*, a container; *haima*, blood). A state of the blood characterized by an excess of (generally red) blood cells. **P. vera**: a blood disease characterized by the presence of an excess of red blood cells.

polydac·tylism (G. *polus*, many; *daktulos*, finger). The presence of more than the normal number of fingers or toes.

polydip·sia (G. *polus*, many; *dipsa*, thirst). Abnormal thirst.

polydon·tia (G. *polus*, many; *odous*, tooth). The presence of more than the normal number of teeth.

polygalac·tia (G. *polus*, many; *gala*, milk). Abnormally increased secretion of milk.

polygă·stria (G. *polus*, many; *gastēr*, stomach). Abnormally increased secretion of gastric juices.

polygē·nesis (G. *polus*, many; *gennan*, to produce). The production of many offspring.

polyglō·bulism (G. *polus*, many; L. *globus*, globe). Polycythaemia, *q.v.*

polygnā·thus (G. *polus*, many; *gnathos*, jaw). A double monster joined at the jaws.

pŏ·lygraph (G. *polus*, many; *graphein*, to record). An instrument for recording, on the same surface, simultaneous tracings of more than one of the arterial pulse, the jugular pulse, the apex beat, and respiratory movements.

polygȳ·ria (G. *polus*, many; *guros*, a ring). The presence of an abnormally large number of convolutions in the brain.

polyhāe·mia. Polyaemia, *q.v.*

polyhē·dral (G. *polus*, many; *hedra*, seat). Many-faceted.

polyhidrō·sis (G. *polus*, many; *hidrōs*, sweat). Excessive sweating.

polyhydram·nios (G. *polus*, many; *hudōr*, water; *amnion*, membrane round the foetus). The presence of abnormally large quantities of liquor amnii.

polymă·stia, polymazia (G. *polus*, many; *mastos* or *mazos*, breast). A condition in which supernumerary breasts are present.

polymē·lia (G. *polus*, many; *melos*, limb). A deformity characterized by the presence of more than the usual number of limbs.

polȳ·melus (G. *polus*, many; *melos*, limb). A monster with supernumerary limbs.

polymenorrh·oea (G. *polus*, many; *mēn*, month; *rhoia*, flow). Too frequent menstruation.

pŏ·lymer (G. *polus*, many; *meros*, part). A polymeric substance.

polymē·ria (G. *polus*, many; *meros*, part). 1. The presence of extra parts of the body. 2. In chemistry, a chain of atoms.

polymer·ic (G. *polus*, many; *meros*, part). 1. Showing polymerism. 2. Deriving from or relating to a number of pigments.

poly·merism (G. *polus*, many; *meros*, part). 1. Having more than the normal number of parts. 2. A form of isomerism in which the compounds are termed polymers, and have molecular weights, which are multiples of each other.

polymyx·in. An antibiotic isolated from *Bacillus polymyxa*, active against gram-negative organisms.

Polymnia. A genus of composite-flowered plants. *P. ovedalia*, leafcup or bearsfoot, is anthelminthic, alterative, and anti-spasmodic.

po·lymorph (G. *polus*, many; *morphē*, form). A polymorphonuclear leucocyte.

polymor·phic (G. *polus*, many; *morphē*, form). Having several forms.

polymor·phism (G. *polus*, many; *morphē*, form). The condition of being polymorphic.

polymor·phocyte. Myelocyte, *q.v.*

polymorphonū·clear (G. *polus*, many; *morphē*, form; L. *nucleus*, kernel). 1. Having nuclei of many forms. 2. A polymorphonuclear leucocyte.

polymor·phous. Polymorphic, *q.v.*

po·lymyal·gia (G. *polus*, many; *mus*, muscle; *algos*, pain). Myalgia present in a number of muscles.

polymyē·rial. A type of arrangement of the muscular system in the Nematoda. The inside cells or plates are numerous, irregular and penetrate into the parenchyma.

polyneuri·tis (G. *polus*, many; *neuron*, nerve). Multiple neuritis.

polynū·clear (G. *polus*, many; L. *nucleus*, kernel). Multinuclear.

polynū·cleate (G. *polus*, many; *nucleus*, kernel). Polynuclear, *q.v.*

polyodon·tia (G. *polus*, many; *odous*, tooth). The presence of more than the normal number of teeth.

polyony·chia (G. *polus*, many; *onux*, nail). The presence of more than the normal number of nails.

polyor·chidism (G. *polus*, many; *orkhis*, testes). The occurrence of one or more supernumerary testes.

polyor·chis (G. *polus*, many; *orkhis*, testes). A person with three or more testicles.

polyō·tia (G. *polus*, many; *ous*, ear). The presence of more than one auricle on one or both sides of the head.

po·lyp, po·lypus (G. *polus*, many; *pous*, foot). A tumour with a pedicle, usually occurring on mucous membranes. (The derivation implies many pedicles, but the term has come to be used of a tumour with one pedicle.)

polypep·tide (G. *polus*, many; *peptein*, to digest). A compound composed of amino-acids joined together through the peptide link -CO-NH-.

polyphā·gia (G. *polus*, many; *phagein*, to eat). Bulimia.

polyphalan·gism (G. *polus*, many; *phalagx*, the bone between two joints of the fingers and toes). The presence of supernumerary phalanges in a finger or toe.

polyphase (G. *polus*, many; *phasis*, appearance). Having several phases. Containing colloids of several types.

polyphrā·sia (G. *polus*, many; *phrasis*, speech). A morbid condition characterized by excessive loquacity; verbigeration.

polypi·ferous (G. *polus*, many; *pous*, foot; L. *ferre*, to bear). Having or producing polyps.

polyplas·mia (G. *polus*, many; *plasma*, anything formed). Abnormal amount of plasma in the blood.

po·lyplast (G. *polus*, many; *plassein*, to form). 1. Composed of a number of different structures. 2. Having passed through many modifications in the course of development.

polyplas·tic (G. *polus*, many; *plassein*, to form). 1. Cells formed of many substances. 2. Passing through many modifications in the course of development.

Polyplax. A sucking louse of rats and mice.

polyploi·dy (G. *polus*, many; *plekein*, to plait; *eidos*, shape). A variation in chromosomal number in which exact multiples of the typical chromosome numbers are present.

polypnoe·a (G. *polus*, many; *pnoia*, breath). Very quick breathing; panting.

polypō·dia (G. *polus*, many; *pous*, foot). The presence of more than the normal number of feet.

po·lypoid (G. *polus*, many; *pous*, foot; *eidos*, form). Resembling a polyp.

Polyporus. A genus of mushrooms or fungi with many species.

polypō·sis (G. *polus*, many; *posis*, a drink). Abnormal thirst; polydipsia.

polypō·sis (G. *polus*, many; *pous*, foot). Affected with polyps.

poly·potome (G. *polus*, many; *pous*, foot; *tomē*, section). A surgical instrument for the cutting away of polyps.

poly·potrite (G. *polus*, many; *pous*, foot; L. *terere*, to crush). A surgical instrument for the crushing of polyps.

polypty·chial (G. *polus*, many; *ptux*, a layer). Arranged in several layers.

polysă·ccharides. A group of carbohydrates which contain more than three molecules of simple carbohydrates combined with each other. They comprise the dextrins, starches and glycogen; also cellulose, gums, insulin and pectose.

polysar·cia (G. *polus*, many; *sarx*, flesh). Obesity.

polysar·cous (G. *polus*, many; *sarx*, flesh). Corpulent.

polyscē·lia (G. *polus*, many; *skelos*, leg). The presence of supernumerary legs.

polyserosī·tis (G. *polus*, many; L. *serum*, the watery part of anything). Inflammation of the pleura, pericardium and peritoneum.

polysinusī·tis (G. *polus*, many; L. *sinus*, a fold). Inflammation of several sinuses conjointly.

polysō·mia (G. *polus*, many; *sōma*, body). A monstrous condition with more than one body.

polysō·mus (G. *polus*, many; *sōma*, body). A monster with one head and two or more bodies.

polysper·mia, **polysper·mism** (G. *polus*, many; *sperma*, seed). Excessive secretion of seminal fluid.

polysper·my (G. *polus*, many; *sperma*, seed). Fertilization of an ovum by more than one spermatozoon.

polysti·chia (G. *polus*, many; *stikhos*, a row). A condition characterized by the appearance of two or more rows of eyelashes on a single eyelid.

po·lytendinī·tis (G. *polus*, many; L. *tendo*, tendon). Inflammation of a number of tendons conjointly.

polythē·lia (G. *polus*, many; *thēlē*, nipple). The presence of more than the usual number of nipples.

poly·tocous (G. *polus*, many; *tokos*, birth). Multiple birth.

polytri·chia, **polytrichō·sis** (G. *polus*, many; *thrix*, hair). Excessive growth of hair.

Poly·trichum (G. *polus*, many; *thrix*, hair). A genus of moss. The *P. juniperinum* yields a diuretic.

polytrō·phia (G. *polus*, many; *trephein*, to nourish). Over-abundant nutrition.

polyū·ria (G. *polus*, many; *ouron*, urine). The passing of an excessive amount of urine.

poly·valent (G. *polus*, many; L. *valēre*, to be worth). Having the power of combining with more than two univalent atoms.

pomade (Fr. *pommade*, from L. *pomum*, apple). A perfumed scalp ointment.

pomā·tum. Pomade.

pom·egrănate (L. *pomum granatum*, grained apple). The fruit of the tree *Punica granatum*.

pom·pholyx (G. *pompholux*, bubble). Any skin disease exhibiting bullae.

pom·phus (G. *pomphos*, a blister). A wheal.

pō·mum (L.). Apple. **P. Adami:** Adam's apple, the prominence in the front of the throat due to the thyroid cartilage.

ponceau B. Biebrich scarlet.

Pond's extract. A fluid extract of *Hamamelis virginiana*.

pon·derable (L. *pondus*, weight). Possessing weight.

Ponfick's shadows (Ponfick, E., German pathologist, 1844–1913). Unpigmented red cells exhibited in the blood in cases of haemoglobinaemia.

pons (L. bridge). 1. Process of tissue joining two sections of an organ. 2. The **P. Varolii,** the eminence at the base of the brain which connects the various divisions.

ponti·cular (L. *pons*, bridge). Relating to the ponticulus.

ponti·culus (L. dim. of *pons*, bridge). A small pons; the propons, a small transverse ridge between the pyramids of the oblongata and the pons.

pon·tile, pon·tine (L. *pons*, bridge). Relating to the pons Varolii.

Pontocaine hydrochloride. Proprietary name for local anaesthetic with actions similar to procaine hydrochloride. Formula: $C_4H_6.NH.C_8H_4.COO.C_2H_4.N(CH_3)_2$, HCl. Syn. Pantocaine. Use: surface anaesthesia of eye, nose and throat and spine.

poplar (L. *pŏpŭlus*). A tree of the genus Populus.

pop·lĕs (L.). The back of the knee.

poplitae·us (L. *poples*, the ham). A muscle at the back of the knee joint.

popli·teal (L. *poples*, the ham). Relating to or situated on the ham, as p. artery, p. nerve, p. space.

poppy. The *Papaver somniferum* plant, from the capsules of which opium is obtained.

Populus. A genus of trees which includes poplars and aspens. The bark of some varieties is tonic, and the leaf buds of *P. balsamifera* yields balm of Gilead.

porcelain. A fused mixture of kaolin, felspar, quartz, and other substances.

porcine (L. *porcus*, pig). Pertaining to or characteristic of swine.

porcupine disease (L. *porcus*, swine; *spina*, spine). Ichthyosis.

pore (G. *poros*). A minute orifice on a surface, as in the skin.

porencephā·lia, porencĕ·phalus (G. *poros*, pore; *egkephalos*, brain). A condition characterized by the presence of cysts or cavities in the cerebral cortex and due either to congenital arrest of development or to an acquired defect.

porencephal·ic, porencĕ·phalous (G. *poros*, pore; *egkephalos*, brain). Affected with porencephalia.

porencĕ·phaly. Porencephalia, *q.v.*

pork. The flesh of the pig.

pornŏ·graphy (G. *pornē*, prostitute; *graphein*, to write). Lewd writing.

Porocephalus. A genus of wormlike arthropods of the order Linguatulida which are parasitic in man and animals.

porokeratō·sis (G. *poros*, pore; *keras*, a horn). A variety of hyperkeratosis, usually affecting the dorsal aspect of the hands and feet, the extensor aspect of the forearms and legs, and the neck, face and scalp.

porŏ·ma (G. *pŏrōma*, callus). A callosity.

poro·scopy (G. *poros*, pore; *skopein*, to inspect). Inspection of the sweat-glands.

pŏrŏ·sis[1] (G. *pŏrōma*, callus). Callus formation.

pŏrŏ·sis[2] (G. *poros*, pore). A porous condition.

porŏ·sity (G. *poros*, pore). The state of being porous.

porous (G. *poros*, pore). Having pores.

por·phin. The fundamental ring structure of four linked pyrrole nuclei around which porphyrins, haemin and chlorophyll are built.

z

por·phyrin (G. *porphura*, purple dye). Any one of **a** group of iron- or magnesium-free pyrrole derivatives which occur universally in protoplasm. They form the basis of the respiratory pigments of animals and plants, e.g., proto-, haemato-, actio-, copro-, uro-porphyrin.

porphy̆·reus (G. *porphura*, purple dye). In biology, showing purple spots on a ground of a different colour.

por·phyrināe·mia (G. *porphura*, purple dye; *haima*, blood). A condition in which the blood contains porphyrin.

porphyrinū·ria (G. *porphura*, purple dye; *ouron*, urine). The passing of urine containing an excess of porphyrin.

porri·go (L.). Ringworm and other scalp diseases.

por·ta (L. gate). The hilum of an organ through which vessels pass.

portal. Relating to the porta or hilum of an organ; applied especially to the porta hepatis or to the p. vein which passes through the porta hepatis.

Portal's muscle (Portal, Baron A., French anatomist, 1742–1832). The capsularis subbrachialis muscle. The fibres of the brachialis muscle inserted to the anterior part of the capsule of the elbow joint.

porte-aiguille (Fr.). A holder for surgical needles.

Porter's fascia (Porter, W. H., Irish physician, 1790–1861). The pretracheal fascia. **P.'s symptom:** tracheal tugging.

por·tio (L. a part). 1. A portion. 2. An abbreviation for p. vaginalis uteri.

port-wine mark or stain. Naevus flammeus.

porus (G. *poros*, pore). 1. A pore, or opening. 2. A callosity. **P. acusticus externus:** the opening of the external ear. **P. acusticus internus:** the internal auditory foramen. **P. opticus:** the optic disc. **P. sudoriferus:** opening of a sweat gland.

position (L. *positio*). Place; attitude; posture. **Fowler's:** head of patient's bed raised 18″–20″, patient sitting with pillow under knees. **Genupectoral:** knee-chest; the patient resting on knees and chest. **Left lateral recumbent:** the patient on left side with right thigh and knee drawn up. **Lithotomy:** the patient on back, legs flexed on thighs, thighs flexed on belly and abducted. **Occipito-anterior:** with the occiput directed anteriorly (said of the foetus in labour). **Occipito-posterior:** with the occiput directed dorsally (said of the foetus in labour). **Sim's:** patient on left side and chest, right knee and thigh drawn up, the left arm along the back.

positive (L.L. *positivus*, from *pōnere*, to place). Actual; existing.

pŏ·sitron. Positive electron; a particle having the mass of the electron but a positive charge.

posolŏ·gical (G. *posos*, how much; *logos*, treatise). Relating to posology.

posŏ·logy (G. *posos*, how much; *logos*, treatise). The science of the dosage of medicines.

postax·ial (L. *post*, after; *axis*, axis). Situated posterior to the embryonic axis of a limb.

postcen·tral (L. *post*, after; *centrum*, centre). 1. Behind a centre. 2. Behind the central fissure of the brain, the fissure of Rolando.

postcerebel·lar (L. *post*, after; *cerebellum*, a small brain). Situated in the posterior part of the cerebellum.

postcĕ·rebral (L. *post*, after; *cerebrum*, the brain). Situated in the posterior part of the cerebrum.

postci·bal (L. *post*, after; *cibus*, food). Occurring after eating.

postcister·na (L. *post*, after; *cisterna*, cistern). The cisterna magna.

postclavĭ·cular (L. *post*, after; *clavicula*, dim. of *clavis*, key). Behind the clavicle.

postclimacter·ic (L. *post*, after; G. *klimax*, ladder). Occurring after the menopause.

postcom·missure (L. *post*, after; *cum*, together; *mittere*, to send). The posterior commissure of the brain.

postcon·dylar (L. *post*, after; G. *kondulos*, knuckle). Situated behind a condyle.

postconnū·bial (L. *post*, after; *connubium*, marriage). Occurring after marriage.

postconvul·sive (L. *post*, after; *convulsio*, cramp). Occurring after a convulsion.

postcor·nu (L. *post*, after; *cornu*, horn). The posterior horn of the lateral ventricle.

postcri·brum (L. *post*, after; *cribrum*, a sieve). The posterior perforated space of the brain.

postdiastol·ic (L. *post*, after; G. *diastole*). Following the diastole.

postdicrot·ic (L. *post*, after; G. *dis*, twice; *krotos*, a beat). Occurring after the dicrotic wave of the pulse.

postdiges·tive (L. *post*, after; *digerere*, to digest). Happening after digestion.

postdiphtherit·ic (L. *post*, after; G. *diphthera*, leather). Happening after diphtheria, as p. paralysis.

postdū·ral (L. *post*, after; *durus*, hard). Situated behind the dura mater.

postembryŏn·ic (L. *post*, after; G. *embruon*, embryo). Happening after the embryonic stage has been passed.

postencephali·tis (L. *post*, after; G. *egkephalos*, brain). The condition which sometimes remains after recovery from epidemic encephalitis marked by troublesome freakish behaviour.

post-epilep·tic (L. *post*, after; G. *epilēpsia*, epilepsy). Occurring after an attack of epilepsy.

poste·rior (L. *posterior*, comp. of *posterus*, following). Placed behind or towards the dorsal aspect. **P. chamber:** the area between the iris and the lens.

postĕ·rula (L. *posterus*, following). A small space posterior to the turbinal bones of the nose.

posteth·moid (L. *post*, after; G. *ethmos*, sieve; *eidos*, form). Posterior to the ethmoid bone.

postex·ion. Backwards flexion.

postfeb·rile (L. *post*, after; *febris*, fever). After a fever.

postgangliŏn·ic (L. *post*, after; G. *gagglion*, tumour under the skin). Behind a ganglion.

postgĕ·minum (L. *post*, after; *geminus*, twin). Posterior corpora quadrigemina.

postglē·noid (L. *post*, after; G. *glēnē*, a cavity; *eidos*, form). Situated posterior to the glenoid fossa.

postgră·cile (L. *post*, after; *gracilis*, delicate). Posterior to the slender lobe of the cerebellum.

postgră·duate (L. *post*, after; *gradus*, a step). After graduating.

post-haē·morrhage (L. *post*, after; G. *haima*, blood; *rhegnunai*, to burst forth). An attack of haemorrhage succeeding another.

post-hemiplē·gic (L. *post*, after; G. *hemi*, half; *plēgē*, a stroke). Following an attack of hemiplegia.

posthepat·ic (L. *post*, after; G. *hēpar*, liver). Situated behind the liver.

posthe·tomy (G. *posthē*, prepuce; *tomē*, a cutting). Circumcision.

posthī·tis (G. *posthē*, prepuce). Inflammation of the prepuce.

pŏ·sthumous (L. *postumus*, coming after). After death. **P. child:** one born after the death of its father, or removed by Caesarean section from the dead body of its mother.

posthȳ·oid (L. *post*, after; G. *huoides*, like the letter y). Situated posterior to the hyoid bone.

posthypnot·ic (L. *post*, after; G. *hupnos*, sleep). Following hypnotism.

posthypŏ·physis (L. *post*, after; G. *hupophusis*, growth under). The posterior section of the pituitary body.

pos·ticus (L.). Posterior.

postis·chial (L. *post*, after; G. *iskhion*, hip). Situated posterior to the ischium.

postmala·rial (L. *post*, after; It. *malaria*, bad air). Succeeding an attack of malaria.

postmas·toid (L. *post*, after; G. *mastos*, breast; *eidos*, form). Situated posterior to the mastoid process.

postmē·dian (L. *post*, after; *medius*, middle). Posterior to the middle transverse line of the body.

postmediasti·nal (L. *post*, after; *in medio stare*, to stand in the centre). Situated behind the mediastinum.

postmeiŏ·tic. At the stage following the reduction of the chromosomes in the meiotic cycle.

postmenopau·sal (L. *post*, after; G. *mēn*, month; *pauein*, to stop). After the menopause.

postmesentĕ·ric (L. *post*, after; *mesos*, middle; *enteron*, intestine). Situated posterior to the mesentery.

post mortem (L.). 1. After death. 2. An examination of the dead body; a necropsy.

postnā·sal (L. *post*, after; *nasus*, nose). Behind the nose. **P. catarrh:** catarrh of the nasopharynx.

postnā·tal (L. *post*, after; *natus*, born). After birth has taken place.

postnŏ·dular (L. *post*, after; *nodulus*, dim. of *nodus*, node). Situated behind the nodulus.

postŏ·cular (L. *post*, after; *oculus*, eye). Behind the eye.

post-operative (L. *post*, after; *operatio*, from *operari*, to perform). After an operation, e.g., p.-o. insanity.

postoesophă·geal (L. *post*, after; G. *oisophagos*, gullet). Situated posterior to the oesophagus.

postparalyt·ic (L. *post*, after; G. *paralusis*, paralysis). Occurring after an attack of paralysis.

post-partum (L. after parturition). Occurring after delivery of the infant; e.g., p.-p. haemorrhage.

postpon·tile (L. *post*, after; *pons*, bridge). Behind the pons Varolii.

post-pran·dial (L. *post*, after; *prandium*, dinner). After a meal.

postrolan·dic (L. *post*, after; Rolando, L., Italian anatomist, 1773–1831). Behind the fissure of Rolando.

postsā·cral (L. *post*, after; *sacer*, sacred). Behind the sacrum.

postscalē·nus (L. *post*, after; G. *scalēnos*, unequal). The posterior scalenus muscle.

postscap·ular (L. *post*, after; *scapula*, shoulder blade). Behind the scapula.

postscapulā·ris (L. *post*, after; *scapula*, shoulder blade). The infraspinatus muscle.

postscarlat·inal (L. *post*, after; It. *scarlatto*, scarlet). Following and resulting from scarlet fever.

pŏ·stulate (L. *postulare*, to demand). A well-known law; a basic assumption.

pŏ·stural (L. *positura*, position). Relating to posture or position; carried out by using a special posture, as p. treatment. **P. reflexes:** a group of reflexes serving to maintain posture or attitude.

pŏ·sture (L. *positura*, position). Position. **P. sense:** the power of perceiving, without seeing, the position in which a limb has been placed.

postū·terine (L. *post*, after; *uterus*, womb). Behind the uterus.

postvac·cinal (L. *post*, after; *vacca*, a cow). Following and resulting from vaccination.

postver·mis (L. *post*, after; *vermis*, worm). The inferior vermis of the cerebellum.

Pot. Abbreviation for potash.

pŏ·table (L. *pōtare*, to drink). Fit to drink.

Potain's apparatus (Potain, P. C. E., French physician, 1825–1901). An apparatus used for aspirating air or fluid from, or injecting air into the pleural cavity.

potash. 1. Potassium hydroxide; caustic potash. 2. Potassium carbonate.

potas·sa. Potash.

potas·sium (Latinisation of potash). An element belonging to the alkali group. Symbol K (from L. *kalium*). Sp. gr. 0·865. Atomic weight 39·096.

pō·tency (L. *potens*, powerful). 1. Power; efficiency. 2. In homoeopathy, the extent of the dilution of a drug.

potentia coeundi (L.). Ability to cohabit sexually.

poten·tial (L. *potens*, able). Capacity for action, but not yet performing an act. In electricity, electric tension or pressure as measured by the capacity of producing electric effects in bodies of a different state of electrification. When bodies of different potentials are put in communication an electric current passes between them. If they are of the same potential no current passes.

potentiŏ·meter (L. *potens*, powerful; G. *metron*, measure). An apparatus for measuring voltage.

potion (L. *potio*, draught). A drink.

potomā·nia (L. *pōtare*, to drink; G. *mania*, madness). Delirium tremens.

Pott's aneurysm (Pott, P., English surgeon, 1713–88). Aneurysmal varix. **P.'s boss:** in tuberculous disease of the spine the spinous processes in the region of the disease are prominent. **P.'s curvature:** the gibbus produced in tuberculous disease of the spine. **P.'s disease:** tuberculous disease of the spine. **P.'s fracture:** fracture of the lower quarter of the fibula. **P.'s gangrene:** senile gangrene. **P.'s paralysis:** paraplegia due to tuberculous disease of the spine. **P.'s puffy tumour:** swelling produced by osteomyelitis of the skull.

pouch (Old Fr. *poche*, bag). A sac. **P. of Douglas:** the recto-uterine pouch of peritoneum in the pelvis. **P., perineal:** a pouch containing the crura penis, the bulb of the penis, superficial perineal muscles, nerves and vessels. **P. of Prussak:** the inferior pouch of the outer attic of the tympanum. **P., Rathke's:** a diverticulum of buccal ectoderm which passes upwards towards the sella turcica of the sphenoid bone. **P., rectovesical:** is formed by a reflection of peritoneum passing from the rectum to the upper part of the base of the bladder. **P. of Tröltsch:** two in number. Anterior and posterior recesses in the attic of the tympanum. They are produced by folds of mucous membrane. **P., recto-uterine:** see p. of Douglas. **P., vesico-uterine:** a small recess in front of the uterus caused by a folding of the pelvic peritoneum.

poultice. Any soft and moist pultaceous mass applied hot to the surface of a part for the purpose of supplying heat and moisture.

powder. An aggregation of small particles obtained by the grinding or trituration of a solid drug.

Pozzi's muscle (Pozzi, S. J., French gynaecologist, 1846–1918). The extensor brevis digitorum manus or layer of deep extensors of the fingers. **P.'s syndrome:** low backache associated with uterine discharge and no uterine enlargement; present in some cases of endometritis.

p.p. factor. Pellagra-preventing factor, pellagra, *q.v.*

Poulet's disease (Poulet, A., French physician, 1848–88). Osteoperiostitis of rheumatic origin.

pound (L. *pondus*, weight). A measure of weight. The Troy pound contains 12 oz. or 5,760 grains and the avoirdupois pound 16 oz. or 7,000 grains. Symbol lb. (from L. *libra*, pound).

Poupart's ligament (Poupart, F., French anatomist, 1616–1708). Ligamentum inguinale. This ligament had been described previously by Falloppius in 1584.

pox. 1. Any disease possessing a vesicular or pustular eruption (pock). 2. Vulgarly applied to syphilis.

P-R interval. The interval from the start of the P-wave, *q.v.*, to the beginning of the Q- or R-wave, *q.v.*

The duration of the spread of excitation from the dicro-auricular node to the ventricle, normally up to 0·2 second.

prac·tise (L. *praticare*, to practise). To perform the work of a physician.

practi·tioner (L. *praticare*, to practise). One who practises medicine.

prae·coid (L. *praecox*, premature, G. *eidos*, form). Like dementia praecox.

praecox (L. premature). Occurring early, as in dementia p.

prae·via (L. *praevius*, going before). Coming before. **P. placenta:** see placenta p.

pragmatism (G. *pragma*, an act). The doctrine that the whole meaning of a conception lies in its practical consequences.

praxis (G.). The doing or performance of an action.

pre-adult (L. *prae*, before; *adultus*, full grown). Before adult life.

pre-ă·gonal (L. *prae*, before; G. *agōnia*, struggle, anguish). Occurring immediately before the death agony.

pre-anaesthē·sia (L. *prae*, before; G. *an*, neg.; *aisthēsis*, feeling). Narcosis induced by the giving of a drug before administration of a general anaesthetic.

pre-aortic (L. *prae*, before; *aorta*). Situated anterior to the aorta.

pre-atax·ic (L. *prae*, before; G. *ataxia*, disorder). Before the setting in of ataxy.

pre-ax·ial (L. *prae*, before; *axis*). Situated in front of the embryonic axis of a limb.

prebrā·chial (L. *prae*, before; G. *brakhiōn*, the arm). Situated on the front of the brachium or upper arm; e.g. the group of p. muscles.

precan·cerous (L. *prae*, before; *cancer*, crab). Before the occurrence of a carcinoma.

precapil·lary (L. *prae*, before; *capillus*, fine hair). A venule or arteriole.

precar·diac (L. *prae*, before; G. *kardia*, heart). In front of the heart.

precā·va (L. *prae*, before; *cavus*, hollow). The vena cava descendens.

precen·tral (L. *prae*, before; *centrum*, centre). In front of the central fissure of the brain.

prechor·dal (L. *prae*, before; G. *khordē*, string). In front of the notochord.

precĭ·pitant (L. *praecipitare*, to throw down). Any agent causing precipitation.

precĭ·pitate (L. *praecipitare*, to throw down). 1. To cause the solid in a solution to settle down. 2. A precipitated deposit. 3. Headlong (as in p. labour).

precipitā·tion (L. *praecipitare*, to throw down). The act of precipitating solids in solution.

precĭ·pitin (L. *praecipitare*, to throw down). An antibody found in the blood of an animal which has been injected with bacterial culture fluids, blood serum, or any other antigenic material. The blood serum of such an animal will produce a precipitate when added to or brought into contact with the antigen which has been used in its production.

precipitin·ogen (L. *praecipitare*, to throw down; G. *gennan*, to produce). Any substance capable, on injection, of producing a specific precipitin.

precō·cious (L. *praecox*, premature). Premature development; a physical or mental state that is normal except for its early onset.

precom·missure (L. *prae*, before; *cum*, together); *mittere*, to send). The anterior horn of the lateral ventricle.

precon·scious (L. *prae*, before; *conscius*, aware). Pychoanalytical term describing mental processes of which the individual is unaware but which he can recall more or less readily, as opposed to 'unconscious' processes which he cannot recall.

preconvul·sive (L. *prae*, before; *convellere*, to convulse). Before a convulsion; usually applied to the stage of epilepsy immediately preceding a seizure.

precor·dia (L. *prae*, before; *cor*, the heart). The section of the chest overlying the heart.

precor·dial (L. *prae*, before; *cor*, the heart). Relating to the precordia.

precor·dium (L. *prae*, before; *cor*, heart). The region over the heart and stomach; the epigastrium and lower part of the thorax.

precor·nu (L. *prae*, before; *cornu*, horn). The anterior horn of the lateral ventricle of the brain.

precŏ·stal (L. *prae*, before; *costa*, rib). Situated in front of the ribs.

precrā·nial (L. *prae*, before; G. *kranion*, skull). Situated in the fore part of the cranium.

precrib·rum (L. *prae*, before; *cribrum*, sieve). The anterior perforated space of the brain.

precū·neal (L. *prae*, before; *cuneus*, wedge). Situated anterior to the cuneus.

precū·neus (L. *prae*, before; *cuneus*, wedge). The quadrate lobule of the cerebellum situated anterior to the cuneus of the occipital lobe.

predias·tolĕ (L. *prae*, before; G. *diastolē*, dilatation). The hiatus in the cardiac rhythm immediately preceding the diastole.

prediastŏ·lic (L. *prae*, before; G. *diastolē*, dilatation). Before the diastole.

predicrot·ic (L. *prae*, before; G. *dikrotos*, double-beating). Preceding the dicrotic wave of the sphygmographic tracing.

predigĕ·sted (L. *prae*, before; *digerere*, to digest). Food partially digested by artificial means before it is consumed.

predigĕs·tion (L. *prae*, before; *digerere*, to digest). The partial artificial digestion of food before it is eaten.

predispŏ·sing (L. *prae*, before; *disponere*, to dispose). Rendering susceptible to disease.

predisposi·tion (L. *prae*, before; *disponere*, to dispose). The condition of being susceptible to disease.

pre-eclamp·sia (L. *prae*, before; G. *eklampein*, to flash forth). The syndrome of nausea, vomiting, headache, dyspnoea, and albuminuria, which precedes the onset of true eclampsia.

pre-epiglot·tic (L. *prae*, before; G. *epi*, on; *glottis*, mouth of windpipe). Situated in front of the epiglottis.

pre-erup·tive (L. *prae*, before; *erumpere*, to burst forth). The stage in any disease characterized by eruptions prior to the appearance of the rash.

prefron·tal (L. *prae*, before; *frons*, forehead). 1. Lying in the anterior part of the frontal lobe of the brain. 2. The middle part of the ethmoid bone. **P. leucotomy**: division of the nerve fibres in the frontal lobe of the brain in cases of schizophrenia.

preganglion·ic (L. *prae*, before; G. *gagglion*, tumour under the skin). Situated in front of a ganglion.

preg·nancy (L. *praegnans*, pregnant). The condition of the woman during the period between conception and the birth of the child. **P. cells**: modified eosinophilic cells of the pituitary gland, found during and after pregnancy.

preg·nant (L. *praegnans*, pregnant). With child; carrying an infant.

Preg·nyl. A proprietary brand of gonadotrophic hormone.

prehemiplē·gic (L. *prae*, before; G. *hemi*, half; *plēgē*, a stroke). Happening before the onset of a hemiplegia, as p. chorea.

prehen·sile (L. *prehendere*, to grasp). Capable of grasping.

prehen·sion (L. *prehendere*, to grasp). The act of grasping.

prehȳ·oid (L. *prae*, before; G. *huoeides*, like the letter upsilon). Situated in front of the hyoid bone.

prehypŏ·physis (L. *prae*, before; G. *hupo*, under; *phusis*, growth). The anterior lobe of the pituitary body.

prelim·bic (L. *prae*, before; *limbus*, a border). Lying in front of a border.

premalig·nant (L. *prae*, before; *malignus*, evil). A condition in which the tissues are predisposed to malignant change, but in which this change cannot yet be shown.

premanī·acal (L. *prae*, before; G. *mania*, madness). Previous to insanity or to an attack of mania.

prĕ·mature (L. *prae*, before; *maturus*, ripe). Occurring before the due time, e.g., p. labour.

premaxil·la (L. *prae*, before; *maxilla*). The intermaxillary bone.

premax·illary (L. *prae*, before; *maxilla*). Anterior to the maxilla.

premedicā·tion (L. *prae*, before; *medicare*, to heal). The giving of a drug to induce a degree of narcosis before administering a general anaesthetic.

premen·strual (L. *prae*, before; *mensis*, month). Occurring before menstruation.

premō·lar (L. *prae*, before; *mola*, mill). 1. Lying in front of the molar teeth. 2. Either of the two bicuspid teeth. 3. A molar tooth of the deciduous set.

premŏ·nitory (L. *prae*, before; *monēre*, to warn). Forewarning. **P. symptoms**: those which herald the onset of disease.

prenā·tal (L. *prae*, before; *natalis*, from *nasci*, to be born). Before birth.

preneoplā·stic (L. *prae*, before; G. *neos*, new; *plassein*, to form). Before the occurrence of a tumour.

pre-occī·pital (L. *prae*, before; *occiput*). Situated in front of the occipital region.

pre-ŏ·perative (L. *prae*, before; *operari*, to perform). Before an operation, e.g., p. treatment.

pre-oper·culum (L. *prae*, before; *operculum*). The frontal operculum of the brain.

pre-op·tic (L. *prae*, before; G. *optikos*, relating to vision). Situated in front of the optic lobes of the brain.

pre-or·al (L. *prae*, before; *os*, mouth). In front of the mouth.

prepal·atal (L. *prae*, before; *palatum*, palate). In front of the palate.

preparā·tion (L. *praeparare*, to prepare). 1. The act of making ready. 2. Anything prepared; applied especially in anatomy to a part of the body made ready for demonstration, etc. 3. In pharmacy, any mixture compounded from a formula.

prepă·rative (L. *praeparare*, to prepare). An amboceptor, *q.v.*

prepatel·lar (L. *prae*, before; *patella*, kneecap). Lying anteriorly to the patella, as the p. bursa.

preponderance, ventricular. Term used in electrocardiography, when there is disproportionate development between the ventricles of the heart.

pre·puce (L. *praeputium*, prepuce). The foreskin of the penis.

prepū·tial (L. *praeputium*, prepuce). Relating to the prepuce.

prepylor·ic (L. *prae*, before; G. *pulōrus*, pylorus). Anterior to the pylorus.

prepyră·midal (L. *prae*, before; G. *puramis*, pyramid). Situated anteriorly to the pyramid.

prerec·tal (L. *prae*, before; *rectus*, straight). In front of the rectum.

prerĕ·nal (L. *prae*, before; G. *rēn*, kidney). Lying anterior to the kidney.

prerĕ·tinal (L. *prae*, before; *rētē*, net). Situated in front of the retina.

presbiat·rics (G. *presbus*, an old man; *iatros*, physician). Geriatrics; the treatment of diseases occurring in old age.

presbycū·sis, presbykou·sis (G. *presbus*, an old man; *akouein*, to hear). Lessening of the power of hearing, occurring in old age.

pres·byope (G. *presbus*, an old man; *ōps*, eye). One who is affected with presbyopia.

presbyō·pia (G. *presbus*, an old man; *ōps*, eye). Long sight and impairment of vision due to old age. The crystalline lens loses its elasticity and powers of accommodation.

presbysphă·celus (G. *presbus*, an old man; *sphakelos*, gangrene). Senile gangrene.

prescrip·tion (L. *praescriptio*, a preface). A written direction from the physician to the chemist for the preparation of a medicine, giving also the dosage and manner of administration.

presē·nile (L. *prae*, before; *senex*, an old man). Prematurely old.

preseni·lity (L. *prae*, before; *senex*, an old man). Premature old age.

present (L. *praesentare*, to present). Said of the part of the foetus to appear first at the mouth of the uterus.

presentā·tion (L. *praesentare*, to present). In obstetrics, that part of the foetus which the examining finger first encounters presenting at the os uteri.

presphēn·oid (L. *prae*, before; G. *sphēn*, a wedge; *eidos*, form). The front part of the body of the sphenoid bone.

presphyg·mic (L. *prae*, before; G. *sphugmos*, pulsation). Relating to the period preceding the pulsewave.

pressor (L. *premere*, to press). Stimulating. **P. substance:** any substance which causes a rise in the blood pressure.

pressure (L. *pressura*). Force or tension. See also blood pressure.

prester·num (L. *prae*, before; G. *sternon*, the chest). The manubrium.

presyl·vian (L. *prae*, before; Sylvius, F., French anatomist, 1614–72). The ascending branch of the Sylvian fissure.

presys·tolē (L. *prae*, before; G. *sustolē*, contraction). The duration of the heart's pause before the systole.

presystol·ic (L. *prae*, before; G. *sustolē*, contraction; *eidos*, form). Preceding the systole of the heart.

pretar·sal (L. *prae*, before; G. *tarsos*, tarsus). In front of the tarsus.

prethy·roid (L. *prae*, before; G. *thureos*, shield). In front of the thyroid gland.

preti·bial (L. *prae*, before; *tibia*, shin). In front of the tibia.

pretră·cheal (L. *prae*, before; *trachea*). Situated in front of the trachea.

pretuberculō·sis (L. *prae*, before; *tuberculum*, tubercle). Preceding the occurrence of tuberculosis.

pretympan·ic (L. *prae*, before; G. *tumpanon*, drum). In front of the tympanum.

preven·tive (L. *praevenire*, to prevent). Warding off; inhibiting. **P. medicine:** that branch of medicine which deals with the prevention of disease.

prever·tebral (L. *prae*, before; *vertebra*). Situated anterior to the vertebrae.

pri·apism (G. Priapos, the god of gardens and fructification). Persistent and abnormal erection of the penis, usually without sexual desire. It is seen in diseases and injuries of the spinal cord and may be caused by vesical calculus or certain injuries of the penis.

Prichard's reticulated membrane (Prichard, U., English aural surgeon, 1845–1925). The intercellular membrane in the ampulla of the semicircular canals.

prickle-cell. A polygonal cell possessing delicate protoplasmic fibres continuous with the spongioplastic network of the cell. **P.-c. layer:** the lowest stratum of the epidermis.

prickly heat. Miliaria papillosa.

primae viae (L. first ways). The alimentary canal.

pri·mary (L. *primarius*, principal). First in order or importance. **P. colours:** red, green and blue, from combinations of which all other colours of the spectrum, as well as white, black and grey, can be obtained. **P. lesion:** the original lesion from which secondary lesions develop. **P. sore:** the initial chancre of syphilis.

Primā·tes (L. *primus*, first). The highest order of mammals, which includes man.

primigrā·vida (L. *primus*, first; *gravidus*, loaded). A woman in her first pregnancy.

primi·para (L. *primus*, first; *parere*, to bear). A woman who has borne her first child.

primipă·rity. The state of being a primipara.

primi·parous (L. *primus*, first; *parere*, to bear). Bearing one child.

pri·mitive (L. *primitivus*). Original.

primor·dial (L. *primordium*, commencement). Existing from the beginning; primitive.

primor·dium (L.). Any structure in its first state.

prin·ceps (L. chief). First; original. Name given to certain arteries, e.g., **P. pollicis:** a branch of the radial artery supplying the palmar surface of the thumb.

Princeteau's tubercle (Princeteau, of Bordeaux; 1892). On the temporal bone at the apex, where superior petrosal sinus commences.

prin·ciple (L. *principium*, a beginning). Law, dogma or tenet. **P., proximate:** next or nearer p. **P., ultimate:** final or last possible, fundamental or basic p.

Pringle's band (Pringle, S. S., Irish surgeon, 1879–1936). A peritoneal band from the mesocolon to the duodenojejunal flexure.

Pringle's disease (Pringle, J. J., English dermatologist, 1855–1922). Adenoma sebaceum.

Prior-Finkler vibrio. The *Vibrio proteus*.

prism (G. *prisma*, anything sawn). A solid with a triangular or polygonal cross section. A triangular glass prism splits up a ray of light into its constituent colours, and turns or deflects light towards its base.

prismat·ic (G. *prisma*, anything sawn). Prism-shaped.

pris·moid (G. *prisma*, anything sawn; *eidos*, form). Like a prism.

pris·mosphere (G. *prisma*, anything sawn; *sphaira*, a ball). A prism and a globular lens combined.

pri·vates. A colloquial name for the genital organs.

Privine. A proprietary powerful synthetic vasoconstrictor, causing decongestion of nasal mucous membrane. Privine, 2(naphthyl-l-methyl)-imidazoline hydrochloride, is available in aqueous solution in two strengths, 1-1000 for adults and 1-2000 for children and those with sensitive nasal mucosa. It is used in nasal congestions of allergic or inflammatory origin, acute rhinitis, etc.

p.r.n. Abbreviation for L. *pro re nata*, as may be required; lit., for the thing arisen.

proăm·nion (G. *pro*, before; *amnion*, membrane round the foetus). That part of the embryonic area at the sides and in front of the head of the developing embryo, which remains for some considerable period without mesoderm.

pro-antithrom·bin (G. *pro*, before; *anti*, against; *thrombis*, a clot). A hypothetical precursor of antithrombin.

proăt·las (G. *pro*, before; *atlas*). A rudimentary vertebra which in some animals lies in front of the atlas. Sometimes seen as an anomaly in man.

probable expectation of life. The time, determined statistically, that a person of given age may expect to live.

prō·bang (L. *probare*, to test). A rod of flexible material used in removing foreign bodies from the oesophagus.

probe (L. *probare*, to test). A slender flexible rod used to explore channels or to introduce into a wound.

probos·cis (G. *pro*, before; *boskein*, to feed). 1. An elephant's trunk. 2. The tubular flexible parts of the mouth of insects and other invertebrates.

procaine hydrochloride. A local anaesthetic given by injection, and regarded as being one of the safest cocaine substitutes. Syn. ethocaine hydrochloride; Novocain.

process. 1. A course of action. 2. A slender prominence, as the spinous p. of a vertebra. **Acromion:** the large flattened portion of bone at the lateral extremity of the spine of the scapula. **Alveolar:** the most dependent part of the body of the maxilla. It lodges the teeth. **Calcaneal:** a backward projection on the outer surface of the cuboid bone. **Clinoid:** three in number: anterior, middle and posterior. **Clinoid, anterior:** a projection from the inner part of the lesser wing of the sphenoid bone to which is attached the anterior end of the tentorium cerebelli. **Clinoid, middle:** a small tubercle on the side of the body of the sphenoid bone. It may ossify. **Clinoid, posterior:** a projection on the anterio-superior border of the dorsum sellae of the sphenoid bone. **Condyloid:** a large ovoid process which surmounts the posterior border of the ramus of the mandible. **Coracoid:** a strong curved portion of the head of the scapula. **Coronoid:** of mandible. A thin flattened portion of bone which surmounts the anterior border of the ramus of the mandible. **Coronoid, of ulna:** a pyramidal portion of bone at the upper end of the ulna. **Dentatus:** see odontoid. **Ensiform:** (xiphoid) the small lower end of the body of the sternum. It may be bony or cartilaginous. **Ethmoidal:** a small projection on the inferior nasal concha which articulates with the uncinate process of the ethmoid bone. **Falciform:** a prolongation of the sacrotuberous ligament in the ischiorectal fossa. **Frontal:** of maxilla which articulates with the frontal bone. **Infraorbital:** a slender pointed process on the anterior surface of the zygomatic bone which articulates with the maxilla near the infra-orbital foramen. **Intrajugular:** a thin piece of bone which passes between the occipital bone and the petrous portion of the temporal in the region of the jugular foramen. **Jugular:** that part of the condylar portion of the occipital bone which lies above the transverse process of the atlas, and is homologous with it. **Lacrimal:** a thin projection of bone on the inferior nasal concha which articulates with the descending process of the lacrimal bone. **Mastoid:** a thick mass of bone on the posterior part of the temporal bone; within it are the mastoid air cells. **Maxillary:** a blunt truncated portion of the zygomatic bone which articulates with the maxilla. **Nasal:** a small portion of the frontal bone which articulates with the nasal bone. **Odontoid** (processus dentatus): a constricted and somewhat circular projection of bone which springs from the superior surface of the body of the axis. It represents the body of the atlas. **Orbital:** a curved portion of the zygomatic bone which articulates with the greater wing of the sphenoid bone. **Palatine:** is situated on the mesial surface of the body of the maxilla from which it projects horizontally inwards and, with its fellow, forms three-fourths of the hard palate. **Papillary, of liver:** is the left eminence of the caudate lobe of the liver. **Paroccipital:** a projection of the jugular process of the occipital bone. **Petrosal, posterior:** a small process at the lower end of the lateral border of the body of the sphenoid. It articulates with the apex of the petrous portion of the temporal bone. **Postauditory:** an embryonic process of the squamosal portion of the temporal bone which forms the outer wall of the tympanic antrum. **Pterygoid:** two processes which project downwards from the body of the sphenoid bone. **Sphenoidal:** the upper process of the palatine bone. **Styloid:** a cylindrical, tapering process of the temporal bone. **Styloid, of fibula:** a blunt projection from the upper end of the fibula, to the tip of which the lateral ligament of the knee-joint is attached. **Styloid, of radius:** a stout conical process which projects downwards from the lower end of the radius. **Styloid, of ulna:** a small projection from the lower end of the ulna, it gives attachment to the medial ligament of the wrist-joint. **Supracondylar:** an inconstant projection of bone which arises from the upper part of the medial supracondylar ridge of the humerus. **Temporal:** the posterior blunt part of the zygomatic bone. **Uncinate:** a thin curved plate of bone which projects downward from the ethmoid bone. **Uncinate, of pancreas:** a projection of the head of the pancreas which is posterior to the superior mesenteric vessels. **Vaginal:** a sharp ridge of bone ensheathing the styloid process of the temporal bone. **Vaginal, of sphenoid:** a thin scale of bone on the side of the rostrum of the sphenoid bone. **Xiphoid:** see ensiform. **Zygomatic:** the outer process of the frontal bone.

processomā·nia (L. *processus*, a law-suit; G. *mania*, madness). A morbid desire to enter into litigation.

proces·sus (L.). A process.

prochorē·sis (G. *prokhōrēsis*, a going forth). Gastric peristalsis.

prochrō·mosomes (L. *pro*, before; G. *khrōma*, colour; *sōma*, body). Localized basichromatin masses in the nucleus, believed to give rise to the chromosomes.

prociden·tia (L. *procidere*, to fall down). Prolapse.

procreā·tion (L. *procreare*, to beget). The act of begetting young.

proctal·gia (G. *prōktos*, anus; *algos*, pain). Pain in the anus or rectum.

proctatrē·sia (G. *prōktos*, anus; *a*, neg; *tresis*, perforation). Imperforation of the anus or rectum.

proctectā·sia (G. *prōktos*, anus; *ektasis*, extension). Dilatation of the anus or rectum.

proctec·tomy (G. *prōktos*, anus; *ektomē*, excision). Surgical removal of the anus or rectum.

proctenclei·sis (G. *prōktos*, anus; *egkleiein*, to shut in). Stenosis of the rectum or anus.

proc·teurynter (G. *prōktos*, anus; *eurunein*, to widen). An instrument used for dilating the anus.

procti·tis (G. *prōktos*, anus). Inflammation of the anus or rectum.

proc·tocele (G. *prōktos*, anus; *kēlē*, hernia). Prolapse of a part of the rectum.

proctō·clysis (G. *prōktos*, anus; *klusis*, a drenching). The slow instillation of a liquid into the rectum.

proctococ·cypexy, proctococcypex·ia (G. *prōktos*, anus; *kokkux*, cuckoo; *pēxis*, fixation). The suturing of the rectum to the coccyx.

proctodae·um (G. *prōktos*, anus; *hodaios*, the cross-roads). A fold of the ectoderm in the embryo which advances towards the cloaca until the ectoderm and entoderm meet; the membrane formed between the two ultimately disappears and the bowel then opens externally.

proctody·nia (G. *prōktos*, anus; *odunē*, pain). Pain in or about the anus or rectum.

proctogen·ic (G. *prōktos*, anus; *gennan*, to produce). Originating from the anus or rectum.

procto·logy (G. *prōktos*, anus; *logos*, treatise). That branch of medical science dealing with the anatomy and diseases of the rectum.

proctoparā·lysis (G. *prōktos*, anus; *paralusis*, paralysis). Paralysis of the anal and rectal muscles.

proc·topexy, proctopex·ia (G. *prōktos*, anus; *pēxis*, fixation). Fixation of the rectum to another part by sutures.

proctophō·bia (G. *prōktos*, anus; *phobos*, fear). The state of nervous apprehension which is often seen in patients with diseases of the rectum.

proc·toplasty (G. *prōktos*, anus; *plassein*, to form). Plastic surgery of the rectum or anus.

proctoptō·ma (G. *prōktos*, anus; *ptōma*, a fall). Rectal prolapse.

proctoptō·sis (G. *prōktos*, anus; *ptōsis*, a falling). Prolapse of the rectum; proctoptoma.

proctorrhā·gia (G. *prōktos*, anus; *rhēgnunai*, to burst forth). Haemorrhage from the anus.

proctor·rhaphy (G. *prōktos*, anus; *rhaphē*, suture). The suturing of the rectum or anus.

proctorrhoe·a (G. *prōktos*, anus; *rhoia*, a flowing). The discharge of mucus through the anus.

proc·toscope (G. *prōktos*, anus; *skopein*, to view.) An instrument designed for the visual inspection of the rectum.

proctŏ·scopy. Inspection of the rectum with the aid of a proctoscope.

proctosigmoidec·tomy (G. *prōktos*, anus; *sigma*, letter S; *eidos*, form; *ektomē*, excision). Operation used in prolapse of rectum, and some cases of cancer of rectum. Rectum and part of sigmoid are excised, and continuity of bowel restored by anastomosis of proximal part of sigmoid colon to the stump of rectum.

proctosigmoidī·tis (G. *prōktos*, anus; *sigma*, letter S; *eidos*, form). Inflammation involving the rectum and sigmoid colon.

proctostenō·sis (G. *prōktos*, anus; *stenos*, narrow). Stricture of the rectum or anus.

proctŏ·stomy (G. *prōktos*, anus; *stoma*, mouth). The making of an artificial opening into the rectum.

proc·totome (G. *prōktos*, anus; *tomē*, a cutting). A surgical knife used in proctotomy.

proctŏ·tomy (G. *prōktos*, anus; *tomē*, a cutting). Surgical incision into the rectum, especially for stricture.

prodrō·mal (G. *prodromos*, a going in advance). Premonitory.

prŏ·drome (G. *prodromos*, going in advance). An advance symptom indicating the approach of a disease.

prŏ·dromous. Prodromal, *q.v.*

product (L. *producere*, to bring forth). Outcome; result; issue.

produc·tive (L. *producere*, to bring forth). Forming; applied especially to the forming of new tissues.

proencĕ·phalus (G. *pro*, before; *egkephalos*, brain). A monster characterized by the protrusion of a part of the brain through a frontal fissure.

prŏĕn·zyme (G. *pro*. before; *en*, in; *zumē*, leaven). The substance which eventually becomes an active ferment.

professional (L. *professio*, declaration). 1. Relating to a profession. 2. Resulting from professional activity; e.g. writer's cramp.

Profeta's law (Profeta, G., Italian dermatologist, 1840–1910). Normal children of syphilitic parents possess a definite immunity to syphilitic disease.

Profichet's disease (Profichet, G. C., French physician, born 1873). Periarticular calcareous nodules.

Proflavine, Neutral. A highly active antiseptic, less active and irritant than Proflavine B.P., and suitable for ophthalmic and brain surgery.

profun·dus (L. deep; f. s. and n. pl. *profunda*). Deepseated.

pro·gaster (G. *pro*, before; *gaster*, belly). The archenteron.

prŏ·geny (G. *pro*, before; *gennan*, to produce). Offspring.

proge·ria (G. *pro*, before; *gerōn*, old man). Senile appearance at an early age, sometimes associated with pituitary dwarfism.

progĕ·sterone. The hormone of the ovarian corpus luteum, inducing premenstrual changes of the endometrium after ovulation and those occurring during the early stages of pregnancy, and probably inhibiting uterine contractions.

progĕ·stin. The name originally given to progesterone, the hormone of the corpus luteum.

proglos·sis (G. *pro*, before; *glossa*, tongue). The tip of the tongue.

proglot·tis (G. *pro*, before; *glōttis*, the mouth of the windpipe). A segment of a tapeworm.

prog·nathism (G. *pro*, before; *gnathos*, jaw). Having an abnormally projecting jaw.

prog·nathous. Having projecting jaws.

prognō·sis (G. *pro*, before; *gnōsis*, knowledge). A forecast of the probable duration, course and termination of a disease.

prognos·tic. Relating to prognosis.

prognos·ticate (G. *pro*, before; *gnōsis*, knowledge). To make a prognosis.

progres·sion (L. *progressio*, advancement). The act of moving forward. **Backward p.**: walking backward, a symptom noted in certain diseases of the nervous system.

progres·sive (L. *progredi*, to advance). Gradually advancing. **P. lenticular degeneration**: a form of hepatolenticular degeneration, *q.v.*, characterized by hypertonia and weakness of muscles, poverty of movement, tremor, dysarthria, absence of pyramidal signs, by pigmentation of the corneal limbus, by cirrhosis of the liver and by p. deterioration of the mental faculties. **P. muscular atrophy**: progressive form of muscular atrophy due to degeneration in cells of anterior horn of spinal cord and consequent degeneration of anterior nerve roots and atrophy of muscles supplied by them. Sometimes called chronic anterior poliomyelitis.

Proguanil. See Paludrine.

prohis·tiocyte (G. *pro*, before; *histion*, a sail; *kutos*, a container). A reticular cell, the precursor of the histiocyte, having a diameter of 12–14μ, irregular outline, a large pachychromatous nucleus and opaque eosinophilic cytoplasm.

projectile vomiting. The forcible projection of the stomach contents due to pyloric stenosis in infants. Seen also in some diseases of the brain.

projec·tion (L. *projectio*, a throwing forward). 1. The act of throwing forward. 2. A part extending beyond the level of the surrounding surface. 3. The referring of mental impressions to the object producing them. **P. fibres**: (*a*) fibres arising in cortical cells and proceeding to areas outside the endbrain: (*b*) fibres arising outside the endbrain and proceeding to the cerebral cortex.

prolā·bium (L. *pro*, before; *labium*, lip). The red outer part of the lip.

prolac·tin (L. *pro*, before; *lac*, milk). The lactogenic hormone of the anterior lobe of the pituitary gland.

prolā·min. Alcohol soluble protein found in cereals.

prō·lan. An activating ovarian hormone from the anterior lobe of the pituitary gland.

prolapse (L. *prolabi*, to slip forward). The falling forward or downward of a part. **P. of the cord**: premature expulsion of the umbilical cord during labour. **P. of the iris**: protrusion of the iris through a tear in the cornea.

prolap·sus (L.). Prolapse. **P. ani**: prolapse of the anus.

prolep·sis (G., preconception). A paroxysm returning before the expected time.

prolep·tic (G. *prolēpsis*). Recurring sooner than expected.

proli·ferate (L. *proles*, offspring; *ferre*, to bear). To multiply.

prolifera·tion (L. *proles*, offspring; *ferre*, to bear). The act of multiplying.

proli·ferating, proli·ferous (L. *proles*, offspring; *ferre*, to bear). Multiplying; characterized by the formation of new tissues or by cell-proliferation.

proli·fic (L. *proles*, offspring; *facere*, to make). Fruitful.

proli·gerous (L. *proles*, offspring; *gerere*, to bear). Germinating.

prō·line. An amino acid containing the pyrrole ring.

prŏ·minence (L. *prominentia*). A projection.

promitō·sis (G. *pro*, before; *mitos*, a thread). A type of mitosis in some protozoa, in which cell division takes place only within the nucleus.

prŏ·montory (L. *promontorium*). A projecting eminence.

pronā·tion (L. *pronare*, to bend forward). 1. The state of being prone, or the act of placing in a prone position. 2. The turning of the hand palm downward.

pronā·tor (L. *pronare*, to bend forward). That which pronates. The term is given to certain muscles, e.g., p. teres.

prone (L. *pronus*, bent forward). Lying face downwards; of the hand, with the palm turned downwards.

pronĕ·phron, pronĕ·phros (G. *pro*, before; *nephros*, kidney). The primitive kidney.

Prontosil. A proprietary preparation of sulphanilamide.

pronū·cleus (L. *pro*, before; *nucleus*, kernel). The nucleus of the male or female gametes during fertilization.

prooe·strum (G. *pro*, before; *oistros*, orgasm). The period preceding the season or "heat" in animals.

prŏŏt·ic (G. *pro*, before; *ous*, ear). In front of the ear.

prop-cells. Purkinje cells.

propaedeu·tics (G. *pro*, before; *paideuein*, to educate, from *pais*, child). Preliminary instruction.

propagā·tion (L. *propagare*, to reproduce). Reproduction.

propa·midine isethi·onate. A synthetic chemical used in jelly or cream for the prevention and treatment of sepsis in wounds and burns.

Propeomy̆·cēs. A genus of fungi, some types of which are capable of causing skin lesions in man.

propep·sin. Pepsinogen, *q.v.*

pro·phase (G. *pro*, before; *phainein*, to show). The first stage of karyokinesis, characterized by formation of the mitotic figure and longitudinal division of the chromosomes.

prophylac·tic (G. *pro*, before; *phulassein*, to guard). 1. Relating to prophylaxis. 2. Any agent which prevents disease.

prophylax·is (G. *pro*, before; *phulassein*, to guard). Prevention of disease.

prō·pione. Diethyl ketone.

propionic acid. CH_3CH_2COOH. A monobasic saturated fatty acid.

prō·ponal. Dipropylmalonyl urea; a hypnotic.

propioni·trile. Ethyl cyanide.

proplex·us (L. *pro*, before; *plexus*, a plait). The choroid plexus of the lateral ventricle of the brain.

proprietary medicine. Any medicine which is trademarked or patented.

prō·priocep·tive (L. *proprius*, one's own; *capere*, to receive). Nerve impulses which receive their stimuli from within the body tissues.

pro·priocep·tor (L. *proprius*, one's own; *capere*, to receive). A receptor which is stimulated by mechanical impulses from organs of mesodermal origin; especially from muscles, joints and bones.

propriospī·nal (L. *proprius*, one's own; *spina*). Belonging to or relating solely to the spinal cord.

pro-prothrom·bin (G. *pro*, before; *thrombos*, a clot). A hypothetical precursor of prothrombin, supposed to be activated on contact with some foreign substance.

proptō·sis (G. *pro*, before; *ptōsis*, a falling). A prolapse. **Ocular p.:** exophthalmus.

propul·sion (L. *propellere*, to propel). 1. The act of pushing forward. 2. A tendency to fall forward in walking; a symptom found in cases of paralysis agitans.

pro re nata (L.). For an occasion as it arises.

pror·sad (L. *prorsum*, forwards; *ad*, to). Forwards; in a forward direction.

prosecrē·tin (L. *pro*, before; *secernere*, to separate). The precursor of secretin, *q.v.*, present in the intestinal mucosa.

prosec·tor (L. *pro*, before; *sectare*, to cut). One who dissects subjects for anatomical lectures and demonstrations.

prosencĕ·phalon (G. *prosō*, forwards; *egkephalos*, brain). The forebrain. The anterior part of the anterior cerebral vesicle.

prosodem·ic (G. *prosō*, forwards; *dēmos*, people). Transmission of disease directly from person to person, as opposed to transmission from one to many by water supply.

prŏ·sogaster (G. *prosō*, forwards; *gastēr*, belly). The foregut.

prosŏ·pagus (G. *prosōpon*, face; *pēgnunai*, to fasten). A monster with a twin attached to its face.

prosopal·gia (G. *prosōpon*, face; *algos*, pain). Neuralgia of the trigeminal nerve. Syn. tic douloureux.

prŏsoponeural·gia (G. *prosōpon*, face; *neuron*, nerve; *algos*, pain). Facial neuralgia.

prŏsopoplē·gia (G. *prosōpon*, face; *plēgē*, stroke). Paralysis of the face.

prosopŏ·schisis (G. *prosōpon*, face; *skhisis*, cleavage). An oblique fissure or cleft of the face in a foetal monstrosity. It passes from the mouth to one of the orbits and is generally associated with malformation of the brain.

prŏ·sopospasm (G. *prosōpon*, face; *spasmos*, spasm). Risus sardonicus.

prŏ·soposternodỹ·mia (G. *prosōpon*, face; *sternon*, chest; *didumos*, twin). A form of double monstrosity in which the twins are united by their faces and chests.

prŏ·sopothoracŏ·pagus (G. *prosōpon*, face; *thōrax*, chest; *pagos*, anything fixed). A double monster united at the upper abdomen, chest and face.

prŏsopotō·cia (G. *prosōpon*, face; *tokos*, birth). Presentation of the face in labour.

prosper·mia (G. *pro*, before; *sperma*, sperm). Ejaculatio praecox.

prostatal·gia (G. *pro*, before; *statos*, standing; *algos*, pain). Pain in the prostate gland.

prostataux·ē (G. *prostatēs*, standing before; *auxein*, to increase). Enlargement of the prostate gland.

prostate (G. *prostatēs*, standing before). **P. gland:** a firm conical organ which surrounds the neck of the bladder in the male. It is of a reddish-brown colour and is subject to much variation in size. It is traversed by the first one and a quarter inches of the urethra and consists of two lateral lobes and a middle lobe.

prostatec·tomy (G. *pro*, before; *statos*, standing; *ektomē*, excision). Excision of part or the whole of the prostate gland.

prostat·ic (G. *pro*, before; *statos*, standing). Relating to the prostate gland.

prostatit·ic (G. *prostatēs*, standing before). Relating to prostatitis.

prostatī·tis (G. *prostatēs*, standing before). Inflammation of the prostate gland.

prostatorrhoē·a (G. *pro*, before; *statos*, standing; *rhoia*, a flow). A urethral discharge of catarrhal character coming from the prostate.

prostă·tomy (G. *pro*, before; *statos*, standing; *tomē*, a cutting). Incision into the prostate.

prŏ·statovesiculec·tomy (G. *pro*, before; *statos*, standing; L. *vesicula*, vesicle; G. *ektomē*, excision). Excision of the prostate and the seminal vesicles.

prŏ·statovesiculi·tis (G. *prostatēs*, standing before; L. *vesicula*, vesicle). Combined inflammation of the prostate gland and the seminal vesicles.

pros·thesis (G. *pros*, to; *thesis*, a putting). An artificial substitute for a part surgically removed or missing; e.g. an artificial limb.

prosthet·ics (G. *pros*, to; *thesis*, a putting). The branch of surgery dealing with prosthesis.

Prostig·mine. Proprietary name for a synthetic alkaloid related to physostigmine, and having a similar action. It is used as a salt.

prostitu·tion (L. *prostituere*, to prostitute). Promiscuous sexual intercourse for pay.

prŏ·strate (L. *pro*, before; *sternere*, to spread). 1. Exhausted; stricken down. 2. Lying at full length.

prostrā·tion (L. *pro*, before; *sternere*, to spread). Great exhaustion of nervous or muscular energy. P.,nervous: neurasthenia.

prŏ·tal (G. *prōtos*, first). Congenital.

protal·bumose. Proto-albumose. *q.v.*

protă·minase. An enzyme which splits protamines.

prŏ·tămines. One class of simple proteins.

prŏ·tămine zinc insulin. A sterile aqueous suspension of the specific antidiabetic principle of mammalian pancreas, together with a suitable protamine and zinc chloride. An injection results in a steady and slow absorption of insulin.

pro·tanope. A person with protanopia.

protanŏ·pia (G. *prōtos*, first; *an*, neg.; *ōps*, eye). A defect in a primary constituent necessary for colour-vision, as in red-blindness.

protar·gin. A silver protein containing 20–25 per cent silver.

protar·gol. A silver protein containing 8 per cent of silver.

prŏ·tēan (G. *Prōteus*, a sea-god). 1. Assuming many shapes, as p. eruption. 2. Any first insoluble derivative of a protein.

prŏ·tēase (G. *prōtos*, first). An enzyme or ferment that digests protein.

protec·tive. Affording a guard against harm, as a p. dressing.

pro·teid. Protein, *q.v.*

prŏ·tein (G. *prōtos*, first). The most important constituent of living protoplasm, usually of large molecular weight, but of simple molecular structure. Proteins are made up of various combinations of amino-acids, and contain oxygen, hydrogen, carbon, and nitrogen, and usually sulphur.

proteinae·mia (G. *prōtos*, first; *haima*, blood). An abnormal amount of protein in the blood.

pro·teinase (G. *prōtos*, first). A protein-splitting enzyme.

protein·ic. Relating to protein.

proteinū·ria (G. *prōtos*, first; *ouron*, urine). Protein in the urine.

proteoclast·ic (G. *prōtos*, first; *klasis*, a breaking). The breaking up of proteins.

proteŏ·lysis (G. *prōtos*, first; *lusis*, dissolution). The changes produced in proteins by ferments which convert them into diffusible bodies.

proteolyt·ic (G. *prōtos*, first; *luein*, to dissolve). Relating to or effecting proteolysis.

proteomorphic theory (G. *prōtos*, first; *morphē*, shape). States that immunity against bacterial infection is due primarily to the haematopoietic system, and secondarily to all the cells of the body.

prŏ·teose (G. *prōtos*, first). Any one of a group of proteins formed in gastric digestion, intermediate in molecular size between the food proteins and the peptones.

proteosū·ria (G. *prōtos*, first; *ouron*, urine). The presence of proteose in the urine.

Proteus (G. *Prōteus*, a sea-god). A genus of Schizomycetes.

prothrom·bin (G. *pro*, before; *thrombos*, a clot). A substance partly associated with the globulin fraction of the plasma protein and activated to thrombin by the combined action of calcium and blood platelets.

Protis·ta (G. *prōtos*, first). A unicellular organism; term originally applied by Haeckel to certain lower organisms which cannot easily be classed as belonging either to the vegetable or to the animal kingdom.

proto-al·bumose. A primary proteose precipitated from albumin by half saturation with ammonium sulphate.

Prŏ·tobacteri·aceae (G. *prōtos*, first; *baktron*, rod). Organisms belonging to the family of Nitrobacteriaceae. They oxidise inorganic compounds of carbon or hydrogen.

prŏ·tobe (G. *prōtos*, first; *bios*, life). A name proposed by d'Herelle, for ultraviruses.

protodiă·stolě (G. *prōtos*, first; *diastolē*, expansion). The first part of the ventricular diastole during which the pressure in ventricle and aorta is falling rapidly.

prŏ·togaster (G. *prōtos*, first; *gastēr*, belly). The foregut.

protŏ·minobacter. An organism (bacterium) found in soil.

Protomonă·dina. An order of Flagellata, which includes Leishmania.

prŏ·ton (G. *prōtos*, first). 1. The rudiment of a part. 2. A particle of one atomic unit of mass and positive charge equivalent to the negative charge on the electron; identical with the nucleus of a hydrogen atom.

protoneph·ron (G. *prōtos*, first; *nephros*, kidney). The primitive kidney; the pronephron, metanephron and mesonephron taken together.

protopath·ic (G. *prōtos*, first; *pathos*, disease). Primary, applied to disease or sensibility.

prŏ·tophyte (G. *prōtos*, first; *phuton*, plant). Any plant of the lowest and simplest type, a single-celled plant organism.

protoplā·sis (G. *prōtos*, first; *plassein*, to form). The primary formation of tissue.

prŏ·toplasm (G. *prōtos*, first; *plasma*, something formed). 1. The active substance of the cell-body exclusive of the nucleus. Syn. cytoplasm. 2. The active substance of the cell inclusive of the nucleus.

protoplas·mic. 1. Relating to protoplasm. 2. Consisting of protoplasm.

protoplas·tin (G. *prōtos*, first; *plassein*, to form). The basic material of protoplasm.

protopor·phyrinū·ria (G. *prōtos*, first; *porphura*, purple dye; *ouron*, urine). The presence of protoporphyrin in the urine.

protopor·phyrin (G. *prōtos*, first; *porphura*, purple dye). A natural porphyrin $C_{34}H_{34}N_4O_4$ found combined with iron, in haemoglobin, myoglobin, etc.

protop·sis (G. *prōtos*, first; *opsis*, vision). Protrusion of the eyeball.

prototox·oid (G. *protos*, first; *toxikon*, poison, *eidos*, form). Protoxoid, *q.v.*

prototroph·ic (G. *prōtos*, first; *trophē*, nourishment). Term given to organisms subsisting on inorganic matter.

prŏ·totype (G. *prōtos*, first; *tupos*, type). An original type; one from which others are copied.

protover·tebra (G. *prōtos*, first; L. *vertebra*). A mesoblastic segment formed on the side of the embryonic notochord.

protox·oid (G. *prōtos*, first; *toxikon*, poison; *eidos*, form). A toxoid having a greater affinity for the antitoxin than is possessed by the corresponding toxin.

Protozō·a (G. *prōtos*, first; *zōon*, animal). The lowest class of the animal kingdom; organisms without nervous or circulatory systems and consisting of a single cell or of cell groups.

protozō·an, protozō·on. A single-celled organism belonging to the Protozoa.

protozoö·logy (G. *prōtos*, first; *zōon*, animal; *logos*, treatise). The study of Protozoa.

protrac·tor (L. *protrahere*, to draw forward). A surgical instrument used for the extraction of foreign bodies from wounds.

protryp·sin. Trypsinogen, *q.v.*

protū·berance (L. *pro*, before; *tuber*, a hump). A projecting part; e.g. the cerebral p., or pons Varolii.

proud flesh. Excessive production of granulation tissue.

Proust's space (Proust, P. T., work published, *Sur le peritonite*, Paris, 1822). The rectovesical pouch.

provī·tamin. A hypothetical precursor of a vitamin.

Prowazek's bodies. See Prowazek-Greeff body.

Prowazek-Greef body (Prowazék, S. J. M. von, German zoologist, 1876–1915; Greeff, C. R., German ophthalmologist, born 1862). Inclusion body found in the cells of conjunctiva in trachomatous eyes; also called trachoma body.

prox·imad (L. *proximus*, next; *ad*, to). Towards the proximal end.

prox·imal (L. *proximus*, next). Nearest to the centre.

prox·imate (L. *proximus*, next). Nearest.

prune. The dried fruit of the *Prunus domestica*. It is laxative in action.

Prunus. A genus of trees of the order Rosaceae, including plums and cherries.

prurī·ginous. Relating to or resembling prurigo.

prurī·go (L. *prurigo*, from *prurire*, to itch). A disease of the skin, affecting mainly the extensor surfaces of the limbs and the trunk, characterized by small, hard, intensely itching papules, leading to lichenification of the affected area.

prurit·ic. Relating to or resembling pruritus.

prurī·tus (L. *prurire*, to itch). Itching. **P. ani**: extreme itching around the anus. **P. vulvae**: intense itching about the vulva.

Prussak's fibres (Prussak, A., Russian otologist, 1839–97). The boundaries of Shrapnell's membrane. **P.'s space**: the recessus membranae tympani superior.

Prussian blue. The name given to the blue compounds resulting from the interaction of ferric salts with potassium ferrocyanide.

prussic acid. Hydrocyanic acid.

Ps. Abbreviation for Pseudomonas.

psă·lis (G., a vault). The cerebral fornix.

psaltē·rium (G. *psaltērion*, harp). The lyra Davidi.

psammō·ma (G. *psammos*, sand). A form of meningioma, characterized by a whorl-like arrangement of cells with hyaline degeneration and central deposition of calcium and iron.

psam·mosarcō·ma (G. *psammos*, sand; *sarx*, flesh). A sarcoma containing calcareous deposits.

psam·mous (G. *psammos*, sand). Sandy.

pselaphē·sis (G., a touching). 1. Groping with the fingers, as observed in fever delirium. 2. Ticklishness.

psel·lism (G. *psellismos*, a stammering). Stuttering or stammering.

pseudacon·itin (G. *pseudēs*, false; *akonīton*, a poisonous plant). A very poisonous alkaloid derived from Aconitum ferox.

pseudacou·sia, pseudacous·ma, pseudacū·sis (G. *pseudēs*, false; *akouein*, to hear). A state in which the patient's perception of sound gives him the impression that pitch and/or quality are altered.

pseudaesthē·sia (G. *pseudēs*, false; *aisthēsis*, sensation). An imaginary sensation for which there is no stimulus; e.g., pain felt in an amputated limb.

pseudarthri·tis (G. *pseudēs*, false; *arthron*, joint). Hysterical affection of a joint simulating arthritis.

pseudarthrō·sis (G. *pseudēs*, false; *arthron*, joint). A false joint.

pseudencě·phalus (G. *pseudēs*, false; *egkephalos*, brain). A monster with a collection of blood-vessels and connective tissue in place of a brain.

pseudo-angī·na (G. *pseudēs*, false; L. *angina*, spasmodic pain). False angina; a syndrome accompanied by cardiac pain and lassitude, seen in neurotic individuals. There is usually no disease of the heart associated with it.

pseudobul·bar (G. *pseudēs*, false; L. *bulbus*, bulb). Term applied usually to a form of paralysis which appears to, but does not in fact, result from a lesion in the bulb of the brain.

pseū·docoxal·gia (G. *pseudēs*, false; *coxa*, hip; *algos*, pain). Coxa plana, Perthes's disease. A disease of the upper epiphysis of the femur. The epiphysis is small, flattened and often fragmented.

pseudocrī·sis (G. *pseudēs*, false; *krisis*, crisis). A false crisis; a sudden but transitory fall of temperature.

pseū·docroup (G. *pseudēs*, false). Laryngismus stridulus, or false croup.

pseudocȳē·sis (G. *pseudēs*, false; *kuēsis*, conception). False pregnancy.

pseudodiphthē·ria (G. *pseudēs* false; *diphthera*, leather). An inflammation accompanied by the formation of a false membrane not due to the Klebs-Loeffler bacillus.

Pseudodis·cus Watsoni. An intestinal parasite found in Africa. It infests humans.

pseudo-epitheliō·ma (G. *pseudēs*, false; *epi*, upon; *thēlē*, nipple). A skin eruption simulating epithelioma.

pseudogang·lion (G. *pseudēs*, false; *gagglion*, a tumour under the skin). A false ganglion; usually a thickened nerve.

pseudo-geusaesthē·sia (G. *pseudēs*, false; *geusis*, taste; *aisthēsis*, sensation). A condition in which colour and taste sensations accompany each other.

pseudogeū·sia (G. *pseudēs*, false; *geusis*, taste). Hallucination of taste.

pseudogliō·ma (G. *pseudēs*, false; *glia*, glue). An organized inflammatory mass in the vitreous humour, due to uveitis and resembling the cat's eye appearance of glioma of the retina.

pseū·dohermaph·roditism (G. *pseudēs*, false; *Hermēs*, messenger of the gods; *Aphroditē*, Venus). A condition in which the external genitalia, the bodily appearance and usually the emotional outlook are largely of a sexual type contrary to that of the gonads; possibly caused by dysfunction of the androgenic tissue of the adrenal cortex during certain stages of foetal life.

pseudoher·nia (G. *pseudēs*, false; L. *hernia*). An inflamed hernia sac resembling strangulated hernia.

pseudohyper·trophy (G. *pseudēs*, false; *huper*, above; *trophē*, nutrition). False hypertrophy; increase in the size of an organ owing to hypertrophy of another than the functionally important tissue, e.g. of fat in a muscle.

pseudo-ic·terus (G. *pseudēs*, false; *ikteros*, jaundice). False jaundice.

pseū·doleukae·mia (G. *pseudēs*, false; *leukos*, white; *haima*, blood). An obsolete term formerly applied to various reticulo-endothelial diseases other than leukaemia. **P., infantile**: von Jaksch's disease, *q.v.*

pseū·domelanō·sis (G. *pseudēs*, false; *melas*, black). Dark staining of the tissues after death with blood pigments.

pseudomem·brane (G. *pseudēs*, false; L. *membrana*). A false membrane.

pseu·domeningi·tis (G. *pseudēs*, false; *mēnigx*, membrane). A collection of symptoms resembling those of meningitis.

pseu·domenstruā·tion (G. *pseudēs*, false; L. *mensis*, month). Bleeding from the uterus not associated with endometrial changes.

pseu·do-methaemoglo·bin (G. *pseudēs*, false; *meta*, beyond; *haima*, blood; L. *globus*, globe). Methaemalbumin.

pseudomnē·sia (G. *pseudēs*, false; *mnasthai*, to remember). Perversion of memory, in which things that never occurred seem to be remembered.

Pseudŏ·monas pyocyanea (G. *pseudēs*, false; *monas*, single). A genus of micro-organisms with polar flagella.

Pseu·domonĭ·lia. A genus of fungi.

pseudomū·cin (G. *pseudēs*, false; L. *mucus*). A type of mucin seen in proliferative ovarian cysts.

pseudomyxō·ma (G. *pseudēs*, false; *muxa*, slime). A gelatinous growth on the peritoneum often resulting from the rupture of a pseudomucinous cyst of the ovary or a mucous cyst of the appendix.

pseudonar·cotism (G. *pseudēs*, false; *narke*, numbness). A hysterical simulation of narcotism.

pseu·doneurō·ma (G. *pseudēs*, false; *neuron*, nerve). A false neuroma.

pseudo-oedē·ma (G. *pseudēs*, false; *oidēma*, swelling). A condition resembling oedema.

pseu·dopară·lysis (G. *pseudēs*, false; *paralusis*, paralysis). Apparent loss of muscle power, without true paralysis, marked by defective co-ordination of movements or repression of movement due to pain.

pseudoparē·sis (G. *pseudēs*, false; *paresis*, a slackening). An hysterical or other condition simulating paresis.

pseudoph·thisis (G. *pseudēs*, false; *phthisis*, a wasting). A wasting disease arising from causes other than tuberculosis.

Pseudophyllĭ·dea. An order of cestodes which have a single terminal or two opposite sucking organs on the scolex.

pseudoplē·gia (G. *pseudēs*, false; *plēgē*, a stroke). Hysterical paralysis.

pseu·dopod, pseudopō·dium (G. *pseudēs*, false; *pous*, foot). Temporary protrusion of the enveloping membrane of an amoeba serving for purposes of locomotion and feeding.

pseudopreg·nancy (G. *pseudēs*, false; L. *praegnans*, pregnant). False pregnancy.

pseudoprō·tein (G. *pseudēs*, false; *prōtos*, first). A protein that lacks one or more of the essential amino-acids.

pseudop·sia (G. *pseudēs*, false; *opsis*, vision). False vision.

pseu·doptery̆·gium (G. *pseudēs*, false; *pterugion*, dim. of *pterux*, a wing). False pterygium.

pseudoptō·sis (G. *pseudēs*, false; *ptōsis*, a falling). Narrowing of the palpebral aperture.

pseudorā·bies (G. *pseudēs*, false; L. *rabies*, rage). A disease resembling hydrophobia.

pseudo-reaction (G. *pseudēs*, false; L. *reagere*, to react). A false or deceptive reaction. A skin reaction in an intradermal test that is due not to the specific protein used but to the protein of the medium employed in producing the toxin.

pseudo-reduction. See synapsis (1).

pseudosclerō·sis (G. *pseudēs*, false; *sklēros*, hard). A form of hepato-lenticular degeneration, *q.v.*, in which a coarse tremor is present, first of the limbs, later of the whole body, in addition to the syndrome of progressive lenticular degeneration, *q.v.*

pseu·do-smallpox (G. *pseudēs*, false). Alastrim.

pseudos·mia (G. *pseudēs*, false; *osmē*, a smell). Delusions of the sense of smell.

pseudo-tū·mour (G. *pseudēs*, false; L. *tumor*, tumour). 1. A phantom tumour. 2. A temporary swelling, generally of inflammatory origin. **P.-t. cerebri:** a condition resembling clinically that of cerebral tumour, usually due to cerebral oedema.

pseudoty̆·phoid (G. *pseudēs*, false; *tuphos*, stupor; *eidos*, form). False typhoid fever.

pseudoxan·thine (G. *pseudēs*, false; *xanthos*, yellow). 1. A leucomaine isolated from fresh beef. 2. A compound isomeric with xanthine, obtained from uric acid.

pseudoxanthō·ma (G. *pseudēs*, false; *xanthos*, yellow). A rare chronic familial disease of the skin characterized by the eruption of raised yellowish plaques, which usually appear on special parts of the skin, e.g., lower abdomen, axilla, sides of the neck. Sometimes seen in association with angioid streaks of the fundus.

psilō·sis (G. *psilos*, bare). Depilation. **P. of intestines:** sprue.

psittacō·sis (G. *psittakos*, parrot). A virus disease of birds, especially parrots, transmissible to man, in whom it runs the course of a severe typhoid fever without abdominal symptoms, but with pulmonary disturbances resembling pneumonia.

psō·as (G. *psoa*, loin muscle). Either of the loin muscles, p. magnus and p. parvus.

psō·dymus (G. *psoa*, loin muscle; *didumos*, twin). A monster with two heads and trunks joined to a single lower part.

pso·ra (G., itch). 1. Scabies. 2. Psoriasis.

psori·asis (G. *psōra*, itch). A chronic, usually relapsing, disease of the skin, affecting especially the extensor surfaces of the limbs and the lumbar region, but also face, scalp, nails, etc.; characterized by proliferation and oedema of the epidermis, mainly of the prickle cells, inflammation and elongation of the papillae in the corium, leading to the development of red, scaly macules or papules, which on spreading form well-defined red patches covered by silvery scales which, scratched off, leave a bright red area dotted over with punctate haemorrhages.

psoriă·tic (G. *psōra*, itch). Affected with or relating to psoriasis.

Psorŏ·phora. A genus of mosquitoes.

psorophthal·mia (G. *psōra*, itch; *ophthalmos*, eye). Ulcerative marginal blepharitis.

psō·rosperm (G. *psōra*, itch; *sperma*, seed). A single-celled micro-organism belonging to the Protozoa.

psō·rospermī·asis (G. *psōra*, itch; *sperma*, seed). A morbid condition caused by the presence of psorosperms.

psorospermō·sis. Psorospermiasis, *q.v.* **P. follicularis vegetans:** Darier's disease, *q.v.*, originally thought to be due to psorosperms.

pso·rous (G. *psōra*, itch). Affected with or relating to the itch.

psȳ·chē (G. *psukhē*, soul). The mind.

psychiăt·ric (G. *psukhē*, soul; *iatros*, physician). Pertaining to psychiatry.

psychiăt·rics (G. *psukhē*, soul; *iatros*, physician). Psychiatry, *q.v.*

psychia·trist (G. *psukhe*, soul; *iatros*, physician). One skilled in psychiatry.

psychĭ·atry (G. *psukhē*, soul; *iatros*, physician). The science of mental disease.

psȳ·chic, psȳ·chical (G. *psukhē*, soul). Pertaining to the mind. **P. blindness:** Mind-blindness, *q.v.* **P. secretion:** salivary or gastric secretion associated with activity of certain cortical cells in the brain, due to stimulation of sensory receptors in mouth, eye, etc.

psȳchoană·lysis (G. *psukhē*, soul; *analusis*, analysis). Method in which knowledge of past emotional experiences and facts of mental life is obtained, in order to elucidate mechanism of production of a pathological mental state and act as a guide in treatment.

psȳchoǎ·nalyst. A specialist in the practice of psychoanalysis.

psȳchoasthē·nia (G. *psukhē*, soul; *a*, priv.; *sthenos*, strength). Feeble-mindedness.

psychocor·tical (G. *psukhē*, soul; L. *cortex*, bark or rind). Relating to the cerebral cortex.

psychogen·esis (G. *psukhē*, soul; *genesis*, from *gennan*, to produce). The development of mental characteristics.

psychogē·nia (G. *psukhē*, soul; *gennan*, to produce). Disease due to faulty psychic activity.

psychogen·ic (G. *psukhē*, soul; *gennan*, to produce). Psychic.

psychognō·sis (G. *psukhē*, soul; *gnōsis*, knowledge). Study whereby, through hypnosis or hypnoidal states, complete knowledge of patient's mind may be obtained.

psȳcholǒ·gical. Relating to psychology.

psȳchǒ·logy (G. *psukhē*, soul; *logos*, word). The study of mental processes or individual behaviour. **P., abnormal:** the study of abnormal mental processes or behaviour. **P., individual:** (*a*) the p. of individual differences, (*b*) the psychological theory of Adler, which concerns the individual mode of striving for superiority or achievement.

psychǒ·meter (G. *psukhē*, soul; *metron*, measure). An apparatus used in psychometry.

psychǒ·metry (G. *psukhē*, soul; *metron*, measure). The measurement of the time occupied by mental processes.

psychomō·tor (G. *psukhē*, soul; L. *movēre*, to move). Relating to voluntary movement.

psychoneurō·sis (G. *psukhē*, soul; *neuron*, nerve). A disorder of the psyche, especially of the subconscious mind, but not severe enough to disrupt the whole psyche (as in psychosis). "Insight," i.e. awareness of symptoms, generally remains.

psychǒ·nomy (G. *psukhē*, soul; *nomos*, law). Science of laws of mental activity.

psychoparē·sis (G. *psukhē*, soul; *paresis*, from *parienai*, to slacken). Feeble-mindedness.

psȳ·chopath (G. *psukhē*, soul; *pathos*, disease). A psychopathic individual.

psychopǎ·thia. Psychopathy, *q.v.*

psychopǎ·thic (G. *psukhē*, soul; *pathos*, disease). Relating to disease of the mind.

psȳ·chopathǒ·logy (G. *psukhē*, soul; *pathos*, disease; *logos*, treatise). The pathology of psychoneuroses and psychoses.

psychǒ·pathy (G. *psukhē*, soul; *pathos*, disease). Any mental disease.

psychoplē·gia (G. *psukhē*, soul; *plēgē*, a stroke). Mind weakness of sudden onset.

psychoplē·gic (G. *psukhē*, soul; *plēgē*, a stroke). 1. Relating to psychoplegia. 2. A drug which acts by an elective affinity for the grey matter of the brain, lessening its excitability and suppressing its receptivity.

psychǒ·sin (G. *psukhē*, soul). A cerebroside found in brain tissue.

psychǒ·sis (G. *psukhē*, soul). A disease of the mind, especially one without any observable organic lesion; generally applied to the more severe forms of mental derangement, in which the patient has no "insight," i.e. awareness of symptoms.

psychosomat·ic (G. *psukhē*, soul; *soma*, body). Descriptive of a mind-body relationship. Bodily symptoms are produced by a psychic, emotional, or mental reaction.

psychotherapeu·tic (G. *psukhē*, soul; *therapōn*, an attendant). Relating to psychotherapy.

psychothě·rapy (G. *psukhē*, soul; *therapeia*, treatment). The treatment of disease by mental factors.

psychot·ic. Relating to or marked by psychosis.

psychro-al·gia (G. *psukhros*, cold; *algos*, pain). A feeling of cold accompanied by pain.

psychrothě·rapy (G. *psukhros*, cold; *therapeia*, treatment). The treatment of disease by the application of cold.

Pt. Abbreviation of pint; symbol for platinum.

ptar·mic (G. *ptarmos*, a sneezing). 1. Relating to the act of sneezing; sternutatory. 2. A material that induces sneezing.

ptē·rion (G. *pteron*, wing). The meeting-point of the frontal, parietal, temporal and sphenoid bones.

pterȳ·gium (G. *pterux*, a wing). A patch of mucous membrane growing on the conjunctiva. The apex of the patch, which tends to grow over the cornea, and which is generally fan-shaped, points towards the pupil, the base towards the canthus of the eye.

ptě·rygoid (G. *pterux*, wing; *eidos*, form). Wing-shaped.

ptě·rygomandǐ·bular (G. *pterux*, wing; L. *mandibula*, jaw). Relating to the pterygoid process and the mandible.

ptě·rygomax·illary (G. *pterux*, wing; L. *maxilla*, jaw). Relating to the pterygoid process and the maxilla.

ptě·rygopǎ·latine (G. *pterux*, wing; L. *palatum*, palate). Relating to the pterygoid plate of the sphenoid bone and the palate bone, as the p. canal.

ptilō·sis (G. *ptilon*, down feathers). Loss of the eyelashes.

ptomaines (G. *ptoma*, carcass). Poisonous amines produced by bacterial decomposition of animal or vegetable proteins.

ptō·sis (G., a falling). 1. Abnormal depression of organs; prolapse. 2. Drooping of the upper eyelid, due to paralysis of the ocular motor nerve.

ptȳǎ·logogue (G. *ptualon*, spittle; *agōgos*, leading). A medicine producing an increased flow of saliva; a sialogogue.

ptȳ·alin (G. *ptualon*, spittle). A diastatic ferment present in saliva, converting starch into dextrin and sugar.

ptȳ·alism (G. *ptualon*, spittle). Excessive salivation.

ptȳǎ·locele (G. *ptualon*, spittle; *kēlē*, tumour). A cyst containing saliva.

ptȳalorrhoe·a (G. *ptualon*, spittle; *rhoia*, a flow). Excessive flow of saliva.

ptȳ·alose (G. *ptualon*, spittle). A sugar obtained from saliva; the same as maltose.

pū·beral (L. *puber*, adult). Relating to puberty.

pū·bertas (L.). Puberty. **P. praecox:** puberty at an early age.

pū·berty (L. *pubertas*). The period at which the reproductive organs become functional. This is shown in the male by a change of voice and discharge of semen, and in the female by appearance of menstruation.

pū·bēs (L.). 1. The pubic hair or the area covered by it. 2. The pubic bone.

pubes·cence (L. *pubes*, hair at puberty). 1. Downiness. 2. Puberty, or the approach of puberty.

pū·bic (L. *pubes*, hair at puberty). Relating to the pubes. **P. bone:** the os pubis.

pubiǒ·tomy (L. *pubes*, hair at puberty; G. *tomē*, a cutting). The operation of dividing the pubic bone.

pū·bis (L.). The pubic bone.

pubofě·moral (L. *pubes*, hair at puberty; *femur*, the thigh). Relating to the os pubis and the femur.

pubotǐ·bial (L. *pubes*, hair at puberty; *tibia*, shin). Relating to the os pubis and the tibia.

pubovesi·cal (L. *pubes*, hair at puberty; *vesica*, bladder). Relating to the os pubis and the bladder.

puden·da (L. *pudere*, to feel shame). Plural of pudendum, *q.v.*

pudendă·gra (L. *pudere*, to feel shame; G. *agra*, seizure). Pain in the reproductive organs. **P. pruriens:** pruritus vulvae.

puden·dal (L. *pudere*, to feel shame). Relating to the pudenda.

puden·dum (L. *pudere*, to feel shame). The external reproductive organs, especially of the female. **P. muliebre:** the vulva.

pū·dic (L. *pudere*, to feel shame). Relating to the pudenda.

puĕ·riculture (L. *puer*, boy; *cultura*, cultivation). The care of children and of the potential mother.

pū·erile (L. *puer*, boy). Relating to childhood; trivial.

puer·pera (L. *puer*, boy; *parere*, to bear). A woman in labour or one recently delivered of the infant.

puer·peral (L. *puer*, boy; *parere*, to bear). Relating to or caused by childbirth, as p. convulsions, p. insanity. **P. fever:** an acute febrile disease of women in childbed, generally due to the *Streptococcus haemolyticus*. **P. insanity:** insanity occurring during the puerperium, generally within five or ten days after delivery.

puer·perant (L. *puer*, boy; *parere*, to bear). A woman in the puerperium.

puerpe·rium (L. *puer*, boy; *parere*, to bear). The condition of being in labour or recently delivered.

puf·finess. Swelling of the tissues.

puking. Vomiting. **P. fever:** milk-sickness.

pū·lex (L. flea). A genus of insects parasitic on the skin of men and animals. **P. irritans:** the common flea.

pū·licide (L. *pulex*, flea; *caedere*, to kill). Any flea-destroying agent.

Pullulă·ria. A genus of fungi.

pullulă·tion (L. *pullulare*, to sprout). The act of sprouting or budding, a reproductive method of some plants.

pul·mo (L.). Lung.

pulmo-aor·tic (L. *pulmo*, lung; G. *aorta*). Relating to the lungs and aorta.

pul·molith (L. *pulmo*, lung; G. *lithos*, stone). A calculus in a lung.

pulmŏ·meter (L. *pulmo*, lung; G. *metron*, measure). An instrument for measuring the volume of the lungs; a spirometer.

pulmŏ·metry (L. *pulmo*, lung; G. *metron*, measure). The estimation of the volume of the lungs.

pul·monary (L. *pulmo*, lung). Relating to or affecting the lungs; e.g. p. arteries, p. tuberculosis.

pulmonec·tomy (L. *pulmo*, lung; G. *ektomē*, excision). Pneumonectomy, *q.v.*

pulmon·ic (L. *pulmo*, lung). 1. Relating to the lungs; pulmonary. 2. Relating to the pulmonary artery, as p. valves.

pulmoni·tis (L. *pulmo*, lung). Syn. of pneumonia.

pulp. The fleshy part of animal or vegetable tissue.

pulpefac·tion (L. *pulpa*, pulp; *facere*, to make). Conversion into pulp.

pulpī·tis (L. *pulpa*, pulp). Inflammation of the dental pulp.

pulpy. Pulp-like.

pulsate (L. *pulsare*, to beat). To beat or throb rhythmically.

pul·satile (L. *pulsare*, to beat). Pulsating.

Pulsatil·la. The flowering herb, *Anemone pulsatilla*, one of the ranunculaceae. From it are obtained anemonia and anemonic acid. It may cause vomiting, it is alterative and depressant, and is used in inflammation.

pulsā·tion (L. *pulsare*, to beat). A beating or throbbing.

pulse (L. *pulsus*, a stroke). The rhythmic throbbing of the arteries caused by the expansion and contraction of the heart. The pulse is generally taken at the wrist (p. radialis) but may be counted at the temporal, brachial, femoral and other arteries. **P. pressure:** the variation in blood pressure occurring in an artery during the cardiac cycle; it is the difference between systolic and diastolic pressure.

pulsĭ·meter (L. *pulsus*, a stroke; G. *metron*, measure). An instrument used for measuring the force or rate of the pulse.

pul·sus (L.). Pulse. **P. alternans:** a condition characterized by alternate differences in pulse pressure, usually a sign of a severe myocardial lesion.

pultă·ceous (L. *puls*, pottage). Pulpy or mushy.

pulverizā·tion (L. *pulvis*, powder). The reduction of a solid to powder.

pulvĕ·rulent (L. *pulvis*, powder). Resembling powder.

pulvī·nar (L. a couch). The posterior tubercle of the optic thalamus.

pul·vis (L.). A powder.

pū·mĭce. The lava from volcanoes.

pump. An apparatus for drawing up a liquid or gas. **P., air-:** one used to draw air out of a container or to force more air into one already air-filled. **P., breast-:** a pump for the removal of milk from the breast. **P., dental:** one for removing saliva during dentistry. **P., stomach-:** one for removing stomach contents, as in cases of poisoning.

punctate (L. *pungere*, to perforate). Dotted; having numerous dots or punctures.

punctum (L.). A point, or small aperture as the opening of sebaceous gland, or lacrimal canaliculus.

puncture (L. *punctum*, point). A piercing with a pointed implement. **P., lumbar:** puncture of the spinal canal in order to withdraw cerebrospinal fluid.

pungent (L. *pungere*, to perforate). Biting or acrid.

P.U.O. Abbreviation for pyrexia of unknown origin.

pupa (L. doll). The second stage of insect development. It follows that of the larva.

pupil (L. *pupilla*, pupil of the eye). The opening in the iris of the eye to allow the passage of light. **P., artificial:** the aperture made by iridectomy. **P., cat's eye:** a narrow slit-like p. **P., pinhole:** one which is extremely miotic.

pūpil·lary (L. *pupilla*, pupil of the eye). Relating to the pupil.

pupillŏ·meter (L. *pupilla*, pupil of the eye; G. *metron*, measure). An instrument for measuring the pupil.

pupil·lostatŏ·meter (L. *pupilla*, pupil of the eye; G. *statos*, standing; *metron*, measure). An instrument for determining the precise distance between the centres of the two pupils.

pure (L. *purus*, clean). Unstained; unalloyed.

purgā·tion (L. *purgare*, to purge). Bowel evacuation produced by the administration of purgatives.

pur·gative (L. *purgare*, to purge). 1. Cathartic. 2. A purge, *q.v.*

purge (L. *purgare*, to purge). 1. To cause the evacuation of the bowels. 2. An agent that produces bowel evacuation.

pū·riform (L. *pus*, pus; *forma*, shape). Resembling pus; having the nature of pus.

purinae·mia (purine; G. *haima*, blood). A condition characterized by the presence of purine bases in the blood.

pū·rinase. An enzyme which brings about changes such as oxidation and deamination in purines.

pu·rine. A heterocyclic compound.

$$\begin{array}{c} \text{N} = \text{CH} \\ \quad | \qquad | \\ \text{CH} \quad \text{C} - \text{NH} \\ \quad \| \qquad \| \qquad \text{CH} \\ \text{N} - \text{C} - \text{N} \end{array}$$

It is not itself found naturally, but is the basic structure of a group of substances known as the purine bodies; e.g. uric acid, xanthine, hypoxanthine, adenine and guanine. Theobromine, caffeine and theophylline are derivatives of xanthine.

Purkinje's cells (Purkinje, J. E. von, Bohemian anatomist, 1787–1869). Large pyriform nerve-cells, with many dendrites, found in the cortex of the cerebellum. **P.'s corpuscles:** the lacunae of bone. **P.'s fibres:** the muscular fibres beneath the endocardium. **P.'s figures:** the dark lines on a yellow background observed when a candle is held a little way away from the eye in a darkened room. They are produced by the retinal vessels. **P.'s granular layer:** Czermak's interglobular spaces, *q.v.* **P.'s images:** three images of a candle-flame obtained by reflection from the cornea and the anterior and posterior surfaces of the crystalline lens, the third image being inverted. **P.'s network:** the network of beaded fibres (P.'s fibres) visible to the naked eye in the subendocardial tissue of the ventricles. **P.'s vesicle:** the nucleus of the ovum.

Purkinje-Sanson's images. Purkinje's images, *q.v.*

pur·pura (G. *porphura*, purple dye). A disease characterized by the presence on the skin of purple patches produced by subcutaneous haemorrhages. It may occur independently or be symptomatic of other diseases. **P., anaphylactoid:** p. precipitated by injection of foreign substances. **P. haemorrhagica:** a severe form with diminution of the blood platelets. **P. rheumatica:** p. characterized by pain in the joints. Syn. Schönlein's disease. **P. simplex:** p. with slight symptoms, the haemorrhages being confined to the skin. See also Henoch's p.

purpū·ric (G. *porphura*, purple dye). Relating to purpura.

pur·purin. 1:2:4-trihydroxyanthraquinone, a substance found with alizarin in the madder root.

pū·rulence, pū·rulency (L. *purulentus*, festering). The state of suppuration.

pū·rulent. Of the nature of or containing pus; marked by the formation of pus.

pu·ruloid (L. *pus*; G. *eidos*, form). Resembling pus.

pus (L.). A liquid consisting of cells and a greenish-creamy albuminous fluid, seen in certain types of inflammation.

pus·tula malig·na (L.). Anthrax.

pus·tulent (L. *pustula*, from *pus*). 1. Causing pustules to form. 2. An agent causing the formation of pustules.

pus·tular. Characterized by the formation of pustules.

pustula·tion. The formation of pustules.

pus·tule (L. *pustula*, from *pus*). A small elevation of the skin containing pus. **P., malignant:** anthrax.

pus·tulocrustā·ceous (L. *pustula*, from *pus*; *crusta*, rind). Marked by the formation of pustules and scabs.

putā·men (L.). The lateral part of the lenticular nucleus.

putrefac·tion (L. *putrefacere*, to cause to rot). The decomposing of animal or vegetable substance, caused in general by the action of micro-organisms. Unpleasant odours arise, due to the production of ammonia, hydrogen sulphide and other gases. Ptomaines and numerous other compounds are also formed. The end-products are water, amino-acids, nitrogen, methane and carbon dioxide.

putrefac·tive. Relating to or producing putrefaction.

pū·trefy. To make or become putrid.

putres·cence (L. *putrescere*, to rot). The condition of putrefaction.

putres·cent (L. *putrescere*, to rot). Rotting.

putres·cine. $H_2N(CH_2)_4.NH_2$-tetramethylene diamine, found with cadaverine or pentamethylene diamine in decomposing proteins and numerous bacilli and moulds. They are called ptomaines and are deadly poisons.

pū·trid (L. *putridus*). Rotten. **P. fever:** Typhus, *q.v.*

putty, Horsley's. See under Horsley.

P. wave. Term applied to the electrocardiographic wave associated with the auricular systole.

Px. Abbreviation for pneumothorax.

pyae·mia (G. *puon*, pus; *haima*, blood). Pyogenic organisms in the bloodstream.

pyarthrō·sis (G. *puon*, pus; *arthron*, joint). Suppuration within a joint.

pycnocar·dia (G. *puknos*, frequent; *kardia*, heart). Tachycardia, *q.v.*

pyc·nolepsy (G. *puknos*, frequent; *lēpsis*, from *lambanein*, to seize). Very frequently recurring epileptiform attacks resembling *petit mal* in children.

pycnophrā·sis (G. *puknos*, thick; *phrasis*, speech). Thickness of speech.

pycnō·sis (G. *puknos*, thick). 1. Thickening. 2. A type of cell degeneration in which the nucleus shrinks thus causing condensation of the protoplasm.

pycnot·ic. Relating to pycnosis.

pyelec·tasis (G. *puĕlos*, a trough; *ektasis*, extension). Dilatation of the pelvis of the kidney.

pyĕl·ic (G. *puĕlos*, a trough). Relating to the renal pelvis.

pyelit·ic. Relating to pyelitis.

pyelī·tis (G. *puĕlos*, a trough). Inflammation of the pelvis of the kidney.

py·elocysti·tis (G. *puelos*, a trough; *kustis*, bladder). Pyelitis accompanied by cystitis.

pyelŏ·graphy (G. *puĕlos*, a trough; *graphein*, to write). Skiagraphy of a kidney and ureter after filling them with a silver salt solution. **P., intravenous:** the radiogram is of a contrast substance which has been injected intravenously and is excreted by the kidney.

py·elolithŏ·tomy (G. *puĕlos*, a trough; *lithos*, stone; *tomē*, a cutting). Removal of stone from renal pelvis.

py·elonephrī·tis (G. *puĕlos*, a trough; *nephros*, kidney). Pyelitis and nephritis combined.

py·elonephrō·sis (G. *puĕlos*, a trough; *nephros*, kidney). Any diseased condition of the kidney and its pelvis.

pyelŏ·pathy (G. *puelos*, a trough; *pathos*, disease). Any disease of the pelvis of the kidney.

pyelŏ·tomy (G. *puelos*, a trough; *tomē*, a cutting). Incision of the renal pelvis.

pyē·sis (G. *puon*, pus). Suppuration.

py·gal (G. *pugē*, rump). Relating to the buttocks.

pygodi·dymus (G. *pugē*, rump; *didumos*, twin). A double monster joined at the buttocks.

pygŏ·melus (G. *pugē*, rump; *melos*, limb). A monster with a parasite attached to the buttock or to the region of the buttocks.

pygŏ·pagus (G. *pugē*, rump; *pagos*, anything fixed). A double monster united at the buttocks or backs.

pyk·nic (G. *puknos*, thick). Of a short and stocky build.

py·la (G. *pulē*, gate). The passage between the third ventricle and the Sylvian aqueduct.

py·lephlebec·tasis (G. *pulē*, gate; *phleps*, vein; *ektasis*, extension). Dilatation of the portal vein.

py·lephlebi·tis (G. *pulē*, gate; *phleps*, vein). Inflammation of the portal vein; the condition is ordinarily secondary to disease of the stomach.

pylethrom·bophlebī·tis (G. *pulē*, gate; *thrombos*, a clot; *phleps*, vein). Inflammation and thrombosis of the portal vein.

py·lethrombō·sis (G. *pulē*, gate; *thrombos*, a clot). Thrombosis of the portal vein.

py·lic (G. *pulē*, gate). Relating to the portal vein.

py·lon (G. *pulōn*, a gateway). An artificial leg.

pylorec·tomy (G. *pulōros*, pylorus; *ektomē*, excision). Surgical removal of the pylorus.

pylor·ic. Relating to the pylorus.

pylŏ·roplasty (G. *pulōrus*, pylorus; *plassein*, to form). Plastic surgery of the pylorus.

pylorŏ·scopy (G. *pulōrus*, pylorus; *skopein*, to inspect). Examination of the pylorus.

pylŏ·rospasm (G. *pulōros*, pylorus; *spasmos*, spasm). Pyloric spasm.

pylorostenŏ·sis (G. *pulōrus*, pylorus; *stenos*, marrow). Stricture of the pylorus.

pylorŏ·stomy (G. *pulōrus*, pylorus; *stoma*, mouth). Formation of an opening through the abdominal wall into the pyloric end of the stomach.

pylorŏ·tomy (G. *pulōrus*, pylorus; *tomē*, a cutting). Incision into the pylorus.

pylor·us (G. *pulōros*, pylorus). The opening of the stomach into the duodenum. It is marked by a thickening of the circular muscle coat in this region.

pyocol·pocele (G. *puon*, pus; *kolpos*, gulf; *kēlē*, tumour). A pus-containing tumour of the vagina.

pyocol·pos (G. *puon*, pus; *kolpos*, gulf). The presence of pus within the vagina.

pyoc·tanin. Pyoktanin, *q.v.*

pyocȳ·anin (G. *puon*, pus; *kuanos*, blue). A blue phenazin pigment found in *B. pyocyaneus*.

pȳ·ocyst (G. *puon*, pus; *kustis*, bladder). Any pus-containing cyst.

pȳ·ocyte (G. *puon*, pus; *kutos*, a container). A pus corpuscle.

pyodermatŏ·sis (G. *puon*, pus; *derma*, skin). Any pyogenic skin affection.

pyodermī·tis (G. *puon*, pus; *derma*, skin). Any inflammatory and pustular skin affection.

pyogĕ·nesis (G. *puon*, pus; *genesis*, from *gennan*, to produce). Pus formation.

pyogen·ic (G. *puon*, pus; *gennan*, to produce). Producing pus. **P. micro-organism:** any pus-producing micro-organism.

pyohae·mia. Pyaemia, *q.v.*

pȳ·ohaemothor·ax (G. *puon*, pus; *haima*, blood; *thōrax*, chest). The presence of blood and pus in the pleural cavity.

pȳ·oid (G. *puon*, pus; *eidos*, form). Resembling pus.

pyok·tanin (G. *puon*, pus; *kteinein*, to kill). A name applied to methyl-violet and crystal-violet by reason of their germicidal properties. P. is used as a skin disinfectant and as a local application for blepharitis.

pyomē·tra, pyomētrium (G. *puon*, pus; *mētra*, womb). An accumulation of pus in the uterus.

pyonephrī·tis (G. *puon*, pus; *nephros*, kidney). Inflammation of the kidney accompanied by the formation of pus.

pȳ·onephrolithi·asis (G. *puon*, pus; *nephros*, kidney; *lithos*, stone). The presence of pus and stones in the kidney.

pyonephrŏ·sis (G. *puon*, pus; *nephros*, kidney). A collection of pus in the renal pelvis.

pyonephrot·ic. Characterized by pyonephrosis.

pyo-ovā·rium (G. *puon*, pus; mod. L. *ovarium*, from *ovum*, egg). An abscess in an ovary.

pȳ·opericardī·tis (G. *puon*, pus; *peri*, around; *kardia*, heart). Pericarditis, accompanied by suppuration.

pȳ·opericar·dium (G. *puon*, pus; *peri*, around; *kardia*, heart). An accumulation of pus in the pericardium.

pȳ·operitonē·um (G. *puon*, pus; *peritonaion*, peritoneum). A collection of pus in the peritoneal cavity.

pyophā·gia (G. *puon*, pus; *phagein*, to eat). The swallowing of pus.

pyophthal·mia (G. *puon*, pus; *ophthalmos*, eye). Suppurative inflammation of the eye.

pyophylac·tic (G. *puon*, pus; *phulax*, guard). Aimed at avoiding suppurative disease; description of any drug or treatment which acts in this way.

pȳ·opneu·mopericardī·tis (G. *puon*, pus; *pneumon*, lung; *peri*, around; *kardia*, heart). Pericarditis accompanied by pus and gas collections in the pericardium.

pȳ·opneu·mopericar·dium (G. *puon*, pus; *pneumon*, lung; *peri*, around; *kardia*, heart). The presence of pus and air or gas in the pericardium.

pȳ·opneu·moperitonē·um (G. *puon*, pus; *pneumon*, lung; *peritonaion*, peritoneum). An accumulation of pus and air in the peritoneal cavity.

pȳ·opneu·moperitonī·tis (G. *puon*, pus; *pneumon*, lung; *peritonaion*, peritoneum). Peritonitis accompanied by pus and air in the peritoneal cavity.

pȳ·opneumothor·ax (G. *puon*, pus; *pneumon*, lung; *thōrax*, chest). A collection of air or gas and pus in the pleural cavity.

pȳ·opoiē·sis (G. *puon*, pus; *poiēsis*, from *poiein*, to make). Suppuration.

pyorrhoe·a (G. *puon*, pus; *rhoia*, a flowing). A discharge of pus. **P. alveolaris:** inflammation of the dental periosteum accompanied by necrosis of the dental alveoli. The condition is a progressive one.

pyorrhoe·al. Relating to pyorrhoea.

pȳ·osalpingi·tis (G. *puon*, pus; *salpigx*, trumpet). Purulent inflammation of the uterine or pharyngotympanic tube.

pyosal·pinx (G. *puon*, pus; *salpigx*, trumpet). The presence of pus in an oviduct.

pȳ·osapraē·mia (G. *puon*, pus; *sapros*, rotten; *haima*, blood). Suppurative infection of the blood.

pyosclerŏ·sis (G. *puon*, pus; *sklēros*, hard). Suppurative sclerosis.

pȳ·osepticaē·mia (G. *puon*, pus; *sēptos*, rotten; *haima*, blood). Pyaemia and septicaemia combined.

pyostat·ic (G. *puon*, pus; *statikos*, causing to stand). 1. Preventing the formation of pus. 2. Any agent capable of inhibiting pus formation.

pyothor·ax (G. *puon*, pus; *thōrax*, chest). A collection of pus in the pleural cavity; empyema. **P., subphrenic:** an abscess underneath the diaphragm.

pyo-ū·reter (G. *puon*, pus; *ourētēr*, ureter). A collection of pus in the ureter.

pȳ·ramid (G. *puramis*). An elevation on the ventral surface of the medulla oblongata produced by the pyramidal tract.

pyră·midal (G. *puramis*, pyramid). Resembling or formed like a pyramid. **P. bone:** the carpal cuneiform bone.

pyramidā·lis muscle (G. *puramis*, pyramid). A small muscle at the lower end of the abdominal wall.

pyrenae·mia (G. *purēn*, fruit stone; *haima*, blood). The presence of nucleated erythrocytes in the blood.

pȳ·rene. A polycyclic hydrocarbon.

pyre·thrine. Syn. Pellitorine. The active principle from *Anacyclus pyrethrum*; a sialagogue and astringent.

pyrē·thrum. The dried flower heads of *Chrysanthemum cineriaefolium*, the active constituents of which are pyrethrin I and II. An insecticide.

pyret·ic (G. *puretos*, fever). Relating to fever.

pȳ·retotyphō·sis (G. *puretos*, fever; *tuphos*, stupor). Fever delirium.

pȳ·retotypō·sis (G. *puretos*, fever; *tupos*, form or type). Fever of intermittent character.

pyrex·ia (G. *puressein*, to be feverish). The rise of the body temperature above the normal level; fever.

pyrex·ial (G. *puressein*, to be feverish). Relating to pyrexia.

pȳ·ridine (G. *pur*, fire). C_5H_5N. A coal tar base.

pyridox·ine. Vitamin B_6. Syn. adermin.

pȳ·riform (L. *pirum* or *pyrum*, pear; *forma*, shape). Pear-shaped.

pyrifor·mis muscle. An intrapelvic muscle with an extrapelvic tendon which is attached to the upper end of the femur.

pyri·midine. A nitrogenous base.

pyrobor·ate. A salt of pyroboric acid.

pyrobŏ·ric acid. A dibasic acid obtained by heating boric acid.

pyrogal·lic acid. 1:2:3-trihydroxybenzene, obtained from gallic acid. Syn. Pyrogallol.

pȳ·rogen (G. *pur*, fire; *gennan*, to produce). Any fever-producing agent.

pyrogen·ic (G. *pur*, fire; *gennan*, to produce). Producing fever.

pyrolig·neous (G. *pur*, fire; L. *lignum*, wood). Relating to the destructive distillation of wood. **P. acid:** wood vinegar.

pyromā·nia (G. *pur*, fire; *mania*, madness). A condition characterized by a recurring impulse to set fire to buildings, etc.

pyrŏ·meter (G. *pur*, fire; *metron*, measure). An instrument for measuring the intensity of heat that is beyond the range of an ordinary thermometer.

pyrophŏ·bia (G. *pur*, fire; *phobos*, fear). A neurotic fear of fire.

pyrŏ·phorus (G. *pur*, fire; *pherein*, to bear). A compound which ignites spontaneously when exposed to air.

pyrophos·phate (G. *pur*, fire; *phōs*, light; *pherein*, to bear). A salt of pyrophosphoric acid.

pyrophosphor·ic acid. An acid formed by the elimination of water on heating two molecules of phosphoric acid to a high temperature.

pyrŏ·sis (G. *pur*, fire). Heartburn.

pyrot·ic (G. *pur*, fire). Caustic or inflammable.

pyrox·ilin. A nitrated cellulose used in preparing collodion.

pyr·role. A five-membered nitrogenous heterocyclic compound which is of importance as a fission product of the porphyrins, e.g. haemin, chlorophyll.

pyrū·vic acid (G. *pur*, fire). $CH_3.CO.COOH$. An intermediate product in the decomposition of sugars during fermentation. Its salts are known as pyruvates.

pythogĕ·nesis (G. *puthein*, to rot; *genesis*, from *gennan*, to produce). Production from decaying matter.

pyū·ria (G. *puon*, pus; *ouron*, urine). The presence of pus in the urine.

Q

q.d. Abbreviation for L. *quater in die*, 'four times daily'.

q.h. Abbreviation for L. *quaque hora*, 'every hour'.

q.2h. Abbreviation for L. *quaque secunda hora*, 'every second hour'.

q.3h. Abbreviation for L. *quaque tertia hora*, 'every third hour'.

q.l. Abbreviation for L. *quantum libet*, 'as much as may be desired'.

q.p. Abbreviation for L. *quantum placet*, 'as much as you please'.

q.s. Abbreviation for L. *quantum sufficit*, 'as much as suffices'.

quack. A medical charlatan.

quackery. The practice of medical charlatanism.

quacksalver. A pedlar of nostrums.

quadrang·ular (L. *quadrangulum*). Having four angles.

quad·rant (L. *quadrans*, quarter). 1. A quarter of a circle, subtending an angle of 90°. 2. Any of the quarters or areas into which the abdomen may be divided for diagnostic purposes.

quad·rate (L. *quadratus*, squared). Square; four-sided. Q. lobe: the part of the right lobe of the liver between the ligamentum teres on the left side, the gall-bladder on the right side and the porta hepatis posteriorly.

quadrā·tus (L., squared). Four-sided; squared. See also muscles.

quadribā·sic (L. *quattuor*, four; G. *basis*, base). Having four atoms of hydrogen that are replaceable.

quad·riceps (L. *quattuor*, four; *caput*, head). Four-headed, See also muscles.

quadrigĕ·mina (L. *quadrigeminus*, fourfold). The corpora quadrigemina.

quadrigĕ·minal (L. *quadrigeminus*, fourfold). Fourfold; having four parts.

quadrigĕ·minum (L. *quadrigeminus*, fourfold). Any one of the corpora quadrigemina.

quadrilă·teral (L. *quattuor*, four; *latus*, side). Four-sided.

quadrilŏ·cular (L. *quattuor*, four; *loculus*, a little space). Having four cells.

quadri·para (L. *quattuor*, four; *parere*, to bear). A woman who has borne her fourth child, or is having her fourth confinement.

quadri·parous. Relating to a quadripara or to a fourth confinement.

quadripar·tite (L. *quattuor*, four; *partire*, to divide). Divided into four.

quadriplĕ·gia (L. *quattuor*, four; G. *plēgē*, a stroke). Paralysis of all four limbs.

quadripō·lar (L. *quattuor*, four; G. *polos*, pole). Having four poles.

quad·risect (L. *quattuor*, four; *secare*, to cut). To section into four parts.

quadriū·rate (L. *quattuor*, four; G. *ouron*, urine). Any hyperacid urate of human urine.

quadri·valent (L. *quattuor*, four; *valēre*, to be worth). In chemistry, having a combining power of four.

quadroon (Sp. *cuarterón*). The offspring of one white and one mulatto parent.

quad·ruped (L. *quattuor*, four; *pes*, foot). A four-footed animal.

quad·ruplet (L. *quadruplus*, fourfold). Any one of four children born at a single birth.

Quain's fatty heart (Quain, Sir R., English physician, 1816–98). Fatty degeneration of the heart muscle fibres.

qual·itative (L. *qualis*, of what kind). Relating to quality.

quan·titative. Relating to quantity.

quan·tity (L. *quantitas*, quantity). Any amount.

quantivā·lence (L. *quantus*, how much; *valēre*, to be worth). The combining power of an element stated in terms of the number of hydrogen atoms with which it will unite.

quan·tum (L., pl. *quanta*). 1. As much as. 2. A stated amount. 3. The smallest unit or ultimate finite quantity of radiation.

quar·antine (Ital. *quaranta*, forty). 1. The time (generally 40 days) during which travellers from infected ports are legally required to be segregated in order to prevent the spread of disease. 2. The place where travellers from suspect ports are detained. 3. The act of detaining ships or travellers for the purpose of examination or disinfection.

quart (L. *quartus*, fourth). One fourth of a gallon.

quar·tan (L. *quartanus*, relating to one-fourth). 1. Recurring every four days. 2. A type of intermittent fever the attacks of which recur every fourth day.

quarter evil. A synonym for symptomatic anthrax.

quarti·para (L. *quartus*, fourth; *parere*, to bear). A woman pregnant for the fourth time, or one who has borne four children.

quarti·parous. Four times pregnant.

quartz. The dioxide of silica.

quassā·tion (L. *quassatio*, a shaking). The reduction of roots and other materials to small fragments before submitting them to further pharmaceutical preparation.

Quas·sia (named from Quassi, a negro slave, who first used the material). The dried stem wood of *Picroena excelsa*, which contains a bitter principle, picrasmin. Surinam quassia from *Quassia amara* (Linn.) contains quassin and neo-quassin, both being used as bitters.

quater·nary (L. *quaterni*, four at a time). Having four elements.

Quatrefages's angle (Quatrefages de Bréau, J. L. A., French anthropologist, 1810–92). The parietal angle employed in craniotomy.

Queckenstedt's sign (Queckenstedt, H., German physician, died 1918). Pressure on one or both internal jugular veins causes rapid rise in c.s.f. pressure of healthy persons, and this falls rapidly on release of the veins. When there is a block in vertebral canal the pressure of the c.s.f. is affected only slightly or not at all.

Queensland fever. An acute febrile disease caused by *Rickettsia burneti*.

Quénu's haemorrhoidal plexus (Quénu, E. A. V. A., French surgeon, 1852–1933). A series of lymphatic plexuses (inferior and middle) in the mucous membrane and skin of the anus.

Quénu-Mayo operation (Quénu, E. A. V. A., French surgeon; Mayo, W. J., American surgeon, 1861–1939). Excision of the rectum and anal canal with their lymphatics for cancer.

Queyrat's erythroplasia (Queyrat, A., French dermatologist, born 1872). Red patches found on penis, labia, mouth, or arms, which are painful and tend to become malignant.

quick. 1. A sensitive part, such as the flesh beneath a nail. 2. Pregnant and feeling the movements of the foetus.

quickening. The first foetal movement perceived by the pregnant woman. This takes place between the fourth and fifth months of pregnancy.

quicklime. Calcium oxide; caustic lime.

quicksilver. Mercury.

Quillaia, Quillaja (Chilian *quillai*). A genus of trees of the order Rosaceae. The dried bark of *Q. saponaria* (called also soap bark) contains saponin and is used as an expectorant and as a sternutatory.

qui·nacrine hydrochloride. An antimalarial substance.

qui·nate. A salt of quinic acid.

quince. A tree belonging to the order Rosaceae, the seeds of which yield a mucilage which is widely used as a demulcent.

Quincke's capillary pulse (Quincke, H. I., German physician, 1842–1922). A perceptible pulsation in capillaries of nail bed, with alternating flushing and blanching, due to aortic insufficiency.

quin·ic (Peruv. *kina*). Relating to quinine. **Q. acid:** an acid found in cinchona bark, and in the bark of several other trees including oaks and elms. **Q. fever:** fever accompanied by skin eruptions, occurring among makers of quinine.

quin·icine. A bitter alkaloid obtained from cinchona.

quinidă·mine. $C_{19}H_{24}N_2O_2$ an alkaloid obtained from cinchona.

quin·idine (Peruv. *kina*). An alkaloid of cinchona bark. It is isomeric with quinine, which it resembles in taste. It is used in the treatment of cardiac arrhythmias.

quinine (Peruv. *kina*). A bitter, amorphous or crystalline alkaloid, obtained from cinchona bark. It is used internally as a bitter stomachic and as a tonic in cases of debility. Although synthetic substances, such as Mepacrine, are now displacing it in the treatment of malaria, it is still used for this purpose. Large doses of quinine produce toxic effects; very large doses can cause death.

quin·ol (Peruv. *kina*). 1:4-dihydroxybenzene $HO.C_6H_4.OH$. A powerful reducing agent used in photographic developers. Syn. hydroquinone.

quin·oline (Peruv. *kina*). A coal-tar base, C_9H_7N, the basic structure of which is found in many different classes of substance, e.g. alkaloids, dyestuffs.

quinqui·valent (L. *quinque*, five; *valēre*, to be worth). Having a valency of five; able to combine with five hydrogen atoms.

quin·sy (G. *kunagkhē*, inflammation of the larynx). Acute tonsillitis, usually with suppuration.

quin·tan (L. *quintus*, fifth). An intermittent fever recurring every five days.

quintes·sence (L. *quintus*, fifth; *essentia*, essence). The strongest concentrated extract of a substance.

quinti·para (L. *quintus*, fifth; *parere*, to bear). A woman who has had five children or is in labour for the fifth time.

quin·tuplet (L. *quintuplex*, fivefold). One of five children born at a single birth.

quiz. 1. Informal answering of questions. 2. To teach by following this method of informal question and answer.

quō·ad vī·tam (gerat) (L.). So long as he lives.

quoti·dian (L. *quotidianus*, daily). 1. Recurring daily. 2. An intermittent fever, recurring each day.

quō·tient (L. *quoties*, how often?). The result of a division sum. **Blood q.:** the amount of haemoglobin in a specimen of blood divided by the number of red cells contained in it. Indicates percentage of haemoglobin in the red cells. **Caloric q.:** the heat evolved in a metabolic process (expressed in calories) divided by the oxygen consumed (expressed in milligrams). **Intelligence q.:** see intelligence. **Protein q.:** the quantity of globulin of the blood plasma divided by the quantity of albumin. **Respiratory q.:** the ratio between volume of carbon dioxide expired and volume of oxygen inspired in a given time.

q.v. Abbreviation for L. (1) *quantum vis*, as much as you wish; (2) *quod vide*, which see.

Q. wave. Term applied to the electrocardiographic wave associated with the contraction of the ventricles.

R

Ra. Chemical symbol of radium.

ră·bid (L. *rabidus*). 1. Affected with rabies or hydrophobia. 2. Relating to rabies.

rā·bies (L. *rabĕre*, to rave). A fatal disease in animals due to a virus, Formidio inexorabilis. It is transmitted to man by direct inoculation such as by the bite of an infected animal. The incubation period is from one to six months. The patient is depressed at the beginning and later passes into tetanic spasms especially increased by drinking or even the sight of water.

RaBr₂. Radium bromide.

race. A genealogic, ethnic or tribal group; hypothetically, a breed or kind of animals or plants with common transmissible characters.

racemose (L. *racemus*, a bunch of grapes). Resembling a bunch of grapes.

rā·diad (L. *radius*; *ad*, to). Towards the radial side.

rā·dial (L. *radius*, ray). 1. Radiating; spreading from a common point, as the rays from the sun. 2. Relating to a radius, or to the radius, the bone in the forearm.

rā·diant (L. *radians*, beaming). To diverge from a common point, or to be arranged in a radiating manner. R. energy: energy which is transmitted in the form of waves from a source of light, heat, or electricity.

radiā·tion (L. *radiare*, to radiate). 1. The act of diverging from a common centre. 2. A structure or process composed of diverging parts. 3. Treatment with radio-active substances.

ră·dical (L. *radix*, root). 1. Belonging to the root or source. 2. A form of treatment, especially an operation, aiming at the eradication of a disease, as in radical mastoid operation. 3. A group of atoms not influenced by entry into and/or exit from chemical combinations, and forming a principal constituent of a molecule.

radi·ciform (L. *radix*, root; *forma*, shape). Root-shaped.

ră·dicle (L. *radicula*, dim. of *radix*, root). 1. The primary root or stem of the embryo. 2. The initial fibril of a nerve; the beginning of a vein.

radicŏ·tomy (L. *radix*, root; G. *tomē*, a cutting). The surgical division of nerve roots.

radi·cula (L.). Radicle, *q.v.*

radi·cular (L. *radicula*, small root). 1. Relating to a radicle. 2. Pertaining to spinal nerve roots.

radiculec·tomy (L. *radicula*, small root; *ektomē*, excision). Surgical removal of nerve roots.

radiculī·tis (L. *radicula*, small root). Inflammation of a nerve-root. The term applies particularly to spinal nerve roots.

radio-active (L. *radius*, ray; *activus*, active). Possessed of the property of radio-activity.

radio-activity. A character of certain substances enabling them to emit spontaneous radiations capable of penetrating materials that cannot be entered by ordinary light rays.

rā·diocar·pal. Relating to the radius and the carpus.

radiochĕ·mistry. The branch of chemistry dealing with radio-active substances and their phenomena.

radio·dermatitis (L. *radius*, ray; G. *derma*, skin). Skin affections produced by exposure to radium rays, or those of other radio-active substances.

rā·dio-diagnō·sis (L. *radius*, ray; G. *dia*, through; *gnosis*, knowledge), Diagnosis by means of radiography.

rā·diodi·gital (L. *radius*, ray; *digitus*, finger). Relating to the radius and the fingers.

radio·element (L. *radius*, ray; *elementum*). Any element possessing radio-active powers.

radiogen·ic (L. *radius*, ray; G. *gennan*, to produce). Produced by radio-active rays.

rā·diograph (L. *radius*, ray; G. *graphein*, to write). 1. An X-ray photograph. 2. To take such a photograph.

radiŏ·grapher (L. *radius*, ray; G. *graphein*, to write). One versed in radiography.

radiŏ·graphy (L. *radius*, ray; G. *graphein*, to write). Photography with X-rays.

rā·dio-hū·meral. Relating to the radius and the humerus.

rādiolŏ·gical. Relating to radiology.

radiŏ·logist. One skilled in the practice of radiology.

radiŏ·logy (L. *radius*, ray; G. *logos*, treatise). 1. The science of radiant energy. 2. The study of radiography and radio-therapeutics.

radi·olus (L. dim. of *radius*, ray). A probe or sound.

rā·dionecrō·sis (L. *radius*, ray; G. *nekros*, corpse). Destruction of tissues caused by exposure to radium rays.

radio-opa·que (L. *radius*, ray; *opacus*, not clear). Does not transmit X-rays.

rā·diophos·phorus (L. *radius*, ray; G. *phos*, light; *pherein*, to bear). Radioactive phosphorus prepared by bombardment of phosphorus by neutrons in a cyclotron.

radio-resistant (L. *radius*, ray; *resistere*, to withstand). Does not respond to irradiation therapy.

rā·diosterĕŏ·scopy (L. *radius*, ray; G. *stereos*, solid; *skopein*, to view). The inspection of the body's internal structures by means of X-rays.

rā·diosur·gery. The surgical use of radium.

rā·diotherapeū·tic (L. *radius*, ray; G. *therapeutikos*, healing). Relating to the therapeutics of radiant energy.

radiotherapeū·tics. Radiotherapy, *q.v.*

rādiothĕ·rapist. One skilled in radiotherapy.

rādiothĕ·rapy (L. *radius*, ray; G. *therapeia*, medical treatment). The treatment of disease by means of X-rays, radium rays, etc.

rā·diothor·ium. A disintegration product of thorium, and has the properties of thorium. Found in pitchblende from Colorado. Gives off thorium X.

radio-ulnar. Relating to the radius and the ulna.

rā·dium (L. *radiare*, to radiate). A rare metal (atomic weight 226) obtained from pitch-blende and first isolated in 1899 by M. and Mme. Curie. A radio-active substance, it undergoes atomic disintegration to yield three types of radiation: 1. Alpha rays (helium atoms which have lost two electrons). 2. Beta rays, composed of electrons. 3. Gamma rays which are short electromagnetic rays similar to X-rays. The half life of radium is 1,600 years: its initial decomposition product being radon or radium emanation. Symbol: Ra.

rā·dius (L.). 1. A ray. 2. The outer of the two forearm bones. 3. A line drawn from the centre to the outer limit of a circle.

ră·dix (L.). 1. A root. 2. Any of the spinal nerve roots.

rage. 1. Violent anger. 2. Any severely painful affection.

ra·don. Symbol: Rn. A gas formed as the initial decomposition product of radium.

ra·ffinose. See melitose.

Rainey's corpuscles (Rainey, G., English anatomist, 1801–84). The calcium nodules deposited in tissues, **R.'s tubes:** the tubules formed in the process of calcification.

raisins. Dried grapes.

râle (Fr. *râler*, to rattle). An abnormal sound heard over the chest in auscultation and indicating some local affection. Râles are either dry or moist—the latter if liquid is present in the air channels. They are classified according to their situation as being tracheal, bronchial, vesicular, cavernous, pleural or pericardial.

Ralfe's test (Ralfe, C. H., English physician, 1842–98). A test for acetone in urine. To 4 cc. of urine in a test-tube add 4 cc. of liquor potassae with 1.5 gm. of potassium iodide; a yellow ring studded with minute particles of iodoform forms at the line of contact.

ra·mal (L. *ramus*, branch). Relating to a ramus; branching.

ramā·lis vena (L. *ramus*, branch; *vena*, vein). The portal vein and its branches.

R.A.M.C. Royal Army Medical Corps.

ra·mi (L. pl. of *ramus*, branch). **R. accelerantes:** the accelerator nerves. **R. musculares:** branches of nerves, arteries or veins supplying muscles.

ramificā·tion (L.L. *ramificare*, to branch). 1. Branching of an organ or part. 2. A branch.

ra·mify (L. *ramus*, branch; *facere*, to make). To branch.

ramisec·tion (L. *ramus*, branch; *sectio*, a cutting). Division or excision of some of the rami of the sympathetic nervous system.

rami·tis (L. *ramus*, branch). Inflammation of the root of a nerve.

ramollissement (Fr.). Softening; applied to the softening of tissues.

Ramon y Cajal's cells. See under Cajal.

ra·mose (L. *ramus*, branch). Having many branches.

Ramsden's ocular (Ramsden, J., English optician, 1735–1800). An eye-piece with two plano-convex lenses.

Ramstedt's operation (Ramstedt, C., German surgeon, born 1867). Incision of the circular muscle coat of the pylorus allowing prolapse of the mucous membrane. Used in cases of congenital pyloric stenosis.

ra·mus (L., pl. *rami*). 1. A branch; particularly one of a nerve or blood-vessel. 2. A slim process projecting from a large bone, such as the r. of the lower jaw.

ran·cid (L. *rancidus*). Foetid or sour; having a rank smell or taste.

Randacio's nerves (Randacio, F., Italian anatomist, 1821–1903). The nerves arising from the spheno-palatine ganglion.

ra·nine (L. *rana*, frog). 1. Relating to a frog. 2. Relating to a ranula. **R. tumour:** ranula, *q.v.*

Ranke's angle (Ranke, J., German physician, 1836–1916). A cephalic angle employed in craniometry. Ranke's angle has elsewhere been wrongly ascribed to H. R. Ranke, 1849–87.

ra·nula (L. *ranula*, dim. of *rana*, frog). A cystic tumour beneath the tongue, due to the occlusion of the duct of the sublingual or submaxillary gland, or of a mucous gland of the floor of the mouth. Syn. frog-tongue.

ra·nular. Relating to a ranula.

Ranun·culus. A genus of plants which includes the buttercup.

Ranvier's crosses (Ranvier, L. A., French pathologist, 1835–1922). Dark cross-shaped markings seen at R.'s nodes on staining longitudinal sections with silver. **R.'s discs:** tactile cup-shaped bodies at the ends of sensory nerve fibres. **R.'s nodes:** the interruptions of the medullary sheaths of nerves.

Raoult's law (Raoult, F. M., French physicist, 1830–99). The depression of the freezing point of a solution is proportional to the molecular concentration of the solution.

rape. Sexual intercourse with a woman without her consent.

ra·phe (G. *rhaphē*, seam). A seam, suture, line, ridge or crease, e.g., the r. of the tongue, a median furrow on the dorsal surface of the tongue corresponding to the fibrous septum which divides it into symmetrical halves.

rap·tus (L. *rapere*, to seize). Any sudden seizure. **R. maniacus:** transient fury.

rarefac·tion (L. *rarus*, thin; *facere*, to make). The act of decreasing the density of a substance; especially applied to air.

rascē·ta (L.). The transverse lines on the inner surface of the wrist.

Rasch's sign (Rasch, H., German obstetrician, born 1875). An early pregnancy sign. Fluctuation obtained by ballottement of the uterus.

rash. A superficial skin eruption, such as nettle-rash, *q.v.*

Rasmussen's aneurysm (Rasmussen, F. W., Danish physician, 1834–81). An aneurysm of an artery in a tuberculous cavity in the lung.

ras·patory (Old Fr. *rasper*, to file). A surgeon's rasp or file.

raspberry mark. Congenital haemangioma.

rasū·ra (L.). Scrapings.

rat. A rodent that haunts inhabited places. Its bite can be dangerous, and it harbours a number of parasites transmissible to man. The commonest species in England is the brown rat, *Mus norvegicus*. Plague is transmitted by a flea of the black rat, *Mus rattus*. The rat is much used as a laboratory animal.

Rathke's pouch, pocket (Rathke, M. H., German anatomist, 1793–1860). A depression in the roof of the embryonic mouth in front of the bucco-pharyngeal membrane.

ra·tio (L.). Degree or proportion.

ra·tion (L. *ratio*, proportion). A fixed allowance of food or other substance.

ra·tional (L. *ratio*, reason). Based upon reason; not empirical.

ratsbane. A common name for arsenic trioxide, or white arsenic.

rattle. Râle, *q.v.*

Rau's apophysis or **process** (Rau, J. J., Dutch anatomist, 1658–1719). The processus gracilis anterior of the malleus.

ray. 1. A beam of light or heat proceeding from a luminous point. 2. One of a number of lines diverging from a common centre. For *alpha*, *beta* and *gamma* rays, see under radium.

Raygat's test. For live birth. Place lungs in water, if inflation has occurred the lungs will float.

Raynaud's disease (Raynaud, A. G. M., French physician, 1834–81). Colour changes produced by vasospasm of the digital vessels, leading in extreme cases to gangrene.

R.C.O.G. Royal College of Obstetricians and Gynaecologists.

R.C.P. Royal College of Physicians.

R.C.S. Royal College of Surgeons of England.

R.C.S.E. Royal College of Surgeons of Edinburgh.

R.C.S.I. Royal College of Surgeons of Ireland.

rēäc·tion (L. *re*, again; *agere*, to act). 1. Counteraction; response to a stimulus. 2. In chemistry, the process by which substances are changed into others. 3. In psychiatry, the mental response to conditions or events.

rĕăc·tivate (L. *re*, again; *agere*, to act). To render active again.

reactivā·tion (L. *re*, again; *agere*, to act). The restoration to activity of a serum that has become inactivated; this is accomplished by the addition of complement.

rēā·gent (L. *re*, again; *agere*, to act). In chemistry, any substance used to provoke a reaction.

rē·agin. An antibody.

re-amputation (L. *re*, again; *amputare*, to lop off). A further amputation on a limb that has already undergone one.

Réaumur's thermometer (Réaumur, A. F., French naturalist, 1683–1757). A thermometer in which the freezing point of water is 0° and the boiling point of water is 80°. Rarely used to-day.

rebound. 1. An outburst of fresh reflex activity following withdrawal of stimulus. 2. The method whereby patient's exhaled carbon dioxide is absorbed in a closed circuit, when under anaesthetic, and the anaesthetic agent and oxygen circulate continuously, small quantities being added to make up that used.

recei·ver. A vessel for receiving distillation products.

receptă·culum chȳ·li (L. *receptaculum*, a receptacle; G. *khulos*, juice). The inferior expanded portion of the thoracic duct.

recep·tor (L. *recipere*, to receive). 1. The atomic lateral chain or haptophorous group in a cell which combines with foreign bodies, toxins, food molecules, etc. 2. Peripheral nerve-endings.

recess, reces·sus (L. *recessus*). A fossa, ventricle or ampulla.

reces·sion (L. *recedere*, to retreat). A drawing away. **R. of the gums:** the shrinking away of the gums from the necks of the teeth.

recessive characteristic. In biology, an inherited character which remains unexpressed when mated with a dominant character.

recessus. See recess.

recidivā·tion (L. *recidivus*, recurring). The relapse of a disease or a return to a life of crime.

reci·divist (L. *recidivus*, recurring). A patient, especially a mental patient, who returns for further treatment; or a criminal who, after punishment, returns to a life of crime.

reci·pient (L. *recipere*). The receiver of a blood transfusion.

recip·rocal (L. *reciprocare*, to move back and forth). Mutual. **R. proportions, law of:** two chemical elements which unite with a third element do so in proportions which are multiples of those in which they unite with each other.

Recklinghausen's canals (Recklinghausen, F. D. von, German pathologist, 1833–1910). The lymph canaliculi, cell spaces in tissues. **R.'s disease:** 1. Multiple neurofibromatosis. 2. Haemochromatosis.

reclinā·tion (L. *reclinare*, to recline). An operation for cataract in which the opaque lens is pushed back into the vitreous chamber.

Reclus's disease (Reclus, P., French surgeon, 1847–1914). Chronic interstitial mastitis.

reconstitū·tion (L. *re*, again; *constituere*, to constitute). The mixing of a dehydrated substance (e.g. dried milk) with water before making use of it.

rĕ·crement (L. *recrescere*, to grow again). Any secretion (such as saliva) that is reabsorbed into the system after it has fulfilled its function.

recrudes·cence (L. *recrudescere*, to break out again). The return of a disease; a relapse.

rec·tal (L. *rectus*, straight). Relating to the rectum.

rectal·gia (L. *rectus*, straight; G. *algos*, pain). Pain in the rectum. Syn. proctalgia.

rectec·tomy (L. *rectus*, straight; G. *ektomē*, excision). Surgical removal of the rectum.

rectificā·tion (L. *rectus*, straight; *facere*, to make). 1. A straightening. 2. The redistillation of a spirit in order to purify it.

rec·tified (L. *rectus*, straight; *fieri*, to become). 1. Corrected. 2. Refined. **R. spirit:** alcohol containing 94 per cent of ethyl alcohol.

recti·tis. Inflammation of the rectum.

recto-abdō·minal (L. *rectus*, straight; *abdomen*). Relating to the rectum and the abdomen.

rec·tocele (L. *rectus*, straight; G. *kēlē*, hernia). 1. Prolapse and protrusion of the rectum. 2. Prolapse of the rectum into the vagina.

rec·tococcȳ·geal (L. *rectus*, straight; G. *kokkux*, coccyx). Relating to the rectum and the coccyx.

rectococ·cypexy (L. *rectus*, straight; G. *kokkux*, coccyx; *pēxis*, a fixation). Suture of the rectum to the coccyx.

rec·topexy (L. *rectus*, straight; G. *pēxis*, a fixation). Fixation by surgical means of the prolapsed rectum.

rectopho·bia (L. *rectus*, straight; G. *phobos*, fear). A sense of foreboding often encountered in patients with rectal disease.

rec·toscope (L. *rectus*, straight; G. *skopein*, to inspect). A speculum for rectal examination.

rectosig·moid (L. *rectus*, straight; G. *sigma*, the letter S; *eidos*, form). The region of the lower sigmoid colon and the upper part of the rectum.

rec·tostenō·sis (L. *rectus*, straight; G. *stenos*, narrow). Stricture of the rectum.

rectŏ·stomy (L. *rectus*, straight; G. *stoma*, mouth). Proctostomy, *q.v.*

rectŏ·tomy (L. *rectus*, straight; G. *tomē*, a cutting). Proctotomy, *q.v.*

recto-urē·thral (L. *rectus*, straight; G. *ourethra*, urethra). Relating to the rectum and urethra.

recto-ū·terine (L. *rectus*, straight; *uterus*). Relating to the rectum and uterus.

rectovagi·nal (L. *rectus*, straight; *vagina*, sheath). Relating to the rectum and vagina. **R. fistula:** an opening connecting the rectum with the vagina.

rectovesi·cal (L. *rectus*, straight; *vesica*, bladder). Relating to the rectum and the bladder.

rec·tum (L. *rectus*, straight). The distal section of the large intestine; from the sigmoid flexure to the anus. It is about five inches in length.

rec·tus (L.). Straight.

recum·bent (L. *recumbere*, to lie down). Reclining; lying down.

recū·perate (L. *recuperare*, to recover). To regain health.

recuperā·tion (L. *recuperare*, to recover). The regaining of health and strength.

recur·rence (L. *recurrere*, to recur). A return of a disease.

recur·rent (L. *recurrere*, to recur). 1. Returning at intervals. 2. In anatomy, a turning back to the source; as r. laryngeal nerve.

recur·ring (L. *recurrere*, to recur). Returning. **R. disease:** one that relapses.

recurved (L. *recurvare*, to curve backwards). Bent backwards.

red. The least refrangible colour of the visible spectrum. **R. fever:** dengue fever. **R. mite:** Chigger. The six-legged red larva of the mite *Trombicula alfreddugesi* (*T. irritans*) known as harvest mite of North America. Lives in long grass and underbrush. The chigger of Europe is *T. autumnalis*. Bites produce a wheal which itches.

redintegrā·tion (L. *redintegrare*, to restore). Full restoration of a part that has been injured or lost.

redressement forcé (Fr.). Forcible correction of a deformity.

reduce (L. *reducere*, to lead back). 1. To return a part to its normal position; as to r. a hernia 2. In chemistry, to cause the gain of one or more electrons by an atom or ion.

redū·cible (L. *reducere*, to lead back). Capable of reduction.

redū·cin. A leucomaine, $C_{12}H_{24}N_6O_9$, present in urine.

reduc·tase. An enzyme that takes part in reduction of chemical processes.

reduc·tion (L. *reductio*). Restoration of a normal situation.

redun·dant. Superfluous; more than is required.

redū·plicated (L. *re*, again; *duplicare*, to double). Doubled, as in r. heart-sounds.

reduplicā·tion (L. *re*, again; *duplicare*, to double). The doubling of the paroxysms in certain forms of intermittent fever. **R. of the heart-sounds:** a doubling of either the first or second sound of the heart.

re-education. The process of training necessary in recovery of use of muscles, limbs, etc., following prolonged disuse, as after poliomyelitis or fracture. May be applied to recovery of any function following prolonged disease.

reference, delusion or idea of. A state of mind in which the patient believes that he is the object of comment.

refine. To free from foreign matter.

reflec·tion (L. *reflectere*, to bend back). A bending or turning backward; the turning back of a ray of light, heat or sound from a surface which it is not capable of penetrating.

reflec·tor (L. *reflectere*, to bend back). A surface that reflects light.

re·flex (L. *reflectere*, to bend back). 1. Anything reflected or thrown back. 2. An involuntary action due to nerve-stimulus. **R., conditioned:** is an acquired reflex which depends for its appearance on the formation of a new functional connection in the c.n.s. and is therefore peculiar to the individual.

reflex·ophil (L. *reflectere*, to bend back; G. *philein*, to love). Marked by reflex activity.

re·flux (L. *refluere*, to flow back). A return flow.

refract (L. *refringere*, to break up). 1. To cause deviation. 2. To estimate the extent of refraction error in an eye.

refrac·ta dosi (L. *refracta*, broken up; G. *dōsis*, a giving). In repeated doses.

refrac·tion (L. *refringere*, to break up). 1. The process of refracting or deviating. 2. The deviation of a ray of light in passing obliquely from one transparent medium to another of different density. 3. The process of correcting errors of ocular refraction by means of glasses.

refrac·tionist. One who corrects errors of ocular refraction.

refrac·tive. Relating to refraction.

refractŏ·meter (L. *refringere*, to break up; G. *metron*, measure). 1. Instrument for estimating the refractive power of the eye. 2. Instrument for determining the refractive indices of liquids.

refrac·tory (L. *refractarius*, stubborn). Resistent to treatment.

refrac·ture (L. *re*, again; *fractura*, a fracture). A rebreaking of fractured bones after faulty union.

refrangibi·lity (L. *refringere*, to break up). Capacity of being refracted.

refran·gible (L. *refringere*, to break up). Susceptible of being refracted.

refresh. To restore the character of a fresh wound to an old lesion.

refri·gerant (L. *refrigerare*, to chill). 1. Cooling; reducing fever. 2. An agent having cooling powers.

refrigerā·tion (L. *refrigerare*, to chill). The therapeutic use of cold. See also under anaesthesia.

refū·sion (L. *refusio*, 1. an overflowing; 2. a restitution). The withdrawing of blood and its subsequent return to the circulatory system after exposure to air oxygen.

regĕ·nerate (L. *regenerare*). To reproduce; to renew.

regenerā·tion (L. *regenerare*, to reproduce). The repair of tissues or structures damaged by disease or injury.

rĕ·gimen (L., guidance). The ordered and guided regulation of habits and/or diet; usually to attain some specific end.

rē·gio (L.). Region, *q.v.*

rē·gion (L. *regio*, region). A part or division of the body possessing either natural or arbitrary boundaries; e.g., ciliary r., femoral r., gastric r., nasal r.

rē·gional (L. *regio*, region). Relating to a region. **R. anatomy:** a subdivision of anatomy which deals with the relations of a particular region of the body.

rē·gister (Mediaeval L. *regestrum*, from *regestum*, registered). In singing, the compass of the voice.

regres·sive (L. *regredi*, to go back). Going back; retreating; subsiding.

rē·gular (L. *regularis*, pertaining to rules). According to rule or custom.

reg. umb. Abbreviation for L. *regio umbilici*, the navel region.

regur·gitant (L. *regurgitare*, to surge back). Flowing backward.

regurgitā·tion (L. *regurgitare*, to surge back). 1. An eructation or throwing back of food from the stomach without the ordinary efforts at vomiting. 2. A flowing back of blood through a defective heart-valve.

rehabi·litate (L. *re*, again; *habilitas*, aptitude, from *habilis*, manageable). To render a handicapped person fit for employment.

Reichel's cloacal duct (Reichel, P., German gynaecologist, born 1858). Embryonic communication between the hind gut and the bladder-anlagen of the entodermal cloaca.

Reichert's cartilage (Reichert, K. B., German anatomist, 1811–83). The cartilage of the second branchial arch. Hensen's canal is sometimes called **R.'s canal.**

Reichmann's disease (Reichmann, N., Polish physician, 1851–1918). Gastrosuccorrhoea, a neurosis of the stomach attended with hypersecretion.

Reid's base line (Reid, R. W., Scottish anatomist, 1851–1939). The anthropometric base line on the skull.

Reil's ansa (Reil, J. C., German anatomist, 1759–1813). A tract of white fibres passing from the optic thalamus to the hemisphere. **R.'s island:** the insula of the cerebral cortex.

reimplantā·tion (L. *re*, again; *in*, in; *plantare*, to plant). The replacement of a tissue or an organ into its previous environment, or into a new one.

reinfec·tion (L. *re*, again; *inficere*, to infect). Infection for a second time with the same type of organism.

reinoculā·tion (L. *re*, again; *inoculare*, to ingraft). A second inoculation with the same kind of organism.

reins (L. *ren*, kidney). The kidneys or their region; the lower part of the back.

reinver·sion (L. *re*, again; *invertere*, to turn over). The replacement of an inverted organ; applied especially to the reduction of an inverted uterus.

Reisseisen's muscle (Reisseisen, F. D., German anatomist, 1773–1828). The smooth muscle fibres of the smallest bronchial tubes.

Reissner's fibre (Reissner, E., German anatomist, 1824–78). A highly refractive cylindrical fibre or rod running through the whole length of the central canal of the spinal cord, first described in the spinal cord of Petromyzon. **R.'s membrane:** the membrana vestibularis of the cochlea.

rejuvenes·cence (L. *re*, again; *juvenescere*, to grow young). A renewal of youth or strength.

relapse (L. *relabi*, to slide back). A recurrence of disease after convalescence has apparently begun.

relapsing fever. An acute infectious fever due to *Spirochaeta obermeieri*. It is characterized by fever, chills, pains in the back and limbs, enlargement of the spleen, sweats and delirium. After about six days the symptoms cease by crisis. A second attack sets in about a week later and may be followed by a third and sometimes even a fourth. Syn. famine fever.

relax·ant (L. *relaxare*, to loosen). 1. Loosening. 2. An agent that reduces tension.

relaxā·tion (L. *relaxatio*, an easing). 1. Diminution of tension. 2. A lessening of functional powers, as r. of the skin. 3. Languor.

relax·in. Hormone produced by corpus luteum which is said to cause relaxation of pelvic ligaments during pregnancy.

relief (L. *relevatio*, alleviation). The alleviation of distress or pain.

Remak's fibres (Remak, R., German neurologist, 1815–65). The unmyelinated nerve fibres. **R.'s ganglia:** the autonomic ganglia in the nerves of the stomach. **R.'s ganglion:** the ganglion of the autonomic system in the inferior vena-caval opening in the diaphragm.

remē·dial (L. *remedium*, remedy). Curative.

rĕ·medy (L. *remedium*, remedy). An agent used in the treatment of disease.

remis·sion (L. *remissio*, sending back). 1. The subsiding of disease symptoms. 2. The period during which such subsidence occurs.

remit·tent (L. *remittere*, to send back). Alternately subsiding and recurring. **R. fever:** a fever characterized by remission periods.

ren (L. pl. *renes*). The kidney.

rē·nal (L. *ren*, kidney). Relating to the kidneys. **R. calculus:** a concretion in the kidney. **R. glands:** the suprarenal capsules.

Renaut's layer (Renaut, J. L., French physician, 1844–1917). A name given to a hypothetical layer of 'perles réfringentes' separating the mucous cells of the Malpighian layer of the skin.

Rendu's tremor (Rendu, H. J. L. M., French physician, 1844–1902). Hysterical tremor.

rĕ·nicapsule (L. *ren*, kidney; *capsula*, a small box). A suprarenal capsule.

renicar·diac (L. *ren*, kidney; G. *kardia*, heart). Relating conjointly to the kidneys and the heart.

rĕ·niform (L. *ren*, kidney; *forma*, shape). Shaped like a kidney.

rē·nin. A hormone released by anoxia of the kidneys that is thought to be responsible for the production of hypertension.

renipor·tal (L. *ren*, kidney; *porta*, gate). Relating to the portal system of the kidney.

rĕ·nipuncture (L. *ren*, kidney; *punctura*, puncture). Surgical puncture of the renal capsule.

reni·tis (L. *ren*, kidney). Inflammation of the kidney.

ren·net. The prepared milk-curdling enzyme obtained from the glandular layer of the fourth stomach of the calf.

rennin. Rennet, *q.v.*

renogas·tric (L. *ren*, kidney; G. *gaster*, stomach). Relating to the kidneys and the stomach.

reno·intestin·al (L. *ren*, kidney; *intus*, within). Relating to the kidneys and the intestine.

renovā·tion (L. *renovatio*, renewal). The repair of damaged tissues or structures.

repercolā·tion (*L. re*, again; *percolare*, to filter through). Percolation repeated once or more often.

repercus·sion (L. *re*, again; *percussio*, a beating). 1. Ballottement. 2. An after-effect.

replantā·tion (L. *re*, again; *plantare*, to plant). The act of planting again.

replē·tion (L. *replēre*, to fill again). The state of being full.

replicā·tion (L. *replicare*, to fold back). Refolding or duplication of a part.

reposi·tion (L. *reponere*, to replace). Return of an abnormally situated part to its correct position.

repres·sion (L. *re*, again, *premere*, to press). The mechanism whereby ideas or perceptions of an unpleasant nature are thrust back from consciousness into unconsciousness.

reproduce (L. *re*, again; *producere*, to bring forth). To bring forth offspring.

reproduc·tion. The production of offspring. **R.,asexual:** that which takes place without sexual connection, e.g., by cell-division.

reproduc·tive. Relating to reproduction.

resect (L. *re*, again; *secare*, to sever). To cut away a section, especially to excise the end of one or more bones entering into a joint.

resec·tion (L. *re*, again; *secare*, to sever). The surgical excision of a part of an organ, especially of part of the structures forming a joint.

rĕ·servoir (Fr. from L. *reservare*, to reserve). A cell or organ for storing assimilated substances.

resi·dual (L. *residuus*, remainder). Remaining. **R. air:** the air remaining in the lungs after the most powerful possible expiration, or the small residue left in a vessel after the use of an air-pump.

rĕ·sidue (L. *residuus*, remainder). That which is left over; a remainder.

resi·duum (L. *residuus*, remainder). The balance or remainder; see also residue.

resi·lience (L. *resilire*, to spring back). Elasticity.

resi·lient (L. *resilire*, to spring back). Elastic.

rē·sin (L. *resina*). The residue left after removal by distillation of the ethereal oil from the crude exudate of various plants such as various species of Pinus. See colophony.

rĕ·sinoid (L. *resina*, resin; G. *eidos*, form). 1. Resembling a resin. 2. A resin-like substance.

rĕ·sinous (L. *resina*, resin). Having the nature of a resin.

resis·tance (L. *resistere*, to resist). 1. Opposition by conductors to the passage of electric currents. 2. In psychoanalysis, the opposition to perception of repressions.

resolū·tion (L. *resolvere*, to loosen). 1. The return of a tissue or part to its normal condition, e.g. after disease or injury. 2. In chemistry, the act of separation of a substance into its optically active isomers.

resol·vent (L. *resolvere*, to loosen). 1. Causing solution or dissipation of a pathological condition or growth. 2. An agent causing the solution of tissue.

rĕ·sonance (L. *resonantia*, an echo). 1. A sound heard on percussing the chest or on auscultating the chest during speech. 2. The voice sounds heard when the ear is applied to the chest.

rĕ·sonant (L. *resonare*, to echo). Producing a quivering or vibrating sound on auscultation.

resor·cin Resorcinol, *q.v.*

resor·cinol (L. *resina*, resin; *Orcus*, the underworld or its god). Metadihydroxybenzene; used as a surface antiseptic and in ointments in irritant skin affections.

resorp·tion (L. *resorbere*, to suck up). The reabsorption of secreted matter, tissues, etc. Applied in dentistry to the processes leading to the disappearance of the roots of deciduous teeth.

res·pirable (L. *respirare*, to breathe). Capable of being breathed.

respirā·tion (L. *respiratio*, breathing). Inspiration and expiration of air by the lungs.

respirā·tor (L. *respirare*, to breathe). An appliance for breathing through, to protect from cold or from the inhalation of volatile substances.

res·piratory (L. *respirare*, to breathe). Relating to respiration.

respire (L. *respirare*). To breathe.

respirŏ·meter (L. *respirare*, to breathe; G. *metron*, measure). An apparatus used in testing the character of the respiration.

response (L. *responsum*, answer). Reaction to a stimulus.

responsibi·lity (L. *respondere*, to answer). In medical jurisprudence, the accountability of a person for an act committed. It generally turns upon the question of whether or not the person was of sound mind and capable of controlling his actions and thoughts.

rest. 1. Repose. 2. Embryonic cells which, having been misplaced in intra-uterine life, remain present in the adult body.

restibrā·chium (L. *restis*, rope; *brachium*, arm). An inferior cerebellar peduncle.

res·tiform (L. *restis*, rope; *forma*, shape). Rope-shaped or cord-like. **R. body:** a part of the medulla oblongata, connecting the cerebellum with the spinal nerve roots.

resting. Quiescent; at rest.

res·tis (L., rope). The restiform body.

restitū·tio ad integ·rum (L.). Complete restoration to health.

restitū·tion (L. *restitutio*). 1. A return to the normal condition. 2. Rotation of the foetal head, or other presenting part, immediately after its delivery.

res·tocythae·mia (L. *restare*, to be left; G. *kutos*, a container; *haima*, blood). The presence of broken-down red cells in the blood.

resto·rative (L. *restaurare*, to restore). A remedy which assists in the restoration of health and strength.

restraint. The condition of being under control; specifically, the circumscription of liberty in the case of the insane.

resuscitā·tion (L. *resuscitatio*, revival). The revival of one apparently dead.

resus·citator (L. *resuscitare*, to revive). An apparatus for giving artifical respiration.

retardā·tion (L. *retardare*, to delay). The delay or prevention of a function; backwardness; slowness of development.

retch, retching. Involuntary attempt to vomit.

rē·te (L. *rete*, net). Any network of fibres or, especially, blood-vessels.

reten·tion (L. *retentio*). The act of holding back; stoppage. **R. of urine:** inability to pass the secreted urine from the bladder.

rē·tial (L. *rete*, net). Relating to a rete.

reti·cular (L. *reticulum*, dim. of *rete*, net). Net-like; full of interstices.

reti·culate (L. *reticulum*, small net). Possessing net-like meshes.

reti·culocyte (L. *reticulum*, small net; G. *kutos*, a container). A net-like or meshed erythrocyte observed during the process of blood regeneration.

reti·culocytō·sis. An excess of reticulocytes in the blood.

reticulo-endothelial system (L. *reticulum*, small net; G. *endon*, within; *thēlē*, nipple). A group of cells which show endothelial and reticular attributes and phagocytic properties. Includes endothelial and reticular of the spleen, lymph glands, Kupffer cells of liver, tissue of the bone marrow. Concerned in formation of blood cells and bile, in destruction of blood cells and in metabolism of iron and blood pigments.

reti·culosarcō·ma (L. *reticulum*, small net; G. *sarx*, flesh). Type of lymphosarcoma composed of large cells with vesicular nuclei. Derived from the reticular cells of lymph glands.

reti·culum (L.). A network.

rĕ·tiform (L. *rete*, net; *forma*, shape). Net-shaped.

rĕ·tina (L. *rete*, net). The light-sensitive internal nervous tunic of the eyeball. It is soft in consistence, translucent, and of a pinkish colour. It consists of eight superimposed layers, seven of which are nervous and one pigmented. The eight layers are as follows, commencing internally: (1) stratum opticum, or layer of nerve-fibres; (2) ganglionic layer, or layer of nerve-cells; (3) inner plexiform (inner molecular) layer; (4) inner nuclear or granular layer; (5) outer plexiform (outer molecular) layer; (6) outer nuclear or granular layer; (7) layer of rods and cones; and (8) pigmented layer.

retină·culum (L. *retinēre*, to retain). A band serving to keep an organ or part in its place.

rĕ·tinal. Relating to the retina.

retinī·tis. Inflammation of the retina.

retinoblastō·ma (L. *rete*, net; G. *blastos*, germ). A tumour originating in the germ cells of the retina.

retinochoroidī·tis (L. *rete*, net; G. *khorion*, an intestinal membrane; *eidos*, form). Inflammation of both retina and choroid.

rĕ·tinoscope (L. *rete*, net; G. *skopein*, to view). An instrument for measuring the refraction of the eye.

retinŏ·scopy (L. *rete*, net; G. *skopein*, to view). The art of measuring the refraction of the eye, so named after the supposed observation of retinal images.

retort (L. *retortus*, bent backwards). A vessel used in distillation. It has a long neck and a globular body.

retrac·tile (L. *retrahere*, to draw back). Capable of being drawn back.

retracti·lity (L. *retrahere*, to draw back). The power of drawing back.

retrac·tion (L. *retrahere*, to draw back). Shortening; drawing back.

retrac·tor (L. *retrahere*, to draw back). An instrument for drawing aside the edges of a wound.

rĕ·trad (L. *retro*, back; *ad*, to). Towards or in the rear.

rĕ·trahens (L. *retrahere*, to draw back). Drawing back. **R. aurem:** muscle drawing back the ear.

retrench·ment (Fr. *retrenchement*). A plastic operation in which superficial tissues are removed so as to obtain contraction of a scar.

retrobron·chial (L. *retro*, backward; G. *brogkhos*, bronchus). Situated behind the bronchi.

retrobul·bar (L. *retro*, backward; G. *bolbos*, bulb). Situated behind the eyeball.

retrocar·diac (L. *retro*, backward; G. *kardia*, heart). Situated behind the heart.

retrocae·cal (L. *retro*, backward; *caecus*, blind). Behind the caecum.

retrocē·dent (L. *retrocedere*, to retreat). Disappearing from the surface.

retroces·sion (L. *retrocedere*, to retreat). A retrograde movement; the act of going back.

retrocŏl·ic (L. *retro*, backward; G. *kolon*, colon). Behind the colon.

retrocol·lic (L. *retro*, backward; *collis*, neck). Relating to the back of the neck.

retrocol·lis (L. *retro*, backward; *collis*, neck). Torticollis, *q.v.*

retrodisplace·ment. Displacement in a backward direction.

retrodū·ral (L. *retro*, backward; *durus*, hard). Behind the dura mater.

rĕ·troflexed (L. *retro*, backward; *flectere*, to bend). Bent backward.

retrofle·xion (L. *retro*, backward; *flectere*, to bend). A bending or flexing backward.

re·trograde (L. *retrogradus*, going backwards). Receding or going backward.

retro·graphy (L. *retro*, backward; G. *graphein*, to write). A reversal of the order of writing; mirror-writing.

retrogres·sion (L. *retrogredi*, to go backward). Degeneration.

retro-infec·tion (L. *retro*, backward; *inficere*, to dye). Infection of the mother by the foetus.

retro-in·sular (L. *retro*, backward; *insula*, island). Situated or occurring behind the island of Reil.

retromam·mary (L. *retro*, backward; *mamma*, breast). Situated at the back of a mammary gland.

retromandi·bular (L. *retro*, backward; *mandibula*, mandible). Situated behind the lower jaw.

retromas·toid (L. *retro*, backward; G. *mastos*, breast; *eidos*, form). Behind the mastoid process.

retromorpho·sis (L. *retro*, backward; G. *morphe*, shape). Retrograde metamorphosis.

retrona·sal (L. *retro*, backward; *nasus*, nose). Behind the nose.

retro-oc·ular (L. *retro*, backward; *oculus*, eye). Behind the eyeball. See also retrobulbar.

retro-oesopha·geal (L. *retro*, backward; G. *oisophagos*). Behind the oesophagus.

ret·roperitone·al (L. *retro*, backward; G. *peri*, around; *teinein*, to stretch). Behind the peritoneum.

ret·roperitone·um (L. *retro*, backward; *peri*, around; *teinein*, to stretch). The space lying behind the peritoneum and anterior to the spinal column and lumbar muscles; the retroperitoneal space.

ret·roperitoni·tis. Inflammation of the retroperitoneum.

ret·ropharyn·geal (L. *retro*, backward; G. *pharugx*, throat). Situated behind the pharynx.

ret·ropharyngi·tis. Inflammation of the posterior section of the pharynx.

ret·ropharynx (L. *retro*, backward; G. *pharugx*, throat). The posterior part of the pharynx.

retropul·sion (L. *retro*, backward; *pellere*, to drive). 1. A driving back, as of the foetal head in parturition. 2. A backward gait; a form of walking sometimes seen in locomotor ataxia.

retrospec·tion (L. *retro*, backward; *spicere*, to look). Morbid exercise of the memory.

retroster·nal (L. *retro*, backward; G. *sternon*, the chest). Situated behind the sternum.

retrosymphy·seal (L. *retro*, backward; G. *sun*, with; *phusis*, growth). Behind the symphysis.

retrotar·sal (L. *retro*, backward; G. *tarsos*, a flat place). At the back of the eyelid.

retro-u·terine (L. *retro*, behind; *uterus*). Located behind the uterus.

ret·rovaccina·tion (L. *retro*, backward; *vacca*, a cow). Vaccination with virus obtained from a cow previously inoculated with the virus of smallpox from a human being.

retrover·sion (L. *retro*, backward; *vertere*, to turn). The turning backward of an organ.

Retzius's cave (Retzius, A. A., Swedish anatomist, 1796–1860). The cavum prevesicale. **R.'s ligament:** the 'schleuderformig' ligament of German, frondiform of French and fundiform of English authors; the deep attachment of the extensor retinaculum in the sinus tarsi that acts as a sling for the extensor tendons. **R.'s gyri:** the callosal convolutions of the brain named by G. M. Retzius in honour of his father as the **Gyri Andreae Retzii.**

Retzius's bodies (Retzius, G. M., Swedish anatomist and neurologist, son of above, 1842–1919). The sensory nerve-endings akin to the corpuscles of Herbst. **R.'s gyrus:** the gyrus intralimbicus of the rhinence-phalon. **R.'s striae:** the 'brown lines' in the enamel of the teeth.

reu·nion (L. *re*, again; *unire*, to join). The uniting of parts that have been divided.

Reuss's colour charts (Reuss, A., Ritter von, Austrian ophthalmologist, 1841–1924). Charts with coloured letters printed on coloured backgrounds. Used for testing colour vision.

re·verie (Fr.). A state of day-dreaming.

Reverdin's graft (Reverdin, J.L., Swiss surgeon, 1842–1908). 'Pinch' graft. Small pieces of epidermis placed on granulating surface to promote healing.

reversal of gradient. A block of the faecal stream due to an area of irritation causing local spasticity of the intestine with higher local tone than the area above.

rever·sion (L. *revertere*, to turn back). The re-appearance of characteristics that existed in distant ancestors.

revive (L. *re*, again; *vivere*, to live). To recover after apparent death.

revi·vifica·tion (L. *re*, again; *vivus*, living; *facere*, to make). 1. Recovery of consciousness, as from a fainting-fit. 2. The refreshing of surfaces before placing them in apposition for the purpose of uniting them.

revul·sion (L. *revulsio*, a tearing off). The withdrawal of blood from a diseased part.

revul·sive (L. *revellere*, to tear off). 1. Causing revulsion. 2. An agent producing revulsion.

Rh. Symbol of rhodium.

Rh. factor. See under Rhesus factor.

Rhabdi·tis (G. *rhabdos*, rod). A genus of nematode worms, species of which are occasionally found in humans.

rhab·dium (G. *rhabdion*, little rod). A striped muscle fibre.

rhab·doid (G. *rhabdos*, rod; *eidos*, form). Rod-shaped.

rhabdomyo·ma (G. *rhabdos*, rod; *mus*, muscle). A type of myoma composed of striated muscular fibres.

rhabdomyosarco·ma. A malignant tumour of striated muscle.

rhachial·gia (G. *rhakhis*, spine; *algos*, pain). Pain in the spine.

rhachianaesthe·sia (G. *rhakhis*, spine; *an*, not; *aisthesis*, feeling). Spinal anaesthesia.

rha·chicente·sis (G. *rhakhis*, spine; *kentesis*, a pricking). Spinal puncture.

rhachi·dial (G. *rhakhis*, spine). Relating to a rhachis.

rhachid·ian (G. *rhakhis*, spine). Relating to the spine; vertebral.

rhachiocamp·sis (G. *rhakhis*, spine; *kampsis*, curve). Spinal curvature.

rhachio·chysis (G. *rhakhis*, spine; *khusis*, a pouring). An accumulation of fluid in the spinal canal.

rhachiody·nia (G. *rhakhis*, spine; *odune*, pain). Pain in the spinal column.

rha·chiokypho·sis (G. *rhakhis*, spine; *kuphosis*, being humpbacked). Kyphosis; hunchback.

rhachio·meter (G. *rhakhis*, spine; *metron*, measure). An instrument for measuring the degree of spinal curvatures.

rhachiomyeli·tis (G. *rhakhis*, spine; *muelos*, marrow). Inflammation of the spinal cord.

rhachiopara·lysis (G. *rhakhis*, spine; *paralusis*, paralysis). Spinal paralysis.

rhachio·pathy (G. *rhakhis*, spine; *pathos*, disease). Any spinal disease.

rha·chiople·gia (G. *rhakhis*, spine; *plege*, a stroke). Paralysis of the spine.

rha·chiotome (G. *rhakhis*, spine; *tome*, a cutting). A surgical instrument for cutting the vertebrae.

rhachio·tomy (G. *rhakhis*, spine; *tome*, a cutting). Cutting into or through the vertebral column. In obstetrics, the cutting of the foetal spine to assist delivery.

rhachi·pagus (G. *rhakhis*, spine; *pagos*, that which is fixed). A twin monster joined by a portion of the spinal column.

rhă·chis (G. *rhakhis*, spine). The spinal column.

rhachi·schisis (G. *rhakhis*, spine; *skhizein*, to cleave). A congenital cleft in the vertebral column.

rhachit·ic (G. *rhakhis*, spine). Affected with, produced by or resembling rhachitis.

rhachi·tis (G. *rhakhis*, spine). Rickets, a deficiency disease of infancy, due to lack of Vitamin D and characterized by poor nutrition and osseous changes. Apart from general symptoms there are slight fever and profuse sweating, together with alterations affecting the skeletal system. Various deformities result from the effect of muscle action upon the softened bones. There is often delay in the appearance of the teeth and in the closure of the fontanelles. Nervous symptoms, such as laryngismus stridulus, may also occur.

rhacŏ·ma (G. *rhakoein*, to tear in strips). 1. Excoriation or chapping. 2. Pendulousness of the scrotum.

rhă·cous (G. *rhakos*, a rag). Lacerated; excoriated.

rhă·gadēs (G. *rhagas*, a rent). Chaps or excoriations of the skin.

rham·nose (G. *rhamnos*, a prickly shrub). A methylpentose, a sugar found in certain types of glycosides, e.g. those of *strophanthus*.

Rham·nus (G. *rhamnos*, a prickly shrub). A genus of trees and shrubs; buckthorns; the source of cascara sagrada.

Rhă·phanus (G. *rhaphanos*, radish). A genus of plants which includes the radish.

rhă·phē (G.). Suture.

rhĕg·ma (G., a fracture). A rupture or fracture.

rhē·obase (G. *rheos*, a stream; *băsis*, basis). The galvanic threshold for striated muscle. The smallest galvanic current acting for an indefinite period required to stimulate the muscle.

rheobā·sic (G. *rheos*, a stream; *băsis*, basis). Relating to rheobases.

rhē·ochord (G. *rheos*, a stream; *khordē*, chord). An instrument for controlling the strength of electric currents. See also rheostat.

rhĕŏ·meter (G. *rheos*, a stream; *metron*, measure). 1. A galvanometer. 2. An apparatus for determining the velocity of the blood current.

rhē·onome (G. *rheos*, a stream; *nōmān*, to distribute). An apparatus for detecting the effect of irritation on a nerve.

rhē·ophore (G. *rheos*, a stream; *pherein*, to bear). An electrode.

rhē·oscope (G. *rheos*, a stream; *skopein*, to view). An instrument for discovering the presence of an electric current.

rhē·ostat (G. *rheos*, a stream; *statos*, placed). An instrument for regulating the strength of an electric current.

rhĕōtax·is. The phenomenon of a body moving in a direction contrary to the current of fluid in which it lies.

rhē·otome (G. *rheos*, a stream; *temnein*, to cut). An instrument used for interrupting a galvanic circuit.

rhē·otrope (G. *rheos*, a stream; *trepein*, to turn). An apparatus for reversing an electric current.

Rhē·sus factor (also called Rh. factor). The blood of some 85 per cent of human beings contains the agglutinogen known as the Rhesus factor because it is present also in the blood of the Rhesus monkey. Presence of the Rh. agglutinogen in the foetus of a mother who does not herself possess it may bring about the syndrome of haemolytic disease of the newborn. **Rh. positive, Rh. negative:** possessing or lacking respectively the Rh. agglutinogen.

rheum (G. *rheuma*, flux). 1. Any watery or catarrhal discharge. 2. The rhizome of *Rheum palmatum* (Linn.) and related varieties—a purgative containing certain anthraquinone derivatives. See rhubarb.

rheumarthri·tis, rheumarthrō·sis (G. *rheuma*, flux; *arthron*, joint). Acute rheumatism of the joints.

rheumatal·gia (G. *rheuma*, flux; *algos*, pain). Pain due to rheumatism.

rheumat·ic. Relating to rheumatism. **R. fever:** acute rheumatism of the joints.

rheu·matism (G. *rheuma*, flux). A specific disease characterized by fever, arthritis of a well-defined type and a tendency to involve the heart. **R., acute articular:** a form of rheumatic fever characterized by swelling of various joints. **R., chronic:** a chronic variety in which the muscles are involved. **R., gonorrhoeal:** an infective arthritis due to gonococci. **R., synovial:** inflammation of the synovial membrane with some serous exudate into the joint.

rheu·matoid (G. *rheuma*, flux; *eidos*, form). Resembling rheumatism. **R. arthritis:** a disease of unknown origin which begins in the synovial membrane and periarticular tissues, which become thickened and proliferated. Later the proliferated synovial membrane becomes adherent to the articular cartilage, which may be destroyed.

rheu·mic (G. *rheuma*, flux). Relating to rheum.

rhex·is (G. *rhēxis*, a breaking). Rupture of a vessel or organ.

rhi·nal (G. *rhis*, nose). Relating to the nose.

rhinal·gia (G. *rhis*, nose; *algos*, pain). Nasal pain.

rhinencĕ·phalon (G. *rhis*, nose; *egkephalos*, brain). The olfactory lobe of the brain.

rhinencĕ·phalus (G. *rhis*, nose; *kephalē*, head). Rhinocephalus, *q.v.*

rhineuryn·ter (G. *rhis*, nose; *eurunein*, to widen). A rubber bag used to dilate the nostril.

rhi·nion (G. *rhis*, nose). The lower part of the suture between the nasal bones.

rhini·tis (G. *rhis*, nose). Inflammation of the mucous membrane of the nose. Syn. coryza.

rhinŏ·byon (G. *rhis*, nose; *buein*, to plug). A nasal plug.

rhinocĕ·phalus (G. *rhis*, nose; *kephalē*, head). A monster in which the nose resembles a head.

rhinoclei·sis (G. *rhis*, nose; *kleisis*, closure). Obstruction of the nose.

rhi·nocoele (G. *rhis*, nose; *koilos*, hollow). The ventricle of the brain's olfactory lobe.

rhinodў·nia (G. *rhis*, nose; *odunē*, pain). Pain in the nose.

rhinolā·lia (G. *rhis*, nose; *lalia*, speech). A nasal tone in the voice. **R. aperta:** caused by undue patency of the posterior nares. **R. clausa:** caused by undue closure of the posterior nares.

rhinolaryngi·tis (G. *rhis*, nose; *larugx*, windpipe). Inflammation of the nasal and laryngeal mucosa.

rhinolaryngŏ·logy (G. *rhis*, nose; *larugx*, windpipe; *logos*, treatise). The science dealing with the structure of the nose and larynx and their diseases.

rhi·nolith (G. *rhis*, nose; *lithos*, stone). A calculus of the nose.

rhinolithi·asis (G. *rhis*, nose; *lithos*, stone). The formation of rhinoliths.

rhinolŏ·gical (G. *rhis*, nose; *logos*, treatise). Relating to rhinology.

rhinŏ·logist (G. *rhis*, nose; *logos*, treatise). An expert in the treatment of diseases of the nose.

rhinŏ·logy (G. *rhis*, nose; *logos*, treatise). The science dealing with the structure and diseases of the nose.

rhinomeiō·sis (G. *rhis*, nose; *meiōsis*, diminution). Surgical reduction of the size of the nose.

rhinommec·tomy (G. *rhis*, nose; *omma*, eye; *ektomē*, excision). Surgical removal of the inner canthus of the eye.

rhinomycō·sis (G. *rhis*, nose; *mukēs*, mushroom). Fungoid infection of the nasal mucosa.

rhinonecrō·sis (G. *rhis*, nose; *nekros*, corpse). Necrosis of the bones of the nose.

rhinŏ·pathy (G. *rhis*, nose; *pathos*, disease). Any nasal disorder or disease.

rhinopharyn·geal (G. *rhis*, nose; *pharugx*, throat). Relating to the nose and the pharynx.

rhinopharyngi·tis (G. *rhis*, nose; *pharugx*, throat). Inflammation of the nasopharynx.

rhinophă·rynx (G. *rhis*, nose; *pharugx*, throat). Nasopharynx, *q.v.*

rhinophō·nia (G. *rhis*, nose; *phōnē*, voice). A nasal tone in the speaking voice.

rhi·nophore (G. *rhis*, nose; *phoros*, bearing). A nasal cannula.

rhinophȳ·ma (G. *rhis*, nose; *phuma*, a growth). A marked hypertrophy of the nose, giving it a lobulated appearance.

rhi·noplasty (G. *rhis*, nose; *plassein*, to form). A plastic operation on the nose for replacing lost tissue with tissue taken from another part of the body.

rhinopolyp, rhi·nopŏ·lypus (G. *rhis*, nose; *polus*, many; *pous*, foot). Polyp of the nose.

rhinorrhă·gia (G. *rhis*, nose; *rhēgnunai*, to burst forth). Haemorrhage from the nose; epistaxis.

rhinorrhoe·a (G. *rhis*, nose; *rhoia*, a flow). The discharge of mucus from the nose.

rhinosalpingi·tis (G. *rhis*, nose; *salpingx*, trumpet). Inflammation of the nasal mucous membrane and that of the auditory tube.

rhinosclerō·ma (G. *rhis*, nose; *skleros*, hard). A growth affecting the skin and mucous membrane of the nose. The growth is very hard and is painful when pressed. There may be a number of distinct nodules or some may coalesce.

rhi·noscope (G. *rhis*, nose; *skopein*, to view). An instrument used in examining the interior of the nose.

rhinŏ·scopy (G. *rhis*, nose; *skopein*, to view). Examination of the nasal passages by means of a rhinoscope.

rhinostenō·sis (G. *rhis*, nose; *stenōsis*, a narrowing). Obstruction of the nose.

rhinŏ·tomy (G. *rhis*, nose; *tomē*, a cutting). Incision into the nose.

rhĭ·zoid (G. *rhiza*, root; *eidos*, form). Root-like.

rhĭ·zome (G. *rhiza*, root). A stem resembling a root and emitting roots below the surface of the ground.

rhizomĕ·lic (G. *rhiza*, root; *melos*, limb). Relating to the hip-joint or the shoulder-joint.

rhĭ·zoneure (G. *rhiza*, root; *neuron*, nerve). A cell forming a nerve-root.

Rhizŏ·poda (G. *rhiza*, root; *pous*, foot). A sub-class of protozoa.

rhizŏ·tomy (G. *rhiza*, root; *tomē*, a cutting). Operation involving section of spinal nerve roots.

Rhodĕ·sian fever. A fever affecting cattle in Africa; it is caused by infection with the *Piroplasma* (*Theileria*) *parva*. It is transmitted by the tick, *Rhipicephalus appendiculatus.*

rhŏ·dium (G. *rhodon*, a rose). A rare metal (atomic weight 102·9) belonging to the platinum group. Symbol Rh.

Rhŏ·dobacteriā·cĕae (G. *rhodon*, a rose; *bakterion*, dim. of *baktron*, a staff). A group of Thiobacteriales.

rhŏ·docyte (G. *rhodon*, a rose; *kutos*, a container). An erythrocyte.

rhodogĕ·nesis (G. *rhodon*, a rose; *genesis*, reproduction). Restoration of the purple colour in rhodopsin after bleaching by light.

rhŏ·dophane (G. *rhodon*, a rose; *phanos*, bright). A red pigment found in the retinal cones of certain birds and fish.

rhŏ·dophylax·is (G. *rhodon*, a rose; *phulaxis*, a guarding). The power of the retinal epithelium to produce rhodogenesis.

rhodop·sin (G. *rhodon*, a rose; *ōps*, eye). Visual purple which is contained in the rods of the retina.

rhombencĕ·phalon (G. *rhombos*, rhomb; *egkephalos*, brain). The metencephalon and myencephalon combined.

rhom·bocoele (G. *rhombos*, rhomb; *koilos*, hollow). A small dilatation of the lower end of the spinal cord.

rhom·boid (G. *rhombos*, rhomb; *eidos*, shape). Shaped like a rhomb; diamond-shaped. **R. fossa:** the fourth ventricle of the brain.

rhomboid·ĕŭs muscle. See muscle.

rhon·chal, rhon·chial (G. *rhegkhos*, a snore). Relating to or having the nature of a rhonchus.

rhon·chus (G. *rhegkhos*, a snore). A rattling sound in the throat or bronchial tubes. See also râle.

rhŏ·tacism (G. *rhō*, the letter r). Over-use of the *r* sound in speech.

rhū·barb. The rhizome of the *Rheum palmatum* and other varieties of the *Rheum* species dried and employed as a stomachic and as a laxative.

Rhus (G. *rhous*, the sumach). A genus of shrubs of the order Anacardiaceae. The leaves of the *Rh. toxicodendron* (Syn. poison-ivy leaves) yield a substance which in the form of a tincture has been much used by homoeopathists in the treatment of rheumatism.

Rhynchō·ta. An order of insects which includes the Pediculidae and Acanthiidae.

rhypophō·bia (G. *rhupos*, filth; *phobos*, fear). A neurotic fear of filth.

rhythm (G. *rhuthmos*, rhythm). Action or function recurring at regular intervals.

rhyth·mic (G. *rhuthmos*, rhythm). Relating to rhythm.

rhyth·mophone (G. *rhuthmos*, rhythm; *phōnē*, voice). An instrument used for the study of heart-beats.

rhytidec·tomy (G. *rhutis*, wrinkle; *ektomē*, excision). A cosmetic operation for the removal of wrinkles.

rhytodō·sis (G. *rhutis*, wrinkle). A wrinkling.

rib. One of the 24 curved, flat bones passing round the upper portion of the trunk from the vertebral column and forming the walls of the thorax. **R., cervical:** an enlarged transverse process of the seventh cervical vertebra. **R., false:** one of the five lower ribs on each side that are not attached to the sternum. **R., true:** one of the seven upper ribs on each side that are directly attached to the sternum.

Ribbert's theory (Ribbert, M. W. H., German pathologist, 1855–1920). That a tumour is formed from the development of cell rests owing to reduced tension in the surrounding tissues.

Ribes's ganglion (Ribes, F., French surgeon, 1800–64). Situated on the anterior communicating artery of the Circle of Willis; the uppermost sympathetic ganglion.

riboflāvine. Vitamin B_2; a water-soluble pigment present inter alia in milk, eggs, malted barley and yeast. Of value therapeutically only in deficiency states.

rice (G. *oruza*, rice). The plant *Oryza sativa* of the order Gramineae; also its seed.

rice-water stools. The bowel discharges in cholera.

Richard's fringe (Richard, F. A., French surgeon, 1822–72). The ovarian fimbria of the ostium of the uterine tube.

Richardson's sign (Richardson, Sir B. W., English physician, 1828–96). A test of death. A tight band is applied to the arm. If veins distal to this fill, life is not extinct.

Richet's canal (Richet, L. A., French surgeon, 1816–91). The canal for the umbilical vein on the anterior wall of the abdomen, made by the passage of some fibres of the transversus deep to the vein. **R.'s fascia:** the fascia covering the canal.

Richter's hernia (Richter, A. G., German surgeon, 1742–1812). A partial obstruction of the bowel in which only a part of the circumference is constricted. Occurs most commonly in femoral herniae.

ri·cinine (L. *ricinus*, the castor oil plant). An alkaloid of the pyridine group isolated from the castor oil seed.

Ri·cinus. A plant of the order Euphorbiaceae. The *R. communis*, or castor oil plant, yields *ricini oleum*, castor oil, which is used as a laxative.

rickets (Etym. dub.; taken by D. Webster (1645) for corruption of rhachitis, which he introduced as its scientific name). See rhachitis.

Rickett·sia (Ricketts, H. T., American pathologist, 1871–1910). A class of large viruses responsible, amongst other affections, for typhus fever, Rocky Mountain spotted fever and trench fever.

rickety. Affected with rickets.

Rideal-Walker coefficient (Rideal, S., English chemist, 1863–1929; Walker, A., contemporary English chemist). A number indicating the disinfecting value of a substance. It is the quotient obtained by dividing the number representing the dilution of a disinfectant which kills an organism in a fixed time by the number representing the degree of dilution of carbolic acid which kills the organism in the same time.

Ridell's operation. An operation for frontal sinusitis, in which the anterior wall of the sinus is removed.

rider's bone. An ossified portion of the adductor longus muscle in the leg due to prolonged pressure during riding on horseback.

ridge. An elevation or crest.

rid·gel, ridg·ling. A male animal with one testicle excised or lacking.

Ridley's sinus (Ridley, H., English anatomist, 1653–1708). The sinus circularis or sinus coronarius. Also called Ridley's bay.

Riedel's lobe (Riedel, B. M. C. L., German surgeon, 1846–1916). A form of 'constriction lobe' of the right side of the liver. **R's struma, R's thyroiditis:** Ligneous thyroiditis, densely hard infiltration of the thyroid gland.

Rieder's cells (Rieder, H., German radiologist, 1858–1932). Lymphoblasts, the nuclei of which are multi-lobulated.

Riegel's pulse (Riegel, F., German physician, 1843–1904). Pulse which is diminished in size during expiration.

right. That side of the body which lies to the east when the face is turned northward; dextral.

ri·gid (L. *rigidus*). Stiff; hard.

rigi·dity (L. *rigiditas*). Stiffness; inflexibility. **R., cadaveric:** rigor mortis, *q.v.*

ri·gor (L.). 1. Coldness; stiffness; chill; rigidity. 2. A sudden chill, especially one accompanied by fits of shivering. Generally prodromal of certain infections. **R. mortis:** the muscular rigidity occurring soon after death. **R. nervorum:** tetanus.

ri·ma (L.). A crack or cleft.

ri·mose, ri·mous (L. *rima*, a crack). Full of cracks or fissures.

ri·mula (L. dim. of *rima*). A small cleft, especially one of the spinal cord or the brain.

ring. A circular opening or organ. See also annulus.

Ringer's solution (Ringer, S., English physiologist, 1835–1910). A solution composed of sodium calcium and potassium chlorides, used for injection to replace water loss due to vomiting or diarrhoea.

ringworm. A contagious skin disease, characterized by circular, pigmented patches and caused by a vegetable parasite, the *Trichophyton*. See also tinea.

Rinne's test (Rinne, F. H., German ear specialist, 1819–68). A tuning-fork test to detect whether air or bone conductivity of the ear is the better.

Riolan's anastomoses (Riolan, J., the second, French anatomist, 1577–1657). Between the superior and inferior mesenteric arteries. **R.'s arcade:** the arterial anastomoses of intestinal vessels. **R.'s bouquet:** the muscles and ligaments arising from the styloid process; 'les fleurs rouges et les fleurs blanches'. **R.'s muscle:** the marginal bundle of the orbicularis palpebrarum.

ri·pa (L., bank). A line indicating the reflection of the ependyma of the ventricle over any plexus or tela of the brain.

R.I.P.H. Royal Institute of Public Health.

risor·ius muscle (L. *risus*, laughter). A muscle of the face which produces the act of laughing.

ri·sus sardŏ·nicus (L.). The sardonic grin; a distortion of the face caused by muscle spasm. It is seen in tetanus.

Ritter's disease (Ritter, G., von Rittersheim, German physician, 1820–83). Exfoliative dermatitis of infants.

Rivinus's ducts (Rivinus, A. Q., German anatomist, 1652–1723). The ducts of the sublingual glands. **R.'s membrane:** Shrapnell's membrane. **R.'s notch:** the incisura tympanica in the sulcus tympanicus, described in connection with a foramen in the membrana tympani noted in 1680.

ri·ziform. Resembling rice.

Rn. The symbol for radon.

Robin's myeloplax (Robin, C. F., French histologist, 1821–85). The osteoclast. **R.'s sheath:** the cellular sheath surrounding nerves. **R.'s spaces:** the lymphatic spaces associated with arteries.

Robinson's abdominal brain (Robinson, F. B., American anatomist, 1855–1910). The ganglion coeliacum. **R.'s cervical loop:** the uterine artery adjacent to the cervix. **R.'s circle:** the utero-ovarian arterial circle. **R.'s menstrual ganglia:** the autonomic ganglia on the uterine walls.

rō·borant (L. *robor*, strength). 1. Tonic. 2. A tonic remedy.

Rochelle salt (named from La Rochelle in France, where it is found). Potassium and sodium tartrate.

rodent ulcer. See under ulcer.

roentgen rays (Roentgen, W. K., German physicist, 1845–1922). See under X-rays.

roent·genism. 1. The therapeutic application of roentgen rays (X-rays). 2. Bad effects produced by misuse of roentgen rays.

roentgenŏ·graphy (Roentgen, W. K.; G. *graphein*, to write). Photography by means of X-rays. Syn. radiography; skiagraphy.

roentgen-therapy (Roentgen, W. K.; G. *therapeia*, treatment). The treatment of disease by means of roentgen rays (X-rays).

rötheln (Ger. from *roth*, red). See rubella.

Rohr's stria (Rohr, K., Swiss embryologist, born 1863). 'Rohrsche Fibrinstreifen'. The layers of the placenta.

Rokitansky's disease. See Budd's jaundice.

Rolando's area (Rolando, L., Italian anatomist, 1773–1831). The excitomotor region of the brain. **R.'s fissure:** the sulcus centralis. **R.'s funiculus:** an elevation on the lateral side of the fasciculus cuneatus of the medulla. **R.'s tubercle:** a prominence on the brain stem marking the upper extremity of the funiculus and overlying the substantia. Also called **Rolandic area, fissure,** etc.

rolandŏ·meter. An instrument for marking out the fissure of Rolando on the head.

Roller's nucleus (Roller, C. F. W., German neurologist, born 1844). 1. A small-celled nucleus of the hypoglossal nerve; nucleus sublingualis. 2. The nucleus lateralis of the accessory nerve. His work has sometimes been wrongly ascribed to his father, also C. F. W. Roller, 1802–78.

Rollet's stroma (Rollet, Austrian physiologist, 1834–1903). The colourless stroma of the erythrocytes.

Rollier's treatment (Rollier, A., Swiss physician, born 1874). Treatment of surgical tuberculosis by systematic exposure of the part to the rays of the sun.

Romberg's disease (Romberg, M. H., German physician, 1795–1873). Facial hemiatrophy. **R.'s sign:** when the eyes are covered and the feet placed together, the body sways about; an early symptom of locomotor ataxia. Syn. Brach-Romberg's sign.

Romberg-Howship sign. Shooting pains down inner aspect of thigh, as far as knee, which are found with incarcerated obturator hernia.

rongeur-forceps (Fr. *ronger*, to gnaw). A strong forceps used for cutting off pieces of bone.

röntgen rays. See roentgen.

root. 1. The part of a plant that is situated below the surface of the ground and conveys nourishment from the soil. 2. That part of an organ that is embedded in the tissues, e.g., the r. of a tooth, nail, hair, etc.

rosā·cĕa (L. *rosa*, rose). A chronic skin disease appearing on the face and characterized by red pigmentation and the formation of pustules. The disease leads to a coarsening of the skin areas affected. Also called acne rosacea.

rosă·nilin, rosă·niline. A colourless crystalline derivative of aniline, used as the basis of various dyes.

rose (L. *rosa*). A plant of the genus *Rosa*. **R., attar of:** a volatile oil obtained by distillation from the petals of *Rosa damascena*, used as a perfume and flavouring agent.

rosemary (L. *ros*, dew; *marinus*, of the sea). A plant of the order Labiatae. See Rosmarinus.

Rosenbach's disease (Rosenbach, A. J. F., German surgeon, 1842–1923). An erysipeloid which occurs in hands of persons who deal with fish.

Rosenmüller's fossa (Rosenmüller, J. C., German anatomist, 1771–1820). The recessus pharyngeus. **R.'s organ:** the epoophoron. See parovarium.

Rosenthal's canal (Rosenthal, I., German physiologist, 1836–1915). The spiral canal of the cochlea.

rosē·ola (L. *roseus*, rosy). 1. Rose-rash; a name given to any rose-coloured eruption. 2. Syn. of rubella.

Roser's line (Roser, W., German surgeon, 1817–88). From the anterior superior spine of the ilium to the tuber ischii.

rŏ·sin. The material remaining after distillation of the volatile oil of turpentine.

rosindol reaction. See Ehrlich's reagent.

Rosmarī·nus (L. *ros*, dew; *marinus*, of the sea). A genus of labiate plants. *R. officinalis* yields the volatile oil of rosemary which is used as a stimulant.

Ross's black spores (Ross, Sir R., British protozoologist, 1857–1932). Degenerated and pigmented malarial oocysts found in the body of a mosquito. **R.'s cycle:** that cycle in the development of *Plasmodium malariae* which is passed in the mosquito.

rostel·lum (L. dim. of *rostrum*, beak). A small beak, especially applied to the hook-bearing part of the head in certain types of worm.

rŏ·strate. Beaked, or having a beaklike process.

rŏ·strum (L., beak). A beak or beaklike projection.

rot. 1. Decay; decomposition. 2. A disease of sheep, sometimes occurring in man and caused by *Distoma hepaticum*.

rotate (L. *rotare*, to turn). To revolve; to turn round.

rotā·tion (L. *rotatio*, a turning). The act of revolving about an axis passing through the centre of the body.

rotā·tor (L. *rotare*, to turn). A muscle rotating a limb.

rŏ·tenone. A poisonous crystalline substance, $C_{23}H_{22}O_6$, obtained from the dried rhizome of *Derris elliptica* and *Derris malaccensis*. It is used as a horticultural and agricultural insecticide.

Roth's spots (Roth, M., Swiss physician, 1839–1914). Small white spots appearing on the retina in septic retinitis. **R.'s vas aberrans:** a tubule of the epididymis, connected with the rete testis but not with the vas deferens.

rŏ·tula (L. *rotula*, dim. of *rota*, wheel). 1. The patella. 2. A troche. 3. Any bone process resembling a disc.

rŏ·tular. Relating to the patella.

Rouget's cells (Rouget, C., French anatomist, 1824–1904). The isolated cells on the outer surface of the walls of capillaries. **R.'s muscle:** the circular fibres of the ciliary muscle.

roughage. The cellulose or fibrous portion of the diet.

Rougnon-Heberden disease (Rougnon, N. F., French physician, 1727-99; Heberden, W., English physician, 1710–1801). Angina pectoris.

rouleau (Fr.). A roll of red blood corpuscles.

Rous's sarcoma (Rous, F. P., American pathologist, born 1879). A sarcoma-like growth found in some fowls. From it can be obtained a filtrable virus which on inoculation into other fowls reproduces similar growths.

Rousseau's bone (Rousseau, F. F. E., French anatomist, 1788–1868). The accessory lacrimal bone situated anterior to the normal bone; external lacrimal bone.

Roux's muscle (Roux, C., Swiss surgeon, 1857–1934). The musculus recto-urethralis.

Rovsing's sign (Rovsing, T., Danish surgeon, 1862–1927). Pressure on the left side over the point corresponding to McBurney's point will elicit typical pain at McBurney's point in appendicitis but not in other abdominal affections.

Ru. Symbol for one atom of ruthenium.

rubber. The coagulated juice of various species of *Hevea*.

rubē·do (L. *rubere*, to be red). Blushing or redness of the skin.

rubefā·cient (L. *ruber*, red; *facere*, to make). 1. Producing a reddening of the skin. 2. An agent causing the skin to redden.

rubel·la (L. *ruber*, red). German measles or epidemic roseola (Ger. *Rötheln*), an acute contagious disease resembling measles, but lasting only a short time and having only mild symptoms.

rubes·cent (L. *rubescere*, to redden). Blushing; becoming red.

rubī·dium (L. *rubidus*, red). A rare alkaline metal; symbol Rb.

rubī·go (L.). Rust.

rū·bor. The redness due to inflammation.

rubrospī·nal (L. *ruber*, red; *spina*). Relating to the red nucleus and the spinal cord.

rū·brum (L.). The red nucleus or nucleus ruber.

Rubus. A genus of plants of the family Rosaceae which includes the raspberry and blackberry. The root-bark of *R. villosus*, *R. nigrobaccus* and *R. cuneifolius* is used as an astringent.

ruc·tus (L.). The eructation of gas from the stomach.

rudimen·tary (L. *rudimentum*, rudiment). Undeveloped.

rudimen·tum (L.). A rudiment; a beginning.

Rudinger's muscle (Rudinger, N., German anatomist, 1832–96). A muscle internal to the circular fibres of the rectum, M. dilator internus.

rue (G. *rhutē*). A plant, *Ruta graveolens*, which produces an oil, oleum rutae. The oil is used as an emmenagogue and abortifacient.

Ruffini's bodies or corpuscles (Ruffini, A., Italian histologist, 1874–1929). The sensory nerve endings, originally found in the subcutaneous tissues of the fingers.

rū·ga (L.). A wrinkle, ridge or fold. **R. palatina:** one of the elevations on the hard palate.

rū·gitus (L. a roaring). Intestinal rumbling.

rū·gose (L. *ruga*, wrinkle). Characterized by folds.

rugŏ·sity (L. *rugosus*, wrinkled). A fold or wrinkle.

rule. A law; an axiom.

rum. A spirit distilled from sugar-cane.

rū·men (L.). The first stomach of ruminant animals, from which they return their food in order to chew the cud. Also called paunch.

rū·minant (L. *ruminare*, to ruminate). Any cud-chewing animal.

rumina·tion (L. *ruminare*, to ruminate). Syn. merycism.

rump. The gluteal region.

run-around. Paronychia, *q.v.*

rū·pia (G. *rhupos*, filth). A skin eruption usually seen in tertiary syphilis and characterized by the formation of large vesicles with scabs.

rupophŏ·bia (G. *rhupos*, filth; *phobos*, fear). Rhypophobia, *q.v.*

rup·ture (L. *ruptura*, a breaking). 1. The tearing of a part by force. 2. Hernia.

rup·tured (L. *rumpere*, to break). 1. Torn. 2. Affected with hernia.

Rusconi's anus (Rusconi, M., Italian biologist, 1776–1849). The blastopore or protostoma.

rust. 1. The oxide and hydroxide of iron, producing a reddish deposit on the surface of iron exposed to moisture. 2. A disease of cereal plants, causing rust-like patches to form on them.

ruthē·nium (named from Ruthenia, a Russian province). A rare, hard metal. Symbol Ru.; atomic weight 101·7.

rutidŏ·sis (G. *rhutis*, wrinkle). A wrinkling; the puckering or shrivelling of the cornea that precedes death.

rū·tin. A crystalline alcohol, $C_{27}H_{32}O_{16}$, from tomato stems, tobacco, rue leaves, and many flowers.

Ruysch's tunic (Ruysch, F., Dutch anatomist, 1638–1731). The capillary network in the deepest part of the choroid; lamina choriocapillaris.

R. wave. Term applied to the electrocardiographic wave due to the action of the ventricles.

rye. The plant *Secale cereale* and its grain.

Ryle's duodenal tube (Ryle, J. A., English physician 1889–1950). A tube, slightly weighted to assist its passage, used in giving a fractional test meal.

S

S. 1. Chemical symbol for one atom of sulphur. 2. Abbreviation (in prescriptions) of *signum*—sign or label.

s. Abbreviation for L. (1) *sinister*, left; (2) *semis*, half (ordinarily ss).

sabadil·la. The dried ripe seeds of *Schoenocaulon officinale*, of the family Liliaceae. The seeds contain cevadine (syn. veratrine), an amorphous alkaloid, and are used in the preparation of a parasiticide particularly effective against *Pediculosis capitis*.

să·badine. A crystalline alkaloid obtained from sabadilla.

sabi·na. The tops of *Juniperus sabina*, which contain an oil (*oleum sabinae*, or oil of savin) which has strong emmenagogue and abortifacient properties.

să·bulous (L. *sabulum*, sand). Gritty; sandy.

sabur·ra (L.). Sordes.

sabur·ral. Relating to saburra.

sac (L. *saccus*, sack). A cyst; a pouch; a bag-like tumour. **Conjunctival s.:** that created by reflection of the palpebral conjunctiva.

sac·cate, sacchă·ted (L. *saccus*, sack). Sac-shaped; within a sac; encysted.

sacchară·ted (G. *sakkharon*, sugar). Containing sugar.

sac·charephidrō·sis (G. *sakkharon*, sugar; *ephidrosis*, perspiration). Hyperidrosis marked by the excretion of sugar in the sweat.

sacchări·ferous (G. *sakkharon*, sugar; L. *ferre*, to bear). Yielding or containing sugar.

saccharificā·tion (G. *sakkharon*, sugar; L. *facere*, to make). Conversion into sugar.

sacchări·meter (G. *sakkharon*, sugar; *metron*, measure). An instrument for ascertaining the amount of sugar in a solution.

sacchări·metry (G. *sakkharon*, sugar; *metron*, measure). The process of determining the quantity or proportion of sugar in a liquid.

sac·charin (G. *sakkharon*, sugar). A crystalline substance nearly 280 times sweeter than cane sugar, for which it is used as a substitute.

sac·charine (G. *sakkharon*, sugar). Containing sugar; sweet as sugar.

sac·charogalactorrhoe·a (G. *sakkharon*, sugar; *gala*, milk; *rhoia*, a flow). Excretion of excessive sugar with milk.

sac·charolў·tic (G. *sakkharon*, sugar; *lusis*, dissolution). Able to produce the chemical splitting up of sugar.

saccharŏ·meter. Saccharimeter, *q.v.*

Saccharomў·cēs (G. *sakkharon*, sugar; *mukēs*, mushroom). A genus of single-celled fungi, including the yeasts.

sac·charomycō·sis (G. *sakkharon*, sugar; *mukēs*, mushroom). Any disease produced by the presence of yeast fungi.

sac·charorrhoe·a (G. *sakkharon*, sugar; *rhoia*, a flow). Glycosuria, *q.v.*

sac·charose (G. *sakkharon*, sugar). Cane sugar. Syn. sucrose.

sac·charosū·ria (G. *sakkharon*, sugar; *ouron*, urine). The presence of saccharose in the urine.

sac·ciform (L. *saccus*, sack; *forma*, shape). Like a sac.

sac·cular (L. *saccus*, sack). Sac-like.

sac·culated (L. *sacculus*, dim. of *saccus*, sack). Separated into small sacs.

sac·cule (L. *sacculus*, dim. of *saccus*, sack). 1. A small bag or sac. 2. That one of the two vestibular sacs of the membranous labyrinth of the ear which connects with the ductus cochlearis.

sac·culococh·lear (L. *sacculus*, small sack; *cochlea*, shell). Relating to the sacculus proprius and the cochlea.

sac·culus (L. *sacculus*, dim. of *saccus*, sack). A saccule or pouch. **S. communis:** the utricle of the ear. **S. lacrimalis:** the lacrymal sac. **S. laryngis:** laryngeal pouch. A membranous sac between the superior vocal cord and the thyroid cartilage. **S. proprius:** the saccule of the ear. **S. ventricularis:** laryngeal pouch. **S. vestibuli:** that one of the two divisions of the membranous labyrinth of the ear which communicates with the ductus cochlearis.

sac·cus (L.). A sac or bursa. **S. lacrimalis:** the lacrimal sac.

Sachs-Georgi reaction (Sachs, H., German bacteriologist, 1877–1945; Georgi, W., German bacteriologist, 1889–1920). A precipitation test for syphilis. Addition of 1 cc. of a solution of cholesterinized alcoholic extract of human or beef heart (1 part) and normal sodium chloride solution 9 parts to 30 cc. syphilitic serum will cause a flocculant precipitate.

să·cra mē·dia (L. *sacer*, sacred; *medius*, middle). The middle sacral artery, which traverses the middle of the anterior surface of the sacrum and typifies the termination of the aorta.

să·crad (L. *sacer*, sacred; *ad*, to). Towards the sacrum.

să·cral. Relating to the sacrum.

sacral·gia (L. (*os*) *sacrum*; G. *algos*, pain). Pain in the sacrum.

sacred bark. Cascara sagrada, *q.v.*

sacrec·tomy (L. (*os*) *sacrum*; G. *ektomē*, excision). Surgical removal of the sacrum; an operation usually performed for cancer of the rectum.

sacrificial operation. An operation in which some organ is sacrificed for the general good of the patient.

sacro-anterior (L. (*os*) *sacrum*; *anterior*, from *ante*, before). Term used of a foetus with the sacrum directed forward in relation to the mother.

să·crococcў·geal (L. (*os*) *sacrum*; G. *kokkux*, coccyx). Relating to the sacrum and the coccyx.

să·crocoxī·tis (L. (*os*) *sacrum*; *coxa*, hip). Inflammation of the sacro-iliac joint.

sacrodў·nia (L. (*os*) *sacrum*; G. *odunē*, pain). Pain in or around the sacrum.

sacro-iliac (L. (*os*) *sacrum*; *ilium*). Relating to the sacrum and the ilium.

să·crolum·bar (L. (*os*) *sacrum*; *lumbus*, loin). Relating to the sacrum and the loins.

să·croperi·neal (L. (*os*) *sacrum*; G. *perinaion*, space between anus and scrotum). Relating to the sacrum and perineum.

să·cropostē·rior (L. (*os*) *sacrum*; *posterior*, from *post*, behind). Term used of a foetus with the sacrum directed backward.

săcrostă·tic (L. (*os*) *sacrum*; *ischium*). Relating to the sacrum and the ischium.

săcrospī·nal (L. (*os*) *sacrum*; *spina*, spine). Relating to the sacrum and the spine.

săcrospinā·lis muscle (L. (*os*) *sacrum*; *spina*, spine). The long muscle running beside the vertebral spines;

arising below from sacrum, inserted above into vertebrae: it gains secondary origin from the lumbar and dorsal vertebrae. Usually considered in its several parts.

sacrŏ·tomy (L. (*os*) *sacrum*; G. *tomē*, a cutting). Surgical removal of the lower part of the sacrum.

sacro-ū·terine (L. (*os*) *sacrum*; *uterus*). Relating to the sacrum and the uterus.

sā·crover·tebral (L. (*os*) *sacrum*; *vertebra*). Relating to the sacrum and the vertebrae.

sā·crum (L.). The curved triangular bone formed of five united vertebrae between the last lumbar vertebra above and the coccyx below, and flanked by the two innominate bones. Called by the ancient Roman medical writers *os sacrum*, the sacred bone.

saddle-nose. A nose with a depressed bridge, sometimes seen in congenital syphilis.

sā·dism (Marquis de Sade, 1740–1814). Sexual perversion in which pleasure is experienced in the infliction of cruelty.

sā·dist. One given to sadism.

sadis·tic. Relating to sadism.

saf·flower (Ital. *saffiore*, saffron flower). See Carthamus.

saf·fron (Sp. *zafaran*). The dried stigmas and tops of *Crocus sativus*, which yield a yellow colouring matter. Saffron has been used as an abortifacient.

saf·ranine (Ar. *zafaran*, saffron). A coal-tar dye employed in microscopy, particularly in studying karyokinesis. It is a cardiac and respiratory poison.

saf·role. The chief constituent of oil of sassafras, but is also obtainable from essential oil of camphor. Formula $C_{10}H_{10}O_n$. It is used in the treatment of pediculosis and also of ringworm. Syn. safril; allyl catechol methylene ether.

sagapē·num (G. *sagapēnŏn*, the *Ferula persica* plant). A gum-resin obtained from *Ferula persica* and having a taste similar to asafetida. Has been used in the treatment of hysteria and amenorrhoea.

sage. The dried leaves of *Salvia officinalis*. They have tonic and astringent properties and are used in treating dyspepsia.

sā·gittal (L. *sagitta*, arrow). 1. Arrow-shaped, as the s. suture of the skull. 2. Relating to the anteroposterior median plane of the body.

sā·go. A starch prepared from the pith of the sago palm.

St. Agatha's disease. Any disease of the breast.

St. Anthony's fire. Erysipelas.

St. Germain tea. *Species laxantes*; a mixture of senna, elder flowers and other ingredients.

St. Gervasius's disease. Rheumatism.

St. Gotthard's disease. Ankylostomiasis.

St. Hubert's disease. Hydrophobia.

St. Ignatius's bean. Ignatia, *q.v.*

St. Sement's disease. Syphilis.

St. Thomas's balsam. Tolu balsam.

St. Vitus's dance. Chorea.

sa·ke. A spirit distilled by the Japanese from rice.

sal (L.). Salt. **S. volatile:** ammonium carbonate.

salacē·tol. An anti-rheumatic and antiseptic compound of acetone and salicylic acid.

salā·cious (L. *salax*, lecherous). Characterized by lust.

salā·city (L. *salax*, lecherous). Strong venereal desire.

sā·lep. The dried tubers of *Orchis mascula* and other species of Orchidaceae. They are first immersed in boiling water and then dried. The tubers contain mucilage and are valuable in the treatment of gastro-intestinal irritation.

sali·cylate. Any salt of salicylic acid.

salicy̆·lic acid. Orthohydroxy-benzoic acid. Used as an antiseptic in ointments and dusting powders and also in corn preparations.

sā·line (L. *sal*, salt). 1. Salty. 2. A salt of an alkali or of alkaline earth. **S. solution,** a 0·9 per cent solution of sodium chloride; physiological ('normal') salt solution.

salipy̆·rin. $C_{11}H_{12}ON_2$, $C_6H_4(OH)(COOH)$; antipyrine salicylate. A sweetish-tasting, white crystalline powder, which is useful in cases of rheumatic fever, sciatica, etc.

salī·va (L. *salivare*, to spit out). The colourless liquid produced by the combined secretions of the salivary and mucous glands of the mouth ; the spittle. Saliva contains digestive ferments.

sā·livant. Promoting the flow of saliva, or any agent that does this.

sal·ivary. Relating to or created from saliva. **S. calculus:** a concretion occurring in a s. duct. **S. fistula:** an opening between a s. gland or its duct with the skin.

sā·livate (L. *salivare*, to spit out). To produce an excessive quantity of saliva.

salivā·tion (L. *salivare*, to spit out). An excessive flow of saliva; a condition that may be caused by mercury, by pilocarpine and by nervous and mental disturbances; ptyalism.

sā·livator. An agent producing salivation.

sā·livatory. Producing salivation.

Salix (L., willow). A genus of trees, the willows. The bark of the common white willow, *S. alba*, contains salicin, which is tonic and antiseptic. It is used as an antipyretic in rheumatic fever.

sal·monella ty̆·phi. One of the group of organisms causing typhoid and the paratyphoid fevers.

sā·lol (L. *salix*, willow; *oleum*, oil). Phenyl salicylate; used as an intestinal antiseptic.

salpingec·tomy (G. *salpigx*, trumpet; *ektomē*, excision). Excision of a uterine tube.

sal·pingemphrax·is (G. *salpigx*, trumpet; *emphraxis*, stoppage). Closure of a pharyngotympanic or uterine tube.

salpin·gian (G. *salpigx*, trumpet). Relating to a pharyngotympanic or uterine tube.

salpin·gion (G. *salpigx*, trumpet). A point at the apex of the petrous bone on its lower surface.

salpingī·tis (G. *salpigx*, trumpet). 1. Inflammation of a uterine (Fallopian) tube. 2. Inflammation of a pharyngotympanic (Eustachian) tube.

salpingocă·theterism (G. *salpigx*, trumpet; *kathetēr*, catheter). Catheterization of a pharyngotympanic tube.

salpin·gocȳe·sis (G. *salpigx*, trumpet; *kuēsis*, conception). Pregnancy in a uterine tube.

salpin·gomal·leus (G. *salpigx*, trumpet; L. *malleus*, a hammer). The tensor tympani muscle.

sal·pingo-ō·ophorec·tomy (G. *salpigx*, trumpet; *ōon*, egg; *phoros*, bearing; *ektomē*, excision). Excision of a uterine tube and ovary.

sal·pingo-ō·ophorī·tis (G. *salpigx*, trumpet; *ōon*, egg; *pherein*, to bear). Inflammation of the uterine tube and the ovary.

salpin·go-ŏōthē·cocele (G. *salpigx*, trumpet; *ōon*, egg; *kēlē*, hernia). Ovarian hernia.

salpin·gopharyn·geal (G. *salpigx*, trumpet; *pharugx*, throat). Relating to the pharyngotympanic tube and the pharynx.

salpin·gopharyn·geus (G. *salpigx*, trumpet; *pharugx*, throat). The levator palati muscle, extending downwards from the pharyngotympanic tube to the pharyngeal constrictors.

salpin·goplasty (G. *salpigx*, trumpet; *plassein*, to form). Plastic operation on a uterine tube.

salpingor·rhaphy (G. *salpigx*, trumpet; *rhaphē*, suture). Suture of a uterine tube.

salpin·gostă·phyline (G. *salpigx*, trumpet; *staphulē*, uvula). Relating to the pharyngotympanic tube and the uvula.

salpin·gostaphylī·nus (G. *salpigx*, trumpet; *staphulē*, uvula). Tensor palati muscle.

salpingŏ·stomy (G. *salpigx*, trumpet; *stoma*, mouth). The establishment of a drainage opening in a uterine tube.

salpingŏ·tomy (G. *salpigx*, throat; *tomē*, a cutting). The surgical incision of a uterine tube.

salpinx (G. *salpigx*, trumpet). A tube; especially a uterine (Fallopian) or pharyngotympanic (Eustachian) tube.

salt. 1. Sodium chloride. 2. Any compound of a base and an acid.

saltă·tion (L. *saltare*, to dance). The dancing, leaping or skipping sometimes seen in chorea.

sal·tative (L. *saltare*, to dance). Skipping, in the sense of abrupt change or variation of a species.

sal·tatory (L. *saltare*, to dance). Relating to or characterized by leaping.

Salter's lines (Salter, Sir J. A., English dentist, 1825–97). The 'incremental lines' of reaction in the substance of the dentine.

saltpetre (L. *sal*, salt; *petra*, a stone). KNO_3; potassium nitrate. **S., Chile:** sodium nitrate.

salts. A saline cathartic such as Epsom salts.

salū·brious (L. *salubris*, healthy). Favourable to health.

să·lutary (L. *salutaris*, wholesome). Beneficial; promoting health.

salvar·san. Dioxy-diaminoarseno-benzol, a sulphur-yellow powder used in the treatment of syphilis and other spirochaetal infections; Ehrlich's '606'. Syn. Arsphenamine.

salvatel·la. The small vein situated on the back of the little finger; the vena salvatella.

salve. Ointment; unguent.

Sal·via. A genus of labiate plants. See under sage.

Salzer's test meal (Salzer, F. A., Dutch surgeon, born 1858). Two different meals given four hours apart. Stomach emptied one hour after second meal. If stomach is normal there should be no remains of first meal.

Salzmann's membrane (Salzmann, M., Austrian ophthalmologist, born 1862). The external vitreous membrane; basal membrane between the vitreous body and the choroid.

samā·rium. A rare metallic element. Symbol Sm.

Samisch's operation (Samisch, E. J., German ophthalmologist, 1833–1909). Transfixion of the cornea and the base of the ulcer for cure of hypopyon. **S.'s ulcer:** an infectious and serpiginous ulcer of the cornea.

să·native, să·natory (L. *sanare*, to heal). Promoting health.

sanator·ium (L. *sanare*, to heal). 1. An establishment for the treatment of (usually) tuberculous patients or invalids. 2. A health resort with a good climate frequented by invalids.

sand. A mass of fine grains of silicic oxide.

san·dalwood (Ar. *sandal*). The heart wood of *Santalum album* (white s.) and of *Pterocarpus santalinus* (red s.). **S. oil** is the *Oleum santali* of the B.P.

san·darac. A resin obtained from the stem of *Tetraclinis articulata*. It is used in pill varnishes.

Sanders's sign (Sanders, J., English physician, 1777–1843). Undulating cardiac impulse seen especially in epigastrium in cases of adherent pericardium.

Sandström bodies (Sandström, I. V., Swedish anatomist, 1852–89). The parathyroids.

Sandwith's bald tongue (Sandwith, F. M., British physician, 1853–1918). An extremely smooth tongue seen in advanced cases of pellagra.

sane (L. *sanus*). Of sound mind.

Sanger's macula (Sanger, M., Austrian gynaecologist, 1853–1903). A red spot at the orifice of the vulvo-vaginal gland in gonorrhoeal vaginitis.

sangui·colous (L. *sanguis*, blood; *colere*, to inhabit). Living in the blood.

sanguifă·cient (L. *sanguis*, blood; *facere*, to make). Forming blood.

Sanguina·ria. A genus of papaveraceous plants. The dried rhizome of *S. canadensis* is a gastric tonic and emetic. Syn. blood-root.

sanguĭ·narin. An alkaloid resin obtained from the blood-root. See Sanguinaria.

san·guine (L. *sanguis*, blood). 1. Bloody; resembling blood. 2. Competent; vigorous, as s. temperament.

sangui·neous (L. *sanguis*, blood). 1. Relating to the blood. 2. Sanguine.

sangui·nolent (L. *sanguis*, blood). Coloured with blood.

san·guinopoiĕ·tic (L. *sanguis*, blood; G. *poiein*, to make). Forming blood.

san·guis (L.). Blood.

sanguisū·ga (L. *sanguis*, blood; *sugere*, to suck). A leech.

sā·niēs (L., diseased blood). A seropurulen discharge from an ulcer or wound.

sā·nious (L. *sanies*, diseased blood). Relating to or like sanies.

sanita·rian (L. *sanitas*, health). An expert in sanitation and public health.

să·nitary (L. *sanitas*, health). Relating to health. **S. cordon:** one set up to control entry to and exit from an infected area.

sanitā·tion (L. *sanitas*, health). 1. The ensuring of healthy conditions. 2. The adoption of sanitary measures.

să·nity (L. *sanitas*, health). Soundness of mind.

Sanocrȳ·sin (L. *sanus*, sound; G. *khrusos*, gold). A proprietary preparation of sodium and gold thio-sulphate. It is used by injection in the treatment of tuberculosis.

Sansom's sign (Sansom, A. E., English physician, 1838–1907). (1) Increased area of dullness in the second and third intercostal spaces due to pericardial effusion. (2) A murmur heard in aneurysms of the thoracic aorta when the stethoscope is applied to the lips.

Sanson's images (Sanson, L. J., French physician, 1790–1841). (Also known as Purkinje-Sanson's images). Three pairs of images of one object seen in obscuring the pupil.

san·talin. The colouring-matter of red sandalwood.

santŏ·nica. The dried heads of the flower of *Artemisia maritima*. Santonica is used as a vermifuge.

san·tonin. A crystalline, poisonous principle from santonica.

san·toninox·ime. A derivative of santonin than which it is less toxic; used as a vermicide.

Santorini's cartilages (Santorini, G. D., Italian anatomist, 1681–1737). The corniculate cartilages of the larynx. **S.'s caruncula:** c. major; vater's papilla. c. minor; orifice of the accessory duct into the duodenum. **S.'s duct:** the accessory duct of the pancreas. **S.'s vein:** the emissary vein through the parietal foramen.

sap. The natural juice of plants.

saphē·na (G. *saphēnēs*, manifest). Two large veins in the leg; the internal (long) s. and the external (short) s.

saphē·nous (G. *saphēnēs*, manifest). Apparent; manifest. Relating to two of the leg veins (see Saphena) and to the nerves accompanying these veins.

saphran·ophile (Ar. *zafaran*, saffron; G. *philein*, to love). Staining readily with safranine.

sap·id (L. *sapere*, to taste). Having a pleasant taste.

sā·po (L.). Soap.

Sapolini's nerve (Sapolini, G., 1812–93). The nervus intermedius, the thirteenth cranial nerve.

saponā·ceous (L. *sapo*, soap). Having a soapy nature.

Sapona·ria (L. *sapo*, soap). A genus of plants belonging to the family Caryophylleae. The root of *S. officinalis* (soapwort) has been used in the treatment of skin diseases. These and other plants, e.g. Quillaia, contain saponins—glycosides having high foaming power.

saponificā·tion (L. *sapo*, soap; *facere*, to make). The process of converting into soap.

sapō·nin (L. *sapo*, soap). A glucoside occurring in the roots of soapwort and some other plants and capable of creating a strong and durable lather in aqueous solution.

Sappey's plexus (Sappey, M. P. C., French anatomist, 1810–96). The plexus of lymphatics in the areolar area of the mamma. S.'s veins: the venous plexus in the falciform ligament of the liver.

sapphism (G. poetess *Sapphō*). Tribadism; unnatural passion between women.

sapraē·mia (G. *sapros*, rotten; *haima*, blood). Intoxication caused by absorption into the blood of the products of putrefaction.

saprae·mic. Relating to sapraemia.

să·prin (G. *sapros*, rotten). A harmless ptomaine, $C_5H_{14}N_2$ from putrefying animal tissues.

saprodŏn·tia (G. *sapros*, rotten; *odous*, tooth). Caries or putrefaction of the teeth.

saprogĕ·nic, saprŏ·genous (G. *sapros*, rotten; *gennan*, to produce). 1. Producing putrefaction. 2. Caused by putrefaction.

sap·rol. A disinfectant composed of 40 per cent of crude cresols in hydrocarbons from petroleum.

Saproleg·nia (G. *sapros*, rotten; *legnon*, edge). A genus of phycomycetous fungi—partially saprophytic.

saprŏ·philous (G. *sapros*, rotten; *philein*, to love). Living upon putrefying matter.

sap·rophyte (G. *sapros*, rotten; *phuton*, plant). A plant subsisting on putrefying matter.

saprophy̆·tic. Relating to a saprophyte.

sapropy̆·ra (G. *sapros*, rotten; *pur*, fire). Putrid fever.

saproty̆·phus (G. *sapros*, rotten; *tophos*, stupor). True or malignant typhus fever.

saprozō·ic (G. *sapros*, rotten; *zōon*, animal). Subsisting on dead matter.

saprozō·ite (G. *sapros*, rotten; *zōon*, animal). Any protozoon subsisting without a living host.

sar·cin (G. *sarx*, flesh). Hypoxanthine.

Sar·cina (L., package). A genus of schizomycetes. Cell division occurs in three planes forming regular packets.

sar·cine (L. *sarcina*, package). A cube of eight bacterial cells.

sarci·tis (G. *sarx*, flesh). Inflammation of fleshy tissues—particularly of muscle.

sar·co-adenō·ma (G. *sarx*, flesh; *adēn*, gland). Adenosarcoma, *q.v.*

sar·coblast (G. *sarx*, flesh; *blastos*, germ). The precursor of the muscle cell.

sar·cocarcinō·ma (G. *sarx*, flesh; *karkinos*, an ulcer). A malignant growth formed of both carcinomatous and sarcomatous cells.

sar·cocele (G. *sarx*, flesh; *kēlē*, hernia). Any fleshy swelling of the testicles.

sar·cocyst (G. *sarx*, flesh; *kustis*, bladder). Cyst in muscle caused by growth of Sarcocystis.

Sarcocys·tis (G. *sarx*, flesh; *kustis*, bladder). A genus of Sarcosporidia, including *S. miescheri*, which is found in beef and pork.

sar·code (G. *sarx*, flesh; *eidos*, form). Protoplasm of animals.

sarco-enchondrō·ma (G. *sarx*, flesh; *en*, in; *khondros*, cartilage). Sarcoma and enchondroma combined.

sarcogen·ic (G. *sarx*, flesh; *gennan*, to produce). Flesh forming.

sarcog·lia (G. *sarx*, flesh; *glia*, glue). The substance composing the eminences of Doyen at the entrance of a nerve into muscle.

sar·coid (G. *sarx*, flesh; *eidos*, form). 1. Resembling or having the nature of flesh. 2. Resembling a sarcoma.

sarcoidō·sis (G. *sarx*, flesh; *eidos*, form). Boeck's disease. Schaumann's disease. A syndrome consisting of the presence of cutaneous nodules, rarefication of the phalanges and pulmonary changes possibly tuberculous in origin.

sarcolac·tate (G. *sarx*, flesh; *lac*, milk). A salt of sarcolactic acid.

sarcolac·tic (G. *sarx*, flesh; *lac*, milk). Dextro-rotatory lactic acid.

sarcolem·ma (G. *sarx*, flesh; *lemma*, husk). The delicate sheath investing all muscle fibres.

sarcō·logy (G. *sarx*, flesh; *logos*, discourse). The section of anatomy dealing with soft tissues.

sarcō·ma (G. *sarx*, flesh). A malignant tumour composed of embryonic connective tissue. It is characterized by having a great number of cells with comparatively little homogeneous or intercellular substance. S., melanotic: a sarcoma containing intracellular melanin; it is highly malignant.

sarcomatō·sis (G. *sarx*, flesh). A condition marked by the formation of sarcomas in various parts of the body.

sarcō·matous (G. *sarx*, flesh). Relating to a sarcoma.

sarcomĕ·lanin (G. *sarx*, flesh; *melas*, black). The black pigment characterizing melanotic sarcoma.

sar·comere (G. *sarx*, flesh; *meros*, part). A segment of a muscle fibrilla which is divided by the lines of Krause.

Sarcop·tes. A genus of acarus including *S. scabiei* which produces scabies.

Sar·coplasm (G. *sarx*, flesh; *plassein*, to form). The substance in which fibrillae of muscle fibres are embedded.

sarcō·sis (G. *sarx*, flesh). 1. Diffuse sarcomatosis. 2. Inordinate increase of flesh.

sar·cosome (G. *sarx*, flesh; *soma*, body). The contractile part of a muscle fibril.

Sar·cospori·dia (G. *sarx*, flesh; *sporos*, seed). A kind of psorosperms occurring in the muscles of cattle and other animals.

sarcostō·sis (G. *sarx*, flesh; *osteon*, bone). The formation of bone in muscle tissues.

sar·costyle (G. *sarx*, flesh; *stulos*, column). A bundle of muscle fibrillae, i.e., a muscle column.

sarcot·ic (G. *sarx*, flesh). Relating to or causing the growth of flesh.

sar·cous (G. *sarx*, flesh). Relating to flesh or muscle.

sardonic grin. See risus sardonicus.

sar·saparil·la (Sp. *zarza*, bramble; *parrilla*, twohandled jar). A genus of plants of the order Liliaceae, including smilax. The dried roots of *Smilax ornata* has been used in the treatment of rheumatism and of skin affections.

sar·tian (From the Sarto of Central Asia). An epidemic skin disease of Central Asia: there are facial nodules which become ulcerated.

sartor·ius (L. *sartor*, a patcher). The tailor's muscle which is so called from its being used to cross one leg over the other.

sas·safras. The dried inner bark of the root of *S. variifolium*, a tree belonging to the order Lauraceae. It is a carminative.

sat. Abbreviation for saturated. Sat. sol.: the abbreviation for saturated solution.

să·tellite (L. *satelles*, an attendant). Any structure which closely accompanies and is subsidiary to a structure of the same kind.

Sattler's 'couche' (Sattler, H., Austrian ophthalmologist, 1844–1928). The middle layer of the choroid; couche intervasculaire. **S.'s glands:** the glandulae ciliares.

sati·ety (L. *satis*, enough). The state of being glutted or satiated.

să·turated (L. *saturare*, to saturate). 1. In chemistry, the state of any substance when it is either charged with or is holding in solution the utmost amount of another substance that it is capable of absorbing. 2. Of a chemical compound, a state in which all the valencies of its atoms are satisfied.

satura·tion (L. *saturare*, to saturate). 1. Solution continued until the solvent can contain no more; the state of being saturated. 2. Of a chemical compound, a state in which the affinities of all its atoms are saturated. **S. of atmosphere:** the condition in which any lowering of temperature will lead to a precipitation of the aqueous vapour mingled with the atmosphere. **S.-point:** The temperature at which the atmosphere contains as much moisture as it is able to hold. 2. The limit of solubility of a solid in a fluid at a given temperature.

să·turnine (L. *saturnus*, lead). 1. Relating to or produced by lead. 2. Of a gloomy disposition.

să·turnism (L. *saturnus*, lead). Lead-poisoning.

satyrĭ·asis (G. *saturos*, satyr). Excessive sexual desire in the male.

saurider·ma (G. *sauros*, lizard; *derma*, skin). Ichthyosis.

sau·roid (G. *sauros*, lizard; *eidos*, form). Lizard-like.

sausage-poisoning. A state of gastro-enteritis caused by the ingestion of decomposed sausage; botulism.

Saussure's hygrometer (Saussure, H. B. de, Swiss physicist, 1740–79). An instrument for measuring the moisture of the atmosphere. Changes in length of a hair, due to influence of moisture, are the means of measurement.

Savage's perineal body (Savage, H., English gynaecologist, 1810–1900). The perineal body; fibromuscular mass intervening between the anus and vulva.

Savill's disease (Savill, T. D., English physician, 1856–1910). Epidemic eczema.

savin, oil of. A volatile oil obtained from the leaves of the evergreen shrub, *Juniperus sabina*. It has emmenagogue and abortifacient qualities, but is a severe irritant and may set up haematuria and gastrointestinal irritation.

să·vory (L. *satureia*, savory). Herb of the mint family, Satureia; used as a carminative.

să·voury (L. *sapere*, to taste). Having an agreeable odour or flavour.

saw. An instrument consisting of a slender blade with sharp teeth on the cutting edge. It is used for cutting bones and other hard materials. **S. Gigli's:** a wire saw used in opening the skull.

Saxer's cells (Saxer, F., German pathologist, 1864–1903). The 'primary emigrant corpuscles'; a primitive form of leucocyte in the embryonic mesenchymal tissues.

Sb. The symbol for an atom of Antimony (stibium).

scab. 1. The crust produced by the desiccation of secretions from any superficial ulcer or sore. 2. Congealed exudate on the skin. 3. Scabies.

scā·bies (L. *scabere*, to scratch). Itch; a contagious skin disease produced by the parasite *Sarcoptes scabiei* or itchmite, which burrows into the skin and causes intense irritation.

scā·bious (L. *scabere*, to scratch). Scabby; scaly.

scabri·tĭĕs (L. *scaber*, rough). Roughness; scabbiness. **S. unguium:** abnormal roughness and thickness of the nails.

sca·la (L.). A staircase or ladder. **S. media:** the space between the membrane of Reissner and the basilar membrane, containing the essential peripheral organs of hearing. **S. tympani:** the canal lying below the osseous lamina and the basilar membrane of the internal ear. **S. vestibuli:** the canal confined by the osseous lamina and the membrane of Reissner.

scald (L. *ex*, intensive prefix, *calidus*, hot). The burn caused by hot fluids or vapours.

scale[1]. 1. The lamina of horny epidermis cast from the skin in health and in various diseases. 2. To scrape tartar from the teeth.

scale[2]. 1. Anything bearing marks placed at regular intervals and used as a standard in measuring; e.g., barometric s. 2. A weighing machine.

scā·lene (G. *skalēnos*, uneven). 1. Having three unequal sides. 2. Relating to a scalenus muscle.

scalē·nus muscle. Four in number: anterior, medius, posterior and pleuralis. **S. anterior:** (s. anticus) arises by four short tapering tendons from the anterior tubercles of the transverse processes of the third, fourth, fifth and sixth cervical vertebrae. It is inserted into the scalene tubercle of the first rib. **S. medius:** arises by six short tapering tendons from the anterior tubercles of the transverse processes of the lower six cervical vertebrae. It is inserted into the superior surface of the first rib. **S. pleuralis:** (s. minimus or s. quartus) a small muscle not always present. It is attached above to the anterior tubercle of the transverse process of the seventh cervical vertebra and below to the first rib. **S. posterior:** (s. posticus) arises by two or three short tendons from the posterior tubercles of the transverse processes of the lower two or three cervical vertebrae. It is inserted into the outer surface of the second rib.

scalenŏ·tomy. Operation in case of cervical rib syndrome. The scalenus anterior is divided at its insertion.

scā·ling. 1. Desquamating. 2. Removing tartar from the teeth.

scall (Old Norse *scalli*, a bald head). Any scabforming disease of the skin, e.g. psoriasis, impetigo, scabies, etc.

scalp. The integument of the upper part of the head which is covered with hair.

scal·pel (L. *scalpellum*, dim. of *scalprum*, a knife). A surgeon's small knife with a convex edge.

scal·prum (L. *scalprum*, knife). 1. A toothed raspatory. 2. A large scalpel.

scā·ly. 1. Like scales. 2. Characterized by scales.

scam·monin (G. *skammōnia*, the scammony plant). A glucoside, $C_{34}H_{56}O_{16}$, from scammony.

scam·mony (G. *skammōnia*, the scammony plant). The dehydrated juice of the root of *Convolvulus scammonium*. It is cathartic.

scanning speech (L. *scandere*, to scan). A peculiar slow and measured form of speech observed in various diseases of the nervous system, especially in multiple sclerosis.

scā·phocephal·ic (G. *skaphē*, boat; *kephalē*, head). Possessing a boat-shaped head.

scā·phocĕ·phalus (G. *skaphē*, boat; *kephalē*, head). A boat-shaped appearance of the cranium, caused by a premature union of the sagittal suture or by abnormal development.

scā·phoid (G. *skaphē*, boat; *eidos*, form). Boat-shaped. **S. bone;** the boat-shaped bone of the tarsus and of the carpus.

scaphoidi·tis. Inflammation of a scaphoid bone.

scă·pula (L. *scapulae*, the shoulder-blades). The shoulder-blade; the large flat triangular bone composing the back of the shoulder.

scapulal·gia (L. *scapulae*, the shoulder-blades; G. *algos*, pain). Pain in the proximity of the shoulder-blade.

scă·pular (L. *scapulae*, the shoulder-blades). Relating to the shoulder-blade.

scă·pulary (L. *scapulae*, the shoulder-blades). A two-tongued bandage, of which the two ends are brought over the shoulders and the single end is drawn down the back; all three ends are then secured to a body-bandage.

scapulec·tomy (L. *scapulae*, the shoulder-blades; G. *ektomē*, excision). The excision of the scapula or of a part of it.

scă·puloclavi·cular (L. *scapulae*, the shoulder-blades; *clavicula*, dim. of *clavis*, key). Relating to the scapula and the clavicle.

scapulodỹ·nia (L. *scapulae*, the shoulder-blades; G. *odunē*, pain). Pain in the shoulder.

scă·pulohū·meral (L. *scapulae*, the shoulder-blades; *humerus*, shoulder). Relating to the scapula and the humerus.

scă·pulopexy (L. *scapulae*, the shoulder-blades; G. *pēxis*, fixation). The surgical fixation of the scapula to the ribs.

scă·pulothŏră·cic (L. *scapulae*, the shoulder-blades; G. *thōrax*, chest). Relating to the scapula and the thorax.

scă·pulover·tebral (L. *scapulae*, the shoulder-blades; *vertebra*, a joint). Relating to the scapula and the spine.

scar (G. *eskhara*, scab). The connective tissue automatically substituted for a localized loss of substance.

scarf-skin. The cuticle or epidermis.

scarificā·tion (G. *skariphaomai*, from *skariphos*, a pencil). The making of a quantity of small superficial incisions in the skin.

scarificā·tor (G. *skariphos*, a pencil). An instrument formed of a number of small lancets operated by a spring, used for scarification.

scă·rify (G. *skariphos*, a pencil). To make many small superficial incisions.

scarlati·na (It. *scarlattina*, from *scarlatto*, scarlet). Scarlet fever, *q.v.*

scarlăti·nal. Relating to scarlet fever.

scarlăti·noid. Resembling scarlet fever.

scarlet. A bright red colour. **S. Biebrich's:** scarlet red, a dye used in the treatment of wounds. **S. fever:** an acute contagious disease accompanied by pyrexia and characterized by a punctiform bright red eruption appearing on the first or second day. The papillae of the tongue are generally prominent (strawberry tongue). Healing is accompanied by a scaly shedding of the skin. Nephritis is an occasional complication.

Scarpa's fascia (Scarpa, A., Italian anatomist, 1748–1832). A fibrous layer of superficial fascia of the abdomen. **S.'s ganglion:** the ganglion on the vestibular nerve in the internal auditory meatus. **S.'s triangle:** the femoral triangle.

scavenger-cells. Wandering cells pervading the nervous system which carry off debris.

Scedospor·ium. A genus of fungi; the cause of Madura foot.

Schacher's ganglion (Schacher, P. G., German physician, 1674–1737). The ganglion ciliare.

Schachowa's irregular tubule (Schachowa, S., Russian histologist of the 19th century). Of the kidney.

Schaefer's method (Sharpey-Schaefer, Sir E. A., English physiologist, 1850-1935). A method of artificial respiration used in the treatment of the apparently drowned. The patient is placed face downwards and

intermittent pressure is made on the lower part of the thorax.

Schäffer's reflex (Schäffer, S. M., German neurologist, 1852–1923). Flexion of the foot and toes on pinching mid-third of Achilles tendon. Found in hemiplegia.

Schaudinn's bacillus (Schaudinn, F. R., German bacteriologist, 1871–1906). The *Treponema pallidum* or *Spirochaeta pallida*, the organism of syphilis.

Schaumann's disease (Schaumann, J., Swedish dermatologist, born 1879). See sarcoidosis.

Schede's method (Schede, M., German surgeon, 1844–1902). Treatment of caries of bone by removal of the dead bone and allowing the cavity to fill with blood-clot, which may become organized.

schē·ma (G. *skhēma*, figure). 1. An elementary design to illuminate a complicated mechanism. 2. The outline of a theme.

schemat·ic (G. *skhēma*, figure). Relating to a schema. **S. eye:** one exhibiting the proportions of a normal eye.

Scheuermann's disease (Scheuermann, H. W., Danish surgeon, born 1877). Osteochondritis of epiphyses of vertebral bodies.

Schick's test (Schick, B., Austrian paediatrician, contemporarily working in New York). A test to measure immunity to diphtheria. Intracutaneous injection of a quantity of diphtheria toxin equal to one fiftieth of the minimal lethal dose diluted in salt solution. An inflammatory response occurs if the patient cannot neutralize it.

Schiefferdecker's intermediate disc (Schiefferdecker, P., German anatomist, 1849–1931). The substance assumed to fill in the space existing at Ranvier's nodes between Schwann's sheath and the axis cylinder of nerves. **S.'s theory:** that there is a symbiosis between the tissues of the body, so that products of metabolism of one part stimulate other parts.

Schilder's disease (Schilder, P. F., Austrian neurologist, 1886–1940). Progressive subcortical encephalopathy.

schindylē·sis (G. *skhindulēsis*, a cleaving into small pieces). A type of articulation in which one bone is received into a fissure in another.

schis·tasis (G. *skhistos*, cloven). A splitting; usually applied to a congenital split appearing in some part of the body, e.g. schistomelia.

schistocě·phalus (G. *skhistos*, cloven; *kephalē*, head). A monster foetus with a cleft skull.

schistocoe·lia (G. *skhistos*, cloven; *koilia*, stomach). A congenital split in the abdomen.

schistocor·mia (G. *skhistos*, cloven; *kormos*, a log). A congenital fissure of the torso.

schistocys·tis (G. *skhistos*, cloven; *kustis*, bladder). A congenital cleft of the bladder.

schisto·cyte (G. *skhistos*, cloven; *cyton*, cell). Fragmented blood cell.

schistocytō·sis (G. *skhistos*, cloven; *kutos*, a container). The presence of many schistocytes in the blood.

schistoglos·sia (G. *skhistos*, cloven; *glōssa*, tongue). A fissure of the tongue.

schistomē·lia (G. *skhistos*, cloven; *melos*, limb). Congenital fissure of a limb.

schis·toprosō·pia (G. *skhistos*, cloven; *prosōpon*, face). A congenitally cleft condition of the face.

schistoprŏ·sopus (G. *skhistos*, cloven; *prosōpon*, face). A monster foetus with a cleft face.

schistor·rhachis (G. *skhistos*, cloven; *rhakhis*, spine). Spina bifida, *q.v.*

Schistosō·ma (G. *skhistos*, cloven; *sōma*, body). A genus of trematode flukes; the blood flukes.

schistosomī·asis (G. *skhistos*, cloven; *sōma*, body). A condition characterized by invasion with Schistosoma.

schistosō·mus (G. *skhistos*, cloven; *sōma*, body). A monster foetus with a cleft abdomen.

schistotho·rax (G. *skhistos*, cloven; *thōrax*, chest). A congenital cleft of the chest.

schizogĕ·nesis (G. *skhizein*, to cleave; *genesis*, formation). Asexual reproduction, i.e., by fission.

schizŏ·gony (G. *skhizein*, to cleave; *gŏnē*, generation). Schizogenesis, *q.v.*

schi·zoid (G. *skhizein*, to cleave; *eidos*, form). Like schizophrenia.

Schizomȳcē·tēs (G. *skhizein*, to cleave; *mukēs*, mushroom). A class of microorganisms of vegetable composition, the fission fungi.

schizomycō·sis (G. *skhizein*, to cleave; *mukēs*, mushroom). Any disease due to invasion by schizomycetes.

schiz·ont (G. *skhizein*, to cleave). The mother cell in coccidia which, by multiple division, gives rise to the crescentic swarm spores named merozoites.

schizonȳ·chia (G. *skhizein*, to cleave; *ōnux*, nail). Fissuring of the nails.

schizophrē·nia (G. *skhizein*, to cleave; *phrēn*, mind). Chronic progressive mental disorder usually starting in early adult life and characterised by inability to adjust the personality to the stresses of the outer world, with consequent progressive withdrawal from reality into a world of fantasy.

schizophrē·nic (G. *skhizein*, to cleave; *phrēn*, mind). Relating to schizophrenia, or one affected with schizophrenia.

schizophȳ·ta (G. *skhizein*, to cleave; *phuton*, plant). Fission-plants; dried but viable schizomycetes.

Schlatter's disease (Schlatter, C., Swiss surgeon, 1864–1934). An enlargement and often fragmentation of the anterior tubercle of the tibia. It is an epiphysitis and often causes considerable pain. It is treated by rest.

Schlemm's canal (Schlemm, F. S., German anatomist, 1795–1858). The canal at the junction of the cornea and the sclera.

Schmidt's clefts (Schmidt, H. D., American pathologist, 1823–88). The intersegmental clefts in the medullary sheath of peripheral nerves.

Schmiedel's ganglion (Schmiedel, K. C., German anatomist, 1716–92). The inferior carotid ganglion in the cavernous plexus.

Schmorl's nodes (Schmorl, C. G., German pathologist, 1861–1932). Rarified areas seen in X-rays of the spine. They are caused by prolapse of the nucleus pulposus into the adjacent part of the vertebral body.

Schneider's membrane (Schneider, C. V., German physician, 1610–80). The pituitary membrane of the nasal chamber and sinuses.

Schönlein's disease (Schönlein, J. L., German physician, 1793–1864). Thrombocytopenic purpura.

Schreger's line (Schreger, B. G., German anatomist, 1766–1825). A line caused by bending of the dentinal tubules near the surface of the dentine.

Schreiber's manoeuvre (Schreiber, J., German physician, 1848–1932). A method of reinforcing the patellar and ankle jerks by rubbing the skin of the thigh and leg.

Schröder's fibres (Schröder van der Kolk, J. L. C., Dutch physiologist, 1797–1862). The 'formatio reticularis' of the medulla.

Schüffner's granules (Schüffner, W., contemporary German pathologist, born 1867). Coarse red granules seen in parasitized red blood cells in tertian malarial fever on staining with polychrome methylene blue.

Schüle's sign (Schüle, H., German psychiatrist, 1839–1916). Melancholic facies in which vertical folds appear between the eyebrows.

Schüller's disease (Schüller, A., Austrian neurologist, born 1874). Christian-Schüller's disease. Transformation of bones, especially of the skull, into xanthomatous material.

Schüller's ducts (Schüller, K. H. M., German surgeon, 1843–1907). The ducts of Skene's glands.

Schultz-Charlton reaction (Schultz, W., German physician, born 1878). When scarlet fever antitoxin or scarlet fever convalescent serum is injected into an area of the skin showing a bright red rash, a blanching of the skin at the site of the injection occurs.

Schultze's bundle (Schultze, M. J., German biologist, 1825–74). The comma tract. S.'s cells: the cells of the olfactory mucous membrane. S.'s membrane: the olfactory mucous membrane.

Schultze's folds (Schultze, B. S., German gynaecologist, 1827–1919). The folds of the amnion at the origin of the umbilical cord from the placenta. S.'s method: a way of inducing a new-born infant to breathe by swinging it.

Schutz's bundle (Schutz, H., work published in 1902). The dorsal longitudinal bundle of fibres—'fasciculus longitudinalis dorsalis' (*not* the same as the fasciculus longitudinalis medialis).

Schwabach's test (Schwabach, D., German otologist, 1846–1920). Measurement of time difference in hearing tuning forks by air and bone conduction.

Schwalbe's convolutions (Schwalbe, G., German anatomist, 1844–1916). The anterior occipital gyrus. S.'s fissure: the fissura choroidea. S.'s nucleus: the principal vestibular nucleus. S.'s pocket: the depressions between the arcus tendineus and the pelvic wall. S.'s space: the subvaginal space of the optic nerve.

Schwann's sheath (Schwann, T., German anatomist, 1810–82). Neurilemma.

schwannoma. A tumour formed by proliferation of cells of the sheath of Schwann.

Schwartze's operation (Schwartze, H., German otologist, 1837–1910). Conservative operation in which external auditory meatus is preserved; performed in mastoiditis.

sciage (Fr. *scie*, saw). A to-and-fro sawing movement performed in massage.

sciăt·ic (G. *iskhion*, ischium). 1. Relating to the ischium, as the s. notch. 2. Relating to the s. nerve, as s. neuralgia.

sciăt·ica (G. *iskhion*, ischium). Inflammation of the sciatic nerve.

sci·ence (L. *scire*, to know). Co-ordinated, arranged and systematized knowledge.

scienti·fic (L. *scientia*, knowledge; *facere*, to make). Relating to science; based upon science.

sci·entist (L. *scientia*, knowledge). One versed in science; a savant.

scil·la (L.). White squill, obtained from the bulb of *Urginea scilla* and closely resembling digitalis in its action. It is a powerful gastro-intestinal irritant and diuretic.

scil·laren (L. *scilla*, squill). A preparation of the total glycosides of squill. It is given for valvular lesions, cardiac oedema and chronic myocarditis.

scillipic·rin (L. *scilla*, squill; G. *pikros*, bitter). A bitter diuretic principle obtained from squill and used in dropsy and as a diuretic.

scil·lism (L. *scilla*, squill). Poisoning from extracts or tinctures of squill, caused by the glucoside *scillitoxin;* marked by vomiting, retarded pulse and stupor.

scillitox·in (L. *scilla*, squill; *toxikon*, poison). An amorphous, light brown, bitter, active principle of squill, resembling digitalis in action; also used as a diuretic.

scintillā·tion (L. *scintilla*, a spark). 1. To send forth sparks; to twinkle. 2. A subjective visual sensation, as of seeing emissions of sparks.

scir·rhoid (G. *skirrhos*, hard tumour; *eidos*, form). Like a scirrhus.

scirrhō·ma (G. *skirrhos*, hard tumour). A scirrhus.

scirrhō·sis (G. *skirrhos*, hard tumour). The formation of scirrhous carcinoma.

scir·rhous (G. *skirrhos*, hard tumour). Hard.

scir·rhus (G. *skirrhos*, hard tumour). A hard carcinoma, especially of the breast.

scis·sion (L. *scindere*, to cut). Fission.

scissor-leg. A deformity sometimes succeeding double hip-joint disease; the legs are crossed in walking.

scis·sors (L. *scindere*, to cut). An instrument consisting of two blades held together in the centre by a rivet and crossing each other so that in closing they cut the object between them from opposite sides. S., artery: s. with one blade probe-pointed, for insertion into a duct or canal. S., iris: s. with flat blades so bent that they may be applied to the eyeball; also s. used in iridectomy.

scissū·ra (L.). A splitting.

Sclavo's serum (Sclavo, A., Italian physician, 1861–1930). A bactericidal serum used in treatment of anthrax. It is prepared by inoculation of anthrax bacilla into asses.

sclē·ra (G. *sklēros*, hard). The firm, fibrous outer membrane of the eyeball ; the sclerotic coat of the eye.

sclē·ral (G. *sklēros*, hard). Relating to the sclera.

sclerectā·sia (G. *sklēros*, hard; *ektasis*, extension). Localized protuberance of the sclera ; scleral staphyloma.

sclerec·tome (G. *sklēros*, hard; *ektomē*, excision). A surgical knife used in the performance of sclerectomy.

sclerec·tomy (G. *sklēros*, hard; *ektomē*, excision). 1. Surgical excision of the sclera. 2. A cutting away of the sclerosed and ankylosed parts following severe inflammation of the middle ear.

sclerē·ma (G. *sklēros*, hard;) Sclerosis, or hardening particularly of the skin. S., neonatorum: a disease of early infancy, associated with hardening of subcutaneous tissues due to presence of an abnormally large proportion of fat of high melting point.

sclerencephā·lia (G. *sklēros*, hard; *egkephalos*, brain). Hardening of the brain tissue.

sclerit·ic (G. *sklēros*, hard). Sclerous.

scleri·tis (G. *sklēros*, hard). Inflammation of the sclera.

sclē·rochoroidī·tis (G. *sklēros*, hard; *khorion*, an intestinal membrane; *eidos*, form). Inflammation of both the sclera and choroid coats of the eye.

scleroconjunctivī·tis (G. *sklēros*, hard; L. *conjungere*, to join together). Inflammation both of the sclera and the conjunctiva.

sclerocor·nea (G. *sklēros*, hard; L. *corneus*, from *cornu*, horn). The sclera and cornea considered as one.

sclerodactў·lia, sclerodac·tyly (G. *sklēros*, hard; *daktulos*, finger). An ailment of the fingers and toes resembling scleroderma. It is ordinarily symmetrical, occurs mostly in women and results in considerable deformity.

scleroder·ma (G. *sklēros*, hard; *derma*, skin). A disease marked by progressive hardening of the skin, taking place either in patches (see morphoea) or diffusely. The skin becomes hard and pigmented and firmly adherent to the underlying tissues; destructive ulceration may occur and joints may become fixed from adhesions of the skin.

sclerodermati·tis (G. *sklēros*, hard; *derma*, skin). Inflammation and induration of the skin.

sclerodes·mia (G. *sklēros*, hard; *desmos*, a ligature). Hardening of the ligaments.

sclerǒ·genous (G. *sklēros*, hard; *gennan*, to produce). Producing hard tissues.

sclē·roid (G. *sklēros*, hard; *eidos*, form). Hard; of a hard consistency.

sclero-irī·tis. Inflammation of both the sclera and the iris.

sclerokeratī·tis (G. *sklēros*, hard; *keras*, horn). Inflammation both of the sclera and the cornea.

sclerō·ma (G. *sklēros*, hard). Any induration of a part or tissue.

scleromalā·cia (G. *sklēros*, hard; *malakia*, softness). Softening of the sclera.

scleromē·ninx (G. *sklēros*, hard; *mēnigx*, membrane). The dura mater.

sclē·romere (G. *sklēros*, hard; *meros*, part). Any skeletal metamere or segment.

sclerǒ·meter (G. *sklēros*, hard; *metron*, measure). An instrument for measuring the hardness of a substance.

scleronў·chia (G. *sklēros*, hard; *onux*, nail). Induration and dryness of the nails.

scleronyx·is (G. *sklēros*, hard; *nuxis*, a pricking). Perforation of the sclera.

sclero-ōǒphorī·tis (G. *sklēros*, hard; *ōon*, egg; *pherein*, to bear). Induration and inflammation of an ovary.

scleroprō·tein (G. *sklēros*, hard; *prōteion*, from *prōtos*, first). Albuminoids, a class of proteins including keratin, elastin and collagen. They are insoluble in all neutral solvents.

sclerosarcō·ma (G. *sklēros*, hard; *sarx*, flesh). A hard tumour of fleshy tissue. See also epulis.

sclerose (G. *sklēros*, hard). To harden.

sclerose en plaques (Fr.). Multiple sclerosis.

sclerosed (G. *sklēros*, hard). Affected with sclerosis.

sclerō·sing (G. *sklēros*, hard). Undergoing an indurating process. S. phlebitis: induration of the veins.

sclerō·sis (G. *sklēros*, hard). Induration of a part from inflammation, degeneration or fibrosis; applied specially to loss of elasticity of arterial walls (arteriosclerosis) and to gliosis resulting from a specific form of degeneration of the nervous system. (disseminated sclerosis).

scleroskě·leton (G. *sklēros*, hard; *skeleton*, skeleton). In biology, all those sections of the skeleton formed by the ossification of ligaments or tendons.

sclerostenō·sis (G. *sklēros*, hard; *stenos*, narrow). Hardening with contracture of a part.

Sclerostō·ma (G. *sklēros*, hard; *stoma*, mouth). A genus of nematode worms. S. duodenale: the same as *Ankylostoma duodenale*.

sclerot·ic (G. *sklēros*, hard). 1. Hard; indurated. 2. Relating to the outer coat of the eye. 3. Connected with or obtained from ergot. See sclerotis.

sclerǒ·tica (G. *sklēros*, hard). See sclera.

scleroticec·tomy (G. *sklēros*, hard; *ektomē*, excision). Excision of a part of the sclera.

scleroticǒ·tomy (G. *sklēros*, hard; *tomē*, a cutting). Incision into the sclera.

sclerō·tis (G. *sklēros*, hard). Ergot of rye.

sclerotī·tis (G. *sklēros*, hard). Scleritis, q.v.

sclerō·tium (G. *sklēros*, hard). The hard mass forming a resting stage in the growth of certain fungi, such as ergot of rye.

sclē·rotome (G. *sklēros*, hard; *tomē*, a cutting). 1. A surgeon's knife employed in sclerotomy. 2. The hard tissue of the embryo which develops into the bony skeleton.

sclerǒ·tomy (G. *sklēros*, hard; *tomē*, a cutting). The operation of cutting into the sclera. S., anterior: incision making an opening into the anterior chamber of the eye. S., posterior: incision making an opening into the vitreous chamber of the eye.

sclē·rous (G. *sklēros*). Hard.

scolecoidec·tomy (G. *skōlex*, a worm; *eidos*, form; *ektome*, excision). Appendicectomy.

scō·lecoidī·tis (G. *skōlex*, a worm; *eidos*, form). Appendicitis, q.v.

scolecŏ·logy (G. *skōlēx*, worm; *logos*, discourse). Helminthology, *q.v.*

scō·lex (G. *skōlēx*, worm). The head of a tape-worm from which grows the chain of proglottides.

scoliŏ·ma (G. *skolios*, crooked). Scoliosis, *q.v.*

scoliŏ·meter (G. *skolios*, crooked; *metron*, measure). An instrument used in the measurement of spinal curvatures.

scoliopathex·is (G. *skolios*, crooked; *pathos*, disease). Malingering.

scoliorhachit·ic (G. *skolios*, crooked; *rhakhis*, spine). Relating to scoliosis and rickets.

scoliosiŏ·metry (G. *skolios*, crooked; *metron*, measure). The measurement of spinal curvatures.

scoliō·sis (G. *skolios*, crooked). A curvature, especially a lateral one, of the spine.

scoliŏt·ic (G. *skolios*, crooked). Relating to scoliosis.

scoop. An instrument like a spoon employed for the clearing out of cavities, as a lithotomy s..

scopa·rin. $C_{22}H_{22}O_{11}$, a phenolic substance obtained from broom tops. It is diuretic in action.

scopā·rius (L. *scopa*, a twig). The tops of *Cytisus s.*, a shrub of the family Leguminosae. The dried tops contain the alkaloid sparteine and scoparin. Scoparius is diuretic and cathartic.

scopŏ·lamine. The active principle of *Scopolia carniolica*, an alkaloid apparently identical with hyoscine. It is used with morphine in order to induce anaesthesia. **S. hydrobromide:** hygroscopic crystals used as a sedative; externally in ophthalmology, subcutaneously as premedication in anaesthesia. **S. narcophine anaesthesia:** twilight sleep. *q.v.* S. occurs also in other solanaceous drugs, e.g. hyoscyamus stramonium.

Scopolia (Scopoli, G. A., Italian naturalist, 1723–88). The dried rhizome of *Scopolia carniolica* (solanaceae). Contains hyoscyamine, hyoscine and probably atropine.

scopŏ·meter (G. *skopein*, to view; *metron*, measure). An instrument used in measuring the turbidity of solutions.

scopophŏ·bia (G. *skopein*, to inspect; *phobos*, fear). A neurotic fear of being seen.

scoracrā·tia (G. *skōr*, dung; *akratia*, incontinence). The involuntary release of the faeces from the bowels.

scorbū·tic (Ger. *Scharbock*, scurvy). Relating to or affected with scorbutus or scurvy.

scorbū·tus (Ger. *Scharbock*, scurvy). Scurvy, *q.v.*

scorings. Small transverse lines caused by increased density of bone and seen in X-rays of metaphyses of long bones. Due to temporary cessation of growth.

scor·pion. A widely distributed arthropod, which has a venomous sting at the end of its tail.

scotodi·nia (G. *skotos*, darkness; *dinos*, a whirling). Vertigo, accompanied by headache and the appearance of black spots before the eyes.

Scott's dressing. Compound ointment of mercury applied to produce counter-irritation.

scō·tograph (G. *skotos*, darkness; *graphein*, to write). An X-ray photograph.

scotŏ·graphy (G. *skotos*, darkness; *graphein*, to write). X-ray photography.

scotŏ·ma (G. *skotos*, darkness). A blind spot in the visual field.

scotō·matous (G. *skotos*, darkness). Relating to or affected with scotoma.

scotō·meter (G. *skotos*, darkness; *metron*, measure). An instrument used for detecting and measuring scotomata.

scotophŏ·bia (G. *skotos*, darkness; *phobos*, fear). A neurotic fear of darkness.

Scr. Abbreviation for scruple.

scrā·per. An instrument used to produce an abrasion or to remove coated material.

screen. To examine radiologically by means of a fluorescent screen. **S., bjerrum:** screen used in ophthalmology for mapping out visual fields. **S., fluorescent:** sheet of glass treated so as to render visible the appearances produced by X-rays.

screw-worm. The larva of the fly *Chrysomyia macellaria*, found in tropical America, where it may cause death in man by burrowing into the nasal or aural cavities.

scrobi·culate (L. *scrobiculus*, small ditch). Pitted.

scrobi·culus (L. *scrobiculus*, small ditch). Any small hollow or cavity.

scrŏ·phula (L. *scrofula*, a swelling of the glands of the neck). Term formerly applied to a variety of conditions said to arise from a scrophulous diathesis. Most of these conditions are now considered to be manifestations of non-pulmonary tuberculosis.

scrŏ·phulide (L. *scrofula*, a swelling of the glands of the neck). Scrofuloderma, *q.v.*

scrophuloder·ma (L. *scrofula*, a swelling of the glands of the neck; G. *derma*, skin). A disease of the skin due to scrophula and usually marked by the presence of superficial ulcers of irregular shape. It is of tuberculous origin.

scrŏ·phulophȳ·ma (L. *scrofula*, a swelling of the glands of the neck; G. *phuma*, a growth). A skin growth of tuberculous origin.

scrophulō·sis (L. *scrofula*, a swelling of the glands of the neck). A scrophulous diathesis.

scrŏ·phulous (L. *scrofula*, a swelling of the glands of the neck). Of the nature of or affected with scrophula.

scrō·tal (L. *scrotum*). Relating to or contained in the scrotum, as s. hernia.

scroti·tis (L. *scrotum*). Inflammation of the scrotum.

scrō·tocele (L. *scrotum*; G. *kēlē*, hernia). Hernia of the scrotum.

scrō·tum (L.). The sac containing the testicles and comprising skin, dartos, spermatic fascia and parietal tunica vaginalis.

scruff. The nape of the neck.

scruple (L. *scrupulus*, dim. of *scrupus*, a rough stone). In apothecaries' weight, 20 grains; symbol ℈.

scrupulŏ·sity (L. *scrupulosus*). Over-precision or morbid conscientiousness.

scultē·tus bandage (Scultetus, J., German surgeon 1595–1645). A many-tailed bandage in which adjacent strips overlap each other.

scurf. A bran-like desquamation of the epidermis, particularly of the scalp; dandruff.

scur·vy. A deficiency disease, due to lack of vitamin C.

scute (L. *scutum*, a shield). A curved portion of bone which forms the outer wall of the attic in the ear.

scū·tiform (L. *scutum*, a shield; *forma*, shape). Shaped like a shield.

scū·tulum (L., dim. of *scutum*, a shield). Round sulphur-yellow crusts with a central depression seen in typical cases of favus.

scū·tum (L. a shield). 1. Any shield-shaped bone. 2. The thyroid cartilage. 3. The patella.

scȳ·balous (G. *skubalon*, dung). Having the nature of or resembling a scybalum.

scȳ·balum pl. scybala (G. *skubalon*, dung). A collection of abnormally hard faecal material in the intestines.

scȳ·phoid (G. *skuphos*, cup; *eidos*, form). Having the shape of a cup.

scȳ·thian disease. Atrophy of penis and testicles resulting from sexual perversion.

scyti·tis (G. *skutos*, a skin). Dermatitis. *q.v.*

scy̆·toblastē·ma (G. *skutos*, a skin; *blastēma*, a sprout). The embryonic stage of skin growth.

Scytonē·ma (G. *skutos*, a skin; *nēma*, a thread). A genus of schizomycetes.

Se. The symbol for an atom of Selenium.

seal. A body of water or other material placed in the trap of a house-drain to prevent the ingress of sewer air.

seam. Raphe or suture, *q.v.*

searcher. A sound used for the location of calculi in the bladder.

sea-sickness. A state occurring in persons on board ship, produced by the rolling of the ship and characterized by vertigo, nausea, retching and prostration. A similar condition may be induced by riding in trains or motor-coaches and by flying.

sea-tangle. Laminaria, *q.v.*

seaweed. A seaplant, especially one of the Algae.

sebā·ceous (L. *sebum*, suet). Relating to sebum. S. cyst: a tumour formed by the blocking of the duct of a sebaceous gland. S. glands: glands found in connection with the hair follicles. They are very numerous in the scalp.

se̤·bastomā·nia (G. *sĕbastos*, reverend; *mania*, madness). Religious madness.

Sebileau's hollow (Sebileau, P., French surgeon, born 1860). The sublingual depression between the tongue and the sublingual glands. S.'s muscle: the deep layer of the scrotal septum. S.'s suspensory ligaments: the suspensory ligaments of the lung; the costopleural ligaments.

sebī·parous (L. *sebum*, suet; *parĕre*, to bear). Producing sebum.

se̤·bolith (L. *sebum*, suet; G. *lithos*, stone). A concretion within a sebaceous gland.

seborrhā·gia (L. *sebum*, suet; G. *rhēgnunai*, to burst forth.) Seborrhoea, *q.v.*

seborrhōē·a (L. *sebum*, suet; G. *rhoia*, a flow). A condition marked by an excessive secretion of the sebaceous glands. This secretion (sebum) forms an oily coating on the skin and becomes crusty or scaly when dry.

seborrhōē·al (L. *sebum*, suet; *rhoia*, a flow). Relating to seborrhea.

seborrhōē·ic (L. *sebum*, suet; *rhoia*, a flow). Affected with seborrhoea.

se̤·bum (L., suet). The secretion from the sebaceous glands.

Sē·cale. A genus of gramineaceous plants. *S. cereale*, rye. *S. cornutum*—the ergot of rye.

se̤·calin. One of the active principles of ergot.

se̤·calose. A carbohydrate obtained from rye.

secer·nent, secer·ning (L. *secernere*, to separate). Secreting; term used of the function of a gland.

second intention. See under healing. S. nerve: the optic nerve.

secondaries (L. *secundus*, second). Term sometimes given to the metastatic deposits of malignant tumours.

se̤·condary (L. *secundus*, second). 1. Second in order of time or place. 2. Subordinate. 3. A metastasis from a malignant tumour.

secrē·ta (L. *secretio*, a separation). Secretions.

secrē·tagogue (L. *secernere*, to separate; G. *agōgos*, leading). Stimulating secretion, or an agent that does this.

Secretan's disease (Secretan, H. F., Swiss physician, 1856–1916). Severe oedema produced by injury.

secrete (L. *secernere*, to separate). To separate; specifically to separate from the blood by vital processes as distinct from physical processes such as dialysis or filtration.

secrē·tin. A hormone obtained from the duodenal membrane. Conveyed by the blood, it stimulates the secretion of pancreatic juices.

secrē·tion (L. *secretio*, a separation). 1. The function of separating materials from the blood, which are either eliminated from the system or used to perform special functions. 2. Any secreted material. S.,external one that is ejected upon a surface which may be either outside or inside the body, S., internal: one that is not ejected but is absorbed into the blood.

secrē·tomotor (L. *secernere*, to separate; *movēre*, to move). Term applied to a nerve which carries fibres causing secretion, and contraction of the vessels, in a gland.

secrē·tory (L. *secernere*, to separate). 1. Relating to secretion. 2. Performing secretion.

sec·tion (L. *sectio*, a cutting). 1. The act of cutting or dividing. 2. A cut; a cut surface. 3. A part cut off. 4. One of the parts into which anything is divided arbitrarily or may naturally be considered as divided.

sec·tor (L., for *secare*, to cut). The area between two radii of a circle and an arc.

secun·digrā·vida (L. *secundus*, second; *gravida*, pregnant). A woman pregnant for the second time.

secun·dines (L. *secundus*, second). The placenta.

secundī·para (L. *secundus*, second; *parere*, to bear). A woman who has produced two children that are not twins.

secun·dum artem (L. *secundum*, following; *ars*, art). In the approved or professional way.

sed. Abbreviation for L. *sedes*, a seat.

sedā·tion (L. *sedatio*, an assuaging). The production of a condition of decreased functional activity; the process of calming.

se̤·dative (L. *sedare*, to assuage). 1. Quieting or decreasing excitement. 2. An agent that does this.

sedentaria ossa (L.). The ischia and coccyx; the bones supporting the seated body.

se̤·dentary (L. *sedentarius*, sedentary). 1. Used in sitting. 2. Related to the habit of sitting.

se̤·diment (L. *sedimentum*, subsidence). The precipitate subsiding to the bottom of a liquid.

sedimentā·tion (L. *sedimentum*, subsidence). The act of producing a precipitate.

seed. 1. A fertilized ovum. 2. Seminal fluid; sperm. 3. A generic term for fertilizers.

Seeligmüller's sign (Seeligmüller, O. L. G. A., German neurologist, 1837–1912). Mydriasis occurring on the side of the face affected by neuralgia.

seepage. Percolation.

Seessel's pocket (Seessel, A., American embryologist, 1850–1910). A diverticulum of the embryonic pharynx anterior to the cranial attachment of the buccopharyngeal membrane.

Séglas's type of paranoia (Séglas, J. E., French psychiatrist, 1856–1939). The psychomotor type of paranoia.

seg·ment (L. *segmentum*, a slice or strip). 1. A piece cut off or marked off. 2. A natural division effected by segmentation. 3. A subdivision, or a metamere of an articulated body.

segmen·tal (L. *segmentum*, a slice or strip). Relating to or composed of segments.

segmentā·tion (L. *segmentum*, a slice or strip). Cleavage into a number of similar sections.

segregā·tion (L. *segregare*, to set apart). 1. Isolation. 2. Separation of unlike genes at meiosis.

segregā·tor (L. *segregare*, to set apart). An instrument enabling urine to be separately obtained from each kidney without mixing together.

Séguin's symptom (Séguin, E., French neurologist, 1812–80). Involuntary contraction of muscles occurring just before the onset of an epileptic attack.

Seidel's scotoma (Seidel, E., German ophthalmologist, born 1882). A scotoma which is a wing or wedge-shaped extension of the blind spot.

Seidelin's bodies (Seidelin, H., contemporary British physician). Bodies discovered in the red blood cells in cases of yellow fever and believed to be the parasites which cause the disease.

Seidlitz powder (Seidlitz in Bohemia). Pulvis effervescens compositus.

Seignette's salt (Seignette, P., French apothecary, 1660–1719). Rochelle salt, *q.v.*

Seiler's cartilage (Seiler, C., Swiss laryngologist settled in America, 1849–1905). A small cartilaginous rod attached to the vocal process of the arytenoid cartilage.

seismothĕ·rapy (G. *seismos*, earthquake; *therapeia*, treatment). Treatment of disease by mechanical vibration.

seizure. A sudden attack or recurrence of a disease.

selection (L. *selectio*, choice). The act of making a choice. **S., artificial:** the s. for further breeding made by the breeder because of specially desirable and inheritable characters. Applied to animals and plants. **S., natural:** this term was used by Darwin to indicate the method whereby evolution was brought about in the animal kingdom, by a process of survival of those best adapted to their environment.

selē·nium (G. *selēnē*, moon). A rare non-metallic element grouped with sulphur and tellurium and with special uses due to difference in its electric resistance under light and darkness. Usually bivalent, sometimes quadrivalent or hexivalent. Symbol Se.; atomic weight 78·96.

self-abuse. Masturbation, *q.v.*

sella (L. saddle). A chair, **S. turcica:** the pituitary fossa of the sphenoid bone in which the hypophysis is situated.

seltzer water (Selters in Prussia). A sparkling mineral water obtained from Selters.

seman·tic (G. *semainein*, to signify). Pertaining to or affecting the significance or meaning of words.

semeiŏ·graphy (G. *sēmeion*, a sign; *graphein*, to write). A description of disease symptoms.

semeiŏ·logy (G. *sēmeion*, a sign; *logos*, a discourse). Symptomatology.

semeiŏ·sis (G. *sēmeion*, sign). The observation of disease symptoms.

semeiŏ·tic (G. *sēmeion*, sign). Relating to symptoms.

semeiŏ·tics (G. *sēmeion*, sign). Symptomatology, *q.v.*

semelin·cident (L. *semel*, once; *incidere*, to happen). Occurring once only to the same person.

sē·men (L., seed). 1. A seed. 2. The external secretion of the testes combined with prostatic secretion.

semenū·ria. Seminuria, *q.v.*

semicanal (L. *semi*, half; *canalis*, channel). A furrow or canal open on one side.

sĕ·micartilă·ginous (L. *semi*, half; cartilage). Partly composed of cartilage.

semicircular canal (L. *semi*, half; *circulus*, circle). Long canals found in the labyrinth of the ear, an external, superior and posterior on each side. They open into the vestibule at each end (one pair showing a common opening at one end). They are concerned with maintenance of balance and posture.

semidiagrammat·ic (L. *semi*, half; G. *diagramma*). An illustration modified in order to show the principle rather than to represent an exact copy.

semiflex·ion (L. *semi*, half; *flectere*, to bend). A position between flexion and extension.

semilū·nar (L. *semi*, half; *luna*, moon). Crescent-moon-shaped. **S. bone:** carpal lunate. **S. cartilage:** two half-moon intra-articular cartilages of the knee. **S. ganglia:** see Gasserian ganglion. **S. valves:** the valves guarding the commencement of the aorta.

semimembranō·sus muscle (L. *semi*, half; *membrana*). One of the hamstring muscles at the back of the thigh.

sĕ·minal (L. *semen*, seed). 1. Relating to the semen, as s. fluid. 2. Fertilizing.

seminā·tion (L. *seminatio*, propagation). The introducing of semen into the vagina or uterus.

seminī·ferous (L. *semen*, seed; *ferre*, to bear). Carrying semen.

semi-normal (L. *semi*, half; *norma*, a rule). Half normal. **S. solution:** one which holds in solution half the aggregate of the material contained in the normal solution.

seminū·ria (L. *semen*, seed; G. *ouron*, urine). The passing of semen in the urine.

semis (L.). Half; abbreviated for the purpose of prescription-writing to ss.

semispinā·lis muscle (L. *semi*; half; *spina*). An extensor muscle of the back.

semisul·cus (L. *semi-*, half; *sulcus*, furrow). A half-sulcus which combining with an opposing one forms a whole sulcus.

semitendinō·sus muscle (L. *semi*, half; *tendo*). A hamstring muscle extending from the ischial tuberosity to the tibia.

Semmelweis, Ignaz Philipp, a physician of Vienna, 1818–65. In 1847–9 he showed that puerperal fever was a form of septicaemia.

sĕ·nega. *Polygala senega*, a plant of the family Polygalaceae. The root (*Senegae radix*, B.P.) contains two saponins, senegin and polygalic acid, or polygalin. It is used as an expectorant and diuretic and in large doses is purgative and emetic.

sĕ·negin. A glucoside from senega.

senes·cence (L. *senescere*, to grow old). The condition of growing old.

senes·cent (L. *senescere*). Growing old.

sē·nile (L. *senilis*). Relating to or produced by old age.

sē·nilism (L. *senilis*, aged). A state of premature old age. See also progeria.

senī·lity (L. *senilis*, aged). The condition, in animate beings, of being old, especially the enfeebled mental and bodily state characteristic of old age.

senna. The dried leaflets of *Cassia acutifolia* or *C. angustifolia*. They contain aloe-emodin, kaempferol, *iso*rhamnetin, etc. It is used in the treatment of constipation.

sensā·tion (L. *sentire*, to feel). An impression caused by the stimulation of an afferent nerve.

sense. Any of the faculties capable of converting received stimuli into sensations. These faculties are the powers of sight, hearing, touch, smell and taste.

sensibă·mine. A molecular compound of the alkaloids ergotamine and ergotaminine.

sensibi·lity (L. *sensibilis*, capable of perceiving). The capacity to feel; exceptional delicacy and susceptibility of perception.

sen·sible (L. *sentire*, to feel). 1. Capable of being perceived by the senses. 2. Furnished with sensation.

sen·sitive (Fr. *sensitif*, from L. *sensus*, sensation). Capable of accepting or transmitting a sensation.

sen·sitized (L. *sensus*, sensation). Rendered sensitive, especially to bacteria or proteins by preliminary infection with such substances.

sensiti·zer (L. *sensus*, sensation). An agent used in sensitization; an amboceptor.

sensor·ial (Late L. *sensorium*, from L. *sensus*, sensation). Relating to the sensorium.

sen·sorimō·tor (L. *sensus*, sensation or perception; *movēre*, to move). Sensory and motor; concerned with the perceiving of both sensory and motor impulses.

sensor·ium (Late L. *sensorium*, from L. *sensus*, sensation). A sensory nerve centre; particularly that section of the brain concerned with receiving and transmitting sensations to the individual sensory nerve centres.

sen·sory (L. *sensus*, sensation). Relating to or conducting sensation.

sen·sualism (Late L. *sensualis*, from L. *sensus*, sensation). The state of being controlled by animal passions.

sen·tient (L. *sentire*, to feel). Capable of feeling; sensitive.

separā·tor (L. *separare*, to separate). Anything capable of effecting a separation, particularly an apparatus used in dentistry to separate the teeth.

separator·ium (L.L.). A surgical instrument for separating the pericranium from the skull.

sep·sis (G. putrefaction). Poisoning caused by the absorption of putrefactive material. S., **puerperal**: that occurring immediately after childbirth.

septae·mia. Septicaemia, *q.v.*

sep·tal (L. *septum*, a wall). Relating to a septum.

sep·tan (L. *septem*, seven). Recurring every seventh day.

sep·tate (L. *septum*, a wall). Separated by a septum.

septec·tomy. (L. *septum*, a wall; G. *ektomē*, excision). Surgical removal of part of the nasal septum.

sep·tic (G. *sēptikos*, from *sēptos*, rotten). Relating to sepsis; caused by putrefaction. S. **fever**: septicaemia. S. **tank**: a drainage device consisting of a large closed vessel through which sewage is made to pass slowly undergoing anaerobic decomposition.

septicae·mia (G. *sēptikos*, septic, from *sēptos*, rotten; *haima*, blood). An infection marked by the presence of pathogenic bacteria in the blood.

septicae·mic (G. *sēptikos*, septic, from *sēptos*, rotten; *haima*, blood). Relating to or affected with septicaemia.

sep·ticine. A ptomaine from rotting flesh.

sep·ticopyae·mia (G. *sēptikos*, septic, from *sēptos*, rotten; *puon*, pus; *haima*, blood). Septicaemia combined with pyaemia.

septigrä·vida (L. *septem*, seven; *gravida*, pregnant). A woman pregnant for the seventh time.

sep·timetrī·tis (G. *sēptos*, rotten; *mētra*, uterus). Metritis caused by septic poisoning.

septi·para (L. *septem*, seven; *parere*, to bear). A woman who has had seven children.

septi·valent (L. *septem*, seven; *valēre*, to be worth). Having a valency of seven.

septŏ·meter (L. *septum*, wall; G. *metron*, measure). An instrument used in measuring the thickness of the nasal septum.

septonā·sal. Relating to the nasal septum.

sep·totome (L. *septum*; G. *tomē*, a cutting). A surgical instrument for use in operations on the nasal septum.

septŏ·tomy (L. *septum*; G. *tomē*, a cutting). Surgical incision into the nasal septum.

sep·tum (L. a wall). A partition; a dividing wall. S., **interventricular**: the partition between the two ventricles of the heart. S., **nasal**: the division between the two cavities of the nose.

sep·tuplet (L. *septuplum*, a group of seven). One of seven children produced at a single birth.

seq. luce. Abbreviation for L. *sequenti luce*, on the following day.

sē·quel, sequē·la (L. *sequi*, to follow). An abnormal state or lesion following a disease and directly or indirectly due to it.

sequē·stral. Relating to a sequestrum.

sequestrā·tion (L. *sequestrare*, to separate). 1. The production of a sequestrum. 2. The isolation of the sick, either for treatment or in order to protect others.

sequestrec·tomy (L. *sequestrare*, to separate; G. *ektomē*, excision). The operation of cutting out a sequestrum.

sequestrŏ·tomy (L. *sequestrare*, to separate; G. *tomē*, a cutting). The cutting away of diseased bone.

sequĕ·strum, pl. **sequestra** (L. *sequestrare*, to separate). A necrosed fragment of bone that has detached itself from healthy bone.

seralbu·min (L. *sērum*; *albumen*). Serum-albumin; albumin present in the blood.

se·rial (L. *series*). Arranged or following in regular order.

sĕ·riflux (L. *sērum*, whey; *fluxus*, a flow). A watery discharge.

sĕ·rine. A white amino-acid which is not indispensable to growth, alpha-amino-beta-hydroxy-propionic acid.

serious (L. *sērius*, grave). An epithet applied to such severe states or symptoms as give rise to grave prognoses.

seriscis·sion (L. *sēricum*; silk; Late L. *scissio*, from *scindere*, to cut). The separation of soft tissues by a silk ligature.

sĕ·ro-albū·minous. Containing both serum and albumin.

sero-albuminū·ria (L. *sērum*, whey; G. *ouron*, urine). The presence of serum albumin in the urine.

serobac·terins (L. *sērum*, whey; G. *baktērion*, dim. of *baktron*, a staff). Emulsions of dead bacteria sensitized by treatment with the corresponding immune serum.

serocoli·tis (L. *sērum*, whey; G. *kolon*, colon). Inflammation of the serous coat of the colon.

sĕ·roculture (L. *sērum*, whey; *cultura*, culture). A bacterial culture on blood serum.

serodermatŏ·sis (L. *sērum*, whey; G. *derma*, skin). A skin disease marked by serous effusion into the skin.

sĕ·rodiagnŏ·sis (L. *sērum*, whey; G. *dia*, through; *gnosis*, knowledge). Diagnosis founded on the blood-serum reactions of patients.

sero·enterī·tis (L. *sērum*, whey; G. *enteron*, intestine). Inflammation of the serous coat of the intestine.

sero-enzyme (L. *sērum*, whey; G. *en*, in; *zumē*, yeast). An enzyme of blood serum.

serofi·brinous (L. *sērum*, whey; *fibra*, fibre). Consisting of both serum and fibrin.

seroflu·id (L. *sērum*, whey; *fluere*, to flow). A fluid of serous character.

sĕ·rogas·tria (L. *sērum*, whey; G. *gastēr*, stomach). A condition in which blood serum is present in the stomach.

seroglŏ·bulin (L. *sērum*, whey; *globulus*. small ball). The globulin of blood serum.

sĕrohepati·tis (L. *sērum*, whey; G. *hēpar*, liver). Inflammation of the peritoneum covering the liver.

sero-immū·nity (L. *sērum*, whey; G. *immunis*, free). Immunity obtained by the introduction into the system of antiserum.

sĕ·rolin (L. *sērum*, whey; *oleum*, oil). A neutral, fatty, crystallizable compound from blood.

serŏ·logy (L. *sērum*, whey; G. *logos*, treatise). The study of sera, especially immune and haemolytic sera.

serŏ·lȳsin (L. *sērum*, whey; G. *lucin*, to loosen). A lysin contained in blood serum and having bactericidal properties.

seromem·branous (L. *sērum*; *membrana*). Composed of serous membrane.

seromū·cous (L. *sērum*, whey; *mucus*, mucus). Comprising both serum and mucus.

seronĕ·gative (L. *sērum*, whey; *negare*, to deny). Negative to serological tests.

sē·ropneumothor·ax (L. *serum*, whey; G. *pneumon*, lung; *thōrax*, chest). Pleurisy accompanied by serous effusion and associated with pneumothorax.

seropŏ·sitive (L. *serum*; *positivus*). Positive to a serologic test.

seropū·rulent (L. *serum*, whey; *purulentus*, purulent). Consisting of serum and pus.

sē·ropus (L. *serum*, whey; *pus*, pus). A fluid of combined serum and pus.

serŏ·sa (L. *serum*, whey). Any serous membrane.

serosanguī·neous (L. *serum*, whey; *sanguis*, blood). Relating to or comprising both serum and blood.

serosē·rous (L. *serum*, whey). Relating to two or more serous surfaces.

serosi·tis (L. *serum*, whey). Inflammation of a serous membrane.

serŏ·sity (L. *serum*, whey). The quality of being serous.

serosynō·vial (L. *serum*, whey; G. *sun*, with; L. *ovum*, egg). Serous and synovial combined.

sē·rosynovī·tis (L. *serum*, whey; G. *sun*, with; L. *ovum*, egg). Synovitis with a serous effusion.

serother·apy (L. *serum*, whey; G. *therapeia*, treatment). The treatment of disease by the injection of blood serum obtained from immune persons or animals.

seroti·na (L. *serotinus*, late). See decidua serotina.

sē·rous (L. *serum*, whey). 1. Relating to or characterized by serum. 2. Yielding serum, as a s. gland; containing serum, as a s. cyst.

serovaccinā·tion (L. *serum*, whey; *vacca*, a cow). A method of securing mixed immunity by injecting serum to obtain passive immunity and by vaccinating with bacteria to obtain active immunity.

ser·pens (L.). Winding; sinuous. S., ulcus: a fistulous ulcer; a sinuous ulcer of the cornea, generally due to pneumococcal infection.

serpentā·ria. The dried rhizome and roots of *Aristolochia reticulata* (Texan Serpentary); a bitter tonic.

serpī·ginous (L. *serpere*, to creep). Creeping. S. ulcer: one that spreads in one direction while healing in another. See serpens.

serpī·go (L. *serpere*, to creep). A creeping eruption such as herpes.

serra (L.). A saw or a saw-like structure.

serrā·ted (L. *serra*, saw). Having an edge toothed like a saw.

Serrā·tia (L. *serra*, saw). A genus of saprophytic Bacteriaceae.

serrā·tion (L. *serra*, saw). The condition of being toothed or serrated.

serrā·tus (L. *serra*, saw). Applied to muscles arising or inserted by a series of processes resembling the teeth of a saw.

serre·fine (Fr. *serrer*, to press; *fin*, slender). A small spring forceps for seizing and compressing blood-vessels.

serre·noeud (Fr. *serrer*, to press; *noeud*, a knot). An instrument used for tightening ligatures.

Serres's angle (Serres, A. E. R. A., French anatomist, 1786–1868). The metafacial angle of anthropometry. S.'s glands : the gingival 'glands'; islands of epithelium present in the gums of infants.

ser·rulate (L. *serrula*, dim. of *serra*, saw). Minutely serrated.

Sertoli's cells (Sertoli, E., Italian histologist, 1842–1910). The 'supporting' cells of the testicular epithelium.

sē·rum (L. *serum*, whey). 1. The clear liquid separating from the blood after the fibrin has coagulated. 2. Any liquid containing an antitoxin for therapeutic use. S. gonadotrophin : gonadotrophic hormone from pregnant mare's serum. Available as 'Gestyl', 'Serogan', etc. S. sickness: a form of anaphylactic or allergic reaction following the injection of foreign serum. S. therapy: the treatment of disease by the injection of blood serum from immune animals or human beings.

serumū·ria (L. *serum*, whey; G. *ouron*, urine). Albuminuria.

Servetus, M. Spanish theologian and physician, 1509–53. Noted that blood passed into the heart after being aerated in the lung.

sē·samĕ. See under Sesamum.

sē·samoid (G. *sēsamē*, sesame; *eidos*, form). Like a sesame seed. S. bone: a small bone evolved in a tendon upon which much pressure has been exerted. S. cartilage: a small cartilage situated in the nasal alae.

Sĕ·samum (G. *sēsamē*, sesame). A genus of plants of the order Pedaliaceae. Oil of sesamum or sesame oil is expressed from the seeds of *Sesamum indicum*.

sesqui- (L. *sesqui-* one half more). A prefix meaning more by a half.

sesquiox·ide (L. *sesqui-*, one half more; G. *oxus*, sharp). A compound having three parts of oxygen with two of another element.

ses·quisalt (L. *sesqui-*, one half more; *sal*, salt). A salt having one and a half times as much of the acid as of the radical.

ses·sile (L. *sessilis*, with a broad base). Secured by a broad base; without a stalk.

set. 1. To reduce a fracture. 2. To harden.

setā·ceous (L. *seta*, bristle). Bristling or shaped like a bristle.

sē·ton (L. *seta*, bristle). 1. A thread or strip of silk or linen passed through a fold of skin in order to make a fistula. 2. The fistula thus produced.

seven-day fever. Relapsing fever.

seventh nerve. The facial nerve.

sewage. The heterogeneous material composing the excreta and waste matter of domestic economy and the contents of drains. It consists mainly of putrescent animal and vegetable matter and urine, the last in a condition of ammoniacal fermentation. Sewage is mixed with water or dissolved in it. S. farming: the use of s. as manure.

sewer (Old Fr. *essuier*, to drain). A large pipe or canal for the removal of sewage. S.-air gas: the mixture of air, vapours and gases which emanates from sewers; it varies greatly in pathogenic qualities.

sex (L. *sexus*). The state of being male, female or hermaphrodite. S.-limited: occurring only in one sex. S.-linked: a term applied to those characteristics that are not inherited equally by both sexes.

sexdī·gital, sexdī·gitate (L. *sex*, six; *digitus*, finger). Having six fingers or six toes on one hand or foot.

sexi·valent (L. *sex*, six; *valēre*, to be worth). Having a valency of six.

sex·tan (L. *sextus*, sixth). Recurring on every sixth day.

sextigrā·vida (L. *sextus*, sixth; *gravida*, pregnant). A woman who is pregnant for the sixth time.

sexti·para (L. *sextus*, sixth; *parere*, to bear). A woman who has produced six children.

sex·tuplet (L. *sex*, six). One of six young born at a single birth.

sex·ual (L. *sexualis*, from *sexus*, sex). Relating to sex. S. diseases: venereal diseases. S. intercourse: coitus. S. organs: the genitalia.

sexuă·lity (L. *sexualis*, from *sexus*, sex). The collective characteristics rendering an individual male or female.

shadow. 1. A term used in radiography to indicate abnormal opacity. 2. A colourless erythrocyte.

shaft. The diaphysis of any long bone.

shank. 1. The leg from knee to ankle. 2. The shin-bone or tibia.

share-bone. The os pubis.

Sharpey's fibres (Sharpey, W., English anatomist, 1802–80). The connective tissue fibres between periosteum and bone.

sheath. A sac; an envelope. Applied in anatomy to the outer coverings of arteries, nerves, etc.

shed. To cast off.

shedding. Casting off.

sheet. A large oblong of linen or cotton used as bed covering. **Draw-s.**: a folded s. placed under the patient in bed and so arranged as to be withdrawn with a minimum of inconvenience.

shell-shock. Shock affecting soldiers in action; characterized by severe nervous disturbances.

Shenton's arch or line (Shenton E. W. H., contemporary English radiologist). The curved line seen in a skiagram which passes from the neck of the femur to the upper part of the obturator foramen. This line is broken or deformed in fractures or diseases of the hip.

Shepherd's fracture (Shepherd, F. J., Canadian surgeon, 1851–1929). A fracture of the external part of the astragalus.

Sherrington's law (Sherrington, Sir C. S., English physiologist, 1859–1952). States that every posterior spinal nerve root supplies a special region of the skin, although there is a region of overlap in adjacent areas.

sherry. A wine from Spain.

Shiga's bacillus (Shiga, K., contemporary Japanese physician). The *Shigella dysenteriae*.

Shigel·la. A genus of the Salmonelleae tribe containing the dysentery-causing bacilli.

shin. The sharp anterior edge of the tibia. **S.-bone**: the tibia.

shingles (L. *cingulum*, girdle). Herpes zoster.

shiver. A slight tremor caused by cold, etc.

shock. 1. A sudden and serious depression of the system, usually produced by injury, operations, etc. **Anaphylactic s.** : s. produced by the injection of a foreign protein in a sensitized subject. **S. therapy**: the induction of general disturbance as a method of treatment, applied especially in certain types of mental disorder.

shoemaker's spasm. A neurosis analogous to writer's cramp and affecting shoemakers.

short circuit. An anastomosis between the stomach and small intestine, or between small intestine and large.

short-circuiting. The making of openings in the intestine above and below a point of obstruction.

short-sightedness. Myopia.

short-windedness. Dyspnoea.

shotgun prescription. One containing several ingredients written in the anticipation that at least one of them will prove therapeutic. Syn. blunderbuss prescription.

shoulder. The junction point of the arm and the trunk.

show. The discharge of blood preceding the onset of labour or menstruation.

Shrapnell's membrane (Shrapnell, H. J., English anatomist of the nineteenth century). The membrana flaccida of the membrana tympani.

Si. The symbol for an atom of Silicon.

sĭă·laden (G. *sialon*, saliva; *adēn*, gland). A salivary gland.

sĭ·aladenī·tis (G. *sialon*, saliva; *adēn*, gland). Inflammation of a salivary gland.

sĭ·aladenon·cus (G. *sialon*, saliva; *adēn*, gland; *ogkos*, mass). A tumour of a salivary gland.

sĭă·lagogue (G. *sialon*, saliva; *agōgos*, leading). See sialogogue.

sĭ·alapor·ia (G. *sialon*, saliva; *aporia*, difficulty). Saliva deficiency.

sĭă·lic, si·aline (G. *sialon*, saliva). Relating to or like saliva.

sĭ·alism, sialis·mus (G. *sialon*, saliva). Ptyalism; salivation.

sĭ·alo-adenec·tomy (G. *sialon*, saliva; *adēn*, gland; *ektomē*, excision). The surgical removal of a salivary gland.

sĭ·alo-adenŏ·tomy (G. *sialon*, saliva; *adēn*, gland; *tomē*, a cutting). Incision into a salivary gland.

sĭ·alo-aerŏ·phagy (G. *sialon*, saliva; *aēr*, air; *phagein*, to eat). The habit of continually swallowing, and thus conveying saliva and air into the stomach.

sĭ·alo-angĭĕc·tasis (G. *sialon*, saliva; *aggeion*, vessel; *ektasis*, extension). Dilatation of the salivary ducts.

sĭ·alo-angiī·tis (G. *sialon*, saliva; *aggeion*, vessel). Inflammation of the salivary ducts.

sĭ·alocele (G. *sialon*, saliva; *kēlē*, tumour). A cyst of the salivary vessels.

sialŏ·genous (G. *sialon*, saliva; *gennan*, to produce). Producing a flow of saliva.

sĭă·logogue (G. *sialon*, saliva; *agōgos*, leading). 1. Exciting a flow of saliva. 2. A drug exciting a flow of saliva.

sĭ·aloid (G. *sialon*, saliva; *eidos*, form). Relating to or of the nature of saliva.

sĭă·lolith (G. *sialon*, saliva; *lithos*, stone). A salivary calculus.

sĭ·alolithi·asis (G. *sialon*, saliva, *lithos*, stone). The formation of salivary calculi.

sĭ·alolithŏ·tomy (G. *sialon*, saliva; *lithos*, stone; *tomē*, a cutting). Incision into a salivary vessel for the purpose of removing a sialolith.

sialon·cus (G. *sialon*, saliva; *ogkos*, mass). A tumour beneath the tongue, sometimes due to the obstruction of a salivary gland by a calculus.

sialorrhœ·a (G. *sialon*, saliva; *rhoia*, a flow). A flow of saliva.

sialŏ·schesis (G. *sialon*, saliva; *skhĕsis*, retention). Suppression of salivary secretion.

sib (Anglo-Saxon). 1. Related; akin. 2. In genetics a member of the same fraternity; a sibling.

sĭ·bilant (L. *sibilare*, to whistle). Hissing.

sĭ·bilus (L. *sibilare*, to whistle). A hissing râle.

sibling. One of two or more children having the same parents.

Sibson's fascia (Sibson, F., English physician, 1814–76). The septum covering the apical pleura, attached to the first rib. **S.'s muscle** : the scalenus quartus, scalenus pleuralis or scalenus minimus.

sick. 1. Ill; not in health. 2. Affected with nausea. **S. headache**: headache accompanied with nausea; migraine. **S.-list**: a list of persons, especially in the armed forces, who are disabled by illness. **S.-room**: a room occupied by an invalid.

sickle cell. A crescentic or sickle-shaped red blood cell. **S.-c anaemia**: a hereditary anaemia in which the red blood cells of the patient acquire a sickle-like or crescentic shape in vitro; usually found only in negroes.

sickness. The condition of being out of health.

side. A lateral aspect of the body. **S.-chain**: see receptor.

siderŏ·genous (G. *sidēros*, iron; *gennan*, to produce). Iron forming.

sĭ·deropē·nia (G. *sidēros*, iron; *pĕnia*, poverty). Iron deficiency.

siderŏ·philous (G. *sidēros*, iron; *philein*, to love). Term applied to cells tending to absorb iron.

sĭ·deroscope (G. *sidēros*, iron; *skopein*, to view). A magnet or other appliance for determining the presence of metallic iron in the eye.

siderŏ·sis (G. *sidēros*, iron). 1. Pneumoconiosis set up by inhalation of iron particles. 2. An excess of iron in the blood. 3. Pigmentation due to deposition of iron particles. 4. Degenerative changes in the eye arising from a retained intra-ocular foreign body containing iron.

si·derous (G. *sidēros*, iron). Containing iron.

Siebenmann's canals (Siebenmann, F., Swiss oto-laryngologist, 1852–1928). The small vascular canals, probably for lymphatics, in the aqueduct of the cochlea.

Siebold's operation (Siebold, K. K. von, German surgeon, 1736–1807). Pubiotomy.

sieve. A vessel with a meshed bottom used for sifting. The gauge of a s. is generally indicated by the number of meshes per linear inch, e.g. a no. 6 sieve would contain 36 holes per square inch. **S.-bone:** the ethmoid bone.

sig. (L. *signare*, to mark). Abbreviation for L. *signa*, 'label it', or for *signetur*, 'let it be labelled.'

sigh. A prolonged inspiration succeeded by a short expiration.

sight. The act or power of seeing.

sig·ma (G. the letter 's'). It is used to signify one-thousandth of a second. **S. reaction:** a flocculation reaction used in the diagnosis of syphilis.

sig·matism (G. *sigma*, the letter 's'). Faulty or too frequent use of the 's' sound in speech.

sig·moid (G. *sigma*, the letter 's'; *eidos*, form). 1. Shaped like the letter 's'. 2. Relating to the sigmoid flexure of the colon. **S. flexure:** an s-shaped curve in the colon between the iliac crest and the rectum. **S. valves:** the semilunar valves.

sigmoidec·tomy (G. *sigma*, the letter 's'; *ektōme*, excision). Surgical removal of a portion of the sigmoid flexure of the colon.

sigmoidi·tis (G. *sigma*, the letter 's'; *eidos*, form). Inflammation of the sigmoid flexure of the colon.

sigmoi·dopexy (G. *sigma*, the letter 's'; *eidos*, form; *pēxis*, fixation). Fixation of sigmoid colon for prolapse of the rectum.

sigmoi·doproctŏ·stomy (G. *sigma*, the letter 's'; *eidos*, form; *prŏktos*, anus; *stoma*, mouth). The surgical making of an opening between the sigmoid flexure and the rectum.

sigmoi·doscope (G. *sigma*, the letter 's'; *eidos*, form; *skopein*, to view). An instrument for examining the sigmoid flexure.

sigmoidŏ·scopy (G. *sigma*, the letter 's'; *eidos*, shape; *skopein*, to view). Visual examination of the sigmoid flexure with a sigmoidoscope.

sigmoidŏ·stomy (G. *sigma*, the letter 's'; *eidos*, form; *stoma*, mouth). The surgical creation of an artificial anus in the sigmoid flexure.

sign. Any mark or indication providing objective evidence of disease.

sig·na (L. *signare*, to mark). 'Mark' (label) in prescriptions; usually written 'S' or 'Sig' and placed before the physician's directions to the patient.

sig·nature (L. *signare*, to mark). 1. That part of a prescription appearing on the label. 2. Any distinguishing character or feature.

sig·natures, doctrine of (L. *signare*, to mark). Ancient theory that the medicinal use of a plant may be determined by some external characteristic or mark. **Signaturist:** one who believes this.

si·kamin. A poisonous principle obtained from the Japanese *Illicium religiosum* (Magnoliaceae).

Silex's sign (Silex, P., German ophthalmologist, 1858–1929). The furrows radiating from the angles of the mouth in congenital syphilis.

si·lica (L. *silex*, flint). SiO_2, silicon dioxide, present in many precious and other stones and also in quartz and sand.

si·licate (L. *silex*, flint). Salt of silicic acid.

sili·cic acid (L. *silex*, flint). An acid in which silicon is the base; forms silicates. Occurs in various forms: Orthosilicic, H_4SiO_4; Metasilicic, H_2SiO_3; Parasilicic, H_6SiO_6.

si·licon (L. *silex*, flint). A non-metallic element found only in combination, as silica, *q.v.*, and in the form of silicates.

silicŏ·sis (L. *silex*, flint). A deposit of particles of silica in the tissues; specifically a variety of pneumoconiosis, a chronic fibroid condition of the lung or the bronchial lymphatic glands. It is caused by the inhalation of silica particles.

silkworm gut. A suture material made from the fluid silk in a silkworm.

sillonneur (Fr. *sillon*, furrow). A surgical knife with three blades, used in ophthalmological operations.

silver. A soft, white, precious metal; symbol Ag.; atomic weight 107·88. **S. arsenobenzol:** used in the treatment of syphilis. **S. arsphenamine:** used in the treatment of syphilis. **S. gelatose:** albargin. **S. nitrate:** lunar caustic. **S. protein** and **S. proteinate:** solutions used as caustics. **S. trinitrophenolate:** silver picrate.

Silvester's method (Silvester, H. R., English physician, 1829–1908). A form of artificial respiration in which the arms are raised above the patient's head and then pressed against the thorax.

Simmonds's disease (Simmonds, M., German physician, 1855–1925). Premature senility caused by complete atrophy of the hypophysis. Syn. hypophyseal cachexia.

Simon's posture (Simon, G., German surgeon, 1824–76). See position, lithotomy.

simple (L. *simplex*). 1. Not complex or compound; consisting of one substance only. 2. Of weak intellect. 3. A medicinal herb.

simples (L. *simplex*, simple). Term for herbs used medicinally.

sim·plex (L.). Simple.

Sims's position (Sims, J. M., American gynaecologist, 1813–83). See under position. **S.'s speculum:** a form of duck-billed vaginal speculum.

si·mul (L.). At once.

simulā·tion (L. *simulare*, to simulate). The counterfeiting of disease; malingering.

Simū·lium A genus of dipterous insects which are known as black flies, sand flies or buffalo gnats. They are widely distributed and may become a pest at times.

sinal·bin (G. *sināpi*, mustard; L. *albus*, white). The crystalline glycoside, $C_{30}H_{44}N_2S_2O_{16}$, found in white mustard seeds.

Sinā·pis (G. *sināpi*, mustard). A genus of cruciferous plants; mustard.

si·năpism (G. *sināpi*, mustard). A mustard plaster.

si·năpize (G. *sināpi*, mustard). To mix with mustard.

sinci·pital (L. *semi*, half; *caput*, head). Relating to the sinciput.

sin·ciput (L. *semi*, half; *caput*, head). The anterior and top part of the head.

sinew. A tendon.

singers' nodes, or **nodules.** The formation of small pale-coloured nodules on the vocal cords. Syn. chorditis tuberosa.

singul·tus (L.). A hiccup.

si·nigrin (G. *sināpi*, mustard; L. *niger*, black). The crystalline glycoside found in black mustard seeds.

sinis·trad (L. *sinister*, left; *ad*, to). To the left.

si·nistral (L. *sinister*, left). 1. Relating to the left side. 2. A left-handed person.

sinistră·lity (L. *sinister*, left). The condition of being left-handed.

sinistrau·ral (L. *sinister*, left; *auris*, ear). Having better hearing in the left ear than in the right.

sinistrocar·dial (L. *sinister*, left; G. *kardia*, heart). With the heart to the left of the median line.

sǐ·nistrocě·rebral (L. *sinister*, left; *cerebrum*, the brain). Relating to or lying in the left cerebral hemisphere.

sinistrŏ·cular (L. *sinister*, left; *oculus*, eye). Seeing better with the left eye than with the right.

sinistromǎ·nual (L. *sinister*, left; *manus*, hand). Left-handed.

sinistrŏ·pedal (L. *sinister*, left; *pes*, foot). Left-footed; preferring to use the left foot.

sǐ·nistrous (L. *sinister*, left). Unskilled; clumsy.

sǐ·nuous (L. *sinuosus*, from *sinus*, a curve). Undulating; winding in and out.

sǐ·nus (L.). 1. A hollow or cavity, especially the nasal sinuses 2. A large channel containing blood, especially one containing venous blood. 3. Any suppurating tract or channel. 4. A recess or cavity within a bone. 5. The space between the breasts. **Anal:** see crypt of Morgagni. **Aortic:** sinuses of Valsalva. Three well-marked recesses in the interior of the wall of the ascending aorta each of which is placed opposite a segment of the valve. **Basilar:** or transverse venous sinus lies under the central basal dura mater, and is in the form of a network joining the inferior petrosal sinuses. **Cavernous:** is placed on the side of the body of the sphenoid where this joins the greater wing, and formed by the junction of the superior ophthalmic vein and the spheno-parietal sinus. **Circular:** is a spongy venous network that surrounds the pituitary body and connects the two cavernous sinuses. **Coronary:** is the dilated terminal part of the great cardiac vein. It is about one inch in length and opens into the right atrium. **Ethmoidal:** air sinuses contained within the labyrinth of the ethmoid bone. **Frontal:** air sinus in the upper part of the frontal bone. It opens by means of the infundibulum into the middle meatus of the nose. **Inferior petrosal:** passes backwards from the apex of the petrous temporal bone to the jugular foramen through which it passes to join the internal jugular vein. **Inferior sagittal:** a small venous sinus situated in the lower border of the falx cerebri over its posterior two-thirds. **Intercavernous:** small venous channel joining the two cavernous sinuses. **Marginal:** (inferior occipital) small sinuses on each side of the foramen magnum which join to form the occipital sinus. **Maxillary:** an air sinus situated within the body of the maxilla. It opens into the middle meatus of the nose. **Oblique pericardial:** a cul de sac behind the ventricular portion of the heart. **Of larynx:** a recess bounded superiorly by a vestibular fold and inferiorly by a vocal cord. **Of Morgagni:** an interval between the superior, concave border of the superior constrictor of the larynx and the base of the skull. **Of Valsalva:** see aortic sinuses. **Paranasal:** these are hollow cavities lined with mucous membrane, which are contained within the frontal, sphenoid, ethmoid, maxillae and mastoid portions of the temporal bones. **Petrosquamous:** small venous sinus situated along the junction of the petrous and squamous parts of the temporal bone. **Pocularis:** (prostatic utricle) a blind recess in the prostatic urethra. **Portal:** an enlargement of the portal vein as it reaches the right extremity of the porta hepatis. **Prostatic:** see pocularis. **Pulmonary:** recesses in the wall of the pulmonary artery opposite the semilunar valves. **Renal:** the cavity within the kidney. **Sigmoid:** venous sinus, the continuation of the transverse sinus of the skull after it has received the superior petrosal sinus. **Sphenoparietal:** a small venous sinus situated on the inferior surface of the lesser wing of the sphenoid bone. **Sphenoidal:** two large air sinuses situated within the body of the sphenoid bone. **Straight:** is situated at the junction of the falx cerebri with the tentorium cerebelli and is formed by the union of the inferior longitudinal sinus and the great cerebral vein. **Superior sagittal:** is situated in the median line within the superior convex border of the falx cerebri. It extends from the crista galli of the ethmoid bone to the internal occipital protuberance where it opens into the right transverse sinus. **Superior petrosal:** passes backwards along the upper edge of the petrous bone at the base of the tentorium cerebelli to join the transverse sinus. **Tarsi:** the tarsal tunnel on the upper surface of the calcaneum. **Transverse:** extends on each side from the internal occipital protuberance to the postero-lateral compartment of the jugular foramen, through which it passes. **Transverse pericardial:** the space on the posterior surface of the pericardium between the arterial and venous mesocardia. **Tympani:** is a depression posterior to the promontory of the middle ear. **Venosus:** a groove on the inner wall of the right atrium of the heart.

sǐ·nusal (L. *sinus*, a curve or hollow). Relating to a sinus.

sinusi·tis (L. *sinus*, a curve or hollow). Inflammation of a sinus, especially a nasal sinus.

sǐ·nusoid (L. *sinus*, a curve or hollow; G. *eidos*, form). 1. Like a sinus. 2. One of the comparatively large spaces comprising the embryonic circulatory system in the liver and other viscera.

sinusoi·dal (L. *sinus*, a curve or hollow; G. *eidos*, form). Relating to a sinusoid. **S. alternating currents:** electric currents in which the rise from zero to maximum and the fall from maximum to zero are accomplished gradually. There is no interval when zero is reached, but a second rise to maximum and fall to zero on the other side.

sǐ·phon (G. *siphon*, tube). A tube of angular form with one arm longer than the other, used for the purpose of draining fluid from a cavity, wound or vessel.

sǐ·phonage (G. *siphōn*, tube). The use of a siphon for stomach ablutions or for wound drainage.

Siphonap·tera. An order of small, wingless insects which are laterally compressed and adapted to sucking blood. Fleas.

Siphunculā·ta. An order of insects which includes lice.

Siphunculī·na funǐ·cola. The oriental 'eye fly' which some think may transmit yaws.

Sippy diet (Sippy, B. W., American physician, 1866–1924). For the treatment of gastric ulcer and in conditions in which the patient is wasted and unable to take ordinary foods. Milk only for the first few days, cereals and eggs added on the fourth day. Amounts are increased gradually until puréed vegetables are included. Normal diet usually taken by the 24th day. At first two-hourly frequency of small feeds is essential.

sirenŏ·melus (G. *seirēn*, siren; *melos*, limb). A monster with the lower extremities fused and having no feet.

sistomen·sin (L. *sistere*, to arrest; *mensis*, month). A hormone from the corpus luteum; it confines menstruation within the normal limits.

site (L. *situs*). Situation; location.

sitǐer·gia (G. *sition*, food; *eirgein*, to exclude). Hysterical anorexia.

sitiŏ·logy (G. *sition*, food; *logos*, discourse). Sitology, *q.v.*

sitiophŏ·bia (G. *sition*, food; *phobos*, fear). See sitophobia.

sitŏ·logy (G. *sitos*, food; *logos*, discourse). The science of nourishment or dietetics.

sitomā·nia (G. *sitos*, food; *mania*, madness). 1. A neurotic craving for food. 2. Sitophobia.

sitophŏ·bia (G. *sitos*, food; *phobos*, fear). Morbid aversion to food.

sitothĕ·rapy (G. *sitos*, food; *therapeia*, treatment). Treatment by dieting; the therapeutic regulation of food.

sitotox·in (G. *sitos*, food; *toxikon*, poison). Any basic poison generated in a cereal food by a plant microorganism.

sitŏ·tropism (G. *sitos*, food; *tropos*, a turning). Response of living cells to the attractive or repulsive influence of food.

situā·tion. The pattern of the stimulus or the sum total of all factors, internal and external, which affect an organism at any given time.

sī·tus (L.). Site; position. **S. perversus**: displacement or abnormal position of a viscus or of two or more viscera. **S. viscerum inversus**: an anomaly in which the viscera take up a position in the body opposite to the normal.

sitz-bath (Ger. *sitzen*, to sit). A bath taken sitting; a hip-bath.

sixth nerve. The abducent nerve. **S. disease**: see exanthema subitum.

skă·tole (G. *skōr*, *skatos*, dung). Methyl indole, C_9H_9N, a nitrogenous compound yielded by decomposition of protein material in the intestinal tract.

skatŏ·phagy (G. *skōr*, *skatos*, dung; *phagein*, to eat). Coprophagy; the eating of excrement.

skein. 1. A length of yarn or silk thread repeatedly doubled and knotted. 2. Spirem, *q.v.*

skĕ·letal (G. *skeleton*, skeleton). Relating to the skeleton.

skĕ·letins (G. *skeleton*, skeleton). Term applied to a number of insoluble epithelial products found principally in invertebrates.

skĕ·letizā·tion (G. *skeleton*, skeleton). 1. The process of converting into a skeleton. 2. Gradual wasting away of the soft parts, the skeleton only being left.

skeletŏ·genous (G. *skeleton*, skeleton; *gennan*, to produce). Producing bony structures.

skeletŏ·logy (G. *skeleton*, skeleton; *logos*, a discourse). That branch of anatomy that treats of the skeleton.

skĕ·leton (G.). A supporting structure, especially the bony framework (osseous s.) sustaining and protecting the soft tissues of the body.

Skene's tubules or **glands** (Skene, A. J. C., Scottish physician practising in America, 1838–1900). The para-urethral glands of the female.

ski·agram (G. *skia*, shadow; *gramma*, a picture). The print of an X-ray picture.

ski·agraph. Skiagram, *q.v.*

skĭā·graphy (G. *skia*, shadow; *graphein*, to write). Photography by means of X-rays; radiography.

skĭalў·tic (G. *skia*, shadow; *luein*, to dissolve). Destroying shadows.

skĭā·meter (G. *skia*, shadow; *metron*, measure). An instrument for measuring the intensity of X-rays.

skĭā·metry (G. *skia*, shadow; *metron*, measure). Measurement of the accommodation of the eye by skiascopy.

ski·ascope (G. *skia*, shadow; *skopein*, to view). An instrument used in carrying out retinoscopy.

skĭā·scopy (G. *skia*, shadow; *skopein*, to view). 1. Refraction of the eye by illumination of the retina with a mirror, i.e. retinoscopy. 2. Examination of the body by X-rays, i.e. fluoroscopy.

skin. The outer covering of the body, comprising the epidermis, scarf skin or cuticle and the corium or true skin. **S. graft**: see graft.

skleri·asis (G. *sklēros*, hard). See scleroderma.

Skoda's râle (Skoda, J., Austrian physician, 1805–81). A bronchial râle heard in consolidated tissue especially in pneumonia. **S.'s sign**: a tympanic sound heard when the chest is percussed above a large pleural effusion or over consolidation in pneumonia.

skopophŏ·bia (G. *skopos*, a watcher; *phobos*, fear). Morbid dread of spies.

scō·tograph (G. *skotos*, darkness; *graphein*, to write). The same as skiagraph.

skotŏ·graphy. The same as skiagraphy.

skull. The bony framework of the head, comprising the cranium and the face. The cranium is composed of the occipital, frontal, sphenoid and ethmoid bones and two parietal and two temporal bones. The face is formed of two nasal, two superior maxillary, two lacrimal, two malar, two palate and two inferior turbinated bones and the vomer and the inferior maxillary bone.

slā·ver (Old Norse *slafra*). Drivel; saliva, especially if involuntarily discharged.

sleep. The periodic condition of rest, during which voluntary consciousness is in abeyance.

sleeping sickness. 1. African lethargy, a disease marked by increasing somnolence, due to trypanosomiasis. 2. Encephalitis lethargica, a virus infection.

slide. A piece of glass, usually three inches by one inch, on which objects are examined under the microscope.

sling. A supporting bandage, usually applied to one suspended from the back of the neck to rest an injured arm or hand.

slippery elm. The dried inner bark of *Ulmus fulva*, which contains much mucilage and is useful as a demulcent in cases of catarrh or dysentery.

slit. Any narrow opening.

slit·lamp of Gullstrand (Gullstrand, A., Swedish ophthalmologist, 1862–1930). An apparatus which, in combination with the corneal microscope, enables the physician to observe magnified optical sections of the anterior segment of the eye.

slough. The necrosed matter separating in cases of ulceration and the like.

sloughing. Relating to or characterized by sloughs.

Sm. The symbol of Samarium.

smallpox. Variola. A contagious and infectious disease starting with severe febrile symptoms, which are followed two or three days later by a papular eruption spreading all over the body. In the course of about a fortnight the eruption goes through a vesicular and pustular stage after which there is a formation of crusts. When the crusts separate, the skin is often much marked and pitted (pock-marks). The period of incubation is twelve to fourteen days, but may be a little longer.

smear culture. A bacteriological culture made by smearing the organisms on the surface of the culture medium.

Smee cell (Smee, A., English surgeon, 1818–77). An electric battery cell consisting of two plates—one zinc and the other platinized silver—in a dilute solution of sulphuric acid.

smeg·ma (G. *smēgma*, soap). A thick cheesy secretion found under the prepuce and around the labia minora.

smegmat·ic. Relating to smegma.

smell. 1. Odour perception. 2. Odour.

smelling salts. Various preparations of ammonium carbonate scented with aromatic substances.

Smith's disease (Smith, E., English physician, 1835–1914). Mucous colitis. **S.'s sign**: a murmur heard in cases of enlarged bronchial glands on auscultation over the manubrium with the patient's head thrown back.

Smith's dislocation (Smith, R. W., Irish surgeon, 1807–73). Upward and backward dislocation of the metatarsals and the internal cuneiform bone. **S.'s fracture**: fracture of lower end of radius with forward

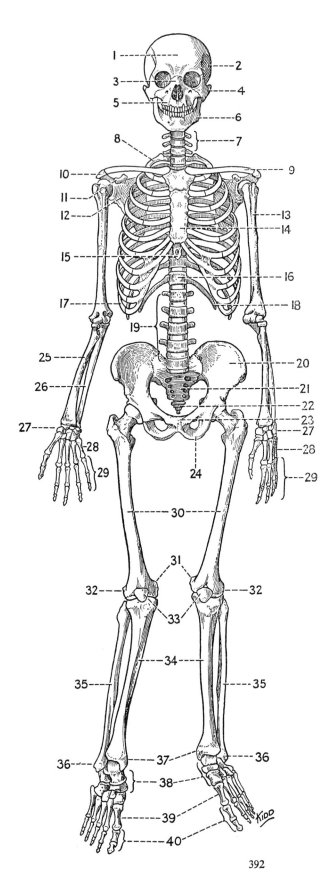

THE SKELETON

1. FRONTAL BONE
2. PARIETAL BONE
3. NASAL BONE
4. ZYGOMA
5. MAXILLA
6. MANDIBLE
7. CERVICAL VERTEBRAE (3 of)
8. 1st RIB
9. CLAVICLE
10. ACROMION PROCESS OF SCAPULA
11. CORACOID PROCESS OF SCAPULA
12. SCAPULA
13. HUMERUS
14. STERNUM
15. XIPHOID
16. 12th THORACIC VERTEBRA
17. 10th RIB
18. 12th RIB
19. THE FIVE LUMBAR VERTEBRAE
20. ILEUM
21. SACRUM
22. COCCYX
23. PUBIS
24. ISCHIUM
25. RADIUS
26. ULNA
27. CARPUS OR CARPAL BONES
28. METACARPAL BONES
29. PHALANGES (carpal)
30. FEMUR
31. MEDIAL CONDYLE OF FEMUR
32. LATERAL CONDYLE OF FEMUR
33. PATELLA
34. TIBIA
35. FIBULA
36. LATERAL MALLEOLUS
37. MEDIAL MALLEOLUS
38. TARSUS OR TARSAL BONES
39. METATARSAL BONES
40. TARSAL PHALANGES

displacement of lower fragment, sometimes called a reverse Colles fracture.

Smith's operation (Smith, H., English surgeon, in India, 1823–94). 1. Crushing of haemorrhoids with clamps and subsequent application of cautery. 2. Extraction of an immature cataract with an intact capsule.

Smith's test (Smith, W. G., Irish physician, born 1844). An iodine test for bile pigments.

Smith-Petersen nail (Smith-Petersen, M. N., American orthopaedic surgeon, born 1886). A tri-flanged nail used to fix the head of the femur in cases of fracture.

Smith-Pitfield method (Smith, J. B., contemporary English surgeon; Pitfield, R. L., American physician, 1870–1942). A method of staining to show flagella.

smoker's patch. The chronic inflammation of a small area of the mucous membrane of the mouth, due to irritation by the stem of the tobacco-pipe.

smoker's sore throat. A condition of pharyngeal and laryngeal catarrh accompanied by hoarseness, common in heavy smokers.

Sn. The symbol for tin.

snakeroot, black. The dried rhizome and roots of *Cimicifuga racemosa*. It is a bitter tonic and has mild expectorant and emmenagogue properties. It is used in cases of bronchitis, rheumatism, dysmenorrhoea and amenorrhoea.

snare. A small, light wire-loop for removing polypi and other small protruberances.

sneezing. The act of ejecting air violently through the nose.

Snell's law (Snell, S., English ophthalmologist, 1851–1909). The sine of the angle of incidence bears a constant relation to the sine of the angle of refraction for two given media.

Snellen's reform eye (Snellen, H., Dutch ophthalmologist, 1834–1908). An artificial eye composed of two concavo-convex plates with an empty space between. **S.'s test types:** lines of letters constructed from small squares used to ascertain the acuteness of a person's vision.

snore. 1. Breathing in such a way as to cause vibration of the soft palate, producing a harsh sound. 2. The sound thus made.

snow, carbon dioxide. Solid CO_2, used in the treatment of warts and naevi.

snow-blindness. Photophobia and conjunctivitis caused by exposure of the eyes to the reflection of sunlight from snow.

snuffles. A cararrhal affection of infants, generally due to inherited syphilis.

SO₂. Sulphur dioxide.

Sŏä·min. A proprietary preparation of sodium *p*-aminophenylarsonate, useful in cases of syphilis and some chronic skin diseases.

soap. A metallic salt of one or more of the higher fatty acids. Soaps of metals other than potassium and sodium are usually insoluble in water.

sob. A short, convulsive inspiration.

sŏ·bee. A mixture of soya bean flour and barley flour with olive oil, sodium chloride and calcium. It is used as a milk substitute for infants with milk idiosyncrasy.

sobis·minol mass. A complex substance obtained by interaction of sodium bismuthate, *triiso*-propanolamine and propylene glycol. It is used for the treatment of syphilis and is taken orally. **S. solution:** is a solution of sobisminol mass in mixture of propylene glycol and water. It is given intramuscularly for all types of syphilis.

sŏ·cia parŏ·tidis (L. *socius*, companion; G. *parōtis*, the gland beside the ear). A small detached lobe of the parotid gland.

cc

sŏ·cial (L. *socius*, companion). Gregarious; growing in groups. **S. evil:** prostitution. **S. medicine:** the study of the social factors making for health and disease.

sociŏ·logy (L. *socius*, companion; G. *logos*, discourse). Science of the development and nature and laws of human society.

socket. A cavity or depression into which another part fits. **S., tooth:** the alveolus in which a tooth inheres.

sŏ·da (It., from L. *solidus*, substantial). A vague term usually meaning sodium carbonate, Na_2CO_3, or its decahydrate, $Na_2CO_310H_2O$ (washing soda), but sometimes applied to caustic soda, NaOH, or its solution.

sodae·mia (It. *soda*, from L. *solidus*, substantial; G. *haima*, blood). The presence of soda in the blood.

sodium (It. *soda*, from L. *solidus*, substantial). A metallic element belonging to the alkaline metals. It melts at 95·6° C.; its specific gravity is 0·97 and atomic weight 23; it has a valence of one. Symbol Na., from L. *natrium*. S. occurs widely in nature and is an important constituent of animal tissues and of many medicinal compounds. **S. amytal:** a sedative. **S. bicarbonate:** an antacid (baking powder). **S. biphosphate** (acid sod. phosphate): a urinary antiseptic. **S. bisulphate:** used in the preparation of effervescing baths. **S. carbonate:** washing soda. **S. chloride:** common salt. **S. citrate:** an antacid. **S. iodide:** used for treatment of syphilis. **S. salicylate:** used in the treatment of rheumatism and rheumatic fever. **S. silicate:** waterglass. **S. sulphate** (Glauber's salt): a purgative.

sŏ·doku (Japanese *so*, rat; *doku*, fever). The Japanese term for ratbite fever.

sŏ·domist, sŏ·domite (Sodom in ancient Palestine). One practising sodomy.

sŏ·domy. Copulation by the anus between male persons.

Soemmering's ligament (Soemmering, T. von, German physician, 1755–1830). The suspensory ligament of the lacrimal gland. **S.'s muscle:** musculus levator glandulae thyroidae. **S.'s nerve:** the 'long pudendal nerve'; perineal branch of cutaneus femoris posterior or small sciatic nerve. **S.'s substance:** the substantia nigra intervening between the tegmentum and basis penduculi in the mesencephalon.

soft. Easily yielding; not hard.

softening. The act or process of becoming soft. **S. of the bones:** osteomalacia. **S. of the brain:** encephalomalacia.

soil. The ground; earth.

soil-pipe. The discharge pipe of the plumbing system of a house.

Sol. Abbreviation for solution.

sŏ·lanism (L. *sōlanum*, nightshade). Poisoning from ingestion of *Solanum dulcamara* or *Solanum nigrum*. It is characterized by symptoms similar to belladonna poisoning.

sŏ·lanoid (L. *sōlanum*, nightshade; G. *eidos*, form). Resembling a raw potato.

solanŏ·ma (L. *sōlanum*, nightshade). A solanoid cancer, i.e. having the texture of a raw potato.

Solā·num (L., nightshade). A genus of plants including the potato.

sŏ·lar (L. *sol*, sun). Relating to the sun. **S. plexus** (coeliac plexus): A large prevertebral sympathetic plexus.

solarizā·tion (L. *sol*, sun). Exposure to sunlight.

Solayres's obliquity (Solayres de Renhas, F. L. J., French gynaecologist, 1737–72). Descent of the child's head by its occipitomental diameter into the oblique diameter of the pelvis.

sole (L. *solea*). The bottom, or plantar, surface of the foot.

ō·l enoid. A coil of wire equally spaced between turns. When a current flows through the wire a magnetic field is set up round the wire.

sō·leus (L. *solea*, sole). A muscle of the calf of the leg.

solid (L. *solidus*, substantial). 1. Firm; compact; not gaseous, fluid or hollow. 2. Any tissue or substance that is not gaseous or fluid.

solidă·rity (L. *solidus*, substantial). The unitary nature of the several parts of a body, whereby these contribute to the wellbeing of the whole organism.

sŏ·lidism (L. *solidus*, substantial). An obsolete doctrine that changes in the solids of the body are the causes of every disease.

sō·lipsism (L. *solus*, alone; *ipse*, self). The belief that the world exists only in the mind of the individual or that it consists solely of the individual himself and his own experiences.

sŏ·litary (L. *solus*, alone). Single; existing separately; not aggregated.

Solium (L. *sol*, sun). A species of tapeworm. *Taenia solium*, a tapeworm in pork.

solubi·lity (L. *solubilis*, from *solvere*, to dissolve). The condition of being soluble.

sŏ·luble (L. *solubilis*, from *solvere*, to dissolve). Susceptible of being dissolved.

sō·lum tym·pani (L.). The floor of the tympanic cavity. **S. ventriculi quarti:** floor of the fourth ventricle.

sōlū·tion (L. *solutio*, from *solvere*, to dissolve). 1. The act or process of dissolving. 2. A liquid in which a solid has been dissolved. 3. A severance or break.

sol·vent (L. *solvere*, to dissolve). 1. Dissolving. 2. A liquid that is capable of dissolving.

sō·ma (G., body). 1. The whole body, excluding the germ-cells. 2. The body alone, without the limbs.

sō·macule (G. *sōma*, body). The smallest possible fragment of protoplasm.

somaesthet·ic (G. *sōma*, body; *aisthētikos*, sensitive). Relating to the general sensory structures.

somasthē·nia (G. *sōma*, body; *a*, neg.; *sthenos*, strength). Bodily weakness, poor appetite and sleep; the patient is easily exhausted.

somat·ic (G. *sōmatikos*, from *sōma*, body). 1. Relating to the body. 2. Relating to the body's framework, excluding the viscera. 3. Possessing two sets of chromosomes.

somă·toblast (G. *sōma*, body; *blastos*, germ). Any plastidule from which cell-material (as distinguished from nuclear material) is developed.

somă·toceptor (G. *sōma*, body; L. *capere*, to take). A receptor concerned in receiving stimuli of the skeletal and somatic musculature.

somă·tochrome (G. *sōma*, body; *khrōma*, colour). A nerve-cell having a cell-body completely enveloping the nucleus, its protoplasm possessing a distinct contour and readily staining.

somă·toderm (G. *sōma*, body; *derma*, skin). The somatic layer of mesoderm.

sō·matodi·dymus (G. *sōma*, body; *didumos*, twin). A twin monster foetus with trunks united.

somatodŷ·mia (G. *sōma*, body; *duein*, to enter). A twin monstrosity with united trunks.

somatŏ·logy (G. *sōma*, body; *logos*, discourse). The anatomical and physiological study of the body.

sō·matome (G. *sōma*, body; *tomē*, a cutting). 1. An instrument used in obstetrics for cutting the body of the foetus. 2. A somite.

sō·matomě·galy (G. *sōma*, body; *megas*, large). Gigantism.

somatŏ·metry (G. *sōma*, body; *metron*, measure). Measurement of the body.

somatŏ·pagus (G. *sōma*, body *pegnunai*, to fix). A double monster with separated trunks.

somatopath·ic (G. *sōma*, body; *pathos*, disease)· Bodily disordered.

somatŏ·pathy (G. *sōma*, body; *pathos*, disease). Any bodily disease or disorder.

somatophrē·nia (G. *sōma*, body; *phrēn*, mind). A mental state in which bodily disorders are imagined or exaggerated.

somă·toplasm (G. *sōma*, body; *plasma*, something formed). The protoplasm of the body-cells as distinguished from the germ-plasm.

somă·topleure (G. *sōma*, body; *pleura*, side). The somatic mesoblast.

somatopsȳ·chic (G. *sōma*, body; *psukhē*, mind). Relating to both the body and the mind.

somatŏ·tomy (G. *sōma*, body; *tomē*, section). Anatomy or dissection.

sō·matotri·dymus (G. *sōma*, body; *tridumos*, threefold). A monster having three trunks.

sō·mite (G. *sōma*, body). A primitive segment; sometimes called mesodermal segment.

somit·ic (G. *sōma*, body). Relating to or resembling a somite.

somnam·bulism (L. *somnus*, sleep; *ambulare*, to walk). 1. Sleep-walking. 2. A hypnotic condition in which the subject retains full possession of his senses but has his will and consciousness under the control of the hypnotizer. The subject has no subsequent recollection of what has happened.

somnam·bulist (L. *somnus*, sleep; *ambulare*, to walk). A sleep-walker.

somnifā·cient (L. *somnus*, sleep; *facere*, to make). 1. Causing sleep. 2. Any agent that causes sleep; a hypnotic.

Som·nifaine. A proprietary preparation of the diethylamine salts of diethylbarbituric acid (barbitone) and ally*liso*propyl-barbituric acid. It is a powerful sedative and hypnotic.

somni·ferous (L. *somnus*, sleep; *ferre*, to bring). Inducing sleep.

somni·loquence, somni·loquism, somni·loquy (L. *somnus*, sleep; *loqui*, to talk). The act or habit of speaking during sleep.

som·nolence (L. *somnus*, sleep). A state of drowsiness or sleepiness.

som·nolent (L. *somnus*, sleep). Inclined to sleep; drowsy.

somnolen·tia (L. *somnolentus*, sleepy). Sleep-drunkenness; a state of incomplete sleep in which some of the faculties are abnormally active while others are passive.

sonde coudé (Fr.). A catheter with an elbow or sharp beak-like bend near the end.

Sŏ·neryl. A proprietary hypnotic containing butylethylbarbituric acid. **S. sodium:** a sodium derivative of Soneryl, used for basal narcosis in obstetrics.

sō·nitus (L., sound). Tinnitus, *q.v.*

Sonne dysentery (Sonne, C., Danish bacteriologist, born 1882). Inflammation of the bowel, especially the colon, caused by the Sonne strain of *Shigella dysenteriae*.

sonŏ·meter (L. *sonus*, sound; G. *metron*, measure). 1. An apparatus for measuring the pitch of sounds. 2. An instrument for testing the acuity of hearing.

sŏ·norous (L. *sonorus*, from *sonor*, a noise). Resonant.

soot-cancer. Epithelioma of the scrotum, often affecting chimney sweeps.

sophi·stication (G. *sophistikos*, from *sŏphistēs*, a wise man or, ironically, a deceiver). The adulteration or counterfeiting of food or drugs.

sō·por (L.). A profound sleep.

sopori·ferous (L. *sopor*, sleep; *ferre*, to bring). Inducing profound sleep.

sopori·fic (L. *sopor*, sleep; *facere*, to make). 1. Causing deep sleep. 2. A sleep-inducing agent.

sō·porose, sō·porous (L. *sopor*, sleep). Relating to or affected with sound sleep.

s. op. s. Abbreviation for L. *si opus sit*, if required.

sorbefā·cient (L. *sorbere*, to suck in; *facere*, to make). 1. Inducing absorption. 2. An agent promoting absorption.

sor·bitol (Sorbite). $CH_2OH(CHOH)_4CH_2OH$. A hexahydric alcohol made by reducing grape-sugar (glucose).

sor·dēs (L.). Filth, dirt; particularly the brown crusts that collect on the lips and teeth in fevers.

sore. 1. Painful. 2. An ulcer or skin lesion.

Sorensen's reagent (Sorensen, S. P. L., Danish chemist, 1868–1939). An acetate buffer solution for combining with Pandy's test for albumin.

sor·ghum. 1. Indian millet. 2. Chinese sugar-cane.

Soret's band (Soret, C., French physicist, died 1931). A band in the violet end of the spectrum of haemoglobin. **S.'s effect**: when a solution is maintained for some time in a temperature gradient, the upper part being warmer than the lower, a difference in concentration between the two parts is set up.

Sorgius's gland (Sorgius, W.; work published in Strassburg, 1880). The paramammary lymphatic gland. **S.'s glands**: the anterior group of the axillary lymphatic glands.

sorŏ·che (Sp., antimony). Mountain sickness of the Andes ascribed (incorrectly) to metallic exhalations.

s.o.s. Abbreviation for L. *si opus sit*, if necessary.

souffle (Fr. *souffler*, from L. *sufflare*, to puff). A puffing sound; an auscultatory murmur.

sound (¹). (L. *sonus*, sound). The effect produced by stimulation of the auditory nerve through aerial vibrations.

sound (²). (Fr. *sonder*, to plumb). An instrument used for insertion into a cavity or canal in order to ascertain whether constrictions, foreign bodies, etc., are present.

sour. Acid to the taste; fermented.

Sousa's nerve (Sousa, M. B. de, Portuguese anatomist, 1835–99). The gustatory nerve fibres contained in the petrosal system.

Southey's tubes (Southey, R. S., English physician, 1835–99). Cannulas of small calibre pushed by means of a trocar into the tissues to drain them.

soya bean. The bean of the *Soja hispida*, the Chinese bean. It is rich in albuminoids and contains little starch.

sō·zin (G. *sōzein*, to save). Any of the defensive proteins occurring naturally in the animal body. A sozin able to destroy micro-organisms is called a mycosozin; one counteracting bacterial poisons, a toxosozin.

sp. Abbreviation for L. *spiritus*, spirit.

space. Term given to a number of enclosed or partly circumscribed areas in or about the body. **Axillary,** is situated between the upper part of the arm and the upper part of the thoracic wall. **Burns's** (suprasternal): interfascial interval just above the sternum. **Deep forearm** (of Parona): situated in the distal third of the forearm. **Distal pulp:** is a closed fascial compartment situated on the palmar aspect of the terminal phalanx. **Fascial palmar:** three in the palm of the hand: the thenar, middle palmar, and hypothenar. **Hypothenar:** a small space confined to the volar surface of the fifth metacarpal bone. **Middle palmar:** a space situated on the ulnar side of the third metacarpal bone. **Of Parona:** see deep forearm. **Palmar:** see fascial palmar. **Pelvocrural:** is the interval between the inguinal ligament anteriorly and the pubis and ilium posteriorly, through which the false pelvis communicates with the thigh.

Retropharyngeal: the interval between the buccopharyngeal and prevertebral fascial. **Retropubic:** prevesical space. Syn. Retzius' space. **Suprasternal:** see Burns's. **Thenar:** situated to the radial side of the third metacarpal bone.

spagi·ric (G. *spaein*, to tear or pluck; *ageirein*, to collect). Relating to the obsolete chemical, alchemistic or Paracelsian school of medicine.

Spahlinger's treatment (Spahlinger, H. A., Swiss bacteriologist, born 1882). A treatment of pulmonary tuberculosis consisting of: first, a destruction of tuberculous toxins by injecting various bacteriolytic and antitoxic serums; secondly, a therapeutic vaccination with a series of tuberculins.

Spallanzani's law (Spallanzani, L., Italian anatomist, 1729–99). That regeneration is more complete in younger individuals than in older ones.

spanae·mia (G. *spanis*, scarcity; *haima*, blood). Inadequacy of the blood; anaemia.

Spanish fly. Cantharides, *q.v.*

spanō·gyny (G. *spanis*, scarcity; *gunē*, woman). A decline in the number of female births and thus of the female population.

spanopnoē·a (G. *spanis*, scarcity; *pnein*, to breathe). Infrequency of respiration.

spargō·sis (G. *spargan*, to swell). Expansion of a part; especially the distension of the mammae with milk.

spar·tĕine (L. *spartium*, the Spanish broom plant). An alkaloid present in scoparius and resembling digitalis in its action.

spasm (G. *spasmos*). A sudden, involuntary muscular contraction.

spasmoder·mia (G. *spasmos*, spasm; *derma*, skin). Spasm of the skin.

spasmod·ic (G. *spasmos*, spasm). Relating to or characterized by spasm.

spas·modism (G. *spasmos*, spasm). A spasmodic condition due to medullary excitation.

spasmŏ·logy (G. *spasmos*, spasm; *logos*, discourse). The sum of what is known of the nature and causes of convulsions and spasms.

spasmophi·lia (G. *spasmos*, spasm; *philein*, to love). A morbid inclination to convulsions.

spasmophil·ic (G. *spasmos*, spasm; *philein*, to love). Characterized by a tendency to spasms.

spasmotox·in (G. *spasmos*, spasm; *toxikon*, poison). The toxin of tetanus.

spas·mous (G. *spasmos*, spasm). Of the nature of a spasm.

spas·mus (G. *spasmos*). A spasm. **S. nutans:** nodding movements of the head due to clonic contraction of sternomastoid muscles.

spas·tic (G. *spastikos*). Relating to or characterized by spasm; produced by spasms. **S. paralysis:** paralysis of central origin in which the muscles affected have increased tone.

spasti·city. The condition of being spastic.

spa·tia zonula·ria. Petit's canal, *q.v.*

spā·tial Relating to space.

spă·tula (L. dim. of *spatha*, from G. *spathē*, a blade). A blunt instrument, shaped like a knife and used for spreading ointments and plasters.

spă·tulate. Resembling a spatula.

spay (L. *spădo*, eunuch). To excise the ovaries.

spē·cialist (L. *specialis*, from *species*, a particular sort). One who confines his practice to a certain disease, or to the diseases of a particular organ or type.

spē·cies (L.). A subdivision of a genus, either animal or vegetable, of which the members are identical or vary only in unimportant details.

speci·fic (L. *species*, a particular sort; *facere*, to make). 1. Of or relating to a species, or the distinguishing mark or essential feature of a species. 2. A medicine with a distinct influence on a particular disease. 3. Produced by a single micro-organism.

specifi·city (L. *species*, a particular sort; *facere*, make). The condition of being specific.

specil·lum (L. *specere*, to look at). A probe.

spĕ·cimen (L.). A sample.

spec·tacles (L. *spectaculum*, a show). Lenses in a frame or mount to assist vision and to correct defects of the eyes.

spec·tral (L. *spectrum*, image). Relating to a spectrum.

spec·trograph (L. *spectrum*, image; G. *graphein*, to write). An apparatus for photographing a spectrum.

spectrŏ·meter (L. *spectrum*, image; G. *metron*, measure). An instrument used for measurement of the deviation of light rays caused by a prism, or for determining the wavelength of a light ray.

spectrŏ·metry (L. *spectrum*, image; G. *metron*, measure). The employment of the spectrometer.

spectrophŏ·bia (L. *spectrum*, image; G. *phobos*, fear). Neurotic fear of mirrored images.

spectrophotŏ·meter (L. *spectrum*, image; *phōs*, light; *metron*, measure). An instrument used for determining the degree of absorption of light of any particular wavelength by a liquid or a solution.

spec·troscope (L. *spectrum*, an image; G. *skopein*, to view). An instrument for forming and examining the spectra of luminous bodies so as to determine their composition.

spectrum (L., image; pl. *spectra*). The stripe of rainbow colours (red, orange, yellow, green, blue, indigo, violet) formed by decomposing light by means of a prism.

spĕ•culum (L., a mirror). 1 (Optics). A reflector usually made of polished metal. 2 (Surgical). An instrument for bringing into view parts otherwise hidden, e.g., aural speculum for ear, vaginal speculum for vagina.

speech. The faculty of speaking; the power of conveying meaning through vocal sounds. **S. centre:** that part of the brain controlling speech; it lies in the third left frontal convolution.

Spence's axillary tail (Spence, J., Scottish surgeon, 1812–82). A process of the mammary gland passing upwards to the axilla.

Spencer Wells facies (Spencer Wells, Sir T., English surgeon, 1818–97). The facial expression of ovarian disease.

Spengler's fragments (Spengler, C., Swiss physician, 1860–1937). Small round bodies seen in tuberculous sputum. **S.'s immune bodies:** immune bodies extracted from the red blood corpuscles of animals immunized against tuberculosis. **S.'s method:** a method of examining the sputum for tuberculosis by treating it with sodium carbonate solution, pancreatine and carbolic acid. **S.'s tuberculin:** a preparation from the bacilli of bovine tuberculin.

Spens's syndrome (Spens, T., Scottish physician, 1764–1842). The same as Adams-Stokes disease, *q.v.*

sperm (G. *sperma*, seed). Abbreviation for spermatozoon.

spermacē·ti (G. *sperma*, seed; *kētos*, whale). A brittle, white, semi-transparent fat (cetaceum, B.P.C.) obtained from the head of the sperm whale. It consists chiefly of cetyl palmitate and is used in ointments and cold creams.

spermacrā·sia (G. *sperma*, seed; *akratein*, to be impotent). 1. Seminal deficiency of spermatozoa. 2. Spermatorrhoea.

sper·matemphrax·is (G. *sperma*, seed; *emphraxis*, stoppage). An impediment to the discharge of semen.

spermat·ic (G. *sperma*, seed). Relating to semen. **S. cord:** the spermatic cord consists of the vas deferens, blood vessels, lymphatics and nerves, covered by three layers of fascia. The blood vessels are the pampiniform plexus of veins, external spermatic artery and the internal spermatic artery. The nerves are the external spermatic nerve and numerous sympathetic nerves from the aortic plexus. The three layers of fascia are: internal spermatic fascia, cremasteric muscle and fascia, and external spermatic fascia.

sper·matid (G. *sperma*, seed). A cell formed by fission of a secondary spermatocyte.

sper·matin (G. *sperma*, seed). An albuminoid, mucilaginous substance occurring in semen.

sper·matism (G. *sperma*, seed). An emission of semen.

spermatī·tis (G. *sperma*, seed). Funiculitis, *q.v.*

sper·matoblast (G. *sperma*, seed; *blastos*, germ). Spermatid, *q.v.*

sper·matocele (G. *sperma*, seed; *kēlē*, hernia). Swelling of the testicle arising from part of the epididymis or the mediastinum testis—usually a retention cyst.

sper·matoclem·ma (G. *sperma*, seed; *klemma*, a theft). An involuntary discharge of semen.

sper·matocyst (G. *sperma*, seed; *kustis*, bladder). A seminal vesicle.

sper·matocystī·tis (G. *sperma*, seed; *kustis*, bladder). Inflammation of the seminal vesicles.

sper·matocyte (G. *sperma*, seed; *kutos*, cell). The germ-cell from which the spermatozoon develops.

sper·matogĕ·nesis (G. *sperma*, seed; *genesis*, production). The production of spermatozoa.

sper·matogen·ic (G. *sperma*, seed; *gennan*, to produce). Producing spermatozoa.

sper·matogō·nium (G. *sperma*, seed; *gonē*, generation). A formative seminal cell.

sper·matoid (G. *sperma*, seed; *eidos*, form). Like semen.

spermatŏ·lysis (G. *sperma*, seed; *lusis*, dissolution). Destruction of spermatozoa.

sper·matomĕ·rite (G. *sperma*, seed; *meros*, part). One of the granules of chromatin into which the sperm nucleus splits up after entrance of the spermatozoon.

sper·matomi·crons (G. *sperma*, seed; *mīkros*, small). Minute particles found in the semen of various animals.

spermatŏ·pathy (G. *sperma*, seed; *pathos*, disease). Any disease or disorder of the sperm-cells.

sper·matophō·bia (G. *sperma*, seed; *phobos*, fear). A neurotic dread of spermatorrhoea.

sper·matophore (G. *sperma*, seed; *pherein*, to carry). (1) Synonym for spermatogonium. (2) A capsule containing a number of spermatozoa.

sper·matoplă·nia (G. *sperma*, seed; *plănē*, a wandering). Seminal metastases.

sper·matopoiĕt·ic (G. *sperma*, seed; *poiein*, to make). Relating to the production or secretion of semen.

sper·matorrhoē·a (G. *sperma*, seed; *rhoia*, a flowing). The involuntary ejaculation of semen without coitus.

spermatŏ·schesis (G. *sperma*, seed; *skhesis*, retention). Suppression of seminal secretion.

spermă·tospore (G. *sperma*, seed; *sporos*, a sowing). A primitive cell producing spermatoblasts by fission.

spermatŏ·vum (G. *sperma*, seed; L. *ovum*, egg). A fertilized ovum.

spermatozō·an. Relating to spermatozoa.

sper·matozoid (G. *sperma*, seed; *zōon*, animal; *eidos*, form). Spermatozoon, *q.v.*

sper·matozō·on (G. *sperma*, seed; *zōon*, animal). Pl. spermatozoa. The male germ cell capable of impregnating the ovum. It has an oval-shaped head, a centre portion and a long flagellum. It is the essential element of semen.

spermatū·ria (G. *sperma*, seed; *ouron*, urine). The existence of semen in the urine.

spermec·tomy (G. *sperma*, seed; *ektomē*, excision). Surgical removal of a part of the spermatic cord.

sper·moblast (G. *sperma*, seed; *blastos*, germ). Spermatoblast, *q.v.*

sper·molith (G. *sperma*, seed; *lithos*, stone). A concretion in the spermatic duct.

spermŏ·lysis (G. *sperma*, seed; *lusis*, dissolution). The destruction of spermatozoa. Syn. spermatolysis.

sper·moneural·gia (G. *sperma*, seed; *neuron*, nerve; *algos*, pain). Neuralgia of the spermatic cord.

sper·moplasm (G. *sperma*, seed; *plassein*, to form). The protoplasm of spermatozoa.

sper·mosphere (G. *sperma*, seed; *sphaira*, a ball). A group or collection of spermatoblasts.

sper·mospore (G. *sperma*, seed; *sporos*, a sowing). Spermatospore, *q.v.*

sp. gr. Abbreviation for specific gravity.

sphă·celate (G. *sphakelos*, gangrene). To become gangrenous or mortified.

sphacelā·tion (G. *sphakelos*, gangrene). Gangrene; necrosis.

sphă·celoder·ma (G. *sphakelos*, gangrene; *derma*, skin). Gangrene of the skin.

sphă·celous (G. *sphakelos*, gangrene). Gangrenous.

sphă·celus (G. *sphakelos*, gangrene). A slough.

sphagī·tis (G. *sphagē*, throat). Any inflammation affecting the throat.

sphē·nion (G. *sphēn*, wedge). The point of the cranium at the sphenoid angle of the parietal bone.

sphenocĕ·phalus (G. *sphēn*, wedge; *kephalē*, head). A variety of monster in which the two eyes are well separated, the ears united under the head, the jaws and mouth distinct and the sphenoid bone altered in shape, so that it is analogous in form to what is usually found in birds.

sphēno-ethmoid (G. *sphēn*, wedge; *ēthmos*, a strainer; *eidos*, form). Relating conjointly to the sphenoid and ethmoid bones.

sphenofron·tal (G. *sphēn*, wedge; L. *frons*, the forehead). Relating to the sphenoid and frontal bones.

sphē·noid (G. *sphēn*, wedge; *eidos*, form). 1. Shaped like a wedge. 2. The os sphenoidale or sphenoid bone.

sphenoi·dal (G. *sphēn*, wedge; *eidos*, form). Relating to the sphenoid bones.

sphenoidi·tis (G. *sphēn*, wedge; *eidos*, form). Inflammation of the sphenoid sinus.

sphenomā·lar (G. *sphēn*, wedge; L. *mălă*, the jaw). Relating to the sphenoid and malar bones.

sphenomax·illary (G. *sphēn*, wedge; *maxilla*, the jawbone). Relating to the sphenoid and maxillary bones.

spheno-occi·pital. Relating conjointly to the sphenoid and occipital bones.

sphenopă·latine (G. *sphēn*, wedge; L. *palatum*, palate). Relating to the sphenoid bone and the palate.

sphē·noparī·etal (G. *sphēn*, wedge; L. *parietalis*, from *paries*, a wall). Relating to the sphenoid and parietal bones.

sphenot·ic (G. *sphēn*, wedge; *ous*, ear). A portion of the sphenoid bone present in the foetus as a distinct bone and composing those parts next to the carotid groove.

sphenotrē·sia (G. *sphēn*, wedge; *trēsis*, a boring). Perforation or boring into the skull of the foetus in performing craniotomy.

sphē·notribe (G. *sphēn*, wedge; *tribein*, to rub). An instrument for crushing the basal part of the skull of the foetus.

sphē·notripsy. The operation of crushing the foetal skull with a sphenotribe.

sphenotur·binal (G. *sphēn*, wedge; L. *turbo*, a spinning-top). 1. Relating conjointly to the sphenoid and turbinate bones. 2. The sphenoidal turbinate bones or bones of Bertin. They fuse after childhood with the presphenoid, the ethmoid and palate bones.

sphere (G. *sphaira*, a ball). A globe.

spheraesthē·sia (G. *sphaira*, a ball; *aisthēsis*, feeling). Neurotic sensation as of contact with a globe.

sphĕ·rical (G. *sphaira*, a ball). Having the form of or relating to a sphere.

spherobactē·ria (G. *sphaira*, a ball; *baktērion*, dim. of *baktron*, a staff). A group of bacteria to which the micrococci belong.

sphĕ·rocyte (G. *sphaira*, a ball; *kutos*, cell). A red blood cell which is more spherical and more fragile than normal. These cells occur in acholuric jaundice.

sphĕ·roid (G. *sphaira*, a ball; *eidos*, form). Shaped like a sphere.

spherō·ma (G. *sphaira*, a ball). Any spherical tumour.

spherŏ·meter (G. *sphaira*, a ball; *metron*, measure). An instrument used for measuring surface curvatures, particularly those of optic lenses.

sphinc·ter (G. *sphigktēr*, binder). Any muscle surrounding and serving to close an orifice, such as the anal s.

sphinc·teral (G. *sphigktēr*, binder). Relating to a sphincter.

sphincteral·gia (G. *sphigktēr*, sphincter; *algos*, pain). Pain in the anal sphincter.

sphincterec·tomy (G. *sphigktēr*, binder; *ektomē*, excision). Excision of a sphincter, especially of the pyloric sphincter.

sphincterī·tis. Inflammation of a sphincter.

sphinc·teroplasty (G. *sphigktēr*, binder; *plassein*, to form). The creation of an artificial sphincter or the plastic surgical repair of one that is damaged.

sphincterŏ·tomy (G. *sphigktēr*, binder; *tomē*, a cutting). Surgical incision into a sphincter.

sphin·gosine (G. *sphiggein*, to bind). $C_{18}H_{27}O_2N$, amino-alcohol found in brain tissue.

sphyg·mic (G. *sphugmos*, pulsation). Relating to the pulse.

sphyg·mocar·diogram (G. *sphugmos*, pulsation; *kardia*, heart; *gramma*, a mark). The record made by a sphygmocardiograph.

sphygmocar·diograph (G. *sphugmos*, pulsation; *kardia*, heart; *graphein*, to write). An instrument registering simultaneously the pulse and heart beats.

sphygmochrŏ·nograph (G. *sphugmos*, pulsation; *khronos*, time; *graphein*, to write). A special type of self-registering sphygmograph.

sphyg·mogram (G. *sphugmos*, pulsation; *gramma*, a mark). The tracing produced by the sphygmograph.

sphyg·mograph (G. *sphugmos*, pulsation; *graphein*, to write). An instrument used to make graphic recordings of the pulse.

sphygmŏ·graphy (G. *sphugmos*, pulsation; *graphein*, to write). A record of pulse tracings.

sphyg·moid (G. *sphugmos*, pulsation; *eidos*, form). Resembling a pulse.

sphyg·momanŏ·meter (G. *sphugmos*, pulsation; *manos*, thin; *metron*, measure). An instrument for measuring arterial blood pressure.

sphyg·mophone (G. *sphugmos*, pulsation; *phōnē*, voice). An instrument by which pulse vibrations are made audible.

sphyg·moscope (G. *sphugmos*, pulsation; *skopein*, to view). A contrivance which indicates visually the pulsations of an artery.

sphygmŏ·scopy (G. *sphugmos*, pulsation; *skopein*, to inspect). Examination of the pulse.

sphygmosys·tolĕ (G. *sphugmos*, pulsation; *sustolē*, a contraction). That portion of sphygmographic tracing that records the systolic movement of the heart.

sphyg·motonŏ·meter (G. *sphugmos*, pulsation; *tonos*, tone; *metron*, measure). An apparatus for determining the elasticity of the arterial walls.

sphyg·mous (G. *sphugmos*, pulsation). Relating to a pulse.

sphў·ra (G. *sphura*, a hammer). The malleus.

sphyrec·tomy (G. *sphura*, a hammer; *ektomē*, excision). Excision of the malleus.

sphyrŏ·tomy (G. *sphura*, a hammer; *tomē*, section). Surgical removal of a part of the malleus.

spī·ca (L., a spike or ear of corn). A bandage in the form of a figure of eight.

spī·cule (L. *spicula*, dim. of *spica*, a spike or ear of corn). A needle-like body.

spider-cells. In biology (1) bacilli with numerous flagellae giving them the appearance of spiders; (2) the cells of neuroglia, which are furnished with a number of delicate extensions.

Spieghel's line (Spieghel (Spigelius), A. van der, Flemish anatomist, 1578–1625). The linea semilunaris of the muscles of the abdominal wall. **S.'s lobe:** the lobus caudatus hepatis.

Spiegler's tumours (Spiegler, E., Austrian dermatologist, 1860–1908). Multiple papillomata of the scalp.

Spigē·lia. A genus of loganiaceous plants (named after A. Van der Spieghel, Flemish anatomist, 1578–1625). The rhizome and roots of *S. marilandica* (pinkroot) yield an effective anthelmintic.

spī·kenard. A name for the plant *Nordostachys jatamansi* and other plants which contain valerian.

spilō·ma (G. *spilos*, spot). Naevus, *q.v.*

spiloplā·nia (G. *spilos*, spot; *planē*, a wandering). A condition marked by wandering skin maculae.

spiloplax·ia (G. *spilos*, spot; *plax*, a plain). 1. The appearance of spots symptomatic of pellagra. 2. A red spot seen in leprosy.

spī·lus (G. *spilos*, spot). A naevus, *q.v.*

spī·na (L.). 1. A thorn. 2. Any spinous process. **S. bifida:** a protrusion of the spinal membranes through a congenital fissure in the lower part of the spine. **S. dorsalis:** the spinal column. **S. ventosa:** enlargement and thinning of a bone which is the seat of a neoplasm or caries.

spī·nal (L. *spina*, thorn). Relating to the spine or the spinal cord or column. **S. analgesia:** regional analgesia produced by intrathecal administration of suitable agents. **S. column:** the vertebral column, consisting of vertebrae, cartilages and ligaments. **S. cord:** the nerve structures within the vertebral canal, extending from the atlas to the second lumbar vertebra.

spinā·lis muscle (L. *spina*, thorn). **S. capitis:** upper part of the semi-spinalis capitis. **S. cervicis:** muscle extending from lower cervical and upper dorsal spines to spine of axis and upper cervical vertebrae. **S. dorsi:** muscle extending from lower thoracic and lumbar spines to the upper thoracic spines.

spī·nate (L. *spina*, thorn). Thorny or shaped like a thorn.

spindle. 1. A tapering rod. 2. A fusiform body.

spine (L. *spina*, thorn). 1. A slender, sharp bone process. 2. The spinal column.

spinobul·bar (L. *spina*, thorn; *bulbus*, bulb). Relating conjointly to the spinal cord and the medulla.

spī·nocerebel·lar (L. *spina*, thorn; *cerebellum*). Relating conjointly to the spinal column and the cerebellum.

spinoneū·ral (L. *spina*, thorn; G. *neuron*, nerve). Relating to the spinal cord and the peripheral nerves.

spī·nous (L. *spina*, thorn). Relating to the spine. **S. process:** the apophysis at the back portion of a vertebra.

spin·therism (G. *spinthēr*, a spark). A sensation as of sparks before the eyes.

spintherŏ·meter. Spintometer, *q.v.*

spintherŏ·pia. Spintherism, *q.v.*

spintŏ·meter (G. *spinthēr*, spark; *metron*, measure). Apparatus for measuring changes which occur in the vacuum of an X-ray tube.

spi·ral (G. *speira*, a coil). Winding, as the thread of a screw or as a coil.

spi·rem, spi·reme (G. *speira*, a coil). The same as skein; the skein of chromatin fibrils in a cell undergoing mitosis.

Spīrillā·cĕae (G. *speira*, a coil). A family of Schizomycetes which includes the Vibrio and Spirillum.

spirillae·mia (G. *speira*, a coil; *haima*, blood). The presence of spirilla in the blood.

spirillō·sis (G. *speira*, a coil). 1. Any disorder caused by Spirillum. 2. A cattle disease occurring in the Transvaal. 3. A fatal disease of poultry and some other birds.

spiril·lum (L. dim. from G. *speira*, a coil). A genus of Spirillaceae. Rods of spiral form, usually motile by means of a tuft of polar flagella.

spirit (L. *spiritus*). 1. Alcohol. 2. An alcoholic solution of one or more volatile substances, usually prepared by a process involving distillation.

spi·rituous (L. *spiritus*). Alcoholic; relating to alcohol.

spi·ritus (L.). Spirit.

spi·robactē·ria (G. *speira*, a coil; *baktēria*, a staff). A group of bacteria including the Spirillum, Spirochaeta and Vibrio.

Spirochāe·ta (G. *speira*, a coil; *khaitē*, hair). A genus of bacteria distinguished by slender, spiral filaments. **S. pallida:** the organism responsible for syphilis. See *Treponema pallidum.*

Spirochaetā·lēs (G. *speira*, a coil; *khaitē*, hair). An order of Schizomycetes including the Spirochaeta, Treponema and Leptospira, amongst others.

spi·rochaete (G. *speira*, a coil; *khaitē*, hair). An organism of the order Spirochaetales.

spirochaetae·mia (G. *speira*, a coil; *khaitē*, hair; *haima*, blood). A condition in which spirochaetes are found in the blood.

spirochaetō·sis (G. *speira*, a coil; *khaitē*, hair). A generalized infection with spirochaetes.

spirochaetū·ria (G. *speira*, a coil; *khaitē*, hair; *ouron*, urine). A condition in which spirochaetes are present in the urine.

Spirocid. A proprietary preparation used in the early treatment of syphilis and in the treatment of amoebiasis, lambliasis and malaria. It has low toxicity.

spi·rograph (L. *spirare*, to breathe; G. *graphein*, to write). An instrument used for recording respiration.

spirogră·phidin (G. *speira*, a coil; *graphein*, to write). A hyalin obtained from spirographin.

spirŏ·graphin (G. *speira*, a coil; *graphein*, to write). A substance occurring in the cartilage and skeletal structures of the Spirographis, a wormlike organism.

spī·roid (G. *speira*, a coil; *eidos*, form). Resembling a spiral.

spirŏ·meter (L. *spirare*, to breathe, G. *metron*, measure). An instrument used for measuring the amount of air inhaled and exhaled by the lungs.

spirŏ·metry. The measurement of respiration.

Spiromō·nas (G. *speira*, a coil; *monas*, unit). A type of spirillum.

Spironē·ma (G. *speira*, a coil; *nēma*, thread). See Borrelia.

spi·rophore (L. *spirare*, to breathe; G. *pherein*, to bring). An apparatus for performing artificial respiration.

spiruli·na (L. *spirula*, dim. of *spira*, from G. *speira*, a coil). A spindle-shaped spiral micro-organism.

spissä·ted (L. *spissare*, to thicken). Inspissated, *q.v.*

spis·situde (L. *spissare*, to thicken). The condition of being inspissated.

spit. 1. To eject sputum from the mouth. 2. Saliva.

spittle. Saliva, *q.v.*

Spitzka's bundle (Spitzka, E. C., American embryologist and neurologist, 1852–1914). The fibres of the posterior longitudinal bundle connecting the third and sixth nerve nuclei.

Spix's ossicle or spine (Spix, J. B., German naturalist, 1781–1826). The lingula of the mandible.

splanch·na (G. *splagkhna*, the inward parts). 1. The intestines. 2. The viscera.

splanchnapo·physis (G. *splagkhna*, the inward parts; *apo*, from; *phusis*, growth). A skeletal element, like the lower jaw, connected with the alimentary canal.

splanchnecto·pia (G. *splagkhna*, the inward parts; *ektopos*, displaced). Abnormal location or dislocation of a viscus.

splanchnemphrax·is (G. *splagkhna*, the inward parts; *emphraxis*, stoppage). Intestinal obstruction.

splanch·nic (G. *splagkhna*, the inward parts). Relating to or supplying the viscera. S. nerves: three in number, originating in the sympathetic system.

splanchnicec·tomy (G. *splagkhna*, the inward parts; *ektomē*, excision). Excision of a part of a splanchnic nerve.

splanchnico·tomy (G. *splagkhna*, the inward parts; *tomē*, section). Surgical division of a splanchnic nerve.

splanch·nocele (G. *splagkhna*, the inward parts; *kēlē*, hernia). Hernial protrusion of any abdominal viscus.

splanch·nocoele (G. *splagkhna*, the inward parts; *koilos*, hollow). That part of the coelom, retained in the adult organism, which produces the pericardial, pleural and abdominal cavities.

splanchnodȳ·nia (G. *splagkhna*, the inward parts; *odunē*, pain). Abdominal pain.

splanchnŏ·graphy (G. *splagkhna*, the inward parts; *graphein*, to write). A description of the visceral anatomy.

splanch·nolith (G. *splagkhna*, the inward parts; *lithos*, stone). An intestinal concretion.

splanch·nolithi·asis (G. *splagkhna*, the inward parts; *lithos*, stone). The formation of calculi in the intestines.

splanchnŏ·logy (G. *splagkhna*, the inward parts; *logos*, discourse). That branch of medicine which deals with the viscera.

splanch·nomĕ·galy (G. *splagkhna*, the inward parts; *megas*, large). Abnormal increase in the size of the viscera.

splanch·nomī·cria (G. *splagkhna*, the inward parts; *mikros*, small). Unusual smallness of the viscera.

splanchnŏ·pathy (G. *splagkhna*, the inward parts; *pathos*, disease). Any disease of the viscera.

splanch·nopleure (G. *splagkhna*, the inward parts; *pleura*, side). The innermost or visceral layer of the mesoderm.

splanchnoptō·sis (G. *splagkhna*, the inward parts; *ptōsis*, a falling). Prolapse of the viscera. The condition includes gastroptosis, enteroptosis, nephroptosis, and occasionally hepatoptosis and splenoptosis.

splanch·nosclerō·sis (G. *splagkhna*, the inward parts; *skleros*, hard). Hardening of the viscera.

splanchnŏ·scopy (G. *splagkhna*, the inward parts; *skopein*, to inspect). Visual inspection of the viscera.

splanchnoskĕ·leton (G. *splagkhna*, the inward parts; *skeleton*, skeleton). The part of the skeleton relating to the viscera.

splanchnŏ·tomy (G. *splagkhna*, the inward parts; *tomē*, a cutting). Dissection of the viscera.

splanch·notribe (G. *splagkhna*, the inward parts; *tribein*, to crush). A surgical instrument for crushing the intestine.

splash fremitus. A noise heard in certain cases of pleural effusion.

splash in the stomach. A sound symptomatic of atony in that organ.

splashing. Giving a splashing sound.

splay-foot. Talipes planus or flat-footedness.

spleen (G. *splēn*). One of the abdominal viscera, a large organ resembling a gland and lying just below the diaphragm on the left side.

splenadenō·ma (G. *splēn*, spleen; *adēn*, gland). Hyperplasia of the spleen tissues.

splenae·mia (G. *splēn*, spleen; *haima*, blood). Splenic leukaemia.

splenal·gia (G. *splēn*, spleen; *algos*, pain). Neuralgia of the spleen.

splenä·trophy (G. *splēn*, spleen; *atrophia*, atrophy). Atrophy of the spleen.

splenaux·ē (G. *splēn*, spleen; *auxē*, increase). Abnormal increase in the size of the spleen.

splenec·tasis (G. *splēn*, spleen; *ektasis*, extension). Enlargement of the spleen.

splenec·tomy (G. *splēn*, spleen; *ektomē*, excision). Surgical removal of the spleen.

splenectō·pia (G. *splēn*, spleen; *ektopos*, out of place). Displacement of the spleen.

splenelcō·sis (G. *splēn*, spleen; *helkōsis*, ulceration). Ulceration of the spleen.

splenemphrax·is (G. *splēn*, spleen; *emphraxis*, stoppage). Congestion of the spleen.

splenet·ic (G. *splēn*, spleen). 1. Relating to the spleen. 2. Peevish.

splē·nic (G. *splēn*, spleen). Relating to or affecting the spleen.

spleni·culus (L. dim. from G. *splēn*, spleen). An accessory spleen.

spleni·tis (G. *splēn*, spleen). Inflammation of the spleen.

splē·nium (G. *splēnion*, bandage). 1. A bandage. 2. The rounded posterior end of the corpus callosum.

splē·nius muscle. S. capitis: muscle extending from ligamentum nuchae and spines of upper cervical vertebrae to mastoid process and occiput. Rotates and extends head and neck and flexes sideways. S. cervicis: muscle extending from spines of mid-dorsal vertebrae to transverse processes of upper cervical vertebrae. Extends, flexes spine laterally, and rotates head and neck.

splenizā·tion (G. *splēn*, spleen). The change in an organ, particularly the lung, produced by congestion. This causes it to resemble in appearance the tissue of the spleen.

splē·noblast (G. *splēn*, spleen; *blastos*, germ). The precursor of the splenocyte.

splē·nocele (G. *splēn*, spleen; *kēlē*, hernia). Splenic hernia.

splenocŏ·lic (G. *splēn*, spleen; *kolon*, colon). Relating to both the spleen and the colon.

splē·nocyte (G. *splēn*, spleen; *kutos*, cell). A large phagocytic cell which is peculiar to splenic tissue.

splenodȳ·nia (G. *splēn*, spleen; *odunē*, pain). Pain in the spleen.

spleno·graphy (G. *splēn*, spleen; *graphein*, to write). A description of splenic anatomy.

splenohae·mia (G. *splēn*, spleen; *haima*, blood). Hyperaemia of the spleen.

splē·noid (G. *splēn*, spleen; *eidos*, form). Resembling the spleen.

splenokeratō·sis (G. *splēn*, spleen; *keras*, horn). Hardening of the spleen.

splenō·ma (G. *splēn*, spleen). Tumour of the spleen.

splenomalā·cia (G. *splēn*, spleen; *malakia*, softness). Softening of the spleen.

splenomegā·lia, splenomĕ·galy (G. *splēn*, spleen; *megas*, large). Enlargement of the spleen. **S., tropical:** kala-azar.

splenon·cus (G. *splēn*, spleen; *ogkos*, mass). Splenoma, *q.v.*

splenŏ·pathy (G. *splēn*, spleen; *pathos*, disease). Any disease of the spleen.

splenopex·ia, splē·nopexis, splē·nopexy (G. *splēn*, spleen; *pēxis*, fixation). Attachment of a wandering spleen to the abdominal wall by suturing.

splenophrē·nic (G. *splēn*, spleen; *phrēn*, midriff). Relating to the spleen and the diaphragm.

splenophthī·sis (G. *splēn*, spleen; *phthisis*, a wasting away). A wasting or atrophy of the spleen.

splenopneumō·nia (G. *splēn*, spleen; *pneumōn*, lung). Pneumonia marked by splenization of the lung.

splenoptō·sia, splenoptō·sis (G. *splēn*. spleen; *ptosis*, a falling). Prolapse of the spleen.

splenorrhā·gia (G. *splēn*, spleen; *rhēgnunai*, to burst forth). Splenic haemorrhage.

splenor·rhaphy (G. *splēn*, spleen; *rhaphē*, suture). Suture of the spleen.

splenŏ·tomy (G. *splēn*, spleen; *tomē*, section). Incision into the spleen.

splĕ·nulus (L. dim. from G. *splēn*). An accessory spleen.

splenun·culus (L. dim. from G. *splēn*). Lienunculus, *q.v.*

splint (Swedish *splint*, splints). A piece of wood or other material for maintaining the ends of fractured bones or other movable parts in a fixed position.

splinter. 1. Sequestrum, *q.v.* 2. A small sharp fragment of wood or metal that passes into the skin.

split. A longitudinal cleft.

splitting. A chemical change in which a compound is changed into one or more simpler bodies; hydrolysis.

Spondli's foramen (Spondli, H., Swiss anatomist; work published in Zurich in 1846). A small opening in the base of the skull between the ethmoid and the sphenoid cartilages.

spondylal·gia (G. *spondulos*, vertebra; *algos*, pain). Pain in a vertebra.

spon·dylarthrī·tis (G. *spondulos*, vertebra; *arthron*, joint). Inflammation of a vertebral joint.

spondylarthrŏ·cacē (G. *spondulos*, vertebra; *arthron*, joint; *kakē*, wickedness). Vertebral tuberculosis or caries.

spon·dyle (G. *spondulos*). A vertebra.

spon·dylexarthrō·sis (G. *spondulos*, vertebra; *ex*, from; *arthron*, joint). Dislocation of a vertebra.

spondylī·tis (G. *spondulos*, vertebra). Inflammation of one or more vertebrae; applied especially to Pott's disease. **S. deformans:** chronic rheumatic inflammation of the vertebrae, ending in ankylosis and deformity. **S. tuberculosa:** Pott's disease.

spon·dylodŷ·nia (G. *spondulos*, vertebra; *odunē*, pain). Vertebral pain.

spon·dylolisthē·sis (G. *spondulos*, vertebra; *olisthēsis*, a slipping). Deformity caused by the sliding forward of the lumbar vertebrae over the basal part of the sacrum.

spondylŏ·pathy G. *spondulos*, vertebra; *pathos*, disease). Any disease of the vertebra.

spon·dylopyō·sis (G. *spondulos*, vertebra; *puon*, pus). Any suppurative affection of the vertebrae.

spondylŏ·schisis (G. *spondulos*, vertebra; *skhisis*, cleavage). A congenital cleft of a vertebral arch.

spondylŏ·sis (G. *spondulos*, vertebra). Locking or ankylosis of a vertebral joint.

spon·dylosyn·desis (G. *spondulos*, vertebra; *sundĕsis*, a tying together). An operative procedure by which vertebrae are fused together.

sponge (G. *spoggia*, a sponge). 1. A marine animal, with a porous, horny, absorbent skeleton. 2. The skeleton itself of (1).

spongia (L., from G. *spoggia*). Sponge.

spon·giform (G. *spoggia*, a sponge; L. *forma*, shape). Resembling a sponge.

spon·gioblast (G. *spoggia*, sponge; *blastos*, germ). An embryonic cell originating in the ectoderm of the embryonic neural tube, the precursor of the neuroglia.

spon·gioblastō·ma (G. *spoggia*, sponge; *blastos*, germ). A tumour which contains spongioblasts. **S. multiforme:** a tumour containing spongioblasts arranged irregularly.

spon·gioid (G. *spoggia*, sponge; *eidos*, form). Spongiform.

spongiopī·line (G. *spoggia*, sponge; L. *pila*, hair). A thick felt material with a waterproof indiarubber backing. It is used for applying to warm, moist dressings.

spon·gioplasm (G. *spoggia*, sponge; *plassein*, to form). The fine, protoplasmic fibrils composing the reticulum of cells.

spon·giose (G. *spoggia*, sponge). Porous like a sponge.

spon·gy (G. *spoggia*, sponge). Of the nature of a sponge.

spontā·neous (L., from *sponte*, voluntarily). Voluntary; automatic.

spoon. An instrument with a shallow bowl attached to a handle. A surgical spoon is used for scraping away necrosed tissues, etc. **S.-nail:** see koilonychia.

sporad·ic (G. *sporadikos*, scattered). Singly; occurring in scattered instances.

sporă·doneure (G. *sporadikos*, scattered ; *neuron*, nerve). An isolated nerve cell.

sporan·gia. Plural of sporangium.

sporan·giophore (G. *sporos*, seed; *pherein*, to bear). The threadlike stalk which bears at its tip the sporangium of moulds.

sporan·gium (G. *sporos*, seed). Any encystment containing spores or sporelike bodies as in the larval state of trematode parasites or certain of the mould fungi.

spore (G. *sporos*, seed). 1. The reproductive part of a lower organism such as a cryptogam. 2. Any reproductive element that does not represent a genuine cell.

sporicī·dal (G. *sporos*, seed; L. *caedere*, to kill). Destructive of spores.

sporī·ferous (G. *sporos*, seed; L. *ferre*, to bear). Bearing spores.

sporī·parous (G. *sporos*, seed; L. *parere*, to produce). Spore-producing.

spor·oblast (G. *sporos*, seed; *blastos*, germ). A spherical body produced by endogenous cell-formation in a coccidium.

spor·ocyst (G. *sporos*, seed; *kustis*, bladder). 1. The mother-cell of a spore. 2. The development stage of a sporozoon subsequent to the production of a sporoblast and preceding the production of two sporozoites.

sporogĕ·nesis (G. *sporos*, seed; *genesis*, production). Reproduction by means of spores.

sporogen·ic (G. *sporos*, seed; *gennan*, to produce). Producing spores.

sporŏ·geny (G. *sporos*, seed; *gennan*, to produce). Sporogenesis, *q.v.*

spor·ont (G. *sporos*, seed; *ōn*, being). The mature phase of the sexual cycle of protozoa.

spor·ophore (G. *sporos*, seed; *pherein*, to bear). The spore-bearing part of an organism, e.g. of a fungus.

spor·ophyte (G. *sporos*, seed; *phuton*, plant). The diploid or asexual stage in the antithetic alternation of generation.

spor·oplasm (G. *sporos*, seed; *plasma*, something formed). The protoplasm of reproductive cells.

Spor·othrix (G. *sporos*, seed; *thrix*, hair). Sporotrichum, *q.v.*

spor·otrichō·sis (G. *sporos*, seed; *thrix*, hair). Infection by Sporotrichum fungi, which causes subcutaneous abscesses of an indolent nature.

Sporŏ·trichum (G. *sporos*, seed; *thrix*, hair). A genus of fungi, certain varieties of which cause sporotrichosis in man.

Sporozō·a (G. *sporos*, seed; *zōon*, animal). A class of parasitic protozoa reproducing by means of cell-formation.

sporozō·ite (G. *sporos*, seed; *zōon*, animal). 1. The nucleated protozoan organism formed by the division of a sporocyst. 2. An animal, as distinct from a vegetable spore.

sporozō·on (G. *sporos*, seed; *zōon*, animal). Any member of the class Sporozoa.

sport. An animal or plant deviating conspicuously from the normal.

sporulā·tion (G. *sporos*, seed). Spore formation.

spor·ule (G. *sporos*, spore). A minute spore.

spot. The same as macula, *q.v.*

sprain. The wrenching of a joint, causing forcible extension or laceration of the ligaments.

spray. A liquid vaporized by a strong jet or current of air.

Sprengel's deformity (Sprengel, O. G. K., German surgeon, 1852–1915). A congenital condition in which upward displacement of the scapula is found.

spring conjuncti·vitis. Vernal conjunctivitis, *q.v.*

sprue. A chronic intestinal disorder, with fatty diarrhoea, soreness of mouth and tongue, wasting, and blood picture resembling pernicious anaemia.

spud. 1. A surgical instrument used in detaching the mucosa in flaps during operations requiring the removal of bone. 2. A short blade used to detach foreign substances from the cornea.

spur. 1. Any sharp point or projection. 2. The angle made by the branching off of a subsidiary artery or vein.

spū·rious (L. *spurius*, false). Counterfeit; not genuine; simulated.

spū·tum (L. *spuere*, to spit). The material ejected from the mouth in spitting; it consists of saliva and mucus or muco-pus. **S., rusty:** s. stained with blood.

squā·ma (L.). A scale, or scale-like material.

squā·mate (L. *squama*, scale). Scaly.

squā·mopari·etal (L. *squama*, scale; *paries*, a wall). Relating to the squamous part of the parietal bone.

squamō·sa (L. *squama*, scale). The squamous part of the temporal bone.

squamō·sal (L. *squama*, scale). Squamosa, *q.v.*

squā·mosphē·noid (L. *squama*, scale; G. *sphēn*, a wedge; *eidos*, form). Relating to the squamous part of the temporal bone and to the sphenoid bone.

squamotem·poral (L. *squama*, scale; *temporalis*, from *tempus*, the temple of the head). Relating to the squamous part of the temporal bone.

squā·mous (L. *squama*, scale). 1. Shaped like a scale, as the s. part of the temporal bone. 2. Scaly. **S. epithelium:** the thickened epithelium consisting of more than one layer of cells. Found in the skin, etc.

square lobe. The lobus quadratus of the liver.

squar·rious, squar·rose, squar·rous (L. *squarrosus*). Scurfy.

squaw root. The rhizome and roots of *Caulophyllum thalictroides*, which are diuretic and emmenagogue.

squill. The inner portion of the bulb of *Urginea maritima* or *U. scilla*, sliced and dried. It has a similar cardiac action to that of digitalis, but its action is weaker, and it is mainly used for its expectorant properties.

squint. Strabismus, *q.v.*

squirting cucumber. Elaterium, *q.v.*

Sr. The symbol for strontium.

ss. Abbreviation for L. *semis*, one-half.

stā·ble (L. *stabilis*, stable). Stationary; fixed, **S. current:** an electric current produced by maintaining the electrodes in a fixed position.

stacca·to speech (It. *staccato*, detached). A jerky manner of speaking.

stactŏ·meter (G. *staktos*, dropping; *metron*, measure). An instrument for measuring drops.

Staderini's nucleus (Staderini, R., contemporary Italian neuro-anatomist). The nucleus intercalatus; a small nucleus lying dorsal to the nucleus of the twelfth nerve.

stā·dium (G. *stadion*, race-course). Stage or period of a disease, e.g. s. acmes, the period during which the disease is at its height.

staff. An instrument for inserting into the bladder through the urethra and used as a guide for incisions in bladder operations.

stage (L. *stare*, to stand). 1. A definite phase of a disease marked by certain symptoms. 2. The platform of a microscope on which the slide is supported.

staggers. One of several forms of functional and organic disease in the brain and spinal cord of domestic animals, especially horses, cattle and sheep.

stagnā·tion (L. *stagnare*, to stagnate). 1. Slowing of any fluid in the body, e.g. blood or lymph. 2 (Dental). The accumulation of debris on a tooth, whose antagonist in the other jaw has been removed.

Stahr's gland (Stahr, H., German pathologist, born 1869). The lymphatic gland on the facial artery.

stain. 1. A discoloration. 2. A dye or pigment used to colour tissues being examined microscopically or to produce certain reactions.

staining. The dyeing of tissues in order to study them under the microscope. **S. vital:** the injection of dyes into the intact animal or man.

staircase sign. A difficulty in walking down stairs is an early symptom of the onset of locomotor ataxia.

stalagmŏ·metry (G. *stalagmos*, a dropping; *metron*, measure). A method of diagnosis based on an estimation of the relative degree of surface tension exhibited by the body fluids.

stā·mina (L. *stamina*, pl. of *stamen*, a thread, the male organ in plants). 1. Natural strength of constitution. 2. Staying power.

stammer. To hesitate or falter in speaking.

stammering. Hesitating, defective articulation in speech.

stanch (L.L. *stancare*, from *stagnare*, to stagnate). To restrain or stop a flow, especially of blood from a wound or a haemorrhage.

standard. 1. An established rule or method. 2. That which serves for comparison. **S. solution:** one that contains a fixed amount of a reagent.

standardizā·tion. Control by a standard; reference to or employment as a basis of comparison; the compounding of a preparation to a definite standard.

Stanley's cervical ligaments (Stanley, E., English surgeon, 1791–1861). The reflected capsular fibres on the neck of the femur; retinacular fibres.

stan·nate (L. *stannum*, tin). Any salt of stannic acid.

stan·nic (L. *stannum*, tin). Relating the compounds of tetravalent tin. **S. acid:** a gelatinous hydrated form of stannic oxide, i.e. SnO_2,H_2O.

Stannius's ligature (Stannius, H., German biologist, 1805–83). A ligature tied round a frog's heart between the sinus venosus and the auricle. It cuts off the auricle and ventricle from their pacemaker (the sino-auricular node) so that they contract independently of this.

stan·nous (L. *stannum*, tin). Relating to the compounds of divalent tin, e.g. s. chloride, $SnCl_2$.

stan·num (L.). Tin.

stapedec·tomy (L.L. *stapes*, stirrup; G. *ektomē*, excision). Excision of the stapes.

stapē·dial (L.L. *stapes*, stirrup). Relating to or shaped like the stapes.

stapē·diovestī·bular (L.L. *stapes*, stirrup; *vestibulum*, a forecourt). Relating to both the stapes and the vestibule.

stapē·dius muscle (L.L. *stapes*, stirrup). Arises from interior of pyramid of tympanum, inserted into neck of stapes. Retracts stapes.

stā·pēs (L.L., stirrup). The stirrup-shaped innermost ossicle of the ear, articulating at its head with the incus and at its base with the fenestra ovalis.

staph. Abbreviation for staphylococcus.

staphysā·gria (G. *staphis*, raisins; *agrios*, wild). The poisonous seeds of *Delphinium staphisagria*, used chiefly as ingredients for lotions and ointments for destroying pediculi.

stā·phyle (G. *staphulē*). The uvula.

staphylec·tomy (G. *staphulē*, uvula; *ektomē*, excision). Surgical removal of the uvula.

staphyloedē·ma (G. *staphulē*, uvula; *oidēma*, swelling). Oedema of the uvula.

stā·phyline (G. *staphulē*, uvula). Relating to the uvula. **S. glands:** the palatine glands.

staphy̆·lion (G. *staphulē*, uvula). The central point of the posterior nasal spine.

staphylī·tis (G. *staphulē*, uvula). Inflammation of the uvula.

stā·phylo-angī·na (G. *staphulē*, uvula; L. *angĭna*, quinsy). Pseudomembranous inflammation of the throat, through staphylococcal infection.

stā·phylococ·cal (G. *staphulē*, bunch of grapes *kokkos*, berry). Relating to staphylococci.

stā·phylococcae·mia (G. *staphulē*, bunch of grapes; *kokkos*, berry; *haima*, blood). A morbid condition caused by the presence of staphylococci in the blood.

stā·phylococ·cic (G. *staphulē*, a bunch of grapes; *kokkos*, berry). Relating to or caused by staphylococci.

stā·phylococ·cus (G. *staphulē*, a bunch of grapes; *kokkos*, berry). A micrococcus; a genus of Schizomycetes in which the cocci form irregular clusters or bunches. Staphylococci are the bacteria usually present in boils and other suppurative lesions.

stā·phylodermatī·tis (G. *staphulē*, a bunch of grapes; *derma*, skin). Dermatitis caused by staphylococci.

stā·phylohae·mia (G. *staphulē*, a bunch of grapes; *haima*, blood). Staphylococcaemia, *q.v.*

staphylō·ma (G. *staphulē*, a bunch of grapes). A swelling out of the cornea or sclera of the eye as a result of inflammation.

staphylŏ·matous. Relating to a staphyloma.

stā·phylomycō·sis (G. *staphulē*, a bunch of grapes; *mukēs*, mushroom). A morbid condition caused by staphylococcal infection.

staphylon·cus (G. *staphulē*, uvula; *ogkos*, mass). Swelling of the uvula.

stā·phyloplasty (G. *staphulē*, uvula; *plassein*, to form). A plastic operation on the uvula.

stā·phylopharyn·geus (G. *staphulē*, uvula; *pharugx*, pharynx). The palatopharyngeus.

staphyloptō·sis (G. *staphulē*, uvula; *ptōsis*, a falling). Unusual elongation of the uvula.

staphylor·rhaphy (G. *staphulē*, uvula; *rhaphē*, suture). The suturing of a cleft soft palate.

staphylŏ·schisis (G. *staphulē*, uvula; *skhĭsis*, cleavage). A cleft of the uvula.

stā·phylotome (G. *staphulē*, uvula; *tomē*, a cutting). A surgeon's knife used in operations on the uvula.

staphylŏ·tomy (G. *staphulē*, uvula; *tomē*, section). 1. The operation of incising or detaching a part of the uvula. 2. Incision into a staphyloma.

star. In biology, a term applied to a number of radiating structures, cells or organisms. **S.-cells:** endothelial cells of vessels; they are capable of enclosing various granules.

star-anise fruit. The ripe fruit of *Illicium verum*. One of the sources of aniseed oil, of which it contains about 5 per cent.

starch. An insoluble carbohydrate $(C_6H_{10}O_5)_n$ widely distributed throughout the vegetable kingdom, of which it is the most important carbohydrate food reserve. It occurs in characteristically-shaped grains, the size and shape of the grains varying from one plant to another. On boiling with water the grains burst and a colloidal solution is formed which 'gels' on cooling to form starch paste. On boiling with dilute mineral acid it is converted first into glucose syrup and finally into grape-sugar or glucose, $C_6H_{12}O_6$, of which it is the chief source.

starvā·tion. Deprivation of food; also the condition resulting from such deprivation. **S. treatment:** a treatment given to diabetic patients in which some days of fasting are followed by a restricted diet containing very little carbohydrate.

stā·simorphy (G. *stasis*, a standing; *morphē*, shape). The deformity of an organ or part caused by arrested development.

stasiphō·bia (G. *stasis*, a standing; *phŏbos*, fear). Neurotic fear of standing upright.

stā·sis (G., a standing). Cessation of the flow of any of the fluids of the body, particularly of the blood. **S., intestinal:** atony of intestinal muscle. **S., venous:** s. caused by venous congestion.

state (L. *status*). A condition.

stat·ic (G. *statikos*, causing to stand). Quiescent; not moving; in equilibrium.

stat·ics (G. *statikos*, causing to stand). The science treating of forces in equilibrium.

stā·tion (L. *statio*, from *stare*, to stand). 1. Standing posture. 2. In obstetrics, the location of the head or other presenting part. **S. test:** the patient stands with feet together and eyes shut; abnormal swaying of the body indicates ataxia.

stati·stics (G. *stătos*, standing). 1. A collection of facts which admit of numerical statement. 2. The science dealing with such collections. **S., medical or S., vital:** the branch of medicine relating to mortality and the distribution of diseases.

stā·tocyst (G. *stătos*, standing; *kustis*, bladder). One of the sacs of the labyrinth to which is attributed an influence in the maintenance of static equilibrium.

stā·tolith (G. *stătos*, standing; *lithos*, stone). See otoconia.

stā·ture (L. *statura*, from *stare*, to stand). The height of any animal body when standing upright.

stā·tus (L., condition). A state, a condition. **S. catarrhalis:** a condition marked by a succession of catarrhal affections. **S. cribrosus:** a sieve-like condition of the brain due to dilatation of the perivascular lymph spaces. **S. epilepticus:** a condition in which epileptic seizures follow each other in rapid succession without the patient recovering consciousness between the paroxysms. **S. lymphaticus:** a condition in which the thymus, spleen and other lymphatic tissues are hyperplastic. Sudden death may occur, particularly if the patient has to undergo anaesthesia. **S. marmoratus:** a condition marked by excessive myelinization of the nerve fibres of the corpus striatum. Clinically—spasticity, hyperkinesis, choreic movements and the condition known as Little's disease.

statū·volence (L. *status*, condition; *volens*, willing). A voluntary self-induced state of hypnotism.

stauroplē·gia (G. *stauros*, cross for crucifixion; *plēgē*, stroke). Crossed hemiplegia.

stĕăp·sin (G. *stear*, fat). A ferment of the pancreatic juice; lipase.

stĕăpsin·ogen (G. *stear*, fat; *gennan*, to produce). A pro-enzyme of steapsin.

stĕă·ric acid (G. *stear*, fat). $C_{17}H_{35}COOH$. A fully-saturated carboxylic acid occurring combined as the glyceride in animal fats. It is a hard, white, pearly solid, and its salts with the sodium, potassium and ammonium ions are used in vanishing creams and shaving soaps.

stĕă·riform (G. *stear*, fat; L. *forma*, shape). Resembling fat.

stē·arin (G. *stear*, fat). Any animal fat composed mainly of the tristearic ester of glycerol.

stē·arine (G. *stear*, fat). Impure stearic acid.

stē·aroder·mia (G. *stear*, fat; *derma*, skin). A skin disease in which the sebaceous glands are affected.

stĕărorrhœ̄·a (G. *stear*, fat; *rhoia*, a flowing). Seborrhoea, *q.v.*

stĕătī·tis (G. *stear*, fat). Inflammation of adipose tissues.

stĕă·tocele (G. *stear*, fat; *kēlē*, hernia). A fatty swelling formed within the scrotum.

stĕătŏ·genous (G. *stear*, fat; *gennan*, to produce). Producing fat; causing steatosis.

stĕătŏ·lysis (G. *stear*, fat; *lusis*, dissolution). The emulsifying process which fats undergo preparatory to their absorption into and assimilation by the system.

stē·atoly·tic (G. *stear*, fat; *lusis*, dissolution). Relating to steatolysis.

stĕătŏ·ma (G. *stear*, fat). 1. A sebaceous cyst. 2. A lipoma.

stĕătomatŏ·sis (G. *stear*, fat). The formation of a large number of sebaceous cysts.

stĕătŏ·pathy (G. *stear*, fat; *pathos*, disease). Any disease of the sebaceous glands.

stē·atopȳ·gia (G. *stear*, fat; *pugē*, buttock). Abnormal fatness of the buttocks; seen in the women of some African races.

stē·atorrhœ·a (G. *stear*, fat; *rhoia*, a flowing). 1. Seborrhoea, *q.v.* 2. Excessively fatty evacuations. **S. idiopathic:** see sprue.

stĕătŏ·sis (G. *stear*, fat). 1. Fatty degeneration. 2. Abnormal fat deposits. **S. cardiaca:** fatty heart.

stē·atozō·on (G. *stear*, fat; *zōon*, animal). The parasite *Demodex folliculorum*, sometimes found in comedones.

steel. Iron combined with a small amount of carbon, forming a strong, durable and tensile metal. **S., tincture of:** tinctura ferri chloridi. **S., wine of:** vinum ferri.

Steell's murmur (Steell, G., English physician, 1851–1942). A murmur caused by relative insufficiency of pulmonary valves. A soft diastolic murmur, heard in the pulmonary area in the third left intercostal space near the border of the sternum and thence propagated down the sternum.

stē·gē (G., roof). The internal layer of the rods of Corti.

stegnō·sis (G. *stegnos*, costive). Stenosis, *q.v.*

Stegomȳ·ia (G. *stegein*, to cover; *muia*, a fly). A genus of mosquitoes or Culicidae existing in most tropical and sub-tropical countries. **S. calopus** or **S. fasciata:** the agent spreading the virus of yellow fever.

Steinach's operation (Steinach, E., Austrian physician, 1861–1944). Ligation of the vas deferens with re-section of part of the vas.

Steinmann's pin (Steinmann, F., Swiss surgeon, 1872–1932). Stainless steel pin which can be inserted through distal bone fragment in cases of fracture of the lower limb in order to provide extension.

stel·late (L. *stella*, star). Shaped like a star; arranged in clusters.

stellec·tomy (L. *stella*, star; G. *ektomē*, excision). Surgical removal of the stellate ganglion.

Stellwag's sign (Stellwag, C., Austrian ophthalmologist, 1823–1904). Found in exophthalmic goitre. Retraction of the upper eyelids producing apparent widening of the palpebral opening with which is associated infrequent and incomplete blinking.

stench. An offensive smell.

stē·nion (G. *stenos*, narrow). A craniometric point at the extremity of the smallest transverse diameter in the temporal bone.

stenocar·dia (G. *stenos*, narrow; *kardia*, heart). Angina pectoris.

stĕ·nocephā·lia, stenocĕ·phaly (G. *stenos*, narrow; *kephalē*, head). Abnormal narrowness of the head.

stenocĕ·phalous (G. *stenos*, narrow; *kephalē*, head). Possessing a narrow head.

stenochor·ia (G. *stenos*, narrow; *khōros*, a space). Narrowing; stenosis; partial obstruction, especially of the lacrimal duct.

stĕ·nokorī·asis (G. *stenos*, narrow; *korē*, pupil of the eye). Narrowing or contraction of the pupil of the eye.

stenopāe·ic (G. *stenos*, narrow; *ōpē*, opening). Having a narrow slit.

stenosed (G. *stenos*, narrow). Narrow; affected with a constriction.

stenō·sis (G. *stenos*, narrow). The constriction of a channel or aperture. **S., aortic:** constriction of the aortic orifice of the heart, or of the aorta itself. **S., pyloric :** a (usually) congenital hypertrophic obstruction of the pyloric orifice of the stomach.

stenostŏ·mia (G. *stenos*, narrow; *stoma*, mouth). Narrowing of the mouth.

stenother·mal (G. *stenos*, narrow; *thermē*, heat). Capable of withstanding only a small range of temperature.

stenothor·ax (G. *stenos*, narrow; *thōrax*, chest). Unusual narrowness of chest.

stenot·ic (G. *stenos*, narrow). Marked or caused by stenosis.

Stensen's canals (Stensen, N., Danish anatomist and physician, 1638–86). The canals leading to the foramen incisivum. **S.'s duct:** the ductus parotideus.

stephā·nial (G. *stephanos*, a crown). Relating to the stephanion.

stephā·nion (G. *stephanos*, a crown). The point on the head where the temporal ridge and the coronal suture meet.

steppage-gait. The peculiar high-stepping gait observed in tabes dorsalis and in certain forms of multiple neuritis.

stercobi·lin (L. *stercus*, dung; *bilis*, bile). A brown colouring matter present in all normal stools, but which is absent or deficient when there is obstruction to the entry of bile into the intestinal tract.

ster·colith (L. *stercus*, dung; G. *lithos*, stone). A concretion of faeces.

stercorā·ceous (L. *stercus*, dung). Faecal.

ster·coral. Stercoraceous, *q.v.*

stercorāē·mia (L. *stercus*, dung; G. *haima*, blood). A toxic condition of the blood caused by the absorption of poisons from the faeces.

ster·corous (L. *stercus*, dung). Faecal.

ster·cus (L.). Dung.

stere (G. *stereos*, solid). A kilolitre.

stereo-agnō·sis (G. *stereos*, solid; *a*, neg.; *gnosis*, knowledge). Astereognosis, *q.v.*

stĕ·reochĕ·mistry (G. *stereos*, solid; *khēmia*, chemistry). That aspect of chemistry which deals with the arrangements of atoms in the molecule in three dimensions.

stĕ·reognō·sis (G. *stereos*, solid; *gnōsis*, knowledge). The faculty of perceiving and recognizing the nature of objects by touch and manipulation.

stĕ·reognŏ·stic. Relating to stereognosis.

stĕ·reogram (G. *stereos*, solid; *gramma*, a mark). A stereoscopic X-ray picture.

stĕ·reograph (G. *stereos*, solid; *graphein*, to write). A stereoscopic radiograph.

stereo-isŏ·merism (G. *stereos*, solid; *isos*, equal; *mĕros*, a part). Isomers in which atoms are arranged as mirror images in space, i.e., in three dimensions.

stereo-ī·somers (G. *stereos*, solid; *isos*, equal; *mĕros*, a part). Two or more chemical compounds having the same structural formulae but different spatial arrangements of the atoms in the molecule.

stereŏ·meter (G. *stereos*, solid; *metron*, measure). An apparatus for carrying out stereometry.

stereŏ·metry (G. *stereos*, solid; *metron*, measure). The measurement of the cubic contents of solids or of the capacity of a space.

stereo-orthop·ter (G. *stereos*, solid; *orthos*, straight; *opter*, a spy). A mirror-reflecting instrument for treating strabismus by orthoptic methods.

stĕ·reoplasm (G. *stereos*, solid; *plassein*, to form). The solid portion of cell protoplasm.

stĕ·reoscope (G. *stereos*, solid; *skopein*, to inspect). An instrument by means of which two similar pictures of an object can be combined, thereby rendering an appearance of solidity and relief.

stĕ·reoscop·ic. Relating to stereoscopy.

stereŏ·scopy (G. *stereos*, solid; *skopein*, to inspect). The combination of two pictures by means of the stereoscope.

stĕ·reoskiă·graphy (G. *stereos*, solid; *skia*, a shadow; *graphein*, to write). Stereographic photography by means of X-rays.

stereŏtrop·ism (G. *stereos*, solid; *trōpos*, a turn). The movement of an organism brought about by contact with another organism or other body towards that organism or other body.

stĕ·rile (L. *sterilis*, barren). 1. Barren; infertile. 2. Aseptic; free from germs.

steri·lity (L. *sterilis*, barren). The condition of being sterile; incapable of producing young.

steriliză·tion (L. *sterilis*, barren). 1. The process of rendering anything sterile; the destruction of micro-organisms. 2. The process of rendering an individual incapable of reproduction.

stĕ·rilize (L. *sterilis*, barren). To make sterile.

stĕ·rilizer (L. *sterilis*, barren). An apparatus for destroying micro-organisms adhering to instruments, bedding and other infected objects, especially by means of heat.

ster·nad (G. *sternon*, breast; L. *ad*, to). Towards the sternal aspect.

ster·nal (G. *sternon*, the breast). Relating to the sternum.

sternal·gia (G. *sternon*, the breast; *algos*, pain). Pain in the sternum.

Sternberg-Reed cell (Sternberg, K., German pathologist, 1872–1935; Reed, D., contemporary American pathologist). Large multinuclear cells seen in lymph nodes in Hodgkin's disease.

ster·nebra (G. *sternon*, the breast; L. *vertebra*). Any one of the segments of the sternum.

ster·noclavĭ·cular (G. *sternon*, the breast; L. *clavicula*, dim. of *clavis*, key). Relating to the sternum and the clavicle.

ster·nocleidomas·toid (G. *sternon*, the breast; *kleis*, a key; *mastos*, a breast; *eidos*, form). Relating to the sternum, the clavicle and the mastoid process. S. muscle: a long muscle in the neck.

ster·nocleidomastoi·deus (G. *sternon*, the breast; *kleis*, a key; *mastos*, a breast; *eidos*, form). A muscle in the neck.

sternocos·tal (G. *sternon*, the breast; L. *costa*, rib). Relating to the sternum and the ribs.

sternŏ·dymus (G. *sternon*, the breast; *didumos*, twin). Twin monsters joined at the chest.

sternohȳ·oid (G. *sternon*, the breast; *huoeidēs*, shaped like the letter y). Relating to the sternum and the hyoid bone.

ster·nohȳoi·deus muscle (G. *sternon*, breast; *huoeidēs*, y-shaped). Arises from manubrium sterni and clavicle. Inserted into body of hyoid bone. Depresses the hyoid and larynx.

ster·noid (G. *sternon*, the breast; *eidos*, form). Like the sternum.

sternomas·toid (G. *sternon*, the breast; *mastos*, a breast; *eidos*, form). Relating to the sternum and the mastoid process of the temporal bone.

sternŏ·pagus (G. *sternon*, the breast; *pagos*, anything fixed). Twin monsters joined at the sternum.

sternothȳ·roid (G. *sternon*, the breast; *thureos*, a shield; *eidos*, form). Relating to the sternum and the thyroid cartilage. S. muscle: Arises from back of manubrium sterni and first rib; inserted into ala of thyroid cartilage. Depresses the larynx.

sternotră·cheal. Relating to the sternum and the trachea.

ster·num (G. *sternon*, the breast). The breast-bone; a flat, narrow bone in the centre of the front of the chest. It is composed of three parts, the manubrium, the gladiolus and the ensiform or xiphoid appendix.

sternū·tament (L. *sternutamentum*, from *sternuere*, to sneeze). An agent causing sneezing.

sternuta·tio (L.). Sneezing. S. convulsiva: paroxysmal sneezing like that seen in hay fever.

sternuta·tion (L. *sternutatio*, a sneezing). The act of sneezing.

sternū·tatory. An agent producing sneezing.

stĕ·roid (G. *stereos*, solid; *eidos*, form). A group of compounds which resemble cholesterol chemically and which also contain a hydrogenated cyclopentophenanthrene ring system. The group includes sex hormones, bile acids, sterols and some carcinogenetic hydrocarbons. Ketosteroids are steroids in which ketone groups are attached to functional carbon atoms. Found in the urine of normal men and women and are increased in the presence of certain adrenal cortical and ovarian tumours.

stĕ·rol (G. *stereos*, solid). A class of monohydroxy-alcohols of high molecular weight which are widely distributed in nature. Their solubilities are similar to fats. Cholesterol is a well-known sterol.

ster·tor (L. *stertere*, to snore). Snoring; the sonorous type of breathing heard when the respiratory passages are obstructed with mucus.

ster·torous (L. *stertere*, to snore). Marked by stertor.

stĕ·thograph (G. *stēthos*, the chest; *graphein*, to write). An instrument for registering the respiratory movements of the chest.

stethokyr·tograph (G. *stēthos*, the chest; *kurtos*, curved; *graphein*, to write). An instrument for measuring the curves of the chest.

stĕ·thoscope (G. *stēthos*, the chest; *skopein*, to view). An instrument used to ascertain the state of circulatory and respiratory organs through the sounds made by them. The stethoscope consists of a hollow tube of which one end is placed over the area to be examined and the other at the ear of the examiner. S., binaural: a Y-shaped tube, the two branches of which are applied to the ears of the examiner.

stethoscop·ic (G. *stēthos*, the chest; *skopein*, to inspect). Relating to a stethoscope.

stethŏ·scopy (G. *stēthos*, the chest; *skopein*, to view). Examination by means of the stethoscope.

sthē·nia (G. *sthenos*, strength). Normal strength and activity.

sthen·ic (G. *sthenos*, strength). Strong; active.

stibamine glucoside. Nitrogen-glucoside of sodium *p*-amino-phenylstibonate, which is recommended for the treatment of kala-azar. The proprietary preparations include Neostam and Neostibosan.

sti·bine. Antimony hydride, SbH_3.

sti·bialism (L. *stibium*, from G. *stibi*, antimony). Poisoning with antimony.

sti·bium (L.). Antimony.

stibophě·num. Sodium-antimony-bispyrocatechol-3:5-sodium disulphonate, occurring as a colourless, odourless, crystalline powder. It is used in the treatment of schistosomiasis and is generally given intra-muscularly in the form of a 6·3 per cent solution.

sticking-plaster. Adhesive plaster.

stictac·ně (G. *stiktos*, spotted). Acne punctata, in which the pustules have a raised, red base and a black spot in the centre.

stiff. Rigid; inflexible. The term is particularly applied to parts that are normally capable of movement. **S.-neck:** see torticollis.

stig·ma (G., a mark; pl. *stigmata*). 1. A small mark on the skin. 2. Any mark symptomatic of a morbid condition; generally used in the plural, e.g., hysterical stigmata, or s. of congenital syphilis.

stigmat·ic (G. *stigma*, a mark). Relating to a stigma.

stig·matism (G. *stigma*, mark). The condition of having stigmata.

stig·matism. The condition of having stigmata.

stigmatizā·tion (G. *stigma*, a mark). The formation of stigmata.

stilboestrol. Syn. diethylstilboestrol. $HO.C_6H_4C$ $(C_2H_5)=C(C_2H_5)C_6H_4OH$. A synthetic oestrogen, active by oral administration and given in doses of 0.1 to 5.0 mg.

stilboestrol dipropionate. Obtained by the action of propionic anhydride on stilboestrol.

stilet, stilette (Fr.). A probe.

Still's disease (Still, Sir G. F., English paediatrician, 1868–1941). Chronic polyarthritis which affects children and is marked by enlargement of lymph nodes and spleen and by irregular fever.

stillbirth. The birth of a dead child.

stillborn. Born dead.

stillicǐ·dium (L. *stilla*, a drop; *cadere*, to fall). The drop by drop flowing of a liquid. **S. lacrimarum:** epiphora. **S. narium:** coryza. **S. urinae:** the dribbling of urine.

Stilling's canal (Stilling, B., German surgeon, 1810–79). The canalis hyaloideus. **S.'s column:** Clarke's column. **S.'s fibres:** the formatio reticularis of the medulla.

Stilling's root (Stilling, J., German ophthalmologist, 1842–1915, son of B. Stilling). A prolongation of the optic tract passing to the third nerve nuclei, the cerebellum and the pons.

Stillingia. The dried root of *Stillingia sylvatica*, which contains a volatile oil. In large doses it is emetic and cathartic, in small doses sialogogue and expectorant. Syn. Queen's root; Yaw root.

sti·mulant (L. *stimulare*, to stimulate). 1. Stimulating. 2. An agent serving to stimulate.

sti·mulate (L. *stimulare*, to stimulate). To excite; to quicken; to promote functional activity.

stimulā·tion (L. *stimulare*, to stimulate). The act of stimulating or the effect thus produced.

sti·mulus (L.). A goad; an impulse; anything capable of causing stimulation.

stir·piculture (L. *stirps*, a stem or root; *cultura*, cultivation). The attempt to improve a race, especially man, by giving attention to the laws of breeding.

stirrup. The stapes.

stitch. 1. A sudden, sharp pain. 2. To sew with a needle and thread; a suture.

stock. A quantity of material kept available for casual use. **S. vaccine:** a bacterial vaccine prepared from any of the species and not from a single strain as is the case with an autogenous vaccine.

Stoerk's blennorrhoea (Stoerk, C., Austrian laryngologist, 1832–99). Blennorrhoea associated with profuse chronic suppuration producing hypertrophy of the nasal, pharyngeal and laryngeal mucosae.

Stohr's cellules (Stohr, P., German anatomist, 1849–1911). The cells in the pyloric gastric glands.

stoicheiŏ·logy (G. *stoikheion*, element; *logos*, a treatise). The science of the elements.

stoicheiŏ·metry (G. *stoikheion*, element; *metron*, measure). The mathematical aspects of chemical molecules and atoms.

stoke. The unit of kinematic viscosity.

Stokes's disease (Stokes, W., Irish physician, 1804–78). Exophthalmic goitre. **S.'s law:** a muscle lying above an area affected with inflammation is often paralysed. **S.'s sign:** a pronounced throbbing in the abdomen to the right of the umbilicus is seen in cases of acute enteritis.

Stokes's lens (Stokes, G. G., English physician, 1819–1903). A combination of a concave cylindrical and a convex cylindrical lens, used in the diagnosis of astigmatism.

Stokes-Adams disease (Stokes, W., Irish physician, 1804–78; Adams, R., Irish physician, 1791–1875). Slowing of pulse, attacks of vertigo, epileptiform or apoplectic attacks, the result of auriculo-ventricular block.

stōma (G.). 1. A mouth. 2. A pore providing communication between neighbouring lymph-cells. 3. An opening of variable size supported by two guard cells, occurring on the epidermis of aerial parts of plants, but mainly on the leaves. Stomata control the rate of respiration and photosynthesis.

stomă·cacě (G. *stoma*, mouth; *kakos*, bad). 1. Canker of the mouth. 2. Ulcerative stomatitis.

stomach (G. *stomakhos*, from *stoma*, mouth). The bag-like organ that forms the most distended part of the alimentary canal, lying below the diaphragm. It is connected at the cardiac end with the oesophagus and at the pyloric end with the duodenum. The stomach wall is composed of four coats —serous, muscular, submucous and mucous.

stomachal·gia (G. *stomakhos*, stomach; *algos*, pain). Pain in the stomach.

stomă·chic (G. *stomakhos*, stomach). 1. Relating to the stomach. 2. Any agent promoting the functional activity of the stomach.

stomatal·gia (G. *stoma*, mouth; *algos*, pain). Pain in the mouth.

stomati·tis (G. *stoma*, mouth). Inflammation of the mouth. **S., gangrenous:** cancrum oris, noma, *q.v.* **S., ulcerative:** that marked by the formation of ulcers on the lips, tongue and the inside of the cheeks.

stomatŏ·cacě (G. *stoma*, mouth; *kakos*, bad). Ulcerative stomatitis.

stomatŏ·logy (G. *stoma*, mouth; *logos*, treatise). That branch of medical science dealing with the mouth and its diseases.

stō·matomycŏ·sis (G. *stoma*, mouth; *mukēs*, mushroom). Any disease of the mouth caused by fungi, especially that due to *Oidium albicans*.

stō·matonecrō·sis (G. *stoma*, mouth; *nekros*, corpse). Cancrum oris, *q.v.*

stō·matonō·ma (G. *stoma*, mouth; *nŏmē*, an eating ulcer). Gangrene of the mouth.

stomatŏ·pathy (G. *stoma*, mouth; *pathos*, disease). Any disease of the mouth.

stō·matoplasty (G. *stoma*, mouth; *plassein*, to form). Plastic surgery of the mouth.

stō·matorrhā·gia (G. *stoma*, mouth; *rhēgnunai*, to burst forth). Haemorrhage from the mouth.

stomatŏ·schisis (G. *stoma*, mouth; *skhĭsis*, cleavage). Harelip.

stomocĕ·phalus (G. *stoma*, mouth; *kephalē*, head). A monster having the same deformity as a rhinocephalus, but with malformation of the maxillary bones so that the skin hangs in folds about the mouth.

stomodae·um (G. *stoma*, mouth; *hŏdaios*, adj. form of *hŏdos*, a road). A depression in the embryonic ectoderm which later composes the mouth and upper part of the pharynx.

Stomox·ys cal·citrans. The common horse-fly, a dangerous pest to humans as well as animals. It is able to transmit anthrax.

stone. 1. A concretion. See also calculus. 2. A measure of weight—14 pounds.

stool. The faecal evacuation of the bowels. S., pea soup: the liquid evacuations of typhoid fever. S., rice-water: the thin, watery evacuations of cholera.

stop. To plug up; to restrain; to impede.

storax. Styrax, *q.v.*

Stovaine. A proprietary preparation of the hydrochloride of the benzoyl ester of methylethyldimethylaminomethylcarbinol. It is used as a local anaesthetic and also as a spinal anaesthetic.

Stovarsol. A proprietary preparation of acetarsone, useful in amoebiasis, lambliasis, malaria and the early treatment of syphilis.

str. Abbreviation for streptococcus.

strabis·mal, strabis·mic (G. *strabismos*, from *strabos*, squinting). Relating to strabismus.

strabisŏ·meter. Strabometer, *q.v.*

strabis·mus (G. *strabismos*, from *strabos*, squinting). Squint; an abnormality of the eye in which the optic axes do not coincide at the objective because action of the external ocular muscles is not co-ordinated.

strabŏ·meter (G. *strabos*, squinting; *metron*, measure). An apparatus for measuring the optical deviation in strabismus.

Strachan's disease (Strachan, W. H. W., Scottish physician of the 19th century). Pellagra.

strain. 1. Excessive use of a part; injurious stretching. 2. The condition resulting from excessive or unsuitable use of a part. 3. To overtask. 4. A sub-variety of an animal. 5. In pharmacy, to filter.

strait. The superior or inferior opening of the pelvis.

stramō·nium. The dried leaves and flowering tops of the *Datura stramonium* (or thorn-apple) and of *D. tatula*, which contain the alkaloids hyoscyamine, hyoscine and atropine. The action of stramonium is similar to that of belladonna leaf. It is used to relieve bronchial spasm in asthma.

strangalaesthē·sia (G. *straggalē*, a halter; *aisthēsis*). Zonaesthesia, *q.v.*

strangle (L. *strangulare*, to strangle). To choke by compressing the windpipe.

strang·ulated (L. *strangulare*, to strangle). 1. Strangled. 2. Constricted in such a way as to stop the circulation, as in s. hernia.

strangulā·tion (L. *strangulare*, to strangle). 1. The act of strangling or choking. 2. Occlusion causing the arrest of circulation to a part.

strangū·ria, strang·ury (G. *stragx*, that which is squeezed out, a drop; *ouron*, urine). Painful and slow excretion of urine.

strap. 1. A strip, as of adhesive tape or plaster. 2. To bind securely, as with bands of adhesive plaster.

stră·tificā·tion (L. *stratum*, a bed-covering; *facere*, to make). Arrangement in layers.

stră·tified (L. *stratum*, a bed-covering; *fieri*, to become). Arranged in layers.

stră·tified. Arranged in layers.

stră·tiform (L. *stratum*, a bed-covering; *forma*, shape). Formed in layers.

strā·tum (L., a bed-covering). A layer, as the s. of Malphigi in the skin.

strawberry gallbladder. See cholesterolosis. S. tongue: The characteristic tongue of scarlet fever, where in the first day or two the tip and edges are red with prominent papillae and the rest of the tongue is coated.

streak. A groove or line. S. culture: a bacterial culture in streaks.

strĕ·phosymbō·lia (G. *strephein*, to twist; *sumbolon*, symbol). 1. Difficulty in learning to read; word-blindness. 2. A disorder of the perceptive faculties in which there is a tendency to read in the reverse direction and to see objects reversed, as in a mirror.

strep·tobacil·lus (G. *streptos*, twisted; L. *bacillus*, dim. of *baculus*, a staff). A type of bacillus forming twisted chains.

strep·tobactē·ria (G. *streptos*, twisted; *baktērion*, dim. of *baktron*, a staff). Short, rod-shaped bacteria grouped together in twisted chains.

streptococ·cal (G. *streptos*, twisted; *kokkos*, berry). Relating to a streptococcus.

strep·tococcae·mia (G. *streptos*, twisted; *kokkos*, berry; *haima*, blood). A condition in which streptococci are present in the blood.

Streptococ·cĕae (G. *streptos*, twisted; *kokkos*, berry). A tribe of the family Lactobacteriaceae. Includes diplococcus, leuconostoc and streptococcus.

streptococ·cus (G. *streptos*, twisted; *kokkos*, berry). A genus of schizomycetes in which the cocci are disposed in chains. They are pathogenic to man.

streptomȳ·cin (G. *streptos*, twisted; *mukēs*, mushroom). An antibiotic agent used particularly in the treatment of tuberculosis. It is also effective against other organisms which are not attacked by penicillin or sulpha-drugs. It is given by intramuscular injection. It is obtained by extraction of metabolic products of a mould.

streptomycō·sis (G. *streptos*, twisted; *mukēs*, mushroom). A diseased condition caused by streptococcal infection.

strep·tosepticae·mia. Septicaemia caused by streptococcal infection.

streptothrī·cial. Relating to a streptothrix.

streptothricō·sis (G. *streptos*, twisted; *thrix*, hair). A condition of streptothricial infection.

Strep·tothrix (G. *streptos*, twisted; *thrix*, hair). A class of schizomycetes.

stretcher. A litter or couch for transporting the sick or wounded.

strī·a (L. *stria*, a furrow; pl. *striae*). A streak or line.

strī·ae (pl. of L. *stria*, a furrow). Streaks or lines. S. atrophicae: whitish wrinkles on the skin caused by later contraction of skin that has been stretched by fat, pregnancy, or other cause. S. gravidarum: the atrophic s. seen on the abdomen in women who have borne children.

strī·tal. Relating to the corpus striatum.

strī·ate, strī·ated (L. *stria*, a furrow). Striped or streaked. S. body: the corpus striatum.

strī·tion (L. *stria*, a furrow). 1. The condition of being striped or streaked. 2. Any striated structure.

strī·tum (L. *stria*, a furrow). The corpus striatum.

stric·ture (L. *strictura*, from *stringere*, to draw tight). The constriction of a duct or canal by means either of outside pressure or by inflammatory or other changes in its walls.

stri·dor (L. *stridor*, from *stridere*, to hiss). A harsh, vibrating sound of the respiratory system. **S., laryngeal**: that caused by stenosis of the larynx.

stri·dulous (L. *stridulus*, from *stridere*, to hiss). Affected with stridor.

stripe. A streak.

strobi·la (G. *strobilos*, anything twisted up). 1. A developmental stage of certain Hydrozoa. 2. A whole tapeworm.

strobilā·tion (G. *strobilos*, anything twisted up). The formation of segments in certain Hydrozoa and tapeworms.

strŏ·biloid (G. *strobilos*, anything twisted up). Like tapeworm segments.

strō·boscope (G. *strobos*, a whirling; *skopein*, to inspect). An instrument by which a series of slightly different pictures presented rapidly in succession is made to appear as an object in continuous motion; a zoetrope.

stroke. 1. A sudden and severe attack, as of apoplexy. 2. To rub the hands gently over the body.

strō·ma (G. *strōma*, a mattress). The tissue which makes the framework or matrix of an organ.

strō·mal. Relating to a stroma.

stromatŏ·lysis (G. *strōma*, a mattress; *lusis*, dissolution). Destruction of a stroma.

stromuhr (Ger. *strom*, tide; *uhr*, clock). Ludwig's instrument for measuring the velocity of the blood stream.

Strongyloi·dēs (G. *stroggulos*, round; *eidos*, shape). A genus of roundworms found in the intestinal tract of many mammals.

strongyloidō·sis (G. *stroggulos*, round; *eidos*, shape). Infestation with strongyloides.

Stron·gylus (G. *stroggulos*, round). A genus of nematodes present in the intestines of animals, and occasionally found in man.

stron·tium. A metal similar to calcium. **S. bromide**: formerly used in place of potassium bromide as a sedative.

strophan·thin (G. *strophos*, a cord; *anthos*, a flower). A mixture of glucosides obtained from strophanthus soluble in water and alcohol. This mixture is diluted with lactose so as to possess 40 per cent of the activity of anhydrous ouabain. It is given by intravenous or intramuscular injection as a heart tonic but it should be used with great care.

Strophan·thus (G. *strophos*, a cord; *anthos*, a flower). A genus of plants of the order Apocynaceae. The mature seed of *S. kombe* yields strophanthin.

strophocĕ·phalus (G. *strephein*, to twist; *kephalē*, head). A monster foetus with a deformed head and face.

strŏ·phulus (G. *strophos*, a cord). A type of miliaria seen in infants.

Stroud's pecten or **pectinated area** (Stroud, B. B., American physiologist; work published in 1896). The area between Hilton's white line and the lower edge of the valves of Morgagni.

struc·tural (L. *structura*, from *struere*, to build). Relating to or affecting a structure.

strū·ma (L. from *struere*, to build). 1. Scrofula. 2. Goitre.

strumīpri·vous (L. *struma*, a scrofulous tumour; *privare*, to deprive). Caused by the excision of the thyroid gland.

strumi·tis (L. *struma*, a scrofulous tumour). Inflammation of a thyroid gland affected with goitre.

strumoder·ma (L. *struma*, a scrofulous tumour; G. *derma*, skin). Scrofuloderma, *q.v.*

strū·mous. 1. Scrofulous. 2. Goitrous.

Struthers's ligament (Struthers, Sir J., Scottish anatomist, 1823–99). Ligament of the humerus, passing to the medial condyle.

strych·nine (G. *strukhnos*, nightshade). A white, crystalline highly poisonous alkaloid, $C_{21}H_{22}O_2N_2$, obtained principally from the seeds of *Strychnos nux vomica*. Under the British Poison Rules of 1935 strychnine may not be sold except under certain conditions. In small doses it is used as a stomachic and stimulant to the central nervous and circulatory systems.

strych·ninism (G. *strukhnos*, nightshade). Poisoning by strychnine.

strych·ninomā·nia (G. *strukhnos*, nightshade; *mania*, madness). Delirium caused by strychnine poisoning.

Strych·nos (G. *strukhnos*, nightshade). A genus of loganiaceous trees found in the tropics. It includes *S. nux vomica*, from the seeds of which strychnine is obtained.

stump. The distal portion of a limb remaining after an amputation. **S. of the eyeball**: what is left of the globe after evisceration.

stun. To deprive temporarily of consciousness, as by a blow; to knock out.

stupe (L. *stupa*, tow). A cloth or sponge soaked with hot water, rung out practically dry and used to apply heat to a part. A stupe may be medicated by sprinkling it, e.g. with turpentine, and then used as a counter-irritant.

stupefā·cient (L. *stupēre*, to be stunned; *facere*, to make). Narcotic.

stupefac·tion (L. *stupēre*, to be stunned; *facere*, to make). Stupor or the progress towards that state.

stū·por (L. *stupor*, from *stupēre*, to be stunned). The condition of being only partially conscious.

stū·porous. Relating to or affected with stupor.

stutter. A hesitating form of speech characterized by repeated attempts to articulate a syllable.

stuttering. A type of stammering; hesitating speech caused by inability to utter syllables without repeated efforts. **S., urinary**: involuntary pauses during the process of urination.

sty, stye. Suppuration at a lash follicle.

stȳ·let (L. *stilus*, a pointed instrument). 1. A small probe. 2. A wire passed into a cannula to stiffen or clear it. Syn. stilette.

styloglos·sus (L. *stilus*, a pointed instrument; G. *glossa*, tongue). A muscle rising from the styloid process and inserted into the tongue.

stylohȳ·oid (L. *stilus*, a pointed instrument; G. *huoeidēs*, shaped the like letter y). 1. Relating to the styloid process of the temporal bone and the hyoid bone. 2. Relating to the s. muscle.

stȳ·lohȳoi·deus (L. *stilus*, a pointed instrument; G. *huoeidēs*, shaped like the letter y). A muscle connecting the styloid process and the hyoid bone.

stȳ·loid (L. *stilus*, a pointed instrument; G. *eidos*, form). Like a stylus.

styloidī·tis (L. *stilus*, a pointed instrument; G. *eidos*, form). Inflammation of the structures around the styloid process.

stȳ·lomandi·bular ligament (L. *stilus*, a pointed instrument; *mandibula*, a jaw). Passes from the styloid process of the temporal bone to the lingula of the mandible.

stylomas·toid (L. *stilus*, a pointed instrument; G. *mastos*, a breast; *eidos*, shape). Relating to the styloid and the mastoid processes.

stylomax·illary (L. *stilus*, a pointed instrument; *maxilla*, the jawbone). Relating to the styloid process and the maxilla.

stȳ·lopharyn·geus muscle (L. *stilus*, a pointed instrument; G. *pharugx*, the throat). Arises from the styloid process of the temporal bone, inserted into side of pharynx. Raises and dilates the pharynx.

stȳ·lus (L. *stilus*, a pointed instrument). A pointed instrument for making applications; a stylet.

stymatō·sis (G. *stuma*, priapism). A violent erection of the penis accompanied by haemorrhage.

stype (G. *stuppē*, tow). A tampon or pledget.

styp·sis (G. *stuphein*, to contract). 1. Astringency. 2. The use of a styptic.

styp·tic (G. *stuptikos*, from *stuphein*, to contract). 1. Astringent; stopping haemorrhage by means of an astringent contracting the blood vessels. 2. Any agent capable of arresting haemorrhage by its astringent properties.

Styp·ven. A proprietary preparation of Russell's viper venom, recommended for topical application in the control of external haemorrhages.

stȳ·racin. Cinnamyl cinnamate, a crystalline principle, obtained from styrax.

stȳ·rax (Storax). The purified balsam obtained from the trunk of the hamamelidaceous tree, *Liquidambar orientalis*. It is generally purified by solution in alcohol, followed by filtration and evaporation. Used in antiseptic applications.

subabdō·minal (L. *sub*, below; *abdōmen*, abdomen). Below the abdomen.

subacetă·bular (L. *sub*, below; *acetabulum*, a vinegar cup). Below the acetabulum.

subă·cetate (L. *sub*, below; *acetum*, vinegar). Any basic acetate.

subacid (L. *sub*, below; *acidus*, acid). Moderately acid.

subaci·dity (L. *sub*, below; *acidus*, acid). A condition of moderate or deficient acidity.

subacrō·mial (L. *sub*, below; G. *akron*, highest point; *ōmos*, shoulder). Beneath the acromion.

subacute (L. *sub*, below; *acutus*, sharp). Moderately acute; a stage between acute and chronic sickness.

subaponeurot·ic (L. *sub*, below; G. *apo*, from; *neuron*, tendon). Beneath an aponeurosis.

subarach·noid (L. *sub*, below; *arakhnē*, spider; *eidos*, form). Located beneath the arachnoid.

subarachnoidī·tis (L. *sub*, below; *arakhnē*, spider; *eidos*, form). Inflammation of the lower portion of the arachnoid.

subar·cuate (L. *sub*, below; *arcus*, arch). Slightly arched.

subarē·olar (L. *sub*, below; *areola*, dim. of *area*, an open space). Lying or taking place beneath the areola.

subastră·galar, subastră·galoid (L. *sub*, below; G. *astragalos*, the ball of the ankle-joint). Beneath the astragalus.

subastrin·gent (L. *sub*, below; *astringere*, to tighten). Slightly astringent.

subau·ral (L. *sub*, below; *auris*, ear). Located beneath the ear.

subaxil·lary (L. *sub*, below; *axilla*, armpit). Situated or occurring below the armpit.

subcartilă·ginous (L. *sub*, below; *cartilago*, cartilage). 1. Located beneath a cartilage. 2. Partly cartilaginous.

subcerebel·lar (L. *sub*, below; *cerebellum*, a small brain). Beneath the cerebellum.

subcĕ·rebral (L. *sub*, below; *cerebrum*, the brain). Beneath the cerebrum.

subchon·dral (L. *sub*, below; G. *khondros*, cartilage). Situated beneath a cartilage.

subchor·dal (L. *sub*, below; *khordē*, a string). Lying below the vocal cords.

subchoriŏ·nic (L. *sub*, below; *khorion*, an intestinal membrane). Beneath the chorion.

subclă·vian (L. *sub*, below; *clavis*, key). Situated under the clavicle, as s. artery.

subclavĭ·cular (L. *sub*, below; *clavicula*, dim. of *clavis*, key). Located beneath the clavicle.

subclă·vius muscle (L. *sub*, below; *clavis*, key). Arises from first rib and its cartilage. Inserted into lower surface of clavicle. Draws clavicle down and forwards.

subcli·nical (L. *sub*, below; *kline*, bed). Term applied to an infection which is so mild that it does not give rise to clinical signs and symptoms which would allow of diagnosis.

subconjuncti·val (L. *sub*, below; *conjunctivus*, connective). Lying beneath the conjunctiva.

subcon·scious (L. *sub*, below; *conscius*, knowing, from *cum*, with, and *scire*, to know). Partially conscious.

subcon·sciousness (L. *sub*, below; *conscius*, knowing). Imperfect or partial consciousness.

subcor·acoid (L. *sub*, below; G. *korax*, raven; *eidos*, form). Lying beneath the coracoid process.

subcor·tical (L. *sub*, below; *cortex*, rind). Lying beneath the cortex.

subcos·tal (L. *sub*, below; *costa*, rib). Beneath a rib.

subcostā·lēs (L.). The infracostal muscles.

subcrā·nial (L. *sub*, below; G. *kranion*, skull). Beneath the cranium.

subcrĕ·pitant (L. *sub*, below; *crepitare*, to creak). Slightly crepitant.

subcrū·reus muscle (L. *sub*, below; *crus*, leg). Syn. articularis genu.

subculture (L. *sub*, below; *cultura*, cultivation). A secondary bacterial culture made from a primary one.

subcutā·neous (L. *sub*, below; *cutis*, skin). Lying or occurring beneath the skin.

subcuti·cular (L. *sub*, below; *cuticula*, dim. of *cutis*, skin). Lying beneath the epidermis.

subdeli·rium (L. *sub*, below; *delirare*, to rave). Mild delirium.

sub·diaphragmat·ic (L. *sub*, below; G. *diaphragma*, diaphragm). Beneath the diaphragm.

subdor·sal (L. *sub*, below; *dorsum*, back). Below the dorsal area.

subdū·ral (L. *sub*, below; *durus*, hard). Beneath the dura.

subencĕ·phalon (L. *sub*, below; *egkephalos*, brain). The medulla oblongata, pons and corpora quadrigemina considered as one.

subendocar·dial (L. *sub*, below; G. *endon*, within; *kardia*, heart). Lying beneath the endocardium.

sub·endothē·lial (L. *sub*, below; G. *endon*, within; *thēlē*, the nipple). Lying or taking place beneath an endothelial structure.

sub-endothē·lium (L. *sub*, below; G. *endon*, within; *thēlē*, the nipple). The stratum of connective tissue cells situated between the mucosa and epithelium of the bladder, intestines and bronchi; Débové's membrane.

subepider·mal, subepider·mic (L. *sub*, below; G. *epi*, upon; *derma*, skin). Beneath the epidermis.

subepiglot·tic (L. *sub*, below; G. *epi*, upon; *glōttis*, mouth of windpipe). Situated below the epiglottis.

subepithē·lial (L. *sub*, below; G. *epi*, upon; *thēlē*, nipple). Beneath an epithelial surface.

subepithē·lium (L. *sub*, below; G. *epi*, upon; *thēlē*, nipple). 1. A structure lying beneath an epithelial surface. 2. Débové's membrane.

subfal·cial (L. *sub*, below; *falx*, a sickle). Situated beneath the falx cerebri.

subfas·cial (L. *sub*, below; *fascia*, a bandage). Lying beneath a fascia.

subfeb·rile (L. *sub*, below; *febris*, fever). Moderately febrile.

subflā·vus (L. *sub*, below; *flavus*, yellow). Slightly yellow. **S. ligament:** the ligament of yellowish substance lying between neighbouring vertebrae.

subfron·tal (L. *sub*, below; *frons*, the forehead). Beneath the frontal lobe of the brain.

subgin·gīval (L. *sub*, below; *gingīva*, a gum). Situated beneath the gums.

subglē·noid (L. *sub*, below; G. *glēnē*, the socket of a joint; *eidos*, form). Located beneath the glenoid fossa.

subglos·sal (L. *sub*, below; *glōssa*, tongue). Sublingual, *q.v.*

subglot·tic (L. *sub*, below; G. *glōttis*, mouth of windpipe). Situated below the glottis.

subhepat·ic (L. *sub*, below; G. *hepar*, liver). Beneath the liver.

subhȳ·oid (L. *sub*, below; G. *huoeidēs*, shaped like the letter y). Lying or taking place beneath the hyoid bone.

subictē·ric (L. *sub*, below; G. *ikteros*, jaundice). Slightly jaundiced.

subi·culum (L. *subices*, supports, from *subicere*, to bring under). The uncinate gyrus.

subi·lĭăc (L. *sub*, below; *ilium*, the groin). Lying below the ilium.

subi·lĭŭm (L. *sub*, below; *ilium*, the groin). The lowest part of the ilium.

subinfec·tion (L. *sub*, below; *infectio*, taint). 1. Slight infection. 2. A chronic intoxication caused by repeated small doses of a toxin received from outside, or from toxins generated within the organism.

sub·inflammā·tion (L. *sub*, below; *inflammare*, to kindle). A slight degree of inflammation.

subin·trant (L. *subintrare*, to enter by stealth). Entering secretly; applied to malarial and other fevers in which a fresh attack starts before the one preceding it has ended.

sub·involū·tion (L. *sub*, below; *involvere*, to envelop). Incomplete involution; e.g., s. of the uterus when that organ fails to return to its normal state after parturition.

subī·odide (L. *sub*, below; G. *iodēs*, from *ion*, a violet). That iodide of a series containing the least iodine.

sub·ject (L. *subicere*, to bring under). 1. An individual or animal serving, under observation, for the purposes of experiment and study. 2. A cadaver for dissection. 3. The theme of a discourse.

subjec·tive (L. *subicere*, to bring under). 1. Relating only to the individual concerned. 2. Applied to symptoms experienced by the patient and not susceptible of physical examination.

subjū·gal (L. *sub*, below; *jugum*, a yoke). Lying below the malar bone.

sublā·tio (L.). Removal or ablation. **S. retinae:** detachment of the retina.

sub·limate (L. *sublimare*, to raise). A substance obtained by sublimation. **S. corrosive:** mercuric chloride.

sublimā·tion (L. *sublimare*, to raise). 1. The act of vaporizing and condensing a solid. 2. Term used by Freud to denote the deviation of sexual feelings to aims and objects of a non-sexual character.

subli·minal (L. *sub*, below; *limen*, threshold). Beneath the threshold of consciousness.

sublin·gual (L. *sub*, below; *lingua*, tongue). 1. Beneath the tongue. 2. Relating to the parts beneath the tongue.

sublŏ·bular (L. *sub*, below; *lobulus*, lobule). Beneath a lobule.

sublum·bar (L. *sub*, below; *lumbus*, loin). Beneath the lumbar area.

subluxā·tion (L. *sub*, below; *luxare*, to dislocate). A sprain; an incomplete dislocation.

submam·mary (L. *sub*, below; *mamma*, breast). Beneath the breast.

submandi·bular (L. *sub*, below; *mandibula*, a jaw). Situated below the mandible.

submar·ginal (L. *sub*, below; *margo*, edge). Beneath a marginal area.

submaxil·la (L. *sub*, below; *maxilla*, the jawbone). The lower jaw.

submax·illary (L. *sub*, below; *maxilla*, the jawbone). 1. Beneath the lower maxilla. 2. Relating to the s. gland.

submē·dial (L. *sub*, below; *medius*, middle). Beneath the middle.

submem·branous (L. *sub*, below; *membrana*). Consisting partly of membranous substance.

submenin·geal (L. *sub*, below; G. *mēnigx*, membrane). Beneath the meninges.

submen·tal (L. *sub*, below; *mentum*, chin). Below the chin.

submerge (L. *sub*, below; *mergere*, to dip). To plunge below the surface of a liquid.

submi·cron (L. *sub*, below; G. *mikros*, small). A particle visible with the aid of the ultramicroscope.

sub·microscŏ·pical (L. *sub*, below; G. *mikros*, small; *skopein*, to view). Too minute to be seen with the aid of a microscope.

submor·phous (L. *sub*, below; G. *morphē*, shape). Partaking of the natures both of a crystalline and of an amorphous body.

submucō·sa (L. *sub*, below; *mucus*, mucus). The stratum of areolar connective tissue attaching the mucous membrane to the adjacent structures.

submū·cous (L. *sub*, below; *mucus*, mucus). Lying beneath a mucous membrane.

subneū·ral (L. *sub*, below; *neuron*, nerve). Lying beneath a nerve.

subnor·mal (L. *sub*, below; *norma*, a rule). Below normal.

subnū·cleus (L. *sub*, below; *nucula*, dim. of *nux*, nut). A secondary or smaller collection of cells into which a large nerve-nucleus may be divided.

subnutri·tion (L. *sub*, below; *nutrire*, to nourish). Defective or insufficient nutrition.

suboccī·pital (L. *sub*, below; *ob*, at; *caput*, head). Beneath the occiput.

suboper·culum (L. *sub*, below; *operculum*, a lid). The section of the occipital gyrus lying between the presylvian and sub-sylvian fissures.

subor·bital (L. *sub*, below; *orbita*, from *orbis*, an orbit). Lying beneath the orbit.

subordinā·tion (L. *sub*, below; *ordinare*, to regulate). The state of being under subjection or control; the condition of those organs which depend upon or are controlled by others.

subox·ide (L. *sub*, below; G. *oxus*, sharp). That oxide of a series which contains the least oxygen.

subparī·etal (L. *sub*, below; *paries*, a wall). Beneath the parietal bone, convolution or fissure.

subpatel·lar (L. *sub*, below; *patella*, the patella). Beneath or below the patella.

subpec·toral (L. *sub*, below; *pectus*, the breast). Beneath the chest.

subpedun·cular (L. *sub*, below; *pedunculus*, from *pes*, foot). Beneath a peduncle.

subpericar·dial (L. *sub*, below; G. *peri*, around; *kardia*, heart). Beneath the pericardium.

subperiŏ·steal (L. *sub*, below; G. *peri*, around; *osteon*, bone). Beneath the periosteum.

subperitonē·al (L. *sub*, below; G. *peritonaion*, the peritoneum). Beneath the peritoneum.

subpetrō·sal sinus (L. *sub*, below; *petrosa*, stony). The inferior petrosal sinus.

subpharyn·geal (L. *sub*, below; G. *pharugx*, the throat). Beneath the pharynx.

subphrĕ·nic (L. *sub*, below; *phrēn*, the midriff). Beneath the diaphragm; subdiaphragmatic.

subpitū·itarism (L. *sub*, below; *pituita*, phlegm). Hypopituitarism.

subplacen·ta (L. *sub*, below; *placenta*, from G. *plakous*, a flat cake). The decidua vera.

subplacen·tal (L. *sub*, below; *placenta*, from G. *plakous*, a flat cake). 1. Beneath the placenta. 2. Relating to the decidua vera.

subpleu·ral (L. *sub*, below; G. *pleura*, a rib). Lying beneath the pleura.

subplex·al (L. *sub*, below; *plexus*, a braid). Beneath a plexus.

subpon·tine (L. *sub*, below; *pons*, a bridge). Lying or taking place beneath the pons.

subprepū·tial (L. *sub*, below; *praeputium*, the prepuce). Situated beneath the prepuce.

subprostat·ic (L. *sub*, below; G. *pro*, before; *statos*, standing). Beneath the prostate gland.

subpū·bic (L. *sub*, below; *pubes*, hair at puberty). Beneath the pubic arch or symphysis.

subpul·monary (L. *sub*, below; *pulmo*, lung). Situated beneath or below the lungs.

subpyrä·midal (L. *sub*, below; G. *puramis*, pyramid). Below a pyramid.

subrec·tal (L. *sub*, below; *rectus*, straight). Situated below the rectum.

subrĕ·tinal (L. *sub*, below; *rete*, a net). Lying below the retina.

sub-salt (L. *sub*, below; *sal*, salt). A basic salt.

subsartor·ial plexus (L. *sub*, below; *sartor*, tailor). A nerve plexus situated beneath the sartorius muscle in the thigh.

subscă·pular (L. *sub*, below; *scapulae*, the shoulderblades). 1. Beneath the scapula. 2. Relating to the subscapularis muscle.

subscapulä·ris muscle (L. *sub*, below; *scapulae*, shoulder blades). A muscle on the anterior surface of the scapula.

subsclē·ral (L. *sub*, below; G. *sklēros*, hard). Taking place beneath the sclera.

subscrip·tion (L. *subscriptio*, a legal subscription). That section of a prescription comprising the instructions to the pharmacist as to how the ingredients are to be prepared and mixed.

subsē·rous (L. *sub*, below; *sĕrum*, serum). Beneath a serous membrane.

sub·sidence (L. *subsidere*, to settle down). The gradual abatement and disappearance of disease symptoms.

sub-soil (L. *sub*, below; *sŏlum*, soil). The under-soil. **S. water:** water which has entered the soil and is present above the first impenetrable stratum.

subspi·nous (L. *sub*, below; *spina*, thorn). 1. Beneath or below a spine. 2. Beneath the spinal column.

sub-stage (L. *sub*, below; *stare*, to stand). The parts of a microscope situated beneath the stage.

sub·stance (L. *substantia*, substance). 1. The material of which anything consists. 2. A tissue.

substan·dard (L. *sub*, below; *stare*, to stand). Below the normal or the required standard.

substan·tia (L.). Substance. **S. alba:** the white matter of the brain and nerves. **S. cinerea:** the grey matter of the brain and spinal cord. **S. propria:** the essential tissue of a structure, especially the connective tissue. E.g. substantia propria corneae, the connective tissue of the cornea.

subster·nal (L. *sub*, below; G. *sternon*, the breast). Situated beneath the sternum.

substitū·tion (L. *substituere*, to substitute). 1. The act of replacing one thing by another. 2. In chemistry, the replacement of one element or group of elements by another. **S. therapy:** treatment of a disorder by a

chemical normally produced in sufficient amount by the patient himself, e.g. the use of insulin in diabetes mellitus.

subsul·tory (L. *subsultare*, to jump). Twitching.

subsul·tus ten·dinum (L.). A twitching movement of the muscles and tendons in a typhoid state.

subsyl·vian. Located beneath the fissure of Sylvius.

subtar·sal (L. *sub*, below; G. *tarsos*, a flat surface). Lying below the tarsus.

subter·tian fever (L. *sub*, below; *tertius*, third). Remittent malarial fever.

subthalam·ic (L. *sub*, below; G. *thalamos*, an inner chamber). Situated beneath the optic thalamus.

subthă·lamus (L. *sub*, below; G. *thalamos*, inner chamber). Hypothalamus, *q.v.*

subtrochantĕ·ric (L. *sub*, below; G. *trochantēr*, runner). Lying below a trochanter.

subtrŏ·chlear (L. *sub*, below; G. *troikhilia*, sheaf of a pulley). Lying beneath the trochlea.

subtrŏ·pical (L. *sub*, below; G. *tropikos*, the tropic circle). Relating to regions having an almost tropical climate.

subtympan·ic (L. *sub*, below; G. *tumpanon*, drum). Situated below the tympanum.

subtў·pical (L. *sub*, below; G. *tupos*, type). Below or less than what is the typical condition.

subū·berēs (L. *sub*, below; *uber*, a teat). Children at the breast; sucklings.

subumbili·cal (L. *sub*, below; *umbilicus*). Lying beneath the umbilicus.

subun·gual (L. *sub*, below; *unguis*, a fingernail). Lying beneath a nail.

suburē·thral (L. *sub*, below; G. *ourēthra*, urethra). Situated beneath the urethra.

subvagi·nal (L. *sub*, below; *vagina*, (1) sheath (2) the female vagina). Located beneath a sheath or below the vagina. **S.-space:** lymph space along the outer surface of dural sheath of optic nerve.

subver·tebral (L. *sub*, below; *vertebra*, vertebra). Situated beneath a vertebra.

subzŏ·nal (L. *sub*, below; G. *zōnē*, a girdle). Beneath a zone.

subzygomat·ic (L. *sub*, below; G. *zugōma*, bolt). Below the zygoma.

suc·cagogue (L. *succus*, juice; G. *agōgos*, leading). Stimulating secretion, or an agent that stimulates the flow of gastric juices.

succedä·neous (L. *succedere*, to follow). Relating to or resembling a succedaneum.

succedä·neum (L. *succedere*, to follow). A substitute. **S., caput:** oedematous swelling developing during labour over the presenting part of the foetus.

suc·cinate. A salt of succinic acid.

succin·ic acid. Ethylene 1:2-dicarboxylic acid (COOH $(CH_2)_2COOH_2$. It is a cathartic.

succi·nimide. $(CH_2CO)_2NH$, a compound produced by the action of gaseous ammonia on succinic anhydride.

suc·cinous (L. *succinum*, amber). Relating to amber.

suc·cinum (L.). Amber.

succinyl-sulpha·thiazole.   COOH.CH$_2$.CH$_2$.CONH.

$C_6H_4.SO_2NH.C:N.CH:CH.S.H_2O$. A derivative of sulphanilamide, used for infection of the gut, from which it is only slowly absorbed. One proprietary name is Sulphasuxidine.

succorrhoē·a (L. *succus*, juice; G. *rhoia*, a flow). Excessive flow of a secretion.

suc·cus (L., juice). An animal or vegetable secretion or juice. **S. citri:** lime juice. **S. entericus:** the intestinal juice. **S. gastricus:** the gastric juice. **S. pancreatis:** the digestive juice of the pancreas.

Sucquet's canals (Sucquet, J. P. Work published in Paris between 1860–82). The communications between small arteries and small veins without the intervention of capillaries.

su·crase (Fr. *sucre*, sugar). An enzyme capable of converting many times its own weight of cane sugar into glucose and fructose. It is obtained from intestinal juice and from yeast. Syn. invertase.

sucrosae·mia (Fr. *sucre*, sugar; G. *haima*, blood). The presence of sugar in the blood.

sū·crose (Fr. *sucre*, sugar). Sugar from sugar-cane or beet; saccharose.

sucrosō·ria (Fr. *sucre*, sugar; G. *ouron*, urine). The excretion of sugar in the urine.

sudā·mina (L. *sudor*, sweat). Small whitish vesicles brought about by the collection of sweat in the sweat-glands caused by copious sweating, especially in certain fevers.

sudā·minal (L. *sudor*, sweat). Relating to sudamina.

sudan. A diazo-compound in the form of a brown powder used as a stain for fat.

sudā·nophile. A leucocyte which, as a result of fatty degeneration, stains readily with sudan III.

sudā·tion (L. *sudatio*, from *sudare*, to sweat). Sweating, or excessive sweating.

sudato·ria (L. *sudor*, sweat). Ephidrosis, *q.v.*

sudato·rium (L. *sudatorium*, from *sudare*, to sweat). A hot air bath or the chamber used for the purpose of giving hot air baths.

Sudeck's atrophy. (Sudeck, P. H. M., German surgeon, 1866–1938). Acute atrophy of a bone of traumatic origin. **S.'s critical point:** the region of the bowel between the areas supplied by the last sigmoid artery and the superior haemorrhoidal artery.

sudokeratō·sis (L. *sudor*, sweat; *keras*, a horn). Keratosis affecting the sweat-glands.

su·dor (L.). Sweat. **S. anglicus:** miliaria, *q.v.* **S. sanguineus:** the sweating of blood.

sū·doral (L. *sudor*, sweat). Marked by disorder of the function of sweating.

sudori·ferous (L. *sudor*, sweat; *ferre*, to bear). Secreting sweat.

sudori·fic (L. *sudor*, sweat; *facere*, to make). 1. Diaphoretic. 2. An agent promoting sweating.

sudori·parous (L. *sudor*, sweat; *parĕre*, to bring forth). Secreting sweat.

sū·dorous (L. *sudor*, sweat). Sweaty.

sudorrhoē·a (L. *sudor*, sweat; *rhoia*, a flow). Excessive production of sweat.

suet. Fat from the abdomina of cattle and sheep. Mutton suet (sevum praeparatum, B.P.) is used as an emollient in the preparation of ointments.

suffocā·tion (L. *suffocare*, to choke). The stoppage of respiration.

suffumigā·tion (L. *suffumigare*, to fumigate from below). Fumigation or a fumigatory material.

suffūsion (L. *suffundere*, to overspread). The condition of being bloodshot or the spreading of any body fluid into surrounding tissues.

sugar (F. *sucre*, sugar). The generic name for the sweet, soluble carbohydrates obtained (mainly) from plants and animals. **Cane s.:** $C_{12}H_{22}O_{11}$ converted by the enzyme invertase or by dilute acids to glucose, $C_6H_{12}O_6$ (grape- or starch-sugar) and fructose, $C_6H_{12}O_6$ (fruit-sugar or laevulose). **Milk s.:** $C_{12}H_{22}O_{11}$ (lactose or saccharum lactis). **Malt s.:** $C_{12}H_{22}O_{11}$ (maltose).

suggě·stible (L. *suggerere*, to suggest). Submissive to suggestion.

suggě·stion (L. *suggerere*, to suggest). 1. The artificial inducement of a psychic condition in which the patient accepts and acts upon ideas suggested to him. 2. That which is suggested.

suggillā·tio, sugillā·tion (L. *suggillare*, to bruise). A bruise or a livid mark.

suicī·dal (L. *sui*, gen. of *se*, self; *caedere*, to kill). Self-destroying.

sū·icide (L. *sui*, gen. of *se*, self; *caedere*, to kill). 1. Intentional self-killing. 2. One who intentionally kills himself.

sul·cate (L. *sulcus*, a furrow). Furrowed.

sul·cus (L., a furrow). A furrow; used particularly of brain fissures. **Calcarine:** is a deep cleft visible on the medial surface of the hemisphere. It commences near the occipital pole and takes an arched course, at first upwards and then downwards. **Callosal:** separates the cingulate gyrus from the corpus callosum. **Centralis** (fissure of Rolando): begins at the supero-medial border of the hemisphere about half an inch behind its mid-point and passes downwards and forwards on the supero-lateral surface making an angle of about 70 degrees with the median plane. **Centralis insulae:** passes upwards and backwards across the insula, almost in line with the central sulcus, and divides the insula into precentral and postcentral lobules. **Cingulate:** pursues a curved course on the medial surface of the hemisphere, parallel with the corpus callosum and between it and the supero-medial border. **Collateral:** is situated on the tentorial surface of the hemisphere, close to the medial occipital border. It starts near the occipital pole and extends forwards towards the temporal pole. **Dentate** (hippocampal): is situated on the medial surface of the hemisphere, but is obscured by the mid-brain. **Ethmoidal:** a groove on the nasal bone for the anterior ethmoidal (nasal) nerve. **Frontal:** the superior and inferior frontal sulci extend forwards from the precentral sulcus and mark out the superior, middle and inferior frontal gyri. **Hippocampal:** see dentate. **Hypothalamic:** a shallow groove below the thalamus which passes backwards from the interventricular foramen to the entrance to the aqueduct. **Intermedius:** a groove on the stomach which divides the pyloric antrum from the pyloric canal. **Interparietal:** has two parts or rami, known as the horizontal ramus and occipital ramus. The horizontal ramus passes backwards with a downward inclination from a point near the middle of the postcentral sulcus. The occipital ramus, which may be separate, takes a curved course around the external border of the parieto-occipital sulcus, from which it is separated by a curved gyrus known as the arcus parieto-occipitalis. **Lateral** (fissure of Sylvius): is the first sulcus to appear in the course of development, possesses a stem and three diverging branches or rami. The stem is a deep cleft between the orbital surface and the temporal lobe that passes horizontally outwards from the region of the anterior perforated substance. **Limitans:** a sulcus which surrounds the insula. **Lunate:** is situated close to the occipital pole. It is a short, curved sulcus, having its concavity directed backwards. **Marginal:** one of the posterior rami of the cingulate sulcus. **Occipital:** the *transverse* occipital sulcus passes more or less vertically downwards across the occipital cortex from the occipital ramus to the intraparietal sulcus. The *lateral* occipital sulcus passes obliquely forwards and downwards a short distance in front of the occipital pole. It may be joined by the transverse occipital sinus. **Of cerebrum:** may be divided into two groups:— (i) those that are present and fairly constant in position in nearly every brain; and (ii) those that are more subject to a considerable range of variation. **Olfactorius:** a groove on the frontal process of the maxilla. **Olfactory:** a groove on the under surface of the frontal lobe which lodges the olfactory tract and olfactory bulb. **Orbital:** is of very variable form; it is situated on the under surface of the frontal lobe and has three limbs: medial, lateral and transverse. **Paracentral**: the upward termination of the cingulate sulcus on the medial surface of the brain. **Parieto-occipital**: cuts across the supero-medial border of the brain about 2½ inches above the occipital pole and marks the boundary between the parietal and occipital lobes. **Post-central**: lies behind and roughly parallel to the central sulcus, from which it is separated by the post-central gyrus. **Precentral**: is bounded behind by the central sulcus and in front by the superior and inferior parts of the post-central sulcus. **Rhinal** (incisura temporalis): is a shallow groove that separates the anterior extremity, or caput, of the hippocampal gyrus from the temporal pole. **Sagittal**: a faint groove on the internal or cerebral surface of the frontal bone which lodges a part of the superior sagittal venous sinus. **Scleral**: a slight groove in front of the corneo-scleral junction of the eyeball. **Subparietal** (suprasphenoid): one of the terminal rami of the cingulate sulcus. **Temporal**: two in number, superior and inferior, situated on the inferior surface of the temporal lobe of the brain. **Terminalis**: a groove on the right atrium of the heart. **Tympanicus**: a narrow groove on the deep end of the osseous part of the external auditory meatus. **Valleculae**: a furrow which separates the inferior vermis from the two cerebellar hemispheres.

sulpha-drugs. Sulphonamides, a group of chemicals most of which contain the sulphonamido grouping $-SO_2NH$. They are extremely valuable bacteriostatics for systemic infections as well as local. Toxic symptoms, such as granulocytopenia, drug rash, anuria, etc., may possibly occur.

sulphacĕt·amide. $NH_2.C_6H_4.SO_2.NH.COCH_3$. A sulphonamide used in the treatment of *Bact. coli* infections of the urinary tract. In gonococcal infections it is less effective than sulphathiazole or sulphadiazine. Trade name, Albucid. **S. sodium**: the soluble form, is used in ocular infections.

sulphadī·azine. $NH_2C_6H_4.SO_2NH-C:N.CH:CH.CH.N.$ A sulphonamide similar in action to sulphanilamide and sulphathiazole. The soluble sodium derivative is given intravenously.

sulphadi·midine. $NH_2.C_6H_4SO_2NH-C:N.C(CH_3):CH.C(CH_3):N.$ A dimethyl derivative of sulphadiazine. Trade name, Sulphamezathine. It is said to be less toxic than sulphadiazine, which it resembles in its action.

sulphaemoglō·binaēmia. The presence of sulphmethaemoglobin in the blood.

sulphaguăn·idine. $NH_2C_6H_4.SO_2NH.C(NH).NH_2H_2O.$ A sulpha-drug not readily absorbed from the intestine and hence of great use in intestinal infections such as bacillary dysentery.

sulphal·dehyde. A hypnotic substance yielded by the action of hydrogen on ethylic aldehyde.

sulphamĕ·thylthī·azole. A compound, 2-(*p*-amino-benzenesulphonamido)-4-methylthiazole, which is effective against infections due to *Staph. aureus*. Syn. Sulphamethiazole.

sulphamĕr·azine. $NH_2.C_6H_4-SO_2NH.C:N.CH:CH.C(CH_3):N.$ The monomethyl derivative of sulphadiazine. It has the advantage in giving a higher and more persistent blood level than the other sulpha-drugs as it is more rapidly absorbed and more slowly excreted.

sulphamĕz·athine. See sulphadimidine.

sulphă·minol. A compound, thioxydiphenylamine, an antiseptic material yielded by the action of sulphur on salts of methoxydiphenylamine. It is useful in diseases of the antrum and frontal sinuses, being applied by insufflation.

sulphanĭ·lamide. $NH_2.C_6H_4SO_2NH_2.$ The simplest of the sulpha-drugs. Effective against haemolytic streptococci, meningococci, gonococci and some types of staphylococci and pneumococci. Like all drugs of this type it is bacteriostatic rather than bactericidal. Trade name, Prontosil Album.

sulphapȳ·ridine. $NH_2.C_6H_4SO_2NH.C_5H_4N.$ One of the earliest sulpha-drugs and the first really effective chemotherapeutic agent for pneumonia. Now seldom used owing to its toxicity. Trade name, M. & B. 693.

sulpharsenoben·zene,   sulpharsphen·amine. Arsenic compounds given by intramuscular injection in treatment of syphilis and some protozoal infections.

sulphate. A salt of sulphuric acid.

sulphathī·azole. $NH_2.C_6H_4.SO_2.NH.C:N.CH:CH.S.$ More rapidly excreted than most other sulpha-drugs, but more toxic. Trade name, M. & B. 760.

sul·phide. A salt or organic derivative of hydrogen sulphide, H_2S, in which one or both of the hydrogen atoms are replaced by metal atoms or groups of atoms.

sul·phite. A salt of sulphurous acid.

sulphocarbŏ·lic acid. Phenol sulphonic acid, $HO.C_6H_4.SO_2OH.$ Its salts were formerly used as antiseptics, especially zinc sulphocarbolate.

sul·phonal. Diethylsulphone-dimethylmethane, a crystalline substance used as a hypnotic.

sulphon·amides. The sulpha-drugs; a group of drugs developed from sulphanilamide (para-aminobenzenesulphonamide). These drugs are effective against a wide range of bacteria and some viruses. The most commonly used are sulphanilamide, sulphathiazole, sulphamezazine, sulphadiazine and sulphacetamide.

sul·phur (L.). A non-metallic element native in volcanic areas. It is found in combination with a number of metals, especially iron and copper, in the form of sulphides. Sulphur exists in various allotropic forms, ordinary s. being a yellow brittle solid. Sp. gr. 2·07; atomic weight 32·07. Symbol S.

sulphū·ric. Combined with sulphur. **S. acid**: an oily, highly caustic and poisonous acid H_2SO_4.

sul·phurous. Of the nature of or combined with sulphur. **S acid**: a dibasic acid H_2SO_3 produced by combination of sulphur dioxide and water. A bleaching agent.

sulphuret·ted. Combined with sulphur.

sul·phurize. To impregnate with sulphur.

sum. Abbreviation of L. *sumat*, let him take.

sū·mach. The dried fruits of *Rhus glabra*, or poison ivy, used in the treatment of subacute and chronic rheumatism.

sum·bul. The root of *Ferula s.*, or musk root, formerly used as a nerve sedative.

summā·tion (L. *summa*, a sum total). The accumulated effect of muscular, sensory or mental stimuli.

summer diarrhœ·a. An acute cholera-like disease of infants.

sunburn. Superficial skin inflammation caused by exposure to the sun's rays.

sunstroke. Insolation; a state of feverish prostration caused by over-exposure to the rays of the sun.

superă·cid (L. *super*, above; *acidus*). Extremely acid.

superci·liary (L. *supercilium*, eyebrow). Relating to the eyebrow.

superci·lium (L.). The eyebrow.

superdisten·sion (L. *super*, above; *distendere*, to stretch). A marked degree of distension.

superdū·ral (L. *super*, above; *durus*, hard). Situated above the dura mater.

super-ego (L. *super*, above; *ego*, I). Those mental processes which exert a modifying influence over the ego.

superexcita·tion (L. *super*, above; *excitare*, to stimulate). Extreme excitement.

superfecunda·tion (L. *super*, over and above; *fecundare*, to fertilize). The fertilization of two or more ova of one ovulation in consequence of several acts of coitus.

superfi·cial (L. *superficies*, surface). Relating to, located on or confined to a surface.

sū·perficiā·lis (L. *superficies*, surface). At or near a surface, as s. muscle or s. artery.

superfi·cies (L.). Any external surface.

superfoetā·tion (L. *super*, above; *foetus*, offspring). Fertilization of an ovum following on a previous fecundation; conception by a woman already pregnant.

superfunc·tion (L. *super*, above; *fungi*, to perform). Over-activity of any organ or part.

sū·perimpregnā·tion (L. *super*, above; *impraegnare*, to fertilise). 1. Superfecundation. 2. Superfoetation.

superinduce (L. *super*, above; *inducere*, to bring in). To bring on, for example, a complication to an already existent state.

superinfec·tion (L. *super*, above; *inficere*, to infect). A re-infection by the same micro-organism.

sū·perinvolū·tion (L. *super*, over and above; *involutio*, from *involvere*, to envelop). Hyper-involution, *q.v.*

supē·rior (L. *superior*, comp. of *superus*, upper). Higher; the uppermost of two parts or organs.

superlactā·tion (L. *super*, above; *lactare*, to suckle). Excessive or over-prolonged secretion of milk.

supermē·dial (L. *super*, above; *medius*, middle). Above the middle.

supernā·tant (L. *super*, above; *natare*, to swim). To float upon a liquid.

supernor·mal (L. *super*, above; *norma*, a rule). Above the normal.

supernū·merary (L. *super*, above; *numerus*, a number). Exceeding the usual number.

superphos·phate (L. *super*, over; G. *phōsphŏrŏs*, light-bringing). An acid phosphate.

sū·persalt. An acid salt.

supersā·turate (L. *super*, above; *saturare*, to saturate). To add to a liquid more of a material than it is capable of holding in a dissolved state.

supersecrē·tion (L. *super*, above; *secretio*, from *secernere*, to separate). Over-abundant secretion.

superten·sion (L. *super*, above; *tendere*, to stretch). Excessive tension.

supervi·rulent (L. *super*, above; *virus*, poison). Extremely virulent.

supinā·tion (L. *supinus*, lying on the back). 1. The turning of the hand palm uppermost. 2. Lying on the back.

supinā·tor muscle (L. *supinus*, lying on the back). Arises from outer condyle of humerus, ligaments of elbow joint and oblique line of ulna; inserted neck of radius. Supinates the forearm and hand.

supine (L. *supinus*, lying on the back). Lying on the back; turning the palm upward.

supplemen·tal (L. *supplementum*, a filling up). Additional.

suppŏ·sitory (L. *suppositorius*, from *supponere*, to place under). Medicinal substances incorporated into a base made of cocoa-butter or gelatin, and intended for introduction into the rectum.

suppres·sion (L. *suppressio*, from *supprimere*, to hold back). The sudden stopping of a secretion.

sup·purant (L. *suppurare*, to suppurate). 1. Inducing suppuration. 2. An agent inducing suppuration.

suppurā·tion (L. *suppurare*, to suppurate). The formation of pus.

sup·purative (L. *suppurare*, to suppurate). 1. Forming pus. 2. An agent favourable to suppuration.

supra-acrō·mial (L. *supra*, over; G. *akron*, a point; *ōmos*, the shoulders). Above the acromion.

supra-auri·cular (L. *supra*, over; *auricula*, dim. of *auris*, ear). Above the auricle.

supracho·roid (L. *supra*, over; *khorion*, membrane; *eidos*, form). Above the choroid.

suprachoroi·dea (L. *supra*, over; G. *khorion*, membrane; *eidos*, form). The outside layer of the choroid coat, next to the sclera.

supraclavi·cular (L. *supra*, over; *clavicula*, dim. of *clavis*, key). Above the clavicle.

supracon·dylar, supracon·dyloid (L. *supra*, over; G. *kondulos*, a knuckle; *eidos*, form). Located above a condyle.

supracŏ·stal (L. *supra*, over; *cŏsta*, rib). Located above the ribs.

supracŏ·tyloid (L. *supra*, over; G. *kotulē*, the socket of a joint; *eidos*, form). Situated above the cotyloid cavity.

supradiaphragmat·ic (L. *supra*, over; G. *diaphragma*, diaphragm). Located above the diaphragm.

supradū·ral (L. *supra*, over; *durus*, hard). Situated above the dura mater.

supraglē·noid (L. *supra*, over; *glēnē*, the socket of a joint; *eidos*, form). Located above the glenoid cavity.

suprahepat·ic (L. *supra*, over; G. *hēpar*, liver). Above the liver.

suprahȳ·oid (L. *supra*, over; G. *huoeidēs*, shaped like the letter y). Located above the hyoid bone.

suprain·guinal (L. *supra*, over; *inguen*, the groin). Located above the groin.

supralī·minal (L. *supra*, over; *limen*, threshold). Within the field of consciousness. **S. consciousness:** ordinary self-consciousness.

supralum·bar (L. *supra*, over; *lumbus*, loin). Located above the loin.

supramallē·olar (L. *supra*, over; *malleolus*, dim. of *malleus*, hammer). Lying above a malleolus.

supramam·mary (L. *supra*, over; *mamma*, female breast). Located above the mammary gland.

supramar·ginal (L. *supra*, over; *margo*, on edge). Situated above an edge or margin.

supramas·toid (L. *supra*, above; G. *mastos*, a breast; *eidos*, form). Located above the mastoid process of the temporal bone.

supramaxil·la (L. *supra*, over; *maxilla*, jaw). The upper jawbone.

supramax·illary (L. *supra*, over; *maxilla*, jaw). Relating to the superior maxilla.

supraoccĭ·pital (L. *supra*, over; *ob*, at; *caput*, head). 1. Located above the occipital bone. 2. Located in the upper portion of the occipital bone.

supra·orbital (L. *supra*, over; *orbita*, from *orbis*, orbit). Located above the orbit.

suprapel·vic (L. *supra*, over; *pelvis*, a basin). Located above the pelvis.

suprapon·tine (L. *supra*, over; *pons*, a bridge). Located above or in the superior portion of the pons.

suprapū·bic (L. *supra*, over; *pubes*, hair at puberty). Located above the pubic arch.

suprarē·nal (L. *supra*, over; *renes*, kidneys). 1. Above the kidney. 2. Relating to the s. capsule.

suprascā·pular (L. *supra*, over; *scapulae*, the shoulder-blades). Situated above or in the upper portion of the scapula.

suprascle·ral (L. *supra*, over; G. *skleros*, hard). Situated on the external surface of the sclera.

suprasep·tal (L. *supra*, over; *septum*, a fence). Above a septum.

supraspī·nal (L. *supra*, over; *spina*, spine). Located above a spine.

supraspinā·tus muscle (L. *supra*, over; *spina*, thorn). Arises in supraspinous fossa, inserted into greater tuberosity of humerus. Moves shoulder joint, raises and adducts arm.

supraspī·nous (L. *supra*, over; *spina*, thorn). Located above a spinous process.

supraster·nal (L. *supra*, over; G. *sternon*, the breast). Located above the sternum.

suprasyl·vian. Lying above the sylvian fissure.

supraton·sillar (L. *supra*, above; *tonsillae*, the tonsils). Above a tonsil.

supratroch·lear (L. *supra*, over; G. *trokhilia*, the sheaf of a pulley). Located above the trochlea of the superior oblique muscle.

supravagi·nal (L. *supra*, over; *vagina*, a sheath). Located above a sheath or on its external surface; also located above the vagina.

supraver·gence (L. *supra*, over; *vergere*, to incline). The divergence of the two eyes in a vertical plane.

sū·ra (L.). The calf of the leg.

sū·ral (L. *sura*). Relating to the calf of the leg.

suralimentā·tion (Fr. *suralimentation*, from L. *super*, over and above; *alimentum*, food). Forced or excessive supply of food.

suramin. $C_{51}H_{34}O_{23}N_6S_6Na_6$. A complex urea used in the treatment of trypanosomiasis. Trade names: Bayer 205; Naganol; Fourneau 309; Moranyl.

sur·ditas (L.). Deafness.

surdity (L. *surditas*, deafness). Deafness.

sur·domute (L. *surdus*, deaf; *mutus*, dumb). A deaf-mute.

sur·face (L. *super*, upon; *facies*, the face). 1. The outside part of a body. 2. The face or facets of a body; a term commonly used in the anatomical description of bones. **S.-markings:** in anatomy, lines drawn on the skin to show the size and location of deep structures.

sur·fen.   Bis-2-methyl-4-aminoquinoly-6-carbamide hydrochloride, a non-staining antiseptic used for wounds.

surgeon (G. *kheirourgia*, surgery). One skilled in surgery.

sur·gery (G. *kheirourgia*, surgery, from *kheir*, hand; *ergon*, work). 1. That branch of medicine concerned with diseases requiring operative treatment. 2. A physician's or surgeon's consulting room.

sur·gical (G. *kheirourgia*, surgery). Relating to surgery.

sur·rogate (L. *surrogare*, to substitute). Any medicine or ingredient substituted for another.

sursā·nure (L. *super*, above; *sanus*, healthy). An ulcer that has healed superficially but not beneath.

sursumduc·tion (L. *sursum*, up; *ducere*, to lead). 1. The act of elevation of the visual axis of one eye above the other; also the degree to which such elevation can be made. 2. The ability to elevate the axis of either eye above that of the other.

survī·val (L. *super*, above; *vivere*, to live). The persistence of an individual or race after the general extinction of related forms, or through a mortal crisis.

suscep·tible (L. *suscipere*, to undergo). 1. Able to receive an impression; sensitive to an influence. 2. In pathology, apt to be infected by a disease.

susotox·in (L. *sus*, hog; G. *toxikon*, poison). A toxin present in the cultures of the bacillus of hog cholera.

suspen·ded (L. *suspendere*, to hang). Hanging. **S. animation:** term sometimes used to characterize an interruption of vital functions.

suspen·sion (L. *suspensio*). 1. Hanging. 2. Interruption of a function. 3. Undissolved particles in oil or water.

suspen·sory (L. *suspensio*, a hanging). 1. Serving to suspend, as s. bandage. 2. A contrivance for suspending a part.

suspirā·tion (L. *suspiratio*). A sigh.

sustentā·cular (L. *sustentare*, to sustain). Sustaining.

sustentā·culum (L.). A support.

susur·rus (L.). A murmur in cases of aneurysm, etc.

sutū·ra (L.). Suture, *q.v.*

sū·tural (L. *sutura*, suture). Relating to or like a suture.

sū·ture (L. *sutura*). 1. A stitch or row of stitches closing the lips of a wound. 2. In anatomy, a line of junction. **Coronal:** separates the two parietal bones from the frontal bone. **Cranial:** the junctions of the various cranial bones with each other. A synarthrodial joint. **Ethmolacrimal:** a cranial suture between the ethmoid and lacrimal bones. **Fronto-ethmoid:** articulation between the middle of the frontal bone and the perpendicular plate of the ethmoid bone. **Frontolacrimal:** an articulation between the orbits of the frontal bone and the two lacrimal bones. **Frontomaxillary:** a suture between the frontal process of the maxilla and the middle of the frontal bone. **Interalveolar** (of Jarmer): divides the incisor alveoli into rather larger anterior and smaller posterior portions. **Intermaxillary:** is a simple edge to edge suture that extends on the face from the nasal spine and runs down the mid-line of the upper jaw to pass between the two alveoli for the upper central incisors and so reaches the palate to end at the incisive canal. **Internasal:** a suture between the two nasal bones. **Interpremaxillary:** a suture separating the two premaxillae in early life. **Jarmer's:** see interalveolar s. **Lambdoid:** a suture between the occipital and the two parietal bones. **Maxillary-ethmoid:** a suture between the maxilla and the ethmoid bones. **Maxillary-lacrimal:** a simple linear suture between the maxilla and lacrimal bones. **Maxillary-premaxillary:** a suture which starts from the incisive canal and passes laterally and forwards to the alveolar margin between the alveoli for the lateral incisor and the canine. **Median palatine:** separates the two maxillae in the anterior two-thirds and the two palatine bones in the posterior third of the middle line of the hard palate. **Metopic** (frontal suture): is formed at the meeting of the two frontal bones in the middle line. **Nasofrontal:** intervenes between the nasal notch of the frontal and the upper borders of the two nasal bones. **Nasomaxillary:** a serrated squamous suture between the lateral margins of the nasals and the nasal processes of the maxillae. **Neurocentral:** the suture between the centrum and neural arches of a vertebra. **Occipito-mastoid:** is the continuation of the lambdoid suture. **Palatine:** see median palatine and transverse palatine. **Parietomastoid:** runs from the squamous suture in front to the lower end of the lambdoid suture behind. **Petrosquamous:** is a transitory intracranial suture between the petrous and squamous elements of the temporal bone. **Premaxillary-maxillary:** See Maxillary-premaxillary. **Sagittal:** runs between the two parietal bones. **Spheno-ethmoidal:** intervenes between the part of the sphenoid anterior to the optic foramen and the posterior edge of the orbital plate of the ethmoid bone. **Sphenofrontal:** a simple suture between the upper edge of the great wing of the sphenoid and the frontal bone in the orbit. **Spheno-orbital:** is between the upper edge of the lesser wing of the sphenoid and the frontal in the orbit. **Sphenoparietal:** separates the anterior extremity of the lower margin of the parietal from the posterior part of the upper margin of the great wing of the sphenoid. **Sphenosquamosal:** separates the posterior margin of the great wing of the sphenoid from the anterior margin of the squamous portion of the temporal. **Sphenozygomatic:** runs between the anterior edge of the great wing of the sphenoid and the orbital extension of the zygomatic bone. **Squamo-mastoid:** a transient suture between the two parts of the temporal bone. **Squamous:** is continuous with the parieto-mastoid suture and is characterized by the extensive scale-like overlapping of the parietal by the temporal. **Transverse palatine:** separates the maxillae and palatine bones on the surface of the palate.

Zygomaticofrontal: a serrated suture on the outer margin of the orbit. **Zygomaticomaxillary:** commences at the lower margin of the orbit and runs downwards and outwards, usually terminating at a prominence marking the junction of the two bones on the cheek. **Zygomaticotemporal:** a serrated suture between the zygomatic processes of the temporal and the temporal process of the zygomatic.

Suzanne's gland (Suzanne, J. G., French physician, born 1859). The mucous gland found in the floor of the mouth close to the median line.

swab. 1. A piece of soft material or a sponge attached to the end of a short rod, used to make applications to the throat, to cleanse the teeth, etc. 2. Absorbent material used to remove blood from the site at operations.

swallow. To pass food into the first part of the alimentary tract through the throat.

Swammerdam's glands or corpora heterogenia (Swammerdam, J., Dutch physician, 1637–80). The adrenal glands of amphibia.

sweat. Perspiration; the secretion of the sweat glands.

sweating. The act of perspiring. **S. sickness:** miliary fever or English sweat.

Swedish gymnastics. Gymnastics without apparatus.

sweetbread. The popular name for the following organs when used as food: (i) Pancreas, (ii) Thymus of young animals, (iii) Testes.

swelling. Any enlargement or tumour.

swoon. Syncope.

sycō·ma (G. *sukon*, fig). A condyloma or wart.

sycō·siform (G. *sukōsis*, a fig-like ulcer; L. *forma*, shape). Like sycosis.

sycō·sis (G. *sukōsis*, a fig-like ulcer). An inflammatory disorder involving the hair follicles (especially those of the beard) and marked by the appearance of pustules perforated by hairs and by infiltration of the surrounding skin. **S. nuchae:** see dermatitis papillaris capillitii.

Sydenham's chorea (Sydenham, T., English physician, 1624–89). Uncomplicated chorea.

syllable stammering. A type of dysphasia in which syllables can be correctly uttered but the whole word is pronounced with difficulty.

Sylvian aqueduct (Sylvius, F. de la B., French anatomist, 1614–72). The aqueductus cerebri. **S. fissure:** the lateral cerebral fissure.

Sylvius, bone of (Sylvius, J. D., French anatomist, 1478–1555). The lenticular process of the malleolus. **S., muscle of:** the musculus accessorius of foot.

sym·bion, sym·biont (G. *sun*, together; *bios*, life). Either of two organisms existing in intimate association.

symbiŏ·sis (G. *sun*, together; *bios*, life). The intimate association of two organisms not being parent and offspring, male and female, parasite and host, etc. Syn. commensalism.

symbiŏ·tic (G. *sun*, together; *bios*, life). Relating to symbiosis.

symblĕ·pharon (G. *sun*, together; *blepharon*, eyelid). Adhesion of the eyelids to the ball of the eye.

symblepharō·sis (G. *sun*, together; *blepharon*, eyelid). Adhesion of the eyelids to the eyeball or to each other.

sym·bol (G. *sumbolon*). 1. A sign or character used to convey an idea. 2. In chemistry, an abbreviation of the name of an element, generally the initial letter or letters of the name in Latin or English.

sym·bolism (G. *sumbolon*, symbol). An abnormal mental condition in which events or objects are interpreted as having a mystic meaning; a habit often observed in certain forms of insanity.

symbră·chydactў·lia (G. *sun*, together; *brakhus*, short; *daktulos*, finger). A condition characterized by the possession of unusually short and adherent fingers.

Syme's operation (Syme, J., Scottish surgeon, 1799–1870). 1. External urethrotomy. 2. Amputation of the foot at the ankle.

Symington's anococcygeal body (Symington, J., Scottish anatomist, 1851–1924). A fibro-muscular mass situated in the perineum between the coccyx and the anus.

sym·melus (G. *sun*, together; *melos*, limb). A monster characterized by defective development of the pelvis and lower limbs, with more or less close union of the latter.

symmet·ric, symmet·rical (G. *summetria*, symmetry). Relating to or showing symmetry.

sym·metry (G. *summetria*). In anatomy, the due correspondence of parts; the relation of homologous parts at opposite sides or ends of the organism.

sympară·lysis (G. *sun*, together; *paralusis*, paralysis). Conjugate paralysis; term applied to the abolition of certain synkineses of the eye.

sympathec·tomy (G. *sun*, together; *pathos*, disease; *ektomē*, excision). Surgical removal of a portion of the sympathetic nervous system.

sympathet·ic (G. *sumpatheia*, sympathy). 1. Relating to or produced by sympathy. 2. Conveying sympathy, as the s. system. **S. nervous system:** a system of nerves (the s. ganglia) forming a series from the brain to the end of the spinal column, linked together by nerve fibres, and supplying the viscera and blood-vessels. In modern literature the word 'sympathetic' is tending to be replaced by 'thoracolumbar'.

sympathĕ·thicoblast (G. *sumpatheia*, sympathy; *blastos*, germ). The primitive cell from which sympathetic nerve cells are developed.

sympathĕ·ticoparalў·tic (G. *sumpatheia*, sympathy; *paralusis*, paralysis). Caused by paralysis of the sympathetic nerve.

sympathĕ·ticoton·ic (G. *sumpatheia*, sympathy; *tonos*, tension). Term applied to migraine caused by tonic contraction of the arteries due to overaction of the sympathetic.

sympă·thic (G. *sumpatheia*, sympathy). Syn. of sympathetic.

sympă·thoblast (G. *sun*, together; *pathos*, disease; *blastos*, germ). The precursor from which a sympathetic ganglion cell develops.

sympă·thomimet·ic (G. *sumpatheia*, sympathy; *mimēsis*, imitation). Having a similar action to the sympathetic.

sym·pathy (G. *sumpatheia*, sympathy). The relation existing between the various parts of an organism causing a change in one to affect another.

symphă·langism (G. *sun*, together; *phalagx*, the bone between two finger- or toe-joints). An inherited affection marked by stiffness of the fingers or ankylosis of the finger-joints.

symphў·sĕal (G. *sun*, together; *phusis*, growth). Relating to a symphysis.

symphysiĕc·tomy (G. *sumphusis*, a growing together; *ektomē*, excision). Excision of the symphysis pubis.

symphў·sion (G. *sumphusis*, a growing together). The most anterior point of the alveolar process of the lower jaw.

symphysiŏr·rhaphy (G. *sumphusis*, a growing together; *rhaphē*, suture). The suturing of a cleft symphysis.

symphysiŏ·tomy (G. *sumphusis*, a growing together; *tomē*, a cutting). The surgical division of the fibrous cartilage of the symphysis pubis in order to increase pelvic diameter and thus facilitate labour and delivery.

sym·physis (G. *sun*, together; *phusis*, growth). The junction line of two bones. **S. pubis:** a cartilaginous joint between the two pubic bones.

Sym·phytum (G. *sun*, together; *phusis*, growth). A genus of plants belonging to the Boraginaceae. The dried rhizome of *S. officinale* (comfrey root) contains allantoin and is useful for applying to wounds in the form of a decoction.

sympŏ·dia (G. *sun*, together; *pous*, foot). A condition in which the feet are fused together.

symp·tom (G. *sumptōma*). Any change in a patient occurring during a disease and indicating its nature and position.

symptomat·ic (G. *sumptōma*, symptom). Relating to or of the nature of a symptom.

symptomatŏ·logy (G. *sumptōma*, symptom; *logos*, treatise). 1. The study of symptoms. 2. The symptoms of a disease considered as a whole.

symptŏ·sis (G. *sun*, together; *ptōsis*, a falling). The sapping of bodily strength; emaciation, breakdown.

sym·pus (G. *sun*, together; *pous*, foot). A monster with the lower extremities joined together. Syn. sirenomelus.

synadel·phus (G. *sun*, together; *adelphos*, brother). A monster with eight limbs.

synaesthē·sia (G. *sun*, together; *aisthēsis*, feeling). A secondary sensation excited by an actual perception, e.g., sensations of colour or sound aroused by the perception of taste.

synal·gia (G. *sun*, together; *algos*, pain). Pain felt in one part but produced by wound or stimulus to another part.

synal·gic (G. *sun*, together; *algos*, pain). Relating to or characterized by synalgia.

syn·anastomŏ·sis (G. *sun*, together; *anastomosis*, a bringing to a point). The union of a number of blood-vessels.

synanthē·ma (G. *sunanthein*, to blossom together). A cluster of papules on the skin.

sȳ·napse. Synapsis, *q.v.*

synap·sis (G. *sun*, together; *haptein*, to touch). 1. The anatomical relation of one neuron to another; the intertwining of the end branchings of neurons enabling nerve-impulses to pass from one to another. 2. The union of chromosomes.

synap·tase (G. *sun*, together; *haptein*, to touch). Emulsin, *q.v.*

synap·tic. Relating to a synapsis.

synarthrŏ·dia (G. *sun*, together; *arthron*, joint). Synarthrosis, *q.v.*

synarthrŏ·dial. Relating to synarthrosis.

synarthrŏ·sis (G. *sun*, together; *arthron*, joint). A joint in which the bones are immovably fastened together without any interposed synovial tissues.

syncephā·lia (G. *sun*, together; *kephalē*, head). A monster having two bodies and one head.

syncĕ·phalus (G. *sun*, together; *kephalē*, head). A monster with two incomplete and connected heads.

synchei·lia, synchī·lia (G. *sun*, together; *kheilos*, lip). Congenital atresia of the lips.

synchondrŏ·sis (G. *sun*, together; *khondros*, cartilage). A joint the surfaces of which are united by a band of cartilage.

synchondrŏ·tomy (G. *sun*, together; *khondros*, cartilage; *tomē*, a cutting). A cutting of the cartilage uniting bones, particularly applied to that of the symphysis pubis.

syn·chronism (G. *sun*, together; *khronos*, time). Occurrence at the same time of two or more events.

syn·chronous (G. *sun*, together; *khronos*, time). Simultaneous.

syn·chysis scintil·lans (G. *sugkhusis*, confusion; L. *scintilla*, a spark). The existence of bright particles in the vitreous humour of the eye.

syn·clitism (G. *sugklitēs*, a table-companion). A condition characterized by similarity of inclination; parallelism between the planes of the pelvis and those of the foetal head.

syn·clonus (G. *sun*, together; *klonos*, turmoil). 1. The clonic contraction of a number of muscles at the same time; muscular tremor. 2. Any disease marked by muscular tremor, e.g. chorea.

syn·copal (G. *sugkopē*, sudden loss of strength). Relating to or marked by syncope.

syn·copĕ (G. *sugkopē*, sudden loss of strength). A swoon or faint; temporary loss of the respiratory and circulatory functions due to cerebral anaemia.

syncy·tial (G. *sun*, together; *kutos*, container). Relating to a syncytium.

syncytiŏ·ma (G. *sun*, together; *kutos*, container). A uterine tumour consisting of syncytial tissues. **S. malignum:** see deciduoma malignum.

syncȳ·tium (G. *sun*, together; *kutos*, container). 1. A protoplasmic mass with many nuclei. 2. The totality of epithelial cells composing the exterior covering of the chorionic villi.

syn·cytoid (G. *sun*, together; *kutos*, container; *eidos*, form). Like a syncytium.

syndactȳ·lia, syndac·tylism, syndac·tyly (G. *sun*, together; *daktulos*, finger). Adhesion between fingers and toes; webbed fingers; webbed toes.

syndac·tylus (G. *sun*, together; *daktulos*, finger). A person affected with syndactylia.

syndec·tomy (G. *sun*, together; *deein*, to bind; *ektomē*, excision). Removal of a piece of conjunctiva as a treatment for a pannus. Syn. peritomy.

syndel·phus (G. *sun*, together; *adelphos*, brother). A double monster with a single head and pelvis, united thoraces and eight limbs.

syn·desis (G. *sundesis*, a binding together). The condition of being fastened together.

syndesmec·tomy (G. *sundesmos*, ligament; *ektomē*, excision). Surgical removal of a ligament, in part or in whole.

syndesmī·tis (G. *sundesmos*, ligament). 1. Inflammation of a ligament. 2. Conjunctivitis.

syndesmŏ·graphy (G. *sundesmos*, ligament; *graphein*, to write). A written description of the ligaments.

syndesmŏ·logy (G. *sundesmos*, ligament; *logos*, a discourse). That branch of anatomy concerned with the ligaments.

syndesmŏ·ma (G. *sundesmos*, ligament). A new growth mainly composed of connective tissue.

syndes·mopexy (G. *sundesmos*, ligament; *pexis*, fixation). Surgical fixation of a dislocation by using the ligaments of the joint.

syndesmor·rhaphy (G. *sundesmos*, ligament; *rhaphē*, suture). The suturing of a ligament.

syndesmŏ·sis (G. *sundesmos*, ligament). Fixed articulation between bones where fibrous tissue holds together the opposing surfaces.

syndesmŏ·tomy (G. *sundesmos*, ligament; *tomē*, a cutting). The dissection or incision of a ligament.

syndes·mus (G. *sundesmos*). A ligament.

syn·drome (G. *sun*, together; *dromos*, a running). All the symptoms of a disease; a symptom complex.

syndrŏ·mic. Relating to a syndrome.

synē·chia (G. *sun*, together; *ekhein*, to hold). A morbid union of parts, especially adhesion of the iris to the lens capsule or the cornea.

synechŏ·tomy (G. *sun*, together; *ekhein*, to hold; *tomē*, a cutting). Cutting of a synechia.

syn·echtenterŏ·tomy (G. *sun*, together; *ekhein*, to hold; *enteron*, bowel; *tomē*, a cutting). The cutting of an intestinal adhesion.

syneidē·sis (G. *suneidēsis*, consciousness). In biology, the self-regulating principle which unconsciously differentiates between the various instincts.

synêr·esis (G. *sunairein*, to bring together; whence *sunairesis*, a contracting). The condition in which a gel contracts and some of its fluid separates.

synerget·ic (G. *sun*, together; *ergon*, work). Showing synergy; working together.

syn·ergist (G. *sun*, together; *ergon*, work). An agent acting jointly with another agent.

syn·ergy (G. *sun*, together; *ergon*, to work). Co-operation or joint action of two or more organisms or agents.

Syn·gamus (G. *sun*, together; *gamos*, marriage). A genus of nematode worms.

syn·gamy (G. *sun*, together; *gamos*, marriage). Sexual reproduction.

syngĕ·nesis (G. *sun*, together; *genesis*, production). 1. The theory that the embryo results from the union of male and female elements. 2. The theory that the embryo contains the germs of all future generations springing from it. 3. Reproduction by male and female elements.

syngig·noseism (G. *sun*, together; *gignōskein*, to get to know). Hypnotism; so called from the mental agreement involved between two minds.

synezē·sis (G. *sun*, together; *hezesthai*, to sit). Closure or occlusion. S. pupillae: closing of the pupil.

synka·ryon (G. *sun*, together; *karuon*, net). A nucleus produced by the fusion of two pronuclei.

synkinē·sia, synkinē·sis (G. *sun*, together; *kinēsis*, movement). An involuntary movement occurring simultaneously with a voluntary movement in another part of the body.

synneurō·sis (G. *sun*, together; *neuron*, tendon). Syndesmosis, *q.v.*

syn·ocha, syn·ochus (G. *sun*. together; *ekhein*, to hold). Continued fever.

synophthal·mia (G. *sun*, together; *ophthalmos*, eye). The more or less complete fusion of the eyes into one.

synophthal·mus (G. *sun*, together; *ophthalmos*, eye). Cyclops, *q.v.*

synop·sia (G. *sun*, together; *ōps*, eye). Congenital fusion of the two eyes.

synop·sis (G. *sun*, together; *opsis*, vision). A methodical comparison; a general outline or view.

syn·orchism (G. *sun*, together; *orkhis*, testicle). A fusion of the testes.

synō·scheos (G. *sun*, together; *oskheos*, scrotum). A condition of adherence between the skin of the penis and that of the scrotum.

synostĕŏ·logy (G. *sun*, together; *osteon*, bone; *logos*, treatise). The total of what is known of the joints.

synostĕŏ·sis, synostō·sis (G. *sun*, together; *osteon*, bone). The junction by osseous matter of bones that are normally separate.

synostĕŏ·tomy (G. *sun*, together; *osteon*, bone; *tomē*, a cutting). The dissection of joints.

synō·tus (G. *sun*, together; *ous*, ear). A monster with fused ears.

synovec·tomy (G. *sun*, together; L. *ovum*, egg; G. *ektomē*, excision). Surgical removal of synovial membrane.

synō·via (G. *sun*, together; L. *ovum*, egg). The clear fluid of a joint cavity.

synō·vial (G. *sun*, together; L. *ovum*, egg). Relating to or secreting synovia. S. membrane: that covering the articular surfaces of bones and the inner surfaces of ligaments forming a joint. S. sheath: the s. membrane lining the cavity of a bone through which the tendon passes.

sy·novin (G. *sun*, together; L. *ovum*, egg). The variety of mucin that is present in synovia.

synovi·parous (G. *sun*, together; L. *ovum*, egg; *parere*, to give birth). Yielding or secreting synovia.

synovi·tis (G. *sun*, together; L. *ovum*, egg). Inflammation of a synovial membrane.

synō·vium (G. *sun*, together; L. *ovum*, egg). A synovial membrane.

synpneumŏ·nic (G. *sun*, together; *pneumon*, lung). Occurring at the same time as pneumonia.

syntax·is (G. *sun*, together; *tassein*, to arrange). Articulation, *q.v.*

syn·thesis (G. *sun*, together; *thĕsis*, a placing). 1. In chemistry, the artificial production of a compound by means of the combining of its various constituents. 2. A comprehensive view of disjointed knowledge.

syn·thesize. To develop or produce anything by means of synthesis.

synthet·ic (G. *sun*, together; *thĕsis*, a placing). Relating to or produced by synthesis; artificial.

syntox·oid (G. *sun*, together; *toxikon*, poison; *eidos*, form). A toxoid with the same affinity as the associated toxin for an antitoxin.

syntrip·sis (G. *sun*, together; *tribein*, to crush). Comminuted fracture.

syn·trophus (G. *suntrophos*, congenital). Any disease of an inherited or congenital nature.

syntrop·ic (G. *sun*, together; *trepein*, to turn). Alike and turned in the same direction; e.g., the ribs of one side are s.; those of the other side are antitropic.

synulō·sis (G. *sun*, together; *oulē*, a scar). Cicatrization.

synulot·ic (G. *sun*, together; *oulē*, a scar). Leading to cicatrization, or an agent that does this.

sy̆·philelcō·sis (syphilis; G. *helkos*, ulcer). Syphilitic ulceration; the condition of having a chancre.

syphilel·cus (syphilis; G. *helkos*, ulcer). A syphilitic ulcer.

sy̆·philid, sy̆·philide (syphilis). Any skin disease caused by syphilis.

sy̆·philine (syphilis). An extract of the liver of a syphilitic foetus used in testing for syphilis.

sy̆·philĭon·thus (syphilis; *ionthos*, an eruption on the face). Any copper-coloured, scaly, syphilitic eruption.

sy̆·philiphō·bia. syphilophobia, *q.v.*

sy̆·philis (name invented by the Italian physician Fracastoro in 1530). An infectious and contagious venereal disease, characterized by many structural and cutaneous lesions. The primary lesion is the hard chancre, which may make its appearance up to forty days after infection. The cause is invasion by a micro-organism, the *Spirochaeta pallida* or *Treponema pallidum*.

syphilit·ic (syphilis). Relating to or affected with syphilis.

syphilizā·tion (syphilis). Infection with syphilis.

sy̆·philioderm, syphiloder·ma (syphilis; G. *derma*, skin). See syphilide.

sy̆·philogĕ·nesis, syphilŏ·geny (syphilis; G. *genesis*, production). Development of syphilis.

sy̆·philoid (syphilis; G. *eidos*, form). Like syphilis.

syphilŏ·logist (syphilis; G. *logos*, a treatise). One skilled in the treatment of syphilis.

syphilŏ·logy (syphilis; G. *logos*, a discourse). All that is known of the origin and nature of syphilis.

syphilŏ·ma (syphilis). A syphilitic gumma.

syphilomā·nia (syphilis; G. *mania*, madness). Syphilophobia, *q.v.*

syphilŏ·pathy (syphilis; G. *pathos*, disease). Any disease of a syphilitic nature or origin.

syphilophō·bia (syphilis; G. *phŏbos*, fear). A neurotic state in which the patient supposes himself to be infected with syphilis, or a morbid dread of syphilis.

syphĭŏn·thus. The same as syphilionthus, *q.v.*

syr. Abbreviation for syrupus.

syrigmophō·nia (G. *surigmos*, a hissing; *phōnē*, voice). A high, whistling sound in the voice.

syrig·mus (G. *surigmos*, a hissing). A ringing sound in the ears.

sy̆·ringe (G. *surigx*, a pipe). An instrument for injecting fluids into a cavity.

syringec·tomy (G. *surigx*, a pipe; *ektomē*, excision). The surgical removal of the walls of a fistula.

syringī·tis (G. *surigx*, a pipe). Inflammation of the pharyngotympanic (Eustachian) tube.

syringobul·bia (G. *surigx*, a pipe; *bolbos*, a bulbous root). Abnormal cavitation in the medulla oblongata due to an enlargement of the central canal.

syrin·gocoele (G. *surigx*, a pipe; *koilos*, hollow). The central canal of the spinal cord.

syrin·gocystadenō·ma (G. *surigx*, a pipe; *kustis*, bladder; *adēn*, gland). A papular disease of the skin originating in the sweat-glands.

syrin·gocystō·ma (G. *surigx*, a pipe; *kustis*, the bladder). A cystic tumour in the sweat-glands.

syrin·gomȳē·lia (G. *surigx*, a pipe; *muelos*, marrow). A neurological disease marked by the appearance of cavities in the substance of the spinal cord.

syrin·gomyelī·tis (G. *surigx*, a pipe; *muelos*, marrow). Inflammation accompanying or preceding syringomyelus.

syrin·gomȳ·elocele (G. *surigx*, a pipe; *muelos*, marrow; *kēlē*, tumour). A type of spina bifida in which the cavity of the projecting mass communicates with the central canal of the spinal cord.

syrin·gomȳ·elus (G. *surigx*, a pipe; *muelos*, marrow). Abnormal dilation of the central canal of the spinal cord, the grey matter changing into connective tissue.

syrin·gotome (G. *surigx*, a pipe; *tomē*, a cutting). A surgical knife used for cutting a fistula.

syringŏ·tomy (G. *surigx*, a pipe; *tomē*, section). The operation of incising a fistula; applied particularly to an anal fistula.

sȳ·rinx (G. *surigx*, a pipe). 1. A fistula. 2. The pharyngotympanic (Eustachian) tube.

sȳ·rup (Arab. *sharab*). A concentrated solution of sugar often medicated.

syspā·sia (G. *suspăsis*, contraction). Spasmodic inability to speak.

syssarcō·sis (G. *sun*, together; *sarx*, flesh). The uniting of bones by means of muscular tissue.

syssō·mus (G. *sun*, together; *sōma*, body). A double monster joined at the trunks and with two heads.

systal·tic (G. *sustellein*, to draw together). Systolic; contracting and expanding alternately.

sys·tem (G. *sustēma*). 1. A methodical scheme. 2. A connected series of parts, such as the nervous s. or the circulatory s.

systemat·ic (G. *sustēma*, system). Relating to or affecting a system.

systē·mis (G. *sustēma*, system). 1. Of or relating to a system. 2. Relating to the whole organism.

sys·tolĕ (G. *sustolē*, contraction). The period during which the heart contracts; the contraction itself.

systol·ic (G. *sustolē*, contraction). Relating to or occurring during the systole.

systolŏ·meter (G. *sustolē*, contraction; *metron*, measure). An apparatus for measuring cardiac sounds.

systrem·ma (G. *sustremma*, anything twisted). Cramp in the calf muscles of the leg.

syzȳ·gial (G. *suzugia*, a combination). Relating to syzygy.

sȳ·zygy (G. *suzugia*, a combination). 1. A fusion of two organisms without loss of identity. 2. A zygote formed by the coalition of two similar gametes.

T

Ta. The symbol for tantalum.

T.A.B. vaccine. Anti-typhoid-paratyphoid vaccine, made from cultures of typhoid and paratyphoid A. and B. organisms.

tă·bacum (Latinised form of the American word *tobacco*). Tobacco; the dried leaves of *Nicotiana tabacum*.

tă·bagism (Sp. *tabaco* (a word of American origin), tobacco). The tobacco habit.

tabatière anatomique (Fr.). Anatomical snuffbox. A hollow at the base of the thumb bounded in front by the tendon of abductor pollicis longus and extensor pollicis brevis and behind by extensor pollicis longus.

tabefac·tion (L. *tabefacere*, to melt). A wasting away; emaciation.

tabel·la (L., a writing-tablet). A tablet or troche.

tă·bēs (L., a wasting away). Progressive emaciation; a wasting away or consumption. The term is generally used to mean **tabes dorsalis** (locomotor ataxia), a disease caused by sclerosis of the dorsal columns of the spinal cord as a later result of syphilitic infection.

tabet·ic (L. *tabes*, a wasting away). 1. Relating to or affected with tabes. 2. Relating to or affected with tabes dorsalis.

tabĕ·tiform (L. *tabes*, a wasting away; *forma*, shape). Resembling tabes.

tă·bic. Tabetic, *q.v.*

tabificā·tion. Tabefaction, *q.v.*

tă·ble. 1. A flat-topped article of furniture, e.g., an operating table. 2. A layer of bone.

tab·let (L. *tabula*, a writing-tablet). A lozenge or troche.

tab·loid (L. *tabula*, a writing-tablet; G. *eidos*, form). A trade name for drugs or other substances compressed into a convenient shape and size.

tabopară·lysis (L. *tabes*, a wasting away; G. *paralusis*, paralysis). Taboparesis.

taboparē·sis (L. *tabes*, a wasting away; G. *paresis*, paralysis). Tabes associated with general paralysis.

tă·bular (L. *tabula*, a board). Shaped like a table.

tache (Fr.). A spot. **Taches blanches:** white spots on the liver, particularly on its convex surface, observed in infectious diseases.

tachet·ic (Fr. *tache*, spot). Characterized by the presence of spots.

tachŏ·meter (G. *takhus*, swift; *metron*, measure). Haemotachometer, *q.v.*

tachycar·dia (G. *takhus*, swift; *kardia*, heart). Abnormal rapidity of the heart's action.

tachycar·diac. Relating to tachycardia.

tachylā·lia (G. *takhus*, swift; *lalia*, talk). Abnormal rapidity of speech.

tachyphrā·sia (G. *takhus*, swift; *phrasis*, speech). Abnormal volubility; sometimes a symptom of mental aberration.

tachyphrē·nia (G. *takhus*, swift; *phrēn*, mind). Abnormal activity of the mental processes.

tachypnoē·a (G. *takhus*, swift; *pnoē*, breath). Abnormal rapidity of breathing.

tac·tile (L. *tactilis*, tangible). Relating to the sense of touch.

tac·tual. Tactile, *q.v.*

tac·tus (L.). Touch.

tae·dium vī·tae (L.). A morbid weariness of life which may lead to suicidal tendencies.

Tae·nia (G. *tainia*, a riband). A genus of worms of the class Cestoda; tapeworms.

tae·nia (G. *tainia*, a riband). A flat band or strip.

tae·niacide (G. *tainia*, a riband; L. *caedere*, to kill). Destroying tapeworms, or an agent that does this.

tae·niafuge (G. *tainia*, a riband; L. *fugare*, to put to flight). Expelling tapeworms, or an agent that does this.

taeniŏ·la cinē·rea (L.). Band of grey matter in the floor of the fourth ventricle of the brain.

Tagliacotian operation (Tagliacozzi, G., Italian surgeon, 1546–99). A plastic operation to form a new nose. Syn. rhinoplasty.

tail. A cauda; the projecting termination of the spinal column of an animal. Also applied to anything resembling a tail, e.g. the t. of a muscle; the t. of the pancreas.

Taillefer's valve (Taillefer, L. T., French physician, 1802–68). In the nasolacrimal duct.

taint (L. *tingere*, to wet). An infection; a spot or blemish.

Tait's knot (Tait, L., English surgeon, 1845–99). Syn. Staffordshire knot. A knot used in tying off pedicles. **T.'s law:** states that laparotomy should be performed in all cases of abdominal and pelvic diseases endangering life, except those known to be malignant. **T.'s operation:** an operation for the repair of a torn perineum.

taka-diastase. A preparation of an amyolytic enzyme derived from species of *Eurotium oryzae* cultivated on wheat bran.

talal·gia (L. *talus*, ankle; G. *algos*, pain). Any pain in the heel or the ankle.

talc·cum (Arab. *talq*). A preparation of magnesium silicate; used as a dusting powder.

tă·lipĕd (L. *talus*, ankle; *pes*, foot). A club-footed person.

ta·lipēs (L. *talus*, ankle; *pes*, foot). Club-foot; due to the contraction of certain muscles or tendons, either congenital or acquired. **T. calcaneus:** in which the deformity is a dorsiflexion of the foot. **T. calcaneovalgus:** a combination of talipes calcaneus and talipes vagus. **T. calcaneovarus:** a combination of talipes calcaneus and talipes varus. **T. cavus:** talipes in which the deformity is an exaggeration of plantar flexion. Syn. pes cavus. **T. equinovalgus:** talipes in which the deformity is a combination of plantar flexion, external inversion and abduction of the foot. **T. equinovarus:** talipes in which the deformity is a combination of plantar flexion, internal rotation and adduction of the foot. **T. equinus:** in which the deformity is plantar flexion.

talipŏ·manus (L. *talus*, ankle; *pes*, foot; *manus*, hand). Club-hand; a deformity somewhat resembling club-foot.

Tallerman's apparatus (Tallerman, L. A., contemporary English scientist). Apparatus for applying dry heat to an extremity. Used in the treatment of rheumatism.

tal·low. The fat obtained from suet.

Talma's disease (Talma, S., Dutch physician, 1847–1918). Myotonia acquisita. **T.'s operation:** the formation of artificial adhesions between the omentum, liver and spleen and the abdominal wall. Used in cases of ascites due to cirrhosis of the liver.

tā·localcā·nean (L. *talus*, ankle; *calcaneum*, heel). Relating to the talus and the calcaneum.

talocrū·ral (L. *talus*, ankle; *crus*, leg). Relating both to the talus and the leg-bones.

tā·lofi·bular (L. *talus*, ankle; *fibula*, a buckle). Relating both to the talus and the fibula.

taloti·bial (L. *talus*, ankle; *tibia*, shin). Relating both to the talus and the tibia.

tal·pa (L.). A mole.

tālus (L.). 1. The astragalus or ankle bone. 2. The ankle.

tă·marind (Arab. *tamr*, date; Pers. *Hind*, India). The leguminous tree, *Tamarindus indica*, also its laxative fruit, which is an ingredient of confection of senna.

tambour (Fr., drum). A drum-like apparatus employed in physiological experiments for transmitting movements.

tam·pon (Fr.). 1. A plug of lint or other soft material for inserting into a cavity, usually to check haemorrhage. 2. To stop up with a tampon.

tank. A vessel, usually of metal, for containing fluids.

tan·nate (Fr. *tan*, oak bark). Any salt of tannic acid.

tannic acid. A highly astringent yellow powder obtained from oak galls and other sources. Its composition approximates to that of penta-m-digalloyl glucose $C_{76}H_{52}O_{46}$, and it is used as a styptic, haemostatic and astringent. Its use in burn dressings has been discontinued as a result of many cases of permanent disfigurement.

tan·nin (Fr. *tan*, oak bark). The name given to two types of astringent substance. 1. The pyrogalloyl tannins, such as tannic acid. 2. The pyrocatechol tannins, such as occur in catechu and krameria.

tan·sy. A herb, *Tanacetum vulgare*, of the order Compositae. The leaves and tops yield a bitter principle, tanacetin, tannic acid and an essential oil, *Oleum tanaceti*. Tansy has diuretic, emmenagogue and anthelmintic properties.

tan·talum (L. *Tantalus*, a mythical king of Phrygia). A hard, very resistant metal, somewhat similar to vanadium, and used in surgery. Symbol Ta; atomic weight 180.88.

tan·trum. A violent outburst of temper.

tap. 1. A light blow. 2. To draw off fluid. 3. A mechanism for drawing off fluid.

tă·peinoce·phaly (G. *tapeinos*, low; *kephalē*, head). Condition in which there is flattening of the skull.

tapē·tum (G. *tapēs*, carpet). 1. The layer composing the ceiling of the posterior and middle cornua of the lateral ventricles of the brain; it consists of fibres from the corpus callosum. 2. The glittering greenish layer of the eyes of night-prowling animals, which are thus visible in the dark. Syn. tapetum lucidum.

tapeworm. One of the Cestoda, a class of worms parasitic in warm-blooded vertebrates.

taphophō·bia (G. *taphos*, tomb; *phobos*, fear). A morbid terror of being buried alive.

tapinoce·phaly. Tapeinocephaly, *q.v.*

tapiō·ca (Native Braz. *tipioca*). A starch prepared from the cassava or manioc plant; it is used as food.

tā·pir mouth (Native Braz. *tapira*). A disjunction and thickening of the lips with degeneration of the orbicularis oris muscle, so that the lips have the appearance of those of the tapir.

tapotement (Fr. *tapoter*, to tap). The tapping movement in massage.

tapping. 1. Paracentesis, *q.v.* 2. Tapotement, *q.v.*

tar. A dark-coloured or black viscous liquid mainly obtained from the distillation of pine-wood. It has antipyretic and antiseptic properties. Coal-t.: a black viscous liquid distilled from bituminous coal.

taran·tism (Taranto, a town in southern Italy). 1. Dancing mania. 2. A choreic malady supposed to be caused by the bite of the tarantula and popularly believed to be cured by dancing.

taran·tula (Taranto, a town in southern Italy). A species of spider, *Lycosa tarantula*, similar to the trap-door spider, *Mygale henzii*, for which it is often mistaken. Its bite is poisonous.

Tarax·acum (Latinised form of Arab. *tarashagun*). A genus of plants including the *T. officinale*, or common dandelion, the dried roots of which yield a principle that is diuretic and stomachic in action.

Tardieu's spots (Tardieu, A. A., French physician, 1818–79). Petechial haemorrhages beneath the pleura which are seen following death by suffocation.

Tarin's valves (Tarin, P., French anatomist, 1700–61). The thickenings of the velum medullare posterius joining the vermis of the cerebellum (valvulae et scrobes ventriculi cerebri quarti).

Tarnier's forceps (Tarnier, E. S., French obstetrician, 1828–97). Axis-traction midwifery forceps. **T.'s sign:** a sign of abortion in which the angle between the upper and lower uterine segments becomes obliterated.

tarsadeni·tis (G. *tarsos*, a broad, flat surface; *adēn*, gland). Inflammation both of the tarsus of the eyelid and of the Meibomian glands.

tar·sal (G. *tarsos*, a broad, flat surface). 1. Relating to the instep. 2. Relating to the tarsus of an eyelid.

tarsal·gia (G. *tarsos*, a broad, flat surface; *algos*, pain). Neuralgic pain in the tarsus of the foot.

tarsec·tomy (G. *tarsos*, a broad, flat surface; *ektomē*, excision). 1. Excision of the tarsus or a portion of it. 2. Excision of a tarsal cartilage or a portion of it.

tarsectŏ·pia (G. *tarsos*, a broad, flat surface; *ektopos*, distant). Tarsal dislocation.

tarsī·tis (G. *tarsos*, a broad, flat surface). Inflammation of the tarsus of an eyelid. See also blepharitis.

tarsomalā·cia (G. *tarsos*, a broad, flat surface; *malakia*, softness). Abnormal softening of the tarsus of an eyelid.

tarsomě·galy (G. *tarsos*, a broad, flat surface; *megas*, great). Enlargement of the heel-bone, or os calcis.

tar·sometatar·sal (G. *tarsos*, a broad, flat surface; *meta*, after). Relating to the tarsus and the metatarsus.

tarso-or·bital (G. *tarsos*, a broad, flat surface; L. *orbis*, orbit). Relating conjointly to the tarsus and the orbit.

tar·sophalan·geal (G. *tarsos*, a broad, flat surface; *phalagx*, bone between joints of fingers and toes). Relating conjointly to the tarsus and the phalanges.

tarsophȳ·ma (G. *tarsos*, a broad, flat surface; *phuma*, a growth). Any tumour of the tarsus.

tar·soplasty (G. *tarsos*, a broad, flat surface; *plassein*, to form). Plastic repair of an eyelid; blepharoplasty.

tarsoptō·sis (G. *tarsos*, a broad, flat surface; *ptōsis*, a falling). Flatfootedness.

tarsor·rhaphy (G. *tarsos*, a broad, flat surface; *rhaphē*, suture). An operation for reducing the width of the aperture between the eyelids; sewing the eyelids together for part or the whole of their extent.

tarsoti·bial (G. *tarsos*, a broad, flat surface; L. *tibia*, shin). Relating conjointly to the tarsus and the tibia.

tarsŏ·tomy (G. *tarsos*, a broad, flat surface; *tomē*, a cutting). Incision into the tarsus of the foot or into an eyelid.

tar·sus (G. *tarsos*, a broad, flat surface). 1. The instep. 2. The connective tissues forming the eyelid.

tar·tar (Late L. *tartarum*, perhaps from Arab. *durd*, dregs). 1. Acid potassium tartrate, deposited on the inside of winecasks. 2. The calcareous substance deposited on teeth.

tartă·ric acid. $H_2C_4H_4O_6$. An astringent acid of frequent occurrence throughout the vegetable kingdom, but principally obtained from the juice of grapes which deposit it after fermentation as acid potassium tartrate (argol). Its main uses are in cooling drinks and as a constituent of baking powder.

tar·trate (L.L. *tartarum*, wine deposit). Any salt of tartaric acid.

tar·trated. Containing tartar or tartaric acid.

tar·trazine. $C_{16}H_9O_9N_4S_2Na_3$. A dye used to impart a yellow colour to foodstuffs and to medicines.

Tashkend ulcer (Tashkend in Soviet Turkistan). A variety of oriental sore.

tasikinē·sia (G. *tăsis*, a straining; *kinēsis*, movement). An abnormal desire to walk.

taste. 1. The sensation resulting from stimulation of the taste buds situated in the tongue by soluble substances. 2. The sense which perceives flavours.

tattoo·ing (Tahitian *tatau*). 1. Permanent colouring of the skin through the introduction of foreign substances by means of a needle. 2. The restoring of natural colours in faded pigmented parts by the introduction of foreign substances.

tau·rine (L. *taurus*, bull). $NH_2.CH_2.CH_2SO_2OH$. An acid decomposition product of taurocholic acid, and found in the faeces.

taurochō·late (L. *taurus*, bull; G. *kholē*, bile). Any salt of taurocholic acid.

taurochol·ic acid (L. *taurus*, bull). One of the two main bile acids, $C_{26}H_{46}NO_7$. On hydrolysis it splits into taurine and cholic acid.

tauropho·bia (L. *taurus*, bull; *phobos*, fear). Neurotic fear of bulls.

tauto·meral, tautomer·ic (G. *tauto*, the same; *meros*, part). Relating to tautomerism.

tautŏ·merism (G. *tauto*, the same; *meros*, part). The phenomenon exhibited by a compound existing in two or more forms differing only in the position of a hydrogen atom, and existing in a state of dynamic equilibrium, one or other form predominating according to the conditions.

Tavel's serum (Tavel, E., Swiss surgeon, 1858–1912). An anti-streptococcal serum.

Tawara's node (Tawara, S., Japanese pathologist, born 1873). The auriculo-ventricular node.

tax·is (G.). 1. Arrangement. 2. The correction by manipulation of a prolapsed uterus or other structure.

taxŏ·nomy (G. *taxis*, arrangement; *nomos*, a law). Classification; especially its laws and principles.

Tay's disease (Tay, W., English physician, 1843–1927). Tay choroiditis: choroiditis occurring in old age and probably due to atheromatous changes in the arteries. T.'s spot: a red spot seen in the fovea centralis in cases of amaurotic familial idiocy.

Tay-Sachs disease. Amaurotic idiocy.

Tb. The symbol for terbium.

Te. The symbol for tellurium.

tea (Chinese *ch'a*). The dried leaves of *Thea sinensis* (*Camellia thea*) used to prepare the drink known as tea. The word 'tea' is also applied to infusions of other vegetable substances, e.g. 'dandelion tea.'

teaberry. Gaultheria, *q.v.*

Teale's amputation (Teale, T. P., English surgeon, 1801–68). Amputation with rectangular flaps of different size.

tears. The secretions of the lacrimal glands.

tease. To divide a tissue into shreds.

teat. The nipple.

technē·tium. Chemical element No. 43, the first artificially produced chemical element not found in nature. Symbol Tc.

technic (G. *tekhnē*, skill). Technique, *q.v.*

tech·nical (G. *tekhnikos*, workmanlike). Relating to technique.

techni·cian (G. *tekhnē*, skill). One skilled in technical arts.

technique (G. *tekhnē*, skill). The mode of procedure in mechanical or surgical operations of all kinds.

technocau·sis (G. *tekhnē*, skill; *kausis*, a burning). Mechanical cauterization as opposed to that produced by chemicals.

tecnotō·nia (G. *teknon*, child; *ktonos*, murder). Infanticide.

tec·tiform (L. *tectum*, roof; *forma*, shaped). Like a roof.

tectocĕ·phaly (L. *tectum*, roof; G. *kephalē*, head). Having a roof-shaped head.

tectŏ·logy (G. *tektōn*, craftsman; *logos*, treatise). A sub-science of morphology, dealing with the structure of the organism.

tectō·rial (L. *tectorium*, a covering). Acting as a roof.

tectō·rium (L.). A covering.

tec·tum (L., roof). Any structure resembling a roof.

tē·dious (L. *taedium*, weariness). Unduly prolonged, as t. labour.

teel oil. Sesamum, *q.v.*

teeth. The organs of mastication.

teething. The emergence of the teeth; dentition.

teg·men (L. *tegimen*, a cover). A roof; a cover; e.g., t. mastoideum, the roof of the mastoid cells.

tegmen·tal (L. *tegimen*, a cover). Relating to the tegmentum.

tegmen·tum (L. *tegumentum*, a covering). A covering; specifically, the posterior superior portion of the crus cerebri and pons varolii.

tegumen. Tegmen, *q.v.*

tĕ·gument (L. *tegumentum*, a covering). The integument.

tegumen·tal (L. *tegumentum*, a covering). Relating to the skin or tegument.

Teichmann's crystals (Teichmann, L. K. Stawiarski-, German pathological anatomist, 1823-95). Crystals of haemin. T.'s networks: the superficial and deep lymphatic plexuses in the wall of the stomach.

teichop·sia (G. *teikhos*, a wall; *opsis*, vision). Temporary amblyopia with subjective images, often an accompaniment of migraine.

teinody·nia (G. *tenōn*, a tendon; *odunē*, pain). Tenodynia, *q.v.*

tē·la (L. web). Any tissue of webbed structure.

telaesthē·sia (G. *tēle*, at a distance; *aisthēsis*, feeling). Perception at a distance; perception not due to the recognized channels of sense.

telal·gia (G. *tēle*, at a distance; *algos*, pain). Pain felt in a site distant from the actual lesion.

telan·giectă·sia, tel·angĭec·tasis (G. *telos*, end; *aggeion*, vessel; *ektasis*, extension). Dilation of the capillaries or smaller blood-vessels.

telangii·tis (G. *telos*, end; *aggeion*, vessel). Inflammation of the capillaries.

telangiō·sis (G. *telos*, end; *aggeion*, vessel). Any disorder or disease of the capillaries or small blood-vessels.

teledac·tyl (G. *tēlĕ*, at a distance; *daktulos*, finger). A device used to pick up objects from the ground without stooping; used in certain spinal diseases.

telegrapher's cramp. A neurosis of telegraph workers.

telencĕ·phalon (G. *telos*, end; *egkephalos*, brain). The hindbrain.

teleneu·ron (G. *telos*, end; *neuron*, nerve). Any nerve ending.

teleolŏ·gic (G. *teleios*, finished; *logos*, discourse). Relating to final causes.

telĕŏ·logy (G. *teleios*, finished; *logos*, discourse). The theory of final causes.

telĕ·pathist (G. *tēle*, at a distance; *pathos*, experience). A thought-reader.

telĕ·pathy (G. *tēle*, at a distance; *pathos*, experience). Thought-reading; thought-transference.

telesỹ·philis (G. *tēle*, at a distance; *syphilis*). Meta-syphilis.

telesystol·ic (G. *telos*, end; *sustolē*, contraction). Relating to the end of the systole.

teletac·tile. Relating to the teletactor.

teletac·tor (G. *telos*, end; L. *tactus*, to touch). An apparatus enabling the deaf to hear by means of a vibrating plate.

tel·lurate (L. *tellus*, earth). Any salt of telluric acid.

tellū·ric (L. *tellus*, earth). 1. Obtained from the soil. 2. Relating to the hexavalent compounds of tellurium. **T. acid:** H_2TeO_4, an acid which, with bases, forms tellurates.

tel·lurism (L. *tellus*, earth). The influence of the soil in promoting or causing disease.

tel·lurate (L. *tellus*, earth). A salt of telluric acid, H_2TeO_4.

tellurite (L. *tellus*, earth). A salt of tellurous acid, H_2TeO_3.

tellū·rium (L. *tellus*, earth). A non-metallic element. Symbol Te.; atomic weight 127·5.

teloden·dron (G. *telos*, end; *dendron*, tree). The terminal arborization of a nerve-cell process.

telolĕ·cithal (G. *telos*, end; *lekithos*, yolk). Having a large-sized yolk eccentrically disposed.

telolem·ma (G. *telos*, end; *lemma*, husk). The membrane sheathing the eminence of Doyère, or the point at which a motor nerve enters a muscular fibre.

tĕ·lophase (G. *telos*, end; *phasis*, phase). The final stage of cell-division or of any process.

tem·perament (L. *temperamentum*). Individual peculiarity of mental or physical organization.

tem·perature (L. *temperatura*). The degree of intensity of heat of a body or of the atmosphere, especially as measured by a thermometer.

tem·plate. A pattern.

tem·ple (L. *tempora*, the temples). The flat, depressed portion of the head behind the eye and above the ear.

tem·pora (L.). The temples.

tem·poral (L. *temporalis*, from *tempus*, time). 1. Relating to the temple, as the t. bone, etc. 2. Relating to time.

temporā·lis muscle (L.). One of the muscles of mastication, arising from the temporal fossa and temporal fascia and inserted into the coronoid process of the mandible.

temporizā·tion (L. *tempus*, time). Expectant treatment of a disease.

temporo-auri·cular (L. *tempora*, temples; *auris*, ear). Relating to the temporal and auricular areas.

temporofā·cial (L. *tempora*, temples; *facies*, face). Relating conjointly to the temples and the face.

temporofron·tal tract (L. *tempora*, temples; *frons*, forehead). Tract connecting the temporal and frontal lobes of the brain.

temporomandĭ-bular (L. *tempora*, temples; *mandibula*, lower jaw). Relating to the temporal bone and the mandible.

tem·poromaxil·lary (L. *tempora*, temples; *mandibula*, jaw). Relating to the temporal bone and the upper jaw.

temporo-occĭ·pital (L. *tempora*, temples ; *occiput*). Relating to the temporal and occipital regions.

tem·porosphē·noid (L. *tempora*, temples; G. *sphēn*, wedge). Relating to the temporal and sphenoid bones.

tĕ·mulence (L. *temulentia*, intoxication). Drunkenness.

tenā·cious (L. *tenax*, gripping). Adhesive; tough.

tenā·city (L. *tenax*, gripping). Toughness.

tenā·culum (L. *tenaculum*, a holder). A hook-shaped implement for seizing and holding parts.

tenal·gia (G. *tenōn*, tendon; *algos*, pain). Any pain in a tendon.

ten·derness. Abnormal susceptibility to touch; soreness.

tendini·tis (L. *tendere*, to stretch). Inflammation of a tendon.

tendinō·sus (L. *tendere*, to stretch). The semitendinosus muscle.

ten·dinosū·ture (L. *tendere*, to stretch; *sutura*, suture). The suturing of a tendon.

ten·dinous (L. *tendere*, to stretch). Relating to a tendon.

ten·do (L.L.). A tendon. **T. Achillis:** the Achilles tendon of the gastrocnemius and soleus muscles.

ten·don (L.L. *tendo*). White, fibrous tissue forming the termination of a muscle and attaching the muscle to the bone.

ten·doplasty (L. *tendere*, to stretch; G. *plassein*, to form). A plastic operation on a tendon.

tendovagī·nal (L. *tendere*, to stretch; *vagina*, sheath). Relating conjointly to a tendon and its sheath.

ten·dovagini·tis (L. *tendere*, to stretch; *vagina*, sheath). Inflammation of a tendon and its sheath.

tenes·mic (G. *teinein*, to strain). Relating to a tenesmus.

tenes·mus (G. *teinein*, to strain). A straining; particularly a painful effort to empty the bladder or bowel, without success.

tennis elbow. A strain of the elbow occurring in tennis-players due to an incomplete rupture of muscular fibres arising from the external condyle of the humerus.

tenŏ·desis (G. *tenōn*, tendon; *desis*, a binding together). Fixation of a joint by shortening the tendons passing about the joint.

tenodỹ·nia (G. *tenōn*, tendon; *odunē*, pain). Pain in a tendon.

Tenon's capsule (Tenon, J. R., French surgeon, 1724–1816). The fascia bulbi of the orbit. **T.'s space:** the spatium interfasciale of the orbit.

tenonec·tomy (G. *tenōn*, tendon; *ektomē*, excision). The surgical shortening of a tendon.

tenoni·tis[1] (Tenon, J. R., French surgeon, 1724–1816). Inflammation of Tenon's capsule.

tenoni·tis[2] (G. *tenōn*, tendon). Inflammation of a tendon.

tenontā·gra (G. *tenōn*, tendon; *agra*, seizure). Gouty pain in a tendon.

tenonti·tis (G. *tenōn*, tendon). Inflammation of a tendon.

tĕ·nophyte (G. *tenōn*, tendon; *phuton*, a plant). An osseous or cartilaginous growth on a tendon.

tĕ·noplasty (G. *tenōn*, tendon; *plassein*, to form). A plastic operation on a tendon.

tenor·rhaphy (G. *tenōn*, tendon; *rhaphē*, suture). The suturing of a tendon.

tenostō·sis (G. *tenōn*, tendon; *osteon*, bone). Ossification of a tendon.

tenosū·ture (G. *tenōn*, tendon; L. *sutura*, suture). Tenorrhaphy, *q.v.*

tĕ·nosynovi·tis (G. *tenōn*, tendon; *syn*, with; L. *ovum*, egg). Inflammation of a tendon and its sheath.

tĕ·notome (G. *tenōn*, tendon; *tomē*, section). An instrument for performing tenotomy.

tenŏ·tomy (G. *tenōn*, tendon; *tomē*, section). The section of a tendon.

tenovagini·tis (G. *tenōn*, tendon; L. *vagina*, sheath). Inflammation of the sheath of a tendon.

tense (L. *tensio*, tension). Rigid.

tensiŏ·meter (L. *tensio*, tension; G. *metron*, measure). An instrument for determining the surface tension of liquids.

ten·sion (L. *tensio*). 1. The act of stretching; the condition of being stretched. 2. In electricity, the power of surmounting resistance; voltage.

ten·sor (L. *tendere*, to stretch). Any muscle stretching or tensing a part.

tent (L. *tendere*, to stretch). A roll of material that increases in volume by the absorption of water; used to dilate a canal or to keep open a wound.

ten·tative (L. *tentare*, to test). Experimental.

tenth nerve. The vagus nerve.

tenti·ginous (L. *tentigo*, tension or lust). Lecherous.

tenti·go (L. tension or lust). Lecherousness. **T. prava:** syn. of lupus. **T. venerea:** syn. of nymphomania.

tentor·ium (L. tent). The process of the dura lying between the cerebrum and the cerebellum.

ten·tum (L.). The penis.

tĕ·nuis (L.). Slight; thin.

tenū·ity (L. *tenuis*, thin). The state of being thin.

tĕ·nuous (L. *tenuis*, thin). Thin; slight.

tephromalā·cia (G. *tephros*, ash-coloured; *malakia*, softness). Morbid softening of the grey matter of the brain or spinal cord.

tephromўěli·tis (G. *tephros*, ash-coloured; *muelos*, marrow). Inflammation of the grey matter of the spinal cord; poliomyelitis.

tephrō·sis (G. *tephra*, ashes). Cremation.

tĕ·pid (L. *tepidus*, luke-warm). At about blood heat.

ter in die (L.). Three times daily; abbreviated to t.i.d.

tĕ·ras (G.; pl. *terata*). A monster.

terat·ic (G. *teras*, monster). Monstrous.

tĕ·ratism (G. *teras*, monster). Any anomaly of conformation, whether congenital or acquired.

tĕ·ratoblastō·ma (G. *teras*, monster; *blastos*, germ). Syn. teratoma.

tĕ·ratogĕ·nesis (G. *teras*, monster; *genesis*, production). The bearing of foetal monsters.

tĕ·ratoid (G. *teras*, monster; *eidos*, form). Like a monster.

teratō·logy (G. *teras*, monster; *logos*, treatise). The study of monstrosities.

teratō·ma (G. *teras*, monster). A complex congenital tumour containing teeth, hair or other substance not found normally in the part where the tumour is located; resulting from an embryonic malplacement or from the enclosure of parts of a rudimentary foetus.

teratophō·bia (G. *teras*, monster; *phobos*, fear). A neurotic fear of monsters, or the morbid dread of giving birth to a monstrosity.

teratō·sis (G. *teras*, monster). Teratism, *q.v.*

ter·bium. A metallic element; symbol Tb; atomic weight 159·2.

terchlor·ide (L. *ter*, three times; G. *khlōros*, green). See trichloride.

tĕ·rebene (G. *terebinthos*, turpentine). A mixture of hydrocarbons mainly dipentene $C_{10}H_{16}$, obtained by shaking oil of turpentine with sulphuric acid, and then distilling. It is used in the treatment of bronchitis.

tĕ·rebinth (G. *terebinthos*, turpentine). 1. The tree *Pistacia terebinthus*, which yields China turpentine. 2. Turpentine.

terebin·thina (G. *terebinthos*, turpentine). Turpentine.

terebin·thinate (G. *terebinthos*, turpentine). Containing turpentine.

terebin·thism (G. *terebinthos*, turpentine). Turpentine poisoning.

tĕ·rebrant, tĕ·rebrating (L. *terebrare*, to pierce). Piercing; e.g., t. pain.

terebrā·tion (L. *terebrare*, to pierce). Trephining.

tĕ·rĕs (L. *tĕrĕs*, round). 1. Round and smooth, as the ligamentum t. 2. Any muscle of cylindrical shape, as the t. major and t. minor.

term (L. *terminus*, a boundary). A definite period, as the full t. of gestation.

ter·ma (G. *terma*, a boundary). The lamina cinerea of the brain.

termat·ic (G. *terma*, a boundary). Relating to the terma.

ter·minad (L. *terminus*, a boundary; *ad*, to). Towards a terminal.

ter·minal (L. *terminalis*, from *terminus*, a boundary). 1. Placed at or forming the end; relating to the end. 2. In the plural, the poles of a battery or any source of electricity, or the ends of conductors attached to it.

terminā·tion (L. *terminatio*, from *terminus*, a boundary). A terminus; an end.

terminŏ·logy (G. *terminus*, a boundary; G. *logos*, treatise). Nomenclature.

ter·minus (L.). The end.

ter·nary (L. *ter*, thrice). Consisting of three elements or radicals; said of chemical compounds.

terni·trate. Trinitrate.

terox·ide (L. *ter*, thrice; G. *oxus*, sharp). Trioxide.

ter·pene (a modified form of Terebene, from G. *terebinthos*, turpentine). A group of hydrocarbons of the formula $C_{10}H_{16}$ and derived theoretically from isoprene, $CH_2{:}CH.C(CH_3){:}CH_2$.

ter·pin hydrate. $C_{10}H_{20}O_2$. A dihydric alcohol obtained from oil of turpentine and used in bronchitis. Crystalline solid, M.Pt. 116–119° C.

terpi·neol. $C_{10}H_{18}O$. A mixture of unsaturated monohydric alcohols obtained from terpin hydrate and smelling of lilac. It is used as a solvent for various antiseptics containing chlorocresol.

ter·ra (L.). Earth. **T. alba:** white clay. **T. foliata:** sulphur. **T. japonica:** catechu.

terracing a suture. Closing a wound by suturing in successive tiers.

terrain-cure (Fr. *terrain*, earth). Treatment of adiposity and certain other conditions by mountain-climbing, etc.

Terrier's valve or promontory (Terrier, L. F., French surgeon and veterinarian, 1837–1908). The 'proximal valve' of the gall bladder, between the gall bladder and the cystic duct.

Terson's glands (Terson, A., French ophthalmologist, 1867–1935). The conjunctival glands; glands of Krause.

ter·tian (L. *tertianus*, from *tertius*, third). Occurring every third day as t. fever, a form of intermittent fever.

ter·tiary (L. *tertiarius*, from *tertius*, third). Third in order. **T. syphilis:** the third stage of syphilis.

tertigrā·vida (L. *tertius*, third; *gravida*, pregnant). A woman in her third pregnancy.

terti·para (L. *ter*, thrice; *parere*, to bear). A woman who has produced three children.

tes·sellated (L. *tessellatus*, from *tessella*, dim. of *tessera*, a square). Chequered. **T. epithelium:** flattened epithelial cells with united edges.

test (L. *testum*, an earthen vessel for assaying). 1. A trial. 2. A characteristic reaction distinguishing one body or circumstance from another. 3. A reagent producing such an effect.

tes·ta (L.). A shell. **T. ovi:** an egg-shell.

testā·ceous (L. *testa*, shell). Relating to a shell.

testec·tomy (L. *testis*, testicle; G. *ektomē*, excision). The excision of a testicle; castration.

testibrā·chial (L. *testis*, testicle; *brakhiōn*, arm). Relating to the testibrachium.

testibrā·chium (L. *testis*, testicle; *brakhion*, the arm). The superior peduncle of the cerebellum.

tes·ticle (L. *testiculus*, dim. of *testis*, testicle). See testis.

tes·ticond (L. *testis*, testicle; *condere*, to hide). Having the testicles undescended.

testi·cular (L. *testiculus*, dim. of *testis*, testicle). Relating to the testicles. **T. fluid:** the semen. **T. therapy:** the therapeutic use of testicular extracts.

tes·tis (L. testicle). 1. One of the two semen-secreting glands of the male animal. 2. One of the two posterior tubercles of the corpora quadrigemina.

testŏ·pathy (L. *testis*, testicle; *pathos*, disease). Any disease of the testicles.

testŏ·sterone. $C_{19}H_{28}O_2$. An androgen, or testicular hormone. **T. proprionate:** $C_{22}H_{32}O_3$ prepared by treating t. with propionic anhydride and administered in oily injection.

Testoviron. A proprietary preparation of testosterone propionate.

tetā·nia (G. *tetanos*, tetanus). Tetany.

tetan·ic (G. *tetanos*, tetanus). 1. Relating to or resembling tetanus. 2. Causing tetanus.

tetā·niform (G. *tetanos*, tetanus; L. *forma*, form). Similar to tetanus.

tetanil·la (G. *tetanos*, tetanus). Tetany.

tĕ·tanine (G. *tetanos*, tetanus). A ptomaine from cultures of the bacillus of tetanus and from the tissues of patients affected with tetanus.

tetanizā·tion (G. *tetanos*, tetanus). The inducing of tetanic spasms.

tĕ·tanoid (G. *tetanos*, tetanus; *eidos*, form). Like tetanus.

tetanolȳ·sin (G. *tetanos*, tetanus; *lusis*, dissolution). The ingredient of tetanus-toxin which produces haemolysis.

tĕ·tanospas·min (G. *tetanos*, tetanus; *spasmos*, seizure). A specific neurotoxin which can be obtained from the toxin of tetanus.

tĕ·tanus (G. *tetanos*). 1. Lockjaw; an infectious disease marked by tonic spasms of voluntary muscles and extreme exaggeration of the reflexes. It is caused by the *Clostridium tetani.* 2. A tense tonic muscular spasm, especially such a spasm produced experimentally. **T. toxin:** a poisonous ptomaine formed from cultures of the *Clostridium tetani.* It causes tremor, paralysis and severe convulsions. **T. toxoid:** t. toxin after the removal of its toxicity by the action of chemical agents, but still retaining its immunizing properties.

tĕ·tany (G. *tetanos*, tetanus). A syndrome marked by intermittent, bilateral and painful tonic spasms of the muscles. It occurs most often in the upper extremities.

tetartanop·sia (G. *tetartos*, fourth; *an*, neg.; *opsis*, vision). Defect of vision in the corresponding quadrant of visual field of each eye.

tetrabā·sic. An acid having four replaceable hydrogen atoms.

tetrabrā·chius (G. *tetra*, from *tessara*, four; *brakhiōn*, arm). A four-armed monster.

tĕ·tracaine. Amethocaine hydrochloride, $C_{15}H_{24}O_2N_2$. HCl. The hydrochloride of *p-n*-butylaminobenzoic ester of β-dimethyl-aminoethanol. It is used as a local anaesthetic and for surface anaesthesia.

tetrachei·rus (G. *tetra*, from *tessara*, four; *kheir*, hand). A four-handed monster.

tetrachrō·mic (G. *tetra*, from *tessara*, four; *khroma*, colour). Able to perceive four colours only.

tetracoc·cus (G. *tetra*, from *tessara*, four; *kokkos*, berry). A micrococcus occurring in clusters and forming groups of four.

tĕ·trad (G. *tetras*, quadrant). 1. A group of four bodies. 2. An element with a valency of four.

tetra-ethyl lead. An organic compound of lead of a poisonous nature used in petrol as an 'anti-knock' substance.

tĕ·tragon (G. *tetra*, from *tessara*, four; *gōnia*, a corner). A quadrangle.

tĕtraiō·dophenolphthā·lein. Iodophthalein $C_{20}H_8O_4I_4$ $Na_2,3H_2O$. An iodine compound used in cholecystography.

tetrā·logy of Fallot (Fallot, L. A., French physician, 1850–1911). Congenital cardiac lesion consisting of: (1) Stenosis of pulmonary artery. (2) Patent interventricular septum. (3) Dextroposition of aorta so as to receive blood from right as well as left ventricle. (4) Hypertrophy of right ventricle.

tetramā·zia (G. *tetra*, from *tessara*, four; *mazos*, breast). The condition of having four breasts.

tetramĕ·thyl (G. *tetra*, four; *methu*, wine). Containing four methyl groups.

tetra-op·sis (G. *tetra*, from *tessara*, four; *opsis*, vision). A condition in which the visual field is limited to one quadrant.

tĕ·trose (G. *tetra*, from *tessara*, four). A sugar containing four carbon atoms in its molecule.

tetraplē·gia (G. *tetra*, from *tessara*, four; *plēgē*, stroke). Paralysis of the four extremities.

tĕ·trapus (G. *tetra*, from *tessara*, four; *pous*, foot). 1. Four-footed. 2. A monster with four feet.

tetrā·scelus (G. *tetra*, from *tessara*, four; *skēlos*, leg). A four-legged monster.

tetrā·ster (G. *tetra*, from *tessara*, four; *astēr*, star). The karyokinetic figure when there is a fourfold division of the nucleus, characterized by an arrangement of four stars.

tĕ·trastichī·asis (G. *tetra*, from *tessara*, four; *stikhos*, a row). The presence of four rows of eyelashes.

Tetrastō·ma (G. *tetra*, from *tessara*, four; *stoma*, mouth). A genus of trematodes.

tetrā·valent (G. *tetra*, from *tessara*, four; L. *valēre*, to be worth). Having a valency of four. See also quadrivalent.

tĕ·tronal. Diethylsulphondiethylmethane. A hypnotic.

tetronĕ·rythrin (G. *tetra*, from *tessara*, four; *eruthros*, red). A pigment existing in certain animals, e.g. the lobster.

tetrophthal·mos (G. *tetra*, from *tessara*, four; *ophthalmos*, eye). A monster with two faces and having two ears and four eyes.

tetrox·ide (G. *tetra*, from *tessara*, four; *oxus*, sharp). A compound of a base and four oxygen atoms.

Teutleben's ligament (Teutleben, F. E. K. von, German anatomist, born 1842). The pleuro-diaphragmatic ligament; ligamentum pulmonale.

tex·is (G., a child-bearing). Parturition.

textō·ma (L. *textus*, tissue). A tumour composed of undifferentiated cells.

textō·meter (L. *textus*, tissue; G. *meter*, mother). Protoplasm.

textoblā·stic (L. *textus*, tissue; G. *blastos*, germ). The formation of regenerative tissue.

tex·tural (L. *textura*, a web). Relating to a tissue.

texture (L. *textura*, tissue). The structure or substance of the body tissues.

Th. The symbol for thorium.

thā·lamencephā·lic (G. *thalamos*, chamber; *egkephalos*, brain). Relating to the thalamencephalon.

thā·lamencĕ·phalon (G. *thalamos*, chamber; *egkephalos*, brain). The posterior portion of the anterior embryonic brain-vesicle; the part of the brain derived from this portion of the anterior vesicle.

thalam·ic (G. *thalamos*, chamber). Relating to the optic thalamus.

thā·lamocoele (G. *thalamos*, chamber; *koilia*, a hollow). The third ventricle of the brain.

thā·lamocor·tical (G. *thalamos*, chamber; L. *cortex*, rind). Relating to the optic thalamus and the cortex of the brain.

thā·lamocrū·ral (G. *thalamos*, chamber; L. *crus*, leg). Relating to the optic thalamus and the crus cerebri.

thā·lamolentī·cular (G. *thalamos*, chamber; L. *lenticula*, lentil). Relating to the optic thalamus and the lenticular nucleus.

thă·lamus (G. *thalamos*, chamber). The great basal ganglion of the brain through which practically the whole of the sensory tracts must pass before diverging to the sensory area in the cortex. The primary visual centres are situated in its posterior portion.

thalassanae·mia (G. *thalassa*, sea; *an*, neg.; *haima*, blood). Anaemia occurring mainly in the Mediterranean area. Associated with splenomegaly, mongoloid facies, and changes in the bones.

thă·lassophō·bia (G. *thalassa*, sea; *phŏbos*, fear). Neurotic fear of the sea.

thă·lassothĕ·rapy (G. *thalassa*, sea; *therapeia*, treatment). Treatment by means of sea-bathing, sea-voyages, sea-air, etc.

thal·line (G. *thallos*, a green shoot). A liquid basic material, tetrahydroparamethyloxychinolin.

thal·lium (G. *thallos*, green shoot). A metallic element with an atomic weight of 204 and a specific gravity of 11·19. Symbol Tl. Salts of thallium are poisonous.

Thal·lophyte (G. *thallos*, green shoot; *phuton*, a plant). One of the lower groups of spore-forming plants.

thă·natognomon·ic (G. *thanatos*, death; *gnōmōn*, an indicator). Suggesting death.

thanato·graphy (G. *thanatos*, death; *graphein*, to write). 1. A disquisition on death. 2. A description by the patient of his feelings while dying.

thă·natoid (G. *thanatos*, death; *eidos*, form). Similar to death.

thă·natomā·nia (G. *thanatos*, death: *mania*, madness). Suicidal mania.

thanatŏ·meter (G. *thanatos*, death; *metron*, measure). An instrument used to prove that death has occurred by the reduction of bodily temperature.

thă·natophō·bia (G. *thanatos*, death; *phŏbos*, fear). A neurotic fear of death.

thă·natopsy (G. *thanatos*, death; *opsis*, vision). Necropsy.

thanatŏ·sis (G. *thanatos*, death). Gangrene.

thaumă·tropy (G. *thauma*, a wonder; *tropos*, a turn). The transformation of a structure into another structure.

thaumatur·gic (G. *thauma*, a wonder; *ergon*, a work). Miraculous.

thē·a (L.). Tea. The infused dried leaves of *Thea sinensis* make a stimulating and agreeable beverage.

thebā·ine (Named after the Greek town, Thebes). A poisonous alkaloid from opium, a powerful tetanizer. It is also called paramorphine.

thē·baism (G. town Thebes). Poisoning by opium; the condition induced by thebaine or paramorphine; opiumism.

Thebesius's foramina (Thebesius, A. C., Dutch anatomist, 1686–1732). The openings of the venae minimae of the heart. **T.'s valve**: the valvula sinus coronarii. **T.'s veins**: the venae minimae of the heart.

thē·ca (G. *thēkē*, a case). A sheath or enclosing membrane, especially of a tendon.

thē·cal (G. *thēkē*, a case). Relating to a sheath.

thē·cate (G. *thēkē*, a case). Sheathed; having a sheath.

theci·tis (G. *thēkē*, a case). Inflammation of a tendon sheath.

thē·ic (Fr. *thé*, tea). One who is immoderately addicted to tea.

Theile's canal (Theile, F. W., German anatomist, 1801–79). The space produced by the reflection of the pericardium on the aorta and pulmonary artery. **T.'s glands**: glandular formations in the walls of the gall-bladder and the cystic duct. **T.'s muscle**: m. transversus perinei superficialis, an inconstant subcutaneous muscle described also by Lesshaft.

Theilĕ·ria (Theiler, Sir A., Swiss biologist, 1867–1936). A genus of minute protozoal parasites.

thē·ine (F. *thé*, tea). The active principle of tea; the same as caffeine.

EE

thē·ism (F. *thé*, tea). The morbid condition due to excessive tea-drinking, characterized by headache, palpitation, tremor, insomnia, cachexia, etc.

thelal·gia (G. *thēlē*, nipple; *algos*, pain). Any pain of the nipple.

Thelā·zia. A genus of worms, some varieties of which are parasitic in the eyes of animals.

thē·leplasty (G. *thēlē*, nipple; *plassein*, to form). A plastic operation on the nipple.

theli·tis (G. *thēlē*, nipple). Inflammation of the nipple.

thē·lium (G. *thēlē*, nipple). 1. A papilla. 2. A nipple.

thelorrhā·gia (G. *thēlē*, nipple; *rhoia*, a flow). Haemorrhage of the nipple.

thē·lothism (G. *thēlē*, nipple; *ōtheein*, to push). Jutting out of the nipple.

thē·lyblast (G. *thēlus*, feminine; *blastos*, germ). The active centre of the female generative cell.

thelygĕ·nic (G. *thēlus*, feminine; *gennan*, to produce). Producing only female children.

thē·lyplasty (G. *thēlē*, nipple; *plassein*, to form). Plastic surgery of the nipple.

thē·nad (G. *thĕnar*, palm of the hand; L. *ad*, to). Towards the thenar eminence.

thē·nal (G. *thĕnar*, palm of the hand). Relating to the palm or the thenar eminence.

thē·nar (G. *thĕnar*, palm of the hand). 1. The palm of the hand or sole of the foot. 2. The fleshy mound situated at the base of the thumb.

Theobaldia (Theobald, F. V., English zoologist, 1868–1930). A genus of mosquito found in the temperate zones of both Eastern and Western Hemispheres.

Theobrō·ma (G. *theos*, god; *brōma*, food). A genus of trees including the *T. cacao*, the seeds of which are used in the preparation of chocolate and cocoa. They also yield an oil (cacao-butter) which is useful in the making of ointments, pills, etc.

theobrō·mine (G. *theos*, god; *brōma*, food). $C_7H_8O_2N_4$. 3:7: dimethylxanthine. A purine base closely related to caffeine and obtained from theobroma seeds.

theomā·nia (G. *theos*, god; *mania*, madness). Religious mania, especially the type in which the person believes himself to be divine.

theomā·nic (G. *theos*, god; *mania*, madness). A person affected with theomania.

theophyl·line (F. *thé*, tea; G. *phullon*, leaf). $C_7H_8O_2N_4$. 1:3: dimethylxanthine. A purine base closely related to caffeine and usually prepared by synthesis. Used as a diuretic.

theorĕ·tical (G. *theōrētikos*, contemplative). Depending upon theory; speculative.

thē·ory (G. *theōria*, theory). 1. The general principles of a science. 2. A reasonable assumption; a supposition broader and more probable than a hypothesis.

therapeu·tic (G. *therapeutikos*, from *therapeuein*, to attend). Relating to therapeutics; remedial. **T. test**: diagnosis by administration of remedies known to affect the supposed disease.

therapeu·tics (G. *therapeutikē*, treatment). The branch of medical science concerned with the application of remedies and the treatment of disease.

therapeu·tist (G. *therapeuein*, to attend). One skilled in therapeutics.

thē·rapist (G. *therapeia*, treatment). The same as therapeutist.

thē·rapy (G. *therapeia*, treatment). Therapeutics, *q.v.*

theri·aca (G. *thēriakē*, an antidote). Treacle. **T. andromachi**: Venice treacle, a compound comprising 64 ingredients and formerly used as an antidote against poisons.

theri·acal (G. *thēriakē*, an antidote). Useful as a snake-bite antidote.

therm (G. *thermē*, heat). A unit of heat, 100,000 British thermal units (B.T.U.). The latter is the amount of heat required to raise the temperature of one pound of water through 1° Fahrenheit.

ther·mea (G. *thermē*, heat). Hot springs.

thermaesthē·sia (G. *thermē*, heat; *aisthēsis*, feeling). The power of perceiving heat.

thermaesthesĭŏ·meter (G. *thermē*, heat; *aisthesis*, feeling; *metron*, measure). An instrument used to measure sensitivity to heat.

ther·mal (G. *thermē*, heat). Relating to or marked by heat.

thermalgē·sia (G. *thermē*, heat; *algos*, pain). A state in which heat causes pain.

thermanaesthē·sia (G. *thermē*, heat; *an*, neg.; *aisthesis*, feeling). Thermo-anaesthesia, q.v.

ther·mic (G. *thermē*, heat). Relating to heat.

thermo-anaesthē·sia (G. *thermē*, heat; *an*, neg.; *aisthesis*, feeling). Loss of the normal powers of the heat-sense. This condition is sometimes seen in cases of syringomyelia.

thermo-analgē·sia (G. *thermē*, heat; *an*, neg.; *algos*, pain). Insensibility to heat; caused by cerebral lesion.

ther·mocauterec·tomy (G. *thermē*, heat; *kautērion*, a branding iron; *ektomē*, excision). Extirpation by means of a cautery.

thermocau·tery (G. *thermē*, heat; *kautērion*, a branding iron). 1. A hollow point, usually made of platinum, maintained at a high temperature by means of a benzene vapour current. 2. Any instrument heated to act as a cautery.

thermochĕ·mistry (G. *thermē*, heat; Arab. *al-qimia*, chemistry). The branch of chemical science concerned with the relations between heat and chemical changes.

ther·mo-electri·city (G. *thermē*, heat; *ēlektron*, amber). Electricity generated by heat.

thermogĕ·nesis (G. *thermē*, heat; *genesis*, production). The production of heat.

thermogenet·ic, thermogēn·ic (G. *thermē*, heat; *gennan*, to produce). Relating to thermogenesis; producing heat.

ther·mograph (G. *thermē*, heat; *graphein*, to write). An instrument for automatically recording temperature variations.

ther·mohyperaesthē·sia (G. *thermē*, heat; *huper*, over; *aisthēsis*, feeling). Excessive acuity of the heat-sense.

ther·mohyperalgē·sia (G. *thermē*, heat; *huper*, over; *algos*, pain). A state in which severe pain is felt on the application of only moderate heat.

thermo-inhĭ·bitory (G. *thermē*, heat; L. *inhibēre*, to restrain). Inhibiting the production of heat.

thermolā·bile (G. *thermē*, heat; L. *labilis*, from *labi*, to slip). Capable of being changed or destroyed by heat.

thermŏ·lysis (G. *thermē*, heat; *lusis*, dissolution). 1. The dissipation of bodily heat. 2. Chemical decomposition produced by heat.

thermolyt·ic (G. *thermē*, heat; *lusis*, dissolution). Relating to thermolysis.

thermŏ·meter (G. *thermē*, heat; *metron*, measure). An instrument for measuring temperatures.

thermŏ·metry (G. *thermē*, heat; *metron*, measure). The use of the thermometer.

thermoneurō·sis (G. *thermē*, heat; *neuron*, nerve). Pyrexia of vasomotor origin.

ther·mophile (G. *thermē*, heat; *philein*, to love). A micro-organism which is unable to flourish unless it is kept at a very high degree of heat.

thermophil·ic (G. *thermē*, heat; *philein*, to love). Term applied to micro-organisms requiring great heat for growth.

thermophō·bia (G. *thermē*, heat; *phŏbos*, fear). Neurotic fear of heat.

ther·mophore (G. *thermē*, heat; *pherein*, to bear). 1. Any device for holding heat. In local treatment, e.g., a hot water-bottle. 2. A vessel containing chemicals

which absorb a considerable amount of heat and give it off by degrees during the process of crystallization.

thermoplē·gia (G. *thermē*, heat; *plēgē*, stroke). Heat-stroke.

ther·mopolypnoē·a (G. *thermē*, heat; *polus*, many; *pnoia*, breath). Rapid breathing due to high temperature.

thermostā·ble (G. *thermē*, heat; L. *stabilis*, firm). Not affected by heat.

ther·mostat (G. *thermē*, heat; *statos*, standing). A device for automatically registering the temperature and keeping it constant.

thermotac·tic (G. *thermē*, heat; *tassein*, to arrange). Relating to thermotaxis; regulating body heat.

thermotax·is (G. *thermē*, heat; *tassein*, to arrange). 1. The regulation or adjustment of body temperature. 2. Thermotropism.

thermothĕ·rapy (G. *thermē*, heat; *therapeia*, treatment). The treatment of disease by the application of heat.

thermŏ·tropism (G. *thermē*, heat; *tropos*, a turn). The peculiarity of certain cells and organisms which bend towards or away from a source of heat.

thē·sis (G. a position). A theory; usually a philosophical discussion concerning original research, and presented by a candidate for a higher university degree, such as that of Master or Doctor.

thiaē·mia (G. *theion*, sulphur; *haima*, blood). A condition in which sulphur is present in the blood.

thi·amin chloride. Thiamine hydrochloride, q.v.

thi·amine hydrochlor·ide. Aneurine hydrochloride, $C_{12}H_{17}ON_4SCl.HCl.H_2O_1$. Vitamin B_1, water-soluble, fat-soluble, thermolabile. The richest sources are whole cereal grains, yeast and pork. The anti-beri-beri vitamin.

Thiă·zamide. A proprietary brand of sulphathiazole.

thi·azole. The chemical ring system:

Thielmann's koleradraa·ber (Thielmann, K. H., German physician, 1802–72). A mixture of oil of peppermint 3, alcohol 90 per cent., 22, tincture of opium with saffron 10, tincture of ipecacuanha 25, ethereal tincture of valerian 40, used in the treatment of diarrhoea.

Thiersch's graft (Thiersch, K., German surgeon, 1822–95). A thin graft consisting of epidermis, rete and part of the cutis vera.

thigh. That portion of the lower limb which lies between the pelvis and the knee. **T.-bone:** the femur. **T.-joint:** the hip-joint.

thigmaesthē·sia (G. *thigma*, touch; *aisthēsis*, feeling). Sensitiveness to touch.

thĭ·ochrome (G. *theion*, sulphur; *khroma*, colour). The compound which gives the yellow colour to yeast.

thiogen·ic (G. *theion*, sulphur; *gennan*, to produce). Capable of transforming hydrogen sulphide into higher sulphur compounds.

thiopen·tone sodium.

$$CH_3(CH_2)_2.CH(CH_3)(C_2H_5).C.C(ONa){:}N.C(S).NH.CO.$$

A barbiturate derived from thiobarbituric acid; used intravenously for general anaesthesia.

thi·onin stain. $NH_2C_6H_3(NS).C_6H_3NH_2$. A dark green stain used in microscopy.

thi·ophene. The chemical ring system:

thī·osină·mine. (NH₂)CS.NHCH₂CH:CH₂, allyl thiourea. Used in an endeavour to resolve some of the scarring in certain skin conditions, e.g. lupus, dermatitis, etc.

thiou·racil. 2-mercapto-4-hydroxypyrimidine, prepared by the condensation of ethyl formylacetate with urea; used in the treatment of thyrotoxicosis. T. methyl and T. propyl are derivatives of thiouracil which are used in cases of thyrotoxicosis.

thio-ū·rea (G. *theion*, sulphur; *ouron*, urine). Sulphocarbamide; urea in which sulphur replaces oxygen.

third nerve. The oculomotor nerve.

thirst. A desire for water or other drink.

thlipsencě·phalus (G. *thlipsis*, pressure; *egkephalos*, brain). A monster in which there is extensive exposure of the base of the brain owing to the upper part of the skull being deficient or lacking.

Thomas's splint (Thomas, H. O., English surgeon, 1834–91). A splint designed primarily for first aid treatment of fractured femur. A leather-padded ring surrounds the upper part of the thigh and transmits weight through the ischial tuberosity. From this ring, on either side of the limb, metal bars extend, these being longer than the limb and joined by a cross-piece below the foot. Slings lie under the limb from the inner metal bar to the outer and extension to the limb may be attached to the lower cross-piece.

Thomsen's disease (Thomsen, A. J., Danish physician, 1815–96). See myotonia congenita.

Thomson's fascia (Thomson, A., Scottish anatomist, 1809–84). The ilio-pectineal fascia and septum.

Thiry's fistula (Thiry, J. H., Belgian physician, 1817–97). An artificial intestinal fistula for obtaining pure intestinal juices.

thrix annulā·ta (G. *thrix*, hair; L. *annulatus*, ringed). Ringed hair—a condition in which bands of light and dark colours are seen on the hair.

thŏ·racal (G. *thōrax*, the chest). Thoracic, *q.v.*

thoracentě·sis (G. *thōrax*, the chest; *kentēsis*, a pricking). Perforation of the thorax for the tapping of fluid.

thoră·cic (G. *thōrax*, the chest). Relating to or situated in the chest.

thoră·cico-abdŏ·minal (G. *thōrax* the chest; L. *abdōmen*). Relating to both the chest and the abdomen.

thŏ·racocoelŏ·schisis (G. *thōrax*, the chest; *koilia*, a hollow; *skhisis*, a cleaving). Fissure of the chest and the abdomen.

thŏ·racocyllŏ·sis (G. *thōrax*, the chest; *kullōsis*, a crippling). Malformation of the thorax.

thŏ·racocyrtŏ·sis (G. *thōrax*, the chest; *kurtos*, curved). Abnormal prominence of the chest.

thŏ·racodel·phus (G. *thōrax*, the chest; *adelphos*, brother). A double monster joined at a point above the navel. It has one head and two arms but four lower limbs.

thŏ·racodĭ·dymus (G. *thōrax*, the chest; *didumos*, twin). A double monster united at the chest.

thŏ·racodў·nia (G. *thōrax*, the chest; *odunē*, pain). Pain in the chest.

thŏ·racogastrŏ·schisis (G. *thōrax*, the chest; *gastēr*, belly; *skhisis*, a cleaving). Thoracocoeloschisis, *q.v.*

thoracoplă·sty (G. *thōrax*, the chest; *plassein*, form). Operation which is designed to collapse the chest wall and allow obliteration of pulmonary cavities in tuberculosis. It involves the excision of ribs.

thoracŏ·scopy (G. *thōrax*, the chest; *skopein*, to view). Examination of the chest, particularly by means of the endoscope.

thoracostenŏ·sis (G. *thōrax*, the chest; *stenos*, narrow). Compression of the thoracic walls.

thoracŏ·stomy (G. *thōrax*, the chest; *stoma*, mouth). The making of an aperture in the thorax, usually for drainage purposes.

thoracŏ·tomy (G. *thōrax*, the chest; *tomē*, section). Incision into the thoracic wall.

thoradel·phus (G. *thōrax*, the chest; *adelphos*, brother). A double monster joined above the navel, with one head, two arms and four lower limbs. Syn. thoracodelphus.

thor·ascope (G. *thōrax*, the chest; *skopein*, to view). Endoscope for viewing the pleural cavity. It is used also for division of pleural adhesions.

thor·ax (G.). The chest; that section of the body situated between the neck and the abdomen. It is bounded by the diaphragm below, anteriorly by the ribs and sternum and posteriorly by the ribs and the vertebral column and above by the neck. It contains the heart enveloped in the pericardium, the lungs enclosed in the pleura and the mediastinal structures.

Thorel's bundle (Thorel, G., German physician, 1868–1935). A bundle of muscle fibres found in the heart. This bundle passes round the opening of the inferior vena cava and connects the sino-auricular and auriculoventricular nodes.

thor·ium (Thor, one of the Nordic gods). A rare metal allied to tin. Symbol Th; atomic weight 234·4. It has radio-active properties.

Thormählen's test (Thormählen, J., German physician, qualified 1885). The production of a deep blue colour by addition of solution of sodium nitroprusside, potassium hydroxide and acetic acid to urine, when melanuria is present.

thornapple. Stramonium, *q.v.*

threadworm. Oxyuris, *q.v.*

three-day fever. Dengue, *q.v.*

thrĕ·onine. CH₃.CH(OH).CH(NH₂)COOH. One of the essential amino acids.

threp·sis (G.). Nutrition.

threpsŏ·logy (G. *threpsis*, nutrition; *logos*, a discourse). Nutritional science.

threshold. 1. The lowest level of stimulus which will produce a reaction; applicable to nervous reaction or to mental processes. 2. The lowest level of concentration of substance, e.g. sugar, in blood, above which excess is excreted in the urine—renal threshold.

thrill. A delicate vibration felt by the hand and perceived over an aneurysm, over a heart which has disease of the valves and also over hydatid cysts.

throat. 1. The front of the neck. 2. The pharynx. 3. The fauces.

throb. A pulsation or beat.

throbbing. A rhythmic pulsation.

throe. A paroxysm of extreme pain, as in parturition or at approaching death.

throm·base (G. *thrombos*, clot). Thrombin.

thrombec·tomy (G. *thrombos*, clot; *ektomē*, excision). The excision of a thrombus.

throm·bin (G. *thrombos*, clot). The fibrin-ferment; the enzyme producing coagulation of shed blood.

thrombi·nogen (G. *thrombos*, clot; *gennan*, to produce). Prothrombin.

thrombo-angii·tis (G. *thrombos*, clot; *aggeion*, vessel). Inflamed intima of a blood vessel with the formation of a clot. T.-a. obliterans: inflammatory and obliterative disease of the blood vessels of the extremities. Syn. Buerger's disease.

thrombo-arterī·tis (G. *thrombos*, clot; *arteria*, artery). Thrombosis accompanied by inflammation of an artery.

thromboclā·sis (G. *thrombos*, clot; *klasis*, a breaking). The breaking up or dispersal of a thrombus.

thrombocys·tis (G. *thrombos*, clot; *kustis*, bladder). The sac which sometimes encloses a thrombus.

throm·bocyte (G. *thrombos*, clot; *kutos*, a container). A blood platelet.

throm·bogen (G. *thrombos*, clot; *gennan*, to produce). Prothrombin, the precursor of thrombin.

thromboge·nesis (G. *thrombos*, clot; *genesis*, production). The forming of a clot.

thrombogen·ic (G. *thrombos*, clot; *gennan*, to produce). Forming a clot.

throm·boid (G. *thrombos*, clot; *eidos*, form). Resembling or having the character of a thrombus.

thromboki·nase (G. *thrombos*, clot; *kinein*, to move). A body tissue substance which can change thrombogen into thrombin.

thrombokine·sis (G. *thrombos*, clot; *kinesis*, movement). The clotting of blood.

throm·bolymphangi·tis (G. *thrombos*, clot; L. *lympha*, water; G. *aggeion*, vessel). Lymphangitis caused by a thrombus.

thrombo·lysis (G. *thrombos*, clot; *lusis*, dissolution). The dispersal of a thrombus.

throm·bophlebi·tis (G. *thrombos*, clot; *phleps*, vein). Thrombosis accompanied by inflammation of a vein.

thrombophthi·sis (G. *thrombos*, clot; *phthisis*, a wasting away). Destruction of blood-platelets produced by a disorder of bone marrow function.

thromboplas·tid (G. *thrombos*, clot; *plassein*, to form). A blood platelet.

thromboplas·tin (G. *thrombos*, clot; *plassein*, to form). A substance contained in the tissues which causes coagulation of blood.

throm·bosed (G. *thrombos*, clot). 1. Affected with thrombosis. 2. Clotted.

throm·bosin (G. *thrombos*, clot). Thrombin, *q.v.*

thrombot·ic (G. *thrombos*, clot). Relating to thrombosis.

throm·bus (G. *thrombos*, clot). A clot of blood in the heart or in a blood vessel, usually caused by slackened circulation or by changes in the blood or in the walls of blood vessels.

throttle. To strangle.

through-drainage. A form of drainage in which a perforated tube is inserted into the cavity, which is then flushed by the introduction of fluid into one end of the tube.

throw-back. The appearance of a characteristic which existed in remote ancestors; an organism exhibiting such characteristics.

thrush. 1. A variety of stomatitis due to fungi of the Oidium, Saccharomyces, or Monilia types, and characterized by the presence of white patches in the mouth. It usually occurs in debilitated children but may also affect adults. 2. A disease affecting the frog of a horse's hoof, marked by a foul discharge.

thryp·sis (G. *thrupsis*, comminution). A comminuted fracture.

thu·lium (*Thulē*, old name of Shetland). A rare element. Symbol Tm; atomic weight 168·5.

thumb. The digit on the extreme radial side of the hand, distinguished by having only two phalanges—all other digits having three. The metacarpal bone of the thumb is capable of separate movement.

thylaci·tis (G. *thulakos*, pouch). Inflammation of the sebaceous glands.

thyme (G. *thumon*). Any plant of the genus Thymus (Labiatae). **T. vulgaris:** a species which produces a volatile oil containing cymene, thymene and thymol.

thymec·tomy (G. *thŭmos*, the thymus gland; *ektomē*, excision). Excision of the thymus gland.

thymelco·sis (G. *thŭmos*, the thymus gland; *helkos*, ulcer). Ulceration of the thymus gland.

thy·mi oleum (G. *thŭmon*, thyme; L. *oleum*, oil). The volatile oil of garden thyme, from which thymol is derived.

thy·mic¹ (G. *thumon*, thyme). Relating to thyme. (Pronounced ti·mik.)

thy·mic² (G. *thŭmos*, the thymus gland). Relating to the thymus gland. (Pronounced thi·mik.)

thy·mion (G. *thumion*). A wart.

thymio·sis (G. *thumion*, a wart). 1. Yaws. 2. A state in which there is an appearance of wart-like growths.

thymi·tis (G. *thŭmos*, the thymus gland). Inflammation of the thymus gland.

thy·mol (G. *thumon*, thyme; L. *oleum*, oil). $C_6H_3(OH)(CH_3,(CH(CH_3)_2)(1:3:6)$. A crystalline phenol obtained from the volatile oil of *Thymus vulgaris* and from the volatile oils of a number of other labiate plants. It melts at 44° C. and is slightly soluble in water. It is used externally in the treatment of ulcers etc., and internally as an anthelminthic.

thymo·lysis (G. *thŭmos*, the thymus gland; *lusis*, dissolution). The destruction of thymus tissue.

thymo·pathy¹ (G. *thŭmos*, the thymus gland; *pathos*, disease). Any disorder of the thymus gland.

thymo·pathy² (G. *thŭmos*, mind; *pathos*, disease). Any mental disease.

thy·mus¹ (G. *thŭmos*, thymus gland). An organ situated in the anterior portion of the superior mediastinum. It grows until about the second year, remains unaffected until about the fourteenth year when it passes through certain fatty changes, after which it atrophies. The thymus consists of lobules consisting mainly of lymphadenoid tissue and contains minute concentric bodies, the corpuscles of Hassall.

Thymus². A genus of labiate plants. See thyme.

thy·rĕin (G. *thureos*, a shield). Iodothyrin, *q.v.*

thyremphrax·is (G. *thureos*, a shield; *emphraxis*, stoppage). Thyroid gland obstruction.

thyreo-arytae·noid. See thyro-arytaenoid.

thyreo-epiglot·tic. See thyro-epiglottic.

thy·reohyroi·deus. See thyro-hyoid.

thyro-adeni·tis (G. *thureos*, shield; *adēn*, gland). Inflammation of the thyroid gland.

thyro-arytae·noid (G. *thureos*, shield; *arutaina*, a ladle; *eidos*, form). Relating to the thyroid and arytenoid cartilages. **T. muscle:** see under muscle.

thy·rocele (G. *thureos*, shield; *kēlē*, hernia). A tumour involving the thyroid gland; a goitre.

thyrochondro·tomy (G. *thureos*, shield; *khondros*, cartilage; *tomē*, section). Incision into the thyroid cartilage.

thyro-epiglot·tic (G. *thureos*, shield; *epi*, upon; *glōttis*, mouth of the windpipe). Relating both to the thyroid cartilage and the epiglottis.

thyro-epiglotti·deus (G. *thureos*, shield; *epi*, upon; *glōttis*, mouth of the windpipe). See under muscle.

thyroglo·bulin (G. *thureos*, shield; L. *globulus*, dim. of *globus*, globe). The iodine protein of the thyroid gland, which secretes it. It settles in the colloid substance.

thyroglos·sal (G. *thureos*, a shield; *glōssa*, tongue). Relating to the thyroid gland and the tongue.

thyrohy·oid (G. *thureos*, shield; *huoeidēs*, shaped like the letter y). Relating to the thyroid gland or cartilage and the hyoid bone.

thy·rohyoi·deus (G. *thureos*, shield; *huoeidēs*, shaped like the letter y). See under muscle.

thy·roid (G. *thureos*, shield; *eidos*, form). 1. Shaped like a shield. 2. Relating to the thyroid gland or cartilage or to the thyroid foramen. 3. The thyroid gland. **T. cartilage:** the shield-shaped structure lying between the hyoid bone and the first ring of the larynx. **T. gland:** see gland. **T. therapy:** the treatment of disease by the administration of thyroid extract.

thyroidec·tomy (G. *thureos*, shield; *eidos*, form; *ektomē*, excision). Removal of the thyroid gland.

thy·roidism (G. *thureos*, shield; *edois*, form). 1. A toxic condition due to over-use of thyroid gland preparations. 2. The disturbances due to hyperthyroidism. 3. The after-effects caused by excision of the thyroid gland.

thyroidi·tis (G. *thureos*, shield; *eidos*, form). Inflammation of the thyroid gland.

thyroidŏ·tomy (G. *thureos*, shield; *eidos*, form; *tomē*, section). Incision into the thyroid gland.

thyro-iodine (G. *thureos*, shield; *iŏdēs*, violet-like). A substance usually found in combination with a protein, but also free, in the thyroid gland. Syn. iodothyrin.

thyron·cus (G. *thureos*, shield; *ogkos*, a mass). Thyrocele, *q.v.*

thyrophy·ma (G. *thureos*, shield; *phuma*, tumour). A tumour of the thyroid gland.

thyropri·val (G. *thureos*, shield; L. *privare*, to deprive). Caused by removal or cessation of function of the thyroid gland.

thyropri·vus (G. *thureos*, shield; L. *privare*, to deprive). 1. Lacking the thyroid gland. 2. A morbid state caused by loss of the thyroid gland.

thyroprō·tein (G. *thureos*, shield; *prōtŏs*, first). A toxic protein obtained from the thyroid gland.

thyroptō·sis (G. *thureos*, shield; *ptōsis*, a falling). Dislodgement of a goitrous thyroid so that it is concealed in the thorax.

thyrō·sis (G. *thureos*, shield). Any disorder or disease resulting from the malfunctioning of the thyroid gland.

thȳ·rotome (G. *thureos*, shield; *tomē*, section). A surgical instrument used for incising the thyroid cartilage.

thyrŏ·tomy (G. *thureos*, shield; *tomē*, section). 1. The operation of dividing the thyroid cartilage. 2. Incising the thyroid gland.

thȳ·rotoxicō·sis (G. *thureos*, shield; *toxikon*, poison). Condition caused by adenoma of the thyroid gland and its toxic activity. Syn. hyperthyroidism.

thȳ·rotrope (G. *thureos*, shield; *tropos*, a turn). One possessing a constitution affected by thyroid gland disorder.

thyrŏ·tropism (G. *thureos*, shield; *tropos*, a turn). A form of endocrine constitution in which the influence of the thyroid gland predominates.

thyroxinae·mia (G. *thureos*, shield; *oxus*, sharp; *haima*, blood). The presence of thyroxine in the blood.

thyrox·ine. $C_{15}H_{11}NO_4I_4$. The active thyrotropic substance of the thyroid gland, now prepared more cheaply by synthesis. Used for thyroid deficiency in humans and to increase lactation in cattle.

Ti. The symbol for Titanium.

ti·bia (L.). The larger of the two bones in the lower part of the leg, popularly called the shinbone. It articulates with the femur, fibula and astragalus.

ti·bial (L. *tibia*, shin-bone). Relating to the tibia.

tibiǎl·gia (L. *tibia*, shin-bone; G. *algos*, pain). Pain in the shinbone.

tibiocalcā·nean (L. *tibia*, shin-bone; *calcaneum*, the heel). Relating to the tibia and the calcaneus.

tibiofē·moral (L. *tibia*, shin-bone; *femur*, thigh). Relating to the tibia and the femur.

tibiofi·bular (L. *tibia*, shin-bone; *fibula*, a clasp). Relating to the tibia and the fibula.

tibiotar·sal (L. *tibia*, shin-bone; G. *tarsos*, the flat of the foot). Relating to the tibia and the tarsus.

tic (Fr.). A spasmodic twitching, especially of the muscles of the face. **T. convulsif:** facial spasms in the area supplied by the seventh nerve. **T. douloureux:** spasmodic neuralgia in the area of the trifacial nerve.

tick. Popular name given to a number of blood-sucking parasites of the genus Acarus. **T. fever:** 1. Texas fever; 2. Rocky Mountain spotted fever; 3. African relapsing fever.

tickle. To titillate; to touch so as to cause a sensation that usually produces laughter and reflex muscular movements.

t.i.d. Abbreviation for L. *ter in die*, three times daily.

tidal breathing. Cheyne-Stokes respiration, in which respirations increase rhythmically up to a certain point, then gradually decrease until they temporarily cease. It is observed in certain disorders of the heart and lungs.

Tiedmann's glands (Tiedmann, F., German anatomist, 1781–1861). Bartholin's glands; Duverney's glands. **T.'s nerve:** a minute sympathetic nerve said to run with the arteria centralis retinae.

tigretier (Fr.). A kind of tarantism caused by the bite of a poisonous spider.

ti·groid (G. *tigroeidēs*, tiger-like). An epithet applied to chromophile corpuscles, finely granular bodies, varying in size and shape, made visible in the cytoreticulum by staining with Nissl's stain. **T. fundus:** the fundus oculi patterned with dark stripes.

til·mus (G. *tilmos*, a plucking). The plucking out of the hair.

timbre (Fr.). The distinctive quality of a sound or tone.

Timofeev's nerve endings (Timofeev, D. A., Russian anatomist; work published in 1894 and 1902). Supposed sympathetic nerve endings of a sensory nature.

tin. A grey-white, metallic malleable element. Symbol Sn. (L. *stannum*); specific gravity 7·3; atomic weight 118.7. **T. chloride:** a compound used as a reagent; also called stannous chloride.

tinct. Abbreviation for tincture.

tinc·tion (L. *tingere*, to dye). 1. A staining agent. 2. The act of staining.

tinctū·ra (L.). Tincture.

tinc·ture (L. *tinctura*, a dyeing). The alcoholic extract of a vegetable drug, usually of such a strength that one part by weight of drug is equivalent to ten parts by volume of tincture. Main exceptions are t. of nux vomica (1:12) and t. of ipecacuanha (1:20).

ti·nea (L., moth). Ringworm; a term characterizing a class of skin diseases due to invasion of parasitic fungi. **T. cruris:** ringworm of the leg. Syn. dhobie itch. **T. versicolor:** pityriasis versicolor. A skin disease caused by Malassezia furfur. Macules appear on the shoulder, chest, back and upper abdomen.

Tinel's sign (Tinel, J., French neurologist, born 1879). A sign indicating a partial lesion or the beginning of regeneration in a divided nerve. Percussion over the site of division produces tingling in region of nerve distribution.

tingle. A pricking sensation; a sudden but not severe pain.

tinkling. A chinking sound heard on auscultation over large pulmonary cavities and also in pneumothorax.

tinni·tus (L. *tinnitus*, a ringing sound). A singing or roaring sound in the ears.

tiqueur (Fr.). One affected with the spasmodic movements designated tics.

tire. To become weary.

tiredness. The state of being weary.

tisane (Fr.). A decoction having slight restorative properties.

tis·sue. A collection of cells or fibres of similar function forming a structure. **T. culture:** a culture of fresh animal tissue in nutrient agar to which has been added one half its volume of ascitic or hydrocele fluid. Paraffin oil floated on the surface favours anaerobic conditions.

titā·nium (G. *Titan*, a mythical giant). A metal related to iron, chromium and tin. Atomic weight 48·1; specific gravity 58. Its medicinal properties are obscure.

titillā·tion (L. *titillatio*). Tickling or the sensation produced by it.

ti'trate (Fr. *titre*, standard). To determine volumetrically by the use of standard solutions of known strength.

titrā·tion (Fr. *titre*, standard). Volumetric analysis by means of standard solutions.

ti·tre (Fr.). A standard of strength or purity.

titubā·tion (L. *titubatio*, a staggering). A reeling gait observed particularly in diseases of the cerebellum.

Tl. The symbol for thallium.

Tm. The symbol for thulium.

TNT. Abbreviation for trinitrotoluene, $CH_3.C_6H_2(NO_2)_3$.

toad-head. A form of head sometimes occurring in acephalous monsters.

tobac·co (Sp. *tabaco*). A plant, *Nicotiana tabacum*, the dried leaves of which (*Tabaci folia*, B.P.) contain a liquid alkaloid, nicotine, one of the most active poisons known. T. is employed as a sedative in most parts of the world, being smoked, chewed or used as snuff. It is a nauseant, anti-spasmodic and depressant. **T.-amblyopia:** amblyopia produced by excessive use of t. **T.-heart:** an irritable heart condition caused by excessive use of tobacco.

tobac·coism (Sp. *tabaco*, tobacco). A morbid state produced by the excessive use of tobacco.

toco·logy (G. *tokos*, birth; *logos*, a treatise). Obstetrical science.

tocophĕ·ryl acetate. $C_{31}H_{52}O_3$. The acetate of α-tocopherol, one form of vitamin E, the antisterility vitamin. The acetate is used as it is far more stable than tocopherol itself. α-tocopherol occurs in wheat germ oil together with β and γ tocopherol.

Tod's muscle (Tod, D., Scottish otologist, work published in 1832). The musculus obliquus auriculae, situated on the posterior aspect of the concha.

Todaro's tendon (Todaro, F., Italian anatomist, 1839–1918). The variable tendinous strand attached to the Eustachian valve in the heart.

Todd bodies (Todd, J. L., Canadian physician, born 1876). Eosinophil structures found in the cytoplasm of the red blood cells of certain amphibians.

Todd's paralysis (Todd, R. B., Irish physician in London, 1809–60). A transient weakness of affected muscles which sometimes follows localized or Jacksonian convulsions.

toe. A digit of the foot.

tokŏ·logy (G. *tokos*, birth; *logos*, a treatise). See Tocology.

tō·kus (G. *tokos*, birth). Childbirth.

Toldt's fascia (Toldt, K., Austrian anatomist, 1840-1920). The fixation of fascial planes behind the body of the pancreas. **T.'s membrane:** the prerenal fascia.

tŏ·lerance (L. *tolerare*, to endure). Capacity to endure the influence of a drug. **T., acquired:** increased resistance to the effects of a drug.

tŏ·lerant (L. *tolerare*, to endure). Withstanding the action of a medicine without suffering harm.

tŏ·lu (Santiago de Tolu, Colombia, where it was first obtained). Balsam of Tolu, obtained from the *Toluifera balsamum*, and used as an expectorant and stomachic.

tŏ·luene. Methylbenzene; a hydrocarbon derived from coal-tar and also from tolu balsam and other resins by distillation.

tolu·idine. A compound homologous with aniline prepared from toluene. It is bactericidal in action.

toma·to (Sp. *tomate*, from Mex. *tomatl*). The fruit of *Lycopersicum esculentum*.

tomen·tum (L. a stuffing for cushions). A network of small blood-vessels of the pia, which enters the cortex of the brain.

Tomes's fibres (Tomes, Sir J., English dental surgeon, 1815–95). The dentinal fibrils. Some works of reference wrongly ascribe the fibres to C. S. Tomes, son of the above.

Tomes's processes (Tomes, C. S., English odontologist, 1846–1928). The processes of the enamel cells; ameloblast processes.

tomomā·nia (G. *tomē*, section; *mania*, madness). 1. An excessive desire to perform surgical operations. 2. An excessive desire to undergo surgical operations.

tonaphā·sis (G. *tonos*, tone; *aphasia*, speechlessness). Musical aphasia.

tone (G. *tonos*, tone). 1. A distinct quality of sound. 2. The proper state of tension of any part or of the whole body.

tongue. The mobile muscular organ situated on the floor of the mouth and used in the processes of tasting, masticating, swallowing and speaking. It is controlled by a number of muscles and enveloped in mucous membrane from which numerous papillae project. In the papillae are located the taste buds.

tŏ·nic (G. *tonikos*, from *tonos*, tone). 1. Relating to tone; causing normal tone. 2. Marked by tension or contraction, as t. spasm. 3. An agent imparting normal tone to a part or to the whole organism.

toni·city (G. *tonos*, tone). The state of normal tone or tension of an organ or of the whole body.

tŏ·nitrophō·bia (L. *tonitrus*, thunder; G. *phŏbos*, fear). Morbid fear of thunder.

ton·ka bean. The seed of *Dipteryx odorata*, an American tree; it contains coumarin and is a useful flavouring agent.

tō·nograph (G. *tonos*, tone; *graphein*, to write). An instrument registering the tension of the arterial blood-current.

tonŏ·meter (G. *tonos*, tone; *metron*, measure). An instrument used for measuring tensions.

ton·sil (L. *tonsillae*, the tonsils). 1. Either of the two small almond-shaped bodies situated on each side of the fauces between the palatal pillars. The tonsil is composed of about 10–18 lymph-follicles and is enveloped in mucous membrane. 2. A small rounded portion of the cerebellar hemisphere, situated on the inferior surface.

tonsil·la (L.). A tonsil. **T. cerebelli:** one of the lobes of the cerebellar hemisphere.

tonsil·lar (L. *tonsillae*, the tonsils). 1. Relating to a tonsil. 2. Acting upon a tonsil, as t. abscess.

tonsillec·tome (L. *tonsillae*, the tonsils; G. *ektomē*, excision). An instrument used in removing a tonsil.

tonsillec·tomy (L. *tonsillae*, the tonsils; G. *ektomē*, excision). The surgical removal of a tonsil.

tonsilli·tis (L. *tonsillae*, the tonsils). Inflammation of a tonsil. **T., Vincent's:** t. resulting from Vincent's spirillum.

tonsil·lolith (L. *tonsillae*, the tonsils; G. *lithos*, stone). A tonsillar calculus.

ton·sillotome (L. *tonsillae*, the tonsils; G. *tomē*, section). Tonsillectome, *q.v.*

tonsillŏ·tomy (L. *tonsillae*, the tonsils; *tomē*, section). The operation of excising the whole or part of a tonsil.

ton·sure (L. *tonsura*, from *tondēre*, to shave). The shaving or clipping of hair away from any part.

tō·nus (G. *tonos*, tone). Tone, *q.v.*

tooth. One of the small bone-like structures situated in the alveolar processes of the jaws and used for the mastication of food.

Tooth's atrophy (Tooth, H. H., English physician, 1856–1926). The peroneal type of progressive muscular atrophy.

toothed. Possessing teeth; dentate.

topaesthē·sia (G. *topos*, place; *aisthēsis*, feeling). Local sensitiveness to touch.

topagnō·sis (G. *topos*, place; *a*, neg.; *gnosis*, knowledge). Loss of sensitiveness to touch localisation.

topal·gia (G. *topos*, place; *algos*, pain). Pain in a limited area. Syn. topo-algia.

Töpfer's test (Töpfer, A. E., German physician, born 1858). A test for HCl in gastric contents, giving a red colour with Töpfer's reagent (dimethyl-amino-azobenzene).

tophä·ceous (L. *tophus*, It. *tufa*, a light, porous stone). Gritty.

tō·phus (L. *tophus*, tufa. Pl. *tophi*). 1. Hard gritty deposits of sodium urate formed in the joints in cases of gout. 2. Dental tartar. 3. A syphilitic node.

tŏ·pical (G. *topos*, place). Local.

Topinard's angle (Topinard, P., French scientist, 1830–1912). The ophryospinal angle. **T.'s line:** that between the glabella and the mental point.

topo-al·gia (G. *topos*, place; *algos*, pain). Local pain; usually experienced in neurasthenia and often felt after emotional disturbances. Syn. topalgia.

topogrǎ·phical (G. *topos*, place; *graphein*, to write). Relating to a locality.

topǒ·graphy (G. *topos*, place; *graphein*, to write). A study of the areas of the body or its parts.

toponeurō·sis (G. *topos*, place; *neuron*, nerve). Any localized neurosis.

topǒ·nymy (G. *topos*, place; *ŏnŏma*, a name). Names pertaining to the position of organs.

topophŏ·bia (G. *topos*, place; *phŏbos*, fear). Neurotic fear of certain places.

tor·cular Herŏ·phili (L., the winepress of Herophilus). The expanded extremity of the superior longitudinal sinus, situated in a depression on the inner surface of the occipital bone.

tor·ic (L. *tŏrus*, a knot). Relating to a torus.

tor·men (L. *tormina*, colic). Tormina, *q.v.*

tormen·til (L. *tormentum*, pain). The rhizome of the plant *Potentilla tormentilla*, which is tonic and astringent in action.

tor·mina (L.). Griping pains in the intestines.

tor·minal, tor·minous (L. *tormina*, colic). Relating to or affected with tormina.

tor·pent (L. *torpēre*, to be inactive). 1. Incapable of normal functioning; inactive. 2. Any agent that allays irritation.

tor·pid (L. *torpidus*, stupefied). Sluggish; inactive.

torpi·dity (L. *torpidus*, stupefied). Torpor, *q.v.*

tor·por. Sluggishness; lack of reaction to normal stimuli.

torrefac·tion (L. *torrefacere*, to parch). Roasting or drying by the application of strong heat.

tor·refy (L. *torrefacere*, to parch). To roast; to parch; to dry by the application of strong heat.

Torres-Teixeira inclusion bodies. Inclusion bodies present in the cells in variola minor.

tor·sion (L. *torquere*, to twist). 1. A twisting, as of the bowel. 2. The rotation of the eye about the visual axis. 3. Inclination of the vertical meridian of the eye. **T. spasm:** spasm produced by torsion.

tor·so (It.). The trunk of the body, excluding the head and limbs.

torso-occlū·sion (L. *torquere*, to twist; *occludere*, to close). The position of a tooth when turned on its long axis out of its proper place.

tort (L. *torquere*, to twist). To incline the vertical meridian of the eye. **Extort:** to incline the v.m. outward. **Intort:** to incline the v.m. inward.

torticol·lis (L. *torquere*, to twist; *collum*, neck). Wry-neck; a contraction of the cervical muscles (usually those on one side), causing the head to be carried in an abnormal posture. Syn. caput obstipum.

tor·tuous (L. *torquere*, to twist). Twisted.

Tor·ula (L. *tŏrŭlus*, a tuft). 1. A genus of fungi, many species of which are alcoholic ferments. 2. A genus of moulds.

torulō·sis (L. *torulus*, a tuft). A state brought about by infection with fungi of the genus Torula.

tor·ulus (L., a tuft). A small prominence or elevation.

tor·us (L., a knot). A swelling; a bulging projection. **T. occipitalis:** external occipital protuberance. **T. palatinus:** a palatine protuberance at the union of the palatomaxillary and intermaxillary sutures. **T. uterinus:** a transverse ridge due to reflection of the peritoneum from the uterus to the posterior vaginal wall.

totaquin. A mixture of alkaloids from cinchona bark. It must contain at least 70 per cent of crystallisable alkaloids of which at least one-fifth must be quinine. Used in malaria.

touch. 1. The tactile sense. 2. The act of judging by the tactile sense; palpation. 3. In obstetrics, digital examination of the female genital adjacent parts through the vagina.

Tourette's disease (Tourette, G. G. de la, French physician, 1857–1904). A neurological condition characterized by incoordination, speech disorders and convulsions.

tour·niquet (Fr.). A bandage or instrument for controlling circulation by compression.

Tourtual's membrane (Tourtual, K. T., German anatomist, 1802–65). The quadrangular membrane; arytaeno-epiglottidean ligaments. **T.'s sinus:** the supratonsillar fossa.

toxae·mia (G. *toxikon*, poison; *haima*, blood). Blood-poisoning, a condition in which the blood contains poisonous substances generally due to the absorption of toxins from a local infection.

toxal·bumin (G. *toxikon*, poison; L. *albumen*, white of egg). A toxic protein.

toxal·bumose (G. *toxicon*, poison; L. *albumen*, white of egg). A poisonous albumose.

toxǎ·mines (G. *toxikon*, poison; G. *ammoniakon*, rock-salt). Poisonous substances in such cereals as oatmeal and wheat which hinder the proper development of bone and produce severe nervous disturbances unless balanced by the addition of vitamins, e.g. butter on bread, or milk with porridge.

toxanae·mia (G. *toxikon*, poison; *an*, neg.; *haima*, blood). Anaemia caused by poison.

Toxas·caris. A genus of nematodes. **T. canis:** the roundworm infesting dogs.

toxen·zyme (G. *toxikon*, poison; *en*, in; *zumē*, a leaven). A poisonous enzyme.

tox·ic (G. *toxikon*, poison). 1. Poisonous; caused by poison. 2. Relating to a toxin.

toxi·city (G. *toxikon*, poison). The quality of being poisonous.

toxicoder·ma (G. *toxikon*, poison; *derma*, skin). Skin disease caused by poison.

toxicodermati·tis (G. *toxikon*, poison; *derma*, skin). Inflammatory skin disease caused by poison.

toxicogen·ic (G. *toxikon*, poison; *gennan*, to produce). Producing a poison.

toxicohae·mia (G. *toxikon*, poison; *haima*, blood). Toxaemia, *q.v.*

tox·icoid (G. *toxikon*, poison; *eidos*, form). Resembling a poison.

toxicǒ·logist (G. *toxikon*, poison; *logos*, a treatise). One skilled in detecting poisons and treating subjects affected with poisoning.

toxicǒ·logy (G. *toxikon*, poison; *logos*, treatise). The study of poisons, their detection and the treatment of their effects.

toxicomā·nia (G. *toxikon*, poison; *mania*, madness). 1. A neurotic desire to take poisonous substances. 2. Toxicophobia.

toxicomū·cin (G. *toxikon*, poison; L. *mucus*). A poisonous albuminoid substance.

toxicǒ·pathy (G. *toxikon*, poison; *pathos*, disease). Any disease produced by poison.

toxicopex·is (G. *toxikon*, poison; *pēxis*, fixation). Neutralization or fixation of poisons.

toxicophō·bia (G. *toxikon*, poison; *phŏbos*, fear). Neurotic fear of being poisoned.

toxicophylax·in (G. *toxikon*, poison; *phulax*, a guard). A phylaxin which counteracts or destroys the toxic products of pathogenic bacteria.

toxicō·sis (G. *toxikon*, poison). A condition of being poisoned.

toxidermi·tis (G. *toxikon*, poison; *derma*, skin). Toxicodermatitis, *q.v.*

toxi·ferous (G. *toxikon*, poison; L. *ferre*, to bear). Producing or transmitting poison.

toxi·genous (G. *toxikon*, poison; *gennan*, to produce). Producing poisons.

tox·in (G. *toxikon*, poison). 1. Any poisonous compound of nitrogenous character derived from animal or vegetable cells. 2. Any poisonous protein from animal or vegetable cells that yields specific antitoxins that may be used in immunization.

toxinae·mia (G. *toxikon*, poison; *haima*, blood). Toxaemia, *q.v.*

toxin-antitoxin. A mixture in which the toxin present is almost neutralized by the appropriate antitoxin.

toxinfec·tion (G. *toxikon*, poison; L. *inficere*, to dye). Infection through a toxin caused by an unseen microorganism.

toxin·ic (G. *toxicon*, poison). Relating to a toxin.

toxi·nicide (G. *toxikon*, poison; *caedere*, to kill). Any agent capable of destroying toxins.

toxinō·sis (G. *toxikon*, poison). Any disease caused by poison.

toxiphō·bia (G. *toxikon*, poison; *phŏbos*, fear). Toxicophobia, *q.v.*

tox·oid (G. *toxikon*, poison; *eidos*, form). A toxin transformation-product without toxicity but still possessing antigenic properties.

toxoid-antitoxoid. A mixture of toxoid and antitoxic serum.

toxoli·poid (G. *toxikon*, poison; *lipos*, fat; *eidos*, form). An antigen obtained by combining a lipoid with a toxin.

toxŏ·lysin (G. *toxikon*, poison; *lusis*, dissolution). Antitoxin, *q.v.*

toxomū·cin (G. *toxikon*, poison; L. *mucus*) Toxicomucin, *q.v.*

toxon, toxone (G. *toxikon*, poison). A diphtheritic poison producing a disease with a prolonged course and having less affinity for antitoxin than has toxin.

tox·ophile (G. *toxikon*, poison; *philein*, to love). Having an affinity for toxins or poisons.

tox·ophore (G. *toxikon*, poison; *pherein*, to bear). The atomic complex of a toxin unit, comprising the poisonous element of a toxin. **T.-group:** that portion of the toxin molecule that produces the poisonous effect.

toxŏ·phorous (G. *toxikon*, poison; *pherein*, to bear). Relating to the toxophore.

toxophylax·in (G. *toxikon*, poison; *phulax*, a guard). Toxicophylaxin, *q.v.*

toxosō·zin (G. *toxikon*, poison; *sōzein*, to save). A sozin acting against bacterial poisons.

Toynbee's corpuscles (Toynbee, J., English otologist, 1815–66). The so-called corneal corpuscles. **T.'s muscle:** m. tensor tympani. This muscle was well known to Eustachius and the older anatomists, and was given its definitive name by Albinus.

trā·bal (L. *trabs*, a timber). Relating to the trabs cerebri or corpus callosum.

trabē·cula (L. *trabecula*, dim. of *trabs*, a timber). Any of the septa passing from the envelope or capsule into the interior of an organ.

trabē·cular (L. *trabecula*, dim. of *trabs*, a timber). Relating to a trabecula.

trabē·culate (L. *trabecula*, dim. of *trabs*, a timber). Relating to or of the nature of a trabecula.

trabs (L., a timber). The corpus callosum or trabs cerebri.

trace 1. A mark. 2. A minute quantity.

trā·cer. A dissecting instrument used to isolate nerves and vessels by lacerating the connective tissue. **T. element:** Syn. radioactive isotope.

trā·chea (G. *trakheia*, fem. of *trakhus*, rugged). The windpipe, the cartilaginous and membranous tube extending from the inferior part of the larynx to the bronchi.

trā·cheĕc·tasy (G. *trakhus*, rugged; *ektasis*, extension). Dilatation of the trachea.

trā·cheal (G. *trakhus*, rugged). Relating to the trachea.

tracheăl·gia (G. *trakhus*, rugged; *algos*, pain). Any tracheal pain.

tracheĭ·tis (G. *trakhus*, rugged). Inflammation of the trachea.

trā·chelaematō·ma (G. *trakhēlos*, neck; *haima*, blood). A haematoma of the neck or of the sternomastoid muscle.

trachelă·gra (G. *trakhēlos*, neck; *agra*, seizure). Gout affecting the neck.

trachelomas·toid (G. *trakhēlos*, neck; *mastos*, the breast; *eidos*, form). Relating to the neck and the mastoid process.

trā·chelectŏ·mopexy (G. *trakhēlos*, neck; *ektomē*, excision; *pēxis*, fixation). Partial excision of the uterus and fixation of the cervix uteri.

trachelis·mus (G. *trakhēlos*, neck). Spasmodic contraction of the neck muscles.

trachelī·tis (G. *trakhēlos*, neck). Inflammation of the cervix uteri; cervicitis.

trachelŏ·logist (G. *trakhēlos*, neck; *logos*, a discourse). A specialist in trachelology.

trachelŏ·logy (G. *trakhēlos*, neck; *logos*, a discourse). The study of the neck and its diseases.

trā·chelomyī·tis (G. *trakhēlos*, neck; *mus*, muscle). Inflammation of the neck muscles.

trā·chelo-occipitā·lis muscle (G. *trakhēlos*, neck; L. *occiput*). The complexus muscle.

trā·chelopex·is, trā·chelopexy (G. *trakhēlos*, neck; *pēxis*, fixation). Fixation of the neck of the uterus.

trā·cheloplasty (G. *trakhēlos*, neck; *plassein*, to form). A plastic operation on the cervix uteri.

trachelor·rhaphy (G. *trakhēlos*, neck; *rhaphē*, suture). Suture of a laceration of the neck of the uterus.

trachelŏ·schisis (G. *trakhēlos*, neck; *skhisis*, a splitting). Congenital cleft in the neck.

trachelŏ·tomy (G. *trakhēlos*, neck; *tomē*, section). Incision of the cervix uteri.

trā·cheo-aerocele (G. *trakhus*, rugged; *aēr*, air; *kēlē*, hernia). An air-containing diverticulum of the trachea.

trā·cheobron·chial (G. *trakhus*, rugged; *brogkia*, the bronchial tubes). Relating to the trachea and the bronchi.

trā·cheobronchī·tis (G. *trakhus*, rugged; *brogkhos*, windpipe). An inflammation involving the trachea and bronchi.

trā·cheolaryn·geal (G. *trakhus*, rugged; *larugx*, larynx). Relating to the trachea and the larynx.

trā·cheolaryngŏ·tomy (G. *trakhus*, rugged; *larugx*, larynx; *tomē*, section). Combined laryngotomy and tracheotomy.

trā·cheomalā·cia (G. *trakhus*, rugged; *malakia*, soft). Morbid softening of the tracheal cartilage.

trā·cheo-oesophă·geal (G. *trakhus*, rugged; *oisophagos*, the gullet). Relating to the trachea and the oesophagus.

tracheopă·thia, tracheŏ·pathy (G. *trakhus*, rugged; *pathos*, disease). Any disease or disorder of the trachea.

trā·cheopharyn·geal (G. *trakhus*, rugged; *pharugx*, the throat). Relating to the trachea and the pharynx.

trachĕŏ·scopy (G. *trakhus*, rugged; *skopein*, to inspect). Examination of the interior of the trachea by a laryngoscopic mirror and reflected light.

tră·cheostenō·sis (G. *trakhus*, rugged; *stenos*, narrow). Abnormal narrowing of the trachea.

trachĕŏ·stōma (G. *trakhus*, rugged; *stoma*, mouth). An artificial opening through the neck into the windpipe.

trachĕŏ·stomy (G. *trakhus*, rugged; *stoma*, mouth). The surgical formation of an opening into the windpipe through the neck.

tră·cheotome (G. *trakhus*, rugged; *tomē*, section). A surgical knife used in performing tracheotomy.

trachĕŏ·tomy (G. *trakhus*, rugged; *tomē*, section). The operation of incising the trachea. **T. tube:** a metal tube placed in the aperture made in t. through which the patient breathes. The principal varieties are Durham's lobster-tailed, Parker's, Fuller's bi-valved and König's tube.

trachi·tis (G. *trakhus*, rugged). Tracheitis, *q.v.*

trachō·ma (G. *trakhus*, rugged). A contagious disease of the eyelids, characterized by small elevations on the conjunctiva and vascular infiltration of the cornea. Sequels are cicatricial contraction of the conjunctiva with consequent deformity of the eyelids, and opacification of the cornea and pannus.

trachō·matous (G. *trakhus*, rugged). Relating to or affected with trachoma.

trachychromă·tic (G. *trakhus*, rugged; *khrōma*, colour). Staining deeply.

trachyphō·nia (G. *trakhus*, rugged; *phōnē*, voice). Roughness or hoarseness of the voice.

tract (L. *tractus*, tract). A more or less limited area of considerable length; particularly of nerves. **Anterior corticospinal** (direct pyramidal): situated in the anterior white column of the spinal cord close to the anterior median fissure. It terminates in the mid-thoracic region. **Anterior spinocerebellar** (tract of Gowers): fibres passing from the spinal cord into the superior peduncle and thence to the cortex of the anterior lobe of the cerebellum. **Anterior spino-thalamic:** a sensory tract, the main pathway by which tactile and pressure impulses pass from the posterior horn cells of the spinal cord to the thalamus. **Bulbo-spinal** (olivospinal of Helweg): a small tract confined to the cervical region of the spinal cord. Its connections are uncertain. **Comma** (fasciculus interfascicularis or semilunar tract): is located in the middle of the posterior white column of the spinal cord. **Corticorubral:** a small pathway from the motor cortex to the nucleus, which is located in the middle of the pyramidal tract. **Crossed pyramidal** (lateral corticospinal): is the great motor pathway through which voluntary movements are executed. Passes from the cerebral cortex to the spinal cord. **Dentato-rubro-thalamic:** arises in the dentate nucleus and passes to the red nucleus. **Direct cerebellar** (posterior spino-cerebellar tract of Flechsig): arises in the posterior horn cells in the thoracic cord and passes to the cortex of the cerebellum. **Direct pyramidal:** see anterior corticospinal. **Fastigiobulbar:** a small pathway arising in the nucleus fastigii and passes to the vestibular nuclei. **Frontopontine:** a descending tract from the frontal cortex to the pontine nuclei in the basal part of the pons. **Iliotibial:** a band-like thickening of the fascia lata of the thigh extending between the tuberosity of the iliac crest and the lateral tibial condyle and the head of the fibula. **Lateral corticospinal:** see crossed pyramidal. **Mamillotegmental:** fibres of the fornix which descend into the tegmentum of the brain stem. **Mamillo-thalamic** (bundle of Vicq d'Azyr): fibres of the fornix which pass upwards and backwards to the anterior nucleus of the thalamus. **Of Flechsig:** see direct cerebellar. **Of Goll** (fasciculus gracilis):

occupies the medial part of the posterior white column in the cervical and upper thoracic parts of the cord. **Of Gowers:** see anterior spinocerebellar tract. **Of Helweg:** see bulbospinal. **Of Lissauer** (postero-lateral fasciculus): lies along the apex of the posterior horn between the postero-lateral sulcus and the substantia gelatinosa Rolandi. **Of spinal cord:** in the white columns of the spinal cord, fibres having a common origin, termination and function are gathered into compact bundles known as tracts or fasciculi. **Olivocerebellar:** fibres from the olivary nucleus going to the cerebellum. **Olivospinal:** see bulbospinal or tract of Helweg. **Optic:** a white band that passes backwards and laterally from the optic chiasma into the interval between the midbrain and the hippocampal gyrus. **Prepyramidal** (rubrospinal): fibres from the red nucleus in the opposite half of the midbrain which decussate and terminate in anterior horn cells. **Pyramidal:** fibres arise in precentral cortex, traverse the corona radiata, decussate in the medulla and terminate in the posterior horn cells where they are linked with the anterior horn cells. **Reticulospinal:** fibres passing from the pons and medulla to the spinal cord. **Rubro-olivary:** afferent fibres from the red nucleus to the olivary nucleus. **Rubroreticular:** arises in the red nucleus and decussates in company with the rubrospinal tract. **Rubrospinal:** see prepyramidal. **Semilunar:** see comma. **Septo-marginal:** lies at the side of the posterior median septum of the spinal cord. **Spinocerebellar:** non-sensory tract situated superficially in the lateral white column of the spinal cord. **Spino-olivary:** a crossed tract of unknown function. **Strio-olivary:** fibres passing from the globus pallidus to the olivary nucleus. **Strio-rubro-olivary:** lies against the dorso-lateral aspect of the olivary nucleus in which its fibres terminate. **Sympathetic:** are of two kinds, ascending and descending, but their position within the spinal cord is not known with certainty. **Tectospinal:** is situated in the anterior white column separated from the anterior surface of the cord by the vestibulospinal and anterior spino-thalamic tracts. **Temporopontine:** fibres arise from the temporal cortex and end in the pontine nuclei. **Vesti-bulocerebellar:** fibres carry impulses from the utricle, saccule and semicircular canals to the nodulo-floccular lobe of the cerebellum. **Vestibulospinal:** fibres from the lateral vestibular nucleus (of Deiters) to the anterior horn cells of the spinal cord.

trac·tion (L. *trahere*, to draw). The act of drawing or dragging. **T., axis:** see under axis. **T., skeletal:** traction on the long bones by means of pins, Kirschner's wire etc., used in orthopaedics. **T. aneurysm:** an aneurysm caused by traction on the aorta by a ductus arteriosus that is not completely atrophied.

tractŏ·tomy (L. *tractus*, tract; G. *tomē*, section). The operation of cutting a nerve tract, especially within the spinal cord. Usually done for relief of pain.

trac·tus (L. *tractus*, tract). A tract. **T. gracilis:** medial portion of dorsal funiculus of the cord; column of Goll. **T. solitarius:** bundle of fibres which connects the internal capsule and lenticular nucleus with parts below.

tră·gacanth (G. *tragos*, goat; *akantha*, thorn). A gum exuded by a number of species of astragalus, shrubs belonging to the order Leguminosae; the trag-acantha of the B.P. It resembles gum-arabic and is used as a demulcent. Added to water it enables insoluble powders to be suspended and it is also useful in the making of troches.

trā·gal (G. *tragos*, goat). Relating to the tragus.

trā·galism (G. *tragos*, goat). Lust; sensuality.

tragophō·nia, tragŏ·phony (G. *tragos*, goat; *phōnē*, voice). A bleating type of voice. See also aegophony.

trā·gus (G. *tragos*, goat). 1. The small cartilaginous protuberance over the meatus of the external ear. 2. One of the hairs growing at the external auditory meatus.

trait (Fr. *trait*, from L. *trahere*, to draw). Any natural distinguishing feature or one peculiar to an individual.

trajec·tor (L. *trajicere*, to throw across). An instrument used to locate the approximate position of a bullet in a wound.

trance. 1. A type of catalepsy marked by abnormally prolonged sleep in which the vital functions are almost completely suspended. 2. Extremely prolonged syncope.

transec·tion (L. *trans*, across; *sectio*, section). Section across the long axis of a part; cross section.

transfer (L. *transferre*). 1. The passing of anaesthesia or hyperaesthesia or of a symptom from one part to another. 2. Experimental inoculation of septic material.

trans·ference (L. *transferre*). 1. Transfer, *q.v.* 2. Telepathy, *q.v.*

transfix (L. *transfigere*). To pierce through.

transforā·tion (L. *transforare*, to pierce through). The act of piercing, especially applied to the perforation of the foetal skull.

transformā·tion (L. *transformare*, to transform). 1. A change of form or substance. 2. Degeneration.

transfū·sion (L. *transfundere*, to transfuse). 1. A transfer of blood from the veins or arteries of one organism to those of another. 2. The introduction of blood, saline solution or other fluid into a vessel of the body.

transĭ·liac (L. *trans*, across; *ilia*, the groin). Crossing from one ilium to the other.

transilluminā·tion (L. *trans*, across; *illuminare*, to light up). Illumination of the walls of a cavity either by means of a light which penetrates them or the projection of brilliant light through the substance of a hollow organ.

transitional epithelium. Name given to a stratified epithelium consisting of only three or four layers of cells. Found in upper part of urethra, urinary bladder, ureter, and pelvis of kidney. Superficial cells large and flattened, then layer of pyriform or columnar cells, then layers of polyhedral cells.

translā·tion (L. *trans*, across; *latus*, borne). A change of place.

translū·cent (L. *trans*, through; *lucēre*, to shine). Partially transmitting light; semi-transparent.

transmigrā·tion (L. *trans*, across; *migratio*, migration). 1. The act of passing across or through anything. 2. Diapedesis.

transmis·sion (L. *trans*, across; *missio*, a sending). 1. Conveyance of anything, especially a disease, from one person or location to another. 2. In genetics, the passing on of normal or abnormal characteristics.

transmutā·tion (L. *trans*, across; *mutare*, to change). The act of changing; the turning of one substance or form into another.

tran·sonance (L. *trans*, across; *sonare*, to sound). Conveyed resonance; the communication of sounds through an organ.

transpa·rent (L. *trans*, through; *parere*, to appear). Having the property of transmitting light rays so that objects beyond the substance are visible.

transpirā·tion (L. *trans*, through; *spirare*, to breathe). 1. The act of emitting fluid or gas through the skin. 2. The material thus exhaled.

transplantā·tion (L. *trans*, across; *plantare*, to plant). The operation of removing tissues from a body and applying them to another body or to another part of the same one.

transposi·tion (L. *trans*, across; *ponere*, to place). Term used in relation to viscera, when due to altered direction of developmental rotation, organs are found on opposite sides of the body from the normal.

tran·sudate (L. *trans*, across; *sudare*, to sweat). A substance produced by transudation.

transudā·tion (L. *trans*, across; *sudare*, to sweat). The passage of liquid through a membrane.

transurē·thral (L. *trans*, across; *urethra*). Applied to resection of prostate. Resection of benign or malignant enlargement of the prostate by means of an instrument passed along the urethra.

transversā·lis (L. *trans*, across; *vertere*, to turn). A muscle or artery running across others.

transverse (L. *trans*, across; *vertere*, to turn). Lying crosswise; at right angles to the long axis of a body.

transversec·tomy (L. *trans*, across; *vertere*, to turn; G. *ektomē*, excision). Excision of the transverse process of a vertebra.

transvē·sical (L. *trans*, across; *vēsica*, the bladder). Through the bladder.

transves·tism (L. *trans*, across; *vestis*, clothes). The wearing of the clothes of one sex by the opposite sex.

transvĕ·stite (L. *trans*, across; *vestis*, clothes). One addicted to transvestism.

transver·sus (L. *trans*, across; *vertere*, to turn). Situated crosswise. **T. abdominis muscle:** arises from inguinal ligament, iliac crest, lower six ribs and lumbar transverse process. Inserted at linea alba, crest of pubis, pectineal line. **T. perinei superficialis muscle:** line arises from tuberosity of ischium, inserted into central tendon or sphincter vaginae. **T. perinei profundus muscle:** arises inferior ramus of ischium. Inserted median raphe of perineum. **T. thoracis muscle:** arises back of xiphoid cartilage and lower portion of sternum. Inserted costal cartilages of second to sixth ribs.

trapē·zium (G. *trapeza*, a table). 1. The first bone of the second row of carpal bones. 2. A band of transverse fibres in the lower part of the pons cerebri.

trapē·zius muscle (G. *trapeza*, table). Arises from superior curved line of the occiput, ligamentum nuchae, spine of C7, and all thoracic vertebrae. Inserted into clavicle, spine of scapula, and acromion. Draws head back or to side. Rotates scapula.

trā·pezoid (G. *trapeza*, a table; *eidos*, form). A geometrical plane; a four-sided figure having none of its opposite sides parallel. **T.-bone:** the multangulum minus, the second bone of the second row of the carpus.

Traube–Hering waves (Traube, L., German physician, 1818–76; Hering, H. E., Austrian physician, born 1866). Rhythmical variations in blood pressure which appear when the medulla is subjected to anoxaemia as in asphyxia, or in head injury or other condition giving rise to increased intracranial pressure.

Traube's space (Traube, L., German physician, 1818–76). The semilunar space; the area on the chest wall over which stomach resonance is obtained.

trau·ma (G., a wound). An injury or wound. **T., psychic:** mental instability produced by shock.

traumat·ic (G. *trauma*, a wound). Relating to or due to a wound or injury.

trau·matism (G. *trauma*, a wound). A state resulting from trauma.

traumatŏ·logist (G. *trauma*, a wound; *logos*, a treatise). One skilled in the treatment of wounds and injuries.

traumatŏ·logy (G. *trauma*, a wound; *logos*, a treatise). The study of wounds.

traumatŏ·pathy (G. *trauma*, a wound; *pathos*, disease). Any disease arising from a wound or injury.

traumatopnoē·a (G. *trauma*, a wound; *pnoē*, a breath). The escape of air through a wound in the thoracic wall.

Trautmann's triangular space (Trautmann, M. F., German aural surgeon, 1832–1902). The area contained between the sigmoid and the superior petrosal sinuses and the seventh nerve.

treat·ment. 1. The means used to remedy a disease. 2. The management of patients.

Treitz's fascia (Treitz, W., Austrian physician, 1819–72). The retropancreatic fascia; behind the head of the pancreas. **T.'s fossa:** the fossa subcaecalis. **T.'s ligament:** the musculus suspensorius duodeni. **T.'s muscle:** the musculus recto-coccygeus.

Trematō·da (G. *trēma*, hole; *eidōs*, form). A class of Platyhelminths, parasitic worms which infest many animals and are sometimes found in man.

trĕ·matode (G. *trēma*, hole; *eidōs*, form). One of the Trematoda.

trem·ble (L. *tremulus*, shaking). To shake or quiver.

trĕ·mor (L. from *tremere*, to quiver). An involuntary quivering or shaking.

trĕ·mulous (L. *tremere*, to quiver). Shaking or trembling.

trend. Tendency to go in a particular direction or following a specific course.

Trendelenburg's operation (Trendelenburg, F., German surgeon, 1844–1925). Ligation of long saphenous vein at its entrance into the femoral vein. **T.'s position:** the patient lies supine on a plane inclined at 45° to the horizontal, with the head at lower end, and the legs flexed at the knees. **T.'s symptom:** a waddling gait due to paralysis of the gluteal muscles. **T.'s test:** (1) for potency of saphenous valves. The leg is raised above the level of the heart until the veins are empty. A finger is placed over the saphenous opening, and the leg lowered. If the veins fill immediately the finger is removed, the valves are incompetent. (2) For hip disease associated with weakness of gluteal muscles. The patient stands with back to examiner. In poliomyelitis, ununited fracture of femoral neck, coxa vara, and congenital dislocations, the pelvis on the sound side falls instead of rising, when the patient is standing on the affected limb.

trepan (G. *trupanon*, a gimlet from *trupa*, a hole). Trephine, *q.v.*

trepan·ning (G. *trupanon*, a gimlet from *trupa*, a hole). Boring; operating with the trephine.

trephinā·tion (G. *trupanon*, a gimlet). Trephining, *q.v.*

trephine (G. *trupanon*, a gimlet). 1. An instrument for excising a circular piece of bone, usually from the skull, or of corneoscleral tissue from the eye. 2. To operate with the trephine.

trĕ·phining (G. *trupanon*, a gimlet). The operation of excising with a trephine.

trĕ·phones (G. *trephein*, to foster). Substances produced by certain body cells and serving to feed other cells.

trepidā·tion (L. *trepidare*, to be agitated). 1. Trembling. 2. Nervous anxiety.

Treponē·ma (G. *trupanon*, a gimlet). A genus of micro-organisms belonging to the order Spirochaetales. The genus includes the *T. pallidum*, the organism causing syphilis; also called Spirochaeta pallida.

treponematō·sis (G. *trupanon*, a gimlet). Yaws, *q.v.*

treponemicī·dal (G. *trupanon*, a gimlet; *caedere*, to kill). Destructive of Treponema.

Treves's bloodless fold (Treves, Sir F., English surgeon, 1853–1923). Of the appendix.

tri·ad (G. *trias*, from *treis*, three). See under quantivalence.

tri·al (Fr. *trier*, to select). The act of testing. **T. lenses:** graduated lenses for testing vision.

tri·angle (L. *triangulum*, triangle). A figure with three sides and three angles. **Anterior:** of the neck, is situated anterior to the sterno-mastoid muscle, and its base is directed superiorly. **Auscultation:** situated on the back, between the superior border of the latissimus dorsi, the inferior border of the trapezius and the base of the scapula. **Carotid:** bounded inferiorly by the superior belly of the omohyoid; superiorly by the posterior belly of the digastric and posteriorly by the anterior border of the sternomastoid. **Deep perineal:** bounded by the crus penis laterally, the bulb of the penis medially and the base is formed by the superficial transverse perineal muscle. **Digastric:** is divided into two parts, anterior and posterior, by the stylo-mandibular ligament. The anterior part contains the superficial part of the submandibular gland. **Femoral (Scarpa's):** the base of the triangle is formed by the inguinal ligament; the inner side by the adductor longus and the outer side by the sartorius muscle. **Hesselbach's (Inguinal):** bounded laterally by the deep epigastric artery, medially by the lateral border of the rectus, the base being formed by the inguinal ligament. **Inguinal:** see Hesselbach's. **Lumbar (Petit's):** situated above the centre of the iliac crest and the margins of the latissimus dorsi and the external oblique muscles form its other boundaries. **Lumbosacral:** is situated on each side of the body of the fifth lumbar vertebra. **Macewen's:** a small depression bounded above by the posterior root of the zygoma, below by the posterosuperior part of the external meatus and behind by the vertical line connecting the upper and lower boundaries. **Marcille's:** see lumbosacral. **Muscular:** bounded anteriorly by the mid line of the neck; posteriorly by the anterior border of the sternomastoid; and superiorly by the superior belly of the omohyoid. **Occipital:** bounded anteriorly by the posterior border of the sternomastoid, posteriorly by the anterior border of the trapezius, inferiorly by the inferior belly of the omohyoid. **Of Lesser:** bounded by the posterior belly of the digastric muscle and the hypoglossal nerve. **Petit's:** see lumbar. **Posterior:** bounded anteriorly by the posterior border of the sternomastoid, posteriorly by the anterior border of the trapezius, inferiorly by the middle third of the clavicle. **Scarpa's:** see femoral. **Subclavian (supraclavicular):** is the inferior division of the posterior triangle of the neck and is separated from the superior division or occipital triangle by the inferior belly of the omohyoid muscle. **Submandibular (submaxillary):** bounded superiorly by the base of the mandible, posteroinferiorly by the posterior belly of the digastric, antero-inferiorly by the mid line of the neck. **Submaxillary:** see submandibular. **Submental:** the base is formed by the body of the hyoid bone, and each lateral boundary is constituted by the anterior belly of the digastric. **Suboccipital:** is situated deep to the superior part of the semispinalis capitis inferior to the occipital bone. **Supraclavicular:** see subclavian. **Suprameatal:** see Macewen's.

triān·gular (L. *tres*, three; *angulus*, angle). Three-cornered. **T. fascia:** is the reflected part of the inguinal ligament and is also known as the ligament of Colles. It is situated behind the spermatic cord and superior crus of the superficial inguinal ring.

triangulā·ris muscle (L. *tres*, three; *angulus*, angle). Arises from the lower border of the mandible, and is inserted into the lower lip near the angle of the mouth. It pulls down the corner of the mouth.

triătom·ic (G. *treis*, three; *atomos*, indivisible). Having three atoms.

tri·badism (G. *tribein*, to rub). Sexual intimacy between women practised by friction of the genitals.

tribā·sic (G. *treis*, three; *basis*, base). Containing three atoms of replaceable hydrogen.

tribrā·chius (G. *treis*, three; *brakhion*, arm). A monster with three arms.

tribrō·mide (G. *treis*, three; *brōmos*, a foetid odour). A bromine compound containing three atoms of bromine in the molecule.

tribrommĕ·thane (G. *treis*, three; *brōmos*, a foetid odour; *methu*, wine). Bromoform.

tribrōmŏe·thanol. $CBr_3.CH_2OH$. A mixture of two parts with one part of amylene hydrate constitutes the basal anaesthetic, bromethol. Trade name Avertin.

tricel·lular (L. *tres*, three; *cellula*, a small store-room). Having three cells.

tricĕ·phalus (G. *treis*, three; *kephalē*, head). A three-headed monster.

tri·ceps (L. *tres*, three; *caput*, head). Three-headed. **T. muscle:** arises by three heads: (1) Lateral; above radial groove of humerus. (2) Medial; below radial groove of humerus. (3) Long; from lower margin of glenoid cavity. Inserted into olecranon process. Extends elbow joint.

trichan·geia (G. *thrix*, hair; *aggeion*, vessel). The capillary blood-vessels.

tri·changiĕc·tasis (G. *thrix*, hair; *aggeion*, vessel; *ektasis*, extension). Distension of the capillary blood-vessels.

trichaux·is (G. *thrix*, hair; *auxēsis*, growth). Hypertrichiasis, *q.v.*

trichi·asis (G. *thrix*, hair). An ingrowing of the eyelashes, causing them to irritate the globe by friction.

Trī·china (G. *thrix*, hair). A genus of very small nematode worms of which the *T. spiralis* is parasitic in pigs and occasionally in man.

trichini·asis (G. *thrix*, hair). Trichinosis, *q.v.*

trichinophō·bia (G. *thrix*, hair; *phŏbos*, fear). Neurotic fear of trichinosis.

trichinō·sis (G. *thrix*, hair). A disease caused by eating pork containing *Trichina spiralis*. Its symptoms are nausea, vertigo, colic and fever in the early stages, and later there is prostration accompanied by muscular swellings, oedema of the face and delirium.

trī·chinous (G. *thrix*, hair). Invaded by or containing trichinae.

trichī·tis (G. *thrix*, hair). Inflammation of the hair bulbs.

trichlor·ide (G. *treis*, three; *khlōros*, green). A compound with three atoms of chlorine to one of a base.

trichloromethylchloroformate (G. *treis*, three; *khlōros*, green; *methu*, wine). Diphosgene, a lethal lung-irritant war gas.

trichlorphĕ·nol (G. *treis*, three; *khlōros*, green; *phoinix*, crimson). A compound obtained from phenol and employed as a disinfectant.

tricho-aesthē·sia (G. *thrix*, hair; *aisthēsis*, feeling). The sensation caused by touching the hair of the subject; hair sensibility.

tricho-anaesthē·sia (G. *thrix*, hair; *an*, neg.; *aisthēsis*, feeling). Absence of hair sensibility.

tri·chobactē·ria (G. *thrix*, hair; *baktron*, a staff). Bacteria which possess flagella, or those of filamentous or threadlike form.

trichobē·zoar (G. *thrix*, hair; *bezoar*). Hair ball. A concretion formed by hair, found in stomach or intestine.

Trichobilhar·zia ocella·ta. A blood-fluke parasitic on ducks.

trichocar·dia (G. *thrix*, hair; *kardia*, heart). 'Hairy heart', inflammation of the pericardium with exudations.

tri·chocephalī·asis (G. *thrix*, hair; *kephalē*, head). A disease caused by infestation with threadworms.

Trichocĕ·phalus (G. *thrix*, hair; *kephalē*, head). A genus of nematode worms, the threadworms.

T. dispar: an intestinal parasite, particularly infesting the large intestine. Also called Trichuris.

trichoclā·sia, trichŏ·clasis (G. *thrix*, hair; *klasis*, a breaking). Trichorrhexis nodosa, *q.v.*

Trichodec·tēs. A genus of parasitic insects.

tricho-epitheliŏ·ma (G. *thrix*, hair; *epi*, upon; *thēlē*, the nipple). A tumour of the skin having its origin in the hair follicles.

trichoglos·sia (G. *thrix*, hair; *glōssa*, tongue). Hairy tongue; a thickening of the papillae giving the tongue appearance of being covered with hair.

trī·choid (G. *thrix*, hair; *eidos*, form). Like hair.

trī·cholith (G. *thrix*, hair; *lithos*, stone). A hairy concretion.

tricholō·gia (G. *thrix*, hair; *legein*, to pick out). Plucking out of the hair.

trichŏ·logy (G. *thrix*, hair; *logos*, a treatise). The study of the hair and its diseases.

trichŏ·matose (G. *trikhōma*, a growth of hair). Matted.

trī·chomatō·sis (G. *trikhōma*, a growth of hair). A fungoid, matted state of the hair.

trichŏ·matous (G. *trikhōma*, a growth of hair). Relating to or affected with trichomatosis.

trichomō·nad (G. *thrix*, hair; *monas*, unit). One of the genus Trichomonas.

trichomō·nal (G. *thrix*, hair; *monas*, unit). Relating to the Trichomonas.

Trichomō·nas (G. *thrix*, hair; *monas*, unit). A genus of ciliate protozoa. **T. intestinalis:** a variety sometimes present in the stools in cases of diarrhoea and enteritis. **T. vaginalis:** a variety that sometimes infests the vagina.

trichomonī·asis (G. *thrix*, hair; *monas*, unit). Invasion with Trichomonas.

Trī·chomycē·tēs (G. *thrix*, hair; *mukēs*, mushroom). A group of organisms found in form of filaments. They appear to be intermediate between the bacteria and higher fungi, and include actinomyces, leptothrix and cladothrix.

trichomycō·sis (G. *thrix*, hair; *mukēs*, mushroom). A disease of the hair caused by any vegetable parasite.

trichonō·sis, trichŏ·nosus (G. *thrix*, hair; *nŏsos*, disease). Any disease affecting the hair.

trichŏ·pathy (G. *thrix*, hair; *pathos*, disease). Any disease of the hair.

trichŏ·phagy, trichophă·gia (G. *thrix*, hair; *phagein*, to eat). The habit of hair-eating.

trichophō·bia (G. *thrix*, hair; *phŏbos*, fear). Neurotic fear of hair.

trichophyt·ic[1] (G. *thrix*, hair; *phuton*, plant). Relating to the genus Trichophyton.

trichophyt·ic[2] (G. *thrix*, hair; *phuein*, to grow). 1. Contributing to the growth of hair. 2. An agent that does this.

Trychŏ·phyton (G. *thrix*, hair; *phuton*, plant). A genus of fungi parasitic upon hair. It is the cause of tinea trichophyton, or ringworm.

trichophytō·sis (G. *thrix*, hair; *phuton*, plant). A contagious disease of the skin and hair and due to infestation with Trichophyton fungi.

trī·chopoliŏ·sis (G. *thrix*, hair; *pŏlios*, grey). Greying of the hair.

trichoptilō·sis (G. *thrix*, hair; *ptilon*, feather-down). Trichorrhexis nodosa.

trichorrhex·is (G. *thrix*, hair; *rhēxis*, a breaking). Abnormal brittleness of the hair, causing it to break off. **T. nodosa:** a hair disease marked by the formation of irregular swellings, resembling nodes, on the hairs. At these node-like points, the hair tends to break off. The disease usually occurs in the beard.

trichorrhoē·a (G. *thrix*, hair; *rhoia*, a flowing). Loss of hair.

trichŏ·schisis (G. *thrix*, hair; *skhisis*, a cleaving). A splitting of hairs.

tricho·scopy (G. *thrix*, hair; *skopein*, to inspect). Inspection of the hair.

trichō·sis (G. *thrix*, hair). Any disease affecting the hair.

Tricho·sporum (G. *thrix*, hair; *sporos*, seed). A genus of fungi which causes trichomycosis.

trichosporō·sis (G. *thrix*, hair; *sporos*, seed). The condition produced by infestation with Trichosporum.

Trichostron·gylus. A genus of nematode worms of the family Strongylidae.

Trichothē·cium. A genus of moulds.

tri·chotillomā·nia (G. *thrix*, hair; *tillein*, to pluck; *mania*, madness). A neurotic impulse to pluck out the hair.

trichrō·ic (G. *treis*, three; *khrŏa*, colour). Exhibiting trichroism.

tri·chroism (G. *treis*, three; *khrŏa*, colour). The property of presenting three different colours under three different aspects.

tri·chromatop·sia (G. *treis*, three; *khrŏa*, colour; *opsis*, vision). Possessing normal colour vision; the power to perceive all three primary colours.

trichuri·asis (G. *thrix*, hair; *oura*, tail). Infestation with Trichuris.

Trichū·ris (G. *thrix*, hair; *oura*, tail). A genus of nematodes that infest the intestinal tract.

trici·pital (L. *triceps*, three-headed). 1. Having three heads. 2. Relating to the triceps.

tricor·nis (L. *tres*, three; *cornu*, horn). Three-horned, or having three processes; said of each of the lateral ventricles of the brain.

tricor·nute (L. *tres*, three; *cornutus*, horned). Possessing three horn-like prominences.

tricrot·ic (G. *treis*, three; *krotos*, a beat). With three waves to one pulse-beat.

tri·crotism (G. *treis*, three; *krotos*, a beat). The quality of being tricrotic.

tricus·pid (L. *tres*, three; *cuspis*, a point). 1. With three cusps. 2. Acting upon or originating at the t. valve. T. valve: the valve found in the opening from the right auricle into the right ventricle.

tridac·tyl (G. *treis*, three; *daktulos*, finger). With three digits.

tri·dent, triden·tate (L. *tridens*, three-toothed). Three toothed or pronged. Trident hand: a hand in which the third and fourth fingers diverge abnormally.

tridermoge·nesis (G. *treis*, three; *derma*, skin; *gennan*, to produce). The stage in embryonic development marked by the formation of the three germ layers.

tridermō·ma (G. *treis*, three; *derma*, skin). An embryo composed of three layers of the blastoderm.

triĕl·con (G. *treis*, three; *helkein*, to pull). A three-pronged surgical instrument for removing bullets and other foreign bodies from the body.

trienc̆·phalus (G. *treis*, three; *egkephalos*, brain). A monster lacking the organs of smell, hearing and sight.

trifā·cial (L. *tres*, three; *facies*, face). The fifth cranial nerve, dividing into three main branches supplying the face; more commonly called the trigeminal nerve.

Trifō·lium (L. *tres*, three; *folium*, leaf). A genus of plants including the clovers.

trigĕ·minal (L. *trigeminus*, triple). 1. Triple; separating into three sections, as the t. nerve. 2. Relating to the t. nerve.

trigĕ·minus (L. *trigeminus*, triple). The fifth cranial nerve; also called the trifacial nerve.

trigger. A device liberating a catch or spring. T.-finger: a condition in which difficulty is at first experienced in flexing or extending a finger, but the movement is later performed with a sudden jerk. T.-knee: a state in which the movement of the knee-joint suddenly ceases during flexion or extension and the leg is jerked sideways.

trigoc̆·phalus (G. *treis*, three; *gōnia*, angle; *kephalē*, head). Trigonocephalus, *q.v.*

tri·gonal (G. *trigōnon*, triangle). Relating to a trigone.

tri·gone (G. *trigōnon*, triangle). A triangle. T. of bladder: a smooth triangular area situated inside the bladder just behind the orifice of the urethra.

trigonoc̆·phalus (G. *trigōnon*, triangle; *kephalē*, head). A triangular-skulled monster with the small end of the triangle in front. The condition is caused by premature junction of the coronal suture.

trigō·num (L. from G. *trigōnon*). 1. A triangle. 2. Interpeduncular space. T. habenulae: a triangular area found in the optic thalamus. It lies between the pulvinar, habenula and midbrain. T. ventriculi: t. collaterale, an irregular triangular area, protruding from the posterior portion of the lateral wall and floor of the lateral ventricle of the brain between the calcar avis and hippocampus. T. vesicae: a triangular area in the floor of the bladder, between the ureteric orifices and the internal urinary meatus, covered by smooth mucous membrane.

trihy·dric (G. *treis*, three; *hudor*, water). The term applied to alcohols possessing three hydroxyl groups to the molecule, e.g. glycerol $CH_2OH.CHOH.CH_2OH$.

tri·labe (G. *treis*, three; *lambanein*, to take). A three-pronged instrument used for removing concretions from the bladder.

trilă·minar (L. *tres*, three; *lamina*, a layer). Having three layers.

trilă·teral (L. *tres*, three; *latus*, a side). Having three sides.

Trilene. A proprietary preparation of the anaesthetic trichlorethylene, $CHCl:CCl_2$, with 0.01 per cent thymol added to stop decomposition and coloured with 1 in 200,000 aniline blue to distinguish it from chloroform.

trilō·bate (G. *treis*, three; *lŏbos*, lobe). Having three lobes.

trilō·cular (L. *tres*, three; *loculus*, a pocket). Having three cells.

trimă·stigate, trimă·stigote (G. *treis*, three; *mastix*, a whip). Possessing three flagella.

trimen·sual (L. *tres*, three; *mensis*, month). Recurring every three months.

trime·thylene. Cyclopropane $\overline{CH_2\text{-}CH_2\text{-}CH_2}$, an anaesthetic.

trimor·phism (G. *treis*, three; *morphē*, shape). 1. The production of hermaphrodite flowers of three kinds (short-, mid- and long-styled) on the same species of plant. 2. The state or property of having three forms, e.g. certain insects are characterized by t.

trini·trate (G. *treis*, three; *nitron*, carbonate of soda). A nitrate having three radicals of nitric acid.

trini·trin (G. *treis*, three; *nitron*, carbonate of soda). Glyceryl trinitrate.

trini·troglў·cerin. Glyceryl trinitrate. $C_3H_5(\text{-}ONO_2)_3$. An oily explosive liquid used in the manufacture of dynamite. In medicine used in angina pectoris for its vasodilator action.

trinitrophĕ·nol. Picric acid. $C_6H_2(OH)(NO_2)_3$.

trinitrotŏ·luene (G. *treis*, three; *nitron*, carbonate of soda). A high explosive, popularly called T.N.T.

trinū·cleate (L. *tri.* three; *nucleus*, dim. of *nux*, nut). Possessing three nuclei.

triocĕ·phalus (G. *treis*, three; *kephalē*, head). A monster without the organs of sight, hearing and smell, and having in place of a head a small, amorphous mass.

tri·onym (G. *treis*, three; *onoma*, name). A name comprising three terms.

trior·chid (G. *treis*, three; *orkhis*, testicle). An individual possessing three testicles.

trior·chidism (G. *treis*, three; *orkhis*, testicle). The condition of having three testicles.

tri·ose (G. *treis*, three). A sugar having three carbon atoms to the molecule.

triox·ide (G. *treis*, three; *oxus*, sharp). A compound with three atoms of oxygen to one of the base.

tri·para (L. *tres*, three; *parere*, to bear). A woman who has had three children.

tripep·tid, tripep·tide (G. *treis*, three; *peptein*, to digest). Substances composed of three amino-acids, formed during the digestion of protein.

triphae·mia (G. *triptos*, pounded; *haima*, blood). The accumulation of waste matter in the blood.

triphā·sic (G. *treis*, three; *phasis*, phase). Passing through three phases or variations.

triple (L. *triplus*). Threefold. **T. phosphate:** ammonio-magnesium phosphate, found in urine and phosphatic concretions.

triplē·gia (G. *treis*. three; *plēgē*, stroke). Hemiplegia with paralysis of one limb on the other side of the body.

trip·let (L. *triplus*, threefold). 1. Any one of three children born at a single birth. 2. In optics, a system composed of three lenses.

tri·pod (G. *tripous*, threefooted). An object supported on three legs. **T., anatomical:** the three supports on which the foot rests in the standing posture: (*a*) the heel; (*b*) the three inner metatarsals; (*c*) the two outer metatarsals. **T., vital:** the heart, brain and lungs: the trilogy supporting the life of an organism.

triquet·rous (L. *triquetrus*, triangular). Three-cornered.

triquet·rum (L. *triquetrus*, triangular). 1. Any of the Wormian bones. 2. The cuneiform bone of the carpus.

trirā·dial, trirā·diate (L. *tres*, three; *radius*, ray). Three-rayed; radiating in three directions.

tris·moid (G. *trismos*, a grinding of the teeth; *eidos*, form). A variety of trismus occurring in new-born infants and believed to be caused by pressure on the occipital bone during labour.

tris·mus (G. *trismos*, a grinding of the teeth). Lock-jaw; the rigid closure of the muscles of the jaw.

trisplanch·nic (G. *treis*, three; *splagkhnon*, an intestine). Serving the three large cavities of the body, e.g., the trisplanchnic nerve (the sympathetic nerve).

tristi·chia (G. *treis*, three; *stikhos*, a row). Having three rows of eyelashes.

tristimā·nia (L. *tristis*, sad; G. *mania*, madness). Melancholia.

tris·tis (L., sad). Melancholy; of dim colour.

trisul·phide (L. *tres*, three; *sulfur*, sulphur). A compound in which there are three atoms of sulphur to one of the base.

tritanō·pia (G. *tritos*, third; *an*, neg ; *ōps* eye). Defectiveness in a third constituent of normal colour vision; e.g. violet-blindness.

triti·ceoglos·sus (L. *triticum*, wheat; G. *glōssa*, tongue). A muscle which is occasionally found extending from the arytenoid cartilage to the side of the tongue.

triti·ceous (L. *triticum*, wheat). Formed like a grain of wheat, as the t. cartilage.

triti·ceum (L. *triticum*, wheat). The triticeous nodule in the thyrohyoid ligament.

tri·topine (G. *tritos*, third; *opion*, opium). An alkaloid derived from opium.

tri·turable (L.L. *triturare*, to thresh). Capable of being reduced to a fine powder.

tri·turate (L.L. *triturare*, to thresh). 1. To rub or grind to a fine powder. 2. A fine powder.

triturā·tion (L.L. *triturare*, to thresh). The process of rubbing or grinding a solid to a fine powder.

tri·valent (L. *tres*, three; *valēre*, to be worth). An element, one atom of which combines with or displaces, directly or indirectly, three atoms of hydrogen.

trō·car (Fr. *trois-quarts*, three-quarters). An instrument consisting of a perforator and a metal tube used in paracentesis or for tapping a cavity.

trochan·ter (G. *trokhantēr*, runner). One of two processes on the upper end of the femur below the neck. The t. major arises on the outer and the t. minor on the inner side of the bone.

trochantĕ·ric (G. *trokhantēr*, runner). Relating to a trochanter.

trochan·tin (G. *trokhantēr*, runner). The lesser trochanter.

trochanti·nian (G. *trokhantēr*, runner). Relating to the trochantin.

troche (G. *trokhos*, a round cake). A lozenge or medicated tablet.

trō·chin (G. *trokhos*, a round cake). The lesser tuberosity of the head of the femur.

trochis·cus (G. *trokhos*, a round cake). Troche, *q.v.*

trŏ·chiter (G. *trokhos*, a round cake). The greater tuberosity of the head of the femur.

trochitĕ·rian (G. *trokhos*, a round cake). Relating to the trochiter.

troch·lea (G. *trokhilia*, the sheaf of a pulley). Any part or process which acts as a pulley; e.g., t. of the humerus.

troch·lear (G. *trokhilia*, the sheaf of a pulley). 1. Acting as or relating to a pulley. 2. Relating to the t. nerve.

trochocar·dia (G. *trokhos*, a wheel; *kardia*, heart). Displacement of the heart due to a rotary movement on its axis.

trochocephā·lia (G. *trokhos*, a wheel; *kephalē*, head). A round-shaped head, due to synostosis of the frontal and parietal bones.

trō·choid (G. *trokhos*, a wheel; *eidos*, form). Acting as a pulley or pivot.

trochoi·dēs (G. *trokhos*, a wheel; *eidos*, form). Any pivot-like joint.

trō·ilism (G. *Trōilŏs*, a son of Priam). A mental disturbance of a sexual nature. The patient desires the sexual partner of the individual for whom he has homosexual desire.

Troisier's syndrome (Troisier, E., French physician, 1844–1919). Cachexia associated with bronzing of skin found in diabetes.

Trolard's net (Trolard, P.. French anatomist, 1842–1910). The venous rete canalis hypoglossi. **T.'s vein:** the great anastomotic vein of the cerebral cortex.

Tröltsch's depressions (Tröltsch, A. F. von, German otologist, 1829–90). The depressions on the inner surface of the membrana tympani. **T.'s folds:** the anterior and posterior malleolar folds of the membrana tympani. **T.'s pockets:** T.'s depressions, *q.v.*

Trombi·cula. A genus of acarine mites.

tromomā·nia (G. *trŏmos*, a trembling; *mania*, madness). Delirium tremens.

tromophō·nia (G. *trŏmos*, a trembling; *phōnè*, voice). A trembling of the voice.

trophē·sial, trophē·sic (G. *trophē*, nourishment). Relating to trophesy.

trŏ·phesy (G. *trophē*, nourishment). An unsatisfactory state of nutrition due to disorder of the trophic nerves.

trŏ·phic (G. *trophē*, nourishment). Relating to or affecting nourishment. **T. centres:** the nerves governing the nutrition of organs or nerves.

trŏ·phoblast (G. *trophē*, nourishment; *blastos*, germ). The external ectodermal layer of the blastodermic vesicle.

trophotax·is (G. *trophē*, nutrition; *taxis*, arrangement). Cell adjustment in relation to food intake.

trophō·tropism (G. *trophē*, nourishment; *trepein*, to turn). The attractive and repulsive effects of various nutritive solutions on certain organic cells.

trophozŏ·ite (G. *trophē*, nourishment; *zōon*, animal). A protozoon parasitic on the cells of its host, from which it takes its nourishment.

trŏ·pine (G. *Atropos* (inflexible), the name of one of the three goddesses of fate). A crystalline substance derived from atropine.

trŏ·pism (G. *tropē*, turn). 1. The efforts of living cells to reach light, darkness, heat or cold. 2. The reactions of organisms without nervous systems.

tropŏ·meter (G. *tropē*, turn; *metron*, measure). 1. A device for measuring the rotations of the eyeball. 2. A device for calculating the amount of torsion in the long bones.

Trousseau's sign (Trousseau, A., French physician, 1801–67). Muscular spasm which occurs in tetany when pressure is applied over large arteries or nerves.

troy ounce. A unit of weight equal to 480 grains.

true. Existing; not false.

Trueta's method (Trueta, J., contemporary Spanish surgeon in England, born 1897). The application of Winett-Orr closed plaster technique to the treatment of war wounds.

trun·cal (L. *truncus*, tree-trunk). Relating to a trunk.

truncā·ted (L. *truncare*, to maim). Deprived of accessory parts, e.g. by the amputation of limbs.

trun·cus (L.). A trunk.

trunk (L. *truncus*, tree-trunk). 1. The torso; the body considered apart from the head and/or limbs. 2. The main stem of a vessel or nerve.

truss. 1. An apparatus for preventing the movement of a hernia. 2. An appliance for exerting pressure.

trypā·gar. A culture-medium containing pea-flour extract and trypsin broth in which the meningococcus is grown.

trȳ·pan blue (G. *trupanon*, a gimlet). A dye of the benzopurpurin series. It is used as a trypanocide.

trȳ·pan red. A reddish-brown dye used in the treatment of trypanosomiasis.

trypă·nocide (G. *trupanon*, a gimlet; L. *caedere*, to kill). Destructive of trypanosomes.

trypanŏ·lysis (G. *trupanon*, a gimlet; *lusis*, dissolution). The destruction of trypanosomes.

Trȳ·panosō·ma (G. *trupanon*, a gimlet; *sōma*, body). A genus of protozoan parasites which infest the blood plasma both of man and animals. It includes the *T. brucei* which produces the tsetse-fly disease of horses.

trȳ·panosomi·asis (G. *trupanon*, a gimlet; *sōma*, body). Any of the various diseases caused by infection with one of the species of Trypanosoma.

tryparsă·mide.
$NH_2CO . CH_2NH . C_6H_4 . AsO (OH) (ONa)_1 \frac{1}{2}H_2O$. Used intravenously in the treatment of trypanosomiasis and syphilis.

trypē·sis (G. *trupēsis*, a boring). The operation of trephining.

tryp·sin (G. *tripsis*, a rubbing). The proteolytic enzmye of the pancreatic juice, which changes proteins to peptones and polypeptides.

trypsi·nogen (G. *tripsis*, a rubbing; *gennan*, to produce). The pancreatic zymogen from which trypsin is produced.

tryp·tic (G. *tripsis*, a rubbing). Relating to or caused by trypsin.

tryptolȳ·tic (G. *tripsis*, a rubbing; *peptein*, to digest; *luein*, to dissolve). Dissolving or splitting up tryptones.

tryp·tone (G. *tripsis*, a rubbing; *peptein*, to digest). Any peptone formed by the action of trypsin.

tryptonae·mia (G. *tripsis*, a rubbing; *peptein*, to digest; *haima*, blood). Peptonaemia; a condition characterized by the presence of tryptones in the blood.

tryp·tophane (G. *tripsis*, a rubbing; *phainein*, to show).

$C_6H_4.NH-CH:C.CH_2CH(NH_2)COOH$. An amino-acid; one of the end-products of tryptic digestion.

tsetse fly. An African fly belonging to the genus Glossina. **T.-fly disease:** a disease affecting horses and cattle resulting from infection by *Trypanosoma brucei*, transmitted by the tsetse fly *Glossina morsitans*.

tsŭ·tsugamŭ·shi disease (Japanese for 'dangerous bug'). A fever caused by *Rickettsia japonica*, and transmitted by the larva of a mite. The disease is endemic in Japan, Sumatra, and New Guinea.

tŭ·ba (L. *tŭba*, a trumpet). A tube. **T. acustica:** the pharyngotympanic or Eustachian tube. **T. root:** derris root; the rhizome of *Derris elliptica* and *Derris malaccensis*; a horticultural and agricultural insecticide. **T. uterina:** the uterine or Fallopian tube.

tŭ·bal (L. *tŭba*, a trumpet). Relating to a tube. **T. pregnancy:** pregnancy in one of the uterine tubes.

tube (L. *tubus*, a tube). Any hollow cylindrical structure. **Carrel's:** small rubber tubes used in Carrel's irrigation treatment of wounds. **Drainage:** used in surgery for drainage of wounds. **Durham's:** jointed tracheotomy tube. **Leiter's:** flexible metal tubes for application of cold water to the surface of the body. **O'Dwyer's:** an intubation tube. **Pharyngotympanic (Eustachian):** a tube about 36 mm. long which passes from the tympanic cavity to the nasopharynx. It is lined with mucous membrane. **Ryle's:** thin rubber tube, for test meal, or introduction of food into the stomach. **Southey's:** small silver tubes for subcutaneous drainage. **Stomach:** for feeding or washing out the stomach. **Uterine (Fallopian):** a long narrow tube, bilateral, extending from ovary to the upper and anterior part of uterus. It serves to conduct ova to the uterus.

tubec·tomy (L. *tubus*, a tube; G. *ektomē*, excision). Excision of a tube.

tŭ·ber (L. *tŭber*, a swelling). 1. A thickened part of an underground stem. 2. Any globular swelling in the body.

tŭ·bercle (L. *tuberculum*, dim. of *tuber*, a swelling). 1. A nodule. 2. A rounded eminence on a bone. 3. The lesion caused by the bacillus of tuberculosis, comprising a collection of round cells and epithelioid cells, sometimes accompanied by giant cells. **Darwin's** (auricular tubercle): a small elevation on the incurved margin of the helix of the ear. **Deltoid:** a bony prominence on the upper surface of the clavicle for the attachment of the deltoid muscle. **Dorsal:** (Lister's tubercle) a prominent elevation on the posterior surface of the lower end of the radius. **Genial:** two in number situated on the medial surface of the symphysis menti. The upper tubercle gives origin to the genio-glossus muscle and the lower to the genio-hyoid. **Hyoid:** a slight projection on the anterior surface of the body of the hyoid bone. **Infraglenoid:** a rough impression on the inferior border of the glenoid cavity, it gives origin to the long head of the triceps muscle. **Lisfranc's** (scalene tubercle): a projection on the internal border of the first rib for the insertion of scalenus anterior muscle. **Lister's:** see dorsal tubercle of radius. **Marginal:** a slight prominence on the frontal process of the zygomatic bone for a strip of the temporal fascia. **Mental:** a prominence on the outer surface of the mandible just lateral to the mental protuberance. **Montgomery's:** irregular projections on the areola of the nipple. These tubercles are due to the presence of large sebaceous glands. **Nonarticular:** small tubercles on the outer surfaces of the ribs, most marked on the sixth rib. **Orbital:** see Whitnall's t.. **Of rib:** a projection on the lateral surface of the rib for articulation with the transverse process of its vertebra.

Of Rolando (trigeminal tubercle): situated on the ventral surface of the restiform body of the medulla oblongata. **Of scaphoid:** a prominent projection at the lower end of the lateral border of the carpal scaphoid, it gives attachment to the flexor retinaculum and abductor pollicis brevis muscle. **Of tibia:** a well marked projection on the anterior surface of the upper end of the tibia for the attachment of the ligamentum patellae. **Palatine:** a projection of bone from the palate bone, which articulates with the lateral pterygoid plate of the sphenoid bone. **Peroneal:** a short oblique ridge on the lateral surface of the calcaneum. **Pharyngeal:** a prominence on the under surface of the basilar process of the occipital bone for the attachment of the superior constrictor of the pharynx. **Postglenoid:** a process of bone which lies between the external auditory meatus and the anterior part of the mandibular fossa. **Preglenoid:** a projection on the outer surface of the zygoma which gives attachment to the temporomandibular ligament. **Pterygoid:** a projection at the posterior border of the medial pterygoid plate of the sphenoid. **Pubic:** a rounded prominence at the outer extremity of the body of the pubis for the attachment of the inguinal ligament. **Quadrate:** an eminence on the posterior surface of the great trochanter of the femur, it gives attachment to the quadratus femoris muscle. **Scalene:** see Lisfranc's. **Supraglenoid:** a small rough elevation on the upper surface of the glenoid cavity of the scapula, it gives origin to the long head of the biceps muscle. **Whitnall's** (orbital t.): a small rounded elevation on the outer wall of the orbit for the attachment of the lateral palpebral ligament. **Woolner's:** see Darwin's.

tuber·cula (L., pl. of *tuberculum*). Tubercles.

tuber·cular. Incorrect form of 'tuberculous.'

tuber·culated (L. *tuberculum*, dim. of *tuber*, a swelling). Bearing or covered with tubercles.

tuber·culid, tuber·culide (L. *tuberculum*, dim. of *tuber*, a swelling). Name given to any skin lesion which is found associated with evident manifestations of tuberculosis.

tuber·culin (L. *tuberculum*, dim. of *tuber*, a swelling). A glycerol extract of cultures of the *Mycobacterium tuberculosis*. The injection of tuberculin causes no reaction in a healthy subject, but in one affected with tuberculosis gives an inflammation at the point of the injection. It is used in various forms for the diagnosis of tuberculous infection in children and cattle.

tuber·culinose. A modified type of tuberculin.

tuberculi·tis. Inflammation of a tuberculous node or of the area surrounding it.

tuber·culocele (L. *tuberculum*, dim. of *tuber*, a swelling; G. *kēlē*, tumour). Tuberculosis of the testicle.

tuber·culocide (L. *tuberculum*, dim. of *tuber*, a swelling; *caedere*, to kill). Destroying the tubercle bacilli.

tuber·culocī·din (L. *tuberculum*, dim. of *tuber*, a swelling; *caedere*, to kill). An albumose obtained from tuberculin by treating it with platinum chloride. It is used in the same way as tuberculin, but is claimed to be free from the injurious after-effects sometimes noted after treatment with tuberculin.

tuber·culoder·ma (L. *tuberculum*, dim. of *tuber*, a swelling; G. *derma*, skin). A tuberculous affection of the skin.

tuber·culofī·broid (L. *tuberculum*, dim. of *tuber*, a swelling; *fibra*, fibre; G. *eidos*, form). Relating to a tubercle after it has been affected with fibroid degeneration.

tuber·culoid (L. *tuberculum*, dim. of *tuber*, a swelling; G. *eidos*, form). Like tuberculosis.

tuberculō·ma (L. *tuberculum*, dim. of *tuber*, a swelling). A tuberculous swelling.

tuberculō·sis (L. *tuberculum*, dim. of *tuber*, a swelling). An infectious disease caused by a specific bacillus, the *Mycobacterium tuberculosis*, and marked by the formation of tubercles. Tuberculous areas are most often situated in the lung, the intestinal tract, the lymphatic glands, the bones, the skin and the brain. The symptoms vary according to the site of the lesion, but wasting, loss of strength, anaemia, fever and sweating are amongst those ordinarily observed.

tuber·culotox·in (L. *tuberculum*, dim. of *tuber*, a swelling; G. *toxikon*, poison). A toxin of the *Mycobacterium tuberculosis*.

tuber·culous (L. *tuberculum*, dim. of *tuber*, a swelling). Relating to, affected with or due to tuberculosis.

tuber·culum (L.). Tubercle, *q.v.* **T. sellae:** a transverse ridge found on the upper surface of the sphenoid bone, lying anterior to the sella turcica, posterior to the sulcus chiasmatis, and between the anterior clinoid processes.

tuberi·ferous (L. *tuber*, a swelling; *ferre*, to bear). Tuberous.

tuberŏ·sity (L. *tuberosus*, lumpy). A prominence on a bone. **Deltoid:** the V-shaped mark on the outer surface of the humerus for the insertion of the deltoid muscle. **Gluteal:** a line on the posterior surface of the upper part of the shaft of the femur for the insertion of gluteus maximus muscle. **Of ischium:** (tuber ischii) the thick dependent part of the ischium, it supports the body in the sitting position. **Of maxilla:** that portion of the posterior surface of the maxilla which is behind the last molar tooth. **Of radius:** an oval eminence below the neck of the radius, gives insertion to the tendon of the biceps muscle.

tū·berous (L. *tuberosus*, lumpy). Resembling a tuber. **T. sclerosis:** a familial disease. Tumours form on the surfaces of the lateral ventricles, and sclerotic patches on the surface of the brain. Clinically there are progressive mental deterioration and epileptic seizures. Adenoma sebaceum, congenital tumour of the eye, and tumours of the kidney and heart muscle may be associated.

tubo-abdŏ·minal (L. *tubus*, tube; *abdōmen*, the paunch). Relating to the uterine tube and the abdomen.

tubocurar·ine. An alkaloid obtained from curare, a species of *Chondrodendron*. The chloride, $C_{38}H_{44}O_6N_2Cl_2,5H_2O$ is used as a muscle relaxant in anaesthesia.

tuboligamen·tous (L. *tubus*, tube; *ligamentum*, a bandage). Relating to the uterine tube and the broad ligament.

tubo-ovā·rian (L. *tubus*, tube; *ovum*, egg). Relating to the uterine tube and the ovary.

tū·boperitonē·al (L. *tubus*, tube; G. *peri*, around; *teinein*, to stretch). Relating to the uterine tube and the peritoneum.

tū·bular (L. *tubus*, tube). 1. Shaped like a tube. 2. Relating to or affecting a tubule. 3. Occurring in a tube.

tū·bule (L. *tubulus*, dim. of *tubus*, tube). A small tube. **T., renal:** the uriniferous tubules which commence at the capsule of Malpighi in the cortex of the kidney and open at the summit of a papilla into the renal pelvis. They form the parenchyma of the kidney. **T., seminiferous:** the minute ducts found in the testicle, which are much twisted and form the body of the testis.

tū·buli (L.). Pl. of tubulus.

tū·bulus (L.). A tubule.

Tuffier's inferior ligament (Tuffier, M. T., French surgeon, 1857–1929). The mesentericoparietal fold; that portion of the enteric mesentery which is inserted into the iliac fossa.

tugging, tracheal. A physical sign elicited in cases of aortic aneurysm. With each heart-beat the trachea is seen to be subjected to a pull.

tular·aēmia. An infectious disease caused by the *Bacterium tularense,* transmitted to man by rodents.

tulle gras (Fr.). Fabric spun in an open network, which is impregnated with soft paraffin, balsam of Peru, and vegetable oils. It is used as a dressing for wounds.

Tulp's valve (Tulp, N., Dutch anatomist, 1593–1674). The ileocaecal valve.

tumefā·cient (L. *tumefacere,* to cause to swell). Causing a swelling.

tumefac·tion (L. *tumefacere,* to cause to swell). The condition of being swollen; a swelling.

tumes·cence (L. *tumescere,* to swell up). The state of becoming tumid; a swelling.

tū·mid (L. *tumidus*). Swollen or distended.

tumi·dity (L. *tumidus*). The condition of being swollen or distended.

tumour (L. *tumor*). 1. A swelling. 2. A neoplasm not due to inflammation. 3. A mass of cells resembling normal ones but atypically disposed and developing at the expense of the body while serving no useful purpose.

tung·sten (Swed. *tung,* heavy; *sten,* stone). A metallic element; specific gravity 19·26, atomic weight 184. Symbol W. (from *Wolframium,* its German name).

tū·nic (L. *tunica,* a shirt). An external coat or membrane.

tu·nica (L.). A tunic. **T. albuginea:** name given to the fibrous capsule of testis, eye (sclerotic coat), ovary, spleen, and corpus cavernosum. **T. vaginalis:** name given to the serous covering of the testis. This is formed by a pouch of peritoneum, which at first communicates with the abdominal cavity, but is later cut off from it. **T. vasculosa:** a covering of loose connective tissue which contains numerous vessels.

Tunicā·ta. A class of small animals with a leathery tunic covering a sac-like body. They are intermediate between invertebrates and vertebrates.

tuning fork. A two-pronged metallic instrument giving, when vibrating, a sound of a certain fixed pitch.

tunnel anaemia. Ankylostomiasis, *q.v.*

tunnel disease. Caisson disease, *q.v.*

tur·bid (L. *turbidus,* troubled (of fluids)). Cloudy.

turbi·dity (L. *turbidus,* troubled (of fluids)). Cloudiness.

tur·binal (L. *turbo,* a spinning-top). 1. Turbinated. 2. Any turbinated bone.

tur·binated (L. *turbo,* a spinning-top). Shaped like an inverted cone. **T. bodies:** the turbinated bones with their coats of vascular and mucous membrane. **T. bone:** one of the three bony protuberances on the external wall of each nasal fossa.

turbinec·tomy (L. *turbo,* a spinning-top; G. *ektomē,* excision). Excision of a turbinated bone.

turbi·notomy (L. *turbo,* a spinning-top; G. *tomē,* section). A surgical knife used in turbinotomy.

turbinŏ·tomy (L. *turbo,* a spinning-top; *tomē,* section). Surgical incision into a turbinated bone.

Turck's column (Turck, L., Austrian neurologist, 1810–78). The direct pyramidal tract. **T.'s tract:** tractus temporo-pontis.

turges·cence (L. *turgescere,* to swell up). A state of being swollen or distended.

tur·gid (L. *turgidus,* inflated). Swollen; distended; congested.

turgidizā·tion (L. *turgidus,* inflated). Causing the distension of a tissue by injecting a fluid.

tur·gor (L.). Turgescence. **T. vitalis:** normal repletion of the blood-vessels.

Turk's stain (Turk, W., Austrian physician, 1871–1916). A weak solution of iodine-potassium iodide.

tur·mĕric. Curcumin, *q.v.*

turn. 1. To cause to rotate on an axis. 2. To shift the position of the foetus in order to facilitate delivery.

turning. See under version.

Turner's membrane (Turner, Sir W., English anatomist, 1832–1916). The subzonal membrane of the amnion within the chorionic vesicle.

Turner's sulcus (Turner, W. A., English neurologist, 1864–1945). The intraparietal sulcus of the cortex cerebri.

tur·pentine (G. *terebinthos,* the turpentine tree). A solidified or liquid oleoresin from various species of *Pinus.* Volatile oil of turpentine is useful as a stimulant, diuretic and, in considerable doses, as a laxative.

tur·pethin (Pers. *turbad*). A resin derived from the root of *Ipomaea turpethum,* an East Indian plant resembling jalap.

turrecĕ·phaly, turricĕ·phaly (L. *turris,* tower; G. *kephale,* head). Syn. oxycephaly.

turun·da (L., a roll of lint). A surgical tent.

tus·sal (L. *tussis,* a cough). Relating to or of the nature of a cough.

tussi·cular (L. *tussis,* a cough). Relating to a cough.

Tussilā·go (L., coltsfoot). A genus of plants including the *T. farfara,* the coltsfoot, the leaves of which are used as a demulcent.

tus·sis (L.) A cough. **T. convulsiva:** whooping-cough.

tus·sive (L. *tussis,* a cough). Relating to or produced by a cough.

tutā·men (L., defence; pl. *tutamina*). A shield or defence. **T. oculi:** the eyelids, lashes, etc.

tū·tocain. $(CH_3)_2N.CH_2.CH(CH_3).CH(CH_3)OCO.C_6H_4NH_2HCl.$ Butamin. A local anaesthetic for surface and infiltration anaesthesia. It is about one-third as toxic as cocaine.

tutty (Arab. *tutiya*). Impure oxide of zinc; used in pulverized form as an external dessicant.

'tween-brain. The portion of the brain containing the optic thalami and the third ventricle; the interbrain.

twelfth nerve. The hypoglossal nerve.

twilight sleep. The production of partial anaesthesia during childbirth; the memory of pain is abolished, but not the pain itself. The process is not without danger.

twin. One of two children born at a single birth.

twinge. A sudden, sharp pain.

twitch. To move or pull with a sudden jerk.

twitching. An irregular spasm of small extent.

Twort's phenomenon (Twort, F. W., British bacteriologist, 1878–1950). The transmission of the power to cause lysis of bacteria, found in filtrates made from faeces of patients. See bacteriophage.

tycal·cin. Calcium acetylsalicylate.

tyle (G. *tulos,* a knot). A callus.

tȳ·lion (G. *tulion,* dim. of *tulos,* a knot). The point on the anterior border of the optic groove in the median line.

tylō·ma (G. *tulos,* a knot). A callus.

tylō·sis (G. *tulos,* a knot). 1. Extreme hyperkeratosis of the soles and palms. 2. A type of blepharitis in which the edge of the eyelid is thickened and hardened.

tym·panal (G. *tumpanon,* a kettledrum). Tympanic ring, *q.v.*

tympanec·tomy (G. *tumpanon,* a kettledrum; *ektomē,* excision). Surgical removal of the tympanic membrane.

tympan·ic (G. *tumpanon,* a kettledrum). 1. Relating to the tympanum. 2. Resonant. **T. annulus:** the circular piece of bone which gives rise to the bony external auditory meatus. **T. antrum** (mastoid): is a large recess placed behind and rather above the tympanum with which it is connected by the large opening (aditus). **T. artery:** a branch of the maxillary, it enters the tympanum through the petro-tympanic fissure and supplies the membrana tympani and anterior part of the tympanum. **T. bone:** the thin plate-like bone situated between the tympanum and the cranial cavity. **T. canaliculus:** a ridge on the inferior surface of the petrous portion of the temporal bone for the tympanic branch of the glossopharyngeal nerve and the tympanic branch of the ascending pharyngeal artery. **T. membrane:** is the membrane which separates the external and inner ears. It contains the handle of the malleus between its two layers. **T. nerve** (N. of Jacobson): is a branch of the glossopharyngeal, it arises from the inferior ganglion and breaks up to form the tympanic plexus. **T. notch:** a small notch in the upper part of the tympanic annulus. **T. plate:** that portion of the temporal bone which is formed from the tympanic ring. **T. plexus:** the termination of the tympanic nerve on the promontory of the temporal bone. **T. ring:** a bony ring forming a portion of the temporal bone at birth and developing into the t. plate. **T. tegmen:** the bony plate constituting the roof of the tympanum.

tym·panism (G. *tumpanon*, a kettledrum). Dilation by gas; tympanites.

tympani·tēs (G. *tumpanon*, a kettledrum). Dilation of the abdominal walls due to the collection of gas in the intestines or the peritoneal cavity. Syn. meteorism.

tympanit·ic (G. *tumpanon*, a kettledrum). Relating to or affected with tympanites. **T. abscess:** an air-containing abscess. **T. resonance:** the sound elicited on percussion of a gas-dilated cavity.

tympani·tis (G. *tumpanon*, a kettledrum). Inflammation of the tympanum; otitis media.

tym·panohȳ·al (G. *tumpanon*, a kettledrum; *huoeidēs*, shaped like the letter y). A small cartilage of the foetus later becoming a part of the temporal bone.

tympanŏ·tomy (G. *tumpanon*, a kettledrum; *tomē*, section). Incision of the tympanic membrane.

tym·panum (G. *tumpanon*, a kettledrum). The middle ear.

tym·pany (G. *tumpanon*, a kettledrum). 1. Tympanites. 2. A resonant or bell-like percussion note.

Tyndall's phenomenon (Tyndall, J., British physicist, 1820–93). The process whereby otherwise invisible particles are rendered visible by reflection or dispersal of light by these particles when a beam of light is passed through a gas or liquid.

type (G. *tupos*, an impression). 1. A distinguishing mark or stamp; an emblem or symbol. 2. A normal or average example. 3. In pathology, the distinctive features of a disease, etc., enabling it to be classified.

Typhā·cĕae. A group of bacteria which includes the *Bacterium typhosum*, formerly called *Bacillus typhosus.*

typhae·mia (G. *tuphos*, stupor; *haima*, blood). The presence of typhoid bacteria in the blood.

tȳ·phic (G. *tuphos*, stupor). Relating to typhoid fever.

typhi·nia (G. *tuphos*, stupor). Relapsing fever.

typhlec·tasis (G. *tuphlon*, the caecum; *ektasis*, extension). Distension of the caecum.

typhlec·tomy (G. *tuphlon*, the caecum; *ektomē*, excision). Surgical removal of the caecum.

typh·lenteri·tis (G. *tuphlon*, the caecum; *enteron*, intestine). Inflammation of the caecum.

typhli·tis (G. *tuphlon*, the caecum). The same as typhlenteritis.

typh·lolithi·asis (G. *tuphlon*, the caecum; *lithos*, stone). The formation of concretions in the caecum.

typhlŏ·logy (G. *tuphlos*, blind; *logos*, a treatise). The study of blindness.

typhlomĕ·galy (G. *tuphlon*, the caecum; *megas*, large). Enlargement of the caecum.

typh·lon (G. *tuphlon*). The caecum.

typhloptō·sis (G. *tuphlon*, the caecum; *ptōsis*, a falling). Downward displacement of the caecum.

typhlor·rhaphy (G. *tuphlon*, the caecum; *rhaphē*, suture). Suture of the caecum.

typhlō·sis (G. *tuphlos*, blind). Blindness.

typh·lostenō·sis (G. *tuphlon*, the caecum; *stenos*, narrow). Abnormal narrowing of the caecum.

typhlŏ·tomy (G. *tuphlon*, the caecum; *tomē*, section). Surgical section of the caecum.

tȳ·phobacillŏ·sis (G. *tuphos*, stupor; L. *bacillus*). Systemic poisoning due to toxins produced by the typhoid bacterium.

tȳ·phoid (G. *tuphos*, stupor; *eidos*, form). Resembling typhus fever. **T. fever:** a continued, acute and infectious fever caused by the *Bacterium typhosum*, with catarrhal inflammation of the mucous membrane of the intestine, enlargement and necrosis of Peyer's patches and enlargement of the spleen and mesenteric glands. Incubation period two to three weeks. An eruption of rose-coloured spots occurs about the eighth day. The most important complications are intestinal haemorrhage, pneumonia and perforation.

typhoi·dal (G. *tuphos*, stupor; *eidos*, form). Resembling typhoid.

typhŏ·lysin (G. *tuphos*, stupor; *lusis*, dissolution). An agent destructive of *Bacterium typhosum*.

tȳ·phomalā·rial (G. *tuphos*, stupor; It. *mal'aria*, bad air). Symptomatic of both typhoid and malaria. **T. fever:** an acute disease presenting the symptoms of both typhoid and malarial fever; generally considered to be purely malarial in origin.

typhomā·nia (G. *tuphos*, stupor; *mania*, madness). Lethargy accompanied by delirium, as observed in typhus and other low fevers.

typhŏ·nia (G. *tuphos*, stupor). The same as typhomania.

typhopă·ludism (G. *tuphos*, stupor; L. *pălus*, a marsh). A type of malarial fever characterized by symptoms of typhoid.

tȳ·phophor (G. *tuphos*, stupor; *phoros*, bearing). A carrier of typhoid.

tȳ·phopneumō·nia (G. *tuphos*, stupor; *pneumōn*, lung). Pneumonia co-existent with typhoid fever.

tȳ·phose (G. *tuphos*, stupor). Resembling typhoid.

typhosep·sis (G. *tuphos*, stupor; *sēpsis*, putrefaction). Systemic poisoning resulting from typhoid fever.

typhŏ·sis (G. *tuphos*, stupor). The typhoid state.

typhotox·in (G. *tuphos*, stupor; *toxikon*, poison). A deadly ptomaine formed by the typhoid bacillus.

tȳ·phous (G. *tuphos*, stupor). Relating to or of the nature of typhus.

tȳ·phus, typhus fever (G. *tuphos*, stupor). An acute infectious and contagious virus disease. The chief symptoms are a petechial rash, nervous disorders and hyperpyrexia ending by crisis in ten to fourteen days. Incubation period may be from a few hours to two weeks. There is an eruption of rose-coloured spots on the fourth or fifth day which later become haemorrhagic. Pneumonia and nephritis are the chief complications.

tȳ·pical (G. *tupos*, an impression). Relating to or of the nature of a type; illustrative; complete.

typing of blood. The procedure whereby the blood group of a patient is determined.

tȳ·rannism (G. *turannos*, tyrant). Cruelty of morbid origin; sadism is a form of it.

tȳ·rĕin (G. *turos*, cheese). Coagulated milk casein.

tyrĕ·mesis (G. *turos*, cheese; *emesis*, a vomiting). The vomiting of caseous material; common among nursing infants.

Tyrŏ·glyphus (G. *turos*, cheese; *gluphein*, to carve). A genus of acarids, including the *T. farinae*, found in flour, and the *T. siro*, or cheese mite.

tȳ·roid (G. *turos*, cheese; *eidos*, form). Resembling cheese.

tyroleu·cine (G. *turos*, cheese; *leukos*, white). A decomposition product of albumin.

tyrō·ma (G. *turos*, cheese). A caseous tumour.

tyromatō·sis (G. *turos*, cheese). Caseation.

tȳ·rosine (G. *turos*, cheese). An amino-acid, $OH.C_6H_4.CH_2.CH(NH_2).COOH$, of crystalline nature. The appearance of tyrosine in the urine is usually in association with bile pigment. Tyrosine is an essential in any diet.

tyrosinō·sis (G. *turos*, cheese). A disease in which metabolism of tyrosine is at fault, and dihydroxyphenylalanine appears in the urine.

tȳ·rosinū·ria (G. *turos*, cheese; *ouron*, urine). A condition in which tyrosine is present in the urine.

tyrō·sis (G. *turos*, cheese). Caseation.

Tȳ·rothrix (G. *turos*, cheese; *thrix*, hair). A genus of Schizomycetes; they cause milk to coagulate.

tyrotox·icon (G. *turos*, cheese; *toxikon*, poison). A ptomaine of highly poisonous character sometimes occurring in stale milk, cheese, ice-cream, etc. It produces serious symptoms, marked prostration and sometimes death.

tyrotox·in (G. *turos*, cheese; *toxikon*, poison). A curare-like poison, a product of bacterial infection of cheese or other milk products.

tyrox·in (G. *turos*, cheese). A decomposition product of albumin.

Tyrrell's fascia (Tyrrell, F., English anatomist, 1797–1843). The prostato-peritoneal aponeurosis.

Tyson's glands (Tyson, E., English anatomist, 1649–1708). Sebaceous and smegma secreting glands of the prepuce and corona glandis.

tysonī·tis. Inflammation of Tyson's glands.

U

U. The symbol for uranium.

ū·la (G. *oulon*, gum). The gum.

ulaemorrhā·gia¹ (G. *oulē*, scar; *haima*, blood; *rhēgnunai*, to burst forth). Haemorrhage from a cicatrix.

ulaemorrhā·gia² (G. *oulon*, gum; *haima*, blood; *rhēgnunai*, to burst forth). Bleeding of the gums.

ulal·gia (G. *oulon*, gum; *algos*, pain). Painful gums.

ulatrō·phia (G. *oulon*, gum; *atrophia*, atrophy). Shrinking of the gums.

ul·cer (L. *ulcus*). A loss of substance on the surface of the skin or mucous membranes. U., callous: (Indolent) occurs most frequently on the legs of women about the middle period of life and is due to poor circulation and lack of cleanliness. U., irritable: occurs about the ankle and may follow a burn or extensive wound. U., rodent: carcinomatous or epitheliomatous ulcer involving soft tissue and bones. U., trophic: occurs in connection with a disturbance of nutrition of the tissues consecutive to a lesion of the central nervous sytem. U., varicose: occurs in the leg of a patient with varicose veins.

ulcerā·tion (L. *ulcus*, ulcer). The formation of ulcers.

ul·cerative (L. *ulcerare*, to cause to ulcerate). Relating to ulceration or characterized by the formation of ulcers. U. colitis: ulceration of the colon giving rise to a discharge of pus and the exfoliation of patches of mucous membrane.

ul·cerous (L. *ulcerare*, to cause to ulcerate). Showing ulceration.

ul·cus (L.). An ulcer. U. molle: see chancroid.

ulec·tomy¹ (G. *oulē*, scar; *ektomē*, excision). The surgical removal of scar tissue.

ulec·tomy² (G. *oulon*, gum; *ektomē*, excision). The surgical removal of gum tissue.

ulegȳ·ria (G. *oulē*, scar; *guros*, a circle). A state in which the convolutions of the brain cortex are distorted by scar-formation.

ulerythē·ma (G. *oulē*, scar; *eruthēma*, redness of the skin). An erythematous disease characterized by the formation of cicatrices.

ulet·ic¹ (G. *oulē*, scar). Relating to scars.

ulet·ic² (G. *oulon*, gum). Relating to the gums.

uli·tis (G. *oulon*, gum). Inflammation of the gums.

Ul·mus (L., elm). A genus of trees including the elms. The inner bark of *U. fulva*, usually known as slippery elm, is useful in the treatment of diarrhoea, dysentery, etc.

ul·na (L. pl. *ulnae*). The larger of the two forearm bones, situated on the inner side. It articulates with the humerus and head of the radius above and with the radius and carpus below.

ul·nad (L. *ulna*; *ad*, to). Towards the ulna.

ul·nar (L. *ulna*, the elbow). 1. Relating to the ulna. 2. Relating to the u. artery, vein, nerve or bone.

ul·naris (L. *ulna*, the elbow). The ulnar muscle situated on the inner side of the forearm.

ulnocar·pal (L. *ulna*, the elbow; G. *karpos*, the wrist). Relating to the ulna and the carpus.

ulnorā·dial (L. *ulna*, the elbow; *radius*, the radius). Relating to the ulna and the radius.

ū·locarcinō·ma (G. *oulon*, gum; *karkinoma*, an ulcer). Carcinoma of the gums.

ū·lodermati·tis (G. *oulē*, scar; *derma*, skin). Inflammation of the skin marked by the formation of scars.

uloglossi·tis (G. *oulon*, gum; *glōssa*, tongue). Combined inflammation of the gums and the tongue.

ū·loid (G. *oulē*, scar; *eidos*, form). 1. Like a scar. 2. A spot resembling a scar and produced by sub-cutaneous degeneration.

ulon·cus (G. *oulon*, gum; *ogkos*, a mass). A tumour of the gum.

ulorrhā·gia (G. *oulon*, gum; *rhēgnunai*, to burst forth). Haemorrhage from the gums.

ulorrhoē·a (G. *oulon*, gum; *rhoia*, a flowing). Bleeding from the gums.

ulō·sis (G. *oulē*, scar). Cicatrization.

ulŏ·tomy (G. *oulon*, gum; *tomē*, section). Surgical incision of the gum.

ulŏ·trichous (G. *oulos*, woolly; *thrix*, hair). Having woolly hair.

ul·timate (L. *ultimus*, last). The last; the most remote.

ul·timum mor·iens (L., 'the last to die'). Term sometimes applied to the right auricle, supposed to be the last part of the heart to cease working.

ul·trabră·chycephal·ic (L. *ultra*, beyond; G. *brakhus*, short; *kephalē*, head). Brachycephaly with a cephalic index exceeding 90°.

ultracen·trifuge (L. *ultra*, beyond; *centrum*, centre; *fugere*, to flee). A very high speed centrifuge which will precipitate molecules of substances of relatively high molecular weight.

ultrafiltrā·tion. Filtration by means of such a fine filter that not only bacteria but also certain colloid particles are removed. Gelatin or collodion may be used as the filter.

ultramī·crobe (L. *ultra*, beyond; G. *mikros*, small; *bios*, life). A micro-organism too small to be seen by the microscope.

ultramī·cron (L. *ultra*, beyond; G. *mikros*, small). An ultramicroscopic particle which is less than a quarter of a micron in diameter.

ul·tramī·croscope (L. *ultra*, beyond; *mikros*, small; *skopein*, to view). A microscope for the viewing of objects too small to be perceived with the aid of an ordinary microscope.

ul·tramicroscop·ic (L. *ultra*, beyond; *mikros*, small; *skopein*, to view). Too small to be seen under a microscope.

ultra-red. The same as infra-red, *q.v.*

ul·trasome (L. *ultra*, beyond; G. *sōma*, body). An ultramicroscopic body.

ultra-violet rays. Waves of luminiferous ether lying beyond the violet rays. They are not perceived by the retina. They are capable of reflection, refraction and polarization, and are able to destroy the vitality of bacteria.

ululā·tion (L. *ululare*, to howl). Hysterical howling.

umbilec·tomy (L. *umbilicus*, navel; G. *ektomē*, excision). Excision of the umbilicus.

umbili·cal (L. *umbilicus*, navel). Relating to the umbilicus, its cord or vessels. U. cord: the cord-like structure connecting the placenta with the navel of the foetus.

umbĭ·licate (L. *umbilicus*, navel). Like the navel.

umbilicā·tion (L. *umbilicus*, navel). 1. A pit or depression resembling that of the navel. 2. The state of being umbilicated.

umbili·cus (L. *umbilicus*, navel). The navel; the round, depressed scar in the midline of the abdomen marking the point of entry of the umbilical cord.

unavoidable haemorrhage. See under haemorrhage, unavoidable.

un·cia (L.). 1. An ounce. 2. An inch.

un·ciform (L. *uncus*, hook; *forma*, shape). Hooked. U. bone: a bone shaped like a hook and situated in the second row of the carpus. Syn. hamate.

Uncinā·ria (L. *uncinus*, dim. of *uncus*, hook). A genus of nematode worms.

un·cinarī·asis (L. *uncinus*, dim. of *uncus*, hook). A disease caused by infestation with worms of the genus Uncinaria; hookworm disease.

un·cinate (L. *uncus*, hook). Hooked.

uncinā·tum (L. *uncus*, hook). The unciform bone. Syn. hamate.

uncon·scious. Insensible; not conscious.

uncon·sciousness. The condition of being insensible and without powers of reflex action.

unc·tion (L. *unctio*). An ointment, or the process of anointing.

unc·tious (L. *unctio*, ointment). Of a greasy or oily nature.

un·cus (L., hook). 1. A hook or hook-like structure. 2. The curved end of the uncinate gyrus of the brain.

under. Beneath. U.-hung: term applied to a prominent lower jaw.

un·dinism (L. *unda*, a wave). A mental state in which water, urine or micturition excites eroticism.

un·dulant (L. *undulans*, wavy). Wavelike. U. fever: an infection caused by infection by the *Brucella melitensis* of goats, the *Brucella abortus bovinus* of cattle or other species of *Brucella*. Man is usually infected by drinking milk from animals attacked by these germs. Syn. Malta fever; abortus fever; Mediterranean fever.

undulā·tion (L. *undulatus*, wavy). A wavelike vibration or movement.

un·dulatory (L. *undulatus*, wavy). Moving in waves; vibratory.

unfruitful. Yielding no fruit; barren.

un·gual (L. *unguis*, finger- or toe-nail). Relating to a nail.

un·guent, unguen·tum (L.). An ointment.

unguī·culate (L. *unguis*, finger- or toe-nail). Possessing nails or claws.

un·guinal (L. *unguis*, finger- or toe-nail). Relating to a nail or to the nails.

un·guis (L., finger- or toe-nail). 1. A nail of a finger or toe. 2. A nail-like part. U. incurvatus: ingrowing toenail. See incarnatio.

un·gula (L. *ungula*, from *unguis*, finger- or toe-nail). 1. A hoof. 2. An instrument employed to deliver a dead foetus.

uniăx·ial (L. *unus*, one; *axis*, axis). Having only one axis.

unibā·sal (L. *unus*, one; *basis*, a base). Having only a single base.

unicel·lular (L. *unus*, one; *cellula*, dim. of *cella*, a store-room). Having only one cell.

unicep·tor (L. *unus*, one; *capere*, to take). A ceptor with only one uniting arm; e.g., the haptophore group.

ū·nicorn (L. *unus*, one; *cornu*, horn). Possessing a single horn.

unilā·teral (L. *unus*, one; *lateralis*, from *latus*, side). Relating to or affecting one side only.

unilō·bar (L. *unus*, one; *lōbus*, lobe). Consisting of only one lobe.

unilŏ·cular (L. *unus*, one; *loculus*, dim. of *locus*, a place). Having only one loculus.

uninū·clear, uninū·cleated (L. *unus*, one; *nucula*, dim. of *nux*, nut). Having only a single nucleus.

uniŏ·cular (L. *unus*, one; *oculus*, eye). Relating to, performed with or affecting only one eye.

ū·nion (Late L. *unio*, from *unus*, one). The joining up of a fractured bone; healing.

uniŏ·vular (L. *unus*, one; *ovum*, egg). Developed from one ovum.

uni·para (L. *unus*, one; *parere*, to bear). A woman who has had only one child.

uni·parous (L. *unus*, one; *parere*, to bear). Having borne only one child.

unipō·lar (L. *unus*, one; G. *polos*, an axis). 1. Possessing only one pole or process. 2. Relating to one pole.

ū·nit (L. *unitas*, from *unus*, one). A single thing or a group considered as a whole.

ū·nitary (L. *unitas*, from *unus*, one). Relating to or formed of one unit.

univā·lent (L. *unus*, one; *valēre*, to be worth). Having a valence of one; capable of replacing or combining with a single hydrogen atom.

univer·sal (L. *universalis*, from *universus*, whole). General; relating to the universe.

Unna's boot (Unna, P. G., German dermatologist, 1850–1929). A dressing of Unna's paste applied on layers of spiral bandage to the leg from knee to toes in varicose ulcerations. U.'s dermatosis: seborrhoeic eczema. U.'s paste: zinc oxide 3, gelatin 3, glycerin 7, distilled water 7.

unoffĭ·cial (A.S. *un*, neg.; L. *officialis*, from *officium*, duty). Not included in the pharmacopoeia.

unor·ganized (A.S. *un*, neg.; G. *organon*, an organ). Without organs; lacking a definite structure.

unpig·mented (A.S. *un*, neg.; L. *pigmentum*, a colour). Without pigment.

unstri·ated (A.S. *un*, neg.; L. *striatus*, from *striare*, to hollow out). Having no striations or striae, as u. muscle.

unwell. 1. Sick; ill. 2. Euphemism for menstruating.

ūrā·chal (G. *ourakhos*, the urinary canal of a foetus). Relating to the urachus.

ūrā·chus (G. *ourakhos*, the urinary canal of a foetus). The stem-like structure connecting the bladder with the allantois in the foetus. In post-natal life it is represented by a cord of fibrous nature situated between the apex of the bladder and the umbilicus.

uracrā·sia (G. *ouron*, urine; *akrasia*, bad mixture). Disorder of the urine.

uracrā·tia (G. *ouron*, urine; *akrateia*, debility). Incontinence of urine.

urae·mia (G. *ouron*, urine; *haima*, blood). The symptom-complex seen in renal failure; characterized by headache, vertigo, vomiting, blindness and later by convulsions and coma. The disease was formerly believed to be due to an excess of urea in the blood.

urae·mic (G. *ouron*, urine; *haima*, blood). Caused by or characterized by uraemia.

urană·lysis (G. *ouron*, urine; *analusis*, analysis). Analysis of the urine.

urā·niscochas·ma (G. *ouraniskos*, palate; *khasma*, a hollow). Cleft palate.

urā·nisconī·tis (G. *ouraniskos*, palate). Inflammation of the uraniscus.

uranis·coplasty (G. *ouraniskos*, palate; *plassein*, to form). An operation for the repair of cleft palate.

uraniscor·rhaphy (G. *ouraniskos*, palate; *rhaphē*, suture). Suture of a cleft palate; staphylorrhaphy.

uranis·cus (G. *ouraniskos*, palate). The palate.

ū·ranism (G. *ouranos*, heaven). Homosexuality.

ū·ranist (G. *ouranos*, heaven). A homosexual individual.

urā·nium (G. *ouranos*, heaven). A heavy white metal, atomic weight 238·2, specific gravity 18·7, symbol U. Its salts are highly poisonous.

ū·ranoplasty (G. *ouranos*, heaven; *plassein*, to form). Uraniscoplasty, q.v.

uranŏ·schisis (G. *ouranos*, heaven; *skhisis*, a cleaving). Cleft palate.

ura·ri. Syn. for curare, q.v.

ū·rase (G. *ouron*, urine). An enzyme associated with bacteria which ferment urea.

uratae·mia (G. *ouron*, urine; *haima*, blood). An excess of urates in the blood.

ū·rate (G. *ouron*, urine). A salt of uric acid.

urat·ic (G. *ouron*, urine). Relating to or characterized by urates.

uratŏ·lysis (G. *ouron*, urine; *lusis*, dissolution). The destruction of urates.

uratō·ma (G. *ouron*, urine). A concretion formed of urates; a tophus.

uratō·sis (G. *ouron*, urine). Deposition of urates in the tissues.

uratū·ria (G. *ouron*, urine). The presence of an excess of urates in the urine.

ūrē·a (G. *ouron*, urine). $NH_2CO.NH_2$. The chief nitrogenous constituent of urine and principal end-product of protein metabolism. Syn. carbamide. **U. concentration test:** a test of renal efficiency, based on the rapid absorption of urea in the stomach and its excretion unaltered by the kidneys. The patient is given 15 gm. urea in 100 cc. water. The concentration of urea in the urine is measured at the end of one hour and at the end of two hours.

ū·real (G. *ouron*, urine). Relating to or containing urea.

urĕă·meter (G. *ouron*, urine; *metron*, measure). An apparatus for estimating the amount of urea contained in urine.

ūrē·apoiē·sis (G. *ouron*, urine; *poiein*, to make). The formation of urea.

ū·rease (G. *ouron*, urine). 1. Urase, *q.v.* 2. An enzyme occurring in the soya bean and used in tests made to ascertain the amount of urine present in the blood.

urē·chysis (G. *ouron*, urine; *khusis*, a pouring forth). The effusion of urine into areolar tissues.

urē·do (L. *urēdo*, a burning itch). 1. A burning sensation of the skin. 2. Urticarcia.

ū·rĕide (G. *ouron*, urine). A compound of urea and an acid or aldehyde formed by eliminating water. Monoureides come from one molecule of urea and diureides from two molecules of urea.

urelcō·sis (G. *ouron*, urine; *helkōsis*, ulceration). Ulceration of the urinary organs.

urĕŏ·meter. Ureameter, *q.v.*

urē·rythrin (G. *ouron*, urine; *eruthros*, red). Uroerythrin, *q.v.*

urē·sis (G. *ourēsis*, urination). Urination.

urē·tal (G. *ourētēr*, ureter). Relating to a ureter.

urē·ter (G. *ourētēr*). A duct conveying the urine from the renal pelvis to the bladder.

urē·teral (G. *ourētēr*, ureter). Relating to the ureter.

ū·reteral·gia (G. *ourētēr*, ureter; *algos*, pain). Pain in the ureter.

ū·reterec·tasis (G. *ourētēr*, ureter; *ektasis*, extension). Dilatation of the ureter.

ū·reterec·tomy (G. *ourētēr*, ureter; *ektomē*, excision). Excision of the ureter.

uretĕ·ric (G. *ourētēr*, ureter). Relating to the ureter.

ū·reterī·tis (G. *ourētēr*, ureter). Inflammation of the ureter.

urē·terocele (G. *ourētēr*, ureter; *kēlē*, hernia). Cystic dilatation of lower end of the ureter.

urē·terocervī·cal (G. *ourētēr*, ureter; L. *cervix*, neck). Relating to a ureter and the uterine cervix.

urē·terocolŏ·stomy (G. *ourētēr*, ureter; *kŏlon*, colon; *stoma*, mouth). Implantation of ureter into colon, usually sigmoid. See ureterosigmoidostomy.

urē·terocystŏ·stomy (G. *ourētēr*, ureter; *kustis*, bladder; *stoma*, mouth). The artificial making of a connection between a ureter and the bladder.

urē·tero-enterŏ·stomy (G. *ourētēr*, ureter; *enteron*, intestine; *stoma*, mouth). The creation of an artificial communication between a ureter and the intestine.

urē·terolith (G. *ourētēr*, ureter; *lithos*, stone). A concretion in a ureter.

urē·terolithī·asis (G. *ourētēr*, ureter; *lithos*, stone). The formation of a concretion in a ureter.

urē·terolithŏ·tomy (G. *ourētēr*, ureter; *lithos*, stone; *tomē*, section). Surgical cutting into a ureter for the removal of a concretion.

urē·teroplasty (G. *ourētēr*, ureter; *plassein*, to form). A plastic operation on a ureter.

urē·teroproctŏ·stomy (G. *ourētēr*, ureter; *prŏktos*, anus; *stoma*, mouth). The creation of a passage between a ureter and the anus.

urē·teropȳĕlī·tis (G. *ourētēr*, ureter; *puelos*, a trough). Inflammation of a ureter and a renal pelvis.

urē·teropȳō·sis (G. *ourētēr*, ureter; *puon*, pus). Inflammation of a ureter accompanied by suppuration.

urē·terorrhā·gia (G. *ourētēr*, ureter; *rhēgnunai*, to burst forth). Haemorrhage from a ureter.

ū·reteror·rhaphy (G. *ourētēr*, ureter; *rhaphē*, suture). Suture of a ureter.

urē·terosigmoidŏ·stomy. Implantation of ureter into sigmoid colon. This operation is performed especially in cases of carcinoma of bladder as first stage of cystectomy.

urē·terostegnō·sis (G. *ourētēr*, ureter; *stegnōsis*, stoppage). Constriction of a ureter.

urē·terostenō·ma (G. *ourētēr*, ureter; *stenōma*, a narrow place). Abnormal narrowing of the ureter.

urē·terostenō·sis (G. *ourētēr*, ureter; *stenosis*, a being narrowed). Ureterostegnosis, *q.v.*

urē·terŏ·stoma (G. *ourētēr*, ureter; *stoma*, mouth). 1. The mouth of the ureter. 2. A ureteral fistula.

ū·reterŏ·stomy (G. *ourētēr*, ureter; *stoma*, mouth). Operation to form a fistula into the ureter through which the ureter may discharge urine.

ū·reterŏ·tomy (G. *ourētēr*, ureter; *tomē*, section). Incision into a ureter.

urē·tero-ū·reterŏ·stomy (G. *ourētēr*, ureter; *stoma*, mouth). The creation of an artificial passage between the ureters or between different sections of the same ureter.

urē·tero-ū·terine (G. *ourētēr*, ureter; L. *uterus*, the womb). Relating to a ureter and the uterus.

urē·terovagī·nal (G. *ourētēr*, ureter; L. *vagina*, a sheath). Relating to a ureter and the vagina.

urē·terovĕ·sical (G. *ourētēr*, ureter; L. *vesica*, bladder). Relating to a ureter and the bladder.

ū·rethane. Ethyl carbamate; $NH_2.CO.OC_2H_5$. It is a colourless crystalline substance and slightly bitter to the taste. It is used as a hypnotic and antipyretic.

urē·thra (G. *ourēthra*). The channel through which the urine is excreted. It extends from the cervix vesicae to the meatus urinarius. In the male it passes through the prostate and penis and is from eight to nine inches long. In the female it is about one and a half inches in length.

urē·thral (G. *ourēthra*, urethra). Relating to the urethra.

urethral·gia (G. *ourēthra*, urethra; *algos*, pain). Pain in the urethra.

urē·thratrē·sia (G. *ourēthra*, urethra; *atresia*, closure). Imperforate urethra.

urethrec·tomy (G. *ourēthra*, urethra; *ektomē*, excision). Surgical removal of the urethra or a portion of it.

urethremphrax·is (G. *ourēthra*, urethra; *emphraxis*, a stoppage). Obstruction in the urethra. Syn. urethrophraxis.

urethrī·tis (G. *ourēthra*, urethra). Inflammation of the urethra.

urē·throcele (G. *ourēthra*, urethra; *kēlē*, hernia). A thickening of the wall of the female urethra, or prolapse of the female urethra through the meatus urinarius.

urē·throcystī·tis (G. *ourēthra*, urethra; *kustis*, bladder). Joint inflammation of the urethra and the bladder.

urethrody·nia (G. *ourēthra*, urethra; *odunē*, pain). Urethralgia, *q.v.*

urethrŏ·meter (G. *ourēthra*, urethra; *metron*, measure). An instrument used for measuring the urethra.

urethropē·nile (G. *ourēthra*, urethra; L. *penis*). Relating to the urethra and the penis.

urē·throperinē·al (G. *ourēthra*, urethra; *perinaion*, perineum). Relating to the urethra and the perineum.

urē·throperi·neoscrō·tal (G. *ourēthra*, urethra; *perinaion*, perineum; L. *scrotum*, scrotum). Relating to the urethra, perineum and scrotum.

urē·throphrax·is (G. *ourēthra*, urethra; *emphraxis*, a stoppage). An obstruction in the urethra. Syn. urethremphraxis.

urethrophy·ma (G. *ourēthra*, urethra; *phuma*, a growth). A tumour of the urethra.

urē·throplasty (G. *ourēthra*, urethra; *plassein*, to form). A plastic operation on the urethra.

urethrorec·tal (G. *ourēthra*, urethra; L. *rectus*, straight). Relating to the urethra and the rectum.

urethrorrhā·gia (G. *ourēthra*, urethra; *rhēgnunai*. to burst forth). Haemorrhage from the urethra.

urethror·rhaphy (G. *ourēthra*, urethra; *rhaphē*, suture). Suturing of the urethra or of a urethral fistula.

urethrorrhōe·a (G. *ourēthra*, urethra; *rhoia*, a flowing). A morbid discharge from the urethra.

urē·throscope (G. *ourēthra*, urethra; *skopein*, to inspect). An instrument for examining the interior of the urethra.

urethrŏ·scopy (G. *ourēthra*, urethra; *skopein*, to inspect). Examination of the interior of the urethra by means of the urethroscope.

urē·throspasm (G. *ourēthra*, urethra; *spasmos*, spasm). Spasm of the urethral muscles.

urē·throstenō·sis (G. *ourēthra*, urethra; *stenosis*, a being narrowed). A urethral stricture.

urethrŏ·stomy (G. *ourēthra*, urethra; *stoma*, mouth). Making an opening in the urethra.

urē·throtome (G. *ourēthra*, urethra; *tomē*, section). An instrument used for the performance of urethrotomy.

urethrŏ·tomy (G. *ourēthra*, urethra; *tomē*, section). The cutting of a urethral stricture.

urethrovagi·nal (G. *ourēthra*, urethra; L. *vagina*, a sheath). Relating to the urethra and the vagina.

urethrovĕ·sical (G. *ourēthra*, urethra; L. *vesica*, bladder). Relating to the urethra and the bladder.

urēt·ic (G. *ourētikos*, promoting or resembling urine). Relating to urine or promoting the flow of urine.

ū·ric (G. *ouron*, urine). Relating to the urine. U. acid: a product of nuclein metabolism found in blood and urine. A crystalline acid, tri-oxypurine, $C_5H_4N_4O_3$.

ū·ricacidae·mia (G. *ouron*, urine; L. *acidus*, sour; G. *haima*, blood). An excess of uric acid in the blood.

ū·ricacidū·ria (G. *ouron*, urine; L. *acidus*, sour; G. *ouron*, urine). An excess of uric acid in the urine.

uricae·mia (G. *ouron*, urine; *haima*, blood). Uric-acidaemia, *q.v.*

ū·ricase (G. *ouron*, urine). An enzyme found in certain animals, e.g. Dalmatian dog, which converts uric acid into allantoin.

ū·richochō·lia (G. *ouron*, urine; *khŏlē*, bile). The presence of uric acid in the bile.

uricŏ·lysis (G. *ouron*, urine; *lusis*, dissolution). The splitting up of uric acid.

uricoly·tic (G. *ouron*, urine; *lusis*, dissolution). Relating to or producing uricolysis.

uridrō·sis (G. *ouron*, urine; *hidros*, sweat). The presence in the sweat of urea, uric acid or other urinary matter. U. crystallina: a type of u. in which uric acid crystals are deposited on the skin.

urī·na (L.). Urine. U. cruenta: bloodstained urine. U. galactodes: milky urine.

urinae·mia (L. *urina*, urine; G. *haima*, blood). Uraemia, *q.v.*

ū·rinal (L. *urina*, urine). A vessel for the reception of urine.

urinā·lysis (L. *urina*, urine; G. *lusis*, dissolution). Analysis of urine.

ū·rinary (L. *urina*, urine). Relating to the urine. U. organs: those concerned with the secretion and discharge of urine, including the kidneys, ureters, bladder and urethra.

urinā·tion (L. *urina*, urine). The act of discharging urine; micturition.

ū·rine (L. *urina*). The fluid secreted by the kidneys, passed into the bladder and finally discharged by the urethra.

urini·ferous (L. *urina*, urine; *ferre*, to bear). Conveying urine, as a u. tubule.

ū·rinogĕ·nital (L. *urina*, urine; *genitalis*, causing generation). Urogenital, *q.v.*

urinŏ·genous (L. *urina*, urine; G. *gennan*, to produce). Producing or originating in urine.

urinŏ·logist (L. *urina*, urine; G. *logos*, a treatise). Urologist, *q.v.*

urinŏ·ma (L. *urina*, urine). A urine-containing cyst.

urinŏ·meter (L. *urina*, urine; G. *metron*, measure). An instrument for ascertaining the specific gravity of urine.

urinŏ·metry (L. *urina*, urine; G. *metron*, measure). The estimation of the specific gravity of urine with the aid of the urinometer.

ū·rinosanguin·eous (L. *urina*, urine; *sanguis*, blood). Containing both urine and blood.

urinŏ·scopy (L. *urina*, urine; G. *skopein*, to view). Uroscopy, *q.v.*

ū·rinous (L. *urina*, urine). Of the nature of urine, as u. odour.

ur·ning (G. *ouranos*, heaven). A homosexual individual.

ur·nism (G. *ouranos*, heaven). Homosexuality.

Urobacil·lus (G. *ouron*, urine; L. *bacillus*, dim. of *baculus*, a staff). Generic term for bacilli found in urine, especially in decomposing urine.

urobī·lin (G. *ouron*, urine; L. *bīlis*, bile). A yellow-brown amorphous pigment derived from bilirubin and the principal pigment of urine.

urobilinae·mia (G. *ouron*, urine; L. *bilis*, bile; G. *haima*, blood). The presence of urobilin in the blood.

ū·robili·nogen (G. *ouron*, urine; L. *bilis*, bile; G. *gennan*, to produce). A chromogen the decomposition of which produces urobilin.

urobilinū·ria (G. *ouron*, urine; L. *bilis*, bile; G. *ouron*, urine). An excess of urobilin in the urine.

u·rocele (G. *ouron*, urine; *kēlē*, hernia). A swelling of the scrotum caused by extravasation of urine.

urochē·sia (G. *ouron*, urine; *khezein*, to defaecate). The excretion of urine through the anus.

ū·rochrome (G. *ouron*, urine; *khrōma*, colour). A yellow colouring substance found in urine.

uroclep·sia (G. *ouron*, urine; *klepsia*, theft). The unconscious passing of urine.

urocrī·sia (G. *ouron*, urine; *krīsis*, judgment). Diagnosis reached by examination of the urine.

urŏ·crisis (G. *ouron*, urine; *krīsis*, crisis of a disease). 1. Excessive urination. 2. A vesical crisis.

urocy̆·anin (G. *ouron*, urine; *kuanos*, blue). Uro-glaucin, *q.v.*

ū·rocy̆a·nogen (G. *ouron*, urine; *kuanos*, blue; *gennan*, to produce). A blue pigment sometimes appearing in urine; especially in cases of cholera.

ū·rocyanō·sis (G. *ouron*, urine; *kuanos*, blue). Blue discoloration of urine due to the presence of indican; indicanuria.

ū·rocyst (G. *ouron*, urine; *kustis*, bladder). The urinary bladder.

urocys·tic (G. *ouron*, urine; *kustis*, bladder). Relating to the urinary bladder.

urocystī·tis (G. *ouron*, urine; *kustis*, bladder). Cystitis or inflammation of the urinary bladder.

urodāe·um (G. *ouron*, urine; *hodaios*, on the way). That portion of the cloaca into which the ureters and genital ducts empty.

ū·rodiă·lysis (G. *ouron*, urine; *dialusis*, cessation). suppression of the urine.

urodȳ·nia (G. *ouron*, urine; *odunē*, pain). Painful passing of urine.

uro-ĕ·rythrin (G. *ouron*, urine; *eruthros*, red). An amorphous reddish urinary pigment with an acid reaction; it is present in the urine in certain diseases, e.g., in rheumatism.

urofus·cin (G. *ouron*, urine; L. *fuscus*, tawny). A pigment sometimes found in the urine—it is a precursor of haematoporphyrin.

ū·rofuscohāe·matin (G. *ouron*, urine; L. *fuscus*, tawny; G. *haima*, blood). A red pigment derived from haematin and found in urine.

urogĕ·nital (G. *ouron*, urine; L. *genitalis*, causing generation). Relating to the urinary and genital organs.

urŏ·genous (G. *ouron*, urine; *gennan*, to produce). Producing urine.

uroglau·cin (G. *ouron*, urine; *glaukos*, bluish-green). A dark blue pigment occasionally seen in urine.

urŏ·graphy (G. *ouron*, urine; *graphein*, to write). The study of the urinary tract by outlining it with radio-opaque dyes.

urogravi·meter (G. *ouron*, urine; L. *gravis*, heavy; G. *metron*, measure). Urinometer, *q.v.*

urohāe·matin (G. *ouron*, urine; *haima*, blood). Altered haematin in urine.

ū·rohāe·matonephrŏ·sis (G. *ouron*, urine; *haima*, blood; *nephros*, kidney). Dilation of the kidney with an accumulation of urine and blood.

ū·rohāe·matopor·phyrin (G *ouron*, urine; *haima*, blood; *porphura*, purple dye). Urohaematin, an unusual urinary pigment.

urolag·nia (G. *ouron*, urine; *lagneia*, lust). Libido aroused by watching a person micturating.

ū·rolith (G. *ouron*, urine; *lithos*, stone). A concretion occurring in the urine.

ū·rolithī·asis (G. *ouron*, urine; *lithos*, stone). The formation or the presence of urinary calculi.

urŏ·logist (G. *ouron*, urine; *logos*, treatise). One skilled in urology.

urŏ·logy (G. *ouron*, urine; *logos*, treatise). The study of diseases of the urinary tract.

urolū·tēin (G. *ouron*, urine; L. *luteus*, yellow). A yellow pigment occasionally occurring in urine.

u·romancy (G. *ouron*, urine; *manteia*, divination). Prognosis based on the examination of urine.

uromĕ·lanin (G. *ouron*, urine; *mĕlas*, black). A black pigment sometimes occurring in the urine.

urŏ·melus (G. *oura*, tail; *melos*, limb). A monster with the legs more or less completely united and having but a single foot.

urŏ·meter (G. *ouron*, urine; *metron*, measure). Urinometer, *q.v.*

uron·cus (G. *ouron*, urine; *ogkos*, a mass). A urine-containing tumour.

ū·rophan (G. *ouron*, urine; *phainein*, to show). A generic name for those substances which, when ingested, reappear in the urine without having undergone any chemical change.

urophan·ic (G. *ouron*, urine; *phainein*, to show). Occurring in the urine.

ū·rophein (G. *ouron*, urine; *phaios*, grey). A grey-coloured pigment to which is ascribed the distinctive odour of urine.

uropit·tin (G. *ouron*, urine; *pitta*, pitch (tar)). A nitrogenous substance derived from urochrome.

uroplā·nia (G. *ouron*, urine; *plănē*, a wandering). Urine found in parts outside the urinary organs or the discharge of urine from an abnormal exit.

uropoiē·sis (G. *ouron*, urine; *poiēsis*, a making). The secretion of urine.

uropoiē·tic (G. *ouron*, urine; *poiein*, to make). Relating to or promoting uropoiesis.

uropor·phyrin (G. *ouron*, urine; *porphura*, purple dye). $C_{40}H_{38}O_{16}N_4$, a porphyrin found in the urine in porphyrinuria.

uropsam·mus (G. *ouron*, urine; *psammos*, sand). Urinary gravel.

ū·ropȳ·oūrē·ter (G. *ouron*, urine; *puon*, pus; *ourētēr*, ureter). An infected ureter containing a collection of pus.

urorō·sĕin (G. *ouron*, urine; L. *rosa*, rose). A rose-coloured pigment found in urine.

urorrhā·gia (G. *ouron*, urine; *rhēgnunai*, to burst forth). Excessive discharge of urine.

urorrhoē·a (G. *ouron*, urine; *rhoia*, a flow). Involuntary discharge of urine.

urorū·bin (G. *ouron*, urine; L. *ruber*, red). A red pigment obtained by treating the urine with hydro-chloric acid.

urŏ·schĕocele (G. *ouron*, urine; *skhesis*, retention; *kēlē*, hernia). Urocele, *q.v.*

urŏ·schesis (G. *ouron*, urine; *skhesis*, retention). Retention of urine.

urŏ·scopy (G. *ouron*, urine; *skopein*, to view). Examination of urine.

Uroselectan B. A proprietary preparation of the disodium salt of N-methyl-3:5-diiodo-4-pyridone -2:6-dicarboxylic acid. It is in the form of a white, crystalline powder and used as a contrast medium for intravenous pyelography.

urosep·sis (G. *ouron*, urine; *sēpsis*, decay). A toxic state caused by the extravasation of urine.

urosep·tic (G. *ouron*, urine; *sēpsis*, decay). Relating to or marked by urosepsis.

urŏ·sis (G. *ouron*, urine). Any disease of the urinary tract.

urospec·trin (G. *ouron*, urine; L. *spectrum*, an image). A pigment resembling haematoporphyrin found in normal urine when this is shaken up with acetic ether.

urostē·alith (G. *ouron*, urine; *stear*, fat; *lithos*, stone). A fatty material found in certain types of urinary calculi.

urotox·ic (G. *ouron*, urine; *toxikon*, poison). Relating to poisonous substances eliminated in the urine.

urōurē·ter (G. *ouron*, urine; *ourētēr*, ureter). A distension of the ureter by urine.

ū·rous (G. *ouron*, urine). Of the nature of or resembling urine.

uroxan·thin (G. *ouron*, urine; *xanthos*, yellow). A yellow pigment found in urine, which produces indigo blue on oxidation; indigogen.

urŏ·xin (G. *ouron*, urine; *oxus*, sharp). Alloxantin, *q.v.*

Ur·tica (L. *urtīca*, a nettle). 1. A genus of plants including the stinging nettle. 2. A wheal.

urticā·ria (L. *urtīca*, a nettle). An allergic reaction of the skin marked by the development of wheals which induce sensations of burning and itching. A crop of vesicles last from a few minutes to several hours and their onset and disappearance are sudden. Syn. hives; nettlerash. U. papulosa: an urticaria chiefly affecting children, called also lichen urticatus. There is a papular eruption and when this disappears a solid papule is left.

urticā·rial (L. *urtīca*, nettle). Relating to urticaria.

Uskov's pillars (Uskov, N., Russian anatomist of the 19th century). In the embryo, two folds or ridges that grow from the dorso-lateral region of the body wall and unite with the septum transversum to form the diaphragm.

ustulā·tion (L. *ustulare*, to scorch). The act of drying by means of heat.

us·tus (L. *urĕre*, to burn). Burned.

uteral·gia (L. *uterus*; G. *algos*, pain). Pain in the uterus.

uterec·tomy (L. *uterus*, G. *ektomē*, excision). Hysterectomy, *q.v.*

ū·terine (L. *uterus*, the womb). Relating to the uterus.

uterī·tis (L. *uterus*, the womb). Inflammation of the uterus.

ū·tero-abdŏ·minal (L. *uterus*, the womb; *abdōmen*, the paunch). Relating both to the uterus and the abdomen.

ū·terocele (L. *uterus*, the womb; G. *kēlē*, hernia). Uterine hernia.

ū·terocervi·cal (L. *uterus*, the womb; *cervix*, neck). Relating to the uterus and the uterine cervix.

uterodў·nia (L. *uterus*, G. *odunē*, pain). Pain in the uterus.

ū·terofixā·tion (L. *uterus*; *fīgere*, to fix). Hysteropexy, *q.v.*

ū·terogestā·tion (L. *uterus*; *gestatio*, a carrying). Gestation within the uterine cavity; normal pregnancy.

ū·terolith (L. *uterus*; G. *lithos*, stone). A uterine calculus.

uteromā·nia (L. *uterus*; G. *mania*, madness). Nymphomania, *q.v.*

uterŏ·meter (L. *uterus*; G. *metron*, measure). An instrument for the measurement of the uterus.

ū·tero-ovā·rian (L. *uterus*; *ovum*, egg). Relating to the uterus and the ovary.

ū·teropel·vic (L. *uterus*; *pelvis*, a basin). Relating both to the uterus and the pelvic ligaments.

ū·teropexy (L. *uterus*; G. *pēxis*, fixation). Hysteropexy, *q.v.*

ū·teroplacen·tal (L. *uterus*; *placenta*). Referring both to the uterus and the placenta.

ū·teroplasty (L. *uterus*; G. *plassein*, to form). A plastic operation on the uterus.

ū·terosā·cral (L. *uterus*; *sacrum*). Relating both to the uterus and the sacrum.

ū·terosclerŏ·sis (L. *uterus*; G. *sklēros*, hard). Sclerosis of the uterus.

ū·teroscope (L. *uterus*; G. *skopein*, to view). A uterine speculum.

ū·terotome (L. *uterus*; G. *tomē*, section). Instrument used to make an incision into the uterus.

uterŏ·tomy (L. *uterus*; G. *tomē*, section). Hysterotomy, *q.v.*

ū·terotū·bal (L. *uterus*; *tubus*, a tube). Relating both to the uterus and the uterine tubes.

u·terovagi·nal (L. *uterus*; *vagina*). Pertaining both to the uterus and the vagina.

ū·terovĕ·sical (L. *uterus*; *vesica*, bladder). Relating both to the uterus and the bladder.

ū·terus (L., womb) The womb; the organ of gestation into which the ovum is received and where it is sustained after fertilization. The uterus is the principal agent in the expulsion of the foetus at parturition. Anatomically three parts are recognized; the fundus, the body and the cervix. The fundus is the uppermost and broadest part and the body tapers down to the neck, or cervix, which is the narrow part. The mouth (os uteri) communicates with the vagina.

ū·tricle (L. *utriculus*, dim. of *uter*, a bag). 1. The larger of the two membranous sacs of the labyrinth in the bony vestibule of the ear. 2. The uterus masculinus, or prostatic vesicle.

utri·cular (L. *utriculus*, dim. of *uter*, a bag). Relating to the utricle.

utri·culus (L.). Utricle, *q.v.*

utriculī·tis (L. *utriculus*, dim. of *uter*, a bag). Inflammation of the utricle.

ū·vĕa (L. *uva*, grape). The pigmented part of the eye; this includes the iris, ciliary body and choroid.

ū·vĕal (L. *uva*, grape). Relating to the uvea.

uvĕi·tis (L. *uva*, grape). Inflammation of the uvea.

ū·veoparŏ·tid (L. *uva*, grape; G. *para*, beside; *ous*, ear). Relating to the uvea and the parotid gland.

uvifor·mis (L. *uva*, grape; *forma*, shape). The central layer of the choroid coat.

ū·vula (L., little grape). The conical muscular body hanging from the free border of the soft palate.

ūvulaptō·sis (L. *uvula*, little grape; G. *ptosis*, a falling). Uvuloptosis, *q.v.*

ū·vular (L. *uvula*, little grape). Relating to the uvula.

uvulā·ris (L. *uvula*, little grape). The azygos uvulae muscle.

uvulec·tomy (L. *uvula*, little grape; G. *ektomē*, excision). Surgical removal of the uvula.

uvulī·tis (L. *uvula*, little grape). Inflammation of the uvula.

ū·vuloptō·sis (L. *uvula*, little grape; G. *ptōsis*, a falling). A relaxed state of the uvula.

ū·vulotome (L. *uvula*, little grape; G. *tomē*, section). A surgical knife used in performing uvulotomy.

uvulŏ·tomy (L. *uvula*, little grape; G. *tomē*, section). The surgical removal of the whole or a portion of the uvula.

V

V. Abbreviation for vibrio. Symbol for vanadium.

vacci·genous (L. *vacca*, cow; G. *gennan*, to produce). Cultivating vaccine virus.

vac·cinal (L. *vacca*, cow). Relating to vaccination or to vaccine.

vac·cinate (L. *vacca*, cow). To inoculate with vaccinia virus.

vaccinā·tion (L. *vacca*, cow). Inoculation with the virus of cowpox in order to provide protection from smallpox.

vac·cinator (L. *vacca*, cow). One who vaccinates.

vac·cine (L. *vacca*, cow). 1. Lymph from a cowpox vesicle. 2. A preparation of dead or attenuated micro-organisms.

vaccinel·la (L. *vacca*, cow). False vaccinia; a secondary eruption sometimes succeeding an attack of cowpox.

vacci·nia (L. *vacca*, cow). Cowpox, a contagious disease of cows. It can be transmitted to man by vaccination and gives immunity against smallpox.

vacci·nial (L. *vacca*, cow). Relating to or resembling vaccinia.

vacci·niform (L. *vacca*, cow; *forma*, shape). Like vaccinia.

vacciniŏ·la (L. *vacca*, cow). A secondary eruption occasionally following vaccinia and marked by a resemblance to smallpox.

vacciniza·tion (L. *vacca*, cow). Thorough vaccination by the giving of a number of inoculations, repeating these until the virus produces no evident reaction.

vaccinŏ·genous (L. *vacca*, cow; G. *gennan*, to produce). Producing vaccine.

vaccinophŏ·bia (L. *vacca*, cow; G. *phobos*, fear). A neurotic fear of being vaccinated.

vă·cuolā·tion (L. *vacuus*, empty). The development of vacuoles.

vă·cuole (L. *vacuus*, empty). Any clear space formed in the substance of a cell.

vă·cuŭm (L. *vacuus*, empty). A space from which all the air has been withdrawn.

vā·gal (L. *vagus*, wandering). Relating to the vagus nerve.

vagī·na (L.). 1. A sheath. 2. The musculo-membranous canal extending from the opening of the vulva to the neck of the uterus.

vagī·nal (L. *vagina*, sheath). 1. Relating to or resembling a sheath. 2. Relating to the vagina.

vă·ginali·tis (L. *vagina*, sheath). Inflammation of the tunica vaginalis of the testicle.

vă·ginate (L. *vagina*, sheath). Sheathed.

vaginec·tomy (L. *vagina*, sheath; G. *ektomē*, excision). 1. Surgical removal of the tunica vaginalis. 2. Surgical removal of the vagina.

vaginis·mus (L. *vagina*, sheath). Painful spasm of the vaginal walls.

vaginī·tis (L. *vagina*, sheath). 1. Inflammation of the vagina. 2. Inflammation of any ensheathing tissue.

vaginodў·nia (L. *vagina*, sheath; G. *odunē*, pain). Neuralgic pain in the vagina.

vaginofixā·tion (L. *vagina*, sheath; *fīgere*, to fix). Vaginal hysteropexy.

vagī·noperitonē·al (L. *vagina*, sheath; G. *peritonaion*, peritoneum). Relating both to the vagina and the peritoneum.

vagī·noplasty (L. *vagina*, sheath; G. *plassein*, to form). A plastic operation on the vagina.

vagī·noscope (L. *vagina*, sheath; G. *skopein*, to inspect). A speculum for vaginal use.

vaginŏ·tomy (L. *vagina*, sheath; G. *tomē*, section). Surgical incision into the vagina; colpotomy.

vagī·novesī·cal (L. *vagina*, sheath; *vesica*, bladder) Pertaining to the vagina and the bladder.

vagī·tus (L. *vagire*, to cry). The cry of an infant.

vagŏ·tomy (L. *vagus*, wandering; G. *tomē*, section). Surgical division of the vagus nerve, sometimes performed in the treatment of peptic ulcer.

vagotŏ·nia, vagŏ·tony (L. *vagus*, wandering; G. *tonos*, tone). Irritability of the vagus nerve.

vā·gus (L., wandering). The pneumogastric or tenth cranial nerve.

vā·lence, vā·lency (L. *valēre*, to be worth). The relative combining power of an atom as compared with that of a hydrogen atom.

Valentin's ganglion (Valentin, G. G., German physiologist, 1810–83). On the superior dental nerve. V.'s **nerve:** the nerve from the sphenopalatine ganglion to the 6th nerve. V.'s **tubes or cords:** the linear arrangement of the female sex cells in the developing ovary.

valē·rian. Any plant of the genus *Valeriana*. An antispasmodic and nerve stimulant, used in neurasthenia.

Valērĭa·na. A genus of plants. See also valerian.

valē·rianate. A salt of valerianic acid.

valerĭā·nic acid. An organic acid, C_4H_9COOH, found in the roots of valerian.

valetudinā·rian (L. *valetudo*, health, from *valēre*, to be strong). An invalid.

val·gus (L. bow-legged). Bent outwards. V., **hallux:** outward deflection of the great toe. V., **spurious:** (splay-foot) see flat foot. V., **talipes:** a type of club foot in which the foot is turned outwards.

val·late (L. *vallum*, rampart). Having a wall; cup-shaped. See also circumvallate.

vallē·cula (L. *vallecula*, a little valley). Any furrow or fossa.

vallĕ·cular (L. *vallecula*, a little valley). Relating to a vallecula.

Valleix's points douloureux (Valleix, F. L., French physician, 1807–55). Tender point along certain nerves in neuralgia.

val·lis (L., valley). The vallecula of the cerebellum.

val·lum un·guis (L. *vallum*, rampart; *unguis*, finger- or toe-nail). The depression in the skin for the reception of a nail-root.

Valsalva's experiment (Valsalva, A. M., Italian anatomist, 1666–1723). A forced expiratory effort with nose and mouth closed which raises intrathoracic pressure and checks the flow of blood in the great veins. This is manifested by engorged veins in the neck. V.'s **ligament:** the anterior ligament of the auricle. V.'s **muscle:** the muscle of the tragus. V.'s **sinuses:** the sinuses of the aorta.

val·val (L. *valva*, a folding-door). Relating to a valve.

val·vate (L. *valva*, a folding-door). Possessing valves.

valve (L. *valva*, a folding-door). 1. A device placed in a tube so as to permit free passage in one direction but not in the other. 2. A fold of membrane acting as a valve, as v. of the heart or v. of the veins. **Anal:** (valves of Morgagni or valves of Ball) semilunar folds of mucous membrane at the junction of the rectum and anal canal. **Aortic:** three semilunar cusps or segments, consisting of fibrous tissue covered by endocardium which guard the aortic orifice of the heart. The valve prevents regurgitation of blood from the aorta into the left ventricle during the elastic recoil of the arterial wall. **Atrioventricular:** left (mitral or bicuspid valve) is composed of two cusps which guard the mitral orifice of the heart; right (tricuspid) is composed of three cusps and guards the tricuspid orifice of the heart. **Bicuspid:** see atrioventricular left. **Cardiac:** the bicuspid, tricuspid, aortic, and pulmonary valves. **Eustachian:** a small crescentic fold of endocardium which guards the orifice of the inferior vena cava as it enters the right atrium of the heart. **Heister's:** spiral folds of mucous membrane in the interior of the cystic duct, they serve as valves. **Houston's:** horizontal infoldings of the wall of the rectum in certain situations. **Ileocolic** (valve of Tulpius): is situated at the point where the terminal part of the ileum opens into the junction between the caecum and ascending colon. **Mitral:** see atrioventricular left v. **Of Ball:** see anal v. **Of Bauhin:** the ileocolic sphincter. **Of Gerlach:** a fold of mucous membrane which guards the opening of the vermiform appendix into the caecum. **Of Hasner:** a fold of mucous membrane which guards the opening of the nasolacrimal duct into the inferior meatus of the nose. **Of inferior vena cava:** see Eustachian v. **Of Morgagni:** see anal v. **Of Tarin:** the crescentic posterior margins of the nodule of the cerebellum. **Of Tulpius:** see ileocolic v. **Pulmonary:** guards the orifice of the pulmonary trunk, and prevents regurgitation of blood from the trunk into the right ventricle. It is composed of three semilunar cusps. **Pyloric:** an annular fold of mucous membrane at the pyloric sphincter of the stomach. **Rectal:** see Houston's v. **Spiral:** see Heister's v. **Thebesian:** a delicate semilunar fold of the endocardium which guards the orifice of the coronary sinus of the heart. **Tricuspid:** see atrioventricular right v.

valvŏ·tomy (L. *valva*, a folding-door; G. *tomē*, section). Surgical incision into a valve.

val·vula (L. *valvula*, dim. of *valva*, a folding-door). 1. A small valve. 2. The superior medullary velum. **V. of Guerin:** valvula fossae navicularis.

val·vulae conniven·tes (L. *valva*, a folding-door; *connivēre*, to close). The transverse folds of mucous membrane in the small intestine.

val·vular (L. *valva*, a folding-door). Relating to or having the character of a valve.

valvuli·tis (L. *valva*, a folding-door). Inflammation of a valve.

van den Bergh's test (van den Bergh, A. A. H., Dutch physician, 1869–1943). A test for uncombined or combined bilirubin in the blood.

vanil·la (Sp. *vainilla*, dim. of *vaina*, a sheath. Ult. from L. *vagina*, a sheath). A genus of orchidaceous plants. *V. planifolia* grows in Mexico and its beans yield the flavouring agent, vanilla.

vanil·lin (Sp. *vainilla*). A crystallizable principle, $HOC_6H_3(OCH_3)CHO$, obtained from vanilla.

vaporizā·tion (L. *vapor*, vapour). Conversion of a solid or liquid into a vapour.

vā·pour (L. *vapor*, vapour). A gas; the term is applied particularly to the gaseous forms of materials which are either solid or liquid when maintained at ordinary temperatures. **V. bath:** see under bath.

vā·pours (L. *vapor*, vapour). Hysteria.

variā·tion (L. *variare*, to change). Deviation from a specific type as a result of mutation, selection or cultivation.

varicel·la (L. *varius*, mottled). Chickenpox, an acute, contagious disease of children. It is marked by an eruption of transparent vesicles which develop in successive crops on various parts of the body. The disease is usually accompanied by a slight rise of temperature and is of a mild character.

vă·ricēs (L.). Pl. of varix, *q.v.*

varī·ciform (L. *varix*, a dilated vein; *forma*, shape). Resembling a varix.

vă·ricoblĕ·pharon (L. *varix*, a dilated vein; G. *blepharon*, eyelid). Varicose swelling of the eyelid.

vă·ricocele (L. *varix*, a dilated vein; G. *kēlē*, hernia). Dilatation of the veins of the spermatic cord, resulting in the formation of a swelling.

vă·ricocelec·tomy (L. *varix*, a dilated vein; G. *kēlē*, hernia; *ektomē*, excision). Excision of a varicocele.

varicom·phalus (L. *varix*, a dilated vein; G. *omphalos*, navel). A varicosity of the navel.

vă·ricose (L. *varicosus*, from *varix*, a dilated vein). Resembling or having the character of a varix. **V. veins:** a swollen and knotted condition of the veins.

varicō·sity (L. *varix*, a dilated vein). The condition of being varicose.

varicō·tomy (L. *varix*, a dilated vein; G. *tomē*, section). The surgical removal of a varicose vein.

varī·cula (L. *varicula*, dim. of *varix*, a dilated vein). A varicosity of the conjunctiva.

varī·ola (L.L. *variola*, from *varius*, mottled). Smallpox; an acute, contagious and infectious disease. The initially papular eruption becomes vesicular and then pustular, with crust formation. The falling off of the crusts leaves pits in the skin (pock-marks). **V. haemorrhagic:** an almost invariably fatal form, marked by haemorrhage into the vesicles.

vari·olar. Relating to smallpox.

vă·riolate (L. *varius*, mottled). 1. Characterized by the presence of pustules resembling those of variola. 2. To inoculate with smallpox virus.

variolā·tion (L. *varius*, mottled). The inoculation of a subject with the virus of smallpox.

vă·rioloid (L. *varius*, mottled; G. *eidos*, form). A mild form of variola seen in persons who have attained a degree of immunity through vaccination with smallpox virus.

varī·olous (L. *varius*, mottled). Relating to or resembling variola.

varī·olovac·cine (L. *varius*, mottled; *vacca*, cow). A vaccine lymph or crust obtained from a heifer which has been inoculated with smallpox virus.

varī·olovacci·nia (L. *varius*, mottled; *vacca*, cow). Cowpox in the heifer produced by inoculating it with smallpox virus.

vā·rix (L., a dilated vein; pl. *varices*). A swollen and knotted condition of a blood- or lymph-vessel; usually a vein.

Varolius, pons of (Varolius, C., Italian anatomist, 1543–75; L. *pons*, bridge). The mesencephalon; that portion of the brain joining the medulla oblongata with the cerebral peduncles and the cerebellum. It is usually called the Pons Varolii.

vas (L.). A vessel. **V. aberrans** (of Haller): a diverticulum at the point where the epididymis terminates in the vas deferens. **V. deferens:** the excretory duct of the testicle.

vā·sa (L. pl. of *vas*, a vessel). Vessels. **V. efferentia:** the efferent ducts of the rete testis, 12 to 20 in number. **V. recta:** the veins of the renal pyramids. **V. vasorum:** the vessels supplying blood to the arteries and veins.

vā·sal (L. *vas*, a vessel). Vascular, *q.v.*

vasa·lium (L. *vas*, a vessel). True vascular tissue; that of vascular cavities or closed organs.

vas·cular (L. *vasculum*, dim. of *vas*, a vessel). Relating to, consisting of or having vessels.

vasculă·rity (L. *vasculum*, dim. of *vas*, a vessel). The state of being vascular.

vascularizā·tion (L. *vasculum*, dim. of *vas*, a vessel). The act of becoming vascular.

VEINS

1. SUPERIOR SAGITTAL SINUS
2. INFERIOR SAGITTAL SINUS
3. SUPERIOR TEMPORAL
4. TRANSVERSE SINUS
5. ANTERIOR FACIAL
6. POSTERIOR FACIAL
7. INTERNAL JUGULAR
8. EXTERNAL JUGULAR
9. ANTERIOR JUGULAR
10. TRANSCERVICAL
11. R. INNOMINATE
12. SUPERIOR VENA CAVA
13. SUBCLAVIAN
14. L. INNOMINATE
15. AXILLARY
16. BRACHIAL
17. BASILIC
18. CEPHALIC
19. MEDIAN BASILIC
20. MEDIAN CEPHALIC
21. RADIAL
22. POSTERIOR ULNAR
23. ANTERIOR ULNAR
24. SUPERFICIAL MEDIAN
25. PALMAR ARCHES
26. INFERIOR VENA CAVA
27. HEPATIC
28. RENAL
29. PHRENIC
30. SPERMATIC
31. COMMON ILIAC
32. INTERNAL ILIAC
33. EXTERNAL ILIAC
34. SUPERFICIAL CIRCUMFLEX ILIAC
35. MIDSACRAL
36. FEMORAL CIRCUMFLEX
37. PROFUNDA FEMORIS
38. FEMORAL
39. LONG SAPHENOUS
40. POPLITEAL
41. SHORT SAPHENOUS
42. MEDIAN MARGINAL
43. DORSAL VENOUS ARCH
44. DIGITAL

452

vas·cularize (L. *vasculum*, dim. of *vas*, a vessel). To supply with vessels.

vasculī·tis (L. *vasculum*, dim. of *vas*, a vessel). Inflammation of a blood- or lymph-vessel.

vas·culum (L., dim. of *vas*, a vessel). A small vessel.

vasec·tomy (L. *vas*, a vessel; G. *ektomē*, excision). Excision of the vas deferens.

vasifac·tive (L. *vas*, a vessel; *facere*, to make). Forming new vessels.

vā·siform (L. *vas*, a vessel; *forma*, shape). Like a vessel or duct.

vasī·tis (L. *vas*, a vessel). Inflammation of the vas deferens.

vā·soconstric·tion (L. *vas*, a vessel; *constringere*, to tie). The constriction of blood-vessels.

vā·soconstric·tive (L. *vas*, a vessel; *constringere*, to tie). Promoting the constriction of blood-vessels.

vā·soconstric·tor (L. *vas*, a vessel; *constringere*, to tie). 1. Causing the constriction of blood-vessels. 2. An agent causing the constriction of blood-vessels.

vā·socorō·na (L. *vas*, a vessel; *corona*, crown). The system of minute arteries supplying the periphery of the spinal cord.

vasoden·tine (L. *vas*, a vessel; *dens*, tooth). Dentine that is provided with blood-vessels.

vasodepres·sion (L. *vas*, a vessel; *deprĭmĕre*, to press down). Vasomotor depression.

vasodepres·sor (L. *vas*, a vessel; *deprĭmĕre*, to press down). An agent having a depressing influence on the circulation; producing vasomotor depression.

vā·sodilā·tor (L. *vas*, a vessel; *dilatare*, to enlarge). 1. Causing the dilatation of blood-vessels. 2. An agent causing dilatation of the blood-vessels.

vasofac·tive (L. *vas*, a vessel; *facere*, to make). Vasifactive, *q.v.*

vasofor·mative (L. *vas*, a vessel; *formare*, to form). Forming vessels.

vaso-inhĭ·bitor (L. *vas*, a vessel; *inhibēre*, to restrain). An agent tending to inhibit vasomotor activity, especially vaso-constrictors.

vaso-inhĭ·bitory (L. *vas*, a vessel; *inhibēre*, to restrain). Restraining vasomotor action.

vā·soligā·tion (L. *vas*, a vessel; *ligare*, to tie). Ligation of the vas deferens; Steinach's rejuvenation operation.

vasomō·tion (L. *vas*, a vessel; *motio*, a moving). The increase or decrease in the calibre of a vessel.

vasomō·tor (L. *vas*, a vessel; *movere*, to move). Regulating the tension of the vessels. **V. rhinitis:** secretion of mucus from the nose due to vasomotor neurosis.

vā·somotō·rial, vasomō·tory (L. *vas*, a vessel; *movere*, to move). Relating to vasomotor function.

vā·soneurŏ·pathy (L. *vas*, a vessel; G. *neuron*, nerve; *pathos*, disease). Any disorder affecting the blood-vessels and the nerves.

vā·soneurŏ·sis (L. *vas*, a vessel; G. *neuron*, nerve). Angioneurosis; disorder of the vasomotor system.

vasoparē·sis (L. *vas*, a vessel; G. *paresis*, paralysis). A partial paralysis of the vasomotor nerves.

vasopres·sin (L. *vas*, vessel; *premere*, to press). A hormone of the posterior lobe of the hypophysis. Injection of vasopressin is in a sterile aqueous solution prepared by a process of fractionation from the posterior lobe of the pituitary body of oxen and other mammals. It raises blood pressure and promotes peristalsis.

vasor·rhaphy (L. *vas*, a vessel; G. *rhaphē*, suture). Suture of blood-vessels or of the vas deferens.

vasosec·tion (L. *vas*, a vessel; *sectio*, section). Severing of the blood-vessels or of the vas deferens.

vasosen·sory (L. *vas*, a vessel; *sensus*, feeling). Serving as or supplying a sensory apparatus for the blood-vessels.

vā·sospasm (L. *vas*, a vessel; G. *spasmos*, spasm). Spasm of the blood-vessels.

vasosti·mulant (L. *vas*, a vessel; *stimulare*, to incite). Stimulating or promoting vasomotor action.

vasŏ·tomy (G. *vas*, a vessel; *tomē*, section). Operation in which the vas deferens is divided.

vasotrŏ·phic (L. *vas*, a vessel; G. *trophē*, nourishment). Relating to or connected with the nutrition of the vessels.

vasovā·gal (L. *vas*, vessel; *vagus*, wandering). Cardio-vascular reaction due to passage of impulses down the vagus nerve, resulting in slowing of heart rate. **Gower's v. syndrome:** praecordial distress with feeling of impending death and nausea. The attack may last from a few minutes to an hour or more.

vas·tus (L., enormous). Large. **V. intermedius, v. lateralis, v. medialis:** three muscles of the quadriceps femoris group; extensors of the knee-joint.

Vater's ampulla (Vater, A., German anatomist, 1684–1751). The ampulla of the bile duct. **V.'s corpuscles:** the sensory end organs. **V.'s tubercle:** the papilla duodeni; papilla of Santorini.

V.D. Abbreviation for venereal disease.

vec·tion (L. *vectio*, a carrying). The passing of disease germs from the sick to the healthy.

vec·tis (L., a lever, from *vehere*, to carry). An instrument used to expedite the delivery of the foetal head at parturition.

vec·tor (L., a bearer, from *vehere*, to carry). An insect conveying micro-organisms from one host to another, e.g. as malaria-infected mosquitoes.

vĕ·getable (L. *vegetabilis*, animating, from *vegetare*, to animate). A plant, especially one used as food.

vĕ·getal (L. *vegetus*, animated, from *vegēre*, to excite). Of or relating to plants; characteristic of plants. **V. functions:** the vital processes seen in plants and animals: irritability, digestion, excretion, secretion, assimilation, growth, circulation, respiration and reproduction.

vegetā·rian (L. *vegetus*, animated, from *vegēre*, to excite). One who subsists only on vegetable foods.

vegetā·rianism (L. *vegetus*, animated, from *vegēre*, to excite). 1. The theory that vegetable food is the proper diet for man. 2. The habit of subsisting on vegetable foods.

vegetā·tion (L.L. *vegetatio*, an enlivening, from *vegetare*, to animate). A growth resembling a plant, such as the excrescences on the cardiac valves in endocarditis.

vĕ·getative (L. *vegetare*, to animate). Possessing the power of growth.

vĕ·hicle (L. *vehiculum*, a conveyance). A substance serving as a medium for the administration of a drug or other medicine.

veldt sore. An ulceration of the legs and arms occurring in South Africa.

veil (L. *velum*, a cloth). 1. Velum, *q.v.* 2. A caul covering the face of a newly born infant.

vein (L. *vena*). A blood-vessel conveying blood from the tissues to the heart. Veins, like arteries, have three coats, but these, particularly the muscle layer, are less well developed. Many veins are also supplied with valves. **Anastomotic:** 1. Superior of Trolard, a vein which connects the superficial middle cerebral vein with the superior sagittal sinus. 2. Inferior of Labbé, a vein connecting the superficial middle cerebral ¦vein with the transverse sinus. **Anterior caecal:** a small v. on the anterior surface of the caecum; draining into the ileocolic v. **Anterior cardiac:** veins of the heart which ascend on the front of the right ventricle, and open into the small cardiac vein. **Anterior cerebral:** is a slender vessel accompanying the artery of the same name on the medial surface of the brain receiving tributaries from the corpus callosum and cingulate gyrus. It joins the basal vein. **Anterior facial:** is formed by the union of the supratrochlear and supra-orbital veins, it passes across the face and unites with the anterior division of the posterior facial vein to form the common facial vein. **Anterior interventricular:** is part of the great cardiac vein which ascends in the anterior interventricular groove of the heart alongside the anterior interventricular branch of the left coronary artery. **Anterior jugular:** begins in the roof of the digastric triangle where it is formed by the union of radicles that communicate with the submental vein. It descends vertically down the neck into the suprasternal space. It then describes a bend passing beneath the sternomastoid muscle and ends in the external jugular vein. **Anterior vertebral:** begins in a venous plexus anterior to the upper cervical transverse processes. It descends in company with the ascending cervical branch of the inferior thyroid artery and opens into the lower part of the vertebral vein. **Ascending lumbar:** a vein formed by the longitudinal anastomosing branches between the lumbar veins. It communicates by the lumbar azygos vein with the inferior vena cava. On the right side it communicates with the common iliac or internal iliac vein. The vein when traced upwards becomes the vena azygos. **Axillary:** is mainly the continuation upwards of the basilic vein, but results from the somewhat variable junctions of this vein and the two venae comites of the brachial artery. It commences at the lower border of the teres major muscle and ends at the outer border of the first rib. **Azygos:** the azygos veins are three in number—namely, the vena azygos, the inferior vena hemiazygos, and the superior vena hemiazygos. **Azygos vena** (vena azygos major): commences in the right ascending lumbar vein and passes through the aortic opening in the diaphragm and ends in the superior vena cava. **Azygos inferior, hemi-** (vena azygos minor inferior): commences in the left ascending lumbar vein and enters the thorax through the left crus of the diaphragm and ends in the vena azygos. **Azygos superior, hemi-** (vena azygos minor superior): is formed by the union of the fifth, sixth, and seventh left posterior intercostal veins and drains into the vena azygos. **Azygos lumbar:** are two in number, right and left. The right comes back from the back of the inferior vena cava and contributes to the formation of the vena azygos. The left arises from the back of the renal vein and contributes to the formation of the inferior vena hemiazygos. **Basilic:** formed by the union of the median basilic with the anterior and posterior ulnar veins and ends by joining the vena comites of the brachial to form the axillary vein. **Bronchial:** pass from the hilum of the lung into the vena azygos and superior vena hemiazygos. They are not so large as the corresponding arteries. **Cephalic:** is formed by the union of the median cephalic and the radial a little distance from the lateral epicondyle of the humerus. It drains into the axillary vein. **Cerebellar:** these veins are arranged in two sets, superior and inferior. The superior cerebellar veins pass from the cerebellum to the great cerebral vein. The inferior cerebellar veins pass from the cerebellum to the sigmoid, inferior petrosal and occipital sinuses. **Choroid** (deep cerebral): lies in the choroid plexus of the lateral ventricle from which it receives its blood and passes forwards in the lateral ventricle to join the thalamo-striate vein. **Comitans hypoglossi** (Ranine vein): runs from the tip of the tongue and is continued backwards as the lingual vein, which in turn drains into the internal jugular vein. **Common**

facial: is formed by the junction of the anterior and posterior facial veins and opens into the internal jugular vein opposite the body of the hyoid bone. **Common iliac:** formed by the union of the external and internal iliac veins in front of the sacro-iliac articulation. The two veins unite to form the inferior vena cava opposite the upper border of the body of the fifth lumbar vertebra. **Cystic:** passes from the gall-bladder to the right division of the portal vein. **Deep cerebral:** see choroid vein. **Deep cervical:** begins in the suboccipital triangle in the suboccipital plexus, and descends to the lower part of the neck where it joins the vertebral vein. **Deep facial:** issues from the anterior part of the pterygoid plexus and, passing inferiorly and anteriorly, it joins the anterior facial vein on the buccinator muscle. **Deep median:** (black vein) a communicating vein between the deep veins of the forearm and the median vein. **Deep middle cerebral** (deep Sylvian): a tributary of the basal vein of the brain. **Deep Sylvian:** see deep middle cerebral. **Descending pharyngeal:** accompanies the ascending pharyngeal artery and joins the internal jugular vein. **Diploic:** situated in the cancellous tissue between the outer and inner tables of the cranial bones. They terminate partly in extracranial veins and partly in the cranial venous sinuses. **Dorsal lingual:** small veins in the posterior third of the tongue which drain into the lingual vein. **Dorsal, of penis:** two in number, superficial and deep. Superficial dorsal vein drains blood from the glans and skin and opens into the superficial external pudendal vein. Deep dorsal vein drains blood from the glans and corpora cavernosa and opens into the prostatic plexus of veins. **Emissary:** are vessels that pass through foramina in the cranial wall and establish communications between the intracranial venous sinuses and the extracranial veins. **External iliac:** is the continuation of the femoral vein. It extends from the lower border of the inguinal ligament to the sacro-iliac joint where it joins the internal iliac to form the common iliac vein. **External jugular:** is formed by the union of the posterior division of the posterior facial vein and the posterior auricular vein. It descends to the mid-point of the clavicle where it joins the subclavian vein. **Femoral:** extends from the opening in the adductor magnus muscle to the distal border of the inguinal ligament, where it is continuous with the external iliac vein. **Frontal** (supratrochlear vein): A large vein which commences in the scalp and descends towards the orbit where it is joined by the supra-orbital vein forming the angular vein. **Gastric:** small veins in the walls of the stomach which drain into the portal system. **Great cardiac:** commences at the apex of the heart and ascends in the anterior interventricular groove and ends in the coronary sinus. **Great cerebral:** is formed from the right and left internal cerebral veins and it emerges from the transverse fissure to enter the anterior end of the straight sinus. **Hemiazygos:** see Azygos inferior, hemi-. **Hemiazygos, inferior:** see Azygos inferior, hemi-. **Hemiazygos** (inferior vena hemiazygos): is a tributary of the left renal v. and enters the thorax by piercing the left crus of the diaphragm and drains into the vena azygos. **Hepatic:** these veins commence in the centre of each liver lobule as an intralobular or central vein. These open into the sublobular veins which in turn form the hepatic veins. They drain direct into the inferior vena cava. **Inferior cerebral:** small veins which drain the tentorial surface and lower part of the lateral surface of the hemisphere. They end in the transverse sinus, the cavernous sinus and, to a less extent, in the superior petrosal sinus. **Inferior dental:** a small v. which accompanies the inferior dental artery in the mandibular canal and drains into the pterygoid plexus. **Inferior haemorrhoidal** (inferior rectal): commences in a plexus beneath the lining of the anal canal. It drains into the internal pudendal vein which in turn drains into the internal iliac vein. **Inferior mesenteric:** is the continuation of the superior haemorrhoidal veins and receives tributaries that return the blood from the parts of the large intestine supplied by the inferior mesenteric artery. It drains into the splenic vein. **Inferior pudendal:** arise in a plexus of veins which accompany the internal pudendal artery. They form one trunk and open into the internal iliac vein. **Inferior rectal:** see inferior haemorrhoidal. **Inferior striate:** a small tributary which helps to form the basal vein of the brain. **Inferior thyroid:** a small vein or veins which pass from the isthmus of the thyroid gland to the left innominate vein. **Infra-orbital:** a small vein which commences on the face and passes through the infra-orbital canal to end in the pterygoid plexus. **Innominate:** is formed by the junction of the internal jugular vein and the subclavian vein. It lies in the superior mediastinum. **Intercostal:** accompany the corresponding intercostal arteries in the intercostal spaces. **Interlobular:** are the veins of the cortex of the kidney and pass eventually into the renal veins. **Internal auditory:** a small vein draining the labyrinth of the ear, which opens into the inferior petrosal sinus. **Internal cerebral** (vein of Galen): two in number, right and left. Formed by the junction of the thalamo-striate vein and the choroid vein. The two veins join together to form the great vein of Galen. **Internal iliac:** results from the union of tributaries that correspond with branches of the internal iliac artery. It joins the external iliac vein to form the common iliac vein. **Internal jugular:** is the continuation of the intracranial sigmoid sinus. It passes down the neck to the sternoclavicular joint where it joins the subclavian vein to form the innominate vein. **Internal mammary:** formed from the venae comites of the musculophrenic and superior epigastric arteries. They pass up in the thorax and join the innominate vein. **Internal occipital:** a small vein in the suboccipital triangle of the neck, it joins the suboccipital plexus of veins. **Internal pudic:** the internal pudendal v. **Intestinal:** small veins which drain the small intestine and open into the superior mesenteric vein. **Left gastric:** commences on the lesser curvature of the stomach and drains into the portal vein. **Left marginal:** a branch of the great cardiac vein which drains into the coronary sinus. **Lingual:** the vein which drains the tongue, it opens into the internal jugular vein. **Long saphenous:** is the primitive preaxial vein of the lower limb bud. It commences in a plexus on the dorsum of the foot, passes up the leg and thigh and opens into the femoral vein. **Lumbar:** veins on the posterior abdominal wall about four in number on each side. They open into the inferior vena cava. **Maxillary** (internal maxillary vein): a short vessel that issues from the posterior part of the pterygoid plexus. It joins the superficial temporal vein to form the posterior facial vein. **Median:** is formed by the union of radicles of the venous plexus on the anterior part of the wrist. At the elbow it divides into median cephalic and median basilic veins. **Median basilic:** a vein which is formed at the elbow from the median vein; it is joined by the ulnar veins and forms the basilic vein. **Median cephalic:** a branch of the median vein of the arm, it is joined by the radial vein and forms the cephalic vein. **Median sacral:** a small vein which starts at the hollow of the sacrum and ends in the left common iliac vein. **Meningeal:** veins which accompany the meningeal arteries of the brain, they

drain into the pterygoid plexus of veins. **Mental:** a small vein which joins the inferior dental vein which opens into the pterygoid plexus. **Middle cardiac:** commences at the apex of the heart and opens into the right extremity of the coronary sinus. **Middle cerebral:** drains the centre of the brain and opens into the basal vein. **Oblique** (vein Of Marshall): a small vein on the surface of the left atrium of the heart, it opens into the coronary sinus. **Obliterated umbilical:** commences at the anterior border of the interlobar notch of the liver and extends as far back as the left extremity of the porta hepatis. **Occipital:** veins which commence in the muscles of the occipital region and drain into the suboccipital plexus. **Of brain:** the cerebral veins are arranged in two groups, superficial and deep. The superficial drains the cerebral cortex, the deep veins the interior of the brain. **Of clitoris:** is formed from branches which return blood from the glans and prepuce. It passes into the pelvic cavity and enters the internal pudendal vein. **Of Galen:** vide internal cerebral vein. **Of hand:** run between the skin and deep fascia forming a series of large discrete valved channels. **Of kidney:** the cortical veins are known as the interlobular veins. The veins of the medulla are known as the venae rectae. The cortico-medullary venous arches join to form the renal vein which opens into the inferior vena cava. **Of Labbé:** see anastomotic inferior vein. **Of Latarget:** see prepyloric vein. **Of Marshall:** see oblique vein of the left atrium. **Of medulla:** form a plexus on its surface that is drained by an anterior median vein, a posterior median vein and radicular veins. **Of pons:** form a delicate plexus on its ventral surface that drains into the basal vein. **Of spinal cord:** form longitudinal plexuses which drain into the vertebral, intercostal and lumbar veins. **Of Thebesius:** minute veins which return the blood from the wall of the atrium. **Of Trolard:** see anastomotic superior vein. **Oesophageal:** accompany the corresponding arteries and terminate in the vena azygos and the two venae hemiazygos. **Ophthalmic:** two in number, superior and inferior, which drain into the pterygoid plexus. **Ovarian:** arises from pampiniform plexus. The right one opens into the inferior vena cava, the left one into the left renal vein. **Para-umbilical:** small veins within the ligamentum teres of the liver. They anastomose at the umbilicus with the epigastric veins and within the abdomen with the portal vein. **Popliteal:** commences at the distal border of the popliteus muscle and terminates at the femoral opening in the adductor magnus, where it is continuous with the femoral vein. **Portal:** vein about 3 inches long, formed by the junction of the superior mesenteric and splenic veins. **Posterior caecal:** a v. commencing on the posterior surface of the caecum, it receives the appendicular v. and drains into the ileocolic v. **Posterior cardiac:** small veins which ascend upon the posterior surface of the left ventricle, and open into the coronary sinus. **Posterior external jugular:** a vein from the posterior part of the neck which opens into the external jugular. **Posterior intercostal:** eleven in number on each side, and each lies in the costal groove of the rib. They drain into the azygos veins. **Posterior facial:** formed behind the parotid gland and passes through the substance of that gland and divides into two branches, an anterior which passes forwards and unites with the anterior facial v. to form the common facial v., and a posterior which is joined by the posterior auricular v. to form the external jugular v. **Prepyloric** (Latarget): a small vein lying on the pyloric constriction of the stomach, it opens into the right gastric vein. **Profunda femoris:** lies anterior to its companion artery in the thigh, it opens into the femoral vein. **Pulmonary:** four in number, two right and two left. Carry arterial or oxygenated blood from the lungs to the left atrium. **Radial:** commences on the posterior surface of the thumb, drains the radial side of hand and forearm, and joins the median cephalic vein at the elbow. **Ranine** (vena comitans hypoglossi): commences at the tip of the tongue and becomes continuous with the lingual vein. **Rectal:** all rectal veins are destitute of valves; they form plexuses which drain into the inferior mesenteric, internal iliac and internal pudic veins. **Renal:** large veins. Right and left, drain blood from kidneys into inferior vena cava. **Right gastric:** passes from left to right along the lesser curvature of the stomach between the layers of the lesser omentum and opens into the portal vein. **Right gastro-epiploic:** passes from left to right along the greater curvature of the stomach and opens into the superior mesenteric vein. **Short saphenous:** starts in a plexus on the dorsum of the foot, passes up the back of the calf and empties into the popliteal vein. **Small cardiac:** occupies the right atrioventricular groove and opens into the right extremity of the coronary sinus. **Spermatic:** spring from the pampiniform plexus of the spermatic cord. The right drains into the inferior vena cava, the left into the left renal vein. **Splenic:** a large vein passing from the spleen it joins the superior mesenteric vein to form the portal vein. **Subclavian:** a large vein which is the continuation of the axillary vein, it passes over the apex of the lung and ends by joining the internal jugular vein to form the innominate vein. **Subcostal:** small vein below the twelfth rib, it drains into the azygos vein on the right side and into the inferior vena hemiazygos vein on the left. **Suboccipital:** a plexus of veins in suboccipital triangle which drain into the deep cervical vein and the vertebral vein. **Superficial temporal:** drains blood from the lateral surface of the scalp, it enters the parotid gland and joins the maxillary vein to form the posterior facial vein. **Superior cerebral:** six to twelve in number on each side, drain blood from the cortex of the brain. They pass into the superior sagittal sinus. **Superior gluteal:** a vein draining the gluteal region, which passes into the pelvis to join the internal iliac vein. **Superior mesenteric:** is formed by the junction of the appendicular, anterior and posterior caecal veins and receives tributaries that return blood from the parts of the intestinal canal supplied by the superior mesenteric artery. It joins the splenic vein to form the portal vein. **Superior thyroid:** issues from the superior part of the lateral lobe of the thyroid gland and opens into the internal jugular vein. **Supra-orbital:** commences above the orbit and is joined by the supra-trochlear vein to form the angular vein. **Suprarenal:** pass from the suprarenal glands to the inferior vena cava on the right side and into the left renal vein on the left side. **Suprascapular:** passes from the posterior surface of the scapula behind the clavicle to open into the external jugular vein. **Supratrochlear:** a small v. draining the anterior surface of the scalp. It unites with the supra-orbital v. to form the anterior facial v. near the median angle of the eye. **Testicular:** emerge from the testis along its posterior border. The right vein opens into the inferior vena cava, the left into the left renal vein. **Thalamostriate:** passes forwards in the floor of the body of the lateral ventricle of the brain and ends in the internal cerebral vein. **Thyroid:** three in number, superior, middle and inferior. The first two open into the internal jugular vein, the last into the innominate vein. **Transverse cervical:** a vein in the neck which joins the external jugular vein. **Ulnar:** veins on the medial surface of the forearm, which pass upwards and join the median basilic vein at the elbow. **Umbilical:** becomes obliterated, and, lying in the free edge of the falciform fold of peritoneum, is known as the ligamentum teres of the liver. **Uterine:** veins which are destitute of valves, form a plexus in the broad ligament and drain into the internal iliac vein. **Vaginal:** veins which form a plexus and drain into the internal iliac vein. **Vertebral:** commences in the suboccipital venous plexus, passes down the neck and opens into the innominate vein.

velā·men, (L., a covering). A membrane veiling a part.

velamen·tum (L., a veil). A covering membrane.

vĕ·lar (L. *velum*, a cloth). Relating to a velum; applied particularly to the v. palati.

veldt sore. Desert sore, *q.v.*

Vella's fistula (Vella, L., Italian physiologist, 1825–86). An artificial intestinal fistula made to obtain pure intestinal secretions.

vellicā·tion (L. *vellicatio*, a twitching). Spasm of muscular tissue.

velosyn·thesis (L. *velum*, a cloth; G. *sunthesis*, a junction). Suture of a cleft soft palate; syn. staphylorrhaphy.

Velpeau's canal (Velpeau, A. A. L. M., French surgeon, 1795–1867). The inguinal canal. **V.'s fascia propria:** the tela subserosa around the kidney. **V.'s fossa:** the ischio-rectal fossa.

vē·lum (L., a cloth). Any veil-like structure. **V. palati:** the soft palate.

vē·na (L., a vein). A vein. **V. azygos:** see vein azygos. **V. cava, inferior:** commences opposite the upper border of the body of the fifth lumbar vertebra, it is formed by the union of the right and left common iliac veins, it passes through the diaphragm and opens into the right atrium of the heart. **V. cava superior:** is formed by the union of the right and left innominate veins. It is three inches long and opens into the postero-superior angle of the right atrium. **V. salvatella:** a vein situated on the inner side of the hand, it becomes continuous with the ulnar vein. **Venae cordis minimae:** minute veins in the wall of the right atrium. **V. stellatae:** veins of the cortex of the kidney. **V. vorticosae:** veins of the choroid.

venenā·tion (L. *venenum*, a poison). The condition produced by poisoning.

venenĭ·ferous (L. *venenum*, a poison; *ferre*, to bear). Conveying poison.

vĕ·nenose, vĕ·nenous (L. *venenum*, a poison). Poisonous.

venenŏ·sity (L. *venenum*, a poison). The state of being poisoned.

vĕ·nepuncture (L. *vena*, a vein; *punctura*, a pricking). The surgical puncturing of a vein.

venē·real (L. *venereus*, of Venus). Relating to or caused by sexual intercourse. **V. diseases:** gonorrhoea, syphilis, chancroid, etc.

venerĕŏ·logist (L. *venereus*, of Venus; G. *logos*, a treatise). One skilled in the treatment of venereal diseases.

venerĕŏ·logy (L. *venereus*, of Venus; G. *logos*, a discourse). The study of venereal diseases and their treatment.

venē·reophō·bia (L. *venereus*, of Venus; G. *phobos*, fear). 1. Neurotic fear of sexual intercourse. 2. Dread of being infected with venereal disease.

vē·nery (L. *venereus*, of Venus). Copulation.

venesec·tion (L. *vena*, vein; *sectio*, section). The opening of a vein in order to let blood; phlebotomy.

venesū·ture (L. *vena*, vein; *sutura*, a seam). The suturing of a vein; phleborrhaphy.

vĕ·niplex (L. *vena*, vein; *plexus*, a plaiting). A plexus of veins.

venī·tis (L. *vena*, vein). Inflammation of a vein.

ve·nom (L. *venenum*, a poison). Poison, particularly that secreted by certain reptiles and insects.

vĕ·nomosali·vary (L. *venenum*, a poison; *saliva*, spittle). Secreting a venomous saliva.

vĕ·nomous (L. *venenum*, a poison). Poisonous; secreting venom.

venŏ·sity (L. *venosus*, from *vena*, vein). A condition in which arterial blood displays venous characteristics.

vē·nous (L. *venosus*, from *vena*, vein). Relating to the veins. **V. blood:** the dark type of blood found in the veins. **V. hum:** the murmur heard on auscultation of a vein.

vent (L. *ventus*, wind). An outlet; especially the anal opening.

ven·ter (L., belly). 1. The abdomen. 2. Any part shaped like a belly.

ventilā·tion (L. *ventilare*, to fan). The supplying of fresh air; the purifying of air in an enclosed space.

ven·trad (L. *venter*, belly; *ad*, to). Towards any ventral aspect.

ven·tral (L. *ventralis*, from *venter*, belly). Relating to the abdomen or to any venter.

ven·tricle (L. *ventriculus*, dim. of *venter*, belly). A small cavity or sac; particularly the two lower chambers of the heart. **V. of brain:** cystic spaces within the brain filled with cerebrospinal fluid. **V., fifth:** cavity of the brain called also cavum septi pellucidi. **V., fourth:** see under fourth. **V., third:** cavity between and below the central hemispheres, extending from the corpus callosum above to the infundibulum below, and from the pineal body behind to the lamina terminalis in front.

ventri·cular (L. *ventriculus*, dim. of *venter*, belly). Relating to a ventricle.

ventriculā·ris (L.). The thyro-epiglottideus muscle.

ventriculŏ·stomy (L. *ventriculus*, dim. of *venter*, belly; G. *stoma*, mouth). Operation in which a temporary opening is made into one of the cerebral ventricles.

ventri·culus (L., dim. of *venter*, belly). 1. A ventricle. 2. The stomach.

ventricum·bent (L. *venter*, belly; *incumbere*, to recline). Lying with the ventral surface downward.

ven·triduct (L. *venter*, belly; *ducere*, to lead). To bring or convey toward the ventral aspect.

ven·trifixā·tion (L. *venter*, belly; *figere*, to fix). Ventrofixation, *q.v.*

ventri·loquism (L. *venter*, belly; *loqui*, speech). The act or art of speaking in such a way as to make it appear that the voice originated from an enclosed space or from a point away from the speaker.

ventri·meson (L. *venter*, belly; G. *meson*, middle). The middle line on the ventral surface of the body.

ventripy̆·ramid (L. *venter*, belly; G. *puramis*, pyramid). The anterior pyramid of the medulla oblongata.

ven·trocystor·rhaphy (L. *venter*, belly; G. *kustis*, bladder; *rhaphē*, suture). The surgical suturing of the bladder or of a cyst to the abdominal wall.

ven·trofixā·tion (L. *venter*, belly; *figere*, to fix). The suturing of a displaced viscus, especially the uterus, to the abdominal wall.

ven·trose (L. *ventrosus*, from *venter*, belly). Possessed of a belly, or having a belly-like swelling.

ven·trosuspen·sion (L. *venter*, belly; *suspensio*, from *suspendere*, to hang). The cure of uterine retroposition by suturing the uterus to the wall of the abdomen.

ventrŏ·tomy (L. *venter*, belly; G. *tomē*, section). Incision into the abdominal cavity.

ven·trovĕ·sicofixā·tion (L. *venter*, belly; *vesica*, bladder; *figere*, to fix). The fixation of the uterus to the bladder and the abdominal wall.

vē·nula, vē·nule (L. *venula*, dim. of *vena*, vein). A venous radicle or a minute vein.

vē·nular (L. *vena*, vein). Relating to a venule.

Verā·trum (L., hellebore). A genus of liliaceous plants. *V. album* (white hellebore) yields an emetic substance. *V. viride* (green hellebore) yields jervine, which acts as a depressant on the heart and the vasomotor system. Green hellebore further produces veratroidine, a heart stimulant and spinal motor centre depressant. Veratroidine is used in the treatment of pleurisy and certain types of pneumonia.

Verbē·na (L.). A genus of plants of the vervain family. *V. hastata* is sometimes used in the treatment of epilepsy.

ver·bigerā·tion (L. *verbigerare*, to talk). The babbling of senseless words and phrases.

ver·digris (Fr. *vert de Grèce*, Greek green). 1. A mixture of basic copper acetates; astringent. 2. A deposit on copper vessels caused by the formation of cupric salts.

Verga's groove (Verga, A., Italian psychiatrist, 1811–95). A groove below the normal opening of the nasolacrimal duct. **V.'s ventricle:** a space between the corpus callosum and the body of the fornix.

ver·gence (L. *vergere*, to bend). Movement of the eye; see also convergence and divergence.

ver·getures. Striae of the skin occurring in pregnancy, obesity, etc.

Verheyen's stars (Verheyen, P., Flemish anatomist, 1648–1710). The venae stellatae of the kidney.

ver·juice (Fr. *verjus*, sour grapes). The acid juice of green fruits.

ver·micide (L. *vermis*, worm; *caedere*, to kill). An agent destructive of intestinal worms.

vermĭ·cular (L. *vermiculus*, dim. of *vermis*, worm). Resembling a worm in shape or appearance.

vermĭ·culate (L. *vermiculari*, from *vermiculus*, dim. of *vermis*, worm). Resembling a worm.

vermiculā·tion (L. *vermiculatio*, from *vermiculari*, to be worm-eaten). Peristaltic or wormlike movement, as of the intestine; peristalsis.

ver·miform (L. *vermis*, worm; *forma*, form). Shaped like a worm. **V. appendix:** a small diverticulum of the caecum that opens into its medial and posterior part rather more than 1 inch below the ileo-colic orifice. Its diameter is about 5 mm. and its length varies from two to six inches or more.

vermi·fugal (L. *vermis*, worm; *fugare*, to put to flight). Expelling worms.

ver·mifuge (L. *vermis*, worm; *fugare*, to put to flight). An agent that expels worms.

vermĭ·lion (L. *vermiculus*, dim. of *vermis*, a worm). Cinnabar or red mercuric sulphide HgS; a bright red pigment.

ver·min (L. *vermis*, worm). A collective name for animal parasites.

ver·minous (L. *vermis*, worm). 1. Infested with vermin. 2. Relating to vermin.

ver·mis (L.). 1. A worm. 2. The middle lobe of the cerebellum, the v. cerebelli.

ver·m(o)uth (Ger. *Wermuth*, wormwood). A cordial prepared from white wine and flavoured with aromatic herbs; a popular aperitif.

ver·nal (L. *vernalis*, of spring). Relating to the spring. **V. catarrh, V. conjunctivitis:** with seasonal recurrences, usually in the spring or summer.

Verneuil's disease (Verneuil, A. A., French surgeon, 1823–95). Syphilitic bursitis. **V.'s neuroma:** plexiform neuroma. **V.'s operation:** a method of iliac colostomy.

ver·nine. A leucomaine base found in vicia seedlings; when heated with hydrochloric acid it produces guanine.

ver·nix casĕŏ·sa (L. 'cheesy varnish'). A sebaceous substance-covering the skin of the foetus.

Veronal. A proprietary brand of soluble barbitone,

GG

CO.N:C(ONa).C(C$_2$H$_5$)$_2$CO.NH, a white crystalline hypnotic.

Verŏ·nica (L.). A genus of scrophulariaceous shrubs. The root of *V. virginica* (Culver's physic) is purgative and cholagogue.

verrŭ·ca (L.). A wart. **V. acuminata:** a wart usually of venereal origin. **V. necrogenica:** a warty excrescence occurring on the hands of those who frequently perform necropsies or handle the tissues of tuberculous persons.

verrŭ·ciform (L. *verruca*, wart; *forma*, shape). Wartlike.

vĕr·rucose, verrŭ·cous (L. *verruca*, wart). Warty; with many warts.

verrucŏ·sis (L. *verruca*, wart). A condition characterized by the appearance of many warts.

verrŭ·ga peruā·na (Sp. *verruga*, wart). An infectious disease of the skin occurring in Peru; Peruvian wart.

ver·sion (L. *vertere*, to turn). The act of turning; especially the manual turning of the foetus in delivery.

ver·tebra (L.). Any one of the thirty-three bones forming the spinal column.

ver·tebral (L. *vertebra*). Relating to a vertebra.

vertebrā·rium (L.L.). The spinal column.

Vertebrā·ta (L. *vertebra*). A division of the animal kingdom which includes all mammals, birds, reptiles and fish having a vertebral column.

ver·tebrate (L. *vertebra*). Having a vertebral column.

vertebrec·tomy (L. *vertebra*; G. *ektomē*, excision). Surgical removal of a vertebra.

ver·tebrochon·dral (L. *vertebra*; G. *khondros*, cartilage). Relating to the costal cartilages and the vertebrae.

ver·tebrocos·tal (L. *vertebra*; *costa*, rib). Relating to the vertebrae and the ribs.

ver·tebroster·nal (L. *vertebra*; G. *sternon*, the breast). Relating to the spinal column and the sternum.

ver·tex (L.). The crown of the head.

ver·tical (L. *vertex*). Perpendicular; upright.

verti·ginous (L. *vertigo*, from *vertere*, to turn). Relating to or affected with vertigo.

ver·tigo (L. from *vertere*, to turn). A sensation of lack of equilibrium. It may be psychological or due to disease of the ears, eyes, brain, stomach or blood. Vertigo should not be confused with dizziness.

vĕ·rumontā·num (L. *veru*, a roasting spit; *montanus*, mountainous). The caput gallinaginis or colliculus seminalis; a ridge disposed longitudinally on the floor of the prostatic urethra.

Vesalius's bone (Vesalius, A., Belgian anatomist, 1514–64). The separated tuberosity of the base of the fifth metatarsal bone. **V.'s foramen:** a small venous foramen situated immediately anterior to the foramen ovale. **V.'s glands:** the bronchial lymphatic glands; glandulae Vesalanae.

vesā·nia (L.). An obsolete term for insanity.

vesi·ca (L. *vesica*, bladder). The bladder. **V. fellea:** the gall-bladder. **V. urinaria:** the urinary bladder.

vesi·cal (L. *vesica*, bladder). Relating to the bladder.

vĕ·sicant (L. *vesica*, a blister). 1. Causing blisters; blistering. 2. A blistering agent.

vesicā·tion (L. *vesica*, a blister). 1. The formation of a blister. 2. A blister.

vĕ·sicatory (L. *vesica*, a blister). 1. Blistering; causing blisters. 2. A blistering agent.

vĕ·sicle (L. *vesicula*, dim. of *vesica*, a bladder or blister). 1. A small bladder, especially a small sac containing liquid. 2. A skin blister, as in herpes or chickenpox.

vĕ·sico-abdŏ·minal (L. *vĕsica*, bladder; abdomen). Relating both to the bladder and the abdomen.

vĕ·sicocele (L. *vesica*, bladder; G. *kēlē*, hernia). Hernia of the bladder. Syn. cystocele.

vĕ·sicocervĭ·cal (L. *vesica*, bladder; *cervix*, neck). Relating to the bladder and the uterine cervix.

vĕ·sicofixā·tion (L. *vesica*, bladder; *figere*, to fix). 1. Suturing the bladder to the abdominal wall. 2. The surgical fixation of the uterus to the bladder.

vĕ·sicoprostat·ic (L. *vesica*, bladder; G. *prostătēs*, a chief). Relating to the prostate gland and the urinary bladder.

vĕ·sicopū·bic (L. *vesica*, bladder; *pubes*, body-hair). Relating to the bladder and the pubes.

vĕ·sicorec·tal (L. *vesica*, bladder; *rectus*, straight). Relating to the bladder and the rectum.

vĕ·sicorē·nal (L. *vesica*, bladder; *ren*, kidney). Relating to the bladder and the kidney.

vĕ·sicospī·nal (L. *vesica*, bladder; *spina*, spine). Relating to the urinary bladder and the spinal cord.

vēsicŏ·tomy (L. *vesica*, bladder; G. *tomē*, section). Surgical incision into the bladder; cystotomy.

vĕ·sico-urē·teral (L. *vesica*, bladder; G. *ourēter*, ureter). Relating to the urinary bladder and the ureter.

vĕ·sico-urē·thral (L. *vesica*, bladder; G. *ourēthra*, urethra). Relating to the bladder and the urethra.

vĕ·sico-ū·terine (L. *vesica*, bladder; *uterus*, womb). Relating to the bladder and the uterus.

vĕ·sico-vagī·nal (L. *vesica*, bladder; *vagina*, sheath). Relating to the bladder and the vagina.

vēsi·cula (L., dim. of *vesica*, bladder). A vesicle. **V. fellis:** the gall-bladder.

vesi·cular (L. *vesicula*, a small bladder). Relating to or composed of vesicles. **V. breathing:** sound produced by air entering and leaving healthy lung tissue.

vesiculā·tion (L. *vesicula*, a small bladder). The formation of vesicles.

vesiculec·tomy (L. *vesicula*, a small bladder; G. *ektomē*, excision). Complete or partial excision of the seminal vesicles.

vesiculi·ferous (L. *vesica*, bladder; *ferre*, to bear). Having vesicles.

vesi·culiform (L. *vesicula*, small bladder; *forma*, shape). Having the shape of a vesicle.

vĕ·siculī·tis (L. *vesicula*, small bladder). Inflammation of a vesicle, especially of a seminal vesicle.

vesi·culobron·chial (L. *vesicula*, small bladder; G. *brogkhos*, the windpipe). Both vesicular and bronchial.

vesi·culocă·vernous (L. *vesicula*, small bladder; *caverna*, cavern). Both vesicular and cavernous.

vesi·culotympan·ic (L. *vesicula*, small bladder; G. *tumpanon*, drum). Having a quality both vesicular and tympanic.

Vesling's line (Vesling, J., German anatomist, 1598–1641). The raphe or linea media scroti.

ves·sel (L. *vascellum*, dim. of *vas*, vessel). Any one of the tubes or canals conveying blood or lymph.

vesti·bular (L. *vestibulum*, a fore-court). Relating to a vestibule.

vĕ·stibule (L. *vestibulum*, a fore-court). A chamber or cavity at the entrance to a canal. **V., aortic:** that portion of the left ventricle which is immediately below the aortic orifice. **V. of the ear:** the middle part of the internal ear, providing the entrance to the cochlea. **V. of the larynx:** the superior compartment of the larynx above the vestibular cords. **V. of the mouth:** the anterior compartment of the mouth. It is bounded anteriorly and externally by the lips and cheeks, and internally by the alveolar arches and gums. **V. of the nose:** the anterior part of the nose, situated just within the ala of the nostril. **V. of perineum:** the space that is enclosed by the labia minora. It is triangular, the apex which is in front being formed by the glans clitoridis, the lateral boundaries by the labia minora and the base by the posterior margin of the vaginal orifice.

vesti·bulo-ure̅·thral (L. *vestibulum*, a fore-court; G. *oure̅thra*, urethra). Relating to the vulval vestibule and the urethra.

vesti·bulum (L., a fore-court). Any vestibule; usually applied to the vestibule of the ear.

ve̬·stige (L. *vestigium*, a foot-print). 1. A trace of something that has formerly existed. 2. A homologue of an organ or tissue more fully developed in lower forms.

vesti·gial (L. *vestigium*, a foot-print). Having the nature of a vestige; rudimentary.

vesu̅·vine (From the volcano, Mount Vesuvius). Bismarck-brown or phenyl-brown; used for staining in histological preparations.

veterina̅·rian (L. *veterinarius*, a farrier). A practitioner of veterinary medicine.

ve̬·terinary (L. *veterinarius*, a farrier). Relating to domestic animals and their diseases.

vi antigen. One of the typhoid antigens.

vi̅·a (L.). A road or way.

viabi̅·lity (Fr. *vie*, from L. *vita*, life). Ability to live after birth.

vi̅·able (Fr. *vie*, from L. *vita*, life). Capable of living; said of a foetus that has reached such a stage of development that it can live outside the uterus.

vi̅·al (G. *phiale̅*, a pan). A small bottle or phial.

vi̅·bex, vi̅·bix (L. *vibex*, a weal). A narrow linear mark or streak; a linear subcutaneous effusion of blood or ecchymosis.

vibrate (L. *vibrare*, to vibrate). To oscillate; to have a to and fro movement.

vi̅·bratile (L. *vibrare*, to vibrate). Having an oscillatory movement; moving to and fro.

vibra̅·tion (L. *vibrare*, to vibrate). The act of oscillating or moving to and fro.

vi̅·bratory (L. *vibrare*, to vibrate). Marked by vibrations.

Vib·rio (L. *vibrare*, to vibrate). A genus of Schizomycetes. **V. cholerae:** the spirillum of cholera.

vibris·sae (L.). The hairs growing inside the nostrils; also a cat's whiskers.

vi̅·brotac·tile (L. *vibrare*, to vibrate; *tactilis*, tangible). Teletactile, *q.v.*

vi̅·brotherapeu·tics (L. *vibrare*, to vibrate; G. *therapeutike̅*, medical treatment). The use of vibration in treatment.

Vibur·num (L.). A genus of foliaceous shrubs. The bark of *V. opulus* (the cranberry tree) is antispasmodic and is used in the treatment of cramp, etc.

vica̅·rious (L. *vicarius*, substituted). Substitutive; replacing something else. **V. menstruation:** menstruation occurring in an abnormal place.

vice (L. *vitium*, a fault). A defect.

Vichy douche. See bath, Aix. **V. water.** An antacid mineral water with a slightly laxative action; obtained from Vichy in France.

vi̅·cious (L. *vitium*, a fault). Defective. **V. union:** the faulty joining of the ends of a fractured bone.

Vicq d'Azyr's bundle (Vicq d' Azyr, F., French anatomist, 1748–94). The fasciculus mammillothalamicus. **V. d'A.'s stripe:** the same as the stria of Gennari.

Vidal's operation (Vidal de Cassis, A. T., French surgeon, 1803–56). An operation for varicocele consisting of subcutaneous ligation of some of the veins of the pampiniform plexus.

Vi̅·dian canal. The canal in the sphenoid bone for the Vidian artery and nerve. Syn. Guidi's canal. **V. nerve:** nervus canalis pterygoidei. Syn. Guidi's nerve.

viei̅·rin. A principle obtained from the bark of *Remijia vellosii*. It is an amorphous white substance,

is soluble in alcohol and chloroform and is used as a substitute for quinine.

Vieussens's annulus (Vieussens, R. de, French anatomist, 1641–1715). The ansa subclavia of sympathetic nerves. **V.'s scyphus:** the central canal of the cochlear columella. **V.'s valve:** the anterior medullary velum.

Vignal's bacillus (Vignal, G., French physiologist of the nineteenth century). *Leptotrichia buccalis*, a non-pathogenic organism found in the healthy mouth. **V.'s cells:** the embryonic connective-tissue (mesenchymatous) cells lying upon the axis cylinders of which the foetal nerve fibres are made up and eventually forming a complete sheath.

Vigo plaster (Vigo, G. da, Italian surgeon, 1460–1520). A plaster made of mercury, turpentine, wax, lead-plaster, myrrh, saffron and other substances.

Vigouroux's sign (Vigouroux, A., French neurologist of the nineteenth century). Diminished electrical resistance of the skin in thyrotoxicosis.

Villard's button (Villard, E., French surgeon, born 1868). A modification of Murphy's button, used in intestinal anastomosis.

Villemin's sphincter (Villemin, F., French anatomist. Work published in first three decades of the 20th century). The sphincteric fibres or 'muscular valve' at the termination of the duodenum.

vil·li (L. Plural of *villus*, *q.v.*). **V., intestinal:** minute projections of the mucous membrane of the small intestine. They are closely set upon the mucous membrane. Their total number is said to be about four millions.

villi·ferous (L. *villus*, a tuft of hair; *ferre*, to bear). Bearing villi.

vil·lose, vil·lous (L. *villus*, a tuft of hair). Relating to a villus; covered with villi.

villo̬·sity (L. *villus*, a tuft of hair). The state of being villous.

vil·lus (L., a tuft of hair). 1. Any one of the minute projections from the mucous membrane of the intestine. Each villus is composed of a lacteal vessel, an arteriole and a vein and is enveloped in a membrane. 2. Any one of the vascular chorionic tufts.

Vincent's angina (Vincent, H., French physician, born 1862). An infection of the mucous membrane of the mouth, caused by a fusiform bacillus often in association with a spirillum. It affects the tonsils and gums and is very contagious. **V.'s bacillus:** a fusiform bacillus responsible for Vincent's angina. **V.'s serum:** an anti-streptococcal serum. **V.'s sign:** the Argyll-Robertson pupil.

vin·cula aceso̅·ria ten·dinum (L., accessory bands of tendons). The slender, tendinous folds joining the phalanges to the flexor tendons.

vin·culum (L., a band). A ligament.

vi̅·negar (Fr. *vinaigre*, from L. *vinum*, wine; *acer*, acid). 1. An impure solution of acetic acid. 2. A solution of medicinal material in vinegar or acetic acid.

vi̅·nous (L. *vinum*, wine). Of the nature of or containing wine.

vi̅·num (L.). 1. Wine; fermented juice of grapes or other fruit. 2. A solution of medicinal substances in wine.

Vi̅·ola (L., violet). A genus of plants which includes the violets. *V. odorata* and some other varieties have been used in the treatment of bronchitis.

viola̅·tion (L. *violare*, to violate). Rape.

violinist's cramp. A neurosis affecting violin-players and marked by spasm of the fingers.

viper venom. Venom from Russell's viper (a south-eastern Asian snake of the genus *Vipera*) is a useful local haemostatic. It is used in cases of haemophilic bleeding.

vi·perine (L. *viperinus*, of a viper). Relating to a viper.

viragi·nity (L. *virago*, a female of mannish type). A type of sexual perversion in which the female reveals marked male characteristics.

Virchow's disease (Virchow, R. L. K., German pathologist, 1821–1902). Leontiasis ossea. **V.'s spaces:** the spaces between vessels and nerve cells in the spinal cord.

vir·gin (L. *virgo*, virgin). An individual who has had no sexual intercourse.

vir·ginal (L. *virgo*, virgin). Relating to a virgin or to virginity.

virgi·nity (L. *virgo*, virgin). The state of being a virgin.

vi·rile (L. *virilis*). Relating to or characteristic of the male.

virile·scence (L. *virilis*, manly). The appearance of masculine characters in post-menopausal women, e.g., the growth of a beard or the deepening of the voice. Also the development of masculine characteristics in some endocrine disturbances, such as Cushing's syndrome.

viri·lia (L. *virilis*, virile). The male reproductive organs.

viri·lity (L. *virilis*, virile). The state of being virile.

viri·potent (L. *vir*, man; *potens*, fit for). Marriageable; capable of sexual intercourse with a man.

vi·rose (L. *virosus*, poisonous). Poisonous. The term is now rare.

virtual cautery (L. *virtus*, strength; G. *kautērion*, a branding iron). Cauterization by means of the application of caustics.

vi·rulence (L. *virulentus*, poisonous). Malignity; the ability of a micro-organism to cause disease.

vi·rulent (L. *virulentus*, poisonous). Having the nature of a poison.

viruli·ferous (L. *virus*, poison; *ferre*, to bear). Containing or carrying a germ.

vi·rus (L., poison). 1. An ultramicroscopic causal organism of disease. 2. The poison of an infectious disease. **V., attenuated:** a v. the pathogenicity of which has been reduced. **V., filtrable:** a v. so minute that it passes through the pores of a Berkefeld or Chamberland filter; e.g. the virus of variola, mumps, trachoma.

vis (L. force; pl. *vires*). Force or energy. **V. a tergo:** an impelling force. **V. conservatrix:** natural resistance to injury or disease. **V. medicatrix naturae:** nature's healing power.

vi·scera (L.). Plural of viscus, *q.v.*

vi·scerad (L. *viscus*, bowels; *ad*, to). Toward the viscera.

vi·sceral (L. *viscera*, the inner parts). Relating to a viscus or to viscera.

visceral·gia (L. *viscera*, the inner parts; G. *algos*, pain). Pain in a viscus.

vi·sceroptō·sis (L. *viscera*, the inner parts; G. *ptōsis*, a falling). Ptosis of abdominal organs; Glénard's disease.

vi·scid (L. *viscidus*). Sticky; adhesive; glutinous.

visci·dity (L. *viscidus*, sticky). The state of being viscid.

vis·cin (L. *viscum*, mistletoe). A mucilaginous principle from mistletoe.

viscŏ·meter. Viscosimeter, *q.v.*

vis·cose. A viscid solution of cellulose. It is used in the making of artificial silk.

viscosi·meter (L. *viscum*, mistletoe; G. *metron*, measure). An apparatus for measuring the viscosity of fluids.

viscŏ·sity (L.L. *viscosus*, sticky). The condition of being viscous.

vis·cous¹ (L. *viscum*, mistletoe). Viscid, *q.v.*

vis·cous² (L. *viscus*, bowels; pl. *viscera*). Relating to a viscus.

Vis·cum (L., mistletoe). A genus of plants, including mistletoe, of the order *Loranthaceae*, parasitic on trees. The principle viscin is obtained from *V. album* (European mistletoe) and *V. flavescens*.

vis·cus (L., bowels). Any one of the organs situated in one of the three great cavities of the body (thorax, pelvic cavity and abdominal cavity). The term applies particularly to the organs of the abdominal cavity.

visibi·lity (L. *visibilitas*). The quality of being perceived by the eye.

vi·sible (L. *visibilis*). Capable of being perceived by the eye.

vi·sion (L. *visio*). The act of seeing; sight. **Central v.:** v. with the macula lutea. **Peripheral v.:** v. with the periphery of the retina.

vi·sual (L. *visualis*, from *visus*, from *vidēre*, to see). Relating to vision. **V. field:** that portion of space in which objects are visible at the same moment.. **V. purple:** the purple pigment in the retina.

vi·suō-au·ditory (L. *visus*, from *vidēre*, to see; *auditorius*, from *audire*, to hear). Relating to seeing and hearing. **V.-a. nerve fibres:** those connecting the visual and auditory centres.

vi·ta (L.). Life. **V. sexualis:** the sex life.

vi·ta-glass. A type of glass containing quartz which can be penetrated by the ultra-violet rays of the sun.

vi·tal (L. *vita*, life). Relating to life. **V. capacity:** the volume of air that can be exhaled from the lungs after a complete respiration. **V. centre:** the respiratory centre in the medulla oblongata. **V. statistics:** statistics of births, deaths, marriages and diseases.

vi·talism (L. *vita*, life). The doctrine that ascribes all physiological processes to the action of a vital force as distinguished from mechanical or chemical forces.

vitā·lity (L. *vita*, life). 1. The condition of being alive; vigour. 2. The vital force.

vi·talize (L. *vita*, life). To endow with life.

vi·tals (L. *vita*, life). Those organs essential to life.

vi·tamins (L. *vita*, life; amine, organic compound). Organic compounds, present in minute quantities in certain foods and necessary to the normal processes of metabolism. Absence or insufficiency of these substances produces deficiency diseases such as beri-beri, rickets and scurvy. Vitamins are necessary food factors. The most important are: (1) Fat-soluble A, necessary for growth; if not present in the diet in sufficient amount, lack of growth and xerophthalmia will result. It is found in butter, cod-liver oil, cream, egg yolk, milk, spinach. (2) Water-soluble B_1, also necessary for growth; insufficiency results in beri-beri and polyneuritis. B_2 is anti-pellagric and is found in asparagus, beans, spinach, tomatoes, wheat grain, yeast. (3) B complex, a group of water soluble substances including thiamine, riboflavine, nictotinic acid, pyridoxin, folic acid, and B_{12} an anti-pernicious anaemia factor. (4) Water-soluble C (ascorbic acid; hexuronic acid) is antiscorbutic and is found in green cabbage, lettuces, lemon and orange juice, pineapple, raspberries, spinach, tomatoes. (5) Fat-soluble D, antirachitic, is found in cod-liver oil and milk. (6) E, insufficiency results in sterility; found in wheat (oil of germ), hemp seed, legumes (germinated) and wheat grain. (7) K, compound necessary for prothrombin formation; found in spinach, cabbage, fishmeat, liver fat and egg yolk.

vitellā·rium (L. *vitellus*, the yoke of an egg). An accessory gland found in the female reproductive organs of some classes of tapeworms by which the vitellus for the fertilized egg is secreted. Syn. yolkgland; vitelline gland.

vĭ·tellary (L. *vitellus*, the yoke of an egg). Relating to the vitellus.

vitel·lin (L. *vitellus*, the yoke of an egg). A globulin present in egg-yolk.

vitel·line (L. *vitellus*, the yoke of an egg). Relating to the vitellus.

vitellolū·tein (L. *vitellus*, yolk; *luteus*, yellow). A yellow dye obtained from the lutein of eggs.

vitellorū·bin (L. *vitellus*, yolk; *ruber*, red). A reddish pigment obtained from egg-yolk.

vitel·lus (L.). An egg-yolk.

vitili·ginous (L. *vitiligo*, tetter). Relating to or affected with vitiligo.

vitili·go (L. tetter). Piebald skin; a skin affection marked by a loss of the natural pigment. It occurs in patches and leaves whitish areas.

vitiligoi·dea (L. *vitiligo*, tetter; G. *eidos*, form). Xanthoma.

vĭ·tium (L.). Defect.

vitochĕ·mical (L. *vita*, life; ult. G. *kheein*, to pour). Organic.

vitodynă·mic (L. *vita*, life; G. *dunamis*, power). Relating to vital forces.

vĭ·treoden·tine (L. *vitreus*, glassy; *dens*, tooth). An unusually hard and glass-like form of dentine.

vit·reous (L. *vitreus*, glassy). Glass-like or hyaline. V. chamber: the part of the globe of the eye situated posterior to the anterior chamber and crystalline lens. V. humour: the transparent jelly-like substance filling the vitreous chamber of the eye.

vĭ·triol (from L. *vitrum*, glass). 1. Sulphuric acid (oil of vitriol). 2. Any crystalline salt of sulphuric acid.

vit·rum (L.). Glass.

vĭ·tuline (L. *vitulus*, a calf). Relating to a calf.

vĭ·vificā·tion (L. *vivus*, alive; *facere*, to make). The act of assimilating lifeless protein substances and thus converting them into living tissue.

vivĭ·parous (L. *vivus*, alive; *parere*, to bear). Bringing forth living offspring.

vivisec·tion (L. *vivus*, alive; *sectio*, a cutting). Dissection of or experimentation upon a living animal.

vivisec·tionist (L. *vivus*, alive; *sectio*, a cutting). One who practises or defends vivisection; a vivisector.

vivisec·tor (L. *vivus*, alive; *sector*, a cutter). One who practises vivisection.

Vladimirov's operation (Vladimirov, Russian surgeon, 1837–1903). A method of tarsectomy.

vō·cal (L. *vocalis*, sounding). Relating to the voice or the voice-producing organs; loud. V. cord: false vocal cords or vestibular folds are two folds of mucous membrane which extend on each side from the receding angle of the thyroid cartilage to the anterolateral surface of the arytenoid cartilage. True vocal cords or vocal folds are prominent folds on each side which extend from the receding angle of the thyroid cartilage to the vocal process of each arytenoid cartilage.

vod·ka. A spirit distilled in Russia; it is mainly produced from rye.

Voge's test (Voge, C. I. B., contemporary British physician). A test for histidine in the urine of pregnant women.

Vogt's disease (Vogt, O., German neurologist, born 1870). Spastic diplegia. V's syndrome: a syndrome found in lesions of the corpus striatum.

Vogt's point (Vogt, P. F. E., German surgeon, 1847–85). The classical point for trephining the skull in cases of middle meningeal haemorrhage.

voice (L. *vox*). The range of sounds, produced by the speech organs in man.

void (Old Fr. *voidier*, to empty). To evacuate waste products.

Voigt's lines (Voigt, C. A., Austrian anatomist, 1809–90). The hair tracts.

Voillemier's point (Voillemier, L. C., French urologist, 1809–78). A midline point 6·5 cm. below a line joining the anterior superior iliac spines. The point for suprapubic puncture of the bladder.

Voit's nerve (Voit, M., German anatomist, born 1876). A branch of the ramus anterior of the acoustic nerve, supplying the macula sacculi.

Voit's nucleus (Voit, K. von, German physiologist, 1831–1908). The cerebellar nucleus accessory to the corpus dentatum.

voix de Polichinelle (Fr. voice of Punch). A type of aegophony.

vō·la (L.). The palm or the sole.

vō·lar (L. *vola*, palm or sole). Relating to the palm or the sole.

vŏ·latile (L. *volatilis*, winged). Tending to evaporate quickly; converting into vapour at ordinary temperatures; evanescent.

vŏ·latilizā·tion (L. *volatilis*, winged). Conversion into vapour by means of heat.

Volhard's solution (Volhard, J., German chemist, 1834–1910). N/10 potassium thiocyanate.

voli·tion (Mediaeval L. *volitio*, from L. *velle*, to wish). The will to act.

voli·tional (Mediaeval L. *volitio*, from L. *velle*, to wish). Relating to the will.

Volkmann's canals (Volkmann, A. W., German physiologist, 1800–77). The canals in bone-carrying blood vessels from the periosteum. V.'s membrane: the lining membrane of a tuberculous abscess.

Volkmann's deformity (Volkmann, R. von, German surgeon, 1830–89). Congenital dislocation of the ankle. V.'s splint: a splint for fractured tibia and fibula, consisting of guttered back piece, side pieces and foot piece. V.'s spoon: a sharp spoon used for scraping granulations, bone, etc.

vol·ley (Fr. *volée*, ult. from L. *volare*, to fly). A rhythmic succession of muscular twitches artificially produced.

volsel·la (L.). A forceps fitted with one or more hooks at the end of each blade.

volt (Volta, A., Italian physicist, 1745–1827). The electromotive force needed to cause one coulomb of current to perform one joule of work.

voltā·ic. Relating to voltaism.

vol·taism (Italian physicist, Volta; see under volt). Galvanism, q.v.

voltă·meter (Italian physicist, Volta; G. *metron*, measure). An instrument for electrolysing water into hydrogen and oxygen.

Voltolini's disease (Voltolini, F. E. R., German otologist, 1819–89). Acute inflammation of the internal ear.

vŏ·lume (L. *volumen*, a roll of manuscript). The space occupied by a substance; cubic dimension.

volumĕ·tric (L. *volumen*, a roll; G. *metron*, measure). Quantitative analysis by volume.

vŏ·luntary (L. *voluntas*, will). Controlled by the will.

vŏ·luntomō·tory (L. *voluntas*, will; *movēre*, to move). Relating to voluntary motion.

vol·vulus (L. *volvere*, to roll). A twisting of the intestine upon itself which occludes the lumen; this happens most commonly in the sigmoid flexure.

vō·mer (L. *vomer*, ploughshare). The thin plate of bone forming the lower and posterior part of the nasal septum. V., cartilaginous: the cartilaginous plate forming the anterior part of the nasal septum.

vō·merine (L. *vomer*, ploughshare). Relating to the vomer.

voltmeter. An instrument for measuring voltage or electromotive force.

vŏ·mica (L. *vomica*, abscess). 1. A collection of pus in the lungs or neighbouring organs discharged by expectoration. 2. A cavity produced by the breaking down of tissue; especially a lung cavity.

vŏ·mit (L. *vomitus*, from *vomere*, to puke). 1. To cast up from the stomach by vomiting. 2. Vomited substance.

vŏ·miting (L. *vomitus*, from *vomere*, to puke). The forcible expulsion of the stomach contents through the mouth. **V. sickness of Jamaica:** ackee poisoning. A disease caused by poisoning by a fruit known to the natives of Jamaica as Ackee, the fruit of *Blighia sapida*. The disease is characterized by severe vomiting and has a mortality of 80 to 90 per cent in untreated cases. Confined to the West Indies.

vŏ·mito ne·gro (It.). Black vomit.

vŏ·mitory (L. *vomitorius*, from *vomere*, to puke). Any agent acting as an emetic.

vomiturĭ·tion (L. *vomere*, to puke). Repeated, ineffectual efforts at vomiting; retching.

vŏ·mitus (L. from *vomere*, to puke). The matter which is vomited.

vŏ·nulo. A bronchial disease, characterized by considerable pain, occurring in West Africa.

vorā·cious (L. *vorax*). Ravenous.

Voronoff's operation (Voronoff, S., contemporary Russian physician, practising in Paris). A type of "rejuvenation" operation consisting of transplantation of the testes of an ape into a human.

vor·tex (L. a whorl; pl. *vortices*). The whorled arrangement of cardiac muscle fibres.

voussure (Fr. curve). Precordial bulging due to cardiac enlargement in childhood.

vox (L.). The voice.

vul·canite. Vulcanized rubber.

vulcanize: to subject to vulcanization. A process of imparting to caoutchouc, gutta percha, rubber etc., greater elasticity, durability and hardness by heating with sulphur.

vul·nerabĭ·lity (L. *vulnerare*, to wound). Susceptible of injury or infection.

vul·nerary (L. *vulnerarius*, from *vulnus*, a wound). 1. Relating to or healing wounds. 2. An agent promoting the healing of wounds.

vul·nerate (L. *vulnerare*, to injure). To wound.

vul·nus (L.). A trauma or injury.

Vulpian's atrophy (Vulpian, F. A., French physician, 1826–87). Progressive muscular atrophy affecting the shoulder and upper arm. **V.'s law:** on destruction of part of the brain the remainder of the brain carries the function of that part.

vulsel·la, vulsel·lum (L. *volsella*, forceps). See under Volsella.

vul·va (L. womb). The external genitalia of the female.

vul·var. Relating to the vulva.

vulvec·tomy (L. *vulva*; G. *ektomē*, excision). Excision of the vulva.

vulvis·mus (L. *vulva*, womb). Vaginismus, *q.v.*

vulvī·tis (L. *vulva*). Inflammation of the vulva.

vulvŏ·pathy (L. *vulva*; G. *pathos*, disease). Any vulvar disease.

vulvo-ū·terine (L. *vulva*, womb; *uterus*, womb). Pertaining to both the vulva and the uterus.

vulvo-vagī·nal (L. *vulva*, womb; *vagina*, sheath). Relating to both the vulva and the vagina.

vul·vovaginī·tis (L. *vulva*, womb; *vagina*, sheath). Inflammation of the vulva and of the vagina.

W

W. The symbol of tungsten (Wolframium).

Wachendorff's membrane (Wachendorff, E. J., German anatomist of the 18th century). The membrana pupillaris.

wadding. Sheets of cotton or wool used for covering wounds.

wā·fer. A thin layer of moistened flour used to enclose doses of medicine for internal administration.

Wagner's corpuscles (Wagner, R., German physiologist, 1805–64). The tactile nerve endings. **W.'s spot:** the nucleolus of the ovum.

Wagstaffe's fracture (Wagstaffe, W. W., English surgeon, 1843–1910). An adduction (internal rotation) fracture of the ankle.

waist. The narrow part of the trunk situated between the thorax and the hips.

wakefulness. Insomnia.

Wakeley's radium forceps (Wakeley, Sir Cecil, British surgeon, born 1892). Special applicator forceps for inserting tubes of radium into the tissues.

Waldeyer's organ (Waldeyer, W. von, German anatomist, 1836–1921). The paradidymis; organ of Giraldes. **W.'s tract:** the border tract or zone of Lissauer. **W.'s white line:** on the testis at the junction of the germinal epithelium and the peritoneum.

walking typhoid. A mild grade of typhoid fever.

Wallerian degeneration (Waller, A. V., English physiologist, 1816–70). Degeneration of a nerve consecutive upon its section. The myelin becomes segmented and subsequently it and the axis-cylinder disappear.

walnut. A tree of the species Juglans.

Walter's nerve (Walter, J. G., German anatomist, 1734–1818). A branch of the smallest splanchnic nerve passing to the renal plexus.

Walthard's cell rests or islets (Walthard, M., Swiss gynaecologist, born 1867). Squamous cell rests in the ovary.

Walther's canal (Walther, A. F., German anatomist, 1688–1746). The duct of the sublingual salivary gland.

wandering. 1. Moving freely about. 2. Abnormally movable. **W. abscess:** an abscess which "points" at a distance from its origin. **W. cell:** a leucocyte. **W. organ:** an organ which moves from its normal position due to loose attachment.

wane. To decrease; to decline; to fade.

Wanscher's mask (Wanscher, O., Danish physician, 1846–1906). An ether anaesthetic mask.

Warburg's tincture (Warburg, C., Austrian physician of the 19th century). Tinctura antiperiodica; composed of aloes, quinine sulphate, opium and a number of other drugs.

Warburg's factor (Warburg, O. H., German physiologist, born 1883). An enzyme isolated from yeast.

Ward's triangle (Ward, F. O., English osteologist of the 19th century). A triangular area intervening among the trabeculae of the cancellous tissue of the neck of the femur.

wart. A raised portion of the epidermis, produced by hyperplasia of the papillae.

wash. 1. A lotion. 2. To cleanse with a liquid.

washing soda. Sodium carbonate.

Wasmann's glands (Wasmann, A.). The peptic glands.

Wassermann's reaction (Wassermann, A. P. von, German bacteriologist, 1866–1925). A complement fixation test for syphilis.

wasting. Destroying; marasmic.

water. H_2O; hydrogen monoxide. **W. glass:** a strong solution of sodium silicate.

Waterhouse-Friderichsen syndrome (Waterhouse, A., British physician; Friderichsen, C., German physician). A severe form of meningococcal meningitis, accompanied by suprarenal haemorrhage.

watt (Watt, J., Scottish engineer, 1736–1819). A volt-ampere; the amount of pressure developed by a current of one ampere having an electromotor force of one volt.

wave. An oscillating disturbance.

wavemeter. Ondometer, *q.v.*

wax. 1. The material of honeycomb; a mixture of cerotic acid, cerolein and myricin gathered by the honey-bee from the pollen of flowers and the leaves of plants. 2. Cerumen.

waxing. Increasing in size.

waxy. Like wax. **W. degeneration:** amyloid degeneration.

weakness. Loss or lack of strength.

weaning-brash. Severe infantile diarrhoea, popularly ascribed to weaning.

wea·sand. (A.S.). The trachea.

weaver's bottom. Chronic bursitis over the tuberosity of the ischium, due to pressure.

webbed. Joined by a thin band of abnormal tissue, as in w. fingers.

Weber's artery (Weber, M. I., German anatomist, 1795–1875). The external auditory artery; tympanic branch of the external carotid.

Weber's glands (Weber, E. H., German anatomist, 1795–1878). The lateral glands of the tongue. Sometimes called W.'s organ.

Weber's point (Weber, W. E., German physicist, 1804–91). A point about 1 cm. below the promontory of the sacrum that represents the centre of gravity of the body. **W.'s triangle:** the area of the sole of the foot formed by the heads of the first and fifth metatarsals and the mid-point of the plantar surface of the heel.

Weber's syndrome (Weber, Sir H., British physician, 1823–1918). 'Syndrome of cerebral peduncle', consisting of paralysis of the oculomotor nerve on the same side of the brain as the lesion and hemiplegia on the opposite side.

Weber's test (Weber, F. E., German otologist, 1832–91). A tuning fork is held against the vertex; the sound is heard best in the non-affected side in disease of the auditory apparatus and in the affected side in disease of the air passages.

Weeks's bacillus (Weeks, J. E., American ophthalmologist, born 1853). See under Koch's bacillus.

weeping. The shedding of tears.

Wegner's disease (Wegner, F. R. G., German pathologist, born 1843). Separation of the epiphyses in congenital syphilis.

Weigert's method (Weigert, K., German pathologist, 1843–1904). See W.'s stain; Gram's method. **W.'s stain:** Alcohol haematoxylin for myelin sheaths.

weight. 1. Heaviness as determined by a given standard. 2. The force with which bodies tend to approach the centre of attraction.

Weil's basal layer (Weil, L. A., German dentist of the nineteenth century). The layer immediately within the odontoblasts in tooth pulp.

Weil-Felix bacillus (Weil, E., German physician, 1880–1922; Felix, A., Czech bacteriologist, born 1887). A bacillus of the Proteus group found in the urine and faeces of typhus patients. **W.-F. reaction:** an agglutination reaction for typhus.

Weinberg's test (Weinberg, M., French pathologist, 1868–1940). A complement fixation test for hydatid disease.

Weir Mitchell's disease. See erythromelalgia.

Weiss's sign (Weiss, N., Austrian physician, 1851–83). Contraction of the facial muscles following light percussion, seen in cases of tetany.

Weiss's stain (Weiss, L., contemporary German physician). A stain for tubercle bacilli.

Weissmann's bundle (Weissmann, A., German anatomist of the 19th century). The aggregation of striped muscular fibres of a neuro-muscular spindle.

Weitbrecht's fibres (Weitbrecht, J., German anatomist, 1702–47). The retinacular fibres of the neck of the femur. **W.'s foramen ovale:** a gap in the capsule of the shoulder joint between the glenohumeral ligaments. **W.'s ligament:** the chorda obliqua; oblique radio-ulnar ligament.

Welander's treatment (Welander, E. W., Swedish physician, 1840–1917). Treatment for syphilis by the application of mercury ointment on a flannel jacket.

Welch's bacillus (Welch, W. H., American pathologist, 1850–1934). *Clostridium Welchii.* **W.'s stain:** a method of staining the capsule of the pneumococcus.

Welcker's sphenoidal angle (Welcker, H., German anatomist, 1822–98). The angle of the basi-cranial axis.

Wells's facies (Wells, Sir T. S., English gynaecologist, 1818–97). The facies of ovarian disease.

Welsh's cells (Welsh, D. A., Scottish pathologist, born 1875). The cells in the parathyroid gland.

wen. A sebaceous cyst.

Wenckebach's period (Wenckebach, K. F., Dutch cardiologist, 1864–1940). Occasional lengthening of the P–R interval in the electrocardiogram due to an occasional dropped beat in cases of heart block.

Wenzel's ventricle (Wenzel, J., German anatomist, 1768–1808). The ventriculus cerebri primus; cavum septum pellucidi.

Wepfer's glands (Wepfer, J. J., German physician, 1620–95). The duodenal glands better known eponymously by the name of his son-in-law, J. C. Brunner, 1653–1717.

Werdnig-Hoffmann paralysis (Werdnig, G., Austrian neurologist of the nineteenth century; Hoffmann, J., German neurologist, 1857–1919). A type of progressive muscular atrophy.

Wernicke's aphasia (Wernicke, K., German neurologist, 1848–1905). Cortical sensory aphasia. **W.'s centre:** the sensory speech centre on the posterior third of the gyrus temporalis superior. **W.'s disease:** acute haemorrhagic polioencephalitis. **W.'s encephalopathy:** acute haemorrhagic encephalitis. **W.'s fissure:** an inconstant fissure dividing the temporal and parietal lobes from the occipital lobe.

Werniking's commissure (Werniking, F. C. G., German anatomist, 1798–1835). A decussation of the superior cerebellar peduncles or brachia conjunctiva.

Werlhof's disease (Werlhof, P. G., German physician, 1699–1767). Purpura haemorrhagica.

Wertheim's operation (Wertheim, E., German gynaecologist, 1864–1920). An operation for carcinoma of the cervix of the uterus consisting of radical hysterectomy together with the removal of as much of the parametrial tissue as possible.

Westphal's contraction (Westphal, C. F. O., German psychiatrist, 1833–90). Reflex contraction of a muscle on approximating its ends. Seen in certain neurological conditions, paralysis agitans, etc. **W.'s nucleus:** the Edinger-Westphal nucleus; nucleus for accommodation in the 3rd cranial nerve origin. **W.'s sign:** absence of knee jerk in locomotor ataxia.

Wetzel's test (Wetzel, G., German anatomist, born 1871). For carbon monoxide in blood.

Wharton's duct (Wharton, T., English anatomist, 1614–73). The duct of the submaxillary (submandibular) salivary gland.

wheal. A blister produced by urticaria, the sting of a nettle, the stroke of a whip, an insect bite or other irritation.

wheat. The grain of the plant *Triticum vulgare.*

Wheatstone's bridge (Wheatstone, C., English physicist, 1802–75). An apparatus for determining electrical resistance.

Wheelhouse's operation (Wheelhouse, C. G., English surgeon, 1826–1909). External urethrotomy for impassable stricture.

wheeze. The sound heard in partially obstructed breathing, e.g. as in asthma.

whelk. A wheal or pimple.

whey. The liquid portion of milk separating from the curd in coagulation.

whiff, oral. A whiff heard in cases of aortic aneurysm on respiration with the mouth open.

whipworm. Trichuris trichiura, a harmless nematode parasite in the human intestine.

whirl. To revolve repeatedly and quickly. **W.-bone:** 1. The head of the femur. 2. The patella.

whisky. Spirit distilled from barley (usually) or other grains, such as rye.

whisper. Speech produced without vibration of the glottis.

white. 1. The opposite of black; having a colour produced by reflection of all the rays of the spectrum. 2. Any white substance, such as w. of an egg and w. of the eye (sclerotic).

white-spot disease. Syn. morphoea guttata.

Whitehead's operation (Whitehead, W., English surgeon, 1840–1913). 1. A form of haemorrhoidectomy. 2. Excision of the tongue.

whiteleg. Swollen oedematous leg due to thrombosis of the femoral vein. May occur after childbirth.

whites. A popular name for leucorrhoea.

whiting. A preparation of purified calcium carbonate.

whitlow. Inflammatory reaction on finger, especially around the nail; infection of a finger, usually leading to the formation of an abscess. See also paronychia.

Whitnall's tubercle (Whitnall, S. E., English anatomist, born 1876). On the malar (zygomatic) bone.

whole. 1. Hale, hearty; sound. 2. Entire.

whooping-cough. An infectious disease with catarrh of the respiratory tract and paroxysms of coughing ending in whooping respiration. Syn. pertussis.

Whytt's disease (Whytt, R., Scottish physician, 1714–66). Internal hydrocephalus. **W.'s reflex:** failure of the reaction of the pupil to light due to damage to the anterior corpora quadrigemina.

Wiart's duodenal notch. (Wiart, P., French anatomist, born 1870). A mark on the pancreas made by the duodenum.

Wichmann's asthma (Wichmann, J. E., German physician, 1740–1802). Laryngismus stridulus.

Widal's reaction (Widal, F., French physician, 1862–1929). An agglutination reaction for typhoid fever.

Widal-Abrami disease (Widal, F.; Abrami, P., French physician, born 1879). Acquired haemolytic jaundice.

Wiesel's paraganglion (Wiesel, J., Austrian physician, born 1876). The chromaffin body situated in the cardiac plexus of nerves.

Wilde's cone of light (Wilde, Sir W. R. W., Irish surgeon, 1815–76). An optical appearance on the external aspect of the membrana tympani; membrana tensa. **W.'s cords:** transverse striae of the corpus callosum. **W.'s incision:** incision behind the auricle exposing the mastoid process.

Wilkie's artery (Wilkie, Sir D. P. D., Scottish surgeon, 1882–1938). The supraduodenal artery.

Wilkinson's ointment (Wilkinson, J. H., English physician of the nineteenth century). Compound sulphur ointment.

Willan's lepra (Willan, R., English physician, 1757–1812). Psoriasis.

Willett's forceps (Willett, J. A., British obstetrician, died 1932). Forceps designed for applying scalp-traction in obstetrics.

Wil·lia. A genus of fungi, of which some species are parasitic in man.

Williams's tracheal tone (Williams, C. J. B., English physician, 1805–89). Dullness on percussion in the second intercostal space in a large pleural effusion.

Williamson's sign (Williamson, O. K., contemporary English physician). A sign sometimes seen in pneumothorax or pleural effusion in which there is diminished blood pressure in the leg compared with the arm of the same side.

willi·asis. Condition produced in the body by the Willia fungi.

Willis's circle (Willis, T., English anatomist, 1621–75). The arterial circle at the base of the brain; circulus arteriosus. **W.'s cords:** the dural trabeculae in the superior sagittal sinus; chorda transversalis.

willow. Any tree of the genus Salix.

Wilms's tumour (Wilms, M., German surgeon, 1867–1918). Embryoma of kidney.

Wilson's disease[1] (Wilson, S. A. K., British neurologist, 1878–1936). Progressive lenticular degeneration.

Wilson's disease[2] (Wilson, Sir W. J. E., English dermatologist, 1809–84). Exfoliative dermatitis.

Wilson's muscles (Wilson, J., English surgeon, 1765–1821). The muscular fibres surrounding the urethra above the 'triangular ligament' derived from the levator ani; levator prostatae.

Wimshurst machine (Wimshurst, J., English engineer, 1832–1903). A machine for producing static electricity.

windage. Internal contusion without external injury, caused by compression of air through the passage of a missile, shell, etc., near the body.

windpipe. Trachea, *q.v.*

wine. 1. The fermented juice of the grape. 2. A solution of medicinal substance in wine.

Winslow's foramen (Winslow, J. B., Danish anatomist, 1669–1760). The foramen epiploicum. **W.'s ligament:** posterior ligament of the knee. **W.'s pancreas:** the processus uncinatus of the pancreas. **W.'s stars:** capillary whorls in the choroid coat of the eye.

wintergreen. Methyl salicylate. It is useful applied externally in cases of lumbago, rheumatism, etc.

Winterhalter's ganglion (Winterhalter, Elizabeth H., German; work published in 1896). The aggregation of sympathetic nerve cells constituting the ovarian ganglion.

Wirsung's duct (Wirsung, J. G., German anatomist, died 1643). The ductus pancreaticus.

wisdom tooth. The last molar tooth on each side of each jaw.

witch hazel. Hamamelis, *q.v.*

withering. The shrivelling and atrophy of an organ.

Witzel's operation (Witzel, F. O., German surgeon, 1856–1925). A type of gastrostomy.

Woelfler's gland (Woelfler, A., Austrian surgeon, 1850–1917). The aortic gland; accessory thyroid gland.

Wolff's body (Wolff, K. F., German anatomist, 1733–94). The Wolffian body; ren primordialis, **W.'s duct:** the Wolffian duct; ureter primordialis.

Wolff's law (Wolff, J., German anatomist, 1836–1902). That all changes in the function of bones are attended by definite alterations in their internal structure.

Wolfring's glands (Wolfring, E. F. von, Polish ophthalmologist, 1832–1906). The glands of the conjunctiva.

wolfsbane. Aconite.

Wollaston's doublet (Wollaston, T. H., English physician, 1766–1828). A combination of lenses to correct chromatic aberration.

womb. The uterus, *q.v.*

wood. The fibrous substance between the pith and bark of trees. **W. alcohol:** methyl alcohol. **W. sugar:** xylose.

Wood's muscle (Wood, J., English surgeon, 1827–91). The abductor ossis metatarsi quinti pedis.

wool. The hair of sheep. **W. fat:** anhydrous lanolin.

Woolner's tubercle (Woolner, T., English sculptor, 1825–1892). The tubercle on the helix of the auricle, known as Darwin's tubercle. Woolner drew Darwin's attention to it, and it should therefore be called **W.'s** tubercle.

woolsorters' disease. Anthrax, *q.v.*

word blindness. Inability to understand written or printed words.

word deafness. Inability to understand spoken words.

word salad. A term introduced by Forel to describe the meaningless jumble of words uttered by katatonic patients.

worm (L. *vermis*, worm). 1. Any member of the class Vermes. 2. Any anatomical part resembling a worm.

Wormian bones (Worm, O., Danish physician, 1588–1654). Small bones in the cranial sutures; ossa suturalia.

wormwood. The leaves and tops of *Artemisia absinthium*. See absinthium.

Woulfe's bottle (Woulfe, P., English chemist, 1727–1803). Bottle used for passing gas through a liquid.

wound. A trauma caused by an injury. **W., perforating:** a wound penetrating into a cavity.

W.R. Abbreviation for Wassermann reaction.

Wright's method (Wright, Sir A. E., British bacteriologist, 1861–1947). A method of irrigating wounds with saline solution, first hypertonic then isotonic.

Wrisberg's cartilage (Wrisberg, H. A., German anatomist, 1739–1808). The cartilago cuneiformis laryngis. **W.'s ganglion:** the ganglion cardiacum magnum. **W.'s ligament:** the band attached to the posterior cruciate ligament of the knee joint. **W.'s nerve:** the nervus cutaneus internus minor brachii.

wrist. The carpus; the part connecting the forearm and the hand, consisting of eight carpal bones and their ligaments.

wristdrop. Inability to dorsiflex the wrist joint due to paralysis of the extensor muscles.

writer's cramp. An occupational neurosis characterized by painful spasms of the fingers when the patient attempts to write.

wryneck. Torticollis, *q.v.*

Wutz's valve (Wutz, J. B., German anatomist, of the 19th century). A valve said to exist between the lumen of the bladder and the canal of the urachus.

X

xanthae·matine (G. *xanthos*, yellow; *haima*, blood). A bitter, yellow substance obtained from haematin.

xanthae·mia (G. *xanthos*, yellow; *haima*, blood). The presence of yellow pigments in the blood.

xan·thaline (G. *xanthos*, yellow). An alkaloid from opium. Also called papaveraldine.

xan·thate (G. *xanthos*, yellow). A salt of xanthic acid. $S:C(OC_2H_5)SH$. A hypothetical acid whose salts are formed by treating alcoholic solutions of caustic alkalis with carbon disulphide.

xan·thein (G. *xanthos*, yellow). A yellow colouring matter.

xanthelas·ma (G. *xanthos*, yellow; *elasma*, a metal plate). Xanthoma, *q.v.*

xan·thene (G. *xanthos*, yellow). $(C_6H_4)_2$ (O)-CH_2. The compound from which xanthene dyes are derived.

xanthinū·ria (G. *xanthos*, yellow; *ouron*, urine). Excess of xanthine in the urine.

xanthochroi·a (G. *xanthos*, yellow; *khroia*, skin). Yellow-skinned.

xan·thochromat·ic (G. *xanthos*, yellow; *khrōma*, colour). Having a yellow colour.

xanthochrō·mia (G. *xanthos*, yellow; *khroma*, colour). A yellowish discoloration, e.g., of the skin.

xanthŏ·crōous (G. *xanthos*, yellow; *khroia*, skin). Yellow-skinned.

xanthocrē·atine (G. *xanthos*, yellow; *kreas*, flesh). A toxic leucomaine found in muscle. It occurs in yellow crystals and resembles creatinine.

xanthocyanop·sia, xanthocyă·nopsy (G. *xanthos*, yellow; *kuanos*, blue; *opsis*, vision). A defect of colour vision when there is ability to perceive yellow and blue but not red or green.

xanthocy̆·stine (G. *xanthos*, yellow; *kustis*, bladder). A nitrogenous substance found in tubercles from a corpse.

xanthoder·ma, xanthoder·mia (G. *xanthos*, yellow; *derma, skin*). A yellowish discoloration of the skin.

xanthodon·tous (G. *xanthos*, yellow; *odous*, tooth). Having yellow teeth.

xanthokyan·opy (G. *xanthos*, yellow; *kuanos*, blue; *ops*, eye). Xanthocyanopsy, *q.v.*

xanthŏ·ma (G. *xanthos*, yellow). Xanthelasma; a skin affection occurring as patches of nodules of a yellowish colour. On histological examination foam cells, or xanthoma cells, are found. They are large, pale cells with a foamy cytoplasm.

xanthomatŏ·sis (G. *xanthos*, yellow). Disease in which disturbance of lipoid metabolism results in accumulation of an excess of lipoids in the body. Tumours or deposits of high lipoid content are formed in various parts of the body. General bodily health may be adversely affected.

xanthŏ·matous (G. *xanthos*, yellow). Relating to or resembling xanthoma.

xan·thomyĕlō·ma (G. *xanthos*, yellow; *muelos*, marrow). Same as xanthosarcoma.

xanthŏ·pathy (G. *xanthos*, yellow; *pathos*, disease). Xanthoderma, *q.v.*

xan·thophane (G. *xanthos*, yellow; *phainein*, to show). A yellow pigment found in the retina.

xan·thophore (G. *xanthos*, yellow; *pherein*, to bear). A pigment cell found in cold-blooded animals. It contains granules of yellow-red pigment.

xan·thophyll. $C_{40}H_{56}O_2$, 3-3-dihydroxy-alpha-carotene, the yellow colouring matter found in plants. The same as lutein.

xanthopic·rine, xanthopic·rite (G. *xanthos*, yellow; *pikros*, sharp). Berberine; a yellowish pigment from the bark of *Xanthoxylum ceribaeum*.

xanthoprotē·ic (G. *xanthos*, yellow; *prōtos*, first). Derived from or concerning xanthoprotein.

xanthoprō·tein (G. *xanthos*, yellow; *prōtos*, first). A yellowish pigment obtained from proteins by heating these with nitric acid.

xanthop·sia (G. *xanthos*, yellow; *opsis*, vision). Yellow vision, a symptom of jaundice and also occurring in picric acid and santonin poisoning.

xanthrop·sin (G. *xanthos*, yellow; *opsis*, vision). Visual yellow; it is derived from the action of light on rhodopsin.

xanthopuc·cine (G. *xanthos*, yellow). An alkaloid obtained from *Hydrastis canadensis*.

xanthorrhoē·a (G. *xanthos*, yellow; *rhoia*, a flow). A purulent, yellowish discharge from the vagina.

xanthosarcō·ma (G. *xanthos*, yellow; *sarx*, flesh). So-called giant-celled sarcoma of fascial planes and tendon sheaths.

xan·thosine (G. *xanthos*, yellow). $C_{10}H_{12}O_6N_4$, a nucleoside which on hydrolysis gives xanthine and ribose.

xanthŏ·sis (G. *xanthos*, yellow). A yellow discoloration of the skin, seen e.g. in some cases of carcinoma.

xan·thous (G. *xanthos*, yellow). Yellow; yellow-skinned.

xanthū·ria (G. *xanthos*, yellow; *ouron*, urine). Xanthinuria, *q.v.*

x-chromosome. The sex of an organism is dependent on the presence of both members, or of only one member, of a particular pair of chromosomes, the x-chromosomes. The genetic constitution of females is xx. See also y-chromosome.

Xe. The symbol for Xenon.

xĕ·nia (G. hospitality). The appearance of an inherited, dominant factor in seeds during the process of cross-pollination.

xenoge·nesis (G. *xenos*, foreign; *genesis*, production). The generation of something different; the offspring varying in character and life-cycle from the parents. See also heterogenesis.

xenŏ·genous (G. *xenos*, foreign; *gennan*, to produce). Caused by a foreign body.

xenomē·nia (G. *xenos*, foreign; *mēniaia*, menses). Vicarious menstruation.

xĕ·non (G. *xenos*, foreign). A gaseous element found in air; atomic weight, 131·3. Symbol Xe.

xenopă·rasite (G. *xenos*, foreign; *parasitos*, a 'sponger'). A parasite derived from without an organism, which becomes pathogenic on account of lowered resistance of the host.

xenophō·bia (G. *xenos*, foreign; *phŏbos*, fear). Neurotic fear of strangers.

xenophō·nia (G. *xenos*, foreign; *phonē*, voice). Change of accent and intonation of voice.

xenophthal·mia (G. *xenos*, foreign; *ophthalmos*, eye). Conjunctivitis resulting from injury.

xeran·sis (G. a parching). The drying up or desiccation of, e.g., a drug.

xeran·tic (G. *xeros*, dry). Causing or producing dryness.

466

xerā·sis (G. *xēros*, dry). A morbid dryness of the hair with cessation of growth.

xē·rocollỹ·rium (G. *xēros*, dry; *kollurion*, a poultice). An eye salve.

xeroder·ma, xeroder·mia (G. *xēros*, dry; *derma*, skin). 1. Abnormal dryness of the skin. 2. A disease characterized by dryness and hardness of the skin and a fine, scaly desquamation. **X. pigmentosum:** Kaposi's disease, a rare and fatal disease of a neoplastic character.

xē·roform (G. *xēros*, dry; L. *formica*, ant). Bismuth-tribromphenol; used as an intestinal disinfectant.

xerō·ma (G. *xēros*, dry). Xerophthalmia, *q.v.*

xeromē·nia (G. *xēros*, dry; *meniaia*, menses). A condition characterized by bodily disturbances at the menstrual period but without the flow of blood.

xē·rŏnŏsus (G. *xēros*, dry; *nŏsos*, disease). Abnormal dryness of the skin.

xerophā·gia, xerŏ·phagy (G. *xēros*, dry; *phagein*, to eat). The eating of dry food.

xerophthal·mia, xerophthal·mus (G. *xēros*, dry; *ophthalmos*, eye). A dry and thickened state of the conjunctiva and cornea.

xerō·sis (G. *xēros*, dry). A condition of unnatural dryness, especially of the skin or the conjunctiva.

xerostō·ma, xerostō·mia (G. *xēros*, dry; *stoma*, mouth). Dryness of the mouth; sometimes part of the Sjögren syndrome.

xē·rotēs (G.). Dryness.

xerot·ic (G. *xēros*, dry). Marked by dryness.

xerotrip·sis (G. *xēros*, dry; *tribein*, to rub). Dry friction.

xiphicŏ·stal (G. *xiphos*, sword; L. *costa*, rib). Xiphocostal, *q.v.*

xiphister·nal. Relating to the xiphisternum.

xiphister·num (G. *xiphos*, sword; *sternon*, the breast). The metasternum or ensiform cartilage.

xiphocŏ·stal (G. *xiphos*, sword; L. *costa*, rib). Relating to the xiphoid cartilage and the ribs.

xiphŏ·dymus (G. *xiphos*, sword; *didumos*, twin). A double monster united at the pelvis and thorax and having usually two legs.

xiphodỹ·nia (G. *xiphos*, sword; *odunē*, pain). Pain in the ensiform cartilage.

xi·phoid (G. *xiphos*, sword; *eidos*, form). Sword-shaped; ensiform.

xiphoidī·tis (G. *xiphos*, sword). Inflammation of the xiphoid cartilage.

xiphŏ·pagus (G. *xiphos*, sword; *pagos*, fixed). A double monster united by the xiphoid cartilages or the epigastrium.

X-rays (Named thus by the discoverer, Wilhelm Roentgen, German physicist, 1845–1923). Invisible light-rays which penetrate most solids, show fractures, foreign substances, etc., within the body; they are also effective in the treatment of certain diseases. See also under ray.

xyloi·din (G. *xulon*, wood; *eidos*, form). A white inflammable substance resembling pyroxylin, formed by treating starch with nitric acid.

xỹ·lol (G. *xulon*, wood; L. *oleum*, oil). A mixture of about 70 per cent of *m*-dimethyl-benzene, 20 per cent of *p*-dimethyl-benzene and 10 per cent of *o*-dimethyl-benzene. Used in treating respiratory affections and dyspepsia, and as a clearing agent in histology.

xỹ·lose (G. *xulon*, wood). Wood sugar obtained from beechwood and jute. Occasionally found in the urine.

xys·ma (G. *xusma*, scrapings). A flocculent substance, like membrane, occurring in the stools of some patients with diarrhoea.

xỹ·ster (G. *xustēr*, a scraper). A surgeon's file.

xỹ·stus (G. *xustos*, scraped). Scraped lint.

Y

Y. Symbol for yttrium.

Y-angle. Angle formed by line joining the lambda and inion and a line joining the median anterior part of the spheno-occipital bones to the inion.

yard. 1. A measure of length, equal to three feet or thirty-six inches. 2. The penis.

yava-skin. Elephantiasis, *q.v.*

yawn. To gape; to open the mouth widely as an effect of fatigue.

yaws. A disease caused by *Treponema pertenue*. It is contagious and occurs in hot climates. It is characterized by the formation of raspberry-like excrescences on face, hands and feet and external genitals. These run together to form masses, or they may form pustules or ulcers.

Yb. The symbol for ytterbium.

y-chromosome. See also x-chromosome. In some organisms sex is not determined by the presence of both members or of only one member of the pair of x-chromosomes but by the presence of a pair of identical x-chromosomes or the presence of an x-chromosome and a smaller y-chromosome. The genetic constitution of males is xy.

yeast. Any one of the species of fungi of the genus Saccharomyces. Y., brewer's: cerevisiae fermentum (B.P.) produced by *Saccharomyces cerevisiae*. It is used as a stimulant and also as a poultice and deodorant to gangrenous ulcers.

yelk. Yolk, *q.v.*

yellow. One of the primary colours. Y. fever: an acute infectious disease of West Africa and Brazil. It is caused by a filtrable virus, disseminated by the mosquito *Aedes aegypti*. The disease is marked by high temperature, jaundice and other symptoms, and has a high rate of mortality.

Yemen ulcer. Aden boil; furunculus orientalis.

yer·ba (Sp. *yerba*, from L. *herba*, grass), A herb. Y. maté: Paraguay tea.

Yersin's serum (Yersin, A. J. E., Russian bacteriologist, 1863–1943). A serum used to combat plague.

y-ligament. The iliofemoral ligament, a thickened part of the anterior capsular ligament of the hip joint.

yoghurt. See yohourt.

yohim·bine. $C_{22}H_{30}O_4N_2$. An alkaloid obtained from *Corynanthe yohimbé* and used as an aphrodisiac.

yohourt. A preparation of curded milk, much used in the Balkan countries.

yoke-bone. The malar bone.

yolk. The nutritive part of an ovum; applied especially to the yellow portion of a bird's egg.

Young-Helmholtz theory (Young T., English physician, 1773–1829; Helmholtz, H. L. F., German physician and physicist, 1821–92). A theory of colour vision in which the physical stimuli are analysed peripherally into three fundamental types; these have three separate physiological " components " which act on counterparts, giving rise to nervous activities which are integrated centrally.

Young's ligament (Young, R. B., Scottish anatomist, 1858–1927). The trapezo-metacarpal ligament, between the second and third metacarpals and the trapezium.

Young's rule (Young, T., English physician, 1773–1829). A method for determining dosage of drugs in children. Divide the age in years by the age in years plus 12. This gives the fraction of adult dose which should be given to the child.

ytter·bium (Named from Ytterby, in Sweden). A rare metal having the symbol Yb. Its atomic weight is 173·04.

yt·trium (Named from Ytterby, in Sweden). A rare metallic element; symbol Y. Its atomic weight is 89.

Z

Zaglas's ligament. The ligament passing from the posterior superior iliac spine to the second part of the sacrum; the second iliotransverse ligament.

Zahn's lines (Zahn, F. W., German pathologist, 1845–1904). The ridges seen on the exposed surface of a thrombus. They are formed by the projecting edges of the lamellae of blood platelets.

Zambesi fever. A non-malarial fever which occurs in Kaffirs living in the Zambesi valley, S. Africa.

Zambesi ulcer. An ulcer found on leg or foot in natives of the Zambesi valley, S. Africa. Caused by larva of a dipterous fly, which penetrates subcutaneous tissues.

zană·lōin. Aloin from Zanzibar aloes.

Zang's space (Zang, C. B., German surgeon, 1772–1835). Between the two tendons of origin of the sternomastoid in the supraclavicular fossa.

zaran·than (Heb.). Abnormal hardening of the breast tissues.

Zaufahl's fold (Zaufahl, E., Bohemian otologist, 1833–1910). The plica salpingopharyngea.

Zea (G. *zea*, spelt, coarse wheat). A genus of grasses including maize.

ze·doary (Pers. *zadwar*). The aromatic rhizome of *Curcuma zedoaria*. It resembles ginger in odour and taste.

Zeiss's glands (Zeiss, E., German surgeon, 1807–68). The ciliary glands; sebaceous glands in the eyelids.

zeī·mus (G. *zea*, spelt, coarse wheat). A skin disease attributed to the overuse of maize in the diet.

Zeissl's membrane (Zeissl, M., Austrian dermatologist, 1853–1925). The stratum compactum of the subglandular layer of the gastric mucous membrane.

zeloty·pia (G. *zēlos*, rivalry; *tupos*, type). Morbid zeal in any undertaking or occupation.

Zenker's crystals (Zenker, F. A., German pathologist, 1825–1898). Same as Charcot-Leyden crystals. Z.'s **degeneration**: a necrosis and hyaline degeneration which occurs in striated muscle.

Zenker's solution (Zenker, K., German histologist, died 1894). A solution used in fixation of tissues. Corrosive mercuric chloride 6 parts, potassium bichromate 2·5 parts, sodium sulphate 1 part, water 100 parts.

ze·oscope (G. *zeein*, to boil; *skopein*, to view). An apparatus for estimating the alcoholic strength of a liquid by means of its boiling point.

zero (Ital. *zero*, nought). 1. Character denoting 'nil'. 2. The starting-point on a thermometer scale.

Ziehl-Neelsen method (Ziehl, F., German bacteriologist, 1857–1926; Neelsen, F. K. A., 1854–94). Stain for tubercle bacillus. Initially carbol-fuchsin is used and counter-staining is done with methylene blue.

Zimmermann's granules (Zimmermann, G. H. E., German physician, 1817–66). The blood platelets which had been described by Bizzozero three years previously.

zinc, zin·cum. A hard bluish-white metal, symbol Zn. Zinc compounds are toxic and, if ingested, may produce symptoms similar to those of lead poisoning but less severe. Many of the compounds, e.g., z. acetate, z. carbolate, z. iodide, z. oxide and z. sulphate are used therapeutically and as disinfectants.

zin·giber (G. *ziggiberis*, ginger). Ginger. The ginger used in medicine is the scraped and dried rhizome of *Zingiber officinale*, known in commerce as unbleached Jamaica ginger. Used as a carminative.

Zinn's central artery (Zinn, J. G., German anatomist. 1727–59). The central artery of the retina. Z.'s **circle**: the ring of arteries which lies in the sclera around the entry of the optic nerve. Z.'s **ligament**: the annulus tendineus; origin of ocular muscles. Z.'s **zonule**: the portion of hyaloid membrane adjacent to the margins of the lens.

Zinsser inconsistency (Zinsser, H., American bacteriologist, 1878–1940). The local and systemic symptoms of anaphylaxis fail to show quantitative relationship.

zirco·nium (Pers. *zargun*). A metallic element, symbol Zr., resembling titanium and silicon. Its atomic weight is 92 and it is obtained from zircon.

Zn. The symbol for Zinc.

zoăn·thropy (G. *zōon*, animal; *anthrōpos*, man). A type of insanity in which the patient believes that he has been changed into an animal.

zoē·trope (G. *zoe*, life; *trope*, a turning). See stroboscope.

zoiă·tria (G. *zōon*, animal; *iatros*, a physician). The science of veterinary surgery.

zo·ic (G. *zōon*, animal). Relating to animal life.

zo·ism (G. *zōon*, animal). Vitalism, *q.v.*

Zöllner's lines (Zöllner, F., German physicist, 1834–82). An optical illusion based on a constant error of judgment in the bidimensional perception of distance.

zona (G. *zonē*, a girdle). 1. A. girdle. 2. Herpes zoster. Z. **arcuata**: the area enclosed by the arches of Corti. Z. **orbicularis**: the rim of thickened capsular ligament which encircles the acetabulum. Z. **pellucida**: see oolemma.

zonaesthe·sia (G. *zonē*, a girdle; *aisthēsis*, feeling). A sensation of constriction, as of a belt or girdle being drawn round a part or an area.

zo·nal (G. *zōnē*, a girdle). Relating to or resembling a zone.

zone (G. *zōnē*, a girdle). See zona.

zo·nula (G. *zōnē*, a girdle). A small zone. Z. **ciliaris**: syn. for Zinn's zonules, the ring-shaped series of fibres which extend from the ciliary body to the periphery of the lens, and form the suspensory ligament of the lens.

zo·nular. Relating to a zonule. Z. **cataract**: a cataract disposed in alternate layers. Z. **ligament**: zonule of Zinn. Z. **space**: syn. for canal of Petit, space intercommunicating between the fibres of the suspensory ligament of the lens.

zo·nule (L. *zonula*, dim. of *zona*, from G. *zōnē*, a girdle). A little zone or band. Z. **of Zinn**: see under Zinn.

zonuli·tis (L. *zonula*, little girdle). Inflammation of the zonule of Zinn.

zoöĕră·stia (G. *zōon*, animal; *erastēs*, lover). Sexual relations with an animal.

zoögă·mete (G. *zōon*, animal; *gamein*, to marry). In biology, a gamete having the power of locomotion.

zoö·gamy (G. *zōon*, animal; *gamos*, marriage). The sexual generation of animals, mating.

zoögĕ·nesis (G. *zōon*, animal; *genesis*, production). The generation of animal forms.

zoö·genous (G. *zōon*, animal; *gennan*, to produce). Viviparous.

zŏŏ·geny (G. *zōon*, animal; *gennan*, to produce). Zoogenesis, *q.v.*

zŏŏgloe·a (G. *zōon*, animal; *gloios*, oil-lees). A developmental stage of certain bacteria at which they are embedded in a gelatinous matrix.

zŏŏgŏ·nia (G. *zōon*, animal; *gonē*, offspring). Viviparous generation.

zŏŏ·gonous (G. *zōon*, animal; *gonē*, offspring). Viviparous.

zŏ·oid (G. *zōon*, animal; *eidos*, form). 1. Resembling an animal. 2. A zoophyte. 3. An animal cell capable of independent life or movement.

zŏŏlag·nia (G. *zōon*, animal; *lagneia*, lust). Sexual interest in and attraction to animals.

zŏŏ·logy (G. *zōon*, animal; *logos*, a treatise). The science of animal life.

zŏŏmag·netism (G. *zoon*, animal; *Magnesia*, a city in Asia Minor, whence lodestone was first obtained by the Romans). Animal magnetism.

zŏ·onite (G. *zōon*, animal). A cerebrospinal metamere.

zŏŏ·nomy (G. *zōon*, animal; *nomos*, law). The laws governing animal life; syn. zoobiology.

zŏŏsper·mia (G. *zōin*, animal; *sperma*, seed). Indicating the presence of live and active spermatozoa in semen.

zŏŏ·phagous (G. *zōon*, animal; *phagein*, to eat). Living on animal food.

zŏŏ·philism (G. *zōon*, animal; *philein*, to love). 1. The love of animals. 2. Opposition to vivisection.

zŏŏphŏ·bia (G. *zōon*, animal; *phobos*, fear). Morbid fear of animals.

zŏ·ŏphysiŏ·logy (G. *zōon*, animal; *phusis*, nature; *logos*, discourse). Animal physiology.

zŏ·ophyte (G. *zōon*, animal; *phuton*, a plant). 1. A plant-like animal. 2. A member of the lower invertebrates.

zŏ·ŏsperm (G. *zōon*, animal; *sperma*, seed). A spermatozoon.

zŏ·ŏspore (G. *zōon*, animal; *sporos*, seed). A ciliated motile spore.

zŏŏ·sterol (G. *zōon*, animal; *stĕrĕos*, solid). A sterol of animal origin.

zŏŏ·tomy (G. *zōon*, animal; *tomē*, section). The dissection of animals.

zŏŏtox·in (G. *zōon*, animal; *toxikon*, poison). Any poison or venom of animal origin.

zŏ·ster (G., a girdle). Syn. herpes zoster, zona; shingles; an acute, inflammatory, painful disease, showing grouped cutaneous vesicles along the course of the cutaneous nerves, generally the cutaneous branches of the intercostal nerves. **Z. auricularis:** a type of z. affecting the ear. **Z. brachialis:** a type affecting the arm. **Z. ophthalmicus:** herpes affecting the area supplied by the ophthalmic division of the trigeminal nerve.

zostĕ·riform (G. *zōstĕr*, girdle; L. *forma*, shape). Resembling herpes zoster.

Zr. The symbol for Zirconium.

Zuckerkandl's bodies (Zuckerkandl, E., Austrian anatomist, 1849–1910). The aberrant masses of adrenal tissue situated at the side of the aorta; aortic paraganglia. **Z.'s fascia:** the retrorenal fascia.

zwittĕ·rion (Ger. *zwei*, two). Name given to an ion which carries both positive and negative charges.

zy·gal (G. *zugon*, yoke). Yoked or having the form of a yoke.

zygapŏ·physis (G. *zugon*, yoke; *apo*, from; *phusis*, nature). The articular process of a vertebra.

zȳ·gion (G. *zugon*, yoke). A craniometric point at each end of the zygomatic diameter.

zygodac·tyly (G. *zugon*, yoke; *daktulos*, finger). Synonymous with syndactyly, *q.v.*

zȳ·gŏite (G. *zugon*, yoke). The organism formed by the process of zygosis.

zy·golabīā·lis (G. *zugon*, yoke; L. *labium*, lip). Another name for zygomaticus minor muscle.

zygŏ·ma (G. *zugōma*, a bolt). 1. The arch formed by the union of the zygomatic process of the temporal bone and the malar bone. 2. The malar bone.

zygomat·ic (G. *zugōma*, a bolt). Relating to the zygoma. **Z. arch:** the zygoma.

zygomă·tico-auriculă·ric (G. *zugoma*, a bolt; L. *auricula*, dim. of *auris*, ear). Relating to the zygoma and the ear.

zygomă·tico-auriculă·ris (G. *zugōma*, a bolt; L. *auricula*, dim. of *auris*, ear). The attrahens aurem muscle.

zygomă·ticofă·cial (G. *zugoma*, a bolt; L. *facies*, the face). Relating to both the zygoma and the face. **Z. canal:** canal in zygoma through which the zygomaticofacial nerve passes. **Z. foramen:** superficial opening of z. canal. **Z. nerve:** terminal branch of maxillary division of trigeminal nerve, distributed to skin of cheek.

zygomă·ticofron·tal suture (G. *zugoma*, bolt; L. *frons*, forehead). Suture between frontal process of zygomatic and zygomatic process of frontal bones, found in lateral wall of orbit.

zygomă·ticomax·illary suture (G. *zugoma*, bolt; L. *maxilla*, jaw). Suture between zygoma and maxilla, found in inferior wall of orbit.

zygomă·ticotem·poral canal (G. *zugoma*, bolt; L. *tempora*, temples). Canal in zygoma through which passes the zygomaticotemporal nerve. **Z. foramen:** superficial opening of z. canal. **Z. nerve:** terminal branch of the maxillary division of trigeminal nerve, distributed to skin of temple. **Z. suture:** suture between zygomatic process of temporal and temporal process of zygomatic bones.

zygomă·ticus major (G. *zugoma*, bolt; L. *major*, greater). Muscle arising from malar bone anterior to the zygomatic suture and inserted into the angle of the mouth. Draws upper lip upward and outward.

zygomă·ticus minor (G. *zugoma*, bolt; L. *minor*, lesser). Muscle arising from malar bone behind the maxillary suture and inserted into orbicularis oris and levator labii superioris. Draws upper lip backward, upward and outward.

zȳ·gon (G. *zugon*, yoke). The bar joining the two pairs of branches of a zygal fissure.

zȳ·goneure (G. *zugon*, yoke; *neuron*, nerve). A nerve-cell joining other nerve-cells.

zygō·sis (G. *zugōsis*, a balancing). Sexual fusion of two identical unicellular organisms.

zȳ·gosperm (G. *zugon*, yoke; *sperma*, seed). Zygospore *q.v.*

zȳ·gosphere (G. *zugon*, yoke; *sphaira*, sphere). One of the germ cells which unites with a similar cell to form a zygospore.

zȳ·gospore (G. *zugon*, yoke; *sporos*, seed). A spore formed by the fusion of two identical germ cells which show no sexual differentiation.

zȳ·gostyle (G. *zugon*, yoke; *stŭlos*, a pillar). The final caudal vertebra.

zȳ·gote (G. *zugon*, yoke). The cell resulting from the union of two gametes in sexual reproduction.

zygot·ic (G. *zugon*, yoke). Relating to a zygote.

zȳ·lonite (G. *xulon*, timber). A substance closely resembling celluloid.

zȳ·mad (G. *zumĕ*, leaven). The organism causing a zymotic or infectious disease.

zȳ·mase (G. *zumē*, leaven). 1. An enzyme. 2. The active principle of yeast which brings about the process of alcoholic fermentation.

zymā·sis (G. *zumē*, ferment). The extraction of the active principle of yeast by hydraulic pressure.

zyme (G. *zumē*, ferment). A ferment.

zȳ·mic (G. *zumē*, ferment). Of or relating to ferments.

zȳ·mocyte (G. *zumē*, leaven; *kutos*, a container). Any organism causing fermentation.

zȳ·mogen (G. *zumē*, ferment; *gennan*, to produce). 1. Any substance that may give rise to an enzyme. 2. A bacterium which acts as an enzyme in setting up fermentation.

zymogĕ·nic (G. *zumē*, ferment; *gennan*, to produce). 1. Causing fermentation. 2. Relating to or producing a zymogen.

zȳ·moid (G. *zumē*, ferment; *eidos*, form). 1. A toxin from putrid tissues. 2. Resembling an organized ferment.

zymŏ·logy (G. *zumē*, ferment; *logos*, treatise). The science of fermentation.

zymŏ·lysis (G. *zumē*, ferment; *lusis*, dissolution). Fermentation produced by an organized ferment.

zymoly·tic (G. *zumē*, ferment; *luein*, to dissolve). Caused by or relating to zymolysis.

Zymonē·ma. A genus of fungi of the family Eramascaceae.

zȳ·mophore (G. *zumē*, ferment; *pherein*, to bear). That part of the uniceptor, *q.v.*, which carries the lytic ferment.

zymŏ·phorous (G. *zumē*, ferment; *pherein*, to bear). Relating to the zymophore or to that part of an enzyme which is active.

zȳ·mophyte (G. *zumē*, ferment; *phuton*, plant). A micro-organism which causes fermentation.

zȳ·mose (G. *zumē*, ferment). Invertin, *q.v.*

zymosĭ·meter (G. *zumoein*, to leaven; *metron*, measure). An instrument used to determine the extent of a fermentation process.

zymŏ·sis (G. *zumoein*, to leaven). 1. The process of fermentation. 2. The development of zymotic disease 3. Any infectious or contagious disease.

zymot·ic (G. *zumoein*, to leaven). 1. Relating to fermentative changes produced by a zyme. 2. A general term for infective and contagious diseases.

PUBLISHER'S NOTE

THIS Supplement to *The Faber Medical Dictionary* is the work of Dr. J. G. Bate who undertook some of the proof reading of the dictionary before it appeared in 1953. Over the last twelve years Dr. Bate has collected much new material to keep the dictionary up-to-date.

Note: when further definitions of a word which appeared in the original dictionary are given in the Supplement, (add) *appears immediately after the entry in the Supplement.*

A

---

acan·tholy·sis (G. *akantha*, thorn; *luein*, to loose). Degeneration of the intercellular bridges between squamous epithelial cells, leading to formation of intra-epithelial clefts and bullae.

acan·throcyte (G. *akantha*, thorn; *kutos*, cell). Misshapen form of erythrocyte, characterized by thorny surface projections.

acan·throcytosis. Familial syndrome in which the presence of acanthrocytes in the blood is accompanied in childhood by steatorrhoea and in adult life by ataxic neuropathy.

accelerator, linear. Machine used for supervoltage X-ray therapy in which pulses of electrons receive, as a result of passage through devices known as waveguides, an increase of energy equivalent to several million volts.

accel·erin. Convertin, *q.v.*

a·ceprō·mazine măl·eate. $C_{23}H_{26}N_2O_5S$. 2-acetyl-10-(3-dimethylaminopropyl) phenothiazine hydrogen maleate. Drug with similar uses to, but less toxic than, chlorpromazine, *q.v.*

acĕt·azōl·amide. $C_4H_6O_3N_4S_2$. 5-acetamido-1,3,4-thiadiazole-2-sulphonamide. Diuretic given orally for the relief of congestive heart failure.

acĕt·omenaph·thone. $C_{15}H_{14}O_4$. 1,4-diacetoxy-2-methylnaphthalene. Drug used for the prevention of haemorrhagic disease of the newborn.

acĕt·rizo·ic acid. $C_9H_6I_3NO_3$. 3-acetamido-2,4,6-triiodobenzoic acid. Substance used (as sodium salt) as radiographic contrast medium for pyelography and angiography.

Achromycin. Tetracycline, *q.v.*

ă·crokeratō·sis verruciform·is. (G. *akros*, extreme; *keras*, horn; L. *verruca*, wart; *forma*, shape). Presence of large numbers of warty papules on the skin of hands and feet.

Addis count (Addis, T., American physician, born 1881). Count of the number of cells and casts passed in twelve hours' urine by patients with renal disease; a guide to progress and prognosis.

ă·denovī·rus (G. *aden*, gland; L. *virus*, poison). Member of a group of viruses found in tonsils and adenoids of normal children and isolated from throats of patients with febrile catarrh, virus pneumonia and pharyngo-conjunctival fever.

aero·oti·tis. Inflammation of the middle ear in airmen, causing pain, deafness and tinnitus, due to otitic barotrauma, *q.v.*

āer·ospor·in. Polymyxin, *q.v.*

a·ga·mmaglob·ulinaē·mia. More correctly, hypogammaglobulinaemia, *q.v.*

a·gene. Nitrogen trichloride, a gas formerly used as an improver for flour, now discontinued owing to animal toxicity.

akiyami. Leptospiral infection (harvest sickness) occurring in Japan.

Albert's stain (Albert, H., American physician, 1878–1930). Microscopic stain for demonstrating granular structure of diphtheria bacillus.

al·doster·one. 11:21-dihydroxy-3:20 dioxo-4-pregnen-18-al. Adrenal cortical hormone used as substitution therapy to promote sodium retention in Addison's disease.

aldo·ster·onism. Syndrome resulting from excess of aldosterone in the blood, due to adrenal cortical tumour. Interference with sodium, potassium and water transport leads to muscular weakness, tetany, polydipsia and polyuria, and hypertension.

alkalescens-dispar organisms. Non-pathogenic members of the family *Enterobacteriaceae*, serologically related to *Esch. coli*.

all·ēle. Allelomorph, *q.v.*

allox·an. Oxidation product of uric acid. Injection into the body destroys the islets of Langerhans, resulting in diabetes.

Alport's syndrome (Alport, A. C., S. African physician, 1880–1959). Familial deafness associated with albuminuria and chronic nephritis, fatal in early life.

Alzheimer's disease (Alzheimer, A., German neurologist, 1864–1913). Presenile cerebral sclerosis; symptoms of senile dementia appearing in persons of middle-age.

amē·thocai·ne. $C_{15}H_{24}N_2O_2HCl$.2-dimethylamino-ethyl-4-n-butylaminobenzoate. A local anaesthetic.

ami·no-acidu·ria. Urinary excretion of abnormal amino-acids, or of normal amino-acids in excessive amounts.

amin·acrine. $C_{13}H_{11}ClN_2,H_2O$. 9-aminoacridine hydrochloride monohydrate. Use and action as for proflavine sulphate, *q.v.*

aminō·phylline. $(C_7H_8O_2N_4)_2C_2H_4(NH_2)_22H_2O$. Combination of ethylenediamine with theophylline, used as a diuretic and as an antispasmodic in asthma.

am·nio-chorioni·tis (G. *amnion*, caul; *khorion*, membrane). Inflammation of the placenta.

amodi·aquine. $C_{20}H_{22}ClN_3O,2HCl,2H_2O$.7-chloro-4-(3-diethylamino-methyl-4-hydroxyanilino) quinoline hydrochloride. An antimalarial drug.

amphoter·icin. One of a group of antibiotics derived from *streptomyces nodosus*.

ampicill·in. Benzylpenicillin, *q.v.*, modified by substitution of an amino group in the molecule. Antibiotic orally active against the typhoid group as well as against Gram-positive organisms.

amy·lobar·bitone. $CO(NH.CO)_2C(C_2H_5)(CH_2CH_2CH(CH_3)_2)$. 5-isoamyl-5 ethylbarbituric acid. A hypnotic drug.

a·myopla·sia congen·ita (G. *a-*, neg.; *mus*, muscle; *plassein*, to form). Congenital muscular dystrophy leading to rigidity of joints.

anabol·ic steroids. Steroid substances related to testosterone, *q.v.*, which encourage anabolism and promote protein synthesis.

an·albuminaē·mia (G. *an*, neg.; albumin; G., *haima*, blood). Absence of albumin from the blood proteins.

anamnes·tic reaction (G. *anamnesis*, a recalling). Development of agglutinins against some specific infection (previously invoked by infection or immunization) by infection with a different organism.

an·gioten·sin. Angiotonin, *q.v.*

an·gioto·nin (G. *aggeion*, vessel; *tonos*, tone). Substance which induces hypertension when liberated from plasma by an enzyme, renin, produced by kidneys whose blood supply is partially interrupted.

anōv·ulatory cycle. Apparently normal menstrual cycle occurring unaccompanied by ovulation.

Antabuse. Disulfiram, *q.v.*

antazō·line hydrochloride. $C_{17}H_{19}N_3HCl$. 2-N-benzyl-anilinomethyliminazoline. An antihistamine drug.

antibody, blocking. Type of antibody which inhibits the effect of another antibody, *in vitro*, without being able to produce the effect by itself.

antibody, Forssman (Forssman, J., Swedish pathologist, born 1868). Antibody specific for an antigen unrelated to that which provides the immunizing stimulus; e.g. the antibody haemolytic to sheep cells produced in rabbits by the injection of horse serum.

antibody, incomplete. Antibody which will not, by itself, form a precipitate *in vitro* with its corresponding antigen.

antihaemophilic globulin (abbreviation A.H.G.). Member of the globulin fraction of the plasma proteins, deficiency of which forms the basis of haemophilia.

an·tistreptoly·sin O (abbreviation A.S.O.). Antibody to streptococcal toxin found in the blood of patients after streptococcal infections; especially but not exclusively in rheumatic fever.

apoferr·itin. A protein which combines with ferric hydroxide phosphate to form ferritin, *q.v.*

arbor viruses. Abbreviation for arthropod-borne viruses, including those of, e.g., equine encephalomyelitis, Japanese B. encephalitis, yellow fever, dengue, Rift Valley and sandfly fevers.

Arizona organisms. Group of members of genus *Enterobacteriaceae* closely allied to *Salmonella*, and producing similar infections.

Arnold-Chiari malformation (Arnold, J., 1835–1915, Chiari, H., 1851–1916, German pathologists). Herniation of cerebellum through foramen magnum, with elongation of medulla oblongata, in association with spina bifida.

Arthus phenomenon (Arthus, N. M., French bacteriologist, 1862–1945). Tissue necrosis following repeated injections of an antigen, e.g., in anti-rabies vaccination.

Ascoli test (Ascoli, A., Italian serologist, born 1877). Serological precipitation test for detection of anthrax infection in diseased carcases.

Auer bodies (Auer, J., U.S. physiologist, 1875–1948). Blue-staining granules seen in myeloblasts in leukaemia.

auto-immune disease. Group of diseases, including Hashimoto's disease, disseminated lupus erythematosus, rheumatoid arthritis, believed to be due to tissue destruction by antibodies produced within the body itself.

azu·resin. An ion-exchange resin (see Ion-exchange) used for the detection of free hydrochloric acid in the stomach without recourse to the passage of a tube.

B

bar·otrau·ma, otitic (G. *baros*, weight; *trauma*, a wound). Damage to the middle-ear caused by sudden changes in atmospheric pressure, such as may occur in flying.

barrier, blood-brain. Hypothetical obstacle to the passage of certain substances, esp. drugs, from the blood into the cerebro-spinal fluid.

barrier, placental. Layer of placental epithelium which separates maternal from foetal blood.

barrier nursing. Nursing of infectious patients in open wards without recourse to physical isolation.

ba·thymyco·sis (G. *bathus*, deep; *mukes*, mushroom). Any deep-seated fungus infection.

Behçet's syndrome (Behçet, H., Turkish dermatologist, 1889–1948). Virus infection causing ulceration of the mouth and genitalia, with iridocyclitis, sometimes with fatal involvement of the nervous system.

bejel. Non-venereal spirochaetal skin disease found in Arabs of the Euphrates region.

bem·egride. $C_8H_{13}NO_2$. β-ethyl-β-methylglutarimide. Barbiturate antagonist used for the treatment of barbiturate poisoning.

ben·droflu·azide. $C_{15}H_{14}F_3N_3O_4S$. 3-benzyl-3,4-dihydro-6-trifluoromethylbenzo-1,2,4-thiadiazine-7-sulphonamide-1,1-dioxide. A diuretic drug.

benĕ·thamine penicillin. $C_{15}H_{17}N,C_{16}H_{18}N_2O_4S$. N-benzylphenethylamine salt of benzyl penicillin. A slow-acting penicillin, of which a single dose maintains an effective blood level over 3 to 4 days.

ben·zathine penicillin. $C_{16}H_{20}N_2(C_{16}H_{18}N_2O_4S)_2$. Dibenzylpenicillin salt of NN'-dibenzylethylenediamine. A slow-acting penicillin for long-continued prophylaxis against infections.

benzhex·ol. $C_{20}H_{31}ON$. 1-cyclohexyl-1-phenyl-3-piperidino-1-propanol. Drug used for the relief of muscular rigidity in Parkinsonism.

benzthi·azide. $C_{15}H_{14}ClN_3O_4S_3$. 3-benzylthiomethyl-6-chloro-7-sulphamoyl-2H-benzo-1,2,4-thiadiazine-1,1-dioxide. A non-mercurial diuretic.

ben·ztropine mĕ·thanesul·phonate. $C_{21}H_{25}NO,CH_3SO_3H$. Methanesulphonate of 3-diphenylmethoxytropane. Sympathetic antagonist used in Parkinsonism.

ben·zyl penicillin. $C_{16}H_{17}N_2NaO_4S$, or $C_{16}H_{17}KN_2O_4S$. Sodium or potassium salt of 6-phenylacetamidopenicillanic acid. A penicillin ester for administration by intramuscular injection. Syn. penicillin G.

bephĕ·nium hydrox·ynaph·thoate. $C_{28}H_{29}NO_4$. Benzyldimethyl (2-phenoxyethyl) ammonium-3-hydroxynaphthalene-2-carboxylate. An anthelmintic effective esp. against hookworm and roundworm.

Berger rhythm (Berger, H., German neurologist, 1873–1941). The normal wave-form produced by action currents from the cerebral cortex, as observed by electro-encephalography, *q.v.*

bery·llio·sis. Pneumonic condition resulting from the inhalation (usually in industrial processes) of beryllium oxide particles.

bē·ta glŏb·ulin. One of the fractions of the globulin component of the blood proteins.

bē·ta mĕth·asone. $C_{22}H_{29}FO_5$. 9α-fluoro-16β-methylprednisolone. A highly potent chemical variant of cortisone.

bē·tatron. Supervoltage X-ray therapy machine in which electrons are given extreme energy by means of acceleration along a circular path in the field of an electromagnet fed with alternating current.

Bethesda-Ballerup organisms (names of localities in which first isolated). Doubtfully pathogenic members of family *Enterobacteriaceae*, allied to *Salmonella*.

B.H.C. Gamma benzene hexachloride, *q.v.*

bī·alam·icol hydrochloride. $C_{28}H_{42}Cl_2N_2O_2$. 3-3'-diallyl-5,5-di(diethylaminomethyl)4-4'-dihydroxybiphenyl dihydrochloride. Anti-amoebic drug, used as an alternative to emetine, *q.v.*

Bielschowsky-Jansky disease (Bielschowsky, M., German pathologist, 1869–1940; Jansky, I., Czech. physician, 1873–1921). Late infantile form of amaurotic family idiocy. (See idiocy.)

bi·otin. Vitamin of the B complex, found especially in liver and yeast. Deficiency leads to dermatitis and muscular weakness.

bisă·codyl. $C_{22}H_{19}NO_4$. 2-(4,4'-diacetoxydiphenylmethyl)pyridine. A laxative acting on the large intestine.

blue-dome cyst. Cyst appearing in female breast, usually at age 40 to 50, having a bluish colour on the surface. Benign, and associated with fibrous overgrowth of surrounding stroma.

Boeck and Drbohlav's medium (Boeck, W. C.; Drbohlav, J., contemp. American biologists). Culture medium for the growth of pathogenic amoebae.

Bollinger bodies (Bollinger, O. von, German pathologist, 1843–1909). Large inclusion bodies found in cells infected by fowl-pox and molluscum contagiosum viruses.

Bordet-Gengou bacillus. Haemophilus pertussis, *q.v.*

Bordet-Gengou medium (Bordet, J., 1870–1961; Gengou, O., born 1875, Belgian bacteriologists). Culture medium rich in blood for the growth of haemophilus pertussis.

Bordetella (Bordet, J., Belgian bacteriologist, 1870–1961). Generic name for certain respiratory pathogens of *Brucella* family, including *bronchiseptica, parapertussis*.

Bouin's fluid (Bouin, P., French anatomist, born 1870). Histological fixative containing picric acid, acetic acid and formalin.

Bowen's disease (Bowen, J. T., American dermatologist, 1857–1941). Intra-epithelial carcinoma, i.e. carcinoma confined to the natural limits of the epithelium in which it occurs.

Brenner tumour (Brenner, F., German pathologist, born 1887). Fibromatous ovarian tumour containing epithelial cell-nests. Usually benign.

bretÿ·lium tō·sylate. $C_{18}H_{24}O_3NSBr$. (o-bromobenzyl) ethyldimethylammonium tosylate. Hypotensive drug which acts by selective blocking action on adrenergic nerves.

Brewer's medium (Brewer, J. H., contemp. American bacteriologist). Culture medium containing sodium thioglycollate for growth of anaerobic organisms in open vessels.

Brill's disease (Brill, N. E., American physician, 1860–1925). Typhus fever appearing after a long latent period following the original infection.

Brill-Symmers disease (Brill, N. E., American physician, 1860–1925; Symmers, D., American pathologist, born 1879). Chronic disease characterized by proliferation of reticulo-endothelial cells usually in spleen and lymph glands.

Broders' classification (Broders, A. C., American pathologist, born 1885). System for classifying malignant tumours in degrees of malignancy as shown by the extent to which the cells composing them are differentiated.

Browne's splints (Browne, Sir Denis, British paediatric surgeon, born 1892). Metal splints with or without boots attached for the correction of talipes equinovarus.

Brunhilde strain. Type I strain of human epidemic poliomyelitis virus (isolated from chimpanzee of that name).

Budd-Chiari syndrome (Budd, G., 1808–82, British physician; Chiari, H., German pathologist, 1851–1916). Thrombosis of hepatic veins leading to cirrhosis of the liver.

Buerger-Grutz disease. See Hyperlipaemia, idiopathic.

bulbus cordis. Segment of the tubular embryonic heart which develops into the aortic and pulmonary valves, part of the right ventricle, ascending aorta and pulmonary artery.

burr cells. Erythrocytes showing spiny projections round the edge; sometimes seen in haemolytic anaemia.

bū·sul·phan. $C_6H_{14}O_6S_2$. Tetramethylene dimethanesulphonate. Cytotoxic agent for treatment of malignant disease, esp. myeloid leukaemia.

bū·tobar·bitone. $C_{10}H_{16}O_3N_2$. 5-n-butyl-5-ethylbarbituric acid. Barbiturate drug used as a hypnotic and as premedication for general anaesthesia.

C

Caffey's disease (Caffey, J., contemp. American radiologist). Hyperostosis, infantile cortical, *q.v.*

calcă·neo-val·gus (L. *calcaneus*, heel-bone; *valgus*, splayed). Talipes, *q.v.*

Caldwell-Luc operation (Caldwell, G. W., American surgeon, 1834–1918; Luc, H., French surgeon, 1855–1925). Opening of the maxillary antrum through an incision in the gingivo-labial fold.

Call-Exner bodies (Call, F. von, Austrian physician, 1844–1917; Exner, S., Austrian physiologist, 1846–1926). Areas of cystic degeneration surrounded by granulosa cells, seen in the mature Graafian follicle.

Candida. Genus of fungi, of which the species *albicans* is pathogenic. See moniliasis.

caram·iphen hydrochloride. $C_{18}H_{27}NO_2HCl$. Hydrochloride of 2-diethylaminoethyl-1-phenylcyclopentane-1-carboxylate. Parasympathetic antagonist for treatment of Parkinsonism.

carbĭm·azole. $C_7H_{10}O_2N_2S$. 3-ethyl-3-methyl-2-thio-4-imidazoline-1-carboxylate. Drug for the treatment of thyrotoxicosis.

carcinoma in situ. Non-invasive form of squamous-celled carcinoma. Syn. intra-epithelial carcinoma.

car·diolĭpin. Extract of beef heart used as an artificial antigen in serological tests for syphilis.

cat·echolă·mine. Term applied to the mixture of adrenaline and nor-adrenaline produced by the adrenal medulla.

cat-scratch disease. Febrile illness, probably of viral origin, occurring as a sequel to a bite or scratch by a cat.

ceru·loplas·min (L. *caeruleus*, sky-blue; G. *plasma*, formed). Copper-containing protein in plasma,

*

deficiency of which is the basis of Wilson's disease[1], *q.v.*

cĕ·tomac·rogol. Mixture of ethers prepared from cetyl and cetostearyl alcohol, used in pharmacy as an emulsifying agent.

cĕ·tostear·yl alcohol. Mixture of cetyl and stearyl alcohols, used as an emulsifying agent in the preparation of ointments.

cĕt·rimide. See C.T.A.B.

Chediak anomaly (Chediak, A., contemp. S. American physician). Nuclear anomalies of leucocytes with azurophil granules in the cytoplasm. Associated with a fatal form of granulocytopenia.

chela·ting agent (G. *kele*, a claw). Compound which can attach itself to a metallic atom to form a ring structure. In metallic poisoning such toxic substances so treated may be rendered harmless.

chini·ofon. $C_9H_5INNaO_4S$. Sodium-8-hydroxy-7-iodo-quinoline-5-sulphonate. An amoebicide, given orally or by enema for the treatment of dysentery due to *E. histolytica.*

Chi-square test. Statistical test to determine whether a series of values differs significantly (i.e. to a greater degree than by chance) among themselves or from a series of values expected on some hypothetical basis.

chloram·bucil. $C_{14}H_{19}Cl_2NO_2$. γ-*p*-di-(2-chloroethyl) amino-phenylbutyric acid. Cytotoxic substance resembling nitrogen mustard for oral treatment of, esp., lymphatic leukaemia and Hodgkin's disease.

chlorcy·clizine hydrochloride. $C_{18}H_{21}N_2Cl,HCl$. Hydrochloride of 1-(*p*-chlorobenzhydryl)-4-methylpiperazine. An antihistamine drug.

chlor·diazepox·ide hydrochloride. $C_{16}H_{14}ON_3Cl,HCl$. 7-chloro-2-methylamino-5-phenyl-3*H*-benzo-1, 4-diazepine-4-oxide hydrochloride. Sedative and muscle-relaxant drug used in the treatment of neurotic anxiety.

chlorhex·idine. $C_{22}H_{32}Cl_4N_{10}$. 1: 6-di(4'-chlorophenyldiguanido)-hexane. Anti-bacterial agent used for skin disinfection, esp. of the hands.

chlor·ocrĕs·ol. C_7H_7ClO. 2-chloro-5-hydroxytoluene. Antiseptic substance which is the principal ingredient of various proprietary germicides.

chlor·oquine phosphate. $C_{18}H_{26}ClN_3,2H_3PO_4$. Phosphate of 7-chloro-4-(4-diethylamino-1-methylbutylamino)quinoline. Antimalarial drug, used also in the treatment of lupus erythematosus, rheumatoid arthritis and amoebiasis.

chlor·othī·azide. $C_7H_6ClN_3O_4S_2$. 6-chloro-7-sulphamoylbenzo-1: 2 : 4-thiadiazine-1: 1-dioxide. A powerful diuretic.

chlor·otrian·isene. $C_{23}H_{21}ClO_3$. Tri-*p*-anisylchloro-ethylene. A powerful synthetic oestrogen used esp. for relief of menopausal symptoms and in treatment of prostatic carcinoma.

chlor·phenĕ·sin. $C_9H_{11}ClO_3$. 3-*p*-chlorophenoxypropane-1,2-diol. Antibacterial and antifungal drug used for treatment of fungous diseases of the skin.

chlor·phenīr·amine maleate. $C_{16}H_{19}ClN_2,C_4H_4O_4$. Maleate of 1-(4-chlorophenyl)-3-dimethylamino-1-2'-pyridylpropane. An antihistamine drug.

chlorprō·mazine. $C_{17}H_{19}N_2ClS$. 2-chloro-10-(3'-dimethylamino-*n*-propyl) phenothiazine. Sedative drug based on phenothiazine, *q.v.*; other uses include suppression of vomiting, potentiation of analgesics, and as an adjuvant in the production of hypothermia.

chlorprō·pamide. $C_{10}H_{13}O_3N_2SCl$. *N*-*p*-chlorobenzenesulphonyl-*N'*-propylurea. Hypoglycaemic agent given orally in treatment of diabetes mellitus, esp. in elderly patients.

chlor·tetracyc·line. Aureomycin, *q.v.*

chlorthal·idone. $C_{14}H_{11}O_4N_2SCl$. 3-(4-chloro-3-sulphamoylphenyl)-3-hydroxy-iso-indolin-1-one. A diuretic drug.

choă·nal atrĕ·sia (G. *choane*, funnel; *a-*, neg.; *tresis*, boring). Congenital stenosis of the posterior nasal openings.

chocolate cyst. Term usually applied to an ovarian cyst containing chocolate-coloured material, often an endometrial cyst.

chondrodysplasia. Dyschondroplasia, *q.v.*

chor·io-allantō·ic membrane (G. *khorion*, membrane; *allas*, sausage; *eidos*, form). The yolk-sac in a developing egg. Used as a site for the experimental culture of viruses.

chor·io-angiō·ma (G. *khorion*, membrane; *aggeion*, vessel; *-oma*, tumour). Haemangioma of the placenta.

chor·istō·ma (G. *khoristos*, separated; *-oma*, tumour). Tumour arising in misplaced embryonic remnants.

Christmas disease (name of English family in which first reported). Variety of haemophilia in which plasma thromboplastin component (Christmas factor) is deficient. See also P.T.C.

chro·maffino·ma. Chromaffin tumour, *q.v.*

chrō·matŏ·graphy. Method of separation of individual components of mixtures of biological substances in solution by selective adsorption, e.g. on filter paper or in columns of adsorbent material.

chrysī·asis (G. *krysos*, gold). Discoloration of the skin resulting from injections of gold salts.

chȳ·lomi·crons (G. *khulos*, juice; *micron*, small). Microscopic fat particles visible by dark-ground illumination in blood collected during the absorption of fat from the intestine.

cin·eplas·ty, cin·eplas·tic amputation. Shaping of an amputation stump in such a way as to permit the maximum movement of the artificial limb.

cit·rovor·um factor. Folinic acid, *q.v.*

Civatte's poikiloderma reticulare (Civatte, A., French physician, born 1877). Blue-brown pigmentation of the skin of the neck, with telangiectases, *q.v.*

clō·ne (G. *khlon*, a cutting). That group of organisms produced by asexual reproduction from one sexually-produced individual.

clox·acill·in. Sodium chlorophenylmethylisoazolyl penicillin monohydrate. Antibiotic effective, orally or by injection, against penicillin-resistant staphylococci.

coag·ulase (L. *coagulare*, to curdle). Plasma-clotting enzyme produced by pathogenic strains of staphylococci.

co·balt (Germ. *kobold*, goblin living underground). Element of which traces are required for haemopoiesis. Symbol Co.

cobalt 60. Radioactive isotope of cobalt, used as a source of therapeutic ionising radiation in treatment of malignant disease.

cocktail, lytic. Combination of drugs used to promote the action of anaesthetics and the production of artificial hibernation (hypothermia) in surgical operations which demand a prolonged reduction in oxygen uptake by the blood.

cohort isolation (L. *cohors*, division of an army). In obstetric units, the isolation of newborn babies in small groups to reduce colonization with pathogenic organisms.

cōlis·tin. Antibiotic isolated from cultures of *b. colistinus*, having properties similar to polymyxin, *q.v.*

collagen diseases (G. *kolla*, glue; *gennan*, to produce). Group of conditions characterized by breakdown of collagen in connective tissues, e.g. rheumatic diseases, polyarteritis nodosa, disseminated lupus erythematosus.

comĕ·docarcinō·ma. Form of breast carcinoma in which growth fills the ducts, giving the appearance of comedones.

Compound E. Cortisone, *q.v.*

Compound F. Hydrocortisone, *q.v.*

conver·tin. Blood coagulation factor formed by thromboplastin, calcium and proconvertin, which initiates the formation of thrombin.

cō·nus arteriō·sus. Lower part of bulbus cordis, *q.v.*, which takes part in the formation of the right ventricular wall.

Coombs test (Coombs, R., English pathologist, born 1921). Agglutination test to detect the presence of incomplete Rhesus antibody. (See antibody, incomplete.)

cor·ticoster·oids. Generic term for steroid substances found in the adrenal cortex.

cor·ticotrō·phin (G. *cortex*, outer part; *trephein*, to nourish). Anterior pituitary hormone which promotes secretion of corticoid hormones by the adrenal cortex. Syn. adrenocorticotrophic hormone, A.C.T.H.

cor·tisol. See hydrocortisone.

cor·tisone acetate. $C_{23}H_{30}O_6$. 21-acetoxy-17-alpha-hydroxypregn-4-ene-3,11,20-trione. Glucocorticoid secretion of the adrenal cortex produced synthetically and now mainly used in substitution therapy of Simmonds' and Addison's diseases.

coudé (Fr. *coude*, elbow). Of catheters and sounds; having a bend just proximal to the tip.

couvā·de (Fr. *couver*, to brood). Primitive custom in which the father, as well as the mother, takes to bed during childbirth and the puerperium.

Couvelaire uterus (Couvelaire, A., French obstetrician, 1873–1948). Haemorrhagic state of the uterine muscle in severe degrees of concealed accidental antepartum haemorrhage.

Coxsackie viruses (Coxsackie, N. Y., U.S.A.; village in which patients lived from whom first strains were isolated). Group of viruses, most of which are non-pathogenic (Group A). Group B includes five types associated with aseptic meningitis, Bornholm disease, acute myocarditis and various non-specific fevers.

Craigie tube. Small test-tube containing semi-solid culture medium in which stands a smaller tube open at both ends, projecting above the medium. Motile forms of an organism inoculated into the inner tube can be isolated by subculture from the outer tube and thus separated from non-motile forms.

C-reactive protein. Specific protein substance which appears in the blood in the acute phase of various infections and in advanced malignant disease.

cranium bifidum (G. *kranion*, skull; L. *bis*, twice; *findere*, to cleave). Congenital defect in the bony wall of the skull.

crista terminalis (L. *crista*, a crest). Muscular ridge running through the right atrium of the heart, joining the superior to the inferior vena cava.

cross-matching. Direct testing for compatibility of red cells of a blood donor with serum of a recipient as a preliminary to blood transfusion.

crossed laterality. See laterality.

crotam·iton. $C_{13}H_{17}NO$. *N*-crotonoyl-*N*-ethyl-*o*-toluidine. Antipruritic for external application, esp. in scabies.

croup-associated virus. Also known as para-influenza virus; isolated from cases of acute laryngotracheobronchitis in infants.

crush syndrome. Severe shock, with haematuria, resulting from sustained crushing of a limb.

cry·oglob·ulin (G. *kryos*, cold; L. *globulus*, a globule). An abnormal serum protein found especially in myelomatosis, which separates out on exposure to cold.

cry·oglob·ulinae·mia. Presence of cryoglobulin in the blood.

cryp·tobleph·aron (G. *kruptein*, to hide; *blepharon*, eyelid). Congenital deformity in which a continuous layer of skin over the eyeballs replaces the eyelids.

cryp·tococco·sis. Torulosis, *q.v.*

cū·mulus ōö·phorus (L. *cumulus*, a heap; G. *oophoron*, ovary). Small mass of granulosa cells arising from the wall of a developing ovarian follicle to surround the maturing ovum.

cy·anocobal·amin. $C_{63}H_{88}CoN_{14}O_{14}P$. Vitamin B_{12}; contains cobalt and is mainly responsible for the therapeutic effect of liver (in which it occurs) in pernicious anaemia.

cy·clizine hydrochloride. $C_{18}H_{22}N_2HCl$. 1-methyl-4-α-phenylbenzylpiperazine hydrochloride. Drug used in the treatment of nausea and vomiting, especially of pregnancy and motion sickness.

cy·clocou·marol. $C_{20}H_{18}O_4$. 3,4-dihydro-2-methoxy-2-methyl-4-phenyl-2*H*,5*H*-pyrano[3,2-c][1]-benzopyran-5-one. A synthetic anticoagulant.

cy·clometh·ycaine sulphate. $C_{22}H_{33}NO_3,H_2SO_4$. 3-(2-methylpiperidino) propyl - *p* - cyclohexyloxybenzoate hydrogen sulphate. A local anaesthetic for surface application.

cy·clophos·phamide. $C_7H_{15}O_2N_2PCl_2$. *NN'*-di(2-chlorethyl)-*N'*-(3-hydroxy-propyl) phosphorodiamidic acid lactone. Cytostatic agent used for oral or intravenous therapy in malignant disease and to depress immune reactions as a preliminary to organ grafting.

cy·closer·ine. $C_3H_6N_2O_2$. D-4-aminoisoxazolidine-3-one. Antibiotic obtained synthetically or by the growth of *streptomyces orchidaceus*, and used mainly in treatment of pulmonary tuberculosis.

cys·tinosis (G. *kystos*, bladder). Wasting disease of children, similar to Fanconi syndrome, *q.v.*, but with deposits of cystine in liver, spleen and elsewhere.

cy·tology, exfoliative (G. *kutos*, cell; *logos*, a treatise; L. *ex*, out; *folium*, a leaf). Study of cells cast off from internal surfaces of the body, e.g. bronchi, gastric mucosa, cervix uteri, in order to detect early evidence of malignancy, and in gynaecology, also for the study of ovarian endocrine activity.

cy·toly·sate (G. *kutos*, cell; *luein*, to loose). The fluid left after cytolysis, *q.v.*, has taken place.

cy·tomegal·ic inclusion-body disease (G. *kutos*, cell; *megas*, large). Disease occurring usually in neonatal period, characterized by presence of inclusion-bodies, *q.v.*, in, and enlargement of nuclei of, epithelial cells in many organs.

D

dap·sone. $C_{12}H_{12}O_2N_2S$. 4: 4'-diaminodiphenylsulphone. Bacteriostatic drug used specifically for the treatment of leprosy.

Darier-Roussy sarcoid (Darier, F. J., French dermatologist, 1856–1938; Roussy, G., French pathologist, 1874–1948). A subcutaneous form of sarcoidosis, *q.v.*

Darrow's solution (Darrow, D. C., American paediatrician, born 1895). Solution containing sodium and potassium chlorides and molar lactate, used to maintain fluid balance in infantile enteritis.

Debré-deToni-Fanconi syndrome. See Fanconi syndrome.

defib·rillator (L. *de*, from; *fibrilla*, little fibre). Electrical instrument for stopping ventricular fibrillation occurring during general anaesthesia.

dehy·dro-androster·one. Androgenic substance found naturally in male urine and in that of women suffering from adrenal tumours.

de·methylchlor·tetracy·cline. Chemical variant of chlortetracycline, *q.v.*

de·oxycor·tone. $C_{21}H_{30}O_3$. Delta⁴-pregnene-21-ol-3: 20-dione. Steroid hormone derived from adrenal cortex or prepared synthetically; concerned in regulation of salt and water metabolism.

dequalin·ium chloride. $C_{30}H_{40}Cl_2N_4$. Decamethylene bis(4-aminoquinaldinium) chloride. Quaternary ammonium antiseptic used esp. as lozenges for mouth and throat infections.

der·matofibrō·ma (G. *derma*, skin; L. *fibra*, fibre; G. -*oma*, tumour). A fibrous tumour of the skin.

der·matorrhex·is (G. *derma*, skin; *rhexis*, breaking). Ehlers-Danlos syndrome, *q.v.*

de Toni-Fanconi syndrome. See Fanconi syndrome.

dex·ameth·asone. $C_{22}H_{29}FO_5$. 9-α-fluoro-11β,17α,21-trihydroxy-16α-methylpregna-1,4-diene-3,20-dione. Highly potent chemical variant of cortisone.

dex·amphet·amine. $C_6H_5CH_2CH(CH_3)NH_2$. (+)-α-methylphenethylamine sulphate. Similar in effects to amphetamine, *q.v.*

dex·trans. Viscous substances resulting from the fermentation of sucrose by *leuconostoc mesenteroides*; used for the temporary expansion of blood-volume after haemorrhage.

dex·tromethor·phan. $C_{18}H_{25}NO,HBr,H_2O$. Hydrobromide of 3-methoxy-*N*-methyl-morphinan. A cough suppressant.

Diamox. See acetazolamide.

dichlorphen·amide. $C_6H_6Cl_2N_2O_4S_2$. 4-5 dichlorobenzene-1,3 disulphonamide. Drug used in treatment of glaucoma.

dichlor·alphēn·azone. Combination of chloral with phenazone to form a compound in which chloral is retained in a stable form suitable for dispensing in tablets.

dī·cophane. $C_{14}H_9Cl_5$. 1:1:1-trichloro-2:2-di(*p*-chlorophenyl) ethane. Slow-acting and persistent insecticide for large-scale disinfestation in public health and agriculture. More usually known as D.D.T.

dicy·clomine hydrochloride. $C_{19}H_{36}ClNO_2$. 2-diethylaminoethyl 1-cyclohexyl-cyclohexanecarboxylate hydrochloride. Drug used in peptic ulceration to reduce gastric secretion and motility.

dieth·azine hydrochloride. $C_{18}H_{22}N_2S,HCl$. Hydrochloride of 10-(2-diethylaminoethyl) phenothiazine. Parasympathetic antagonist used in relief of Parkinsonism.

diethylcarbamazine citrate. $C_{16}H_{29}O_8N_3$. 1-diethylcarbamoyl-4-methyl piperazine dihydrogen citrate. Compound used for the prophylaxis and treatment of filariasis.

dī·gū·anide. Parent substance of a number of agents which, given orally, reduce blood-sugar in diabetes mellitus.

Di Guglielmo's disease (Di Guglielmo, G., Italian haematologist, born 1886). Erythraemic myelosis, a leukaemia-like condition with abnormal and excessive proliferation of erythroblasts in the bone marrow.

dihy·drotachy·sterol. $C_{28}H_{46}O$. Weakly anti-rachitic synthetic substance resembling calciferol, *q.v.*

di-iō·dohydroxyquï·noline. $C_9H_5ONI_2$. 8-hydroxy-5: 7 di-iodoquinoline. A quinoline derivative for the treatment of amoebiasis.

dī·lox·anide. $C_9H_9Cl_2NO_2$. Dichloroacet-4-hydroxy-*N*-methylanilide. An anti-amoebic used as alternative to emetine, *q.v.*

di·menhy·drinate. $C_{17}H_{21}NO,C_7H_7ClN_4O_2$. 2(benzohydryloxy)-*N*: *N*-dimethylethylamine-8-chlorotheophyllinate. Anti-histamine drug used esp. in motion sickness.

dimercaprol. See B.A.L.

di·methi·sterone. $C_{23}H_{32}O_2,H_2O$. 17β-hydroxy-6α,21-dimethyl-17αpregn-4-en-20-yn-3-one. A progestational steroid.

diox·ane. $C_4H_8O_2$. Diethylene dioxide. Liquid miscible with water and organic solvents, used in histology and as an industrial solvent. The vapour is toxic.

di·phenhȳ·dramine. $C_{17}H_{21}ON$. Benzhydryl 2-dimethylaminoethyl ether. Anti-histamine drug with marked sedative properties.

di·phēn·ylhydan·toin. $(C_6H_5)_2.C:(CONHC:N)OH$. Anti-convulsant drug used in the treatment of major epilepsy.

di·pipanone. $C_{24}H_{31}NO,HCl,H_2O$. Hydrochloride of 4, 4-diphenyl-6-piperidinoheptan-3-one. An analgesic and narcotic, given by injection.

diplō·pagus (G. *diploos*, double; *pagos*, joined). Conjoined twins in whom one or more vital organs are shared.

dis·cus prolig·erus. See cumulus oophorus.

disulfi·ram. $C_{10}H_{20}N_2S_4$. Tetraethylthiuram disulphide. Drug used for the treatment of alcoholism; acts by inducing extreme nausea when alcohol is taken.

di·thranol. $C_{14}H_{10}O_3$. Anthracene-1,8,9-triol. Substance used in an ointment for treatment of psoriasis.

dī·vīn·yl ether. $(CH_2: CH)_2O$. Volatile liquid used for brief general anaesthesia or for induction before other anaesthetics such as ethyl ether.

dōm·iphen bromide. Dodecyldimethyl-2-phenoxyethylammonium bromide. A detergent with antiseptic properties.

Donath-Landsteiner phenomenon (Donath, J., Austrian physician, born 1870; Landsteiner, K., Austrian pathologist, 1868–1943). Presence of a haemolysin active in the cold (5°C.) in the blood of patients with paroxysmal haemoglobinuria.

duc·tus arterio·sus. Embryonic channel between pulmonary artery and aorta; normally closed soon after birth, its persistence constitutes a form of congenital heart disease remediable by surgery.

duc·tus veno·sus. Embryonic channel joining the umbilical vein to the inferior vena cava.

Duffy blood group system (name of patient in whom the specific antibody was first detected). Blood group characterized by possession of an antigen (Fyª), found in 65 per cent of English people.

dȳ·flos. $C_6H_{14}FO_3P$. Di-isopropylfluorophosphonate. Drug used as a meiotic in the treatment of glaucoma.

dys·autono·mia (G. *dus-*, bad; *autos*, self; *nomos*, law). Failure of balance between the sympathetic and parasympathetic nervous systems. Manifested (rarely) as a familial disease.

dyspla·sia, chon·dro-ectoder·mal (G. *dus-*, bad; *plassein*, to form; *khondros*, cartilage; *ectos*, outside; *derma*, skin). Congenital syndrome comprising absence of sweat glands, malformation of face, nails and teeth, polydactyly, congenital heart disease and chondrodystrophy.

E

Earle's solution. Solution of a mixture of inorganic salts with glucose, balanced to form a basis for a medium for tissue culture.

Ebstein's anomaly (Ebstein, W., German physician, 1836–1912). Rare form of congenital heart disease in which the right ventricle is divided into two by a fused and misplaced tricuspid valve.

ECHO viruses (Enteric Cytopathogenic Human Orphan viruses). Large group of viruses isolated from faeces and found in association with outbreaks of aseptic meningitis and various non-specific fevers.

E.D.T.A. Ethylene-diamine-tetra-acetic acid. A chelating agent, *q.v.*

edropho·nium chloride. $C_{10}H_{16}ClNO$. Ethyl-(3-hydroxyphenyl)dimethylammonium chloride. Anticholinesterase drug similar in action to neostigmine, *q.v.*

Ehlers-Danlos syndrome (Ehlers, E., German dermatologist, 1863–1937; Danlos, H. A., French physician, 1844–1912). Rare familial anomaly comprising abnormal elasticity of skin with hyper-extensibility of joints.

Eisenmenger complex (Eisenmenger, V., 19th cent. German physician). Congenital cardiac anomaly comprising interventricular septal defect, dextroposition of aorta and right ventricular hypertrophy.

elec·trophore·sis. Separation of components of protein mixtures (e.g., serum) by means of their differing mobilities in an electric field.

en·terovi·ruses. Viruses which may be isolated from the intestinal tract; these include poliomyelitis, Coxsackie and ECHO viruses, *q.v.*

e·osinophil·ic granulo·ma of bone (eosin, G. *philein*, to love; L. *granula*, a grain). Benign, solitary reticuloendothelial granuloma containing large numbers of eosinophil leucocytes.

ero·sion, cervical (L. *erodere*, to eat away). Extension, usually as result of chronic inflammation, of mucous lining of cervical canal of uterus on to surface of vaginal portion, normally covered by squamous epithelium.

erythraē·mic myelō·sis. See Di Guglielmo's disease.

ery·thromy·cin. Antibiotic produced by the growth of *streptomyces erythreus*, specially effective against penicillin-resistant staphylococci as well as a wide range of activity.

ethanō·lamine. $NH_2CH_2CH_2OH$. 2-aminoethanol. Sclerosing agent for the treatment of varicose veins by injection.

e·thinyloestradi·ol. $C_{20}H_{24}O_2$. 17-ethinyl-3: 17-dihydroxyoestra 1: 3: 5(10)-triene. The most potent of the oestrogens, used for treatment of amenorrhoea due to uterine hypoplasia, menopausal symptoms, and in the male for prostatic carcinoma.

ethi·sterone. $C_{21}H_{28}O_2$. 17β-hydroxy-17α-pregn-4-en-20-yn-3-one. A progestational steroid.

ethoprō·pazine. $C_{19}H_{24}N_2S$. N-(2-diethylamino-*n*-propyl) phenothiazine. Antispasmodic drug chiefly used to relieve motor disturbances in Parkinsonism.

ē·thoto·in. $C_{11}H_{12}N_2O_2$. 3-ethyl-5-phenylhydantoin. Anti-convulsant drug used in treatment of epilepsy.

ethyl biscouma·cetate. $C_{22}H_{16}O_8$. Ethyl 4-4′-dihydroxycoumarin-3: 3-yl-acetate. An anticoagulant providing a rapid effect when given by mouth.

e·thylenedi·amine hydrate. $C_2H_4(NH_2)_2H_2O$. Used in combination with aminophylline as a diuretic in cardiac and renal oedema.

Evans blue (Evans, H., American anatomist, born 1882). Dye which can be injected intravenously in order to estimate blood volume.

F

Fanconi's anaemia (Fanconi, G., Swiss paediatrician, born 1892). Pancytopenia, *q.v.*, with multiple congenital anomalies, skin pigmentation and sometimes mental retardation.

Fanconi syndrome (Fanconi, G., Swiss paediatrician, born 1892). Metabolic disorder in infants and adults, comprising rickets, albuminuria, glycosuria and amino-aciduria, with dwarfing in infants.

fa·vism (It. *fava*, bean). Haemolytic anaemia, after ingestion of fava beans, or inhalation of pollen from their flowers, in persons sensitive to these toxins.

Felty's syndrome (Felty, A. R., American physician, born 1895). Rheumatoid arthritis with neutropenia and splenomegaly occurring in adults (*cf.* Still's disease).

ferr·itin (L. *ferrum*, iron). Iron-containing protein complex concerned with transport and storage of iron in the body. See also apoferritin.

Feulgen reaction (Feulgen, R., German chemist, born 1884). Histochemical reaction to demonstrate deoxyribonucleic acid in cell nuclei.

fi·brin foam (L. *fibra*, a fibre). Porous preparation of human fibrin used as a haemostatic pack.

fi·bro-elasto·sis, endocar·dial (L. *fibra*, a fibre; G. *elaunein*, to beat out). Thickening of endocardium in infancy by deposition of excess of elastic tissue, often in association with a congenital cardiac anomaly.

fibropla·sia, retrolen·tal (L. *fibra*, fibre; G. *plassein*, to form; L. *retro*, backward; L. *lens*, lentil). Growth of fibrous tissue behind the lens as a consequence of exposure to excessive amounts of oxygen given therapeutically in the first few weeks of life.

Fiedler's myocarditis (Fiedler, C. L. A., German physician, 1835–1921). Acute isolated myocarditis, cause unknown, with degeneration of the muscle fibres and interstitial infiltration with leucocytes.

figlu. Formimoglutamic acid, *q.v.*

fixed virus. Naturally acquired ('street') virus of rabies, whose virulence has been exalted by passage through rabbits until its potency is such that it kills in 5 to 6 days from the date of infection.

fla·vonoids. Members of a group of substances having anti-haemorrhagic effects by their actions on the capillary walls.

flu·drocortisone acetate. $C_{23}H_{31}FO_6$. 21-acetoxy-9α-fluoro-11β,17α-dihydroxypregn-4-ene-3,20-dione(9α-fluorohydrocortisone 21-acetate). Adrenocortical steroid for treatment of adrenal cortical insufficiency.

fluoro·sis (L. *fluere*, to flow). Chronic fluorine poisoning, characterized by mottling of the enamel of the teeth.

fluox·ymes·terone. $C_{20}H_{29}FO_3$. 9α-fluoro-11β,17β-dihydroxy-17α-methylandrost-4-en-3-one. Synthetic androgenic hormone similar in action to testosterone, *q.v.* Used in inoperable breast cancer and in male hypogonadism.

flur·andren·olone. 6-fluoro-16 : 17-isopropylidenedioxyhydrocortisone. Steroid substance used by local application for the relief of inflammation in skin disorders.

Foley catheter (Foley, F. E. B., American surgeon, born 1891). Self-retaining catheter, kept in position by a small balloon behind the eye, inflated through a fine passage running in the thickness of the wall.

folin·ic acid. The metabolically active form of folic acid, *q.v.* Also referred to as *citrovorum* factor, being an essential growth factor for the organism *leuconostoc citrovorum*.

follicle-stimulating hormone. Hormone secreted by the anterior pituitary, which stimulates growth of ovarian follicles in the female and of seminiferous epithelium in the male.

formimī·noglutam·ic acid. Substance which, in folic acid deficiency, replaces glutamic acid as the end product of histidine metabolism; may be estimated in urine.

Fox-Fordyce disease (Fox, G. H., 1846–1937, Fordyce, J. A., 1858–1925, American dermatologists). Itching papular eruption in axilla, pubic and perineal regions, and round the nipples, exclusively in women.

fragility, osmotic. Increased tendency of red cells to break up when placed in hypotonic saline solutions. Characteristic esp. of congenital haemolytic anaemia (acholuric jaundice).

framycē·tin. Antibiotic produced by the growth of *aspergillus fumigatus*, esp. active against *entamoeba histolytica*.

Fucidin. Name for sodium salt of fusidic acid, an antibiotic especially active against staphylococci.

furazol·idone. A nitrofuran, *q.v.*, used for treatment of bacterial infections of the bowel.

G

---

galac·tosāe·mia (G. *gala*, milk; *haima*, blood). Hereditary syndrome due to inability to convert galactose to glucose. Characterized by wasting, liver cirrhosis, cataract, mental retardation, galactosuria and aminoaciduria.

gall·amine tri·ethi·odide. $C_{30}H_{60}O_3N_3I_3$. 1:2:3-tri-(2-diethylaminoethoxy) benzene triethiodide. A muscle-relaxant drug used esp. as an aid to muscle relaxation in abdominal surgery.

gamma benzene hexachloride. $C_6H_6Cl_6$. 1:2:3:4:5:6 hexachlorocyclohexane. Insecticide effective against fleas, lice and ticks, and in humans a powerful convulsant poison when taken internally.

gamma globulin (*gamma*, third letter of Greek alphabet; L. *globulus*, a globule). That fraction of the globulin component of the blood proteins which is specially concerned in the processes of immunity.

genodermato·sis (G. *genos*, race; *derma*, skin). Any congenital disease of the skin.

Gerstmann's syndrome (Gerstmann, J., Austrian neurologist, born 1887). Finger-agnosia, *q.v.*, acalculia, *q.v.*, lateral disorientation and other manifestations due to a lesion of the dominant parietal lobe of the brain.

Gey's solution. Solution of a mixture of inorganic salts with glucose, balanced to form a basis for a medium for tissue culture.

Ghon focus (Ghon, A., Czech. pathologist, 1866–1936). Primary tuberculous lesion, as occurring in the lungs of children.

globin zinc insulin. Preparation of insulin with a globin, *q.v.*, and zinc chloride, intended to delay absorption of the anti-diabetic principle, thus prolonging the effect of a single dose.

glu·cagon. Substance secreted by the alpha cells of the islets of Langerhans in the pancreas which raises blood-sugar by breaking down glycogen.

glu·cocort·icoids. Group of steroid hormones secreted by the supra-renals, concerned with carbohydrate metabolism; includes cortisone, corticosterone and hydrocortisone.

glu·curon·ic acid. $CHO(CHOH)_4COOH$. Uronic acid which acts as a detoxicating agent on bilirubin and numerous toxins with which it conjugates to form harmless substances for excretion in the urine.

glu·cur·onides. Salts or esters of glucuronic acid formed by conjugation of that acid with some usually toxic substance.

glutam·ic oxalacet·ic transam·inase. Intracellular enzyme occurring in heart muscle and liver tissue; its presence in increased amounts in blood serum indicates disease of one of these organs.

glutam·ic pyru·vic transam·inase. Intracellular enzyme occurring esp. in liver cells; increased serum level indicates disease of that organ.

glutēth·imide. $C_{13}H_{15}NO_2$. α-ethyl-α-phenylglutarimide. Hypnotic drug whose action resembles that of phenobarbitone, *q.v.*

granulosa cells (L. *granulum*, a little grain). The epithelial cells which line the primordial follicles of the ovary.

granulosa cell tumour. Tumour arising in the granulosa cells of the ovary.

griseoful·vin $C_{17}H_{17}ClO_6$. 7-chloro-4:6-dimethoxy-coumaran-3-one-2-spiro-1'-(2'-methoxy-6'-methylcyclohex-2'-en-4'-one). Substance used for treatment of fungous infections.

gu·aneth·idine sulphate. $C_{10}H_{22}N_4H_2SO_4$. Sulphate of 1-(2-guanidinoethyl) azacyclo-octane. Sympathetic antagonist used in treatment of hypertension.

Guarnieri body (Guarnieri, G., Italian pathologist, 1856–1918). Intracellular inclusion body, seen in exudates from smallpox and vaccinia lesions.

Guillain-Barré syndrome (Guillain, G., French neurologist, born 1876; Barré, J. A., French neurologist, born 1880). More properly, Landry-Guillain-Barré syndrome. Acute infective polyneuritis, with ascending paralysis and increased protein, with no corresponding pleocytosis, in the cerebrospinal fluid.

gynan·droblasto·ma. Ovarian tumour which contains neoplastic elements of both feminizing as well as masculinizing tissues.

H

haem·adsor·ption virus (name derived from method of detection by clumping of guinea-pig red cells on to surface of virus-infected cells). Virus of the para-influenza group recovered from children suffering from acute laryngotracheobronchitis, and capable of inducing symptoms of common cold on injection into adults.

haeman·giopericyto·ma (G. haima, blood; aggeion, vessel; peri, round; kutos, cell). Tumour, usually subcutaneous, made up of contractile cells derived from capillary walls.

hae·modial·ysis. Passage of circulating blood through a dialysing apparatus, e.g. artificial kidney, in order to restore normal balance of chemical components when this has been otherwise irretrievably upset. See dialysis.

haemoglobins, abnormal. Forms of haemoglobin which show genetically determined chemical differences from normal adult haemoglobin, and whose presence in blood of an individual gives rise to specific disease patterns. The varieties of haemoglobin are identified by means of letters, haemoglobin A being normal adult haemoglobin, haemoglobin F foetal haemoglobin. Haemoglobin S is found in sickle-cell anaemia, and many other varieties are known.

haemoglobino·pathy. Any condition resulting from the presence in the blood of an abnormal form of haemoglobin; sickle-cell anaemia and allied conditions, designated by the name of the abnormal haemoglobin responsible, e.g. haemoglobin C disease.

Hagemann factor (named from patient in whom its deficiency was first discovered). Substance present in normal plasma and serum necessary for normal thromboplastin generation in the first stage of blood coagulation.

half-blue baby. Infant showing cyanosis confined to head and arms resulting usually from transposition of aorta and pulmonary artery with patency of ductus arteriosus.

halothane. $CHBrCl,CF_3$. 2-bromo-2-chloro-1:1:1-trifluoroethane. Volatile general anaesthetic given by inhalation.

Hamman-Rich syndrome (Hamman, L., American physician, 1877–1946; Rich, A. R., American pathologist, born 1893). Progressive interstitial fibrosis of the lung, of unknown cause.

Hand-Schuller-Christian disease (Hand, A. J., American physician, 1868–1949; Schuller, A., Austrian neurologist, born 1874; Christian, H. A., American physician, 1876–1951). Metabolic disease of children, characterized esp. by diabetes insipidus and multiple reticulo-endothelial granulomata consisting of lipid-containing histiocytes in skull bones, with enlargement of liver, spleen and lymph nodes.

Hanks' solution. Solution of a mixture of inorganic salts with glucose balanced to form a basis for a medium for growth of cells in artificial culture.

hap·toglobin (G. haptein, to hold fast; L. globus, ball). Plasma protein which binds haemoglobin set free into the plasma.

Hartnup disease (name of English family in which first described). Hereditary syndrome comprising pellagra-like skin rash, periodic ataxia and constant amino-aciduria.

He-La cells. Strain of malignant squamous epithelial cells originating in a carcinoma of the cervix uteri; used in tissue culture as a medium for the growth of certain viruses.

herpangi·na (G. herpein, to creep; agkhein, to throttle). Mild epidemic throat infection in children characterized by vesicles and later ulcers on and around the tonsils and probably due to one or more types of Coxsackie viruses, q.v.

hex·achlor·ophane. $C_{13}H_6Cl_6O_2$. 2, 2'-methylenebis (3,4,6-trichlorophenol). Antibacterial substance which retains activity in presence of soap and is especially used for skin cleansing to prevent cross-infection. Syn. hexachlorophene.

hex·adimeth·rine bromide. Quaternary ammonium compound used to neutralize the anticoagulant properties of heparin.

hex·amethon·ium tartrate. $C_{20}H_{40}N_2O_{12}$. Hexamethylenedi(trimethylammonium hydrogen tartrate). A ganglion-blocking agent used in the treatment of hypertension.

hi·bernō·ma. Tumour made up of fat cells similar to those found in fat accumulations in hibernating animals.

hi·dradeni·tis. Chronic suppuration of apocrine glands, usually those in axilla and pubis.

hi·dradenō·ma (G. hidros, sweat; aden, gland). Benign epithelial tumour of vulva, arising from sweat glands.

his·tiocytō·ma (G. histos, web; kutos, cell). Fibrous tumour of dermis containing nests of histiocytes.

Hurler-Pfaundler syndrome (Hurler, G., 20th-cent. German paediatrician; Pfaundler, M. von, German paediatrician, born 1872). Gargoylism, q.v.

hy·aline membrane, pulmonary. Structureless membrane found post mortem lining the alveolar ducts and bronchioles of infants, esp. premature, dying from anoxia during the first few days after birth.

hydan·toin. Anhydride of hydantoic acid, a derivative of creatinine. Compounds of hydantoin are used as anti-convulsants in treatment of epilepsy.

hydrall·azine hydrochloride. $C_8H_8N_4HCl$. Hydrochloride of 1-hydrazinophthalazine. Vasodilator drug used in treatment of hypertension.

hydrochlor·othi·azide. $C_7H_8ClN_3O_4S_2$. 6-chloro-3,4-dihydro-7-sulphamoyl-$2H$-benzo-1,2,4-thiadiazine-1,1-dioxide. A non-mercurial diuretic, similar to, but more powerful than, chlorothiazide.

hydrocor·tisone. $C_{21}H_{30}O_5$. 11 : 17 : 21-trihydroxy-pregn-4-ene-3 : 20-dione. The most important of the hormones of the adrenal cortex, responsible for maintenance of blood-pressure, water and electrolyte balance, and renal function.

hydroflu·methi·azide. $C_8H_8F_3N_3O_4S_2$. 3,4-dihydro-6-trifluoromethylbenzo-1,2,4-thiadiazine-7-sulphon-amide-1,1-dioxide. A diuretic.

hydrox·ocobal·amin. $C_{62}H_{89}CoN_{13}O_{15}P$. alpha(5,6-dimethylbenzimidazolyl) hydroxocobamide. Cobalt-containing substance used in the treatment of megaloblastic anaemias. See also cyanocobalamin.

hydrox·ytryp·tamine. Toxic substance having an adrenaline-like effect, secreted by Kultschitzky cells of carcinoid tumours, *q.v.*

hy·percalcae·mia(G. *huper*, over; L. *calx*, lime; G. *haima*, blood). Presence of an excess of calcium in the blood.

hy·perlipae·mia (G. *huper*, over; *lipos*, fat; *haima*, blood). Familial disease characterized by persistent increase in serum triglycerides (see glyceride) with abdominal crises and liability to early onset of coronary artery atheroma.

hy·perosto·sis, infantile cortical (G. *huper*, over; *osteon*, bone). Abnormal thickening of the cortex of bones in infants under one year old.

hy·persplēn·ism (G. *huper*, over; *splen*, spleen). Abnormal increase in the destructive power of the spleen against one or more of the cellular elements of the peripheral blood or bone marrow.

hypertē·lorism (G. *huper*, over; *tele*, far; *horizein*, to separate). Developmental anomaly of base of skull producing a broadening and flattening of face and head; sometimes associated with mental defect.

hypocalcāē·mia (G. *hupo*, under; L. *calx*, lime; *haima*, blood). Deficiency of calcium in the blood.

hypo·gammaglŏb·ulināē·mia (G. *hupo*, under; gamma globulin; *haima*, blood). A deficiency of gamma globulin in the blood.

hypomandib·ulism (G. *hupo*, under; L. *mandibula*, mandible). Micrognathia, *q.v.*

hy·poprothrom·binae·mia (G. *hupo*, under; prothrombin; *haima*, blood). Deficiency of prothrombin in the blood.

I

iat·rogĕn·ic (G. *iatros*, physician; *gennan*, to produce). Term applied to disorders supervening in the course of a disease, as a consequence either of the treatment given or of fears engendered by the manners or conversation of the attending physician.

imi·pramine hydrochloride. $C_{19}H_{25}ClN_2$. 5-(3-dimethyl-aminopropyl)-10,11-dihydro-$5H$-dibenz *b,f* azepine hydrochloride. Anti-depressive drug used esp. in treatment of endogenous depression.

inclusion conjunctivitis. Form of conjunctivitis caused by a virus related to that of trachoma; epithelial cells in the exudate contain cell-inclusions like those seen in trachoma. Syn. swimming-bath conjunctivitis.

incontinentia pigmenti. Abnormal skin pigmentation appearing on trunk and legs in infancy.

interference, viral. The action of a virus on cells, as a result of which those cells become unable to support the growth of other viruses, whether related or unrelated to the interfering virus.

interfer·on. Virus-interfering substance produced experimentally by incubation of certain strains of viruses with various kinds of cells. See interference, viral.

intersex. Sex intergrade, *q.v.*

intersexuality. The condition of being intermediate in physical characteristics between male and female types; possessing features of both sexes.

iodine-131. Radioactive isotope of iodine, used esp. as a tracer for estimating thyroid uptake of iodine.

iodip·amide methylglu·camine. *N*-methylglucamine salt of *NN*′-di(3-carboxy-2,4,6-triiodophenyl) adipamide. Radiographic contrast medium given by intravenous injection for cholangiography.

ion-exchange. The process whereby ions of positive or negative charge in a solution may replace ions of similar charge in a material placed in contact with the solution. Ion-exchange resins are synthetic compounds active in this respect and which can be given orally to alter the chemical composition of body fluids.

i·opano·ic acid. $C_{11}H_{12}I_3NO_2$. alpha-(3-amino-2,4,6-triiodobenzyl)butyric acid. Contrast medium to be given orally for cholangiography.

i·ophen·dylate. Ethyl iodophenylundecanoate. Contrast medium for radiographic localization of obstructive lesions of the spinal canal.

i·proniazid phosphate. $C_9H_{13}ON_3H_3PO_4$. *N*-isonico-tinoyl-*N*′-isopropylhydrazine phosphate. Drug originally used for its antituberculous effect; but also found to have anti-depressant effects, for which it is now used.

i·socarbox·azid. $C_{12}H_{13}N_3O_2$. 3-*N*′-benzylhydrazino-carbonyl-5-methylisoxazole. A mono-amine oxidase inhibitor, *q.v.*, used as an anti-depressant drug in the treatment of neurotic or reactive depression.

i·soni·azid. $C_6H_7N_3O$. Pyridine-4-carboxyhydrazide. Bacteriostatic drug used concurrently with other antibacterial drugs in treatment of tuberculosis.

i·sophane insulin. Suspension of insulin crystals with a protamine and zinc. Action is delayed for about two hours and lasts for about 24 hours.

i·soprĕn·aline sulphate. $C_{22}H_{36}N_2O_{10}S,2H_2O$. 1-(3,4-dihydroxyphenyl)-2-isopropylaminoethanol sulphate dihydrate. Synthetic substance having inhibitory actions similar to those of adrenaline. Given orally or by spray inhalation for relief of spasm in bronchial asthma.

i·sopro·panol. See isopropyl alcohol.

ĭ·sopropylarterē·nol. Isoprenaline sulphate, *q.v.*

ĭ·sopropyl myris·tate. $C_{17}H_{34}O_2$. An ester of isopropyl alcohol; an oily liquid used to replace vegetable oils in preparations for external use.

ĭ·sothipen·dyl hydrochloride. $C_{16}H_{20}ClN_3S$. 9-(2-dimethylaminopropyl)-10-thia-1,9-diaza-anthracene hydrochloride. A potent but short-acting anti-histamine drug.

K

kan·amy·cin. $C_{18}H_{36}N_4O_{11}$. Antibiotic produced by the growth of *streptomyces kanamyceticus*. Action and properties are similar to those of neomycin, *q.v.*

Kaposi's sarcoma (Kaposi, M. J., Austrian dermatologist, 1837–1902). Tumour, usually multiple, arising in blood-vessel forming tissues, generally benign, but apt to degenerate into fibro-sarcoma.

Kaposi's varicelliform eruption (Kaposi, M. J., Austrian dermatologist, 1837–1902). Skin disease resulting from accidental inoculation of vaccinia virus into pre-existing eczematous lesions.

Kartagener's syndrome (Kartagener, M., Swiss physician, born 1897). Hereditary syndrome comprising bronchiectasis, maldevelopment of paranasal sinuses and transposition of the viscera.

Kell blood group system (name of family in which first detected). Blood group characterized by the possession of an antigen (K), found in about 10 per cent of the British population.

ker·asin. A cerebroside, *q.v.*, constituent of brain tissue.

Kidd blood group system (name of family in which first detected). Blood group characterized by possession of an antigen (Jk^a), found in about 75 per cent of the English population.

Kimmelstiel-Wilson disease (Kimmelstiel, Paul, American pathologist, born 1900; Wilson, Clifford, British physician, born 1906). Syndrome characterized by glycosuria with nephrotic symptoms, albuminuria and oedema.

King-Armstrong units (King, E. J., Canadian bio-chemist, 1901–1962; Armstrong, A. R., Canadian physician, born 1904). Units in which the activity of alkaline phosphatase is estimated in the blood by the method of King and Armstrong.

Klinefelter's syndrome (Klinefelter, H. F., American physician, born 1912). Infertility in the male, associated with hypogonadism and gynaecomastia.

Klippel-Feil syndrome (Klippel, M., French neurologist, 1858–1942; Feil, A., French neurologist, born 1885). Congenital fusion of the cervical vertebrae, leading to shortening of the neck and restriction of its movements.

Krabbe's cerebral sclerosis (Krabbe, K. H., Danish neurologist, born 1885). Demyelinating disease of central nervous system, usually occurring in infants, and sometimes familial.

Krukenberg tumour (Krukenberg, F. E., German gynaecologist, born 1871). Secondary deposits of carcinoma in the ovaries forming tumours whose epithelial cells are distended with mucus and take on a 'signet-ring' appearance.

Kveim test (Kveim, M. A., Norwegian physician, born 1892). Intradermal test for sarcoidosis, by injection of material from lymph nodes of a known sarcoidosis patient.

L

lach·esine chloride. $C_{20}H_{26}ClNO_3$. (2-benziloyloxy-ethyl) ethyldimethylammonium chloride. A mydriatic and cycloplegic; less powerful and shorter-acting than atropine, and used where there is sensitivity to atropine.

lactic dehydrogenase. Intracellular enzyme whose concentration in the blood rises during active tissue proliferation, e.g. in pregnancy and malignant disease as well as after tissue necrosis esp. of myocardium, liver, pancreas.

Lansing virus. Type II strain of human poliomyelitis virus.

laterality. The dominance of the hand and eye of one side over those of the other side.

laterality, crossed. Condition in which the dominant hand is on the opposite from the dominant eye.

latex fixation test. Serological test used in diagnosis of collagen diseases, esp. rheumatoid arthritis, dependent on agglutination of a suspension of poly-styrene latex particles, coated with human gamma globulin, by abnormal antibodies found in patient's serum.

Laurence-Moon-Biedl syndrome (Laurence, J. Z., English ophthalmologist, 1830–1874; Moon, R. C., American physician, 1844–1914; Biedl, A., Czech. physician, 1869–1933). Form of hypopituitarism associated with polydactyly, retinitis pigmentosa and mental defect.

L.E. cell. Lupus erythematosus cell. Neutrophil leucocyte containing large, deeply staining inclusion body, found in the blood in this disease.

Lederer's anaemia (Lederer, M., American pathologist, born 1885). A variety of acute haemolytic anaemia.

Leon virus. Type III strain of human poliomyelitis virus.

lep·tazol. $C_6H_{10}N_4$. 6,7,8,9-tetrahydro-5*H*-tetrazoloazepine. A cardiac and respiratory stimulant chiefly used in resuscitation after narcotic poisoning, anaesthetic accidents and drowning.

lep·tocyte (G. *leptos*, thin; *kutos*, cell). An erythrocyte of less than normal thickness.

lep·tocytō·sis. The presence of leptocytes in the circulating blood.

Letterer-Siwe disease (Letterer, E., German pathologist, born 1895; Siwe, S. A., contemp. Swedish pathologist). Reticulo-endothelial granuloma composed of histiocytes and eosinophil leucocytes, involving many bones and organs in infants, and invariably fatal.

lev·allor·phan tartrate. $C_{23}H_{31}NO_7$. (–)-*N*-allyl-3-hydroxymorphinan hydrogen tartrate. A morphine antagonist and respiratory stimulant.

levor·phanol tartrate. $C_{21}H_{29}NO_7,2H_2O$. (–)-3-hydroxy-*N*-methylmorphinan hydrogen tartrate dihydrate. An analgesic similar in action to morphine, but effective when given orally.

Lewis blood group system (name of woman in whom the antibody was first detected). Blood group characterized by possession of an antigen (Le^a), found in about 22 per cent of Europeans.

Libman-Sacks syndrome (Libman, E., American physician, 1872–1946; Sacks, B., American physician, born 1896). Progressive anaemia accompanied by fever and a purpuric rash.

Lignac-Fanconi syndrome. Cystinosis, *q.v.*

lig·nocaine hydrochloride. $C_{14}H_{23}ClN_2O,H_2O$. Diethylaminoacet-2, 6-xylidide hydrochloride monohydrate. Local anaesthetic for use by injection and surface application.

li·othy·ronine sodium. $C_{15}H_{11}I_3NNaO_4$. Sodium alpha-amino-beta [4-(4-hydroxy-3-iodophenoxy)-3,5-di-iododiphenyl] propionate. The active principle of the thyroid gland which stimulates cellular metabolism.

Listeria. Erysipelothrix, *q.v.*

listeriosis. Infection with Listeria; see Erysipelothrix.

Löffler's syndrome (Löffler, W., Swiss physician, born 1887). Cough and loss of weight, associated with eosinophilia in the blood.

lucan·thone hydrochloride. $C_{20}H_{25}ClN_2OS$. 1-(2-diethylaminoethylamino)-4-methylthiaxanthone hydrochloride. Synthetic drug used for the treatment of infections with *schistosoma haematobium*.

Lutheran blood group system (name of a blood donor found to possess the antigen responsible). Blood group characterized by possession of an antigen (Lu^a), found in about 7.5 per cent of the English population.

lym·phadenō·pathy (L. *lympha*, water; G. *aden*, gland; *pathos*, disease). Any disease of the lymph glands.

M

McArdle's syndrome (McArdle, B., contemp. British neurologist). Myopathy, *q.v.*, resulting from absence of an enzyme, phosphorylase, from voluntary muscle.

mac·roglobulinae·mia (G. *makros*, large; *globulin*; *haima*, blood). Syndrome associated with presence in the blood of abnormal globulins of high molecular weight; characterized by multiple haemorrhages, dyspnoea and fatigue, esp. in elderly men.

mac·rogols. Polyethylene glycols, used as water-miscible bases for ointments, pessaries and suppositories.

mannomus·tine hydrochloride. $C_{10}H_{24}Cl_4N_2O_4$. 1,6-di (2-chloroethylamino)-1,6-dideoxy-D-mannitol dihydrochloride. Cytotoxic agent used in treatment of various forms of malignant disease.

maple syrup urine disease. Familial cerebral disorder evident from early infancy, associated with urinary excretion of an unidentified substance smelling of maple syrup.

Marchiafava-Micheli syndrome (Marchiafava, E., Micheli, F., 19th–20th cent. Italian physicians). Chronic haemolytic anaemia, with haemoglobinuria occurring during sleep.

Marfan's syndrome (Marfan, B. A. J., French physician, 1858–1942). See arachnodaktyly.

měc·amy·lamine hydrochloride. $C_{11}H_{22}ClN$. 3-methylaminoisocamphane hydrochloride. A ganglion-blocking agent to relieve malignant hypertension.

mec·lozine. $C_{25}H_{27}ClN_2$. 1-*p*-chlorobenzhydryl-4-*m*-methylbenzylpiperazine. Anti-histamine drug used in allergic conditions and to relieve vomiting in pregnancy.

Meigs' syndrome (Meigs, J. V., American gynaecologist, 1892–1963). Hydrothorax and ascites occurring in association with ovarian fibroma.

melars·oprol. $C_{12}H_{15}AsN_6OS_2$. 2-*p*-(4,6-diamino-1,3, 5-triazine-2-ylamino)phenyl-4-hydroxymethyl-1, 3, 2-dithiarsolan. A trypanocide used for the treatment of *trypanosoma rhodesiense* and *t.gambiense* infestations, esp. advanced sleeping sickness.

menadox·ime. Ammonium 2-methylnaphthaquinone-4-oxime O-carboxymethyl ether. A synthetic analogue of Vitamin K.

mephene·sin. $C_{10}H_{14}O_3$. 3-(2-methylphenoxy)propane-1,2-diol. Muscle-relaxing drug used for relief of muscular spasms, as in tetanus and Parkinsonism.

mepro·bamate. $C_9H_{18}N_2O_4$. 2,2-di(carbamoyloxymethyl)pentane. Habit-forming tranquillizer which has muscle-relaxing properties.

měpy·ramine. $C_{17}H_{23}ON_3$. *N*-*p*-methoxybenzyl-*NN'*-dimethyl-*N*-2-pyridylethylenediamine. Anti-histamine drug used to treat allergic conditions.

mercap·topur·ine. $C_5H_4N_4S,H_2O$. 6-mercaptopurine monohydrate. Cytotoxic drug used to procure temporary remissions in acute leukaemia and chronic myeloid leukaemia.

mercur·ialentis. Deposits of metallic mercury in the lens of the eye in persons regularly in contact with mercury or its vapour.

měs·enchymō·ma, feminizing. Group of tumours arising from differentiated ovarian mesenchyme and having feminizing endocrine activity; includes theca-cell and granulosa-cell tumour.

měs·onephrō·ma (G. *mesos*, middle; *nephros*, kidney). Malignant tumours of ovary having structure resembling that of renal glomeruli and tubules.

mesul·phen. $C_{14}H_{12}S_2$. 2, 7-dimethylthianthren. Liquid used for treatment of seborrhoea, acne, scabies and pediculosis.

metform·in hydrochloride. $C_4H_{11}N_5HCl$. *NN'*-dimethyldiguanide hydrochloride. Orally active hypoglycaemic agent used in the treatment of diabetes mellitus.

měth·adone. $C_{21}H_{27}ON$. 2-dimethylamino-4:4-diphenylheptan-3-one. A powerful analgesic, resembling morphine in effect but lacking sedative properties.

methan·dienone. $C_{20}H_{28}O_2$. 17β-hydroxy-17α-methylandrosta-1,4-dien-3-one. A synthetic anabolic steroid derived from testosterone.

meth·icill·in. $C_{17}H_{19}N_2NaO_6S,H_2O$. Sodium-6-(2,6-dimethoxybenzamido) penicillanate. Antibiotic for intramuscular injection, effective against penicillin-resistant staphylococci.

meth·oin. $C_{12}H_{14}O_2N_2$. 5-ethyl-3-methyl-5-phenylhydantoin. An anti-convulsant used especially in the treatment of major epilepsy.

meth·otrex·ate. $C_{20}H_{22}O_5N_8$. 4-amino-*N*-methylpteroylglutamic acid. Folic acid antagonist used to induce remissions in acute leukaemia.

meth·ylcell·ulose. Methyl ether of cellulose. A powder which, when mixed with water, swells to form a viscous liquid. A laxative.

meth·ylpen·tynol. $C_6H_{10}O$. 3-methylpent-1yn-3-ol. An alcohol with short-term tranquillizing and hypnotic properties.

meth·ylprednis·olone. $C_{22}H_{30}O_5$. 11β, 17α, 21-trihydroxy-6α-methylpregna-1, 4-diene-3, 20-dione. An adrenal corticosteroid.

meth·yltestŏ·sterone. $C_{20}H_{30}O_2$. 17β-hydroxy-17α-methylandrost-4-en-3-one. Androgenic substance used as an anabolic steroid and in the palliation of mammary carcinoma.

meth·ylthiou·racil. $C_5H_6N_2OS$. 3,4-dihydro-2-mercapto-6-methyl-pyrimidin-4-one. A thyroid antagonist drug.

methypry·lone. $C_{10}H_{17}NO_2$. 3,3-diethyl-5-methyl-2,-4-dioxopiperidine. A sedative and hypnotic drug.

mi·crospher·ocytes. Spherocytes, *q.v.*

milker's nodules. Painless nodules occurring on the fingers of milkers, resulting from infection with cowpox virus.

Milroy's disease (Milroy, W. F., American physician, 1855–1942). Hereditary oedema of the legs.

mineral·ocor·ticoids. Steroids secreted by the adrenal cortex which regulate sodium and potassium excretion.

MNS blood group system. Blood groups characterized by possession of one or both of the antigens designated M and N. Of the English population, 28 per cent possess M, 22 per cent N and about 50 per cent M and N. The antigen S, usually in association with M, is found in 55 per cent of the population.

Mondor's disease (Mondor, H., contemp. French physician). Superficial phlebitis of the anterolateral chest wall.

mono-amine oxidase inhibitors. Anti-depressive drugs which act by inhibiting the enzyme mono-amine oxidase which is a factor controlling amine metabolism in the central nervous system. e.g. Iproniazid, *q.v.*

Moro reflex (Moro, E., Austrian paediatrician, 1874–1951). Self-protective reflex exhibited, in response to sudden disturbance, by infants up to the age of three months.

Morquio-Brailsford disease (Morquio, L. S., South American physician, 1867–1935; Brailsford, J. F., English radiologist, 1888–1961). A variety of chondrodysplasia.

mu·cormycō·sis (L. *mucor*, mould). Disease caused by infection with fungi of the genus *mucor*.

mucoviscidosis. Fibro-cystic disease of the pancreas, *q.v.*

mustard, nitrogen. Mustine hydrochloride, *q.v.*

mus·tine hydrochloride. $C_5H_{11}NCl_2,HCl$. di(2-chloroethyl)methylamine hydrochloride. Powerful cytotoxic drug producing an effect similar to that of irradiation, and used for the treatment of disseminated forms of malignant disease, e.g. leukaemia, lymphadenoma, lymphosarcoma, where irradiation may be unsuitable.

my·elofibrō·sis (G. *muelos*, marrow; fibrosis). Condition in which the bone marrow becomes infiltrated with fibrous tissue.

my·oepithē·lium (G. *mus*, muscle; epithelium). Stellate, possibly contractile cells which lie, in many forms of externally secreting glands, between the secreting cells and the basement membrane on which they lie.

my·oglo·bin (G. *mus*, muscle; L. *globus*, a globe). Pigment occurring in muscle and resembling haemoglobin in action; acts as an oxygen reservoir within the muscle fibre.

my·xoviruses (G. *muxa*, slime). Group of viruses having certain common features of size, growth and immunological factors.

N

nalor·phine. $C_{19}H_{21}O_3N$. *N*-allylnormorphine. An antagonist to the action of morphine, used as an antidote in poisoning with this and other allied opiates.

nan·drolone phenylpropionate. $C_{27}H_{34}O_3$. 17β-(3-phenylpropionyloxy)oestr-4-en-3-one. An anabolic steroid, *q.v.*

naphăz·oline hydrochloride. $C_{14}H_{14}N_2HCl$. 2-(naphthyl-1-methyl)-iminazole hydrochloride. A powerful vasoconstrictor used for the relief of nasal congestion.

neomȳ·cin. Mixture of antibiotics obtained from the growth of *streptomyces fradiae*. Given orally, it is poorly absorbed and is used for treatment of intestinal infections; also used externally in skin infections.

neph·roblastō·ma (G. *nephros*, kidney; *blastos*, germ). Highly malignant embryonic tumour of the kidney in children. Syn. Wilms' tumour.

neph·rocal·cinosis (G. *nephros*, kidney; L. *calx*, lime). Deposits of calcium in the kidneys, usually resulting from excessive intake of vitamin D.

neur·ilemmō·ma (G. *neuron*, nerve; *lemma*, husk). Benign tumour of a nerve sheath.

Newcastle disease (Newcastle-upon-Tyne, where first reported). Highly infectious disease of fowls due to a virus; transmissible to man in the form of an acute conjunctivitis.

nikěth·amide. $C_{10}H_{14}N_2O$. Diethylamide of pyridine-3-carboxylic acid. A respiratory stimulant.

ni·trofur·ans. Group of antibacterial substances resembling the sulphonamides in action, though chemically distinct from them.

ni·trofuran·toin. $C_8H_6N_4O_5$. 1-(5-nitro-2-furfurylidene-amino)hydantoin. A nitrofuran, *q.v.*, given orally as an antiseptic in urinary infections.

nitrogen mustard. See mustine hydrochloride.

nor·adrěn·aline. $C_{12}H_{17}NO_9,H_2O$. α-(3,4-dihydroxy-phenyl)-β-aminoethanol. Substance closely related to adrenaline and found with it in varying proportions in the secretion of the adrenal medulla. Used for its general vasoconstrictor effect in hypotension.

nor·ethan·drolone. $C_{20}H_{30}O_2$. 17α-ethyl-17β-hydroxy-oestr-4-en-3-one. An anabolic steroid, *q.v.*

nor·ethis·terone. $C_{20}H_{26}O_2$. 17α-ethynyl-17β-hydroxy-oestr-4-en-3-one. A progestational steroid, *q.v.*

nor·ethyn·odrel. $C_{20}H_{26}O_2$. 17α-ethynyl-17β-hydroxy-oestr-5(10)-en-3-one. A progestational steroid, *q.v.*

nos·capine. $C_{22}H_{23}NO_7$. An opium alkaloid used as a cough suppressant.

nos·tras (L. *nostras*, of our country). Adjective used in description of epidemic diseases to stress the difference between the features of the disease as it occurs in one particular country and those of the same disease observed in other countries.

no·vobi·ocin. Antibiotic produced by the growth of *streptomyces niveus*; used esp. for the treatment of penicillin-resistant staphylococcal infections.

ny·statin. Antifungal substance produced by the growth of *streptomyces noursei*. May be applied locally for infections of the skin, or taken orally for alimentary moniliasis.

O

oc·tyl nitrite. $C_8H_{17}NO_2$. 2-ethylhexyl nitrite. A vasodilator drug given by inhalation for relief of, esp., angina of, effort.

oligophrě·nia, phenylpyru·vic. Variety of mental defect associated with an inborn error of metabolism, shown by excretion of phenylpyruvic acid in the urine.

orphan virus. Any virus which is known to exist but has not been established as pathogenic.

orphěn·adrine hydrochloride. $C_{18}H_{23}NO,HCl$. 2-di-methyl[2-(α-*o*-tolylbenzyloxy)ethyl]amine. Drug used to relieve muscle spasm in Parkinsonism.

Osgood-Schlatter disease (Osgood, R. B., American surgeon, born 1873; Schlatter, C., Swiss surgeon, 1864–1934). Osteochondritis affecting the epiphysis of the tibial tuberosity.

ō·valocy·te (L. *ovum*, egg; G. *kutos*, cell). An erythro-cyte of oval shape. Syn. elliptocyte.

P

pan·cytopēn·ia (G. *pan*, all; *kutos*, cell; *penia*, poverty). An abnormal decrease in the number of all forms of cells in the blood.

Papanicolaou's stain (Papanicolaou, G. N., American anatomist, 1883–1962). Haematoxylin, orange G and eosin; staining method used in exfoliative cytology, *q.v.*

para-influenza viruses. Group of respiratory viruses, suspected of being concerned in causation of the common cold. Includes Sendai, haemadsorption 1 and 2 and croup-associated viruses.

paramethadī·one. $C_7H_{11}O_3N$. 5-ethyl-3,5-dimethyl-oxazolidine-2,4-dione. An anti-convulsant drug used, when others fail, in treatment of petit mal.

paravaccĭn·ia. Rash, distinct from that of true vaccinia, which sometimes follows vaccination.

parŏm·omycin. $C_{23}H_{45}O_{14}N_5$. D-glucosaminedeoxy-streptamine-D-ribosediamino-hexose. Antibiotic produced by growth of *streptomyces rimosus* var. *paromomycinus*, effective in amoebic and bacillary dysentery and salmonellosis.

Pelger anomaly (Pelger, K., Dutch physician, 1885–1931). A predominance in the blood of polymor-phonuclear neutrophil leucocytes with unsegmented or bi-lobed nuclei. Inherited as a Mendelian dominant, the anomaly causes no symptoms.

pelvis, frozen. Fixation of female pelvic organs into a single mass by adhesions resulting usually from endometriosis of pelvic peritoneum.

pem·pidine tar·trate. $C_{14}H_{27}NO_6$. 1,2,2,6,6-penta-methylpiperidine hydrogen tartrate. A sympathetic and parasympathetic ganglion-blocking agent used for relief of malignant hypertension.

penicillin V. See phenoxymethylpenicillin.

penicill·amine. $C_5H_{11}O_2NS$. β-β-dimethylcysteine. Degradation product of penicillin, used as a chelating agent, *q.v.*, in metallic poisoning and in Wilson's disease.

penicillinā·se. Penicillin-destroying enzyme secreted by penicillin-resistant bacteria.

pen·taeryth·ritol tetrani·trate. $C_5H_8N_4O_{12}$. 2,2-bishydroxymethylpropane-1,3-diol tetranitrate. Long-acting vasodilator given orally for the relief of angina of effort.

pentam·idine isethī·onate. $C_{26}H_{36}N_4O_{10}S_2$. 1,5-di(*p*-amidinophenoxy)pentane di(2-hydroxyethanesul-phonate). Trypanocidal drug used in African trypanosomiasis, kala-azar and cutaneous leishmaniasis.

pen·tolin·ium tar·trate. $C_{23}H_{42}N_2O_{12}$. NN'-penta-methylenebis(1-methylpyrrolidinium) hydrogen tartrate. Sympathetic and parasympathetic ganglion-blocking agent used for relief of malignant hypertension.

pericyte (G. *peri*, round; *kutos*, cell). Branching cell whose contractile arms embrace capillaries and regulate their calibre.

perphĕn·azine. $C_{21}H_{26}ClN_3OS$. 2-chloro-10,3,4-(2-hydroxyethyl)piperazin-1-yl propyl phenothiazine. Central nervous system depressant used to allay states of mental agitation.

pĕth·idine hydrochloride. $C_{15}H_{22}ClNO_2$. Ethyl-1-methyl-4-phenylpiperidine-4-carboxylate hydrochloride. Analgesic drug used for relief of severe pain; less effective than morphine, but valuable in obstetrics, in which uterine contractions are not affected.

Peutz-Jeghers syndrome (Peutz, J. L. A., contemp. Dutch physician; Jeghers, H., contemp. American physician). Multiple congenital abnormalities including intestinal polyposis, skin pigmentation, and a haemorrhagic tendency, transmitted as a Mendelian dominant.

phan·quone. $C_{12}H_6N_2O_2$. 4,7-phenanthroline-5,6-quinone. Antiamoebic drug used as an alternative to emetine-bismuth iodide.

phenantoin. Methoin, *q.v.*

phenaz·ocine hydrobromide. $C_{22}H_{28}BrNO$. 1,2,3,4,5,6-hexahydro-8-hydroxy-2,6-methano-6,11-dimethyl-3-phenethyl-3-benzazocine hydrobromide hemihydrate. Synthetic analgesic similar in action to, but more powerful than, morphine.

phenel·zine sulphate. $C_8H_{14}N_2O_4S$. Phenethylhydrazine hydrogen sulphate. Monoamine oxidase inhibitor used to combat neurotic and reactive depression.

phen·ethicill·in potassium. $C_{17}H_{19}KN_2O_5S$. Potassium 6-(α-phenoxypropionamido)penicillanate. Antibiotic effective when given orally for the same purpose as phenoxymethylpenicillin.

phenfor·min hydrochloride. $C_{10}H_{15}N_5HCl$. Phenethylbiguanide hydrochloride. Orally active hypoglycaemic agent used in treatment of diabetes mellitus.

phenglūta·rimide hydrochloride. $C_{17}H_{25}ClN_2O_2$. α-2-diethylaminoethyl-α-phenylglutarimide hydrochloride. Atropine-like drug used to control salivation, rigidity and tremor in Parkinsonism.

phenin·damine tartrate. $C_{23}H_{25}NO_6$. 1,2,3,4-tetrahydro-2-methyl-9-phenyl-2-azafluorene hydrogen tartrate. Antihistamine drug used mainly in the treatment of skin diseases.

phenindi·one. $C_{15}H_{10}O_2$. 2-phenylindane-1,3-dione. Anticoagulant drug used in the treatment and prevention of thrombotic diseases.

pheni·odol. $C_{15}H_{12}O_3I_2$. β-(4-hydroxy-3,5-diiodophenyl)-α-phenylpropionic acid. Radio-opaque contrast medium given orally for cholecystography.

phenmet·razine. $C_{11}H_{16}ClNO$. 3-methyl-2-phenylmorpholine hydrochloride. Drug used in the treatment of obesity; acts by reducing the desire for food.

phĕn·olsul·phonphthăl·ein. $C_{19}H_{14}O_5S$. Sulphone of di-(p-hydroxyphenyl)-2-sulphophenylmethanol. A red dye whose rate of excretion in the urine after intramuscular or intravenous injection forms a test of renal function.

phĕn·othi·azine. $C_6H_4S(NH)C_6H_4$. Thiodiphenylamine. Used originally as an anthelmintic, now the parent of a number of drugs having sedative effects on the central nervous system.

phenox·yben·zamine hydrochloride. $C_{18}H_{23}Cl_2NO$. Benzyl(2-chloroethyl)(1-methyl-2-phenoxyethyl)amine hydrochloride. Drug used to reverse the hypertension caused by phaeochromocytoma.

phenox·yeth·anol. $C_8H_{10}O_2$. 2-phenoxyethanol. Antibacterial substance used for external application to lesions caused by infection with bacteria of the *pseudomonas* and *proteus* species.

phenox·ymethylpenicill·in. $C_{16}H_{18}N_2O_5S$. 6-phenoxyacetamidopenicillinic acid. Antibiotic whose spectrum of activity is that of benzylpenicillin, *q.v.* Resists gastric acidity and may therefore be given orally. Syn. penicillin V.

phentō·lamine methanesulphonate. $C_{18}H_{23}N_3O_4S$. 2-(N-m-hydroxyphenyl-p-toluidinomethyl) imidazoline methanesulphonate. Hypotensive drug used esp. to reverse the hypertension caused by phaeochromocytoma.

phē·nylal·anine. $C_6H_5CH_2CH(NH_2)COOH$. Phenylaminopropionic acid. One of the amino acids essential in nutrition.

phē·nylbū·tazone. $C_{19}H_{20}N_2O_2$. 4-butyl-1,2-diphenylpyrazolidine-3,5-dione. Analgesic and antipyretic drug used esp. for relief of rheumatic conditions of joints.

phē·nyleph·rine hydrochloride. $C_9H_{14}ClNO_2$. (-)-m-hydroxyphenyl-2-methylaminoethanol hydrochloride. Vasoconstrictor drug used esp. to prevent hypotension in spinal anaesthesia and to produce vasoconstriction at the site of injection in local anaesthesia.

phē·nylē·thyl alcohol. $C_8H_{10}O$. Bactericide used for the preservation of eye drops.

phenylin·danedi·one. See phenindione.

phē·nylke·tonū·ria. Hereditary form of mental deficiency associated with the presence of phenylpyruvic acid in the urine.

phē·nylmercu·ric nitrate. $C_{12}H_{11}Hg_2NO_4$. Bactericide and fungicide, used in eye drops and as a constituent of some contraceptive substances.

phē·nylpyru·vic acid. Intermediate product in the process of metabolic breakdown of the nutritional amino acid, phenylalanine.

phĕn·ytoin. $C_{15}H_{11}N_2NaO_2$. Sodium derivative of 5,5-diphenyl hydantoin. Anticonvulsant drug used in the treatment of epilepsy.

phol·codine. $C_{23}H_{30}N_2O_4,H_2O$. 3-(2-morpholinoethyl) ether of morphine. A cough-suppressant drug.

phos·phorus 32. Radioactive isotope of phosphorus.

phry·noder·ma (G. *phrunos*, toad; *derma*, skin). Dryness of the skin with papular eruption; an appearance resembling toad skin, resulting from vitamin A deficiency.

phthal·ylsulphathi·azole. $C_{17}H_{13}N_3O_5S_2$. 2-[p-(o-carboxybenzamido)benzenesulphonamido]thiazole. Intestinal bacteriostatic drug used in the treatment of bacillary dysentery and to reduce bacterial content of gut before intestinal operations.

phȳ·saliferous (G. *phusallis*, a bubble). Of cells, filled with vacuoles.

phȳ·tomenadī·one. $C_{31}H_{46}O_2$. 2-methyl-3-phytyl-1,4-naphthaquinone. Naturally occurring vitamin which maintains a normal plasma prothrombin level. Used to treat haemorrhage occurring in the course of anticoagulant therapy. Syn. Vitamin K.

Pick's dementia (Pick, A., Czech. psychiatrist, 1857–1924). Presenile dementia, usually hereditary, due to focal degeneration of nerve cells of frontal or temporal lobes.

picket cells. The tall, narrow, close-set columnar cells lining the glands of the cervix uteri.

pic·rotoxin. $C_{30}H_{34}O_{13}$. Drug obtained from fruit of *anamirta cocculus* L. A nervous system stimulant used esp. in treatment of barbiturate poisoning.

pipam·azine. $C_{21}H_{24}ClN_3OS$. 10-3-(4-carbamoylpiperidino)propyl-2-chlorophenothiazine. An anti-emetic drug.

piper·azine hydrate. $C_4H_{10}N_2,6H_2O$. Drug used for eradication of roundworms and threadworms.

piper·ocaine hydrochloride. $C_{16}H_{24}ClNO_2$. 3-(2-methyl-piperidino)propyl benzoate hydrochloride. Local anaesthetic, also used for surface and spinal anaesthesia.

piperox·ane hydrochloride. $C_{14}H_{20}ClNO_2$. 2-piperidinomethyl-1,4-benzodioxan hydrochloride. Substance used to reduce hypertension caused by phaeochromocytoma, an effect used to differentiate this from other types of hypertension.

pip·radol hydrochloride. $C_{18}H_{22}ClNO$. α-diphenyl-piperid-2-ylmethanol hydrochloride. Stimulant of the cerebral cortex, used in treatment of depressive states.

plas·min. Enzyme found in globulin fraction of blood protein, active against fibrin; concerned in blood coagulation.

plasmin·ogen. Precursor of plasmin.

ple·omor·phic (G. *pleon*, more; *morphe*, shape). Existing in more than one form.

polyarteri·tis nodo·sa (G. *polus*, many; *arteria*, artery; L. *nodus*, knot). Febrile disease characterized by scattered zones of inflammation in the intima of a number of arteries.

Prausnitz-Kustner test (Prausnitz, C. W., German bacteriologist, born 1876; Kustner, H., German gynaecologist, born 1897). Local passive sensitization resulting from intradermal injection of serum from an allergic subject.

prednĭs·olone. $C_{21}H_{28}O_5$. 11β,17α,21-trihydroxy-pregna-1,4-diene-3,20-dione. Synthetic steroid similar in action to cortisone but four times as potent in its anti-inflammatory effect.

pred·nisone. $C_{21}H_{26}O_5$. 17α, 21-dihydroxypregna-1, 4-diene-3,11,20-trione. Synthetic steroid similar in action to prednisolone, *q.v.*

preg·nanedĭ·ol. The reduced form of progesterone, *q.v.*

prim·aquine phosphate. $C_{15}H_{27}N_3O_9P_2$. 8-(4-amino-1-methylbutylamino)-6-methoxy-quinoline-di(dihydrogen phosphate). Anti-malarial drug effective against the exo-erythrocytic stage of *plasmodium vivax*.

prim·idone. $C_{12}H_{14}N_2O_2$. 5-ethylhexahydro-5-phenyl-pyrimidine-4, 6-dione. Anti-convulsant drug used in grand mal and psychomotor epilepsy.

pro·actinomy·cin (G. *pro*, before; *aktis*, ray; *mukes*, fungus). Antibiotic derived from *Nocardia gardneri*, active against Gram-positive bacteria.

prō·band (L. *probare*, to test). Person whose pedigree is investigated to determine the presence and distribution in that pedigree of inherited factors of the disease from which he is suffering.

probĕn·ecid. $C_{13}H_{19}NO_4S$. *p*-(dipropylsulphamoyl)benzoic acid. Drug which promotes the excretion of urates and is used in the treatment of gout.

procain·amide. $C_{13}H_{21}ON_3$. *p*-amino-*N*-(2-diethyl-aminoethyl)benzamide. Myocardial depressant used in the treatment of ventricular and auricular arrhythmias.

procaine penicillin. Salt of penicillin with procaine; sparingly soluble in water, hence having a prolonged period of absorption after injection.

pro·chlorper·azine maleate. $C_{28}H_{32}ClN_3O_8S$. 2-chloro-10 [3-(4-methylpiperazin-1-yl)-propyl] phenothiazine di(hydrogen maleate). Drug used esp. for the suppression of vomiting.

procyc·lidine. $C_{19}H_{29}ON$. 1-cyclohexyl-1-phenyl-3-pyrrolidino-propan-1-ol. Anti-spasmodic drug used to reduce muscular rigidity and increase co-ordination in Parkinsonism.

progesta·tional steroids. Synthetic steroids having pharmacological properties generally resembling those of progesterone; especially used as oral contraceptives by virtue of their effect in suppressing the gonadotrophic function of the pituitary.

progest·ogen. Any substance possessing the same pharmacological properties as progesterone.

progu·anil hydrochloride. $C_{11}H_{17}Cl_2N_5$. *N*-*p*-chlorophenyl-*N*⁵-isopropyldiguanide hydrochloride. Drug used in prevention and treatment of malaria.

prō·mazine hydrochloride. $C_{17}H_{21}ClN_2S$. 10-(3-dimethylaminopropyl)phenothiazinehydrochloride. See chlorpromazine.

prometh·azine. $C_{17}H_{20}N_2S$. *N*-(2-dimethylamino-*n*-propyl)phenothiazine. Anti-histamine drug used in the treatment of urticaria; also as an anti-emetic and to potentiate the action of barbiturate sedatives.

propan·theline bromide. $C_{23}H_{30}O_3NBr$. 2′-diisopropyl-amino-ethylxanthen-9-carboxylate methobromide. Anti-cholinergic drug used to diminish gastric and duodenal motility and to relieve spasm in peptic ulceration.

propŏ·situs. Syn. proband, *q.v.*

prō·pylene glycol. $C_3H_8O_2$. (±)propane-1, 2-diol. A solvent used in the preparation of drops, injections and sprays.

prō·pylhex·edrine. $C_{10}H_{21}N$. (2-cyclohexyl-1-methyl-ethyl)methylamine. Powerful vasoconstrictor, to be inhaled for the relief of nasal congestion.

prō·pylĭ·odone. $C_{10}H_{11}I_2NO_3$. Propyl-1, 4-dihydro-3, 5-diiodo-4-oxypyrid-1-yl acetate. A contrast medium used for bronchography.

prō·pylthioŭ·racil. $C_7H_{10}ON_2S$. 4-hydroxy-2-mercapto-6-*n*-propylpyrimidine. Anti-thyroid substance used in the treatment of thyrotoxicosis.

prō·tamine sulphate. Substance prepared from the sperm or testes of certain fish, which neutralizes the anti-coagulant properties of heparin.

P.T.C. Plasma thromboplastin component; substance essential for prothrombin formation which is absent from serum of patients with Christmas disease. Syn. Christmas factor, Factor IX.

pyrid·ostigmine bromide. $C_9H_{13}BrN_2O_2$. 3-dimethyl-carbamoyloxy-1-methylpyridinium bromide. Drug used for the treatment of myasthenia gravis. Action less effective, but more prolonged than that of neo-stigmine.

pȳr·imethamine. $C_{12}H_{13}N_4Cl$. 2, 4-diamino-5-*p*-chlorophenyl-6-ethylpyrimidine. Anti-malarial drug, used chiefly in prophylaxis.

Q

quin·albar·bitone sodium. $C_{12}H_{17}N_2NaO_3$. Sodium-5-allyl-5-(1-methylbutyl)barbiturate. A short-acting hypnotic drug, similar in action to phenobarbitone.

R

Rauwolfia. Dried roots of *Rauwolfia serpentina* or *R. vomitoria*, containing a number of hypotensive and other alkaloids.

reă·gin. Antibody-like substance considered to be responsible for many of the phenomena of allergy.

Reiter's disease (Reiter, H., German bacteriologist, born 1881). Syndrome comprising abacterial urethritis, conjunctivitis and poly-arthritis; sometimes also enteritis, balanitis and pericarditis. The cause of the condition remains unknown.

Rendu-Osler-Weber disease (Rendu, H. J. L. M., French physician, 1844–1902; Osler, Sir W., Canadian physician, 1849–1919; Weber, F. Parkes, English physician, 1863–1962). Hereditary haemorrhagic telangiectasia.

reser·pine. $C_{33}H_{40}N_2O_9$. Hypotensive alkaloid obtained from *Rauwolfia, q.v.*

resistance (*add*). 3. Of bacterial species: the ability to withstand physical and chemical agents, esp. chemotherapeutic substances. 4. Radio-resistance; the ability of tissues to withstand effects of ionising radiation.

reticulo-endothelial granuloma. Group of diseases in children, characterized by localized accumulations of histiocytes, with or without lipoid content, and eosinophils. See eosinophilic granuloma, Hand-Schuller-Christian disease, Letterer-Siwe disease.

retic·ulo-endothelio·sis (L. *reticulum*, a small net; G. *endon*, within; *thele*, nipple). Abnormal proliferation of the cells of the reticulo-endothelial system as occurs in, e.g., Hodgkin's disease, chronic monocytic leukaemia and reticulo-endothelial granuloma, *q.v.*

retic·ulō·sis (L. *reticulum*, a small net). 1. Reticulo-endotheliosis. 2. Abnormal proliferation of reticulum cells in lymph glands or bone marrow.

rhī·nosporidiō·sis. Endemic infection (esp. in India) of mucous membranes by a fungus, *rhinosporidium Seeberi*, characterized by polypoid growths in mucosae, of esp. eyes, ears and upper respiratory tract.

ri·boflā·vine. $C_{17}H_{20}N_4O_6$. A yellow compound forming part of the vitamin B_2 complex, and of flavoproteins, enzymes of metabolic importance.

Riehl's melanosis (Riehl, G., Austrian dermatologist, 1855–1943). Brown scaly pigmentation, with follicular keratosis, on areas of skin exposed to light.

Roger, maladie de (Roger, H. L., French physician, 1811–1892). Congenital cardiac anomaly comprising a low interventricular septal defect and hypertrophy of the right ventricle.

S

sal·monella. Genus of bacteria of family *Enterobacteriaciae* associated with inflammatory conditions of intestinal tract, e.g. typhoid and paratyphoid infections and many forms of food poisoning.

Schiller's test (Schiller, W., American pathologist, born 1887). Means of diagnosing carcinoma of uterine cervix by painting with tincture of iodine; areas of carcinoma stand out unstained.

scintillation counter. Instrument for the estimation of radio-activity, in which active particles cause, on detection, flashes of light whose energy is multiplied into electric impulses registrable on a suitable meter.

Sendai virus. Virus of the para-influenza group causing epidemic pneumonitis in infants.

ser·otō·nin. Hormone-like substance secreted by chromaffin cells in intestinal mucosa, which increases intestinal motility and diminishes renal blood flow.

sex intergrade. Individual of a physical make-up intermediate between that of the typical male and that of the typical female.

sĭd·eroblasts. Precursors of siderocytes, *q.v.*

sĭd·erocytes. Erythrocytes containing granules of ferric iron. Found in blood after splenectomy and in haemolytic anaemias.

Sjögren's syndrome (Sjögren, H. S. C., Swedish ophthalmologist, born 1899). Deficiency of lacrimal gland secretions, resulting in drying and inflammation of eyes, mouth, and larynx. Usually in postmenopausal women.

slit-sampler. Apparatus for estimating the number of bacteria-carrying particles in a given volume of air.

sodium al·ginate. Extract obtained mainly from *Laminaria* algae and used as a suspending and emulsifying agent.

sodium ami·nosalicylate. $C_7H_6NNaO_3,2H_2O$. Sodium 4-amino-2-hydroxybenzoate dihydrate. Drug used as an adjuvant to streptomycin or isoniazid in the treatment of tuberculosis.

sodium anox·ynaphthonate. $C_{26}H_{16}N_3Na_3O_{10}S_3$. Trisodium 4'-anilino-8-hydroxy-1, 1'-azonaphthalene-3, 6, 5'-trisulphonate. Non-toxic blue dye used in blood-volume measurements.

sodium aur·othiomal·ate. $C_4H_3O_4SAuNa_2$. Organic compound of gold with sulphur, used mainly in the treatment of rheumatoid arthritis.

sodium calciumedetate. $C_{10}H_{12}CaN_2Na_2O_8,2H_2O$. Chelating agent, *q.v.*, used esp. in treatment of lead poisoning.

sodium edetate. $C_{10}H_{14}N_2Na_2O_8,2H_2O$. disodium dihydrogen ethylenediamine-*NNN'N'*-tetra-acetate dihydrate. Chelating agent, *q.v.*, used esp. for removal of calcium; e.g. from corneal opacities.

sodium lauryl sulphate. A mixture of sodium alkyl sulphates used as an emulsifying agent in the preparation of ointments.

sodium radio-iodide. Sodium iodide in which the iodine is in the form of its radioactive isotope, iodine-131.

sodium radiophosphate. Sodium phosphate in which the phosphorus is in the form of its radioactive isotope, phosphorus-32.

sodium stibogluconate (chemical constitution uncertain). Pentavalent antimony compound used in treatment of kala-azar.

solap·sone. $C_{30}H_{28}N_2Na_4O_{14}S_5$. Tetrasodium salt of di[*p*-(3-phenyl-1, 3-disulphopropylamino)phenyl] sulphone. Bacteriostatic agent used in the treatment of leprosy.

sphin·golip·ids (G. *sphiggein*, to bind; *lipos*, fat). Lipids containing sphingosine, *q.v.*, found in excess in certain metabolic diseases; see Niemann, Tay-Sachs, Gaucher.

sphin·gomy̆·elin (G. *sphiggein*, to bind; *muelos*, marrow). A combination of sphingosine with a fatty acid, phosphoric acid and choline, found in Niemann-Pick disease, *q.v.*

spi·ramycin. Antibiotic derived from *streptomyces ambofaciens*, active against many common pathogenic Gram-positive organisms.

spiron·olacto·ne. $C_{24}H_{32}O_4S$. 17α-acetylthio-17β-hydroxy-3-oxo-17α-pregn-4-ene-21-carboxylic acid lactone. Diuretic substance which promotes excretion of sodium without loss of potassium.

Spitz-Holter valve (Spitz, E. B., Holter, J. W., contemp. American neurosurgeon and engineer). Silicone rubber valve inserted beneath scalp to drain lateral ventricles into jugular vein in hydrocephalus.

Stein-Leventhal syndrome (Stein, I. F., Leventhal, M. L., contemp. American gynaecologists). Amenorrhoea, sterility, uterine hypoplasia and masculinization symptoms, associated with presence of polycystic ovaries.

stem cell. Primordial cell from which there arises by division a race of cells having the same structure and function.

Stevens-Johnson syndrome (Stevens, A. M., Johnson, F. C., contemp. American paediatricians). Erythema multiforme with mucosal ulceration affecting especially mouth, conjunctiva, urethra. Allied to Behçet's and Reiter's syndromes, *q.v.*

stib·ophen. $C_{12}H_4O_{16}S_4SbNa_5,7H_2O$. Pentasodium antimony biscatechol-3,5-disulphonate. Antimony compound used in treatment of schistosomiasis.

stiff-man syndrome. Universal muscular rigidity with painful muscular spasm; occurs in late middle life and responds to no known treatment.

stippling, basophilic. Appearance of fine basophilic granules in erythrocytes, seen esp. in lead poisoning.

street virus. Rabies virus found as a naturally acquired infection in dogs; cf. fixed virus, *q.v.*

strontium-90 (*add*). Radioactive isotope of strontium; occurs in fall-out after nuclear explosions. Has a half-life of 28 years and after absorption is incorporated into bone.

stru·ma ovarii (L. from *struere*, to build). Ovarian teratoma in which thyroid elements are present.

Sturge-Weber disease (Sturge, W. A., English physician, 1850–1915; Weber, F. Parkes, English physician, 1863–1962). Form of congenital mental defect with fits and hemiplegia due to an angiomatous malformation of the brain and usually associated with a facial naevus on the affected side. Syn. naevoid amentia.

sulphafur·azole. $C_{11}H_{13}N_3O_3S$. 5-(*p*-aminobenzenesulphonamido)-3,4-dimethylisoxazole. Short-acting soluble sulphonamide with effects similar to sulphadimidine, *q.v.*

sul·phameth·izole. $C_9H_{10}N_4O_2S_2$. 2-*p*-aminobenzenesulphonamido-5-methyl-1,3,4-thiadiazole. Sulphonamide drug soluble in urine and therefore used for treatment of urinary infections.

sul·phamethox·ypyrid·azine. $C_{11}H_{12}N_4O_3S$. 3-*p*-aminobenzenesulphonamido-6-methoxypyridazine. Long-acting sulphonamide drug requiring infrequent dosage.

sul·phinpy·razone. $C_{23}H_{20}N_2O_3S$. 1,2-diphenyl-4-(2-phenylsulphinylethyl)pyrazolidine-3,5-dione. Agent which liberates urates from tissues and lowers blood uric-acid level; used in gout.

sul·phonylure·a. Parent substance of a number of hypoglycaemic agents given orally for the treatment of diabetes mellitus; see chlorpropamide, tolbutamide.

sux·amethon·ium bromide. $C_{14}H_{30}O_4N_2Br_2,2H_2O$. Bis-2-dimethylaminoethyl succinate bismethobromide. A short-acting muscle relaxant drug.

sux·etho·nium bromide. $C_{16}H_{34}O_4N_2Br_2$. 2-dimethylaminoethyl succinate diethobromide. A less potent substance than suxamethonium, *q.v.*, which it resembles.

swimming-bath conjunctivitis. Inclusion conjunctivitis, *q.v.*

syncytiotro·phoblast (G. *syn*, together; *kutos*, cell; *trophe*, nourishment; *blastos*, germ). The outermost layer of syncytial cells covering the chorionic villi.

synō·viō·ma (G. *sun*, together; L. *ovum*, egg; G.-*oma*, tumour). Any tumour arising from synovial tissue.

T

target cell. Erythrocyte having a dark central area and a dark peripheral ring; seen in various forms of anaemia.

tart cell. Macrophage cell found in blood and bone marrow, esp. in disseminated lupus erythematosus.

Terramycin. See oxytetracycline.

tet·rachloroeth·ylene. C_2Cl_4. An anthelmintic for hookworm infestation.

tet·racy·cline. $C_{22}H_{25}ClN_2O_8$. Antibiotic obtained by catalytic reduction of chlortetracycline or oxytetracycline. Chiefly used to combat mixed infections, esp. of bronchi, as well as others, including rickettsial and some virus infections.

thalĭd·omide. Non-barbiturate sedative found to induce foetal malformations when taken by pregnant women.

thecŏ·ma (G. *theke*, a case). Benign tumour of ovarian theca mainly fibromatous but including fatty and sometimes epithelial elements.

thee·lin. Oestrin, *q.v.*

thī·ambū·tosine. $C_{19}H_{25}N_3OS$. *N-p*-butoxyphenyl-*N'*-p'-dimethylaminophenyl thiourea. Chemotherapeutic drug used in treatment of leprosy.

thī·omer·sal. $C_9H_9O_2HgSNa$. Sodium-*o*-(ethylmercurithio)benzoate. Bacteriostatic and fungistatic substance for application to skin, wounds and mucous surfaces.

thīopen·tone sodium. $C_{11}H_{17}N_2NaO_2S$. Short-acting barbiturate drug used for brief periods of anaesthesia, given intravenously.

thī·oprŏ·pazate hydrochloride. $C_{23}H_{30}Cl_3N_3O_2S$. Phenothiazine derivative with effects similar to chlorpromazine, *q.v.*

thī·orĭd·azine hydrochloride. $C_{21}H_{27}ClN_2S_2$. Phenothiazine derivative used mainly in treatment of mental agitation.

thoracŏ·pagus (G. *thorax*, chest; *pagos*, fixed). Conjoined twins united at the sternum.

throm·bocytopē·nia (G. *thrombos*, clot; *kutos*, cell; *penia*, poverty). Deficiency of platelets circulating in the blood.

throm·boplastin·ogen (G. *thrombos*, clot; *plassein*, to form). Precursor of thromboplastin, *q.v.* Probably identical with anti-haemophilic globulin.

thymŏ·ma (G. *thumos*, the thymus gland). A tumour formed by proliferation of cells of the thymus gland.

thy·rotrŏph·ic, thy·rotrŏp·ic (G. *thureos*, shield; *eidos*, form; *trephein*, to nourish; *trepein*, to turn). Influencing the growth of endocrine activity of the thyroid gland.

tolaz·oline hydrochloride. $C_{10}H_{12}N_2HCl$. 2-benzylimidazoline hydrochloride. Anti-histamine drug with dilator effect on peripheral blood vessels.

tolbu·tamide. $C_{12}H_{18}O_3N_2S$. *N*-butyl-*N'*-toluene-*p*-sulphonylurea. Hypoglycaemic agent given orally for treatment of diabetes mellitus, esp. in elderly patients.

tomŏ·graphy (G. *tome*, a section; *graphein*, to write). The radiographic examination of planes of body tissue at any given depth.

tox·ocara canis. A common parasite in the intestine of the dog. Human infections may cause retinal granulomatosis by lodgement of larvae in the eye.

tox·ohormone. A polypeptide isolated from tumour tissue which, on injection into normal mice, causes a reduction in liver catalase, *q.v.*, thus interfering with iron metabolism.

tox·oplas·ma (G. *toxikon*, poison; *plasma*, anything formed). Protozoal parasite of mammals and birds, which causes toxoplasmosis, *q.v.*

tox·oplasmō·sis. Infection with the protozoon *toxoplasma hominis*. Frequently occurs as an intrauterine infection of infants, causing encephalomyelitis and choroido-retinitis; infections in adults are usually less severe.

tranquillizer. Any drug which calms a patient without inducing sleep.

transam·inase. Enzyme which effects the transfer of an amino-group (NH_2) from one compound to another.

transferr·in. An iron-binding globulin in the plasma, which transports iron in the circulation, and from which it is released into the bone marrow and other tissues.

treponema immobilization test. Serological test for syphilis, esp. in later stages. Depends on immobilization of live *treponema pallidum* by syphilitic serum in presence of complement.

trĕt·amine. $C_9H_{12}N_6$. 2,4,6-triaziridin-1-yl-1,3,5-triazine. Cytotoxic agent resembling nitrogen mustard, for oral administration. Syn. T.E.N., triethylene melamine.

tri·amcin·olone. $C_{21}H_{27}FO_6$. 19α-fluoro-11β,16α,17α,21-tetrahydroxypregna-1,4-diene-3,20-dione. Chemical variant of cortisone, six times as potent, and lacking the salt-retaining properties of the parent substance.

tri·fluoper·azine hydrochloride. $C_{21}H_{26}Cl_2F_3N_3S$. 10-[3-(4-methylpiperazin-1-yl)-propyl]2-trifluoromethyl-phenothiazine dihydrochloride. Drug similar to chlorpromazine, *q.v.*, used as a stimulant in treatment of psychoneuroses.

trimĕp·razine tartrate. $C_{40}H_{50}N_4O_6S_2$. 10-(3-dimethyl-amino-2-methylpropyl)phenothiazine tartrate. Antihistamine drug used mainly as an antipruritic.

trimĕt·aphan cam·phorsul·phonate. $C_{32}H_{40}N_2O_5S_2$. 4,6-dibenzyl-5-oxo-1-thia-4,6-diazatricyclo-undecan-ium-β-camphorsulphonate. Ganglion-blocking agent used to induce hypotension in neurological and vascular surgery.

tri·pelenn·amine hydrochloride. $C_{16}H_{22}ClN_3$. *N*-benzyl-*N'*,*N'*-dimethyl-*N*-pyrid-2-ylethylenediamine hydrochloride. Antihistamine drug similar in action to promethazine, *q.v.*

tri·prŏ·lidine hydrochloride. $C_{19}H_{23}ClN_2,H_2O$. trans-1-pyrid-2'-yl-3-pyrrolidin-1''-yl-1-*p*-tolylprop-1-ene hydrochloride. Antihistamine drug similar to, but more powerful than, promethazine, *q.v.*

trisŏ·my (G. *treis*, three; *soma*, body). Condition in which one or more of the chromosomes comprising a set are present three times, the remainder being present twice.

trox·idone. $C_6H_9O_3N$. 3,5,5-trimethyloxazolidine-2,4-dione. Anti-convulsant drug for treatment of *petit mal*.

Turner's syndrome (Turner, H. H., American physician, born 1892). Ovarian agenesis associated with shortness of stature, webbing of the neck and sometimes other deformities.

tyr·othri·cin. Antibiotic derived from *bacillus brevis*, effective against Gram-positive organisms, but suitable only for external use.

Tzanck test (Tzanck, A., contemp. French dermatologist). Finding of nuclear abnormalities in epithelial cells from the floor of bullae as evidence of pemphigus.

U

un·deceno·ic acid. $C_{11}H_{20}O_2$. Undec-10-enoic acid. Antimycotic substance for local application to fungus infections of skin and mucous surfaces.

un·decylĕn·ic acid. Undecenoic acid, *q.v.*

urticar·ia pigmentŏ·sa (L. *urtica*, a nettle; *pigmentum*, paint). Congenital skin disease with widespread urticarial macules containing melanin and mast cells, *q.v.*; occurs usually in children, esp. boys.

V

Vaquez-Osler disease (Vaquez, L. H., French physician, 1860–1936; Osler, Sir W., Canadian physician, 1849–1919). Polycythaemia vera, *q.v.*

vī·nyl ē·ther. C_4H_8O. Divinyl ether. An inhalation anaesthetic, four times as potent as ethyl ether.

vi·omycin. Antibiotic obtained from *streptomyces griseus* var. *purpureus*, bacteriostatic against *mycobacterium tuberculosis*.

W

war·farin. $C_{19}H_{15}NaO_4$. Sodium derivative of 4-hydroxy-3-(3-oxo-1-phenylbutyl)-2 *H*-1-benzopyran-2-one. Substance used therapeutically as an anti-coagulant. Also used as rat-poison.

Weber-Christian disease (Weber, F. Parkes, English physician, 1863–1962; Christian, H. A., American physician, 1876–1951). Nodular, non-suppurative inflammation of superficial fasciae.

Werner's syndrome (Werner, C., contemp. German physician). Hereditary syndrome comprising cataract, osteoporosis, subnormal growth and sexual development, with early onset of arteriosclerosis and premature greying of the hair.

Westergren's method (Westergren, A., Swedish physician, born 1891). Method for determining erythrocyte sedimentation rate by placing citrated blood in a vertical glass tube 200 mm. long, with 2·5 mm. bore and measuring distance through which red cells have fallen after one hour.

von Willebrand's disease (Willebrand, E. A. von, contemp. Finnish physician). Haemorrhagic purpura due to failure of contraction in injured capillaries.

winter vomiting disease. Severe but transitory attacks of vomiting having an epidemic distribution but no obvious cause.

Wintrobe's tube (Wintrobe, M. M., Canadian haematologist, born 1901). Tube used for determination of erythrocyte sedimentation rate and as a haematocrit for determining relative proportions of cells and plasma in blood.

wool alcohols. Alcohol-soluble fraction of sheep's wool grease, used as an emulsifying agent in ointments.

X

Xg blood group. Blood group characterized by presence of an antigen carried on the X-chromosome; the first known sex-linked blood-group antigen.

Z

zinc undeceno·ate. $(C_{10}H_{19}CO_2)_2Zn$. Zinc undec-10-enoate. Fungicide similar in properties and uses to undecenoic acid, *q.v.*

Zollinger-Ellison syndrome (Zollinger, R. M., American surgeon; Ellison, E. H., contemp. American physician). Gastric hypersecretion and peptic ulceration accompanied by hyperplasia or tumour of the pancreatic islet-cells.